EMBRYOGENESIS

Edited by **Ken-ichi Sato**

Embryogenesis
Edited by Ken-ichi Sato

Published by InTech
Janeza Trdine 9, 51000 Rijeka, Croatia

Publishing Process Manager Romina Skomersic

Technical Editor Teodora Smiljanic

Cover Designer InTech Design Team

Additional hard copies can be obtained from orders@intechopen.com

Embryogenesis, Edited by Ken-ichi Sato
p. cm.
ISBN 978-953-51-0466-7

For EU product safety concerns:
IN TECH d.o.o., Prolaz Marije Krucifikse Kozulić 3, 51000 Rijeka, Croatia,
info@intechopen.com or visit our website at intechopen.com.

Meet the editor

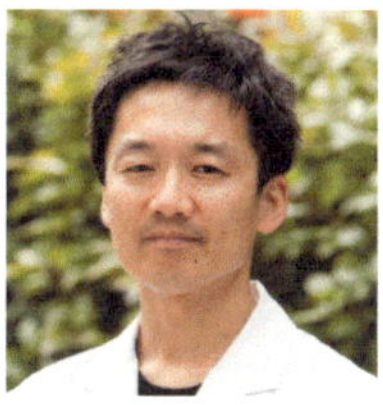

Ken-ichi Sato was born in Hokkaido, Japan. He graduated from Faculty of Science, Kobe University, Kobe, Japan, in 1988. He obtained his Ph.D. degree in biology from the Graduate School of Science and Technology, Kobe University, in 1996. From 1991 to 2007, he worked as an Assistant Professor at the Research Center for Environmental Genomics, Kobe University. In 2007, he launched his own research group of Cell Signaling and Development in Kyoto Sangyo University, Kyoto, Japan. His research interest is the role played by protein-tyrosine kinases in transmembrane signal transduction mechanisms such as in the cancer cells and in the fertilized eggs. Currently, he is a Professor at the Department of Molecular Biosciences, Faculty of Life Sciences, Kyoto Sangyo University.

Contents

Preface

It is my great honor to introduce the bland-new online book entitled "*Embryogenesis*". As has been well appreciated, embryogenesis is the biological process of fundamental importance that governs the production of new life. In human and other animals (and, to some extent, other organisms including plants), embryogenesis is generally considered to be equal to ontogeny that starts from the point of fertilization, an event that involves the union of two gamete cells (i.e. egg and sperm), passes through so-called embryogenic processes such as cleavage, gastrulation, organogenesis, and morphogenesis, and ends at the point of childbirth or the earlier period (i.e. late stage of pregnancy, in the case of human and other mammals). Consequently, embryogenesis also involves production of the gamete cells in an individual organism: this is called gametogenesis where primordial germ cells serve as origins for either eggs or sperm. These events (embryogenesis and gametogenesis) are collectively termed *zygotic* embryogenesis and thought to be a typical feature associated with the sexual reproduction system. On the other hand, cells of many plant species can also undergo *somatic* embryogenesis, where diploid cells, instead of haploid cells, originate to produce embryos. These phenomena witness cellular potential to reproduce or regenerate not only unicellular organisms (e.g. bacterium) but also multicellular one (e.g. ourselves), and the researchers have assumed that this can also be true for the cells of animals. This assumption has been gradually answered in the affirmative by a series of findings, in which, for instance, somatic cell nuclear transfer, embryonic stem cell, and induced pluripotent stem cell have been shown to be (at least potentially) applicable to create not only certain tissues and organs but also a newborn. Taking this background into account, it is certain that study on embryogenesis will continue to be at the center of the research field in biology and medicine. The book "*Embryogenesis*" will provide such a cutting edge view from a variety of studies dealing with animals, plants, and microorganisms. Another intriguing aspect of this book is the line up of the twenty-seven sections that have been contributed from the leading researchers in the field of twenty countries from all over the world (Bangladesh, Belgium, Brazil, Canada, China, Costa Rica, Czech Republic, Germany, Iran, Japan, Mexico, Netherlands, Poland, Russian Federation, Saudi Arabia, South Africa, South Korea, Switzerland, Taiwan/Republic of China, and United States of America). As an editor of this book, I would like to thank to all the contributors. Thanks are also due to Ms. Romina Skomersic, a Publishing Process Manager of InTech who did an excellent, patient, and encouraging job for us to write chapters and manage all necessary things to do in time. Finally, I wish that all readers of this book to enjoy and learn a wonderful array of scientific achievement in *Embryogenesis* and beyond.

Dr. Ken-ichi Sato
Ph.D., Laboratory of Cell Signaling and Development
Department of Molecular Biosciences
Faculty of Life Sciences, Kyoto Sangyo University
Kamigamo-motoyama, Kita-ku Kyoto
Japan

1

Clathrin Heavy Chain Expression and Subcellular Distribution in Embryos of *Drosophila melanogaster*

Georg Petkau[1], Christian Wingen[1], Birgit Stümpges[1] and Matthias Behr*
Life & Medical Sciences Institute University of Bonn Germany

1. Introduction

Tubular organs are essential for organisms to establish transport systems for nutrients, liquids and gases. The development of tubes requires endocytosis of bound ligands, receptors and proteins at the plasma membrane (Bonifacino and Traub, 2003; Nelson, 2009). Clathrin coated vesicles (CCVs) organize major routes of cargo selective endocytosis in higher eukaryotic cells (Conner and Schmid, 2003). The formation of CCVs requires clathrin molecules. During CCV budding, clathrin molecules assemble to form a cage-like coat around the nascent vesicle membrane. Clathrin assembly is assisted by numerous adaptor proteins. After inward budding, CCV scission from the membrane is mediated by the large GTPase Dynamin. Released CCVs diffuse from the membrane and undergo uncoating, whereby Clathrin molecules disassemble from the vesicles. The uncoating process is mediated by the ATPase function of the Heat shock cognate protein (Hsc70), which interacts with Chc and DnaJ adaptor proteins. The released Clathrin molecules reassemble for subsequent rounds of endocytosis while vesicles fuse with acceptor compartments, such as early endosomes (Conner and Schmid, 2003; Kirchhausen, 2000; Ungewickell and Hinrichsen, 2007).

Clathrin is a three-dimensional array of so-called triskelia that possesses the intrinsic ability to form a cage-like lattice around the vesicles (Brodsky et al., 2001). The Clathrin triskelion, a three-legged structure, is composed of three clathrin-heavy chain (Chc) and three Clathrin-light chain (Clc) subunits. Thus, Chc provides a basic component of the Clathrin coat (ter Haar et al., 1998; Kirchhausen, 2000). Evolutionarily, Chc and Clc are highly conserved from yeast to human (Wakeham et al., 2005). In the human genome two isoforms of *chc* and *clc* have evolved by gene duplication (Wakeham et al., 2005). For example the human *clathrin heavy chain* comprises of *CHC17* (genomic location 17q23.2) and *CHC22* (genomic loccation 22q11.21), which show distinct expression patterns (Dodge et al., 1991; Sirotkin et al., 1996; Kedra et al., 1996; Long et al., 1996).

---

* Corresponding Author
[1]These authors contributed equally to this work

Drosophila melanogaster is a well-established model organism to study gene and protein expression and function in tubular organs. During development of the *Drosophila* respiratory system, tracheal tube lumina undergo airway liquid-clearance, to enable liquid-air-transition at the end of embryogenesis. This occurs also in the vertebrate lung (Behr, 2010; Olver et al., 2004). Previously, we demonstrated in *Drosophila* the requirement of clathrin-mediated endocytosis for airway clearance and air-filling at the end of embryogenesis (Behr et al., 2007). However, though *Drosophila chc* gene function has been analyzed in a number of other genetic studies (reviewed in Fischer et al., 2006), the Chc expression, localization and dynamics remained elusive. Recently, we have characterized the *chc* mRNA and protein expression throughout *Drosophila* development (Wingen et al., 2009). In consistence with data of vertebrate Chc (Kirchhausen, 2000), we showed, using a specific purified anti-Chc antibody, Chc overlap with the trans-Golgi network, and co-localization with markers for early endocytosis (Wingen et al., 2009). In summary, the anti-Chc antibody is a new tool to analyze Clathrin heavy chain positive vesicles in *Drosophila.*

In order to analyze subcellular Clathrin distribution, we performed fluorescence labeling studies of endogenous Chc in *Drosophila* embryos. Immunofluorescent co-labeling studies demonstrate asymmetrical Chc distribution in epidermal cells and cells of tubular organs, such as the tracheal system, the salivary glands, and the gut. We show that Chc is enriched at the apical cell cortex and at the apical cell membrane, where it overlaps with the apical membrane organizer Crumbs (Crb). In consistence, we observed Chc mis-localization in airway cells of *crb* null and tracheal specific *crb* knock-down mutants. Furthermore, we show that the Crb-mediated apical membrane organization is involved in Chc-mediated airway-clearance at the end of embryogenesis. As Chc and Crb are highly conserved and broadly expressed in epithelial tissues (Wingen et al., 2009; Bulgakova and Knust, 2009), this new molecular mechanism of *crb* controlling apical Chc endocytosis is of general importance.

2. Results and discussion

In order to characterize Chc expression in *Drosophila* embryos, we used the anti-Chc antibody for immunofluorescent stainings on whole mount embryos. At late embryogenesis, stage 14 until stage 16, Chc was strongly enriched in the epidermis and tube forming organs, such as the foregut, the hindgut, the tracheal system and salivary glands (Fig. 1A-D).

At the end of embryogenesis, additional Chc enrichment was found in other organs, such as the midgut and secretory prothoracic glands (Fig. 1E,F). In *Drosophila,* foregut, hindgut, trachea, salivary glands and epidermis are of ectodermal origin. These organs are primary epithelia, which receive their epithelial character from the blastoderm epithelium (Tepass et al., 2001). Ectodermal epithelial cells display an asymmetric architecture of apical-basal polarity, where the apical cell membrane faces the tube lumen (Tepass et al., 2001).

In order to investigate subcellular Chc distribution, we analyzed immunofluorescent stainings, by using the anti-Chc antibody. In confocal sections of late *wild-type* embryos Chc was found in a vesicle-like punctuate pattern in the cell cortex as well as at distinct sites at the plasma membrane. This pattern was characteristic for cells of the foregut, hindgut, trachea, and salivary glands (Fig. 2A-D). Next, we generated confocal Z-stacks to generate three-dimensional projections of those organs. These projections revealed Chc accumulation at the apical cell cortex and plasma membrane (Figure 2A'-D'). In summary, the

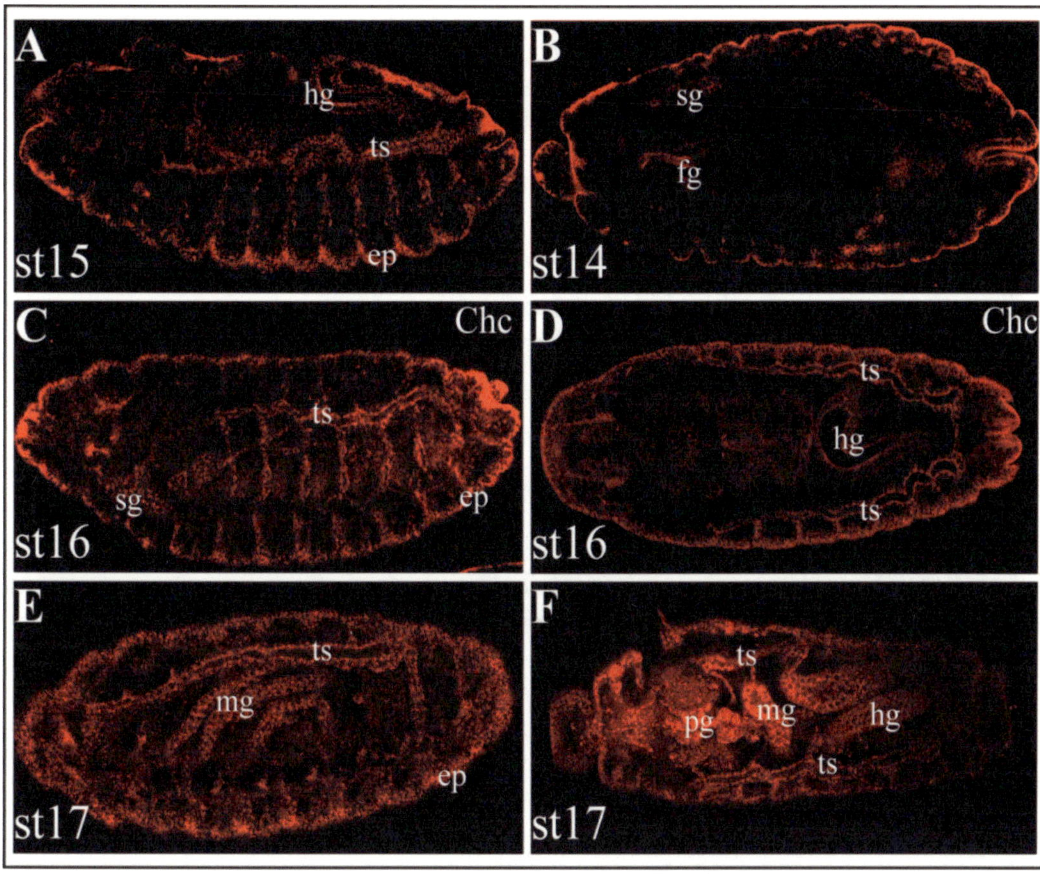

Fig. 1. **Chc is enriched in tube forming organs at late embryogenesis**.
(A-D) Confocal images of whole mount late embryos between stage 14 and stage 16. The left panels illustrate the lateral views, the right panels dorsal views of different embryos. All pictures here and in other Figures show anterior at the left. Immunofluorescent stainings using the anti-Chc antibody revealed strong Chc enrichment in ectodermally derived epidermis (ep) and tube forming epithelial organs, such as the tracheal system (ts), the hindgut (hg), the foregut (fg) and salivary glands (sg). **(E,F)** At the end of embryogenesis, at stage 17, additional Chc enrichment was detectable in the midgut (mg) and the prothoratic glands (pg).

asymmetrical distribution suggests that CCVs are most prominent at the apical membrane of tubular organs at late embryogenesis.

As Chc was apically enriched in tubular organs, we performed double immunofluorescent labeling studies, using anti-Chc together with an anti-Crb antibody, an apico-lateral cell membrane marker (Tepass and Knust, 1990; Wodarz et al., 1995). We analyzed single confocal sections of late *wild-type* embryos. In the cells of tubular organs, Chc accumulated adjacent to the Crb expressing apical cell membranes of foregut, hindgut, trachea, and salivary glands (Fig. 3A-D).

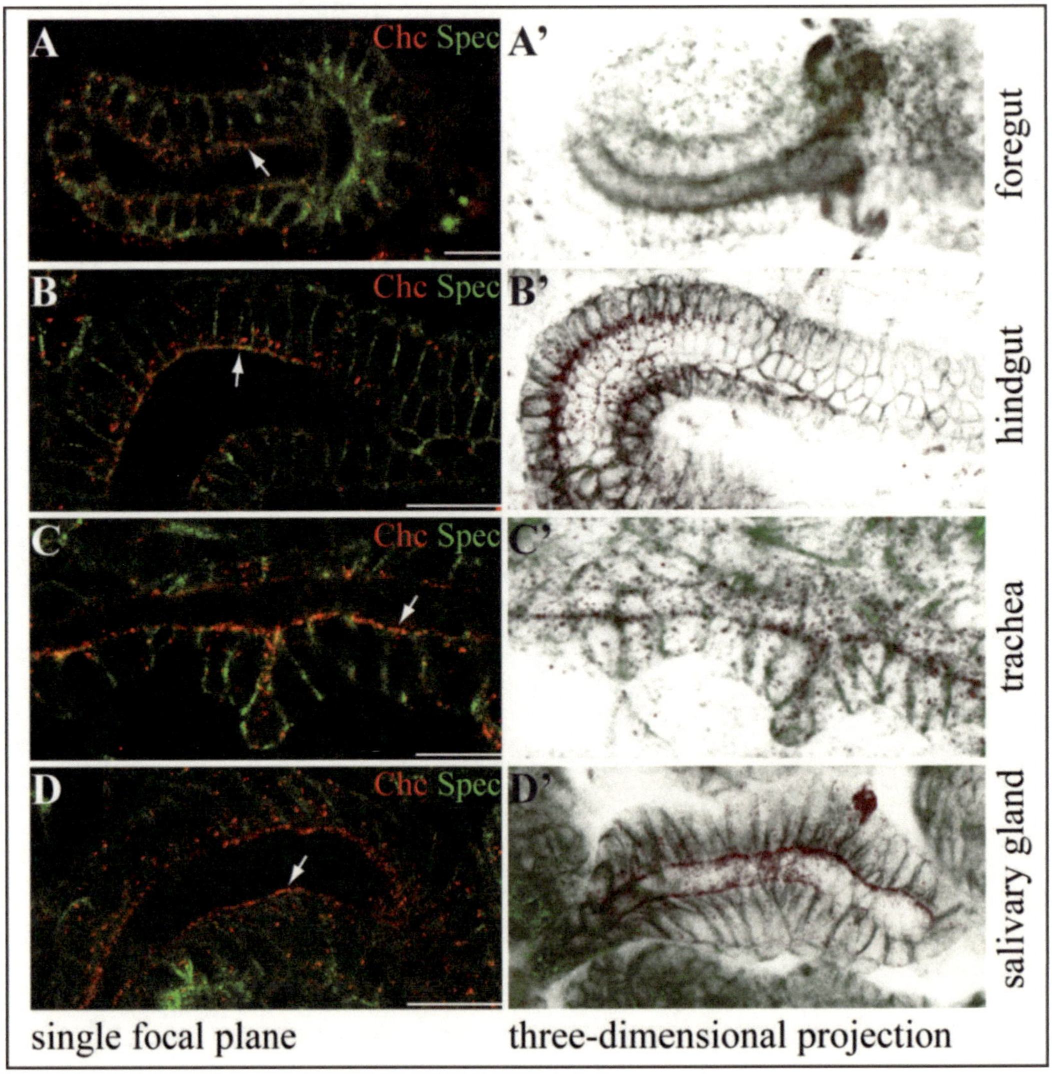

Fig. 2. **Chc vesicles are apically enriched in cells of tubular organs.**
(A-D) The left panels show confocal images of the tubes of foregut (A), hindgut (B), tracheal dorsal trunk (C), and salivary gland (D) of embryos at stage 15 (A,C) and 16 (B,D). **(A'-D')** The right panels illustrate three-dimensional projections of confocal Z-stacks across the tube of foregut (A'), hindgut (B'), tracheal dorsal main trunk (C'), and salivary gland (D'). Using anti-Chc (red) and anti-α-Spectrin (green; Pesacreta et al., 1989; cell membrane marker), images and projections show apical accumulation of Chc vesicles in the tubular organs. Arrows point to the apical membrane. Scale bar = 10μm.

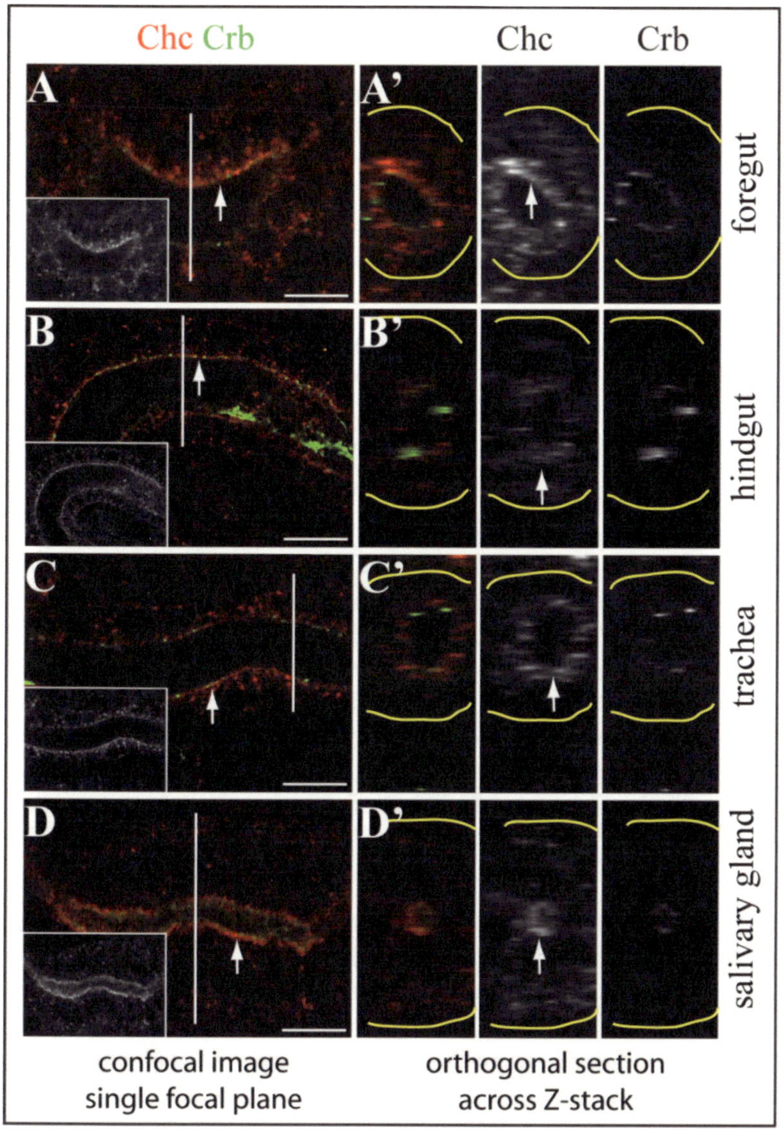

Fig. 3. **Chc vesicles are enriched at the apical cell membrane and apical cell cortex.** **(A-D)** The left panel shows confocal images across the tubes of foregut (A), hindgut (B), tracheal dorsal trunk (C), salivary gland (D) of embryos at stage 15. Arrows point to the apical membrane of tube lumina. The vertical white bars indicate the selected regions which were used for orthogonal projections across the entire tube. Inlays in A-D indicate single Chc stainings in grey. (A′-D′) The right panel illustrates three-dimensional reconstructions of orthogonal section of confocal Z-stacks across the tube of foregut (A′), hindgut (B′), tracheal dorsal trunk (C′), salivary gland (D′). Using anti-Chc (red) and anti-Crb (green) antibodies, which mark the apical cell membrane, images and orthogonal projections, show apical accumulation of Chc positive vesicles (arrows) in the tubular organs. Yellow lines mark the basal cell membrane. Single orthogonal projections of Chc and Crb are indicated in grey in the right pannels. Scale bar = 10μm.

Next, we generated confocal Z-stacks, which were used for orthogonal projections and reconstruction of tube lumen and surrounding cells. Crb function during tracheal development has been recently studied. Crb is involved in determining apical polarity, apical membrane growth, cell-invagination, cell-intercalation, tube size control and airway liquid-clearance (Kerman et al., 2008; Laprise et al., 2010; Letizia et al., 2011; Stümpges and Behr, 2011). The orthogonal projection showed Chc enrichment at the Crb expressing membrane (Figure 3A'-D'). In summary, we have strong evidence, that Chc positive vesicles are asymmetrically distributed and accumulate at the apical cell cortex and cell membrane, which faces the tube lumen.

As *crb* null mutants show severe developmental defects of the tracheal system and other ectodermal tissues (Tepass and Knust, 1990), we tested tracheal specific *crb* knock-down embryos for Chc localization in tracheal cells. In *Drosophila,* organ specific expression experiments can be performed by the use of the UAS-GAL4 system (Brand and Perrimon, 1993).

In order to generate *crb* knock-down mutants, we mated flies bearing a UAS-RNAi-*crb* transgene with flies bearing the tracheal driver line *breathless*GAL4 (*btl*G4). This crossing resulted in a tracheal specific knock-down of *crb* (Stümpges and Behr, 2011) in the offspring. In *wild-type* embryos Chc staining is enriched at distinct sites towards the apical membrane of tracheal cells (Fig. 4A). In contrast, the tracheal *crb* knock-down, led to intracellular accumulation of the Chc staining in tracheal cells (Fig. 4B). Consistently, an intracellular accumulation of Chc staining was also observed in *crb* null mutant tracheal cells (Fig 4C). Next, we tested the Chc localization upon tracheal Crb overexpression, using the *btl*G4 driver and the UAS-*crb* full length transgene. Crb overexpression resulted in strong co-localization of Crb and Chc (Fig. 4D). These findings indicate that Crb is involved in the apical Chc localization.

As Chc and Crb are involved in airway liquid-clearance and air-filling (Behr et al., 2007; Stümpges and Behr, 2011), we tested whether they act together in this process. At the end of embryogenesis, airways undergo lumen clearance, which is accompanied by air-filling in order to enable respiration to conduct oxygen from spiracular openings to the internal tissues (Behr et al., 2007; Stümpges and Behr, 2011; Tsarouhas et al., 2007). Transition from liquid- to air-filled airways can be monitored *in vivo* by bright field microscopy in *wild-type* embryos (Fig. 5 A-A'''', Stümpges and Behr, 2011). In contrast, in *chc* and *crb* null mutants air-filling is defective (Fig. 5B; Behr et al., 2007; Behr et al., 2007; Stümpges and Behr, 2011). Next, we tested *chc* and *crb* genetic interaction for air-filling. One test for genetic interaction is the analysis of trans-heterozygous mutants. A 50% reduction of two genes, which interact in a common process, results in a phenotype, which cannot be observed in individual heterozygous animals. In contrast to *wild-type* and *chc* or *crb* heterozygous mutant embryos (Fig. 5A,D, not shown; Stümpges and Behr, 2011), severe air-filling defects were observed in the trans-heterozygous *chc* and *crb* mutants (Fig. 5 C,D). In summary, we provide evidence that *chc* and *crb* act in a common process for airway liquid-clearance and air-filling. Thus, the Crb-mediated Chc localization is involved in airway clearance and may result in air-filling defects upon mis-localization in *crb* mutants.

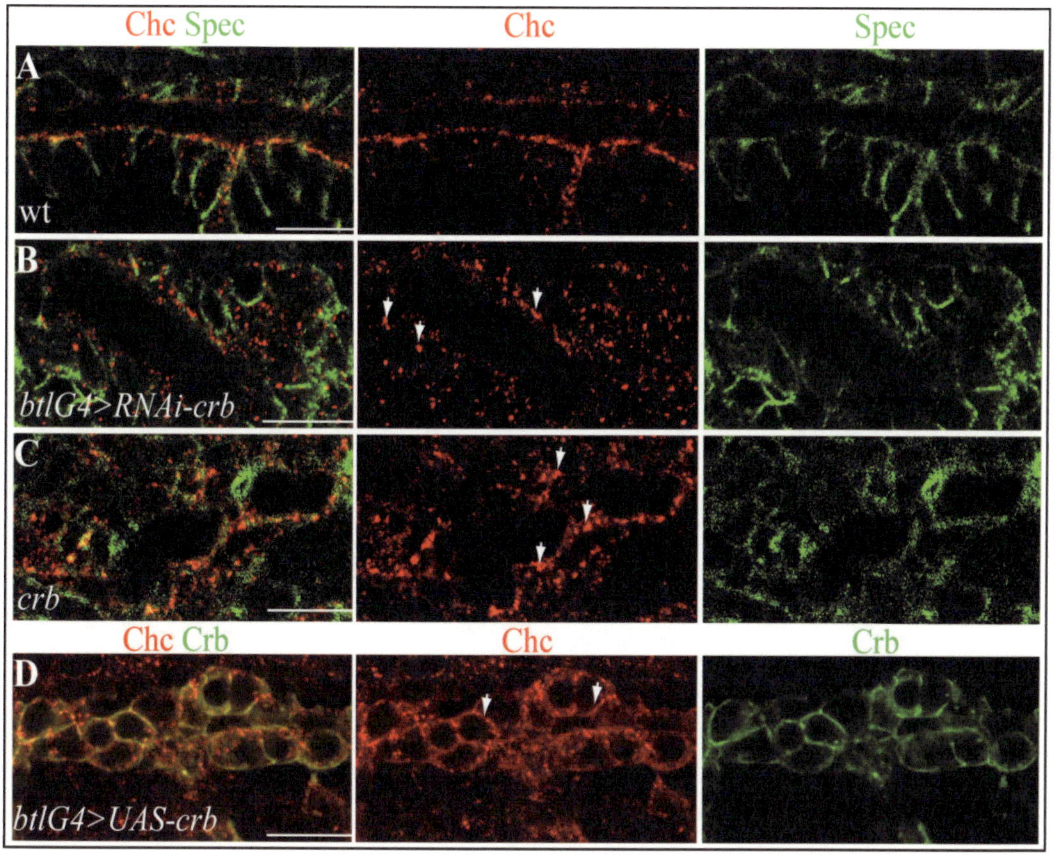

Fig. 4. **Chc mis-localization in *crb* knock-down and *crb* null mutants**.
Confocal immunofluorescent images of tracheal cells using the anti-Chc (red) and the anti α-Spectrin (green) and anti-Crb (green) antibodies. The α-Spectrin marks cell membranes and Crb indicates apical cell membranes. **(A)** In stage 17 *wild-type* embryos Chc (red) is distributed towards the apical cell membrane. **(B,C)** In stage 17 *btl*G4-driven UAS-RNAi-*crb* knock-down embryos and *crb* null mutant embryos, Chc showed intracellular mis-localization in tracheal cells (arrows). **(D)** Tracheal Crb overexpression led to intensive Chc co-localization with Crb (arrows). Scale bars=10μm.

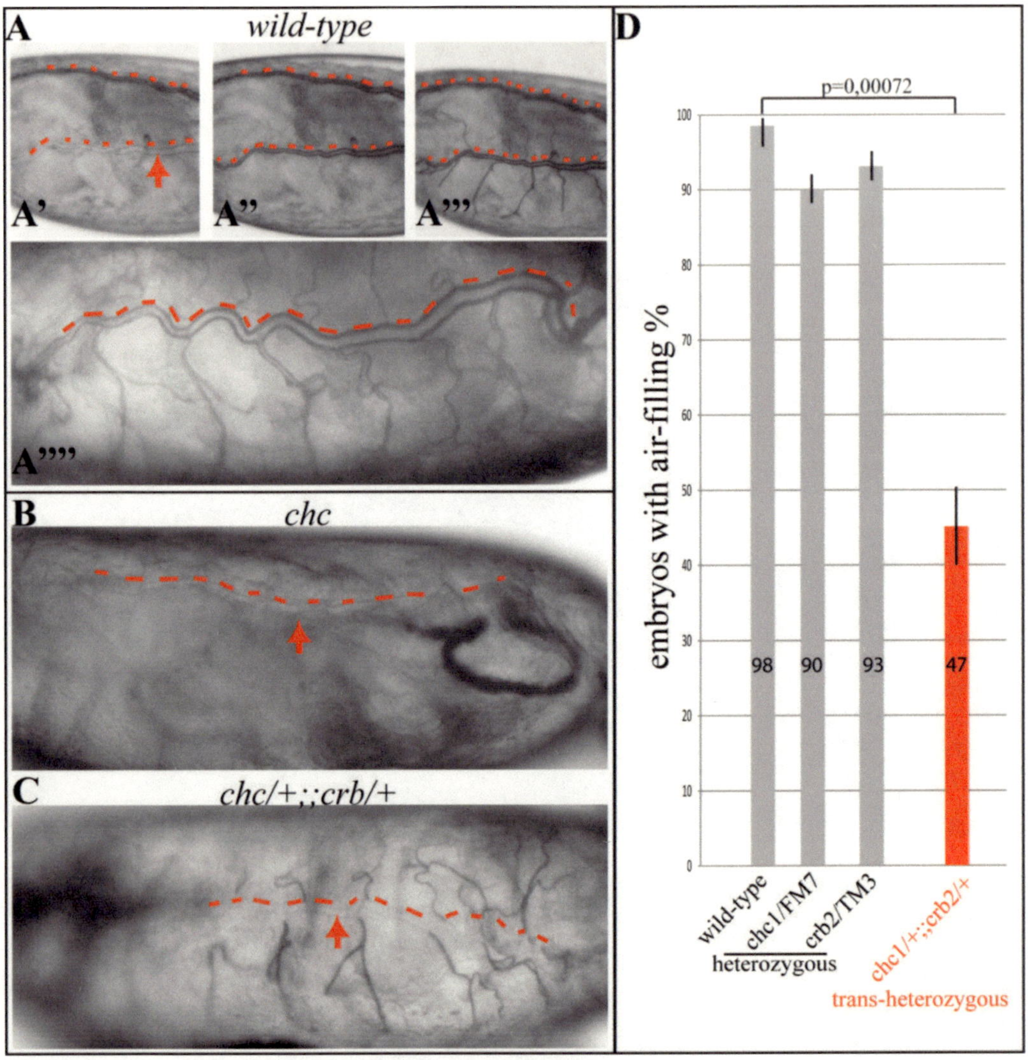

Fig. 5. ***chc*** **and** ***crb*** **trans-heterozygous embryos show defective air-filling.**
(A) Stage 17 *wild-type* embryos undergo airway liquid-clearance and accompanied air-filling. The liquid to air transition can be visualized due to different light diffractions by bright-field microscopy. Images A'-A''' show the air-filling process in a single embryo. Air-filling starts in the main dorsal trunks (indicated with red dashes) and spreads through the other airways. The arrow in A' points to a liquid-filled dorsal airway, where the air transition occurs later on (A''). **(B)** Stage 17 chc^1 null mutant embryos failed for airway liquid-clearance and the accompanied air-filling. The main dorsal trunk is indicated with dashes, the arrow points to the liquid filled airway. **(C)** In stage 17 trans-heterozygous *chc* and *crb* mutant embryos airway liquid-clearance and accompanied air-filling is impaired. Red dashes indicate the main dorsal airways, the arrow points to the liquid filled airway. **(D)** The histogram shows the mean value of quantifications of air-filling in percentage. Standard deviations (bars) and important p-values (p) are indicated; analyzed embryos (n) = 601 (*wild-type*), 85 (*chc*/FM7), 296 (*crb*/TM3), 92 (trans-heterozygous *chc*/+;;*crb*/+).

3. Materials and methods

3.1 Antibodies

The following antibodies were used: anti-Chc (1:40, rat; Wingen et al., 2009), anti-Crumbs (1:10; mouse, Cq4; DSHB; Iowa, USA), anti-α-Spectrin (1:10, 3A9, DSHB; Iowa, USA). Primary antibodies were detected by secondary antibodies obtained from Molecular Probes (Alexa488- and Alexa546-conjugated).

3.2 Immunofluorescent labeling and confocal microscopy

For immunostainings embryos were dechorionated with 2.5% sodiumhypochloride (5 min) and fixed in 2ml 4% PFA (paraformaldehyde) and 3ml heptane for 20 min. Embryos were devitellinized in a mixture of 3ml heptane and 10ml methanol and stored in methanol at -20°C. Afterwards embryos were washed in PBT (PBS, Tween20). Primary antibodies were incubated at 4°C overnight and secondary antibodies were incubated at room temperature for two hours. Finally embryos were mounted in Vectashield (Vector Laboratories) and analyzed with a Zeiss LSM 710 confocal microscope (Zeiss MicroImaging GmbH, Jena, Germany). For confocal sections we used standard settings (Zeiss Zen software, pinhole airy 1 unit). Sequential scans of individual fluorochromes were performed to avoid cross-talk between the channels. Subcellular studies were analyzed by using a Zeiss 63x LCI Plan Neofluar objective. The confocal areas were scanned 16-times using a minimum scan time, suggested by the Zeiss-Zen software. Z-stacks were performed using the suggested optimized distance (between 0,5 - 1μm). The ZEN software was used for the projection of the orthogonal sectioning. Images were cropped and analyzed in Adobe Photoshop CS5; Figures were designed with Adobe Illustrator CS5.

3.3 Airway liquid-clearance and air-filling assay

Embryos were collected for 3 hours and grown at 25°C until stage 17. Embryos were dechorionated in 2.5% sodiumhypochloride for 5min, washed in distilled water and transferred to a thin apple-juice-agar layer. The living embryos were monitored for gas filling by brightfield-microscopy (Zeiss Axiovert) and documented with the Zeiss Axiovision software (release 7.1). The statistical analysis was performed with Microsoft Excel 2010. P-values were determined by using standard setting (2;2) in Excel 2010, which assume two data sets from distribution with same variants.

3.4 Fly stocks

The following fly stocks were obtained from the Bloomington stock center and are described in flybase (http://flybase.bio.indiana.edu/): w^{1118} (here referred to as *wild-type*), *btlG4*, chc^{1}, crb^{2}, UAS-$crb^{wt30.12e}$ were obtained by the Bloomington stock center. The $UAS\text{-}crbRNA^{39178i}$ was obtained by the Vienna *Drosophila* RNAi stock center (Dietzl et al., 2007). For overexpression experiments, we used the Gal4/upstream activator sequence system and the tracheal specific *btl*G4 driver. For all experiments adequate balancer strains (FM7 and TM3) carrying a GFP transgene were used to recognize individual genotypes. For genetic interaction experiments, heterozygous *chc* mutant females, bearing the FM7-actinGFP, were mated with TM3-twistGFP balanced crb^{2} heterozygous males, in order to recognize the non GFP expressing trans-heterozygous animals.

4. Conclusion

We have analyzed the subcellular distribution of Chc in epithelial tube organs in *Drosophila* embryos. Our confocal analysis and three-dimensional reconstructions demonstrate the specific apical accumulation of Chc from stage 14 of embryogenesis onwards when the tracheal system, foregut, hindgut and salivary glands differentiate and mature for physiological functions. Genetic analysis shows that the apical membrane organizer Crb is involved in apical Chc distribution in tracheal cells and that normal Chc localization is required for airway liquid-clearance and air-filling at the end of embryogenesis. This is consistent with previous observations (Behr et al., 2007; Tsarouhas et al., 2007; Stümpges and Behr, 2011), suggesting that apical Clathrin-mediated endocytosis is essential for airway-clearance. Important roles of Clathrin-dependent endocytosis for the internalization of the cystic fibrosis transmembrane conductance regulator (CFTR) and for the activity of the epithelial sodium channels (ENaCs), which are involved in liquid-clearance in the vertebrate lung, have been shown (Lukacs et al., 1997; Shimkets et al., 1997). Thus, up-regulation and apical accumulation of Chc positive vesicles is essential for the development of the tracheal system and other tube forming organs. As Chc and Crb are highly conserved and broadly expressed in epithelial tissues (Wingen et al., 2009; Bulgakova and Knust, 2009), this new molecular mechanisms of *crb* controlled apical Chc endocytosis is of general importance.

5. Acknowledgements

We thank Andreas Fink and Tamara Krsmanovic for critical reading of the manuscript. We thank Michael Hoch for his support. M.B. was supported by the Fritz-Thyssen-Foundation (Az.10.08.2.138) and the Deutsche Forschungsgemeinschaft (SFB645). C.W. was supported by the Boehringer Ingelheim Fonds.

6. References

Behr, M. (2010). Molecular aspects of respiratory and vascular tube development. *Resp Physiol Neurobi,* Vol.173, pp.S33-S36.

Behr, M., C. Wingen, C. Wolf, R. Schuh, and M. Hoch. (2007). Wurst is essential for airway clearance and respiratory-tube size control. *Nat Cell Biol,* Vol. 9, pp.847-853.

Brand, A.H. and Perrimon, N. (1993) Targeted gene expression as a means of altering cell fates and generating dominant phenotypes. *Development,* Vol.118, pp. 401–415.

Bonifacino, J. S., and L. M. Traub. (2003). Signals for sorting of transmembrane proteins to endosomes and lysosomes. *Annu. Rev. Biochem,* Vol.72, pp.395–447.

Brodsky, F. M., C. Y. Chen, C. Knuehl, M. C. Towler, and de Wakeham. (2001). Biological basket weaving: Formation and function of clathrin-coated vesicles. *Annu Rev Cell Dev Bi,* Vol.17, pp.517–568.

Bulgakova, N. A., and E. Knust. (2009). The Crumbs complex: from epithelial-cell polarity to retinal degeneration. *J Cell Sci,* Vol.122. pp.2587–2596.

Conner, S. D., and S. L. Schmid. (2003). Regulated portals of entry into the cell. *Nature* Vol.422 pp.37–44.

Dietzl, G., D. Chen, F. Schnorrer, K.-C. Su, Y. Barinova, M. Fellner, B. Gasser, K. Kinsey, S. Oppel, S. Scheiblauer, A. Couto, V. Marra, K. Keleman, and B. J. Dickson. (2007). A genome-wide transgenic RNAi library for conditional gene inactivation in *Drosophila*. *Nature* Vol.448, pp.151-156.

Dodge, G. R., I. Kovalszky, O. W. McBride, H. F. Yi, M. L. Chu, B. Saitta, D. G. Stokes, and R. V. Iozzo. (1991). Human clathrin heavy chain (CLTC): partial molecular cloning, expression, and mapping of the gene to human chromosome 17q11-qter. *Genomics* Vol.11, pp.174-178.

Fischer, J. A., S. H. Eun, and B. T. Doolan. (2006). Endocytosis, endosome trafficking, and the regulation of *Drosophila* development. *Annu Rev Cell Dev Biol* Vol.22, pp.181-206.

Kedra, D., M. Peyrard, I. Fransson, J. E. Collins, I. Dunham, B. A. Roe, and J. P. Dumanski. (1996). Characterization of a second human clathrin heavy chain polypeptide gene (CLH-22) from chromosome 22q11. *Hum. Mol. Genet*Vol.5, pp.625-631.

Kerman, B. E., A. M. Cheshire, M. M. Myat, and D. J. Andrew. (2008). Ribbon modulates apical membrane during tube elongation through Crumbs and Moesin. *Dev Biol* Vol.320, pp.278-288.

Kirchhausen, T. (2000). Clathrin. *Annu Rev Biochem* Vol.69, pp.699-727.

Laprise, P., S. M. Paul, J. Boulanger, R. M. Robbins, G. J. Beitel, and U. Tepass. (2010). Epithelial Polarity Proteins Regulate *Drosophila* Tracheal Tube Size in Parallel to the Luminal Matrix Pathway. *Curr Biol,* Vol. 20, pp.55-61.

Letizia, A., S. Sotillos, S. Campuzano, and M. Llimargas. (2011). Regulated Crb accumulation controls apical constriction and invagination in *Drosophila* tracheal cells. *J Cell Sci,* Vol.124, pp.240-251.

Long, K. R., J. A. Trofatter, V. Ramesh, M. K. McCormick, and A. J. Buckler. (1996). Cloning and characterization of a novel human clathrin heavy chain gene (CLTCL). *Genomics,* Vol.35, pp.466-472.

Lukacs, G. L., G. Segal, N. Kartner, S. Grinstein, and F. Zhang. (1997). Constitutive internalization of cystic fibrosis transmembrane conductance regulator occurs via clathrin-dependent endocytosis and is regulated by protein phosphorylation. *Biochem J,* Vol.328, pp.353-361.

Nelson, W. J. (2009). Remodeling epithelial cell organization: transitions between front-rear and apical-basal polarity. *Cold Spring Harb Perspect Biol* 1(1):a000513, pp.1-19.

Olver, R. E., D. V. Walters, and S. M Wilson. 2004. Developmental regulation of lung liquid transport. *Annu. Rev. Physiol* 66:77-101. doi:10.1146/annurev.physiol.66.071702.145229.

Pesacreta, T. C., T. J. Byers, R. Dubreuil, D. P. Kiehart, and D. Branton. (1989). *Drosophila* spectrin: the membrane skeleton during embryogenesis. *J. Cell Biol,* Vol.108, pp.1697-1709.

Shimkets, R. A., R. P. Lifton, and C. M. Canessa. (1997). The activity of the epithelial sodium channel is regulated by clathrin-mediated endocytosis. *J. Biol. Chem,* Vol.272, pp.25537-25541.

Sirotkin, H., B. Morrow, R. DasGupta, R. Goldberg, S. R. Patanjali, G. Shi, L. Cannizzaro, R. Shprintzen, S. M. Weissman, and R. Kucherlapati. (1996). Isolation of a new clathrin heavy chain gene with muscle-specific expression from the region commonly deleted in velo-cardio-facial syndrome. *Hum. Mol. Genet, Vol.* 5, pp.617-624.

Stümpges, B., and M. Behr. (2011). Time-specific regulation of airway clearance by the *Drosophila* J-domain transmembrane protein Wurst. *FEBS Letters,* In Press, doi:10.1016/j.febslet.2011.09.018.

Tepass, U., and E. Knust. 1990. Phenotypic and developmental analysis of mutations at the crumbs-locus, a gene required for the development of epithelia in *Drosophila-melanogaster. Roux Arch Dev Biol,* Vol.199, pp.189-206.

Tepass, U., G. Tanentzapf, R. Ward, and R. Fehon. (2001). Epithelial cell polarity and cell junctions in *Drosophila. Annu. Rev. Genet,* Vol.35, pp.747-784. doi:10.1146/annurev.genet.35.102401.091415.

ter Haar, E., A. Musacchio, S. C. Harrison, and T. Kirchhausen. (1998). Atomic structure of clathrin: a beta propeller terminal domain joins an alpha zigzag linker. *Cell,* Vol.95, pp.563-573.

Tsarouhas, V., K.-A. Senti, S. A. Jayaram, K. Tiklová, J. Hemphälä, J. Adler, and C. Samakovlis. (2007). Sequential pulses of apical epithelial secretion and endocytosis drive airway maturation in *Drosophila. Dev Cell,* Vol.13, pp.214-225.

Ungewickell, E. J., and L. Hinrichsen. (2007). Endocytosis: clathrin-mediated membrane budding. *Curr Opin Cell Biol,* Vol.19, pp.417-425.

Wakeham, D. E., L. Abi-Rached, M. C. Towler, J. D. Wilbur, P. Parham, and F. M. Brodsky. (2005). Clathrin heavy and light chain isoforms originated by independent mechanisms of gene duplication during chordate evolution. *Proc Natl Acad Sci USA, Vol.*102, pp.7209-7214..

Wingen, C., B. Stuempges, M. Hoch, and M. Behr. (2009). Expression and localization of clathrin heavy chain in *Drosophila* melanogaster. *Gene Expr Patterns,* Vol.9, pp.549-554.

Wodarz, A., U. Hinz, M. Engelbert, and E. Knust. (1995). Expression of crumbs confers apical character on plasma-membrane domains of ectodermal epithelia of *Drosophila. Cell,* Vol.82, pp.67-76.

2

Human Embryogenesis

Charles E. Boklage
Brody School of Medicine, East Carolina University, Greenville, USA

1. Introduction

The building of the human embryo is a biological process of transcendent complexity. It fails at least three times as often as it succeeds. It takes about six weeks for a 'normal' version of the process to construct a fetus containing all of the differentiated cell types necessary, in the correct numbers and locations, to form all of the tissue and organ systems necessary to become a living, breathing human baby at birth. At the developmental horizon between embryogenesis and the fetal period, the majority of the cellular and molecular work of the developmental biology is done. The rest – the subject matter of obstetrics – is mostly about growing larger.

The business of becoming human thus begun is never complete. You are neither the same today as yesterday nor the same as the person who may awaken wearing your face tomorrow. Most of the time – over two-thirds of the time in optimal conditions for pregnancy – embryogenesis fails and its products become detritus before anyone knows that anything has happened. When the time for full-term birth arrives, fewer than one in four will remain alive and growing. That is, among highly privileged pregnancies: young, healthy mothers, in couples of proven fertility, under research-level medical attention. In the less favorable conditions of most pregnancies in most of the world we may be reasonably certain that the prospects are not that good.

I am here to discuss what we know about how the human embryo builds itself. If you want, you can step aside and waste as much of your own time as you want arguing about what "know" means. However that turns out for you, we actually do know a great deal about the formation of the human embryo, sound inference from sound observational evidence, repeated and reviewed by multiple knowledgeable and competent scientists. In one form of summary, human embryogenesis has a great deal in common with every other kind of embryogenesis we understand at all, and our observations to date also show it is not exactly like any other kind.

First: No part of human embryogenesis is the "beginning of human life." Every human life today is a continuation of something that began a very long time ago. If the sperm and the egg cell are not already very much alive, nothing is going to happen. If the egg and sperm are not both human (the biological definition of which changes with every generation), nothing is going to happen. Even if everything is as it should be when egg and sperm meet, even so, very often nothing very interesting is going to happen. Much more often than not, some part of the awesome complexity of the process does not work.

The sperm and the egg cell bring life forward from the parents, whose lives came from their parents, whose lives came from their parents, etc., etc., etc., all the way back to the very beginning of any form of life on Earth or wherever else it might have begun before coming to Earth. You may, of course, choose not to know that, but that **is** the way **all** living things work, including the human species.

Much of what we know about human embryogenesis we have learned from embryogenesis of other organisms, but there is a wealth of knowledge, specific to the human process, available from the traces left by variations in embryogenesis among living humans with developmental anomalies, and twins and chimeras. By learning how some people have done their embryogenesis differently, we can learn much about the more usual process.

The formation of the human embryo is a complex system of processes of dividing and differentiating cells, very much like every other kind of embryogenesis, but not exactly like any other kind we know anything about. One same nuclear and cytoplasmic genome must be functionally subdivided and sequentially reprogrammed so that each of many thousands of differentiated types of cells may be functionally defined by the expression of a different subset from each of the multiple layers of coded information in that genome.

2. Zygosis and the asymmetric foundations and outcomes of cleavage

That original zygote genome must first be assembled from parts brought forward in the oöcyte, together with parts arriving with the sperm to be reorganized by functions in the egg cell cytoplasm, directed in part by coded settings in and on the hyper-condensed chromatin of the sperm. The cell division machinery necessary to orchestrate the mechanical onset of the differentiating cell divisions of the cleavage stage must be assembled under the direction of components of the centrosome brought by the sperm. [In some other placental mammals, the oöcyte retains its centrosomes through the meiotic cell divisions, but the human oöcyte does not and the structures of the cell's division mechanisms must be brought back from the sperm.] Also arriving with the sperm is a system of *imprints* on the DNA. The *epigenetic* system of imprints on both sperm and oöcyte DNA will play major roles in development - these are relatively new understandings, still unfolding, and there will need to be more said here about that later.

Asymmetry is fundamental. From head to tail, back to belly and left to right, cells form tissues, organs and organ systems specific to their appropriate three-dimensional positions in the organism and specific to the current time in development, from fertilization on to and through senescence.

For decades, my lab and several others have studied embryogenesis from a variety of viewpoints and approaches, hoping to understand the origins of (left, right, etc.) asymmetry and the mechanisms by which it is originated, elaborated and enforced. My original question when I began these studies a few decades ago was *"where do left and right come from?"* That question was triggered by puzzlement over excess nonrighthandedness in twins - more about that later. My conclusions must - like every other piece of science always - be considered preliminary, but it has been a long time building and it has become unlikely to change much further short of a major new influx of observational data. The origin of the developmental asymmetries of living things is enmeshed with the origin of Life itself. Life, as and in the functions of living things, IS - of its chemical and physical essence -

asymmetrical. DNA is physically and chemically asymmetric. Cell structure is fundamentally asymmetric. Cell division in embryogenesis is fundamentally asymmetric, and in general each embryogenic cell division is an event of differentiation for at least one of the daughter cells of that division. Asymmetry is its own mechanism for generating and maintaining asymmetry, all the way forward from the origin of all Life. Asymmetry maintains and propagates itself, and it is a major component of all Life and all the mechanisms of differentiation.

When we see ciliary motion, or heart looping, for example, put forward as the foundation of embryonic asymmetries (each IS one of the earliest *microscopically visible* gross structural asymmetries of the embryonic body) and we determine that certain gene products are essential for that movement to go in the proper direction, and that at least one of those gene product molecules must be in position on the right side of the embryonic midline to make it happen that way ... then we may know with certainty that ciliary motion or heart looping clearly is not the beginning of embryogenic asymmetry. How? How?! did that molecule - that initiated this so-called 'beginning' cascade of events - know which side of the midline he was supposed to be on, at that particular time, to begin this beginning, and make the looping of the heart fall to the normal/usual side? And what does 'side' mean, anyway, in terms of cellular or subcellular structure to which a molecule should respond? Clearly the normal embryo at that stage is long since reliably asymmetric, and the origins of embryogenic asymmetry are much earlier in cellular and developmental Time.

Every vertebrate embryo properly questioned to date is *already reliably asymmetric when it has divided into only three or four cells*, with respect at least to consistent differences among those first few cells in the movements and functions of serotonin (Aw & Levin 2009; Buznikov *et al.*, 1964; Fukumoto *et al.*, 2006; Il'kova *et al.*, 2004). Zeskind and Stephens (2004) report neurobehavioral effects on newborns exposed prenatally to the presently very popular serotonin re-uptake inhibitor antidepressants. If we could find a way to refocus the question on variations around the time of early cleavage, we might have an answer that would be much more to the point.

3. Foundations of embryogenic asymmetry; Introducing chromatin and imprinting

The first few cell divisions of human embryogenesis are visibly asymmetric. One may look at an early cleavage stage human embryo, and know quite confidently which of its cells will divide next - always the largest one among those first few. The first cleavage is asymmetric - one of the daughter cells is larger than the other. That larger cell will be next to divide, leaving the smaller of the first two blastomeres as now the largest of three and now the next to divide. After several such divisions, it becomes impossible to follow in the microphotographs published to date. However, there might be means to follow it further as it has been followed through the entire embryogenesis of *C. elegans* (Begasse & Hyman, 2011).

Every organism yet properly questioned has demonstrated the need and the means to recognize and respond to the differences between old (mother, template) and new (daughter, newly replicated) DNA strands, and between leading and lagging strands, for purposes of cell division and for the control of differentiation of cell function (Huh & Sherley, 2011; Klar 1987; Landsdorp 2007; Merok *et al.* 2002; Pierucci & Zuchowski 1973).

The DNA exists and functions at all times in various degrees of chromatin condensation, wrapping and unwrapping the DNA strands in RNA, histones and other proteins, covering and uncovering the base sequences for varying access to enzyme complexes of replication and transcription. This is the level of control where the effects of imprinting and other epigenetic controls are exerted.

We first learned from mice in the mid-1980s that embryogenesis will fail if the zygote does not contain both maternal and paternal pronuclear half-genomes. If the paternal pronucleus is removed from a zygote and replaced with a maternal pronucleus from another zygote, most of the time the resulting rearranged zygote will die from the effects of the manipulations. When development can continue, the embryo-proper will appear to be well-made, but the extra-embryonic support structures will not. And vice-versa: when development proceeds with two paternal pronuclei and no maternal pronucleus, the extra-embryonic support structures may look wonderful, but the embryo itself will not be at all well put together. The two half-genomes are prepared differently in oögenesis and spermatogenesis for different functions in embryogenesis. DNA base sequences are not changed, but they are marked by chemical modifications in ways that will cause the same DNA sequence in the two half-genomes to be differently expressed (Surani *et al.*, 1984).

We do not know exactly which or how many human genes are involved in the protocols of genomic imprinting. We do know that 'imprinting' in gametogenesis is only a part, and probably a small part, of the whole of epigenetic control of development. Our best guess at the function of imprinting itself has to do with the tug-of-war between the evolutionary long-term best interests of the respective parents. At face value, it seems clearly to be in the male's long-term evolutionary best interest to maximize the number of his offspring. This is not in the long-term best interests of the female, who is better off to husband her reproductive resources, to optimize the strength of her surviving offspring, at the expense of numbers if necessary. That is what we make of the original findings in the mouse ... the paternal imprint in the absence of the maternal imprint maximizes the extra-embryonic support tissues, the better for more of his embryos to maximize their harvesting of uterine resources. The maternal imprint works to moderate all of that, to shepherd her reproductive resources – to save some of her self – for the sake of future as well as the present conceptus. This is a good plausible story, but it does not help us much with the fact that, in addition to placental mammals, at least some plants have found imprinting to the evolutionary advantage of their species. Differential expression of the blocks of 'imprinted' genes is heritable through many cell divisions, until reset in the next generation of gametogenesis (which happens in oögenesis in the first few months of female embryonic and fetal development). Most of the rest of epigenetic control is acted out in the resetting of combinatorial expression codes in each of the asymmetric cell divisions of the rest of embryogenesis.

The hardest thing about understanding human embryogenesis is that we cannot see it experimentally. We must *infer* from what we can see in *'experiments of nature'* and interpolate a testable picture of what is happening when and where we cannot see. Statistically useful samples of the normal real thing are unobtainable. We can stimulate human ovaries to produce large numbers of oöcytes, and we can fertilize them *in vitro*, after which we then may briefly watch their development. We cannot, however, safely assume that what we see in those circumstances is, or even very closely resembles, the normal, natural processes.

Such oöcytes and embryos as those are not entirely normal, as plainly demonstrated by the excesses of anomalous results among the progeny from every form of human reproduction that depends upon artificial ovarian stimulation. Papers in the literature following closely upon the invention of human *in-vitro* fertilization consistently reported "no statistically significant excess" of abnormalities. The sample numbers were too small for statistical significance in the demonstration of sizable increases in those small probabilities. Later studies, when available numbers of ART births are larger, make the risks more clear (examples: Buckett *et al.*, 2007; Green, 2004; Pinborg *et al.*, 2004). Oöcytes from artificially induced ovulation undergo embryogeneses that are less stable, less reliable, less likely to yield a fully 'normal' product. The mechanism most likely as an explanation is disturbance of the integrity of genomic imprinting.

Embryogenesis is all about the differentiation of dividing the single zygote cell and its progeny cells into hundreds of billions of specialized cells in the proper relative positions and growing to form a functional adult body. To the extent that we have come to understand it, human embryogenesis is very much like that of all other placental mammals and not exactly like any of them. The basic elements of this system of processes have much in common with the basic components of embryogenesis in every animal life form since before the radiation of the cnidarians (Morris, 1994). We have learned a great deal from fruit flies, from worms whose adult bodies include 959 cells all of whose paths through embryogenesis have been mapped, and from sea urchins and starfish, and we have learned important things from mice and cattle and sheep and birds and fish - as a far-from-exhaustive list of prominent examples.

In every case, the progeny of successive divisions from the original zygote must be differentiated to use different combinations of the thousands of genes in the one same diploid genome, to take the forms of and assume the functions of thousands of different cell types. The head–tail axis must be defined, and back vs belly, and left vs right; all three mechanical dimensions, and we must not neglect the fact that all of that changes with time. The many different tissues required for proper functioning of a complex body must be built of the right kinds of cells and put in the proper relative positions within the framework thus defined. Otherwise, it fails. In fact, 'otherwise' and 'failure' are the most common results for the human embryo in particular. It is difficult to know quite accurately, but it appears that human embryogenesis must be among the least efficient kinds of embryogenesis in terms of normal live births per fertilization.

From other chapters here, you should be able to form a good vision of the generalized story of embryonic development. This chapter will focus on commonly observed departures of human development from what we understand the "normal" process of human embryogenesis to be. Malformations, aneuploidies, 'birth defects' in general, twinning and chimerism, taken together, comprise a substantial fraction of the outcomes of human prenatal development - even of the small fraction that survives to delivery. From understanding these frequent anomalous outcomes, we can project a vision of the normal process in the light of which we might better claim to understand human embryogenesis.

4. Anomalies and failures of development

'Unusual' or 'anomalous' is of course a matter of perspective. We may prefer to think that the only relevant result of gestation of a human conceptus is a healthy live birth, and to think of anything short of that or other than that as an outcome sufficiently rare and peripheral to ignore. We rarely see what we do not expect to see. We generally believe that we know what we should look for and that we see all of what there is to see.

If, as usual among ordinary folks and obstetricians, we think of pregnancy as beginning with maternal awareness and clinical recognition, then miscarriages and stillbirths qualify as unusual. Only perhaps fifteen to twenty per cent of recognized pregnancies end before live term birth. That IS a minority, but it is a substantial minor fraction. Here today, our concern is for all that happens before they are recognized, the fact that over two-thirds of them typically fail before recognition, and what they were or should have been doing when they failed, how they come to fail.

About half of those spontaneous abortions have a recognizable (cyto)genetic problem in the form of chromosomal anomalies that are big enough to see in a microscope with proper preparation and staining. The other half of them have had no readily diagnosable problem. Recent advances in DNA microarray technology now allow us to see sub-microscopic anomalies in the DNA of some of them, and even to find some of the single-base-pair mutations when we have a reasonable idea of what to look for.

The probability of miscarriage is not uniformly distributed over the population. If a couple has one miscarriage, they are rather more likely to have another one than the couple in the house across the street is to have their first one. Spontaneous abortions are sufficiently common that we seldom investigate before a couple has their second or third one. When we do investigate repeated abortion, we find that the causes tend to repeat, in those broad classes with vs without chromosome anomaly. With very rare exception, the developmental problems that cause failure of recognized pregnancies [spontaneous abortions] are put in place during embryogenesis, before the maternal or clinical recognition of pregnancy.

In the research that led to self-administered pregnancy tests, it became clear that pregnancy can be recognized by biochemical signals (immunoassay of chorionic gonadotropin) from the differentiating trophoblast (in the process of building the chorion and the fetal portion of the placenta) a few weeks ahead of usual maternal awareness or clinical recognition. A much larger fraction of pregnancies discovered this way will disappear than the fraction that will miscarry after more conventional recognition of pregnancy. The majority of failures occur before recognition, during embryogenesis. More than twice as many instances of human embryogenesis end in failure as result in a living fetus carrying a recognized pregnancy forward (Boklage, 1990, 1995).

From the completion of embryogenesis at the recognition threshold [usually about eight weeks since the last normal menses, about six weeks after fertilization] and on through the fetal period [the remaining 30-32 weeks to normal time of birth], the loss rate is much slower than it was during embryogenesis. By the time miscarriages and stillbirths are over, fewer than one in four products of successful syngamy and zygosis remain to be born alive.

5. Secondary and primary sex ratio, imprinting and sex differences in speed and efficiency of embryogenesis

Sex ratio at birth is one of the outcomes from which we can learn some of the facts of embryogenesis. With rare and poorly understood exceptions, the number of males among human live births exceeds the number of females. The 'secondary' (at birth) sex ratio exceeds one (fraction male exceeds 50%) in most samples ever observed. All endings of recognized pregnancies short of live birth (miscarriages and stillbirths) also, with a very few reported exceptions, include an excess of males. If males comprise more than 50% of live births in spite of excess males among all the losses of recognized pregnancies throughout gestation, then ... it has been supposed that the 'primary' sex ratio (at fertilization) must be much higher to supply an excess of males for all prenatal losses and still have an excess of males at birth. This hypotheses has been subjected to many competent tests, and the answer is always no; there is no excess of Y-bearing sperm in the normal ejaculate, nor among the products of fertilization. There is no excess of Y-bearing sperm in the ejaculate after chemotherapy or after any of several efforts at changing the fractions of X-bearing and Y-bearing sperm for purposes of helping a couple influence the likely sex of their next offspring.

There is no significant departure from 50:50::X:Y-bearing sperm at fertilization, but there is a very real excess of males throughout pregnancy from recognition through delivery. What happens in the interval between fertilization and recognition of pregnancy? Embryogenesis - that's what happens between fertilization and recognition of pregnancy. Embryogenesis is approximately complete, with all organs and organ systems in place and needing (almost) only to grow, at about the most usual time of maternal recognition of pregnancy - about eight weeks since the last normal menses, about six weeks since fertilization - when the second consecutive menses goes missing.

Can there be anything about embryogenesis that routinely generates enough of an excess of male conceptuses to last for the remainder of pregnancy? Yes. In a word: speed. Male conceptuses generally do embryogenesis faster. In mouse, human and a few other kinds of embryo so far studied, the presence of a paternally-imprinted X-chromosome slows embryogenesis. Since only female embryos have a paternally-imprinted X-chromosome to slow them down, male embryos (who get not X but Y chromosomes from their fathers) do embryogenesis faster. Because many of the most important cellular achievements of embryogenesis are time-critical chemical signals, to other cells in the embryo or to the placenta, or through the placenta to the maternal physiology, then getting through embryogenesis less quickly very likely means doing it with less success. Since some of the products of every stage of development are signals from cell to cell within the embryo, or from the embryo to the maternal physiology, signals necessary for continuation of the pregnancy, then the establishment and maintenance of viable pregnancy is more efficient in general for male embryos. The extra losses of females because of their slower and less successful embryogenesis can set up an excess of males sufficient to show an excess of males in all losses of recognized pregnancies and still have an excess of males among live births.

6. Imprinting, the rest of epigenetics and major continental subpopulation variations in the epidemiology of embryogenesis

Significantly consistent differences in secondary sex ratio among human major continental subpopulations turn out to match corresponding gradients in several major parameters of the physiology of embryogenesis. The list includes at least: frequency of twinning, same-sex vs opposite-sex fractions of delivered twins, chorionicity fractions of twins, age of females at menarche, age at first birth, age at last birth, and the fraction of births that are premature or of low birth weight. All of these may be seen as arising from differences in relative speed and efficiency of embryogenesis between male and female embryos and among these subpopulations in the strength of the male-female differences. These are reviewed and discussed in Boklage (2005).

Surveys of the genome for gene sequences subject to imprinting have not in general shown a great deal of activity on the X-chromosome in comparison to levels indicated on several of the other chromosomes. It remains likely that the molecular survey criteria used to identify imprinted DNA sequences are imperfect and that there may be any number of different groups or classes of loci subject to imprinting. At least as likely, the 'rest of epigenetics', changes in gene expression mediated by genome markings or modifications other than imprinting, may greatly exceed imprinting in scope.

The parent-specific genome modifications during gametogenesis that we know as 'imprinting' set up only one 'kind' of epigenetic control, wherein the effective developmental difference is not a matter of DNA sequence itself, but a matter of relative expression of the same sequence, differing according to the parent of origin of that particular copy. Epigenetic controls are a means, perhaps the primary means, by which 'environmental' variations can affect all of development, from embryogenesis on through life. The mother's nutrition, the mother's emotional state, the mother's medications, nutrition of the maternal grandmother during the mother's fetal development... all of these have been shown to have effects on prenatal development that are not governed by variations in DNA sequences. Throughout life, physiology can - indeed, must - change to adapt to environmental variation. There are physiological reasons, for example, why losing excess weight or leaving behind any other sort of addiction is so hard. A number of drugs, particularly psychoactive drugs of abuse, and various foods, have been shown to cause changes in physiology mediated by changes in multiple gene functions that may persist long after the drug is withdrawn. Variations in imprinting and other elements of epigenetic control are major functional contributors to variations in the course and outcomes of embryogenesis. Our understanding of those controls is increasing rapidly, but has a long way to go.

7. Twinning

Among the most obvious of the more-or-less 'unusual' outcomes of human embryogenesis is twinning. According to the inferences about prenatal mortality and survival discussed above (Boklage 1990, 1995), twins born as members of live pairs represent no more than about one-in-fifty of all products of twin embryogenesis. Like singletons, over three-fourths of twin conceptions disappear completely (with loss of both conceptuses) before term birth. Most of the remaining one-fourth of twinned embryos arrive at term alone, as sole survivors, outnumbering live-born twins apparently at least ten- to twelve-fold. The strongest indications are that roughly one live birth in eight is a product of a twin embryogenesis, with the great majority of them showing no easily recognized evidence of their origins in twinned embryos. These sole survivors have been totally ignored in all the various literatures about the epidemiology of twinning. Developmental consequences of twin embryogenesis are not terribly hard to find in twins born in pairs (Boklage, 2009) and are therefore to be expected in the lives of those sole-survivor individuals. We do not yet know any simple or inexpensive way to identify all of the sole survivors for an accurate count, but clearly a substantial fraction of all human embryogeneses are twinned and a similar fraction of all live births arise from twinned embryos. I remain satisfied with the estimate of one in eight, with the realization that it may vary considerably up or down with variations in overall efficiency of pregnancies in general.

Since the mid-1960s, from deep within the old orthodoxy [in place since before Galton, 1875], that *'identical'* twins arise from 'splitting' embryos and *'fraternal'* twins arise from double ovulations unfolding into parallel and independent embryogeneses, it seemed obvious that we should be able to learn a great deal about embryogenesis from the ways in which the two 'kinds' of twins differ from each other and/or from singletons in their development.

Just suppose ... that the "common knowledge" is the truth. *Just suppose* that all the unusual things about the development of twins really are due to consequences of 'splitting' the embryos of the 'identical' twins (only) and thereby disturbing the establishment of their embryogenic asymmetries. *Suppose also*, as per the "common knowledge", that 'fraternal' twins arise from separate and independent egg cells, and that their development is the same as that of singletons - except perhaps for any effects specific to living through development - beginning in the cleavage stage or at least no later than the blastula - as twins. If all of that were true, if the common knowledge were the simple truth that it has been assumed and reported to be, we should be able to compare the development of 'identical' twins with singletons and learn a great deal about how embryogenesis generates the doubled three-dimensional body symmetry to make two embryos out of one. Dizygotic twins, from that perspective, would be the obvious 'controls' against any effects of simply being twins. That describes the climate in which these studies of human embryogenesis began, and that has been the outline of the plan of my research for the last few decades.

8. Probing twin embryogenesis

The answers have been surprising and consistent and clear. All "kinds" of twins as groups are about equally different from singleton development, in the same multidimensional directions, at about the same multidimensional distances. Things just are not like the common knowledge would have it. The evidence is clear and ample. *We have no reason to imagine that the cellular processes of embryogenesis in dizygotic twin pairs are any different from those for monozygotic twins.* A single contiguous mass of cells within a single *zona pellucida* confining the mass and substance of a single secondary oöcyte becomes organized by processes of cell differentiation into two complex asymmetric plans to become bodies for two fetuses. The cells may all contain copies of one zygote nucleus (the monozygotic twins), or - if syngamy yields two genetically distinct zygote nuclei, there may be two genetically distinct sibling cell lines (for dizygotic twins).

Like fertilization, or zygosis, or any other proposed definition of conception, the onset of twin embryogenesis, the 'conception' of twins if you will, is not an *event* that can be considered to occur in an instant, but is instead a complex *system process* that occupies space and time. It has no instantaneous beginning or end, but constitutes a developmental horizon, perhaps crisp and clear from a distance, but not subject to clear definition from anywhere within conceptual or temporal proximity.

Whether the twins thus initiated are monozygotic or dizygotic is a genetic distinction, not a cellular one. Two zygotes never had to mean two cells. Cells within an embryogenic cell mass that will generate monozygotic twins all have copies of one nuclear genome. [Keep in mind the occasional occurrence of post-zygotic mutations that may establish a second genetically distinct cell line - even a second embryo. That is the common knowledge explanation of "mosaic" embryos - who may have cytogenetically different cell lines, and are not usually tested for other genetic differences.] Dizygotic twins are built from cells with two different nuclear genomes, most likely different in every chromosome. Syngamy and zygosis have assembled *two zygote nuclei instead of one within the confines of the single secondary oocyte and its zona pellucida*. We must, of course, discuss how that can happen. Very briefly, the frequency of triploidy (the most common of all chromosome anomalies) tells us that tripronuclear zygotes are quite common, more or less equally possessing two paternal contributions or two maternal contributions. Those events are sufficiently frequent that neither can be considered to limit the frequency of their joint occurrence with both two paternal and two maternal pronuclei, to form two zygote nuclei after syngamy (*cf.* Boklage 2009, 2010).

Every trace of embryogenesis we have properly examined, with several independent samples and methods, shows that dizygotic twins differ developmentally from singletons at least as much as the monozygotic twins do, in very similar multidimensional directions and at very similar multidimensional distances (Boklage, 2006, 2009). There are enough differences to significantly distinguish monozygotic from dizygotic twins - as groups of individuals, without any consideration of within-pair similarities or differences. Those differences, however, are very small compared to the common differences of both 'kinds' of twins from singletons.

9. Handedness in twins and their families, and "mirror"-twinning

The minority version of brain function asymmetry (nonrighthanders = lefthanders + 'ambidexters') is more frequent in twins than in the general population. The lore has it that the excess belongs primarily to the 'identical' twins by virtue of 'splitting' their embryos, disrupting the proper asymmetries of ongoing embryogenesis. Actual data, on the other hand, show that the excess occurs *equally* in *both* 'kinds' of twins *and* in the singleton siblings of the twins. The parents of twins are more often nonrighthanded than *their* same-sex siblings - the maternal aunts and paternal uncles of the twins (calculated separately because of the consistent sex difference in frequency of nonrighthandedness in the general population). Each nonrighthanded parent increases probability of nonrighthandedness in the children - regardless of multiplicity - by a factor of about 1.5 (Boklage 1976, 1977a,b, 1981, 1987a).

In all of this, there is no effect of zygosity or chorionicity. Monochorionicity has been thought to indicate exclusively monozygotic twinning events occurring later in embryogenesis than those of dichorionic twins. The 'later splitting' has been imagined to be more likely to disrupt the ongoing establishment of embryogenic asymmetries. In fact chorionicity is not associated with any difference in the distribution of handedness. The excess of nonrighthandedness in twins is not specific to 'identical' twinning. Nor is the excess of nonrighthandedness in twins any greater among monochorionic pairs as proxy for 'late splitting' (Carlier *et al.*, 1996; Derom *et al.*, 1996).

The idea of "*mirror-imaging*" in twins, near and dear to the hearts of twins and their parents though it may be, does indeed mean something special about twin embryogenesis, but what it means is much more complex and fundamental than what they have been thinking (*cf* Boklage 2010), and nowhere near as much fun. In short, twins of both "kinds" are substantially more symmetrical in their craniofacial development than singletons. Dental diameter measurements from left sides and right sides from singletons are quite significantly consistently different - discriminant function calculations can identify the side of a singleton's head from which a set of dental diameter measurements were taken with over 95% accuracy. The same is not true of measurements from twins of either "kind". Discriminant function calculations report probabilities of over 90% that the left- vs right-half-jaw sets of measurements, within statistical error, might as well have been drawn from a single sample.

The excess of nonrighthandedness in twins arises from an inherited tendency to nonstandard brain function asymmetry that is concentrated in families which also have an inherited tendency to deliver live twin pairs. Neither differs as a function of zygosity or chorionicity (Boklage, 1981, 1985, 1987a; Carlier *et al.*, 1996; Derom et al. 1996) Something about establishing an unusual version of motor brain function asymmetry during embryogenesis and something about becoming twins at about that same time in embryogenesis is the same or closely related.

You will find it written in many places that dizygotic twinning and only dizygotic twinning is at all hereditary, and then only in the maternal line, by way of an inherited tendency to double ovulation. The entire literature of the biology of twinning is predicated on variation in the births of live twin pairs being considered a perfect proxy for variation in conceptions of twins - as if every twin conception must generate a live twin birth and that variation in twin deliveries directly reflect variation in double ovulation. Since older mothers for example deliver more twins, so the story goes, it must be because they have more (double ovulations and therefore more) twin conceptions. There is no significant attention paid to the facts 1) that those born alive as members of live twin pairs are a tiny fraction of those conceived as twins and 2) that we know very little about the complexity of the processes that make the differences between those conceived as twins and those born alive as twins. Because the live-born fraction of twin conceptions is so small, very small differences in the determinants of prenatal survival can make large fractional changes in the numbers born alive. For this reason above several others, the use of the Weinberg Difference Method in general is of dubious value, and its application to any population of twins with any significant anomaly is absolute nonsense.

10. Malformations in twins

Malformations, particularly the most common, midline/fusion malformations, are more frequent in twins. Neural tube defects, congenital heart defects, and orofacial clefts are the most common, therefore best known. These all involve structures formed in embryogenesis from the fusion in the midline of bilaterally-approximately-symmetrical half-structures. Following fusion of the asymmetric half-structures, the resulting midline structures are remodeled with and by mesenchyme cells descended from neural crest cells. Like nonrighthandedness, the malformations that are more frequent among twins than among singletons are also more frequent among the sibs and offspring of twins, without zygosity differences except in a few situations where the correlation is in fact stronger among the dizygotics and their families (Boklage 1985, 1987a,b, 2010).

Again like nonrighthandedness, throughout the history of studies of the biology of twinning, it has been reported that the malformations that are excessively frequent in twins are due predominantly to the 'identical' twins because of the 'splitting' required to generate monozygotic twin embryos causing disruptions of embryogenic symmetry operations.

Schinzel *et al.* 1979 provided a reasonably thorough review which is often offered as the standard reference on the relationship between monozygotic twinning and malformations. It included nothing new, being instead a good summary of prevailing prejudices and presumptions as if they were the available "common knowledge" facts of the matter. There are deep and wide problems with the sorting in every one of the sources they gathered to put their review together. With rare exception, none of the twin pairs included in those calculations were actually diagnosed for zygosity, let alone soundly diagnosed. The MZ excesses of the malformations considered there have in general been decided by sorting into same-sex vs opposite-sex twin pairs, under the assumption that the boy-girl pairs are in all ways developmentally representative of all dizygotic twins, and that the apparent concentration of difficulties in the like-sex pairs is due entirely to their concentration among the monozygotic members of the like-sex pairs. I have discussed the severe faults of that idea at length in Boklage 2010. OS-DZ pairs are unique. They are not developmentally representative of any other group. The members of OS-DZ pairs are not representative even of their own respective gender groups, twin or single. Risks of developmental anomaly or pregnancy wastage are in fact at least as great for same-sex DZ twins as for MZ twins (Boklage 1984, 1985, 1987c,d).

11. Blastulation, gastrulation, neurulation, the neural crest and asymmetries of human embryogenesis

The midline/fusion embryonic asymmetry malformations are sufficiently frequent in twins that they can readily be imagined to occur only in twins – if 'twins' properly includes the sole survivors. The numbers would allow it. They all intimately involve the neural crest. The structures in question are built by fusion in the midline, from left- and right-half structures, followed by remodeling with and by mesenchymal cells from the neural crest.

Until about the fourth and fifth days after fertilization, the embryo-in-progress is a solid ball of cells called the *morula* (*L., mul*berry). The outermost layer of cells becomes a membrane and then an epithelium (now the *trophoblast*, the future *chorion*) by forming *tight junctions* between the cells of its outermost layer to replace the *gap junctions* through which the cells of the morula communicated while held together inside the zona pellucida from zygosis through cleavage. Zona-breaker cells of the trophoblast now attack the zona pellucida with enzymes that leave the zona softened and weakened. The outer (trophoblast epithelium) layer of cells pump fluid from outside to inside, and the morula swells (for the first time growing beyond the mass and size of the 'egg cell' secondary oöcyte at ovulation) and sheds the softened zona. This is *hatching*.

The *inner cell mass* remains attached to a patch of the outer layer cells that we will now call the *polar trophoblast*, separated from the *mural trophoblast* (the *wall* of the embryo, exclusive of the *polar* patch) by the fluid pumped in through the trophoblast epithelium. The polar trophoblast will now attach to and penetrate the endometrium, catalyzing the formation of the placenta from interacting fetal and maternal tissues. By separating the *inner cell mass,* attached to the *polar trophoblast,* from the *mural trophoblast* and filling the intervening space with fluid and sloughing the dissolving zona pellucida, the *morula* now becomes the *blastula,* bounded by the trophoblast, containing the inner cell mass in the fluid-filled *blastocyst* cavity - a lump inside a ball.

The inner cell mass will now form and separate a double layer of cells facing the blastocyst cavity, forming another smaller cavity between that new *bilaminar disk* stage of the embryo and the polar trophoblast. The bilaminar disk has one microscopically visible patch of distinctly 'taller' cells in each of its layers. Cells of the *prochordal (sometimes called prechordal) plate,* near the anterior end of the embryo, are longer than their neighbors in the direction of the blastocyst cavity. That direction thereby becomes recognizable as the *ventral* direction. The cells of the *primitive streak,* near the posterior edge of the disk, are taller in the *dorsal* direction, into the newly formed amnionic cavity. The anterior-posterior (head-tail), and dorsal-ventral (back-belly) asymmetries are thereby made visible and the left vs right dimension is also therefore constrained with no dimensional degrees-of-freedom remaining.

The attachment of the inner cell mass to the polar trophoblast has previously identified the dorsal aspect of the embryo. So, the definition of the anterior-posterior axis by the appearance of the prochordal plate and the primitive streak actually constrains the whole system of three axes. It must be remembered that the cells in question began their various biochemical differentiations before those differentiations became microscopically visible in spatial coordinates.

The human blastula does not form a *gastrula* stage exactly like the structures in other embryos to which we usually give that name, but what comes next, the formation of the trilaminar disk stage, is the human homologue of *gastrulation.* From the primitive streak, cells multiply and spread to the anterior and laterally between the layers of the bilaminar disk, forming the third embryonic layer in the middle (the *mesoderm*). The dorsal layer is now the *ectoderm* (which will soon be divided into the neural plate and the non-neural ectoderm that will form the skin), the ventral *endoderm* which will form the gut and associated structures, and the new middle layer will be the *mesoderm,* primarily to build muscle and bone.

When the embryo becomes the trilaminar disk, the process of *neurulation* begins. Most diagrams of this period show the cells of the new middle layer multiplying rapidly from somewhere in or near the anterior end of the primitive streak, diving under the ectoderm just anterior to it, between the ectodermal and endodermal layers, and spreading anteriolaterally, toward the prochordal plate and to the sides. These cells appear to correspond closely in function to the cells of the amphibian *Organizer,* the avian *Hensen's node,* and the zebrafish *shield.*

These cells will induce the formation of the neural plate, the *neurectoderm,* from the portion of the ectoderm lying dorsal to them. The edges of the neural plate– at the border between neural and non-neural ectoderm - begin to roll up and toward the midline in a wavelike structure, led by differentiating cells at the boundary between the neuroectoderm and the non-neural ectoderm. The peaks of those rolls will meet in the midline and fuse to form the neural tube. The cells of the neural crests (of the 'waves') meet in the dorsal midline to differentiate and begin migrating laterally and ventrolaterally to an enormous number of destinations to perform a dazzling array of embryogenic functions on each side of the midline.

12. Formation of the neural crest

Formation of the neural crest is a major watershed moment in embryogenesis. It may well be that no other group of cells comparable in number has more functions to perform in embryogenesis, especially in the realm of the determination and elaboration of embryogenic asymmetries and the formation of midline structures by fusion of bilateral halves.

The autonomic nervous system, the enteric nervous system, the pigment cells, most of the bones of the head and face, the jaws and the teeth, the bones of the ears, the inner structures of the heart, the adrenal medulla ... an incredible variety of specialized cell types will be formed either from, or under influences of, mesenchymal derivatives of the neural crest cells (Chang *et al.,* 2008; Kirby *et al.*, 1983, for examples from a large and varied literature).

The radiation and development of the neural crest cells is driven by a gene regulatory network the complexity of which we have just begun to appreciate. This is a system of interacting signals, transcription factors, and cascades of downstream effector genes that will guide the final migrations and differentiations of the neural crest cells (Betancur *et al.*, 2010; Huang & Saint-Jeanett, 2004); Abnormalities in neural crest development cause '*neurocristopathies*', which include conditions such as frontonasal dysplasia, Waardenburg-Shah syndrome, and DiGeorge syndrome, along with all of the individual non-syndromic midline/fusion malformations.

13. Craniofacial development in twins vs singletons

The developmental anomalies which are more frequent in twins than in singletons are of these kinds: anomalies in the development of midline structures formed from bilaterally-almost-symmetrical half-structures by fusion in the midline, followed by remodeling under influence of neural crest mesenchyme. The excess of nonrighthandedness in twins mentioned above, for example, long assumed and reported to be a certain consequence of monozygotic twinning, but shown here to be equally frequent in dizygotic twins and in the close relatives of all "kinds" of twins, seems to be a clear example. We do not to this day, however, know the cellular bases for the normal asymmetries of the motor functions of the brain, so it is not obvious in molecular terms how they might be disturbed by the cellular events of twinning.

We know a good bit more about the cellular and molecular bases of craniofacial development, as represented in the development of the teeth (Boklage, 1984, 1987d, 2010). Multidimensional structural relationships in craniofacial development, represented in a sub-system model by the covariance matrices of 56 buccolingual and mesiodistal dental diameter measurements, clearly discriminate between twins and singletons, as groups of individuals, with over 95% accuracy. A small fraction of cases entering these analyses identified as singletons are scored as twins by some of the discriminant functions, but no one identified as a twin is ever misclassified as a singleton. This could have been predicted.

Any large enough sample of singletons is highly likely to include some 'sole survivors' of twin embryogenesis. The presently best available estimate is that about one live birth in eight arises from twin embryogenesis (Boklage 1990, 1995). At that rate, the probability that a sample of ten single births will include at least one sole surviving twin is almost 75%.

These results further make it clear that girl-boy pairs are absolutely not developmentally representative of all dizygotic twins. They are different from all other groups. Of course, normal boy-girl pairs are dizygotic. Their developmental patterns are different from singletons and from same-sex twins of either sex. To assume that they are entirely representative of all dizygotic twins, and therefore that every difference between opposite-sex and same-sex twin groups arises entirely from the monozygotic members of the same-sex group, is shortsighted, lazy, baseless and untenable.

If embryogenesis is to be double, to build twin bodies from a single contiguous mass of embryonic cells, then differentiation as twins must begin with a doubling of the definition of the embryonic axes, just as in the simplest of embryos. In the human embryo, the dorsal-ventral direction is the first axis grossly visible, as the bilaminar disc separates from the rest of the inner cell mass attached to the polar trophoblast, before the prochordal plate and the primitive streak appear, to make the anterior-posterior direction apparent. There will need to be two of everything required to induce the formation of primitive streaks, neural tubes and neural crests. It has been proposed that the formation of the primitive streak defines the onset of human individuality because it marks the end of the possibility of twinning and of one conceptus (with one sacred immortal personal human soul) becoming more than one person.

14. Pyloric stenosis, Hirschsprung disease, enteric nervous system, and neural crest: Twins! Yes! But ... No sign of monozygotics!

Pyloric stenosis affects about one in 600 children. It is a disorder of the development of the enteric nervous system, which includes more neurons than the spinal cord, all apparently derived from cells of the neural crest (Farlie et al., 2004, Barlow et al. 2008). Pyloric stenosis is over 30% more frequent in twins than in singletons, four times as frequent in males as in females, rarely concordant in twins, and we really can find no reason to believe that any of the affected twin pairs are monozygotic. The greatest repeat risk is among twin brothers of affected females. This is an intriguing prospect contrary to all of the old background ... a highly heritable multifactorial midline malformation - a neurocristopathy - exclusive to the embryogenesis of dizygotic twins (including sole survivors)?!. If, as it seems, this particular developmental deviation does not in fact occur in liveborn monozygotic twins, then it might be lethal in MZ embryos OR it might require the presence of two different genomes or epigenomes, and singleton cases must all be sole survivors of twin embryogenesis. These results are not yet published - we're thinking of running a contest with a prize for a testable mechanism - that it should also be plausible presently seems too much to ask.

Hirschsprung disease is a less common disorder of the enteric nervous system, affecting the colon in about 1/1500 children, with epidemiology very similar to pyloric stenosis: >80% males, excessive in frequency among twins, even more highly heritable than pyloric stenosis *and* even more rarely concordant in twins (Bolande, 1997; Jones, 1990; Kenny et al. 2010; Martucciello, 1977; Moore, 2006; Shahar & Shinawi, 2003; Tam, 1986; Tam & Garcia-Barceló, 2009; Templeton, 1977).

15. Chimerism and chimeras

Arguably the most intriguing variation on the themes of human embryogenesis is spontaneous embryonic chimerism, and it provides essential insight here. Spontaneous embryogenic chimerism is a branch of the twinning process. A spontaneous embryogenic human chimera is an individual whose body is composed of two embryonic cell lines with different genotypes. For present purposes, this does not include chimerism installed by way of a blood transfusion or other tissue transplant, nor does it include colonization of women by cells transferred into their bodies from a conceptus. It is herein meant to be understood as the embryogenesis of dizygotic twins occurring within a single contiguous mass of cells (Boklage, 2006). Assortment of the cells of two different genotypes into the separate twin body symmetries from a single mass of cells is unlikely to be perfect. Either or both of the cotwins thus derived may incorporate some cells of the other cotwin's genotype (Abuelo, 2009; Boklage, 2006).

According to very nearly everything you will read, human embryogenic chimeras are exquisitely rare. This is quite compatible with chimerism being thought to arise from the fusion of placental circulations of independent dichorionic dizygotic twin fetuses. It does not happen that way. Anastomosis of placental circulation has been found to have happened only a handful of times in examination of several thousand fused dichorionic dizygotic placentas (Foschini et al., 2003).

When directly tested for, chimerism has been found in over eight per cent of a sample of dizygotic twins and 21 per cent of dizygotic triplets (van Dijk et al., 1996), using an exquisitely sensitive test with fluorescent antibodies against five red blood cell antigens. Given that chimerism, when present, need not be present in blood, and the considerable possibility of sib-sib matching for alleles at five loci (so that cells of co-twins would not be detectably different - a negative test for chimerism), these numbers clearly represent a minimal estimate of the chimerism that was there. Remembering that the two cell lines of human embryonic chimeras are by definition the genetic equivalent of dizygotic twins, and that the majority of products of twin conceptions are born single, chimerism found in twins born alive as twin pairs represents a minor fraction of the chimerism that might be found if all cases could be identified.

In another direct study, female cadavers were tested for chimerism in multiple tissues, indicated by fluorescent hybridization histochemistry for Y-chromosome DNA sequences, scored as positive only when labeled in tissue-specific cells to exclude possibility of having captured blood cells 'just passing through'. In about one third of the women tested, chimerism was found in one or more of the tested tissues. History of having borne one or more sons (exposing the woman to the possibility of fetomaternal cell transfer), or of having had one or more transfusions, did not increase the frequency. Since only male 'foreign' cells were visualized, the true frequency of chimerism might have been twice what was observed, closer to two-thirds of the women sampled (Koopmans *et al.*, 2005). The idea that chimerism could be as frequent as two-thirds of live births is hard to believe. Ideally, that study should be extended to similar numbers of virgin females, to control for the possibility of transfers from unrecognized transient conceptions of sons or the transfer of any other types of Y-bearing cells through vaginal mucosa by insemination.

It is abundantly clear that chimerism is not rare. Because of the much greater numbers of twins born alone, chimerism may well be several times as frequent as births of live twins in pairs. Chimerism has no macroscopic phenotype of its own. It has been, and generally still is, called "extremely rare" because it is *discovered* rarely and only by accident. The first reported instance was in 1953, when a unit of blood from a normal, healthy English woman was found to have about a 70:30 mixture of red cells of two different serotypes. Since then, a number of other cases have been found by way of such mixed-field agglutination, but admixtures of less than 15 to 20 per cent are not usually discoverable in standard serological blood typing. Molecular genotyping, as in forensic identification, is - more-or-less as a matter of policy - no better: when a genotyping scan shows an extra allele peak with less than 30 per cent of the strength of the main peak value, it is marked as noise and ignored. When an extra allele peak appears at 30 per cent or more of the main peak value, especially if multiple loci are involved, the sample is declared contaminated and discarded (but see Erlich, 2011). Because "everybody knows" chimerism is exquisitely rare, we do not in general look for it, and we hardly ever find what we do not believe will be there.

The majority of living humans are built of normal cells, and there is every reason to suppose that the great majority of chimeras must have two normal cell lines. A couple of sensational cases were covered in the popular press. Karen Keegan needed a new kidney. Her husband and three sons were tested first. The probability of a match was small, but keeping it in the family has advantages. Her husband proved to be an excellent prospective donor. Almost overshadowing that good news was that the DNA results said two of her three sons [she conceived, carried, delivered and raised them] are not her sons, but cannot be hospital label-switching accidents. The DNA results say they are sons of her husband and another woman. Examination of frozen samples from previous surgeries showed that the "other woman" exists genetically in the form of some cells in her body from her unborn dizygotic twin sister. This woman is a chimera, with no sign in her phenotype, discovered entirely by the accident of carefully genotyping her whole family for purposes unrelated to her chimerism (Yu *et al.*, 2002).

Another case in progress shortly thereafter concerned a young woman who needed public assistance to start over after separating from the father of her two children and her fetus. DNA said the two children were children of her partner and another woman. There were questions of welfare fraud, that she might be seeking public assistance for children who were not her own, and questions as to what she had done with the real mother. Were there crimes rather worse than fraud involved? A representative of the court was in the delivery room to gather samples for DNA on the spot. The newborn is full sibling to the other two - same father, same mother who still is genetically not the woman from whose belly the baby had just been seen to emerge. No old surgical samples were available this time, but samples from various more-or-less accessible parts of her body yielded some cells of "the other woman", the twin sister who was never born and is a perfect genetic candidate for being the mother of all three children. This woman is a chimera, with no sign in her phenotype, discovered entirely by the accident of carefully genotyping her whole family for purposes unrelated to her chimerism. Lydia Fairchild's case never to my knowledge made it into the scientific literature, but can be found in many popular press items on the web.

Some human chimeras are discovered when they are observed to be hermaphrodites and investigation reveals a mixture of XX and XY cells. Experimentally constructed mixed-sex chimeras of mice almost always have a normal male phenotype at delivery. A paternally-imprinted X-chromosome [present only in female embryos], retards the growth of embryonic cells in human as well as in mouse. Faster growth of the XY cells in mixed-sex embryos might reasonably be expected to minimize the fraction of mixed-sex human chimeras that are detectably hermaphroditic. Some chimeras are discovered when twins are observed to be dizygotic (different sex is the easiest, but not the only, way to tell) and monochorionic (*cf* Erlich, 2011; Parva *et al.*, 2009; Walker *et al.*, 2007).

Mixed-sex twins are less often found as chimeras but they are found at sufficient frequency to know they have their place. Because experimental mixed-sex mouse chimeras almost always show up as normal males, I find it plausible that the lower-than-binomially-expected frequency of mixed-sex human chimeras is probably caused by the large growth-rate advantage of XY embryonic cells – reviewed in Boklage, 2005.

16. Monochorionic dizygotic twins are chimeras, and they are common

For most of the history of any analyses of twins, in fact apparently at least since Galton in 1875, monochorionicity has been considered to be absolutely diagnostic of monozygosity. Samples recorded as opposite-sex and monochorionic have been summarily deleted from data bases as obvious errors. It could not be otherwise, since it is clear [so says the common knowledge] that dizygotic twins must come from separate and independent egg cells and could not possibly be from a single embryo as monochorionic twin pairs must be. [Here is one part of the problem: 'monoembryonic' has never been the same as 'monozygotic.' Just as a zygote may become more than one 'embryo', one embryonic cell mass may contain more than one zygote (nucleus).] Over the decades, a few monochorionic dizygotic pairs had been discovered and ignored as meaningless anomalies. A (then-)young physician from Glasgow was publicly declared laboratory-incompetent and shouted down at the Fifth International Congress on Twin Studies in Amsterdam for telling us he had found a few dizygotic pairs among the monochorionic pairs in his practice ["…everyone knows… after all," and the pillars of the Society came down upon his head and shoulders]. I did not know then what I know now and could not defend him.

Recently, the number of reported cases has more than doubled, and the reality of monochorionic dizygotic twins has begun to sink in. Monochorionic dizygotic twins are necessarily chimeric, since they share at least some embryonic cells of one another's genotype in the form of the shared chorion. Monochorionic twins of the same sex were unanimously for decades declared monozygotic without 'wasting the reagents' to genotype them for zygosity – of course it is "well known" that such twin pairs are "always" monozygotic. That 1986 study from Glasgow (Mortimer 1987) and a later and larger one from Taiwan (Yang *et al.*, 2006) agree – about a quarter to a third of consecutive, unselected monochorionic twins are dizygotic, and therefore necessarily chimeric.

A recent paper on the risk of monozygotic twinning in deliveries from artificially assisted pregnancies counted very nearly all of the "monozygotic" pairs included in their analysis merely from ultrasound indications of monochorionicity (Vitthala *et al.*, 2009). The rest were estimated by Weinberg Method calculations, as the excess of same-sex pairs over the number of opposite-sex pairs, with the required unacknowledged assumptions that the pairings were independent at fertilization and stable throughout gestation, in spite of often-reported excess losses of males and of members of same-sex pairs.

The future chorion differentiates, first as the trophoblast, from the outer layer of cells of the morula stage of the 'embryo' before 'hatching' - that is, while still inside the one same *zona pellucida* that came out of the follicle surrounding the egg cell. [Until just before 'hatching' by shedding the zona, as the morula is changing to become the blastocyst, the cell divisions of the cleavage stage of embryogenesis have partitioned the original substance and volume of the oöcyte, increasing in cell number and decreasing in cell size.] Because they are often born as chimeras, and because they are sometimes born monochorionic, we are left with no reason to doubt that naturally-conceived human dizygotic twins can and usually do arise from a single contiguous mass of cells divided from the contents of a single secondary oöcyte. The rest of the background cited above includes no evidence that any naturally conceived dizygotic twins ever develop without the embryogenic differences between singletons and monozygotic twins (Boklage 2009).

Every publication that ever said that dizygotic twins come from double ovulation either just says it as if it-is-a-fact-and-everyone-knows-it, OR provides a reference to another writing as authority for the statement. That reference in its turn either just says it as if it-is-a-fact-and-everyone-knows-it, OR provides a reference to another writing as authority for the statement. Follow each and every such chain as far as you can, you will find no one offering any evidence. There is no evidence anywhere that any spontaneous human twin pair ever came from two egg cells. Once upon a long time ago, someone said it was so, and someone else heard that and thought it made sense and he wrote it down. Someone else read it and then wrote 'it has been written that it is so'. And someone else read that and wrote "it is well and widely known that it is so" and someone else read that and wrote "it is common knowledge that it is so" and so it ever since has been.

17. How can embryogenesis generate two embryos from a single 'egg cell'?

We are left with the question of HOW a single secondary oöcyte can serve as substrate for the embryogenesis of twins with two sibling genomes in the same embryo, differing in both the maternal and paternal contributions.

The paternal part of the story is the simpler part: the orthodox story of 'normal' human embryogenesis includes a very rapid calcium-mediated change in the zona pellucida and the egg-cell cortex after penetration by a sperm cell. This change in the boundaries of the oöcyte is called the *'polyspermy block'*. It is supposed to prevent the entry of a second sperm. One thing we know for certain about it is that it does not work perfectly, maybe not even very well. We know that dispermy is common, because diandric triploidy is common. A triploid embryo has three copies of all chromosomes instead of the normal two; there are three parental half-genomes grown from three pronuclei entering zygosis. The great majority of triploid embryos fail to complete embryogenesis. Most triploids ever seen are seen as spontaneous abortions, of which they constitute one of the largest fractions. Very few are born alive, only to die within at most a few days.

There is disagreement, more apparent than real, in the literature as to the relative frequency of diandric (with two paternal pronuclear contributions) and digynic (with two maternal pronuclear contributions) triploids. There is, however, at least as much variability among the samplings reported as there is in the results. The available data must be reconsidered, the sooner the better, with larger samples to make it possible to fractionate the results by time to failure. Normal diploid embryos grow more slowly with a paternally-imprinted X chromosome (reviewed in Boklage, 2005). There are at least these five possible configurations [xxX xxY xXX xXY xYY] where x represents a maternal X-chromosome, X a paternal X, and Y is Y. There are three configurations with paternally imprinted X-chromosomes, one of which is digynic (xxX) and two diandric (xXX and xXY). The xYY is by far the rarest among triploid spontaneous abortuses, and presumably therefore the least likely to complete embryogenesis. xxX and xXY have one paternally imprinted X; xXX has two of them. We have no reasonable way to examine the progress of embryogenesis to learn about the relative longevity of these various triploid configurations, except by extrapolation and inference from a more thorough study of a larger sample of triploid abortuses.

At any rate, it is clear that dispermy is not rare, nor is the presence of two maternal pronuclei rare, among failures of embryogenesis. Most discussions of possibilities like these have been based on believing that the most likely source of two maternal pronuclei is the failure to sequester the second polar body after the second meiotic division of the oöcyte, which is believed normally to be triggered by, and occur after, penetration of the secondary oöcyte by the sperm. However, several of the papers on the subject suggest that errors of the first oöcyte meiosis are the major source. This may result from the error of believing that the output of Meiosis II is a pair of 'identical' sister chromatids, and that only Meiosis I errors would bring different maternal contributions into a tripronuclear zygote. We all believed that once upon a time, and we thought wrong and did things wrong because of it for a long time. That thinking ignores the effects of recombination … we still expect the centromeres segregating in Meiosis II to be sister centromeres, but the arms of those chromosomes have undergone at least one obligate recombination per arm, and the changes from those rearrangements segregate in the second meiotic division.

18. Conclusions

In every way that we have been able to sample the effects of twin embryogenesis on development, we find monozygotic and dizygotic twins to be equivalent in their clear differences from singletons. The embryogenesis of dizygotic twins is subject to each and all of the anomalies long attributed entirely to monozygotic twin embryogenesis. The twinning mechanism in the embryogenesis of dizygotic twins is the same as that of monozygotic twins, and subtly different from two simultaneous occurrences of singleton embryogenesis (even anencephaly does not represent a very large deviation from the normal developmental protocols – if the product of embryogenesis is not round, at least the basics of the plan has been executed). This is not compatible with the idea of dizygotic twins arising from independent double ovulation. The developmental histories of dizygotic co-twins are not independent and they are not like those of singletons. Whatever happens in embryogenesis to generate dizygotic twins is the same thing that happens to generate monozygotic twins. One embryogenesis becomes two; two body symmetry plans, two sets of axes, are differentiated from a single contiguous mass of cells.

Here it is customary and plausible to fall back on our understanding of these processes drawn from more accessible embryos. Gene products involved in generating the necessary changes in cell shapes and functions are known to serve the same or closely related functions in embryogeneses ranging from flies and worms and tadpoles to fish and birds and mammals. There are genes whose products are synthesized only in anterior cells where head and brain will soon be formed. There are genes whose products are synthesized only in posterior cells that will become germ-line, sperm or egg, cells. There are genes whose products are synthesized to form gradients from anterior to posterior and from dorsal to ventral and vice-versa. For many of those genes, the amino acid sequence of that gene's product, and the DNA sequence encoding it, have been highly conserved across millions to hundreds of millions of years. A favorite of mine is a gene discovered in the fruit fly *Drosophila melanogaster* where it was named *eyeless* because those flies have what looks like burn scars the size of eyes where their eyes should be. The homologous gene from mouse, Pax6, can be patched into transgenic flies whose gametes can then give rise to flies with perfectly good eyes - proper compound insect eyes; not single-chambered ('simple') mouse eyes. Several disorders of eye development in humans are known to be caused by mutations in the homologous human gene, PAX6. Of course, it takes more than one gene product to build an eye, whether the compound insect eye or the single-chambered eyes of mammals and mollusks. But every animal eye the development of which has been properly examined has a close homolog of *eyeless* that it needs to generate a normal functional outcome.

There are many other genes and multigene families involved in embryogenic differentiation, under multiple layers of control. Developmental variations in gene expression to define the myriad cell types of the embryonic and fetal body are combinatorial, rising in number exponentially with the number of genes involved. Potential variation is in fact effectively infinite, because those innumerable combinations of genes are not just binary, on-or-off, but tunable to generate varying amounts of each of their products.

As another layer of control, a great many of the products of developmental genes can be made in multiple forms. At least many, and probably most, of those DNA sequences include multiple *exons* - DNA sequences that can be expressed as amino acid sequences in protein products, alternating with always-one-less-number of *introns* - intervening sequences that will be removed by splicing and will not become part of the messenger RNA to code for the protein product of that gene. The *primary transcript* of RNA copied directly off the DNA sequence of the gene needs to splice out the introns and join the exons to become the mature messenger RNA to be transcribed into protein. In many, maybe most, cases, alternative splicing can make a messenger RNA from any combination of those exons. Ten is not at all an unusually high number of exons for a given gene, and ten exons can yield over 1,000 different versions of that gene product [ten independent binary choices, $(\text{in-or-out})^{10} = 1{,}024$] depending on which exons are included in a given messenger RNA. Instances are also known in which messenger RNAs include exons from more than one gene's primary transcripts.

Remember, furthermore, that all of these developmental variations must occur in the proper place in the embryo and at the proper time. Most of the coding / gene expression changes are most likely to occur in the process of cell divisions, when the chromatin packing of the chromosomes must change with condensation and re-expansion. The DNA is asymmetric in the chemical differences between its strands and in the chromatin changes associated with each round of DNA duplication. The leading and lagging strands for replication are different in their sequence composition and alignment. Each comes through a replication event with an old copy that just served as template, and a new copy. Modifications, such as methylation and demethylation, of DNA bases are realigned in each replication.

DNA in the cell is never naked, and seldom even available for the base-sequence-specific replication or transcription of any given sequence. The DNA is covered in RNA molecules and histones and non-histone proteins, in a constantly moving and changing multidimensional structure. Genes that need to be transcribed in any given cell at any given time must be made available for the RNA polymerase complexes, to reach their promoters, under the influences of their enhancers, silencers, insulators and perhaps other elements of transcriptional control remaining to be discovered.

When replication is due, the entire sequence will become available to multiple replication complexes, no more than a few hundred bases at a time. The five major types of histone molecules that form the bulk of the chromatin structure are subject to modification at multiple amino acid side chains, each with a different effect on the degree to which that region of chromatin sequesters its DNA. Some of the lysines can be acetylated, some of the lysines and some of the arginines can be methylated, some serines and threonines can be phosphorylated, and some lysines can be ubiquitinylated or sumoylated. Some of the modifications occur in the core regions of the histone complexes and some in the amino-terminal tails of histone molecules. Some change the strength of the electrostatic binding between the basic histone proteins and the nucleic acid. Some change the available density of binding sites on the chromatin for non-histone proteins that participate in other ways in the regulation and variation of histone binding. This is the heart of *epigenetic developmental regulation*, where environmental effects ranging from air pollution to mother's moods can reach into embryogenesis and fetal development, where cells can be reprogrammed to reflect an acquired addiction, where proper regulatory control of cell division and differentiation can be lost to cancer.

The structure of every cell's chromatin in fact **must** change over **the whole genome** with every replication of the DNA. Every cell division requires the entire chromatin package to be rearranged, to move aside at least enough to allow DNA replication. Every cell division requires the entire chromatin package to be rebuilt to accommodate the two new DNA strands, each made of one old template strand and one newly replicated strand - the old leading strand is now partnered with a new lagging strand and vice-versa. For all these reasons, by all these means, every cell division is asymmetric in several dimensions and is therefore a perfect place to execute programmatic changes to the combinatorial genetic and epigenetic switches that constitute cellular differentiation.

Caenorhabditis elegans is a nematode worm that is usually about one millimeter long in its adult form. It has 671 cells in its newly hatched larva at the completion of embryogenesis, some of which die, some of which continue to divide, to reach 959 cells in its adult body. Each one is in the exact place it is in by virtue of an invariant developmental history of asymmetric cell divisions - up here, right next, then tailward, then left, now ventral, etc., as the case may be, most of which involve an asymmetric change of epigenetic program. Each adult cell's specialized definition is specified by its history of sequential asymmetric divisions. Many of the genes involved in those differentiations still have homologs with crucial functions in the embryogeneses of placental mammals, including the human. Sidney Brenner, Robert Horvitz and John Sulston won the 2002 Nobel Prize in Physiology or Medicine for explaining this (*cf* Sulston *et al.*, 1983; Sulston, 2003). It took about a hundred years from the start of that project until it reached its present approximation of being finished.

There are millions of cells in the muscles and nerves, skin and bone of my left hand that have to perform exactly the same functions as corresponding millions of cells in my right hand, only in a different direction. Many of them can trace their developmental programs back to neural crest cells that came from opposite sides of the dorsal midline to the periphery to do their jobs, that came to their places in the dorsal midline from exactly opposite positions at the boundary of the neural and non-neural ectoderm, that came to those places at that boundary from a single cell proliferated from the tip of the primitive streak as daughter cells moving in opposite directions. It is reasonable to suppose that their fates have been mirrored throughout the trip.

Embryogenesis of the human is not as strict and precise as that of *C. elegans*. *C. elegans* is more toward the 'mosaic' embryogenesis end of the spectrum and the human more 'regulative'; the cells of *C. elegans* appear to be more, and human embryonic cells less, *determinate*. However, recent work shows more regulative embryonic behavior in *C. elegans* embryogenesis than we have been accustomed to believing. The human body with billions of times more cells than *C. elegans* has, is vastly more complex, but seeing the overlaps of functions to be served and gene products to serve those functions, we are left with little room to doubt that the systems of processes are homologous.

19. Acknowledgments

This work has been supported in part by NIH grants R01-HD-22507 and N01-HG-65403, and by grants from the Children's Miracle Network and the Brody School of Medicine at East Carolina University.

20. References

Aw S, Levin M (2009) Molecular mechanisms establishing consistent left-right asymmetry during vertebrate embryogenesis. In Sommer IEC, Kahn RS (eds) (2009) *Language Lateralization and Psychosis*. Cambridge Univ Press.

Barlow AJ, Wallace AS, Thapar N, Burns AJ (2008) Critical numbers of neural crest cells are required in the pathways from the neural tube to the foregut to ensure complete enteric nervous system formation. Development 135 (9): 1681–1691.

Begasse ML, Hyman AA (2011) The first cell cycle of the Caenorhabditis elegans embryo: spatial and temporal control of an asymmetric cell division. Probl Cell Differ 53:109-133.

Betancur P, Bronner-Fraser M, Sauka-Spengler T. (2010) Assembling neural crest regulatory circuits into a gene regulatory network. Ann Rev Cell Dev Biol 26:581-603.

Boklage CE (1976) Embryonic determination of brain programming asymmetry: A neglected element in twin-study genetics of human mental development. Acta Genet Med Gemellol 25:244-248.

Boklage CE (1977a) Schizophrenia, brain asymmetry development, and twinning: A cellular relationship with etiologic and possibly prognostic implications. Biol Psychiatry 12(1):19-35.

Boklage CE (1977b) Embryonic determination of brain programming asymmetry: A caution about the use of data on twins in genetic studies of human mental development. Annals N Y Acad Sci 299:306-308.

Boklage CE (1981) On the distribution of nonrighthandedness among twins and their families. Acta Genet Med Gemellol; 1981 30:167-187.

Boklage CE (1984) Differences in protocols of craniofacial development related to twinship and zygosity. J Craniofac Genet Devel Biol 4:151-169.

Boklage CE (1985) Interactions between opposite-sex dizygotic fetuses, and the assumptions of Weinberg Difference Method epidemiology. Am J Hum Genet 37(3):591-605.

Boklage CE (1987a) Twinning, nonrighthandedness and fusion malformations: Evidence for heritable causal elements held in common. Invited Editorial Essay, Am J Med Genet 28:67-84.

Boklage CE (1987b) The organization of the oöcyte and embryogenesis in twinning and fusion malformations. Acta Genet Med Gemellol 36:421-431.

Boklage CE (1987c) Race, zygosity, and mortality among twins: Interaction of myth and method. Acta Genet Med Gemellol 36:275-288.

Boklage CE (1987d) Developmental differences between singletons and twins in distributions of dental diameter asymmetries. Am J Phys Anthro 74(3):319-332.

Boklage CE (1990) The survival probability of human conceptions from fertilization to term. Int J Fertil;35:75-94

Boklage CE (1995) The frequency and survival probability of natural twin conceptions In: Keith LG, Papiernik E, Keith DM, Luke B (eds) *Multiple Pregnancy: Epidemiology, Gestation and Perinatal Outcome*. New York: Parthenon, 1995, 41-50.

Boklage CE (2005) The epigenetic environment: secondary sex ratio depends on differential survival in embryogenesis. Hum Reprod 20(3):583-587.

Boklage CE (2006) Embryogenesis of chimeras, twins and anterior midline asymmetries. Hum Reprod 21(3):579-591. Republished in Human Reproduction Indian Edition. May 2006; 2(6): 267-279.

Boklage CE (2009) Traces of embryogenesis are the same in monozygotic and dizygotic twins: not compatible with double ovulation. Hum Reprod 24(6):1255-1266. Epub 2009 Feb 27.

Boklage CE (2010) *How New Humans are Made: Cells and Embryos, Twins and Chimeras, Left and Right, Mind/Self\Soul, Sex and Schizophrenia*. World Scientific Publishers, Singapore, London, Hackensack

Bolande RP (1997) Neurocristopathy: its growth and development in 20 years. Pediatr Pathol Lab Med 17(1):1-25.

Buckett WM, Chian RC, Holzer H, Dean N, Usher R, Tan SL (2007) Obstetric outcomes and congenital abnormalities after in vitro maturation, in vitro fertilization, and intracytoplasmic sperm injection. Obstet Gynecol 110(4):885-891.

Buznikov GA, Chudakova IV, Zvezdina ND (1964) The role of neurohumours in early embryogenesis. I. Serotonin content of developing embryos of sea urchin and loach. J. Embryol exp Morph 12(4)563-573.

Carlier M, Spitz E, Vacher-Lavenu MC, Villéger P, Martin B, Michel F (1996) Manual performance and laterality in twins of known chorion type. Behav Genet 26(4):407-409.

Chang C-P, Stankunas K, Shang C, Kao S-C, Twu KY, Cleary ML (2008) Pbx1 functions in distinct regulatory networks to pattern the great arteries and cardiac outflow tract. Development 135: 3577-3586.

Huang X, Saint-Jeannet JP (2004) Induction of the neural crest and the opportunities of life on the edge. Dev Biol 275(1):1-11.

Derom C, Thiery E, Vlietinck R, Loos R, Derom R (1996) Handedness in twins according to zygosity and chorion type: a preliminary report. Behav Genet 26:407-408.
Erlich Y (2011) Blood ties: chimerism can mask twin discordance in high-throughput sequencing. Twin Res Hum Genet 14(2):137-143.
Farlie PG, McKeown SJ, Newgreen DF (2004) The neural crest: basic biology and clinical relationships in the craniofacial and enteric nervous systems. Birth Defects Res C Embryo Today 72(2):173-189.
Foschini MP, Gabrielli L, Dorji T, Kos M, Lazzarotto T, Lanari M, Landini MP (2003) Vascular anastomoses in dichorionic diamniotic-fused placentas. Int J Gynecol Pathol. 2003 Oct;22(4):359-361.
Fukumoto T, Kema IP, Levin M (2006) Serotonin signaling is a very early step in Patterning of the Left-Right Axis in chick and frog embryos. Current Biol 16:794-803.
Galton F (1875) The History of Twins[1]. *In Inquiries into Human Faculty and its Development*, pp 155-173 .
Green NS (2004) Risks of birth defects and other adverse outcomes associated with assisted reproductive technology. Pediatrics 114(1):256-259.
Huh YH, Sherley JL (2011) Molecular cloaking of H2A.Z on mortal DNA chromosomes during nonrandom segregation. Stem Cells 29(10):1620-1627.
Il'kova G, Rehak P, Vesela J, Cikos S, Fabian D, Czikkova S, Koppel J (2004) Serotonin localization and its functional significance during mouse preimplantation embryo development. Zygote 12:205-213
Jones MC (1990) The neurocristopathies: reinterpretation based upon the mechanism of abnormal morphogenesis. Cleft Palate Journal 27(2):136-140.
Kenny SE, Tam PK, Garcia-Barcelo M (2010) Hirschsprung's disease. Semin Pediatr Surg 19(3):194-200.
Kirby ML, Gale TF, Stewart DE (1983) Neural crest cells contribute to normal aorticopulmonary septation. Science 220(4601): 1059-1061.
Klar AJS (1987) Differentiated parental DNA strands confer developmental asymmetry on daughter cells in fission yeast. Nature 326:466-470.
Koopmans M, Kremer Hovinga CL, Baelde HJ, Fernandes RJ, de Heer E, de Heer E, Bruijn JA, Bajema IM (2005) Chimerism in Kidneys, Livers and Hearts of Normal Women: Implications for Transplantation Studies. Amer J Transplantation 5:11495–11502.
Lansdorp PM (2007) Immortal strands? Give me a break. Cell 129(7):1244-1247.
Levin M, Buznikov GA, Lauder JM (2006) Of minds and embryos: left-right asymmetry and the serotonergic controls of pre-neural morphogenesis. Dev Neurosci 28(3):171-185.
Martucciello G (1997) Hirschsprung's disease as a neurocristopathy. Pediatr Surg Int 12:2-10
Merok JR, Lansita JA, Tunstead JR, Sherley JL (2002) Cosegregation of chromosomes containing immortal DNA strands in cells that cycle with asymmetric stem cell kinetics. Cancer Res 62(23):6791-6795.
Moore SW (2006) The contribution of associated congenital anomalies in understanding Hirschsprung's disease. Pediatr Surg Int 22(4):305-315. Epub 2006 Mar 4

[1] "The reader will easily understand that the word "twins" is a vague expression, which covers two very dissimilar events - the one corresponding to the progeny of animals that usually bear more than one at a birth, each of the progeny being derived from a separate ovum, while the other event is due to the development of two germinal spots in the same ovum. In the latter case they are enveloped in the same membrane, and all such twins are found invariably to be of the same sex."

Morris SC (1994) Why molecular biology needs palaeontology. Development Supplement 1-13.

Pierucci O, Zuchowski C (1973) Non-random segregation of DNA strands in *Escherichia coli* B/r. J Molec Biol 80 (3):477-503.

Pinborg A, Loft A, Nyboe Andersen A (2004) Neonatal outcome in a Danish national cohort of 8602 children born after in vitro fertilization or intracytoplasmic sperm injection: the role of twin pregnancy. Acta Obstet Gynecol Scand 83(11):1071-1078.

Schinzel AA, Smith DW, Miller JR (1979) Monozygotic twinning and structural defects. J Pediatr 95(6):921-930

Shahar E, Shinawi M (2003) Neurocristopathies presenting with neurologic abnormalities associated with Hirschsprung's disease. Pediatr Neurol 28 (5): 385-391.

Sulston JE, Schierenberg E, White JG, Thomson JN (1983) The embryonic cell lineage of the nematode Caenorhabditis elegans. Dev Biol 100(1):64-119.

Sulston JE (2003) Caenorhabditis elegans: the cell lineage and beyond (Nobel lecture). Chembiochem. 4(8):688-696.

Surani MA, Barton SC, Norris ML (1984) Development of reconstituted mouse eggs suggests imprinting of the genome during gametogenesis. Nature 308(5959):548-550.

Tam, P.K.H. (1986) An immunochemical study with neuron-specific-enolase and substance P of human enteric innervation—The normal developmental pattern and abnormal deviations in Hirschsprung's disease and pyloric stenosis. J Pediatr Surg 21(3):227-232.

Tam PK, Garcia-Barceló M (2009) Genetic basis of Hirschsprung's disease. Pediatr Surg Int 25(7):543-558. Epub 2009 Jun 12

Templeton AC (1977) Neurocristopathies in African subjects. Trop Geogr Med 29(1):8-13.

van Dijk BA, Boomsma D and de Man AJ (1996) Blood group chimerism in human multiple births is not rare. Am J Med Genet 61:264–268.

Vandenberg LN, Levin M (2011) Polarity proteins are required for left-right axis orientation and twin-twin instruction. Genesis 2011 Nov 15. doi: 10.1002/dvg.20825. [Epub ahead of print]

Vitthala S, Gelbaya TA, Brison DR, Fitzgerald CT, Nardo LG (2009) The risk of monozygotic twins after assisted reproductive technology: a systematic review and meta-analysis. Hum Reprod Update 15(1):45-55. Epub 2008 Oct 15.

Yu N, Kruskall MS, Yunis JJ, Knoll JH, Uhl L, Alosco S, Ohashi M, Clavijo O, Husain Z, Yunis EJ, Yunis JJ, Yunis EJ. (2002) Disputed maternity leading to identification of tetragametic chimerism. N Engl J Med 346: 1545–1552.

Zeskind PS, Stephens LE (2004) Maternal selective serotonin reuptake inhibitor use during pregnancy and newborn neurobehavior. Pediatrics 113(2)368-375.

3

DM Domain Genes: Sexual and Somatic Development During Vertebrate Embryogenesis

Anna Bratuś
[1]National Research Institute of Animal Production,
Department of Animal Cytogenetics and Molecular Genetics
[2]University Hospital Zurich,
Division of Rheumatology and Institute of Physical Medicine,
Centre of Experimental Rheumatology
[1]Poland
[2]Switzerland

1. Introduction

Sex determination occurs during embryo development in Metazoans that appear as two morphologically distinct sexes. This means that there is a precise time point during embryogenesis when the initial signal starts to act and directs the development of the ambiguous embryo into male or female. What are these primary sex-determination signals? They are different in various vertebrates and can be either genetically or environmentally controlled. Once they appear, they activate the cascade of different genes that respond to these signals and regulate downstream sex-developmental events. Besides the existence of two sexes, which is virtually universal in the animal kingdom, sex-developmental strategies (both the initial signals and the cascade of regulatory genes) vary between phyla and are opposite to somatic-development strategies, which have been found to be more conservative.

Vertebrate sex determination occurs in the gonadal primordium (the genital ridge), and once it takes place, the gonads are differentiated into specific male (testes) and female (ovaries) structures that, mostly because of their hormone-secretion activity, conscript the body into further sexual differentiation (somatic sexual dimorphism).

The revolution in molecular biology technology that started over 50 years ago and continues today has allowed scientists to discover the molecular background of embryogenesis starting from the identification of single genes to the prediction of entire genomic and proteomic regulatory pathways involved in embryo development.

The group of genes that has been found as very important embryogenesis regulators encodes transcription factors, proteins that interact with DNA and regulate the expression of other genes below them in the regulatory hierarchy.

This chapter is dedicated to the fascinating story of one transcription factor family, the family of DM domain genes, which has been discovered in both vertebrate and invertebrate genomes. They all encode the DM (*doublesex* and *mab-3*) domain, possess the highly conservative zing-finger DNA-binding motif and regulate not only sexual, but also somatic developmental pathways in animals. Here, the extensive knowledge of the biology of DM domain genes in vertebrates (from the history of their discovery in different animal genomes to their function in embryo development) is presented. Moreover, the very interesting and slightly contradictory evolutional aspect of DM domain genes is emphasised. So far, they represent the only exception during vertebrate sexual development due to their structural and functional conservation between phyla. On the other hand, the successive discovery of additional vertebrate genes with the DM domain (with their variations in number and function between species) shows how rapidly their evolution took place.

2. The discovery of DM domain genes: The chronological point of view

During the last 13 years, numerous studies of vertebrate DM domain genes have been extensively carried out. Structural analyses of these genes (their genomic organisation, sequence comparisons between species, chromosomal locations, mutational screenings of individuals with developmental abnormalities) as well as their expression profiles in both adult tissues and embryo sections together with functional studies in model organisms have been performed by different research groups all over the world. Here, I present the data that displays how our knowledge of this gene family has been increased over the past decade.

2.1 The DM domain, a link between invertebrates and vertebrates

The first report about the DM domain sequence in the vertebrate genome comes from the studies of Raymond and collaborators (Raymond et al., 1998), who have identified the human locus encoding a DM domain protein. Although the authors primarily named it *DMT1* (for the first DM domain gene expressed in testis), it is now known as *DMRT1* (*doublesex* and *mab-3* related transcription factor 1). The name of the gene reveals its structural homology to sexual regulators: *dsx* (*doublesex*) in *Drosophila melanogaster* and *mab-3* (*male abnormal 3*) in *Caenorhabditis elegans*. These two invertebrate homologs encode the conserved motif similar to the zing-finger DNA-binding domain, first described in both male DSX^M and female DSX^F isoforms of *D. melanogaster* (Erdman & Burtis, 1993) and later, simultaneously with its human homolog, in MAB-3 of *C. elegans* (Raymond et al., 1998). Raymond named this motif DM domain based on its occurrence in fly DSX and worm MAB-3 proteins.

The function of two invertebrate downstream sex regulators, *dsx* and *mab-3*, in somatic sex determination and differentiation was previously well characterised (Burtis &Baker, 1989; Shen & Hodgkin, 1988), and it was found that they are evolutionarily conserved. Both genes control analogous aspects of sexual development: direct regulation of yolk protein gene transcription (Yi & Zarkower, 1999), differentiation of male-specific sense organs (Baker & Ridge, 1980; Shen & Hodgkin, 1988; Yi et al., 2000) and mediation of male mating behaviour (Yi et al., 2000). The studies of Raymond (1998) have additionally emphasised the functional relation between these two evolutionally distinct proteins, showing that they can be functionally interchangeable *in vivo*: The fly dsx^M but not dsx^F could replace *mab-3* during the development of a transgenic *mab-3* mutant *C. elegans* male.

The report of Raymond and co-authors (1998) proved importance in the research field of animal sexual development by giving the first evidence of molecular evolutionary conservation within invertebrates as well as between invertebrate and vertebrate sexual-regulatory mechanisms.

2.2 *DMRT* – Vertebrate DM domain gene family

Although the function of the invertebrate DM domain genes *dsx* and *mab-3* in somatic sexual development was described quite broadly, only little was known about the first vertebrate homolog, *DMRT1*, at the time when Raymond's paper was published (Raymond et al., 1998). His group, however, has provided very convincing data about *DMRT1* as a good candidate gene required in humans for male development. First, it was mapped to the autosomal locus (distal short arm of chromosome 9, band 9p24.3), which has been implicated in human XY sex reversal in numerous previously published reports (Crocker et al., 1988; Bennett et al., 1993; McDonald et al., 1997; Veitia et al., 1997; Veitia et al., 1998; Flejter et al., 1998). Second, *DMRT1* was expressed exclusively in testes among 50 investigated human tissues. Further evidence for *DMRT1* as a male sexual regulator came either from the later studies of its expression in human embryos (Moniot et al., 2000) or from additional reports describing sex-reversed patients with the monosomy of 9p (Raymond et al., 1999a; Calvari at al., 2000; Muroya et al., 2000; Õunap et al., 2004; Privitera et al., 2005; Vinci et al., 2007). In the meantime, the group of Zarkower from the University of Minnesota (Raymond et al., 1999b) and the group of Sinclair from the University of Melbourne (Smith et al., 1999a) published very important data about *DMRT1* expression during mouse, chicken and alligator embryogenesis. They consistently showed that *DMRT1* is unique, in that it is expressed very early and sex specifically in the gonads of three investigated species, regardless of the sex-determining mechanism used (i.e., whether chromosomal (mouse, chicken) or environmental (alligator)). These findings suggested that DM domain genes may play a role in sexual development in a wide range of vertebrate phyla. Indeed, further studies extensively carried out in all vertebrate phyla (from mammals to fish) (Table 1) have supported this hypothesis. Moreover, they have shown the high structural similarity of *DMRT1* across species (protein sequence identity within the DM domain with human DMRT1 ranges from 98% in mice to 87% in fish) as well as the conserved sexually dimorphic pattern of its expression both during early gonadogenesis and in adult tissues (Table 2). These studies, however, needed further confirmation through, for example, functional analyses of the gene (its artificial manipulation in a model organism). For the first time, functional studies were performed in 2000 by Zarkower's group (Raymond et al., 2000), who showed that homozygous *Dmrt1*$^{-/-}$ mutant male mice fail to undergo normal postnatal testis differentiation. From this data, it was clear that *Dmrt1* is a critical regulator of testis development in the mouse.

While Zarkower's group was later mostly concentrated on mouse functional studies providing more and more interesting data about the role of DMRT1 in mammalian sex-developmental pathways (Fahrioglu et al., 2007; Kim et al., 2007a; Krentz et al., 2009; Matson et al., 2010; Murphy et al., 2010; Krentz et al., 2011; Matson et al., 2011), Sinclair and his co-workers were focused on studies in the chicken (Smith et al., 1999b; Smith at al., 2003). They were constantly looking for strong evidence for *Dmrt1* as a male dosage-sensitive sex-determination locus, previously shown to be linked to the Z chromosome (avian males are homogametic ZZ) in the region highly homologous to human 9 chromosome bearing the *DMRT1* locus (Nanda et al., 1999; Nanda et al., 2000). Their long-term studies were finally published in 2009, providing the convincing results that *Dmrt1* is indeed required for testis determination in the chicken and supporting the Z dosage hypothesis for avian sex determination (Smith et al., 2009).

Although *DMRT1* has been studied very intensively during the last decade and its function as the sex-determination/sex-differentiation locus in a wide range of vertebrate species has been very well documented in structural, expression and functional analyses, it has always been known that *DMRT1* is not the only gene with the DM domain in the vertebrate genome. Thus, there was a strong need for further investigations.

Gene Symbol	NCBI Reference mRNA Sequence	Chromosome Localisation	Organism	References
DMRT1/DMT1	AF130728	HSA 9p24.3	*Homo sapiens*	Raymond et al., 1998 Raymond et al., 1999a
Dmrt1	NM_015826.5 AL133300	MMU 19C2-C3	*Mus musculus*	Raymond et al., 1999b De Grandi et al., 2000
Dmrt1	AF379608	RNO 1q51	*Rattus norvegicus*	Chen & Heckert, 2001
Dmrt1	NM_001078060.1	BSA 8q17	*Bos taurus*	Bratuś et al., 2009 Bratuś & Słota; 2009
Dmrt1	AF216651	SSC 1q21	*Sus scrofa domestica*	Bratuś & Słota, 2009
Dmrt1	ENSMEUT00000011422*	MEU 3p	*Macropus eugenii*	Pask et al., 2003 El-Mogharbel et al., 2005
Dmrt1	AJ744848 (exon 1) AJ744847 (exon 3)	OAN X5q	*Ornithorhynchus anatinus*	El-Mogharbel et al., 2007
Dmrt1	NM_001101831.1	GGA Zp21	*Gallus gallus*	Nanda et al., 1999
Dmrt1	-	DNO Zp	*Dromaius novaehollandeae*	Shetty et al., 2002
Dmrt1	AB272609	autosom	*Rana rugosa*	Shibata et al., 2002 Aoyama et al., 2003
Dmrt1	AB201112	autosom	*Xenopus leavis*	Osawa et al., 2005 Yoshimoto et al., 2006
DM-W	AB259777	XLE W	*Xenopus leavis*	Yoshimoto et al., 2008
Dmrt1	AY316537	-	*Trachemys scripta*	Murdock & Wibbels, 2003
Dmrt1	AF335421	-	*Lepidochelys olivacea*	Torres-Maldonado et al., 2002
Dmrt1	-	-	*Chelydra serpentina*	Rhen et al., 2007
Dmrt1	AF464141	-	*Calotes versicolor*	Sreenivasulu et al., 2002
Dmrt1	AF192560	-	*Alligator mississippiensis*	Smith et al., 1999a
Dmrt1	AF209095	Not Y-linked	*Oncorhynchus mykiss*	Marchand et al., 2000 Alfaqih et al., 2009
Dmrt1	AY157562	DRE 5	*Danio rerio*	Guo et al., 2004a Guo et al., 2005
Dmrt1	NM_001037949.1	-	*Takifugu rubripes*	Brunner et al., 2001
Dmrt1	AAN65377	-	*Xiphophorus maculatus*	Veith et al., 2003

Gene Symbol	NCBI Reference mRNA Sequence	Chromosome Localisation	Organism	References
Dmrt1	AY319416	-	*Odontesthes bonariensis*	Fernandino et al., 2006
Dmrt1	AF421347	-	*Monopterus albus*	Huang et al., 2002 Huang et al., 2005a
tDmrt1	AF203489	Not Y-linked	*Oreochromis niloticus*	Guan et al., 2000
tDMO	AF203490	-	*Oreochromis niloticus*	Guan et al., 2000
DMY/Dmrt1bY	AB071534	OLA Y	*Oryzias latipes*	Matsuda et al., 2002 Nanda et al., 2002
Dmrt1/Dmrt1a	-	OLA LG9	*Oryzias latipes*	Brunner et al., 2001 Nanda et al., 2002
DMRT2	NM_001130865.2	HSA 9p24.3	*Homo sapiens*	Raymond et al., 1999a Ottolenghi et al., 2000b
Dmrt2	NM_145831.3	MMU 19C1	*Mus musculus*	Kim et al., 2003
Dmrt2	NM_001192373	BSA 8q17	*Bos taurus*	Bratuś & Słota; 2009
Dmrt2	XM_003480526	SSC 1q21	*Sus scrofa domestica*	Bratuś & Słota; 2009
Dmrt2	ENSOANT00000013193[8]	OAN X5q	*Ornithorhynchus anatinus*	El-Mogharbel et al., 2007
Dmrt2	AY960292	-	*Gallus gallus*	Saúde et al., 2005
Dmrt2	AB264329	-	*Rana rugosa*	Matsushita et al., 2007
Dmrt2	AF209096	-	*Oncorhynchus mykiss*	Marchand et al., 2000
Dmrt2a	AF319992	OLA LG9	*Oryzias latipes*	Brunner et al., 2001
Dmrt2a	NM_001037946.1	-	*Takifugu rubripes*	Brunner et al., 2001
Dmrt2a	AAL83920	-	*Xiphophorus maculatus*	Kondo et al., 2002
Dmrt2a/terra	NM_130952	DRE 5	*Danio rerio*	Meng et al., 1999 Guo et al., 2004a
Dmrt2b	NM_001079976	DRE 6	*Danio rerio*	Zhou et al., 2008
DMRT3/DMRTA3	NM_021240.2	HSA 9p24.3	*Homo sapiens*	Ottolenghi et al., 2002
Dmrt3	NM_177360.3	MMU 19C1	*Mus musculus*	Kim et al., 2003
Dmrt3	XM_001788026	BSA 8q17	*Bos taurus*	Bratuś & Słota; 2009
Dmrt3	-	SSC 1q21	*Sus scrofa domestica*	Bratuś & Słota; 2009
Dmrt3	XM_001507779.2	OAN X5q	*Ornithorhynchus anatinus*	El-Mogharbel et al., 2007
Dmrt3	XP_427822.1	-	*Gallus gallus*	Smith et al., 2002
Dmrt3	AB264330	-	*Rana rugosa*	Matsushita et al., 2007
Dmrt3	AF319993	OLA LG9	*Oryzias latipes*	Brunner et al., 2001
Dmrt3	AY621083	DRE 5	*Danio rerio*	Guo et al., 2004a
Dmrt3	NM_001037945.1	-	*Takifugu rubripes*	Brunner et al., 2001
DMRT4/DMRTA1	NM_022160.2	HSA 9p21-22	*Homo sapiens*	Ottolenghi et al., 2002
Dmrt4/Dmrta1	NM_175647.3	MMU 4C4	*Mus musculus*	Kim et al., 2003
Dmrt4	AY648303	-	*Xenopus leavis*	Huang et al., 2005b
Dmrt4	AF209097	-	*Oncorhynchus mykiss*	Marchand et al., 2000
Dmrt4	-	OLA LG18	*Oryzias latipes*	Kondo et al., 2002
Dmrt4	AB201464.1	-	*Takifugu rubripes*	Yamaguchi et al., 2006
Dmrt4	CAF90474	-	*Xiphophorus maculatus*	Kondo et al., 2002
DMRT5/DMRTA2	NM_032110.2	HAS 1p32.3-33	*Homo sapiens*	Ottolenghi et al., 2002
Dmrt5/Dmrta2	NM_172296.2	MMU 4C7	*Mus musculus*	Kim et al., 2003

Gene Symbol	NCBI Reference mRNA Sequence	Chromosome Localisation	Organism	References
Dmrt5	AB264331	-	*Rana rugosa*	Matsushita et al., 2007
Dmrt5	AY618549	DRE 8	*Danio rerio*	Guo et al., 2004b
Dmrt5	AB201465.1	-	*Takifugu rubripes*	Yamaguchi et al., 2006
Dmrt5	DQ335470	-	*Xiphophorus maculatus*	Veith et al., 2006a
DMRT6/DMRTB1	NM_033067.1	HSA 1p32.2	*Homo sapiens*	Ottolenghi et al., 2002
Dmrt6/Dmrtb1	NM_019872.1	MMU 4C7	*Mus musculus*	Kim et al., 2003
DMRT7/DMRTC2	NM_001040283.1	HSA 19q13.2	*Homo sapiens*	Ottolenghi et al., 2002
Dmrt7/Dmrtc2	NM_027732.2	MMU 7A3	*Mus musculus*	Kim et al., 2003
Dmrt7/Dmrtc2	XM_218456	RNO 1q21	*Rattus norvegicus*	Veith et al., 2006b
Dmrt7	ENSOANT00000021972[8]	-	*Ornithorhynchus anatinus*	Tsend-Ayush et al., 2009
DMRT8/DMRTC1	NM_033053.2	HSA Xq13.2	*Homo sapiens*	Ottolenghi et al., 2002
Dmrt8.1/Dmrtc1a	NM_001038616.2	MMU XD	*Mus musculus*	Veith et al., 2006b
Dmrt8.1/Dmrtc1a	NM_001025288	RNO X	*Rattus norvegicus*	Veith et al., 2006b
Dmrt8.2/Dmrtc1b	NM_001039116.2	MMU XD	*Mus musculus*	Veith et al., 2006b
Dmrt8.2/Dmrtc1b	XM_228580	RNO Xq13	*Rattus norvegicus*	Veith et al., 2006b
Dmrt8.3/Dmrtc1c1	NM_001142691.1	MMU XD	*Mus musculus*	Veith et al., 2006b
Dmrt8.3/Dmrtc1c1	NM_001014222	RNO Xq13	*Rattus norvegicus*	Veith et al., 2006b

[8]the ENSEMBL reference sequence (available at www.ensembl.org),
'-' cDNA sequences published neither in databases nor in given references/unknown chromosome localisation

Table 1. **DM-domain genes in representative vertebrates.** The presented nomenclature of DM domain genes is adopted from Volff (Volff et al., 2003a) or described in given references. The DM domain genes chromosomal localisations linked to sex chromosomes are indicated in grey fields.

The second DM domain gene in humans, *DMRT2*, was first identified by Raymond and co-workers, who mapped it to the same chromosomal band (HSA 9p24.3) as *DMRT1* (Raymond et al., 1999a). Both genes were shown to be deleted in the sex-reversing 9p monosomy, and therefore, *DMRT2* was also considered to be partially responsible for the XY sex-reversal phenotype in humans. Further studies, however, have provided evidence of *DMRT2* as a less likely sex-developmental candidate locus. First, it was mapped outside the deleted region in the newly refined 9p microdeletion in two XY sex-reversed females (Calvari et al., 2000). Second, its expression appeared to be widespread in adult human tissues (not restricted to testis) (Ottolenghi et al., 2000b). Third, DNA sequence analysis showed its high identity (100% in the DM domain) with the previously described DM domain gene in zebrafish, named *terra,* which was evidenced to be involved in somitogenesis but not sex development (Meng et al., 1999). Subsequent studies carried out in other vertebrates and based on both expression and functional analyses have indeed confirmed these preliminary presumptions (Tables 3 and 4).

Interestingly, further detailed screening of PAC/BAC clones overlapping the chromosomal region in humans associated with 46,XY gonadal dysgenesis and mapped to the tip of chromosome 9 (HSA 9p24.3) has revealed an additional (i.e., in addition to *DMRT1* and *DMRT2*) locus with the DM domain named *DMRT3* with a position proximal to *DMRT1* and distal to *DMRT2* (Ottolenghi et al., 2000a). What is more, the newly described human cluster of DM domain genes, *DMRT1-DMRT3-DMRT2*, was later discovered to be a very conservative vertebrate locus. It was surprisingly found to be isolated from different fish species (i.e., medaka *O. latipes*, pufferfish *F. rubripes* (Brunner et al., 2001), zebrafish *D. rerio* (Guo et al., 2004a)) and from mice (Kim et al., 2003), rats (Guo et al., 2004a), platypus (El-Mogharbel et al., 2007), pigs and cattle. However, in these two last species, the order of *DMRT* genes was different (Bratuś & Słota, 2009).

It is now known that eight *DMRT* genes exist in human and mouse genomes (Ottolenghi et al., 2002; Kim et al., 2003; Veith et al., 2006b) (Table 1), which, compared to four and eleven DM domain loci previously isolated from invertebrates *D. melanogaster* and *C. elegans* respectively, is not surprising (reviewed by Volff and collaborators; Volff et al., 2003a). The subsequent expression and selected functional studies in numerous vertebrate species (Tables 3 and 4) have shown the variability in the expression profiles between both DM domain paralogs and homologs. Although the involvement of multiple DM domain genes in vertebrate sexual development was supported and might be considered a general phenomenon in developmental biology, it is obvious that *DMRT* genes also regulate the development of other organs during vertebrate embryogenesis (Tables 3 and 4). The recent data are discussed below in detail.

3. Sexual contra somatic embryo development: The involvement of DM domain genes

In order to determine the role of the genes in sexual development, both expression and functional studies have to be carried out. DM domain genes, as mentioned before, are molecular regulators of developmental processes that take place in the embryo. The embryo is, therefore, the main object used to study the function of *DMRT* genes. However, concerning humans, ethical issues arise. In this respect, performing studies in model organisms is often the only alternative. In the case of DM domain genes, extending investigations to all vertebrate phyla has brought new, interesting data about the evolution of this gene family.

Numerous DM domain genes were studied in different animal models employing various sex-determination strategies: genetic: (male or female heterogamety in XX/XY or ZZ/ZW systems, respectively), environmental (temperature, social factors) or a combination (Table 2). Different molecular biology methods were used to study the spatial and temporal expression of DM domain genes during embryogenesis. Both the mRNA and protein levels were measured either by very sensitive amplification methods (RT-PCR, quantitative RT-PCR) or less sensitive hybridisation techniques (Northern blot, Western-blot). In order to identify the cell type of the developing organ where the gene expression took place, the whole-mount *in situ* hybridisation (using gene-specific RNA probes) and/or immunohistochemistry methods (with specific antibodies) were applied to embryo sections. Since transcription factors, the proteins that regulate the expression of other genes by binding to the DNA sequence in their vicinity, are the final *DMRT* gene expression products, the chromatin immunoprecipitation (ChIP) method was employed to determine the upstream/downstream *DMRT* regulators in the embryo developmental pathways. What is more, both *DMRT* expression and ChIP techniques were supplemented by the next-generation technologies that currently provide tools for whole-genome investigations, such as DNA microarrays (cDNA arrays and ChIP-chip, respectively). Moreover, functional studies, which provide the strongest evidence for gene-role determination, were carried out in different animal models (mostly in mice and in various fish species) and were based on artificial single-gene modifications like the loss of function mutation (e.g., knockout/knockdown of the gene) or the gain of function mutation (e.g., induced gene over-expression).

The function of *DMRT* genes in the developmental pathways of various vertebrate species is here broadly compared and summarised.

3.1 *DMRT1*, vertebrate sexual regulator

There is no doubt that among DM domain genes, *DMRT1* has been the most extensively investigated. A careful on-line search of the PubMed database (http://www.ncbi.nlm.nih.gov/pubmed/) provided the wide collection of data about *DMRT1* expression during vertebrate embryogenesis and in postnatal/adult animal tissues (Table 2).

So far, *DMRT1* appears to have a gonad-specific and sexually dimorphic expression profile during embryogenesis in all vertebrates tested (from mammals to fish). Besides this conservative status of *DMRT1* as the universal vertebrate sexual regulator (which might be considered a new phenomenon in animal developmental biology), several lines of evidence supported its functional variability during vertebrate gonad development. Is this more of a sex determination or a sex-differentiation locus? Is it involved only in male gonad formation, or does it also play a role in ovary development? The expression and functional studies undertaken in a wide range of vertebrate species have resolved some of the above questions.

In most cases, *DMRT1* is up-regulated either late during sex-determination or during the early testis-differentiation period. This subtle difference in its temporal expression during embryogenesis in various vertebrates makes its function vary significantly more among species.

Dmrt1 may be considered a switch sex-determining gene in reptiles employing a temperature-dependent sex-determining strategy. In separate studies of different reptilian species (i.e., crocodiles (*Alligator mississippiensis*) and turtles (*Trachemys scripta, Lepidochelys olivacea, Chelydra serpentine* (Table 2)), it has been shown that *Dmrt1* is the earliest genetic factor whose expression is temperature sensitive: The mRNA level of the gene was higher in embryos incubated in a male-promoting temperature than in embryos incubated in a female-promoting temperature. If the hypothesis that *Dmrt1* is more likely to be itself temperature sensitive and auto-regulatory than to be regulated by another unidentified sensitive-temperature genetic factor is supported, *Dmrt1* may primarily play a male-determining role (Zarkower, 2001). However, no functional studies have been carried out in this vertebrate phylum. That is not the case in birds, where both expression (Table 2) and functional analyses (Table 3) have confirmed the sex-determination status of avian *Dmrt1*. Sex is chromosomally based (ZZ males/ZW females) in birds, but sex determination had been a long-standing mystery. The bird homolog of the previously identified mammalian master-determining *Sry* (Sinclair et al., 1990; Koopman et al., 1991) has not been isolated from the avian genome. Thus, two hypotheses have been proposed regarding the mechanism of sex determination in birds. The primary switch gene may be either a W-linked female dominant factor or a dosage-sensitive gene residing on the Z chromosome and triggering testis development. *Dmrt1*, which has been shown to be Z-linked in different bird species (Nanda et al., 2000; Shetty et al., 2002), is transcribed specifically during chick embryogenesis. Its expression becomes sexually dimorphic before the onset of sex differentiation: It is stronger in developing male than female gonads (Table 2). The elevated expression of *Dmrt1* from two Z chromosomes (unlike the mammalian X chromosome, there is no dosage compensation in birds) in the genital ridge at the time of sex determination may initiate testis differentiation, whereas one gene dosage is insufficient and lets ZW gonads follow a default female pathway. The *Dmrt1* Z dosage hypothesis for chicken sex determination was finally confirmed by the latest functional studies (Table 3), in which *Dmrt1* knockdown ZZ embryos successfully showed significant gonad feminisation (Smith et al., 2009). Although this spectacular finding closes the large gap in the bird sex-determination pathway, further studies of other avian species have to be undertaken in order to confirm/exclude the universal *Dmrt1* status as the bird sex-determining gene.

Phylum	Species	Sex-determination strategy	**Expression** (placement/molecular level/methods)		References
			Embryo	Postnatal/Adult Tissue	
Mammals	Human (*H. sapiens*)	GSD, XX females XY males Dominant Y		T/mRNA/DB	Raymond et al., 1998
			T/mRNA/ISH		Moniot et al., 2000
				T/mRNA/qRT-PCR	Cheng et al., 2006
	Mouse (*M. musculus*)		T+O/mRNA/ISH		Smith et al., 1999a
			T+O/mRNA/ ISH & RT-PCR	T/mRNA/RT-PCR	Raymond et al., 1999b
			T+O/mRNA/ISH	T/mRNA/NB & ISH	De Grandi et al., 2000
				T/protein/IHC	Raymond et al., 2000
				O/protein/IHC	Pask et al., 2003
			T+O/mRNA/ RT-PCR & qRT-PCR	T/mRNA/NB & RT-PCR & qRT-PCR	Lu et al., 2007
			T+O/protein/IHC	T/protein/WB	Lei et al., 2007
	Rat (*R. norvegicus*)		T/mRNA/RPA	T/mRNA/RPA	Chen & Heckert, 2001
	Pig (*S. scrofa*)			T+O+K/mRNA/ RT-PCR	Bratuś & Słota, 2009
	Cattle (*B. taurus*)			T+O+K+L+H+M+L U+S/mRNA/RT-PCR	Bratuś & Słota, 2009
	Tammar wallaby (*M. eugenii*)	GSD, Dominant Y	T+O/protein/IHC	T+O/protein/IHC	Pask et al., 2003
	Platypus (*O. anatinus*)	GSD, 5X+5Y males 2x5X females		T/mRNA/RT-PCR; T+O/protein/IHC	El-Mogharbel et al., 2007 Tsend-Ayush et al., 2009
Birds	Chicken (*G. gallus*)	GSD, ZZ males ZW females Dosage Z	T+O/mRNA/ISH		Smith et al., 1999a Raymond et al., 1999b
			T+O/mRNA/ISH	T/mRNA/NB & RT-PCR	Shan et al., 2000
			T+O/mRNA/ISH & qRT-PCR;		Smith et al., 2003

Phylum	Species	Sex-determination strategy	Expression (placement/molecular level/methods) Embryo	Postnatal/Adult Tissue	References
			T+O/protein/IHC		
			T+O/mRNA/ RT-PCR & ISH	T+H/mRNA/RT-PCR; T/mRNA/NB	Zhao et al., 2007
	Emu (*D. novaehollandeae*)	GSD, Dosage Z?	Embryos of both sexes/mRNA/RT-PCR		Shetty et al., 2002
Reptiles	Alligator (*A. mississippiensis*)	TDS	T+O/mRNA/RT-PCR		Smith et al., 1999a
	Red-eared slider turtle (*T. scripta*)	TDS	T+O/mRNA/ISH & RT-PCR		Kettlewell et al., 2000
			T+O/mRNA/qRT-PCR		Murdock & Wibbels, 2003
	Sea turtle (*L. olivacea*)	TDS	T+O/mRNA/RT-PCR		Torres-Maldonado et al., 2002
	Snapping turtle (*C. serpentine*)	TDS	T+O/mRNA/qRT-PCR		Rhen et al., 2007
	Indian garden lizard (*C. versicolor*)	unknown	T+O/mRNA/ qRT-PCR & ISH	T/mRNA/RT-PCR	Sreenivasulu et al., 2002
Amphibians	Frog (*R. rugosa*)	GSD, XX females XY males	T/mRNA/RT-PCR	T/mRNA/RT-PCR	Shibata et al., 2002
			T/protein/IHC	T/mRNA/ISH; T/protein/IHC	Aoyama et al., 2003
	Clawed frog (*X. laevis*)	GSD, Dosage Z? Dominant W?	T+O/mRNA/RT-PCR	T/mRNA/NB & RT-PCR	Osawa et al., 2005
			T+O/mRNA/ISH & RT-PCR		Yoshimoto et al., 2006 Yoshimoto et al., 2008
Fish	Rainbow trout (*O. mykiss*)	GSD, XX females XY males	T+O/mRNA/NB & RT-PCR	T/mRNA/NB; T+O/mRNA/RT-PCR	Marchand et al., 2000
tDMRT1	Nile tilapia (*O. niloticus*)	GSD, XX females XY males		T/mRNA/NB	Guan et al., 2000
tDMO	Nile tilapia (*O. niloticus*)			O/mRNA/NB	
DMRT1a	Medaka (*O. latipes*)	GSD, XX females XY males Dominant Y	Undetectable/mRNA/RT-PCR	T/mRNA/RT-PCR	Brunner et al., 2001 Nanda et al., 2002
			Undetectable/mRNA/RT-PCR & ISH	T+O/mRNA/ISH	Winkler et al., 2004
			T/mRNA/RT-PCR	T/mRNA/RT-PCR	Kobayashi et al., 2004
DMY/DMRT1BY	Medaka (*O. latipes*)		Detectable in XY embryos/mRNA/RT-PCR	T/mRNA/RT-PCR	Nanda et al., 2002 Kobayashi et al., 2004
	Japanese pufferfish (*T. rubripes*)	Unknown	T/mRNA/RT-PCR & ISH	T+O/mRNA/RT-PCR	Yamaguchi et al., 2006
	Green spotted puffer (*T. nigroviridis*)	Unknown		T+O/mRNA/RT-PCR	Brunner et al., 2001
	Zebrafish (*D. rerio*)	Unknown		T+O/mRNA/RT-PCR & qRT-PCR & NB & ISH	Guo et al., 2005
	Platyfish (*X. maculatus*)	GSD, XX females,	Undetectable/mRNA/ISH	T/mRNA/RT-PCR & ISH	Veith et al., 2006a

Phylum	Species	Sex-determination strategy	Expression (placement/molecular level/methods)		References
			Embryo	Postnatal/Adult Tissue	
		XY males			
	Pejerrey, (*O. bonariensis*)	TDS		T/mRNA/RT-PCR	Fernandino et al., 2006
			T+O?mRNA/qRT-PCR		Fernandino et al., 2008
	Atlantic cod (*G. morhua L.*)			T+O/mRNA/ RT-PCR & qRT-PCR & ISH	Johnsen et al., 2010
	Rice field eel (*M. albus*)			T+O+B/mRNA/ RT-PCR & qRT-PCR; O+T/mRNA/NB	Huang et al., 2005a

Table 2. ***DMRT1* expression in vertebrates**. GSD-genetic sex determination, TDS-temperature dependence sex determination, T-testis/genital ridge in male embryo, O-ovary/genital ridge in female embryo, K-kidney, L-liver, H-heart, M-muscle, LU-lung, S-spleen, ISH-*in situ* hybridisation, RT-PCR-reverse transcription-polymerase chain reaction, qRT-PCR-quantitative RT-PCR, NB-Northern blot, DB-Dot blot, IHC-immunohistochemistry, WB- Western blot, RPA-RNase protection assay.

In fish, it is already known that *Dmrt1* is the unique male sex-determination locus, exclusively identified in a single fish species, medaka *O. latipes*. Medaka, unlike many other fish, uses a simple genetic mechanism similar to that found in mammals, with XX females and XY males. Surprisingly, two research groups simultaneously but independently found that the duplicated copy of previously isolated autosomal *Dmrt1/Dmrt1a* locus (Brunner et al., 2001) is located on the Y chromosome in its sex-determination region. This new paralog was named after the authors: *Dmrt1bY* (Nanda et al., 2002) or *DMY* (Matsuda et al., 2002). Its specific expression pattern during embryogenesis (it is transcribed early and exclusively in XY embryos) (Table 2) and the molecular analysis of XY *DMY* mutants that appeared to be male-to-female sex reversed (Matsuda et al., 2002) are consistent with its sex-determination function. Thus, medaka *Dmrt1bY/DMY* represents the unique non-mammalian vertebrate equivalent of *Sry*; however, it is not described in any other fish species, regardless of their relation to medaka (i.e., whether close or distant) (Kondo et al., 2003; Volff et al., 2003b; Veith et al., 2003).

What is, then, the role of *Dmrt1* in mammals that exhibit a genetic sex-determining mechanism (XX females/XY males) with the well-described Y-borne male-dominant locus of *Sry*? Intriguingly, the latest detailed studies have presented some functional diversity.

The data from humans, similar to that from chicken and medaka, are consistent with the hypothesis that *DMRT1* dosage is crucial for sex determination. Male-to-female sex reversal in XY individuals with monosomic deletion of 9p (bearing *DMRT1*) may be due to haploinsufficiency for expression of this male regulatory factor (either by itself or with nearby genes) (Raymond et al., 1999a). Furthermore, the report of Moniot and others (Moniot et al., 2000) showed co-expression of *SRY* and *DMRT1* in the genital ridge of the human male but not in the female embryo at the time when gonads appear morphologically undifferentiated. This male-specific expression of *DMRT1* in early gonadogenesis prior to sex differentiation suggests a partial (shared with *SRY*) role in human sex determination. Unlike human homolog, murine *Dmrt1*, which has been extensively examined during embryogenesis (Table 2) and in genetically modified mouse models (Table 3), appeared to play an essential role in male gonad differentiation but not sex determination. Its early expression in the genital ridges of both sexes became XY-specific (up-regulated in developing male gonads) after the activation of the *Sry* gene (Smith et al., 1999a; De Grandi et al., 2000). Furthermore, male *Dmrt1* knockout mice were found to have postnatal affected testes but were not sex reversed (Raymond et al., 2000). Murine *Dmrt1*, however, through its expression in premeiotic germ cells and in Sertoli cells of both foetal and postnatal gonads, controls many aspects of testicular development, including differentiation, proliferation, migration and pluripotency of germ cells as well as proliferation and differentiation of Sertoli cells (Fahrioglu et al., 2007; Kim et al., 2007; Krentz et al., 2009).

Despite the well-evidenced redundant function of *Dmrt1* in ovary development due to fully fertile *Dmrt1*$^{-/-}$ XX mouse mutants (Raymond et al., 2000), the latest studies provide some unexpected data suggesting the involvement of mammalian *Dmrt1* in female gonad differentiation. In contrast to humans, both DMRT1 proteins (mouse, tammar wallaby) and *Dmrt1* transcripts (pig, cattle)—together with their expression in testes—were detected in adult ovaries (Table 2). What is more, the latest genome-wide studies have revealed that murine *Dmrt1* is a bi-functional transcriptional regulator that activates some genes and represses others. This not only occurs in juvenile testes, where *Dmrt1* acts differently depending on the testis cell line (Murphy et al., 2010). *Dmrt1* also can regulate the same gene target sex-specifically. *Stra8* (Stimulated by retinoic acid 8), the well-known meiotic inducer, is directly activated by *Dmrt1* in foetal ovary germ cells, which results in oogenesis initiation, whereas in adult testes, *Stra8* is transcriptionally repressed, showing *Dmrt1*-dependant control of spermatogenesis (Krentz et al., 2011). Although *Dmrt1*$^{-/-}$ mutant females were fertile (having reduced but enough functional ovarian follicles), the latest report of Krentz's group has finally demonstrated that *Dmrt1* does indeed function in the foetal ovary (Krentz et al., 2011).

In lower vertebrates, as in mammals, *Dmrt1* mRNA was also expressed in adult ovarian tissue of several fish species (Table 2). Moreover, in addition to the testis-specific *tDmrt1*, the other DM domain gene (*tDMO*) was isolated from one teleost fish, the tilapia (Guan et al., 2000). *tDMO* (tilapia DM domain gene in Ovary), the expression of which is limited to the ovary in adult animals, is the first-described female-specific DM domain gene in vertebrates. In contrast to the alternatively spliced male and female invertebrate *doublesex* (Burtis & Baker, 1989), *tDmrt1* and *tDMO* cDNAs appear to be encoded by two different genes that share little homology outside the DM domain.

However, more spectacular were functional studies carried out by Yoshimoto and co-workers (Yoshimoto et al., 2008; Yoshimoto et al., 2010), who isolated a W-linked *DM-W*. This is a paralog of *Dmrt1* in a single amphibian species, the African clawed frog *Xenopus leavis*, which has a ZZ/ZW-type sex-determining system. Both the *DM-W* transient expression in ZW tadpoles in the period of sex determination and the functional analysis of ZZ transgenic tadpoles carrying a *DM-W* expression vector and showing ovarian cavities and primary oocytes has suggested that *DM-W* is a likely sex (ovary)-determining locus in *X. leavis*, probably acting by antagonising *Dmrt1* (Yoshimoto et al., 2010).

Function	Gene	Species	References
Male sex determination	*Dmrt1*	*Gallus gallus*	Smith et al., 2003 Smith et al., 2009
	DMY/Dmrt1bY	*Oryzias latipes*	Matsuda et al., 2002
Male sex differentiation	*Dmrt1*	*Mus musculus*	Raymond et al., 2000 Boyer et al., 2002 Fahrioglu et al., 2007 Kim et al., 2007a Krentz et al., 2009 Matson et al., 2010 Matson et al., 2011
		Rattus norvegicus	Lei et al., 2009
	Dmrt7	*Mus musculus*	Kawamata & Nishimori, 2006 Kim et al., 2007b
	Dmrt4	*Mus musculus*	Balciuniene et al., 2006
Female sex determination	*DM-W*	*Xenopus laevis*	Yoshimoto et al., 2008 Yoshimoto et al., 2010
Female sex differentiation	*Dmrt1*	*Mus musculus*	Krentz et al, 2011
	Dmrt4	*Mus musculus*	Balciuniene et al., 2006
Muscle development	*Dmrt2*	*Mus musculus*	Seo et al., 2006 Seo, 2007 Sato et al., 2010 Lourenço et al., 2010
	terra/Dmrt2a	*Danio rerio*	Meng et al., 1999 Saúde et al., 2005
	Dmrt2b	*Danio rerio*	Liu et al., 2009
Neurogenesis	*Dmrt4*	*Xenopus laevis*	Huang et al., 2005b

Table 3. **Functional studies of DM domain genes in vertebrates.**

Summarising the presented data, the vertebrate DM domain gene *Dmrt1* and its close paralogs act as primary-sex determining genes in different vertebrate phyla, including fish (*DMY/Dmrt1bY*), amphibians (*DM-W*) and birds (Z-linked *Dmrt1*), each with an independently evolved chromosomal sex-determination mechanism. Unlike sex chromosome-linked *Dmrt1* orthologs, autosomal *Dmrt1* genes appear as critical sex-differentiating (but not sex-determining) factors acting in developing embryonic/postnatal gonads in mammals (mouse), amphibians (frog *Rana rugosa*) and fish (medaka, Nile tilapia).

In species not having sex chromosomes with temperature-dependant sex-determination mechanisms (some reptiles), *Dmrt1* is a likely genetic factor that may play a primary sex-determination role.

From an evolutionary point of view, *Dmrt1* homologs are thought to be frequently recruited or retained to determine/differentiate sex as new sex-determination mechanisms arise.

Despite the wide knowledge about *Dmrt1* as the vertebrate sex-developmental locus, new studies, especially based on recently available high-throughput genome-wide technologies, are being performed in order to better understand its transcriptional regulation in testis/ovary differentiation pathways. Still, little is known about the *Dmrt1* targets or the manner in which their expression is regulated. What is more, the newest intriguing data about the *DMRT1* association with the testicular germ cell tumour (TGCT) in humans also requires further explanation (Kanetsky, et al., 2011; Turnbull et al., 2011).

3.2 DM domain genes, not just a sex issue

It is now well known that besides *Dmrt1,* seven other DM domain genes exist in the vertebrate genome (Table 1) (however, the numbers vary across species). Although they have not been studied as intensively as *Dmrt1,* recent findings provide a great deal of data about their embryonic expression pattern in different vertebrate clades, including mammals (mouse), birds (chicken), amphibians (frogs *R. rugosa, X. leavis*) and broadly investigated fish (medaka, zebrafish, platyfish, Japanese pufferfish). Following the extensive database search (as was done for *Dmrt1*), the newest knowledge about *DMRT* expression in both embryos and adult tissues in a variety of vertebrate species is summarised in Table 4.

A number of general statements can be deduced from this table. In addition to *Dmrt1,* most *Dmrt* genes are expressed in developing gonads during early embryogenesis, and in many cases, their expression is subsequently maintained at higher levels in male than in female gonads. However, in contrast to *Dmrt1,* many *Dmrt* genes are activated in other developing tissues/organs, either before or after the onset of their expression in gonads. This suggests that they may control a broader range of developmental processes. This non-gonad-restricted embryonic expression pattern was observed for *Dmrt2, Dmrt3, Dmrt4, Dmrt5, Dmrt6* and *Dmrt8.1.* In most species, *Dmrt* genes have been detected in mesodermally derived somites (mouse, chick and fish *terra/Dmrt2a* and chick *Dmrt3*), ectodermally derived olfactory placodes (mouse and chick *Dmrt3; Xenopus,* platyfish and medaka *Dmrt4;* and platyfish *Dmrt5*) and neuroectodermally derived developing brain (*Dmrt3, Dmrt4, Dmrt5* and *Dmrt6* in mouse, chicken, *Xenopus* and fish). It is important to emphasise that the expression of some *Dmrt* genes has not been carefully studied besides forming gonads, and therefore, their activation in other tissues may have been overlooked. For example, most murine *Dmrt* genes were analysed in a variety of organs but only at one developmental stage (E 14.5), and subsequent detailed investigations were carried out only in dissected embryonic gonads (Kim at al., 2003). Similarly, the data from the embryonic expression of some *Dmrt* genes in frog *Rana rugosa* were based on cDNA preparations from either whole embryos or gonads of tadpoles (Matsushita et al., 2007). Moreover, the choice of method is also crucial. It was often noticed that transcripts detectable by more sensitive RT-PCR are not visible in embryo sections following the less sensitive *in situ* hybridisation.

Gene	Organism	Expression in embryos	Expression in adult tissues	References
DMRT2	*H. sapiens*	embryos aged 4-7 weeks of both sexes[1]	K, SM, Th, L, I, **T**	Ottolenghi et al., 2000a Ottolenghi et al., 2000b Calvari et al., 2000
Dmrt2	*M. musculus*	*at E9.5* PSM, somites *at E14.5* B, **T**, H, **O**, K, BL, K, L, S, Li	**T**[2]	Meng et al., 1999 Kim et al., 2003
	S. scrofa	-	SM, B, K, **T**, **O**, Sp	Bratuś & Słota, 2009
	B. taurus	-	SM, K, **T**	Bratuś & Słota, 2009
	O. anatinus	-	K, **T**, **O**,	El-Mogharbel et al., 2007 Tsend-Ayush et al., 2009
	G. gallus	PSM, somites[3]	-	Saúde et al., 2005
	R. rugosa	**T, O**[4]	K, **T**, B	Matsushita et al., 2007
	O. latipes	*since day 2*, somites, PSM, *day 4*, somites, B	**T**, **O**, G	Brunner et al., 2001 Winkler et al., 2004
	T. rubripes	-	**T, O,** G, I, E, M	Yamaguchi et al., 2006
	X. maculatus	*since day 3*, somites, head	G	Veith et al., 2006a
terra/Dmrt2a	*D. rerio*	somites, PSM	M, **T**, O, B	Meng et al., 1999
Dmrt2b	*D. rerio*	branchial arches	M, Li, **O, T,** B	Zhou et al., 2008
DMRT3/DMRTA3	*H. sapiens*	-	**T**, B, L, SM	Ottolenghi et al., 2000a Ottolenghi et al., 2002
Dmrt3	*M. musculus*	*at E9.5* forebrain, nasal placodes *at E14.5* B, L, S, **T**, K, I	not expressed in T	Smith et al., 2002 Kim et al., 2003
	S. scrofa	-	**T**	Bratuś & Słota, 2009
	B. taurus	-	**T**	Bratuś & Słota, 2009
	O. anatinus	-	**T**	El-Mogharbel et al., 2007
	G. gallus	*since E1* PSM, somites, at *E2.1* telencephalon, olfactory placodes at E7.5 Müllerian duct	-	Smith et al., 2002
	R. rugosa	**T,O**	B, **T**	Matsushita et al., 2007
	O. latipes	*since day 3*, hindbrain, neural tube	**T**	Brunner et al., 2001 Winkler et al., 2004
	D. rerio	olfactory placodes, neural tube	**T, O**	Li et al., 2008
	T. rubripes	*at 115 days after hatching* **T**	**T, O,** G, B, Li, M,	Yamaguchi et al., 2006
DMRT4/DMRTA1	*H. sapiens*	-	Li, K, P, Pr, L, **T, O**	Ottolenghi et al., 2002
Dmrt4	*M. musculus*	*at E14.5* B, H, **O**, **T**, BL, K, I, L, S	**O,T**, PG, Li, H, K, Sp, Th, L, I	Kim et al., 2003 Balciuniene et al., 2006
	X. laevis	*since stage 17*, olfactory placodes, forebrain, telencephalon	-	Huang et al., 2005b
	O. latipes	*since day 1*, olfactory placodes, telencephalon	**T**, K, G, **O**, E, B	Kondo et al., 2002 Winkler et al., 2004
	T. rubripes	-	**T, O,** Sp	Yamaguchi et al., 2006

	X. maculatus	*since day 3,* olfactory placodes; *day 5*: olfactory placodes, branchial arches, B	G	Veith et al., 2006a
DMRT5/DMRTA2	*H. sapiens*	-	**T**	Ottolenghi et al., 2002
Dmrt5	*M. musculus*	*at E13.5* B *at E14.5* B, **O**, K, H, L, S, **T**	**T**	Kim et al., 2003
	R. rugosa	**T,O**	B, H, **T**, **O**, P, K	Matsushita et al., 2007
	D. rerio	B	B, **T**, **O**	Guo et al., 2004b
	T. rubripes	-	Sp, B	Yamaguchi et al., 2006
	X. maculatus	*since day 3,* olfactory placodes; B, lenses, *day 5*: olfactory epithelium, B	B, E	Veith et al., 2006a
DMRT6/DMRTB1	*H. sapiens*	-	**T**, P, **O**	Ottolenghi et al., 2002
Dmrt6	*M. musculus*	*at E14.5* B	**T**	Kim et al., 2003
DMRT7/DMRTC2	*H. sapiens*	-	**T**, P	Ottolenghi et al., 2002
Dmrt7	*M. musculus*	*at E14.5* **O**, **T**	**T**	Kim et al., 2003 Kawamata & Nishimori, 2006 Kawamata et al., 2007
	O. anatinus	-	**T**	Tsend-Ayush et al., 2009
DMRT8/DMRTC1	*H. sapiens*	-	**T**, **O**, K, P, B, L	Ottolenghi et al., 2002
Dmrt8.1	*M. musculus*	*at E13.5* S, Me, I, **O**, **T**, L, K, H, head, neural tube	**T**	Veith et al., 2006b
Dmrt8.2	*M. musculus*	*at E13.5* **T**, **O**	**T**	Veith et al., 2006b

[1]human *DMRT* genes (with the exception of *DMRT2*) were not investigated in embryos
[2]the expression of murine *DMRT* genes in adult animals was tested only in male gonads (with the exception of *DMRT4*, *DMRT7* and *DMRT8*)
[3]chick *DMRT2* was detected in 2-somite and 14-somite stages of embryo development as well as in the node from stage 4 Hamburger and Hamilton (4HH) to stage 7HH
[4]in frog *Rana rugosa*, the expression of *DMRT2*, -*3* and -*5* was investigated in whole embryos at stages 16, 21, 23 and in the gonad/mesonephros complex of tadpoles at stages I, III, V.

Table 4. **Spatial and temporal expression of *DMRT2-3-4-5-6-7-8* genes during embryogenesis and in adult animals across different vertebrate species.** The order of the indicated tissues in the row correlates with the decreasing level of the detected expression (e.g., the murine *DMRT7* at the E14.5 was enriched in ovaries). B-brain, BL-bladder, E-embryonic day, E-eye, G-gills, H-heart, I-intestine, K-kidney, L-lung, Li-liver, M-muscle, Me-mesonephros, O-ovary, P-pancreas, PG-preputial gland, Pr-prostate, T-testis, PSM-Presomitic mesoderm, S-stomach, SM-skeletal muscle, Sp-spleen, Th-thymus,'-' not reported.

However, based on available data, further observations can be made. While the expression patterns for various *Dmrt* genes have appeared to be conserved across species, there are also some clear differences. For instance, the specific for *Dmrt4* expression profile in nasal placode and in telencephalon in *Xenopus*, medaka and platyfish appears to be *Dmrt3* characteristic in mouse and chicken. What is more, chick *Dmrt3* is additionally expressed in presomitic mesoderm, which is not true for its mouse and fish orthologs but typical for *Dmrt2* is mouse, zebrafish, platyfish and medaka. Additionally, *Dmrt1*, which has been found to be exclusively expressed in developing and adult gonads of all vertebrate phyla, surprisingly appears to be expressed in extragonadal adult tissues in cattle (heart, spleen, skeletal muscle, kidney, lung, liver) and in pig (kidney) (Bratuś & Słota, 2009; Table 2). The bovine *Dmrt1* widespread tissue-expression profile closely resembles the transcription patterns described for *DMRT2*, *DMRT4* and *DMRT8* in adult human tissues (Table 4).

The above observations indicate that the expression patterns and presumably the function of some vertebrate members of the DM-domain gene family may have shifted during evolution (Hong et al., 2007).

It is obvious, however, that in addition to *Dmrt1*, some other DM domain genes are involved in sexual development. This statement was already suggested after the observation of a relatively mild *Dmrt1* mutant phenotype in mice (Raymond et al., 2000). No defects outside the gonads were observed in the *Dmrt1*$^{-/-}$ males, while *Dmrt1*$^{-/-}$ females were not affected. The lack of *Dmrt1*, thus, might have been compensated for by the activation of other DM domain genes during sexual differentiation. Mouse *Dmrt3*, *Dmrt5* and *Dmrt7* exhibit sex-specific expression in the early embryonic gonads (their expression becomes enriched either in developing testes (*Dmrt3*) or in developing ovaries (*Dmrt5*, *Dmrt7*) (Kim et al., 2003). Unlike *Dmrt3* and *Dmrt5*, but similar to *Dmrt1*, *Dmrt7* expression is restricted only to embryonic mouse gonads of both sexes and becomes postnatally testis specific. Although the early XX-enriched expression of *Dmrt7* makes this gene a candidate for a role in early ovary differentiation, further functional studies have shown that it is essential for male fertility (Kawamata & Nishimori, 2006; Kim at al., 2007b; Table 3). While *Dmrt7*-deficient female mice were fertile, adult null males were infertile due to the affected functioning of testicular germ cells. It has been found that the lack of *Dmrt7* in mice is associated with an arrest of spermatogenesis at the late pachyten stage and with abnormal sex chromatin modifications normally required for male meiotic progression (Kim at al., 2007b).

Like *Dmrt7*, another DM domain gene, *Dmrt8* seems to be mammalian specific (so far not described in other vertebrates) and exclusively expressed in the embryonic gonads of both sexes as well as in the testes of adult mice (Veith et al., 2006b). However, unlike *Dmrt7*, its function as a sex regulator is now highly speculated because of at least three reasons: 1) It is widely expressed in human adult tissues including brain, lung, kidney, pancreas and gonads, 2) One of its copy found in mice, *Dmrt8.1*, is expressed in multiple embryonic organs in a non-sex-specific manner, and 3) No functional studies have yet been carried out in order to determine its role in mammalian development.

Conversely, functional studies of another murine *Dmrt* gene, *Dmrt4*, have revealed its involvement in some aspects of sexual development (Balciuniene et al., 2006). Despite its widespread expression in both embryos and adults, *Dmrt4* mutant mice appear to be viable and fertile. However, two potential mutant phenotypes have been observed: 1) *Dmrt4*-deficient females have elevated numbers of polyovular follicles due to affected folliculogenesis, and 2) 25% of mutant males attempt to copulate with other males, suggesting a possible behavioural abnormality. This potential involvement of *Dmrt4* in proper ovary development and male sexual behaviour has not been found in previous functional studies carried out in frog *Xenopus*, suggesting that *Dmrt4* orthologs are not functionally conserved (Huang et al., 2005b). The effects of *Dmrt4* depletion in frog embryos have been shown to be consistent with its early embryonic expression pattern (Table 4). The

Dmrt4-deficient embryos showed specific disruption of the expression of known neuronal differentiation factor (Xebf2) in the olfactory placode. Later, during embryogenesis, mutants exhibited impaired neurogenesis in the olfactory epithelium. Moreover, the forced expression of *Dmrt4* was sufficient to activate neurogenic markers in cultured *Xenopus* explants. Therefore, it was proposed that *Xenopus Dmrt4* is a key regulator in neurogenesis but not in gonad development. Moreover, the maintained activity of some neuronal gene markers in the *Dmrt4* mutant nasal placode may suggest the compensatory activity of other DM domain genes, such as *Dmrt3* and *Dmrt5*.

Similarly, *Dmrt6* and *Dmrt2* have also been shown to be less likely sexual regulators. In contrast to the poorly investigated *Dmrt6*, the expression of which was found to be restricted to the developing brain in mouse embryos (Kim et al., 2003), *Dmrt2* has been extensively studied during vertebrate embryogenesis as well as in genetically modified model organisms (Tables 3 and 4). *Dmrt2* shows a conserved expression pattern during embryogenesis. *Dmrt2* is expressed primarily in the presomitic mesoderm and newly formed somites in various vertebrate clades, including mammals (mouse), birds (chicken) and fish (medaka, platyfish and zebrafish) (Table 4). This suggests its involvement in muscle development across species. The detailed functional analyses, however, performed only in mouse and zebrafish, have indeed confirmed this hypothesis, but they have also revealed that type of developmental processes regulated by *Dmrt2* can differ in these two organisms. In zebrafish, overexpression of *terra/Dmrt2a* (homolog of human and mouse *Dmrt2*) induced rapid apoptosis in the somitic mesoderm both *in vitro* and *in vivo*, suggesting that the *terra* activity needs to be strictly regulated for proper mesoderm development (Meng et al., 1999). Moreover, the depletion of *terra* activity in zebrafish embryos has revealed two important roles of this DM domain gene: 1) It is involved in the active mechanism responsible for the left-right asymmetry formation, fundamental to vertebrate body-plan creation, and 2) It is responsible for proper bilateral synchronisation of the segmentation clock in the mesoderm, essential for the normal development of bilateral structures such as skeletal muscles (Saúde et al., 2005). What is more, it was recently reported that due to a genome duplication event, zebrafish *terra/Dmrt2a* has a paralog named *Dmrt2b* (Zhou et al., 2008). Contrary to *terra/Dmrt2a*, which is present in all vertebrates, *Dmrt2b* duplication exists only in the fish genome. *Dmrt2b*, like *terra/Dmrt2a*, also showed a left-right asymmetry establishment function in zebrafish embryos. However, unlike its paralog, it regulates other aspects of somite differentiation affecting slow muscle development (Liu et al., 2009). Surprisingly, neither the regulation of left-right patterning in the mesoderm nor the involvement in symmetric somite formation has been observed for murine *Dmrt2* (Lourenço et al., 2010). Instead, mouse embryos lacking the *Dmrt2* function showed early somite patterning defects, perturbed somite maturation, abnormal skeletal muscle in myotome and affected onset of myogenesis (Seo et al., 2006; Sato et al., 2010). Thus, murine *Dmrt2* and both zebrafish paralogs, *terra/Dmrt2a* and *Dmrt2b*, appear to be *Dmrt* family members with a well-evidenced role in vertebrate muscle development and not sex determination/differentiation.

4. Conclusion

Summarising the presented story about DM domain genes in vertebrates, it is a privilege for me to adopt one conclusion that has been proposed by professor Zarkower in his excellent review paper about sexual development. "Conservation amidst diversity?" Ten years of further extensive investigations have brought the wide, fascinating knowledge about the DM domain gene family that perfectly reflects the cited conclusion. However, there has been one minor change: The question mark is not needed anymore.

5. Acknowledgment

I would like to thank Stefan for his patience and constant support.

6. References

Alfaqih, M.A.; Brunelli, J.P.; Drew, R.E. & Thorgaard, G.H. (2009). Mapping of five candidate sex-determining loci in rainbow trout (*Oncorhynchus mykiss*). *BMC genetics (electronic resources)*, Vol.10, pp.2, ISSN 1471-2156

Aoyama, S.; Shibata, K.; Tokunada, S.; Takase, M.; Matsui, K. & Nakamura, M. (2003). Expression of Dmrt1 protein in developing and in sex-reversed gonads in amphibians. *Cytogenetic and Genome Research*, Vol.101, No.3-4, pp. 295-301, ISSN 0301-0171

Baker, B.S. & Ridge, K.A.(1980). Sex and the single cell. I. On the action of major loci affecting sex determination in *Drosophila melanogaster*. *Genetics*, Vol.94, No.2, pp.383-423, ISSN 0016-6731

Balciuniene, J.; Bardwell, V.J. & Zarkower, D. (2006). Mice mutant in the DM domain gene DMRT4 are viable and fertile but have polyovular follicles. *Molecular and Cellular Biology*, Vol.26, No.23, pp. 8984-8991, ISSN 0270-7306

Bennett, C.P.; Docherty, Z.; Robb, S.A.; Ramani, P.; Hawkins, J.R. & Grant, D. (1993). Deletion 9p and sex reversal. *Journal of Medical Genetics*, Vol.30, No.6, pp. 518-520, ISSN 0022-2593

Boyer, A.; Dornan, S.; Daneau, I.; Lussier, J. & Silversides, W. (2002). Conservation of the function of DMRT1 regulatory sequences in mammalian sex differentiation. *Genesis*, Vol.34, No.4, pp. 236-243, ISSN 1526-954X

Bratuś, A.; Bugno, M.; Klukowska-Rötzler, J.; Sawińska, M.; Eggen, A. & Słota, E.(2009). Chromosomal homology between the human and the bovine *DMRT1* genes. *Folia biologica (Krakow)*, Vol.57, No.1-2, pp. 29-32, ISSN 0015-5497

Bratuś, A. & Słota, E. (2009). Comparative cytogenetic and molecular studies of DM domain genes in pig and cattle. *Cytogenetic and Genome Research*, Vol.126, No.1-2, pp. 180-185, ISSN 1424-8581

Brunner, B.; Hornung, U.; Shan, Z.; Nanda, I.; Kondo, M.; Zend-Ajusch, E.; Haaf, T.; Ropers, H-H.; Shima, A.; Schmid, M.; Kalscheuer, V.M. & Schartl, M. (2001). Genomic organization and expression of the doublesex-related gene cluster in vertebrates and detection of putative regulatory regions for *DMRT1*. *Genomics*, Vol.77, No.1-2, pp. 8-17, ISSN 0888-7543

Burtis, K.C. & Baker, B.S. (1989). Drosophila *doublesex* gene controls somatic sexual differentiation by producing alternatively spliced mRNAs encoding related sex-specific polypeptides. *Cell*, Vol.56, No.6, pp. 997-1010, ISSN 0092-8674

Calvari, V.; Bertini, V.; De Grandi, A.; Peverali, G.; Zuffardi, O.; Furguson-Smith, M.; Knudtzon, J.; Camerino, G.; Borsani, G. & Guioli, S. (2000). A new submicroscopic deletion that refines the 9p region for sex reversal. *Genomics*, Vol.65, No.3, pp. 203-212, ISSN 0888-7543

Chen, J.K. & Heckert, L.L. (2001). *Dmrt1* expression is regulated by follicle-stimulating hormone and phorbol esters in postnatal Sertoli cells. *Endocrinology*, Vol.142, No.3, pp. 1167-1178, ISSN 0013-7227

Cheng, H.H.; Ying, M.; Tian, Y.H.; Guo, Y.; McElreavey, K. & Zhou, R.J. (2006). Transcriptional diversity of *DMRT1* (*dsx*-and *mab3*-related transcription factor 1) in human testis. *Cell Research*, Vol.16, No.4, pp. 389-393, ISSN 1001-0602

Crocker, M.; Coghill, S.B. & Cortinho, R. (1988). An unbalanced autosomal translocation (7;9) associated with feminization. *Clinical Genetics*, Vol.34, No.1, pp. 70-73, ISSN 0009-9163

De Grandi, A.D.; Calvari, V.; Bertini, V.; Bulfone, A.; Peverali, G.; Camerino, G.; Borsani, G. & Guioli, S. (2000). The expression pattern of a mouse doublesex-related gene is consistent with a role in gonadal differentiation. *Mechanisms of Development*, Vol.90, No.2, pp. 323-326, ISSN 0925-4773

El-Mogharbel, N.; Deakin, J.; Tsend-Ayush, E.; Pask, A. & Graves, J.A.M. (2005). Assignment of the *DMRT1* gene to tammar wallaby chromosome 3p by fluorescence in situ hybridization. *Cytogenetic and Genome Research*, Vol.108, No.4, pp. 362E, ISSN 1424-8581

EL-Mogharbel, N.; Wakefield, M.; Deakin, J.E.; Tsend-Ayush, T.; Grützner, F.; Alsop, A.; Ezaz, T. & Graves, J.A.M. (2007). DMRT1 gene cluster analysis in the platypus: New insights into genomic organization and regulatory regions. *Genomics*, Vol.89, No.1, pp. 10-21, ISSN

Erdman, S.E. & Burtis, K.C. (1993). The *Drosophila* doublesex proteins share a novel zinc finger related DNA binding domain. *The EMBO Journal*, Vol.12, No.2, pp. 527-535, ISSN 0261-4189

Fahrioglu, U.; Murphy, M.W.; Zarkower, D. & Bardwell, V.J. (2007). mRNA expression analysis and the molecular basis of neonatal testis defects in Dmrt1 mutant mice. *Sexual Development*, Vol.1, No.1, pp. 42-58, ISSN 1661-5425

Fernandino, J.I.; Guilgur, L.G. & Somoza, G.M. (2006). *Dmrt1* expression analysis during spermatogenesis in pejerrey, *Odontesthes bonariensis*. *Fish Physiology and Biochemistry*, Vol.32, No.3, pp. 231–240, ISSN 0920-1742

Fernandino, J.I.; Hattori, R.S.; Shinoda, T.; Kimura, H.; Strobl-Mazzulla, P.H.; Strüssmann, C.A. & Somoza, G.M. (2008). Dimorphic expression of *dmrt1* and *cyp19a1* (ovarian aromatase) during early gonadal development in pejerrey, *Odontesthes bonariensis*. *Sexual Development*, Vol.2, No.6, pp. 316-324, ISSN 1661-5425

Flejter, W.L.; Fergestad, J.; Gorski, J.; Varvill, T. & Chandrasekharappa, S. (1998). A gene involved in XY sex reversal is located on chromosome 9, distal to marker D9S1779. *American Journal of Human Genetics*, Vol.63, No.3, pp. 794-802, ISSN 0002-9297

Guan, G.; Kobayashi, T. & Nagahama, Y. (2000). Sexually dimorphic expression of two types of DM (Doublesex/Mab-3)-domain genes in a teleost fish, the tilapia (Oreochromis niloticus). *Biochemical and Biophysical Research Communications*, Vol.272, No.3, pp. 662-666, ISSN 0006-291X

Guo, Y.; Gao, S.; Cheng, H. & Zhou, R. (2004a). Phylogenetic tree and synteny of dmrt genes family of vertebrates. *Acta Genetica Sinica*, Vol.10, pp. 1103-1108, ISSN 0379-4172

Guo, Y.; Li, Q.; Gao, S.; Zhou, X.; He, Y.; Shang, X.; Cheng, H. & Zhou, R. (2004b). Molecular cloning, characterization, and expression in brain and gonad of *DMRT5* of zebrafish. *Biochemical and Biophysical Research Communications*, Vol.324, No.2, pp. 569-575, ISSN 0006-291X

Guo, Y.; Cheng, H.; Huang, X.; Gao, S.; Yu, H. & Zhou, R. (2005). Gene structure, multiple alternative splicing, and expression in gonads of zebrafish *Dmrt1*. *Biochemical and Biophysical Research Communications*, Vol.330, No.3, pp. 950-957, ISSN 0006-291X

Hong, C-S.; Park, B-Y. & Saint-Jeannet, J-P. (2007). The function of *Dmrt* genes in vertebrate development: it is not just about sex. *Developmental Biology*, Vol.310, No.1, pp. 1-9, ISSN 0012-1606

Huang, X.; Cheng, H.; Guo, Y.; Liu, L.; Gui, J. & Zhou, R. (2002). A conserved family of doublesex-related genes from fishes. *Journal of Experimental Zoology*, Vol.294, No.1, pp. 63-67, ISSN 0022-104X

Huang, X.; Guo, Y.Q.; Shui, Y.; Gao, S.; Yu, H.S.; Cheng, H.H. & Zhou, R.J. (2005a). Multiple alternative splicing and differential expression of dmrt1 during gonad transformation of the rice field eel. *Biology of Reproduction.*, Vol.73, No.5, pp. 1017-1024, ISSN 0006-3363

Huang, X.; Hong, C.S.; O'Donnell, M. & Saint-Jeannet, J.P. (2005b). The doublesex-related gene, *XDMRT4*, is required for neurogenesis in the olfactory system. *Proceedings of the National Academy of Sciences of the United States of America*, Vol.102, No.(32), pp. 11349-11354, ISSN 0027-8424

Johnsen, H.; Seppola, M.; Torgersen, J.S.; Delghandi, M. & Andersen, Ø. (2010). Sexually dimorphic expression of dmrt1 in immature and mature Atlantic cod (*Gadus morhua L.*). *Comparative Biochemistry and Physiology Part B: Biochemistry and Molecular Biology*, Vol.156, No.3, pp.197-205, ISSN 1096-4959

Kanetsky, P.A.; Mitra, N.; Vardhanabhuti, S.; Vaughn, D.J.; Li, M.; Ciosek, S.L.; Letrero, R.; D'Andrea, K.; Vaddi, M.; Doody, D.R.; Weaver, J.; Chen, C.; Starr, J.R.; Håkonarson, H.; Rader, D.J.; Godwin, A.K.; Reilly, M.P.; Schwartz, S.M. & Nathanson, K.L. (2011). A second independent locus within DMRT1 is associated with testicular germ cell tumor susceptibility. *Human Molecular Genetics*, Vol.20, No.15, pp. 3109-3117, ISSN 0964-6906

Kawamata, M. & Nishimori, K (2006). Mice deficient in *DMRT7* show infertility with spermatogenic arrest at pachytene stage. *FEBS letters*, Vol.580, No.27, pp. 6442-6446, ISSN 0014-5793

Kawamata, M.; Inoue, H. & Nishimori, K. (2007). Male-specific function of *DMRT7* by sexually dimorphic translation in mouse testis. *Sexual Development*, Vol.1, No.5, pp. 297-304, ISSN 1661-5425

Kettlewell, J.R.; Raymond, C.S. & Zarkower, D. (2000). Temperature-dependent expression of turtle Dmrt1 prior to sexual differentiation. *Genesis*, Vol.26, No.3 pp. 174-178, ISSN 1526-954X

Kim, S.; Kettlewell, J.R.; Anderson, R.C.; Bardwell, V.J. & Zarkower, D. (2003). Sexually dimorphic expression of multiple doublesex-related genes in the embryonic mouse gonad. *Gene Expression Patterns*, Vol.3, No.1, pp. 77-82, ISSN 1567-133X

Kim, S.; Bardwell, V.J. & Zarkower, D. (2007a). Cell type-autonomous and non-autonomous requirements for Dmrt1 in postnatal testis differentiation. *Developmental Biology*, Vol.307, No.2, pp. 314-327, ISSN 0012-1606

Kim S.; Namekawa, S.H.; Niswander, L.M.; Ward, J.; Lee, J.T.; Bardwell, V.J. & Zarkower, D. (2007b). A mammal-specific Doublesex homolog associates with male sex chromatin and is required for male meiosis. *PLoS Genetics*, Vol.3 No.4, pp. 559-571, ISSN 1553-7390

Kobayashi, T.; Matsuda, M.; Kajiura-Kobayashi, H.; Suzuki, A.; Saito, N.; Nakamoto, M.; Shibata, N. & Nagahama, Y. (2004). Two DM domain genes, DMY and DMRT1, involved in testicular differentiation and development in the medaka, Oryzias latipes. *Developmental Dynamics*, Vol.231, No.3, pp. 518-526, ISSN 1058-8388

Kondo, M.; Froschauer, A.; Kitano, A.; Nanda, I.; Hornung, U.; Volff, J.N.; Asakawa, S.; Mitani, H.; Naruse, K.; Tanaka, M.; Schmid, M.; Shimizu, N.; Schartl, M. & Shima, A. (2002). Molecular cloning and characterization of *DMRT* genes from the medaka *Oryzias latipes* and the platyfish *Xiphophorus maculatus*. *Gene*, Vol.295, No.2, pp. 213-222, ISSN 0378-1119

Kondo, M.; Nanda, I.; Hornung, U.; Asakawa, S.; Shimizu, N.; Mitani, H.; Schmid, M.; Shima, A. & Schartl, M. (2003). Absence of the candidate male sex-determining gene *dmrt1b(Y)* of medaka from other fish species. *Current Biology*, Vol.13, No.5, pp. 416-420, ISSN 0960-9822

Koopman, P.; Gubbay, J.; Vivian, N.; Goodfellow, P. & Lovell-Badge, R. (1991). Male development of chromosomally female mice transgenic for *Sry*. *Nature*, Vol.351, No.6322, pp. 117-121, ISSN 0028-0836

Krentz, A.D.; Murphy, M.W.; Kim, S.; Cook, M.S.; Capel, B.; Zhu, R.; Matin, A.; Sarver, A.L.; Parker, K.L.; Griswold, M.D.; Looijenga, L.H.; Bardwell, V.J. & Zarkower, D. (2009). The DM domain protein DMRT1 is a dose-sensitive regulator of fetal germ cell proliferation and pluripotency. *Proceedings of the National Academy of Sciences of the United States of America*, Vol.106, No.52, pp. 22323-22328, ISSN 0027-8424

Krentz, A.D.; Murphy, M.W.; Sarver, A.L.; Griswold, M.D.; Bardwell, V.J. & Zarkower, D. (2011). DMRT1 promotes oogenesis by transcriptional activation of Stra8 in the mammalian fetal ovary. *Developmental Biology*, Vol.356, No.1, pp. 63-70, ISSN 0012-1606

Lei, N.; Hornbaker, K.I.; Rice, D.A.; Karpova, T.; Agbor, V.A. & Heckert, L.L. (2007). Sex-specific differences in mouse DMRT1 expression are both cell type- and stage-dependent during gonadal development. *Biology of Reproduction*, Vol.77, No.3, pp. 466-475, ISSN 0006-3363

Lei, N.; Karpova, T.; Hornbaker, K.I.; Rice, D.A. & Heckert L.L. (2009). Distinct transcriptional mechanisms direct expression of the rat Dmrt1 promoter in Sertoli cells and germ cells of transgenic mice. *Biology of Reproduction*, Vol.81, No.1, pp. 118-125, ISSN 0006-3363

Li, Q.; Zhou, X.; Guo, Y.; Shang, X.; Chen, H.; Lu, H.; Cheng, H. & Zhou, R. (2008). Nuclear localization, DNA binding and restricted expression in neural and germ cells of zebrafish *DMRT3*. *Biology of the Cell*, Vol.100, No.8, pp. 453-63, ISSN 0248-4900

Liu, S.; Li, Z. & Gui, J.F. (2009). Fish-specific duplicated *DMRT2B* contributes to a divergent function through Hedgehog pathway and maintains left-right asymmetry establishment function. *PLoS One*, Vol.4, No.9, pp. e7261, ISSN 1932-6203

Lourenço, R.; Lopes, S.S. & Saúde, L. (2010). Left-right function of DMRT2 genes is not conserved between zebrafish and mouse. *PLoS One*, Vol.5, No.12, pp. e14438, ISSN 1932-6203

Lu, H.; Huang, X.; Zhang, L.; Guo, Y.; Cheng, H. & Zhou, R. (2007). Multiple alternative splicing of mouse *Dmrt1* during gonadal differentiation. *Biochemical and Biophysical Research Communications*, Vol.353, No.3, pp. 630-634, ISSN 0006-291X

Murphy, M.W.; Sarver, A.L.; Rice, D.; Hatzi, K.; Ye, K.; Melnick, A.; Heckert, L.L.; Zarkower, D. & Bardwell, V.J. (2010). Genome-wide analysis of DNA binding and transcriptional regulation by the mammalian Doublesex homolog DMRT1 in the juvenile testis. *Proceedings of the National Academy of Sciences of the United States of America*, Vol.107, No.30, pp. 13360-13355, ISSN 0027-8424

Marchand, O.; Govoroun, M.; D'cotta, H.; McMeel, O.; Lareyre, J-J.; Bernot, A.; Laudet, V. & Guiguen, Y. (2000). DMRT1 expression during gonadal differentiation and spermatogenesis in the rainbow trout, Oncorhynchus mykiss. *Biochimica et Biophysyica Acta*, Vol.1493, No.1-2, pp. 180-187, ISSN 0006-3002

Matson, C.K.; Murphy, M.W.; Griswold, M.D.; Yoshida, S.; Bardwell, V.J. & Zarkower, D. (2010). The mammalian doublesex homolog DMRT1 is a transcriptional gatekeeper that controls the mitosis versus meiosis decision in male germ cells. *Developmental Cell*, Vol.19, No.4. pp. 612-624, ISSN 1534-5807

Matson, C.K.; Murphy, M.W.; Sarver, A.L.; Griswold, M.D.; Bardwell, V.J. & Zarkower, D. (2011). DMRT1 prevents female reprogramming in the postnatal mammalian testis. *Nature*, Vol.476, No.7358, pp. 101-104, ISSN 0028-0836

Matsuda, M.; Nagahama, Y.; Shinomiya, A.I.; Sato, T.; Matsuda, C.; Kobayashi, T.; Morrey, C.E.; Shibata, N.; Asakawa, S.; Shimizu, N.; Hori, H.; Hamaguchi, S. & Sakaizumi, M. (2002). DMY is a Y-specific DM-domain gene required for male development in the medaka fish. *Nature*, Vol.417, No.6888, pp. 559-563. ISSN 0028-0836

Matsushita, Y.; Oshima, Y. & Nakamura, M. (2007). Expression of DMRT genes in the gonads of Rana rugosa during sex determination. *Zoological Science*, Vol.24, No.1, pp. 95-99, ISSN0289-0003

McDonald, M.T.; Flejter, W.; Sheldon, S.; Putzi, M.J. & Gorski, J.L. (1997). XY sex reversal and gonadal dysgenesis due to 9p24 monosomy. *American Journal of Medical Genetics*, Vol.73, No.3, pp. 321-326, ISSN 0148-7299

Meng, A.; Moore, B.; Tang, H.; Yuan, B. & Lin, S. (1999). A Drosophila doublesex-related gene, terra, is involved in somitogenesis in vertebrates. *Development*, Vol.126, No.6, pp.1259-1268, ISSN 0950-1991

Moniot, B.; Berta, P.; Scherer, G.; Südbeck, P. & Poulat, F. (2000). Male specific expression suggests role of DMRT1 in human sex determination. *Mechanisms of Development*, Vol.91, No.1-2, pp. 323-325, ISSN 0925-4773

Murdock, C. & Wibbels, T. (2003). Expression of Dmrt1 in a turtle with temperature-dependent sex determination. *Cytogenetic and Genome Research*, Vol.101, No.3-4, pp. 302-308, ISSN 1424-8581

Muroya, K.; Okuyama, T.; Goishi, K.; Ogiso, Y.; Fukuda, S.; Kameyama, J.; Sato, H.; Suzuki, Y.; Terasaki, H.; Gomyo, H.; Wakui, K.; Fukushima, Y. & Ogata, T. (2000). Sex-determining gene(s) on distal 9p: clinical and molecular studies in six cases. *The Journal of Clinical Endocrinology & Metabolism*, Vol.85, No.9, pp. 3094-3100, ISSN 0021-972X

Nanda, I.; Shan, Z.; Schartl, M.; Burt, D.W.; Koehler, M.; Nothwang, H.; Grützner, F.; Paton, I.R.; Windsor, D.; Dunn, I.; Engel, W.; Staeheli, P.; Mizuno, S.; Haaf, T. & Schmid, M. (1999). 300 million years of conserved synteny between chicken Z and human chromosome 9. *Nature Genetics*, Vol.21, No.3, pp. 258-259. ISSN 1061-4036

Nanda, I.; Zend-Ajusch, E.; Shan, Z.; Grützner, F.; Schartl, M.; Burt, D.W.; Koehler, M.; Fowler, V.M.; Goodwin, G.; Schneider, W.J.; Mizuno, S.; Dechant, G.; Haaf, T. & Schmid, M. (2000). Conserved synteny between the chicken Z sex chromosome and human chromosome 9 includes the male regulatory gene *DMRT1*: a comparative (re)view on avian sex determination. *Cytogenetics and Cell Genetics*, Vol.89, No.1-2, pp. 67-78, ISSN 0301-0171

Nanda, I.; Kondo, M.; Hornung, U.; Asakawa, S.; Winkler, C.; Shimizu, A.; Shan, Z.; Haaf, T.; Shimizu, N.; Shima, A.; Schmid, M. & Schartl, M. (2002). A duplicated copy of DMRT1 in the sex-determining region of the Y chromosome of the medaka, *Oryzias latipes*. *Proceedings of the National Academy of Sciences of the United States of America*, Vol.99, No.18, pp. 11778-11783, ISSN 0027-8424

Osawa, N.; Oshima, Y. & Nakamura, M. (2005). Molecular cloning of Dmrt1 and its expression in the gonad of Xenopus. *Zoological Science*, Vol.22, No.6, pp.681-687, ISSN 0289-0003

Ottolenghi, C.; Veitia, R.; Quintana-Murci, L.; Torchard, D.; Scapoli, L. & Souleyreau-Therville, N. (2000a). The region on 9p associated with 46,XY sex reversal contains several transcripts expressed in the urogenital system and a novel doublesex-related domain. *Genomics*, Vol.64, No2, pp. 170-178, ISSN 0888-7543

Ottolenghi, C.; Veitia, R.; Barbieri, M.; Fellous, M. & McElreavey, K. (2000b). The human doublesex-related gene, *DMRT2*, is homologous to a gene involved in somitogenesis and encodes a potential bicistronic transcript. *Genomics*, Vol.64, No. 2, pp. 179-186, ISSN 0888-7543

Ottolenghi, C.; Fellous, M.; Barbieri, M. & McElreavey, K. (2002). Novel paralogy relations among human chromosomes support a link between the phylogeny of doublesex-related genes and the evolution of sex determination. *Genomics*, Vol. 79, No.3, pp. 333-343, ISSN 0888-7543

Õunap, K.; Uibo, O.; Zordania, R.; Kiho, L.; Ilus, T.; Õiglane-Shlik, E. & Bartsch, O. (2004). Three patients with 9p deletions including DMRT1 and DMRT2: a girl with XY complement, bilateral ovotestes, and extreme growth retardation, and two XX females with normal pubertal development. *American Journal of Medical Genetics*, Vol.130A, No.4, pp. 415-423, ISSN 1552-4825

Pask, A.J.; Behringer, R.R. & Renfree, M.B. (2003). Expression of DMRT1 in the mammalian ovary and testis - from marsupials to mice. *Cytogenetic and Genome Research*, Vol.101, No.3-4, pp. 229-236, ISSN 0301-0171

Privitera, O.; Vessecchia, G.; Bernasconi, B.; Bettio, D.; Stioui, S. & Giordano, G. (2005). Prenatal diagnosis of del(9)(p24): a sex reverse case. *Prenatal Diagnosis*, Vol.25, No. 10, pp. 945-948, ISSN 0197-3851

Raymond, C.S.; Shamu, C.E.; Shen, M.M.; Seifert, K.J.; Hirsch, B.; Hodgkin, J. & Zarkower,D. (1998). Evidence for evolutionary conservation of sex-determining genes. *Nature*, Vol.391, No.6668, pp. 691-695, ISSN 0028-0836

Raymond, C.S.; Parker, E.D.; Kettlewell, J.R.; Brown L.G.; Page, D.C.; Kusz, K.; Jaruzelska, J.; Reinberg, Y.; Flejter, W.L.; Bardwell, V.J.; Hirsch, B. & Zarkower, D. (1999a). A region of human chromosome 9p required testis development contains genes related to known sexual regulators. *Human Molecular Genetics*, Vol.8, No.6, pp. 989-996, ISSN 0964-6906

Raymond, C.S.; Kettlewell, J.R.; Hirsch, B.; Bardwell, V.J. & Zarkower, D. (1999b). Expression of Dmrt1 in the genital ridge of mouse and chicken embryos suggests a role in vertebrate sexual development. *Developmental Biology*, Vol.215, No.2, pp. 208-220., ISSN 0012-1606

Raymond, C.S.; Murphy, M.W.; O'sullivan, M.G.; Bardwell, V.J. & Zarkower, D. (2000). Dmrt1, a gene related to warm and fly sexual regulators, is required for mammalian testis differentiation. *Genes & Development*, Vol.14, No.20, pp. 2587-2595, ISSN 0890-9369

Rhen, T.; Metzger, K.; Schroeder, A. & Woodward, R. (2007). Expression of putative sex-determining genes during the thermosensitive period of gonad development in the snapping turtle, *Chelydra serpentine*. *Sexual Development*, Vol.1, No.4, pp. 255–270, ISSN 1661-5425

Sato, T.; Rocancourt, D.; Marques, L.; Thorsteinsdóttir, S. & Buckingham, M. (2010). A Pax3/DMRT2/Myf5 regulatory cascade functions at the onset of myogenesis. *PLoS Genetics*, Vol.6, No.4, pp. e1000897, ISSN 1553-7390

Saúde, L.; Lourenço, R.; Gonçalves, A. & Palmeirim, I. (2005). *Terra* is a left-right asymmetry gene required for left-right synchronization of the segmentation clock. *Nature Cell Biology*, Vol.7, No.9, pp. 918-920, ISSN 1465-7392

Seo, K.W.; Wang, Y.; Kokubo, H.; Kettlewell, J.R.; Zarkower, D.A. & Johnson, R.L. (2006). Targeted disruption of the DM domain containing transcription factor DMRT2 reveals an essential role in somite patterning. *Developmental Biology*, Vol.290, No.1, pp. 200-210, ISSN 0012-1606

Seo, K.W. (2007). DMRT2 and Pax3 double-knockout mice show severe defects in embryonic myogenesis. *Comparative Medicine*, Vol.57, No.5, pp. 460-468, ISSN 1532-0820

Shan, Z.; Nanda, I.; Wang, Y.; Schmid, M.; Vortkamp, A. & Haaf, T. (2000). Sex-specific expression of an evolutionarily conserved male regulatory gene, *DMRT1*, in birds. *Cytogenetics and Cell Genetics*, Vol.89, No.3-4, pp. 252-257, ISSN 0301-0171

Shen, M.M. & Hodgkin, J. (1988). *Mab-3*, a gene required for sex-specific yolk protein expression and a male-specific lineage in C. elegans. *Cell*, Vol.54, No.7, pp. 1019-1031, ISSN 0092-8674

Shetty, S.; Kirby, P.; Zarkower, D. & Graves, J.A.M. (2002). DMRT1 in a ratite bird: evidence for a role in sex determination and discovery of a putative regulatory element. *Cytogenetic and Genome Research*, Vol.99, No.1-4, pp. 245-251, ISSN 1424-8581

Shibata, K.; Takase, M. & Nakamura, M. (2002). The Dmrt1 expression in sex-reversed gonads of amphibians. *General and Comparative Endocrinology*, Vol.127, No.3, pp. 232-241, ISSN 0016-6480

Sinclair, A.H.; Berta, P.; Palmer, M.S.; Hawkins, J.R.; Griffiths, B.L.; Smith, M.J.; Foster, J.W.; Frischauf, A-M.; Lovell-Badge, R. & Goodfellow, P.N. (1990). A gene from the human sex- determining region encodes a protein with homology to a conserved DNA-binding motif. *Nature*, Vol.346, No.6281, pp. 240-244, ISSN 0028-0836

Smith, C.A.; McClive, P.J.; Western, P.S.; Reed, K.J. & Sinclair, A.H. (1999a). Conservation of a sex-determining gene. *Nature*, Vol.402, No.6762, pp. 601-602, ISSN 0028-0836

Smith, C.A.; Smith, M.J. & Sinclair, A.H. (1999b). Gene expression during gonadogenesis in the chicken embryo. *Gene*, Vol.234, No.2, pp. 395-402, ISSN 0378-1119

Smith, C.A.; Hurley, T.M.; McClive, P.J. & Sinclair, A.H. (2002). Restricted expression of *DMRT3* in chicken and mouse embryos. *Mechanisms of Development*, Vol.119, Suppl 1, pp. S73-S76, ISSN 0925-4773

Smith, C.A.; Katz, M. & Sinclair, A.H. (2003). DMRT1 is upregulated in the gonads during female-to-male sex reversal in ZW chicken embryos. *Biology of Reproduction*, Vol.68, No.2, pp. 560- 570, ISSN 0006-3363

Smith C.A.; Roeszler, K.N.; Ohnesorg, T.; Cummins, D.M.; Farlie, P.G.; Doran, T.J. & Sinclair, A.H. (2009). The avian Z-linked gene *DMRT1* is required for male sex determination in the chicken. *Nature*, Vol.461, No.7261, pp.267-271, ISSN 0028-0836

Sreenivasulu, K.; Ganesh, S. & Raman, R. (2002). Evolutionarily conserved, DMRT1, encodes alternatively spliced transcripts and shows dimorphic expression during gonadal differentiation in the lizard, Calotes versicolor. *Gene Expression Patterns*, Vol.2, No.1-2, pp. 51-60, ISSN 1567-133X

Torres-Maldonado, L.C.; Landa-Piedra, A.; Moreno-Mendozan, N.; Marmolejo-Valencja, A.; Meza-Martines, A. & Merchant-Larios, H. (2002). Expression profiles of Dax1, Dmrt1, and Sox9 during temperature sex determination in gonads of the sea turtle *Lepidochelys olivacea. General and Comparative Endocrinology*, Vol.129, No.1, pp. 20-26, ISSN 0016-6480

Tsend-Ayush, E.; Lim, S.L.; Pask, A.J.; Hamdan, D.D.; Renfree, M.B. & Grützner, F. (2009). Characterisation of *ATRX, DMRT1, DMRT7* and *WT1* in the platypus (*Ornithorhynchus anatinus*). *Reproduction, Fertility, and Development*, Vol.21, No.8, pp.985-991, ISSN 1031-3613

Turnbull, C.; Rapley, E.A.; Seal, S.; Pernet, D.; Renwick, A.; Hughes, D.; Ricketts, M.; Linger, R.; Nsengimana, J.; Deloukas, P.; Huddart, R.A.; Bishop, D.T.; Easton, D.F.; Stratton, M.R.; Rahman, N. & UK Testicular Cancer Collaboration. (2011).Variants near DMRT1, TERT and ATF7IP are associated with testicular germ cell cancer. *Nature Genetics*, Vol.42, No.7, pp.604-607, ISSN 1061-4036

Veith, A.M.; Froschauer, A.; Körting, C.; Nanda, I; Hanel, R.; Schmid, M.; Schartl, M. & Volff, J.N. (2003). Cloning of the dmrt1 gene of *Xiphophorus maculatus*:

dmY/dmrt1Y is not the master sex-determining gene in the platyfish. *Gene*, Vol.317, No.1-2, pp. 59-66, ISSN 0378-1119

Veith, A.M.; Schäfer, M.; Klüver, N.; Schmidt, C.; Schultheis, C.; Schartl, M.; Winkler, C. & Volff, JN. (2006a). Tissue-specific expression of dmrt genes in embryos and adults of the platyfish *Xiphophorus maculatus*. *Zebrafish*, Vol.3, No.3, pp. 325-37, ISSN 1545-8547

Veith, A.M.; Klattig, J.; Dettai, A.; Schmidt, C.; Englert, C. & Volff, J.N. (2006b). Male-biased expression of X-chromosomal DM domain-less *Dmrt8* genes in the mouse. *Genomics*, Vol.88, No.2, pp. 185-195, ISSN 0888-7543

Veitia, R.; Nunes, M.; Brauner, R.; Doco-Fenzy, M.; Joanny-Flinois, O.; Jaubert, F.; Lortat-Jacob, S.; Fellous, M. & McElreavey, K. (1997). Deletions of distal 9p associated with 46,XY male to female sex reversal: definition of the breakpoints at 9p23.3-p24.1. *Genomics*, Vol.41, No.2, pp. 271-274, ISSN 0888-7543

Veitia, R.A.; Nunes, M.; Quintana-Murci, L.; Rappaport, R.; Thibaud, E.; Jaubert, F.; Fellous, M.; McElreavey, K.; Gonçalves, J; Silva, M.; Rodrigues, J.C.; Caspurro, M.; Boieiro, F.; Marques, R. & Lavinha, J. (1998). Swyer syndrome and 46,XY partial gonadal dysgenesis associated with 9p deletions in the absence of monosomy-9p syndrome. *American Journal of Human Genetics*, Vol.63, No.3, pp. 901-905, ISSN 0002-9297

Vinci, G.; Chantot-Bastaraud, S.; El Houate, B.; Lortat-Jacob, S.; Brauner, R. & McElreavey, K. (2007). Association of deletion 9p, 46,XY gonadal dysgenesis and autistic spectrum disorder. *Molecular Human Reproduction*, Vol.13, No.9, pp. 685-689, ISSN 1360-9947

Volff, J-N.; Zarkower, D.; Bardwell, V.J. & Schartl, M. (2003a). Evolutionary dynamics of the DM domain gene family in metazoans. *Journal of Molecular Evolution*, Vol.57, Suppl.1, pp. S241-S249, ISSN 0022-2844

Volff, J-N.; Kondo, M. & Schartl, M. (2003b). Medaka dmY/dmrt1Y is not the universal primary sex-determining gene in fish. *Trends in Genetics*, Vol.19, No.4, pp. 196-199, ISSN 0168-9525

Winkler, C.; Hornung, U.; Kondo, M.; Neuner, C.; Duschl, J.; Shima, A. & Schartl, M. (2004). Developmentally regulated and non-sex-specific expression of autosomal dmrt genes in embryos of Medaka fish (Oryzias latipes). *Mechanism of Development*, Vol.121, No.7-8, pp. 997-1005, ISSN 0925-4773

Yamaguchi, A.; Lee, K.H.; Fujimoto, H.; Kadomura, K.; Yasumoto, S. & Matsuyama, M. (2006). Expression of the DMRT gene and its roles in early gonadal development of the Japanese pufferfish *Takifugu rubripes*. *Comparative Biochemistry and Physiology Part D: Genomics and Proteomics*, Vol.1, No.1, pp. 59-68, ISSN 1744-117X

Yoshimoto, S.; Okada, E.; Oishi, T.; Numagami, R.; Umemoto, H.; Tamura, K.; Kanda, H.; Shiba, T.; Takamatsu, N. & Ito, M. (2006). Expression and promoter analysis of Xenopus DMRT1 and functional characterization of the transactivation property of its protein. *Development, Growth & Differentiation*, Vol.48, No.9, pp. 597-603, ISSN 0012-1592

Yoshimoto, S.; Okada, E.; Umemoto, H.; Tamura, K.; Uno, Y.; Nashida-Umehara, C.; Matsuda, Y.; Takamatsu, N.; Shiba, T. & Ito, M. (2008). A W-linked DM-domain gene, DM-W, participates in primary ovary development in *Xenopus laevis*.

Proceedings of the National Academy of Sciences of the United States of America, Vol.105, No.7, pp. 2469-2474, ISSN 0027-8424

Yoshimoto, S.; Ikeda, N.; Izutsu, Y.; Shiba, T.; Takamatsu, N. & Ito, M. (2010). Opposite roles of DMRT1 and its W-linked paralogue, DM-W, in sexual dimorphism of Xenopus laevis: implications of a ZZ/ZW-type sex-determining system. *Development*, Vol.137, No.15, pp. 2519-2526, ISSN 0950-1991

Yi, W. & Zarkower, D. (1999). Similarity of DNA binding and transcriptional regulation by *Caenorhabditis elegans* MAB-3 and *Drosophila melanogaster* DSX suggest conservation of sex determining mechanisms. *Development*, Vol.126, No.5, pp. 873-881, ISSN 0950-1991

Yi, W.; Ross, J.M. & Zarkower, D. (2000). *Mab-3* is a direct *tra-1* target gene regulating diverse aspects of *C. elegans* male sexual development and behavior. *Development*, Vol.127, No.20, pp. 4469-4480, ISSN 0950-1991

Zarkower, D. (2001). Establishing sexual dimorphism: conservation amidst diversity? *Nature Reviews. Genetics*, Vol.2, No.3, pp. 175-185, ISSN 1471-0056

Zhao, Y.; Lu, H.; Yu, H.; Cheng, H. & Zhou, R. (2007). Multiple alternative splicing in gonads of chicken *DMRT1*. *Development Genes and Evolution*, Vol.217, No.2, pp. 119-126, ISSN 0949-944X

Zhou, X.; Li, Q.; Lu, H.; Chen, H.; Guo, Y.; Cheng, H. & Zhou, R. (2008). Fish specific duplication of DMRT2: characterization of zebrafish *Dmrt2b*. *Biochimie*, Vol.90, No.6, pp. 878-887, ISSN 0300-9084

4

Regulation of Canonical Wnt Signaling During Development and Diseases

Saijun Mo[1] and Zongbin Cui[2,*]
[1]*Department of Basic Oncology, College of Basic Medical Sciences, Zhengzhou University, Zhengzhou,*
[2]*Institute of Hydrobiology, Chinese Academy of Sciences, Wuhan, China*

1. Introduction

Since the discovery of first Wnt gene (*Wnt-1*) in 1982, numerous investigations have focused on the roles of different Wnt proteins in regulation of cellular proliferation, differentiation and apoptosis in a cell-specific and contextual manner (Rao & Kuhl, 2011). Wnts mainly activate intracellular biological processes through one canonical pathway and two well-characterized non-canonical pathways including Wnt/PCP (planar cell polarity) and Wnt/Ca^{2+}. The canonical pathway is also known as Wnt/β-catenin pathway due to the key roles of β-catenin in transcriptional regulation of downstream genes. These pathways play distinct roles in embryonic development, cell fate determination, cell polarity generation and cell movements, cross-talks always occur through a variety of intracellular signal molecules. In this chapter, we mainly focus on the up-to-date understanding of canonical Wnt signaling, including its functions and regulatory mechanisms both in animal development and human diseases.

2. An overview of canonical Wnt signaling

In the canonical Wnt signaling pathway, β-catenin is the key downstream effector. With the absence of Wnt ligands (Fig. 1, right), cytoplasmic β-catenin is associated with adenomatous polyposis coli (APC) and Axin proteins and phosphorylated by glycogen synthase kinase 3β (GSK-3β) and casein kinase I (CKI), resulting in its polyubiquitination and protease- mediated degradation. Under these conditions, the Lymphoid Enhancer Factor/T-cell factor (LEF/TCF) family of transcription factors in the nucleus is able to associate with transcriptional co-repressors to respress the transcription of Wnt target genes. In the presence of Wnt ligands (Fig. 1, left), the binding of a Frizzled (Fz or Fzd) receptor and a low-density lipoprotein related receptor protein (LRP5/6) 5 or 6 co-receptor, and the interaction of Fzd with cytoplasmic protein Disheveled (Dsh or Dvl) results in the phosphorylation of Dsh/Dvl by CKI and binding to GSK-3β with the involvement of Frequently Rearranged in Advanced T-cell lymphomas (FRAT) protein. These events lead to inactivation of the Axin/APC/GSK-

* Corresponding Author

3β/CKI complex and thus the inhibition of β-catenin phosphorylation and degradation, allowing the translocation and accumulation of cytosolic β-catenin into the nucleus. Nuclear β-catenin then interacts with LEF/TCF family transcription factors and several other transcriptional co-activators to initiate transcription of target genes.

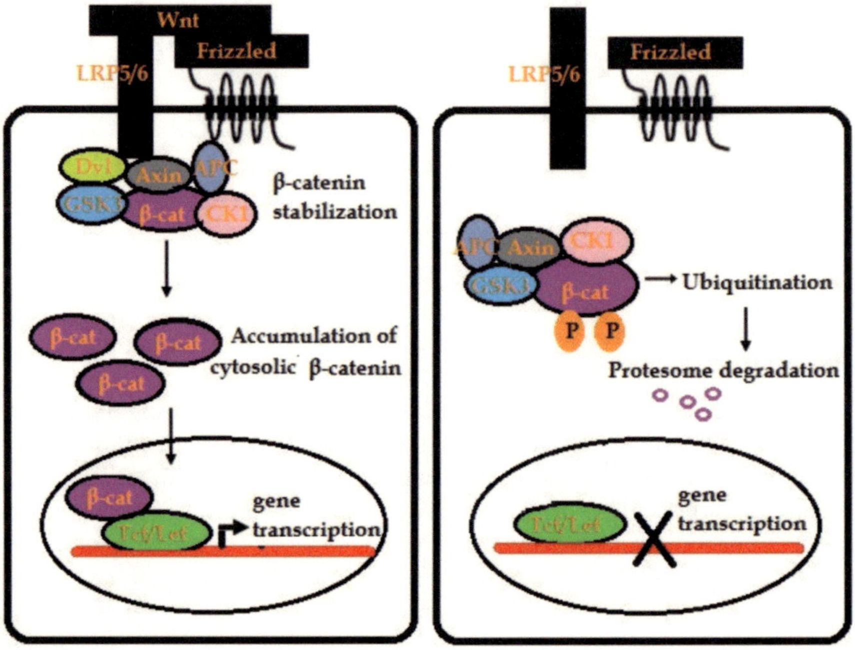

Fig. 1. An overview of Wnt/β-catenin signaling pathway (Modified from Masckauchan & Kitajewski, 2006).

2.1 Components of canonical Wnt signaling

The canonical Wnt signaling pathway mainly consists of multiple components including ligands (Wnts), receptors (Fz and LRP5/6), β-catenin complexes in cytoplasma (GSK-3β/ Axin/APC) and nucleus (TCF/LEF), Dsh (Dvls)/Frat protein, and downstream target genes. Those elements are highly conserved during evolution in species from fly to mammalian. Recent studies have expanded our knowledge of the repertoire of regulatory molecules involved in the Wnt signaling pathway, such as Caveolin-1, Norrin, R-spondin, sFRP, DKK, SOST/Sclerostin, Arrow, Ror, Krm, Lzts2, and so on.

2.1.1 The Wnt family

In general, Wnt genes encode 38- to 43-kDa glycoproteins with features of typical secreted growth factors, including a hydrophobic signal peptide, the absence of additional transmembrane domains, highly conserved cysteine residues, and the presence of *N*-linked glycosylation sites. Up to now, intensive studies have shown that Wnt genes exist in a wide range of species, including *Drosophila, Caenorhabditis elegans (C. elegans*), *Danio rerio*, *Xenopus,* mouse and human (Table 1). The Wnt family members are classically divided into canonical and non-canonical pathway components depending on their ability to transform C57MG mammary cells or induce axis duplication in *Xenopus*. The canonical Wnts include Wnt1, Wnt2, Wnt2a, Wnt3, Wnt3a, Wnt7a, Wnt7b, Wnt-8a, Wnt10a and Wnt10b while Wnt4, Wnt5a and Wnt11 activate the noncanonical Wnt pathways. Generally speaking, the distinction between two groups of ligands is as follows: Canonical Wnts bound to Frizzled and activate the β-catenin/TCF-mediated transcription, whereas non-canonical Wnts bound to Frizzled and activate small Rho GTPases, c-Jun N-terminal kinase (Jnk) and other β-catenin-independent signaling events. However, an increasing number of recent studies have indicated that the two types of Wnts can regulate the canonical and noncanonical pathways each other.

	Wnt proteins	**Frizzled proteins**
Mouse and human	Wnt1, 2, 2B, 3, 3A, 4, 5A, 5B, 6, 7A7B, 8A, 8B, 9A, 9B, 10A, 10B, 11, 16	FZD1–10, Fz, SMO
X. laevis	XWnt1, 2, 2B, 3, 3A, 4, 5A, 5B, 6, 7A, 7B, 7C, 8A, 8B, 10A, 10B, 11, 16	XFz1-9, 10A, 10B, SMO
Danio rerio	Wnt1, 2, 2Bα, 3A, 4A, 4B, 5A, 5B, 7Aα, 7Bα, 8A, 8B, 9A, 9B,10A,10B, 11,16	Fz1-6, 7a, 7b, 8a, 8b, 8c, 9, 10, SMO
C. elegans	CWN-1, 2 and EGL-20	MOM-5, LIN-17, CFZ-2, MIG-1
D. melanogaster	Wg, DWntD, DWnt2, 4, 5, 6, 10	Dfz2, Dfz3, Dfz4, SMO

Table 1. Wnt and Frizzled proteins in mammals (mouse and human), *D. melanogaster*, *X. laevis*, *Danio rerio* (zebrafish) and *C. elegans*. Fz/Dfz, Fz in *D. melanogaster*; XFz, Fz in *X. laevis*; MOM-5, more of mesoderm (MS) family member-5; LIN-17, abnormal cell Lineage family member-17; CFZ-2, *C. elegans* Frizzled homolog family member-2; MIG-1, abnormal cell migration family member-1. For more details, see (van Amerongen & Nusse, 2009; http://www.stanford.edu/ ~rnusse/Wntgenes/zebraf Wnt.html)

2.1.2 Receptors

Both canonical and noncanonical classes of Wnt ligands transduce signals through membrane receptors including FZD1-10, LRP5, LRP6, ROR1, ROR2 and RYK.

2.1.2.1 Frizzled (Fz, FZD) family

The Fz family consists of seven-pass transmembrane proteins that are similar to G protein-coupled receptors. Fz exist in *Drosophila, C. elegans, Danio rerio, Xenopus,* mouse and human (Table 1). Fz exhibit a number of typical features (Huang & Klein 2004): (i) a highly conserved cysteine-rich domain (CRD), which may constitute the orthosteric binding site for Wnts; (ii) a linker region that shows little sequence similarity among family members; (iii) a highly conserved seven- transmembrane domain; and (iv) a cytoplasmic domain of variable size and little sequence homology among family members.

2.1.2.2 LRP5/6 co-receptor and Arrow

The LRP5/6, additional single-pass transmembrane proteins, is low-density lipoprotein receptor-related protein 5/6. *Drosophila* Arrow is homologous to mouse LRP5 and LRP6. LRP5 and 6 contain three ligand-binding repeats, four β-propeller regions and the flanking epidermal growth factor (EGF) repeats. The intracellular domain of LRP5/6 can bind to Axin. The LRP5/6 interaction domain of Dkk has been mapped to the C-terminal domain.

2.1.2.3 Ryk and Ror

Ryk and Ror, also single transmembrane domain Wnt receptors, are not required for, but in some cases may antagonize Wnt/β-catenin signaling. The receptor tyrosine kinases Ror1/2 (Ror in *D. melanogaster;* Cam-1, CAN cell migration defective in *C. elegans*) and Ryk (called Derailed in *D. melanogaster;* Lin-18 in *C. elegans*) should be seen as autonomous Wnt receptors, Fzd coreceptors, or possibly both (Schulte, 2010).

2.1.3 β-catenin complex

2.1.3.1 β-catenin

β-catenin is an essential transcriptional co-activator in the canonical Wnt pathway and exists as an unstable monomer in the cytoplasm. Cytoplasmic β-catenin (not binging to Wnts) is rapidly turned over through the action of multi-component protein phosphorylation machinery consisting of GSK-3β, Axin, and APC protein (formed GSK-3β/Axin/APC complex). Phosphorylated β-catenin is targeted for degradation by proteosome. The binding of Wnts to their receptors results in the nuclear translocation and accumulation of β-catenin and thus activation of LEF/TCF transcription factors by formation of the LEF/TCF complex to initiate the expression of target genes. β-catenin homolog in *Drosophila* is called Armadillo. The Armadillo and β-catenin consist of 13 Armadilllo (Arm) repeat domains, which are essential for interaction with other proteins. Vertebrates have two Armadillo/β-catenin homologs, β-catenin and plakoglobin (also called gamma-catenin).

2.1.3.2 GSK-3β/Axin/APC complex

GSK-3 was first identified as a consequence of its phosphorylation activity toward glycogen synthase. The mammalian GSK3 contains two members GSK-3α and GSK-3β. GSK-3β, also known as human tau protein kinase (TPK I), is a multifunctional serine-threonine kinase discovered in 1980 and originally identified as a regulator of glycogen metabolism. Phosphorylation of the tyrosine 216 residue results in the constitutive activity of GSK-3β, suggesting this residue is important for signal transduction. GSK-3β contains three groups of binding sites: ATP site, Axin binding site and Priming site.

There are two vertebrate Axin genes. Axin1 is constutively expressed, but Axin2 (also called Conductin or Axil) is induced by activation of Wnt signaling and therefore functions in a negative feedback loop. Several functional domains in Axin have been mapped, including an RGS-box (or RGS domain) for the Axin and APC interaction, two binding domains for β-catenin and GSK, and a DIX domain for Axin and Dishevelled interacion. Axin also binds to the phosphatase PP2A.

Both mammals and *Drosophila* carry two APC genes: APC and APC2 (APCL) in mammals, and dAPC1 and dAPC2/E-APC in Drosophila. There is a natural mouse apc1 mutant called *min1*. Mammalian APC contains multiple binding sites for numerous proteins (Aoki & Taketo, 2007), including microtubules (a basic domain), β-catenin (15-aa or 20-aa repeats), Axin (SAMP repeats), cytoskeletal regulators EB1 and IQGAP1 (C-terminal domains), and the Rac guanine-nucleotide-exchange factor (GEF) Asef1 (an armadillo repeat-domain). An oligomerization domain is also found at the N-terminal of APC.

2.1.3.3 TCF/LEF complex

In invertebrates, there is one TCF gene rarely displaying alternative transcripts. However, vertebrates have four TCF genes (*Tcf-1, Lef-1, Tcf-3* and *Tcf-4*), and each of them gives rise to a variety of alternative transcripts (Nusse, 1999; Arce et al, 2006). Four domains are existed in an invertebrate TCF: (i) an N-terminal β-catenin-binding domain (BCBD); (ii) a central domain; (iii) a well-conserved high-mobility group (HMG) DNA-binding domain, including a nuclear localization signal (NLS); and (iv) a long C-terminal tail. The general structures are conserved in vertebrate TCF/LEFs: TCF-1E isoforms are remarkably similar in overall domain structure to invertebrate TCFs; other vertebrate TCF isoforms have lost parts of these domains and/or included novel peptide motifs.

2.1.4 Dishevelled (Dvl/Dsh)

Three Dsh proteins Dsh-1, Dsh-2, and Dsh-3 have been found in mammals, while only Dsh in *Drosophila* and mig-5 in *C.elegans*. The Dsh family members in all organisms are comprised of three highly conserved domains (Habas & Dawid, 2005): (i) an amino-terminal DIX domain (named for Dsh and Axin), which is essential for the interaction between Dsh and Axin; (ii) a central PDZ domain (named for Postsynaptic density-95, Discs-large and Zonula occludens-1); and (iii) a carboxy-terminal DEP domain (for Dsh, Egl-10 and Pleckstrin).

2.1.5 Target genes (http://www.stanford.edu)

The canonical Wnt pathway controls biological processes via the regulation of target gene expression, including direct and indirect target genes. The expression of direct Wnt target genes, e.g. cyclin D1 and Myc, multidrug transporter P-glycoprotein (MDR1/ABCB1), is activated by the transcription factor TCF, which binds to specific sequence motifs in the promoter. Indirect target genes are regulated via transcription regulators, which are also targets of the Wnt pathway. Wnt signaling can promote the expression of several Wnt pathway components, including Fz, LRP5/6, DKK, Axin, Tcf, Lef and so on. The results indicate that feedback controls are key features of Wnt signaling regulation.

2.1.6 Other factors

1. β-arrestin

β-arrestins are originally identified as negative regulators of G protein-coupled receptors (GPCR). β-arrestin-1 and -2 are required for cellular communication by means of Wnts and FZDs. In canonical pathway, β-arrestins participate in the formation of a ternary complex composed of phosphorylated Dvl, β-arrestin and Axin, and affect the transcriptional activity of TCF/LEF (Schulte et al, 2010). It is not clear whether β-arrestin serves only as a scaffolding protein or whether β-arrestin-dependent endocytosis is required.

2. CKI

The CKI family is highly conserved monomeric serine–threonine protein kinases. Mammalian contain several CKI isoforms, which are α, β, γ, δ and ε. CKI prefer substrates primed by prior phosphorylation and works closely with other kinases in the Wnt pathway (Cheong & Virshup, 2011): First, CKI is itself regulated by posttranslational modification including autophosphorylation; Second, CKI plays a role in phosphorylation of Dvl in the Wnt signaling pathway; Finally, CKI also regulate the Wnt signaling pathway by interacting with the Wnt receptor LRP.

2.2 The regulatory mechanism of canonical Wnt signaling

The regulatory mechanisms of canonical Wnt signaling pathway are very complicated. It is well established that components of Wnt/β-catenin pathway include Wnts, Fz, LRP5/6, APC, Axin, Dvl, GSk3β, CKI, TCF/LEF and so on. These components can form different complex and play distinct regulatory roles in canonical Wnt signaling: some components exert their roles as activators, such as canonical Wnts, Dvl, while some components act as inhibitors, such as GSK-3β. The canonical Wnt pathway can be regulated by other molecules such as R-spondins, Dkk, Wise, Caveolin-1, Neucrin, sFRP, and Wif and this pathway also can crosstalk with multiple signaling pathways including BMP, TGF-β, Notch, FGF signaling, and so on.

2.2.1 Activators of canonical Wnt signaling pathway

Many signal molecules can activate the canonical Wnt signaling pathway, leading to stabilization of β-catenin (Nusse, 1999; Bejsovec, 2005; http://www.stanford.edu/group/nusselab/cgi-bin/Wnt/activators_detectors). Approaches to activate this pathway include: (i) increased expression of Wnt ligands, receptors, β-catenin and Axin; (ii) phosphorylation of Dvl and LRP tail; (iii) inhibition of GSK-3β activity by factors such as LiCl and Akt; (iv) blocking the negative regulators of Wnt signaling, such as Axin and APC; (v) increased expression of Dsh (Dvls) to inhibit the function of the degradation complex and phosphorylation of β-catenin through its binding to GSK-3β and then promote the target gene transcription. Some other activators are described below.

1. Norrin

Norrin serves as a ligand and binds to FZD4 to activate the Wnt signaling pathway dependenting on the presence of cell surface LRP5. The CRD of FZD4 has been shown to play a critical role in Norrin-FZD4 binding and is associated with canonical Wnt signaling.

2. R-spondins

R-spondins are a family of cysteine-rich secreted proteins and consist of four homologs (Rspo-1, 2, 3, and 4) in vertebrates. No representative is found in *C elegans, D. melanogaster,* or *Saccharomyces cerevisiae.* All R-spondins contain two furin-like cysteine-rich domains at the N-terminus followed by a thrombospondin domain and a basic charged C-terminal tail. The furin domain of R-spondins is sufficient to synergize with Wnt3a and antagonize DKK1 function. Similar to the activity of Wnts, R-spondins activate Wnt/β-catenin signaling through binding to LRP6, inducing its phosphorylation, and promoting β-catenin stabilization. However, R-spondins do not directly activate LRP6 and require the presence of Wnts to block Dkk-induced endocytosis of LRP6 and thus ensure an appropriate receptor density in the membrane for Wnt signaling. Although all four R-spondins activate the canonical Wnt pathway, R-spondin-2 and -3 are more potent than R-spondin1, whereas R-spondin-4 is relatively inactive. In addition to LRP6, R-spondin-2 interacts with FZD8 to activate the canonical Wnt signaling (Kim et al, 2008).

3. CBP (CREB-binding protein) and P300

CBP or its closely related homolog p300, contains multiple functional domains including CREB binding domain, Bromo-domain, three zinc finger, Gluarrine-rich domain and HAT. Despite the high degree of homology, CBP and p300 are not completely redundant and have unique critical roles: CBP but not p300 is essential for hematopoietic stem cell self-renewal, whereas p300 is critical for proper hematopoietic differentiation (Teo & Kahn, 2010). The C-terminal domain of β-catenin has been found to interact with the histone acetyltransferases CBP/p300, which have distinct functions in the regulation of TCF/β-catenin-mediated survivin/BIRC5 transcription. ICG-001, a selective CBP/Catenin Antagonist, can modulate the canonical Wnt Signaling.

4. Ubiquitin ligase RNF146 (RING finger protein 146)

RNF146 is a RING-domain E3 ubiquitin ligase. RNF146 can act as a positive regulator of Wnt signaling through ubiquitylating and destabilizing Axin and tankyrase (Callow et al, 2011).

5. C/EBPβ, Shikonin and Testosterone

CCAAT/enhancer binding protein β (C/EBPβ) is rapidly induced in early stages of adipogenesis and is responsible for transcriptional induction of Peroxisome proliferator-activated receptor γ (PPARγ) and C/EBPα by maintaining active Wnt/β-catenin signaling, after addition of adipogenic inducers. C/EBPβ is involved in the expression of Wnt10b, a major Wnt ligand in preadipocytes, while C/EBPβ is not an essential factor for the regulation of Wnt10b expression during adipogenesis.

Shikonin is a natural naphthoquinone compound and inhibits adipogenesis through the activation of the Wnt/β-catenin pathway. Shikonin induces the upregulation and nuclear translocation of β-catenin.

Testosterone supplementation in men decreases fat mass. Testosterone and dihydrotestosterone inhibit adipocyte differentiation *in vitro* through an AR-mediated nuclear translocation of β-catenin and activation of downstream Wnt signaling.

6. Frat protein/GBP

Three homologs (Frat1, Frat2 and Frat3) are found in vertebrates. The Frat homolog is called GBP in *Xenopus*, which is essential for embryonic axis formation. No protein similar to FRAT/GBP has been found in *Drosophila*. Frat proteins are potent activators of canonical Wnt-signal transduction: First, the binding of Frat to GSK3 can induce signaling through β-catenin/TCF; Second, Frat can bind to Dishevelled and advocate as the "missing link" that bridges signaling from Dishevelled to GSK3 in the canonical Wnt pathway.

2.2.2 Antagonists of canonical Wnt signaling pathway

2.2.2.1 Antagonists that bind to Wnt ligands

When antagonists bind to Wnt, they prevent Wnts from binding their receptors and presumably block the activity of Wnt signaling pathway. Antagonists in this group include sFRP, WIF-1 and Cerberus (Rubin et al, 2006).

1. Soluble Frizzled-related proteins (sFRPs)

The sFRPs family consists of a group of Wnt binding proteins including a frizzled-type cysteine-rich domain (CRD). Unlike the Frizzled, the C-terminus of sFRPs contains a netrin (NTR) domain and has no transmembrane segments. The sFRPs are encoded by FRP/FrzB genes, including sFRP1-2, FrzB, sFRP4-5 and Sizzled. sFRP1 and sFRP2 are identified to antagonize the Wnt activity. FrzB interacts with Wnt-8 and block the Wnt-8 signaling in *Xenopus* embryos development. In mammalian cells, FrzB can bind to Wnt1 and inhibit the β-catenin accumulation induced by Wnt1.

2. Wnt inhibitory factor-1 (WIF-1)

WIF-1 is a unique Wnt antagonist with differences in structure from sFRP and Dkk families. WIF-1 contains a highly conserved N-terminal domain named WIF domain (WD) and five epidermal growth factor repeats and the WD domain is sufficient for Wnt binding and signaling inhibition.

3. Cerberus

Cerberus belongs to the Cerberus/Dan gene family and lacks the FZD-CRD and WD. The identified members of Cerberus include mouse cerberus-like gene (mCer-1) and cerberus-like-2 (mCer2), chick Cerberus (ccer), *Xenopus* Cerberus (Xcer) and Coco, zebrafish Charon. However, the mCer-1 does not encode a Wnt antagonist and the antagonist activity of mammalian Coco has not been confirmed.

4. Wingful (Wf)/Notum

Notum, formerly called Wf in *Drosophila*, is a secreted hydrolase and has orthologs in mice and human. A number of studies have shown that Notum can also regulate Wnt signaling. For example, overexpression of *Drosophila* Wf severely inhibits Wg signaling activity and serves as a potent feedback inhibitor of Wg and complements the embryonic Naked cuticle (Nkd) system. In addition, Notum is a novel target of β-catenin/TCF4 and high levels of Notum are significantly associated with intracellular (nuclear or cytoplasmic) accumulation of β-catenin protein.

2.2.2.2 Antagonists that bind to LRP5/6

1. Dickkopfs (DKK) family

DKKs were the first glycoproteins reported to block the β-catenin pathway by binding to LRP5/6 and disrupting the formation of LRP5/6–FZD complexes. DKKs include DKK1–4 (no counterpart in *D. melanogaster*) and the DKK-like protein 1 (Dkk-3-related protein which is named Soggy in *D. melanogaster*). There are two conserved cysteine-rich domains (Cys-1 and Cys-2) in DKKs, while Sgy lacks cysteine-rich domains.

DKK-1 and DKK-4 display a Wnt antagonist mechanism, while the mechanism for the antagonizing effect of DKK-1 or -4 on LRP6 and Wnt/β-catenin pathway remains unclear. Results from several studies indicate that the Cys-2 domain of DKK-1 binds to LRP6 and Krm, forming a ternary complex and inducing LRP6 internalization. However, another reseach group has reported that DKK-1 blocks Wnt signaling but does not promote LRP6 internalization and degradation. The mechanism for DKK-2 activity is also disputable. Two groups have reported that DKK-2 is a poor inhibitor of Wnt signaling similar to DKK-1, while another group has found the Wnt antagonizing activity of Dkk-2. There are two possible explanations for this discrepancy: (i) DKK-2 binds to LRP6 with a lower affinity and the binding Kd value is approximately 2 folds of that for DKK-1 (0.73 nM vs 0.34 nM); (ii) Dkk-2 is suggested to play the role as an agonist in low-Wnt/high-LRP6 condition, and acts as an antagonist in environment with high-Wnt levels. DKK-3 does not bind to LRPs or Krm1/2 and can not inhibit Wnt signaling.

2. Neucrin

Neucrin consists of a cysteine-rich domain in its carboxyl terminal region, similar to two domains of DKKs. Neucrin as well as DKKs bind to LRP6 and inhibit the stabilization of cytosolic β-catenin, indicating that Neucrin is also an antagonist of canonical Wnt signaling.

3. Wise/sclerostin

Wise (also known as *Sostdc1*, *ectodin* and *USAG-1*) is a member of Dan family of glycoproteins including Cerberus, gremlin, Dan, Coco, and protein-related-to-Dan-and - Cerberus. Recently, Wise and the related protein sclerostin were identified as inhibitors since they bind to the extracellular domain of the Wnt co-receptors LRP5 and LRP6. Sost shares 36% amino acids identity with Wise. They share a "cysteine knot" domain that occupies the central part of proteins. Sost behaves exclusively as an antagonist for Wnt/LRP5/6 signaling in mammalian cells and *Xenopus* embryos, whereas Wise alone can function as a weak agonist to activate β-catenin signaling to a limited extent. Unlike DKK1, Sost inhibition of Wnt signaling is insensitive to the presence of Krm2, a transmembrane protein that binds to DKK1.

4. CTGF (Connective tissue growth factor)

CTGF, a CCN family member, is a multi-domain protein and each domain can interact with several ligands, such as growth factors (e.g. TGF-β, BMP-4), cell surface proteins (e.g. LRP) and extracellular matrix proteins. CTGF can suppress Wnt signaling through binding to LRP6. This interaction is likely to occur through the C-terminal domain of CTGF.

5. SERPINA3K

SERPINA3K is a member of the serine proteinase inhibitor (SERPIN) family. The interaction between SERPINA3K and the extracellular domain of LRP6 blocks the Fz/LRP6 (receptor/co-receptor) dimerization induced by a Wnt ligand. Reseachers have also found that SERPINA3K binds to LRP6 with a Kd of 10 nM.

6. Adenomatosis polyposis coli down-regulated 1 protein (APCDD1)

APCDD1 is a membrane-bound glycoprotein that is abundantly expressed in human hair follicles. Former studies have found two Tcf-binding motifs in the 5′-flanking region of *APCDD1* and indicated that APCDD1 is directly regulated by the β-catenin/Tcf4 complex. However, recent functional studies show that APCDD1 inhibits Wnt signaling in a cell-autonomous manner and functions upstream of β-catenin. *In vitro* analysis indicates that APCDD1 can interact with Wnt3a and LRP5, two essential components of Wnt signalling. These results suggest that APCDD1 is a novel Wnt inhibitor.

2.2.2.3 Factors binding to Fz

1. Shisa

Homologues of Shisa are found in human, rat and chick, *Xenopus* and Zebrafish. However, no Shisa homologues are identified in *Ciona intestinalis, C.elegans* or *Drosophila*. All Shisa proteins contain two CRD and an N-terminal signal peptide. Shisa proteins represent a distinct family of Wnt antagonists, which trap Fz proteins in the ER and prevent Fz from reaching the cell surface.

2. Other factors

sFRP and Insulin-like growth factor (IGF) binding protein-4 (IGFBP-4) can also antagonize Wnt signaling via binding to both Fz and LRP6 (MacDonald et al, 2009).

2.2.2.4 Factors binding to β-catenin

1. Chibby (Cby)

Cby physically interact with β-catenin and compete with the TCF/LEF family for binding to β-catenin. The coiled-coil motif of Cby is responsible for its specific binding to the armadillo repeats 10−12 and the C-terminal region of β-catenin. And phosphorylated Cby plays an essential role in the intracellular distribution of β-catenin in conjunction with 14-3-3 protein.

2. ICAT (Inhibitor of β-catenin and TCF4)

Orthologs of ICAT are highly conserved in vertebrate except frogs. ICAT inhibit β-catenin to bind to TCF/LEF and functions as a negative regulator of Wnt signaling. The crystal structure data indicate that ICAT bound to the armadillo repeat domain of β-catenin, since ICAT contains an N-terminal helilical domain that binds to repeats 11 and 12 of β-catenin, and an extended C-terminal region that binds to repeats 5-10 in a manner similar to that of Tcfs and other β-catenin ligands.

3. Caveolin-1 (Cav-1)

Cav-1 is an integral membrane proteins and accumulates of β-catenin within caveolae membranes and thus inhibits the β-catenin/Lef-1 signaling activated by Wnt-1 or the overexpression of β-catenin itself. Recent findings indicate that Cav-1 inhibits Wnt signaling by directly interacting with β-catenin depending on its scaffolding domains (Mo et al, 2010).

4. Lzts2

Lzts2 previuosly called LAPSER1 is a putative tumor suppressor that can directly interact with and mediate the nuclear export of β-catenin. We have recently shown that Lzts2 plays important roles in the dorsoventral patterning and embryonic cell movements in zebrafish (Li et al, 2011).

2.2.2.5 Factors associated with LEF/TCF

1. Groucho

Long Groucho/TLEs are transducin-like-enhancer of Split orthologs that function as the inhibitor of canonical Wnt pathway. The β-catenin and LEF/TCFs activation complexes are opposed by the LEF/TCF•Groucho repressor complexes. The C-terminal WD repeat domain in Groucho/TLE is responsible for binding to LEF/TCFs.

2. Endostatin

Endostatin is a C-terminal fragment of collagen XVIII and blocks the canonical Wnt mediated transcription depending on TCF.

2.2.2.6 Dvl inhibitors

1. Naked cuticle (Nkd)

The insects typically have a single Nkd gene, whereas there are two Nkd genes, Nkd1 and Nkd2, in human, mouse and zebrafish (have additional homology Nkd3). Nkd1 and Nkd2 contain a most conserved region of the EFX domain in species from fly to vertebrate. The EFX domain is required for the interaction of Nkd with the basic/PDZ domains of Dsh or Dvl in fly and vertebrate, thus inhibiting Wnt/β–catenin signaling.

2. Protease-activated receptors (PARs)

PARs belong to a large family of seven-transmembrane-spanning G protein-coupled receptors (GPCRs), which can couple to $G\alpha_{i/o}$, $G\alpha_q$, or $G\alpha_{12/13}$ within the same cell type. PAR1-$G\alpha_{13}$ associations inhibit the canonical Wnt signaling pathway by the recruitment of Dvl, an upstream Wnt signaling protein via the DIX domain.

3. Dapper/Frodo

Dapper (Dpr) is also called Frodo or Dact. A conserved C-terminal PDZ-binding motif in Dpr is responsible for the interaction with the PDZ domain of Dvl. This interaction depends on the phosphorylation of Dpr by CKIδ/ε.

2.2.3 Context-dependent agonists/antagonists

1. CKI

CKI family plays a complicated role in Wnt/β-catenin signaling in a context-dependent manner: CKIα acts as a potent negative regulator of β-catenin for interacting with Axin and phosphorylates serine 45 of β-catenin, while CKIε and CKIδ are found to be positive regulators and act upstream of Axin and GSK3 to stabilize β-catenin.

2. sFRPs

Indeed, biphasic effects of SFRPs were reported: low sFRP1 concentrations promote, whereas high sFRP1 concentrations decrease Wingless-induced β-catenin stabilization.

3. DKK-2

The N-terminal domains in DKK-1 and DKK-2 have different functions. The N-terminal fragment of DKK-2 synergies with LRP6 to induce Wnt signaling activation, while the N-terminal domain of DKK-1 appears to have no such function. Together with other evidence, DKK-2 is suggested to play the role as an agonist in low-Wnt/high-LRP6 condition, and acts as an antagonist in environment with high-Wnt levels.

4. Wise

It is known that Wise is an inhibitor of canonical Wnt pathway and first identified as its ability to alter the antero-posterior characterstic of neuralized *Xenopus* animal caps by promoting the activity of the Wnt pathway. Thus, Wise appears to have a dual role in modulating Wnt pathway. It remains unclear how the Wise interacts with components in the Wnt signaling. One explanation is that Wise competes with Wnts for binding to LRP6 in the presence of Wnts, Wise and Dkk, and results in a weak Wnt-dependent activity or a complete block of receptor activity.

5. CBP (cAMP response-element binding protein)/P300

CBP and P300 are bimodal Wnt regulators with conserved roles in organisms from flies to vertebrates (Li et al, 2007). CBP/P300 can negatively regulate canonical Wnt signaling through directly binding and acetylating TCF, thus reducing TCF ability to bind with β-catenin. In contrast, CBP acts as a co-activator by directly interacting with the β-cateinin (Arm in fly). The interaction domain has been mapped to the N-terminal region of CBP and the C-terminal region of β-catenin. A recent study has identified that the phosphorylation of a Proline-directed Serine 92 residue modulates the selective binding of CBP with β-catenin.

2.2.4 Epigenetic regulation

Epigenetic regulation including DNA methylation of promoter CpG islands and/or histone modification often leads to the activation or amplification of aberrant Wnt/β-catenin signaling. Many genes endocing components in this pathway can be modified by DNA hypermethylation, thus being closely associated with tumorgenesis (Fig.2). In addition,

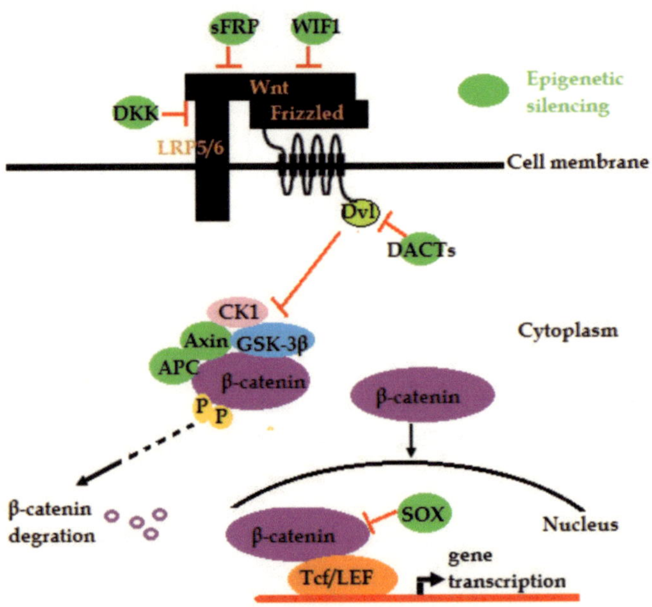

Fig. 2. Several Epigenetic silencing of regulators contribute to the aberrant activation of Wnt/β-catenin signaling in human cancers. Through promoter methylation or histone modification, epigenetic silencing of certain nuclear proteins (SOX) and many antagonists (SFRP, WIF, Dkk, APC and DACT) disrupt individual levels of the Wnt/β-catenin pathway, resulting in constitutive activation of TCF/LEF-β-catenin-dependent transcription of target genes. (Ying & Tao, 2009)

methylation or histone modification of promoters for some inhibitors including Long Groucho/TLEs and Pygopus also affect the activity of canonical Wnt signaling.

2.2.5 Crosstalk among signaling pathways

2.2.5.1 Crosstalk with noncanonical Wnt pathway

There are a number of noncanonical Wnt signaling pathways such as Wnt/PCP, Wnt/Ca^{2+}, Wnt/ROR and Wnt/RYK. Among these pathways, Wnt/PCP and Wnt/Ca^{2+} are well characterized and ligands activating the non-canonical pathways mainly include Wnt4, Wnt5a and Wnt11. The components of canonical Wnt pathway such as Wnts, β-catenin, Fz and Dsh, play roles both in canonical and non-canonical Wnt pathways through distinct mechanisms (Grumolato et al, 2010). The molecular mechanisms underlying the interatction of two Wnt signaling pathways are shown by a model in Fig.3. The canonical and noncanonical Wnts exert reciprocal inhibition at the cell surface by competition for Fzd binding: canonical Wnt3a and noncanonical Wnt5a ligands specifically trigger completely unrelated endogenous coreceptors LRP5/6 and Ror1/2, respectively through a common mechanism that involves their Wnt-dependent coupling to the Frizzled (Fzd) coreceptor and recruitment of shared components, including Dvl, Axin and GSK3.

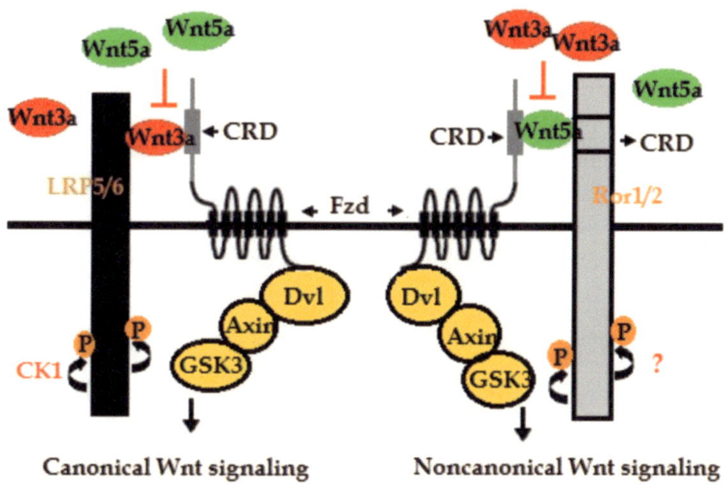

Fig. 3. A model for molecular mechanisms underlying the interatction between canonical and noncanonical Wnt signaling. (Details in Grumolato et al, 2010)

2.2.5.2 TGF-β (Transforming growth factor-β) signaling pathway

TGF-β signaling pathway includes subfamilies of TGF-β, BMPs, Nodal and activin/inhibin . Wnt and BMP pathways cooperate or attenuate each other, thus causing effects that cannot be achieved by either alone in many biological events. The componets of Wnt signaling, including CK, Wise, sFRPs, are associated with their interaction. For example, the molecular mechanisms underlying the interaction between Wnt and BMP signaling are very complex (Itasaki & Hoppler, 2010). First, by mutual regulation of each other's gene expression, activation of the Wnt pathway leads to up- or down-regulation of BMP pathway components, or vice versa. The second mechanism is, extracellular signaling of both pathways can cause either activation or inhibition of signaling; several secreted molecules, including Wise, sFRPs, CK and Cerberus, can bind to extracellular components of both the BMP and Wnt pathways. Third, the interactions between signal transduction components of the pathways can interfer with or enhance one pathway by signal transduction components of the other pathway; the components include Dvl and Smad1 (or Smad3), GSK3 and Smad1, β-catenin and Smad, Smad7 and Axin. The forth mechanism is the regulation at the promoter or enhancer level.

2.2.5.3 Crosstalk with Notch signaling

Notch signaling pathway possesses four different Notch receptors, including Notch1, 2, 3 and 4. During somite differentiation, the interaction of Wnt and Notch signaling are required for activation of the downstream gene *cMESO1/mesp2*. Notch intracellular domain (Notch ICD or NICD) can directly or indirectly interact with several Wnt components including Dvl, β-catenin, APC, Axin and GSK-3β, thus controlling the activity of Wnt signaling (Andersson et al, 2011). Furthermore, the crosstalk is also seen between sFRPs and Notch signaling. The sFRPs bind to ADAM10, downregulating its activity and thus inhibiting Notch signaling.

2.2.5.4 Crosstalk with FGF signaling pathway

FGFs (22 members) signal enter into the nucleus by binding to FGFR (*fgfr1-4*) and activate multiple signal transduction pathways. There are several models of Wnt-FGF signaling interactions. Canonical Wnt pathway can meidiate the expression of FGF16, FGF18 and FGF20 genes as well as the regulation of SPRY4 gene transcription. Within the 5'-promoter region of human *SPRY4* gene, double TCF/LEF binding sites were identified. FGF signaling also can affect Wnt signaling. For example, the activation of Wnt pathway by FGF-2 is mediated by PI3K/Akt signaling to maintain undifferentiated hESC. In addition, Wnt componets, including β-catenin, GSK-3β, Axin, antagonist of Wise, are associated with the interaction between canonical Wnt and FGF pathways.

2.2.5.5 Crosstalk with TNF (Tumor necrosis factor) signaling pathway

TNF is a cytokine involved in systemic inflammation and is a member of cytokines that stimulate the acute phase reaction. The cooperation of Wnt and TNF signaling pathways play important roles in the regulation of many biological events. Early signals induced by TNF-α via the death domain of TNFR1 are required for the mediation of downstream effects on β-catenin/TCF4 activity and for TNF-α-induced antiadipogenesis. A recent study has indicated TNF-α enhances the Wnt/β-catenin signaling by induction of Msx2 expression. In addition, TNF signaling regulated by Wnt pathway is essential for tooth organogenesis.

2.2.5.6 Crosstalk with Hedgehog (Hh) signaling

The vertebrate Hh family is represented by at least three members: Desert Hh (Dhh), Indian Hh (Ihh) and Sonic Hh (Shh). The Hh pathway is able to interact with canonical Wnt pathway. Hh signaling inhibits the canonical Wnt signaling and proliferation in intestinal epithelial cells meidiated by Hh repressor Gli1. However, different mechanisms are found in the development of spinal cord: dorsal Gli3 expression might be directly regulated by canonical Wnt activity; In turn, Gli3, by acting as a transcriptional repressor (mediated by TCf), restrictes graded Shh/Gli ventral activity to properly pattern the spinal cord.

Although Shh is an inhibitor of the Wnt/β-catenin pathway, activation of Wnt/β-catenin signaling upregulates Shh expression during normal development of fungiform papillae. Thus, the positive and negative feedback loop that coordinates Wnt and Shh pathways is essential for fungiform papillae development. Recent findings indicate that Shh is a downstream target of Wnt signaling and acts as a negative-feedback regulator of Wnt signaling via *Dkk1* and other targets.

2.2.5.7 Crosstalk with retinoic acid (RA) signaling

RA is a lipophilic molecule and a metabolite of vitamin-A (all-trans-retinol). Most of studies have suggested that RA can inhibit canonical Wnt signaling pathway. For example, the RA activity in the perioptic mesenchyme is required for expression of Pitx2 and Dkk2, which affects Wnt/β-catenin signaling during eye development. Retinoic acid can downregulate the expression of Wnt-3a in mouse development and repress the expression of Wnt8a and Wnt3a in the developing trunk. Depending on the presence of RA or not, recent findings suggest a dual activity for RA interaction with Wnt signaling: RARγ regulates Wnt/β-catenin signaling in chondrocytes positively or negatively depending on retinoid ligand availability. RARγ enhances the Wnt/β-catenin signaling under retinoid-free conditions, but inhibits the signaling in RA-treated cells.

3. Roles of canonical Wnt signaling in animal development

Canonical Wnt signaling is a highly conserved pathway involved in a variety of biological processes for animal development and homeostasis. Here, we mainly focus on three aspects: (i) Its roles in the embryogenesis, especially the establishment of Spemann organizer and the patterning of body axes. (ii) Its roles in the regulation of mammalian stem cell fate and somatic cell reprogramming. (iii) Its roles in the development of organs, such as nervous system, cardiovascular system, reproductive system, digestive system and skeletal system.

3.1 Invertebrate development

3.1.1 *Drosophila* development

In the *Drosophila* embryo, *wg* is required for formation of parasegment boundaries and for maintenance of *engrailed* (*en*) expression in adjacent cells (Wodarz & Nusse, 1998). Embryos with mutations in genes *porcupine* (*porc*), *dsh*, *armadillo* (*arm*) and *pangolin* (*pan*), exhibit a very similar phenotype. By contrast, mutations in *zeste-white 3* (*zw3*) demonstrate an opposite phenotype, a naked cuticle.

3.1.2 *C.elegans* development

In the *C. elegans* embryo, molecular analysis of three mutants revealed that they encode proteins similar to *porc* (*mom-1*), *mom-2*, and *frizzled* (fz), a Wnt receptor (*mom-5*). Similar to the *pan* mutant, mutation of *pop-1*, an HMG box protein results in an opposite effect of *mom* mutations: both EMS daughters adopt the E fate and produce exclusively gut (Wodarz & Nusse, 1998).

3.1.3 Cnidarians development

Wnt signaling is also essential for cnidarian embryogenesis (Guder et al, 2006). Recent works have revealed that almost all bilaterian Wnt gene subfamilies (except Wnt9) are present in cnidarians. An additional Wnt (WntA) is present in cnidarians. Therefore, the hydroid and sea anemone are used to discuss the roles of canonical Wnt signaling in cnidarians development. The important example is that the formation of *Hydra* head organizer is known to be activated by Wnts. HyWnt3a is expressed in a small cluster of ectodermal and endodermal epithelial cells at the apical tip of the hypostome and at the site of the head organizer. HyTcf is expressed in the hypostome, but in a broader domain than Wnt3a and shows a graded distribution highest at the apex. HyDsh and hyGsk-3β are uniformly expressed throughout the polyp at low levels, although hyGsk-3β transcripts are absent in the foot region cells. The hypostome have much higher levels of nuclear β-catenin than cells in the body column, indicating that Wnt signaling is active in the hypostome.

3.2 Vertebrate development

3.2.1 Embryogenesis

The role of Wnt/β-catenin signaling during embryogenesis has been well characterized in *Xenopus*, zebrafish and mouse.

3.2.1.1 The fate of *Xenopus* body axis

In *Xenopus*, the canonical Wnt signaling acting through β-catenin functions both in establishing the dorsoventral axis and in patterning the anterior–posterior axis. During early cleavage, preferential localization of maternal β-catenin to nuclei of cells on the future dorsal side of the embryo establishes the dorso-ventral axis. However, this nuclear localization of β-catenin, which sends a transient dorsal signal to neighboring cells, disappears briefly about the time the blastopore begins to form. While several maternally expressed Wnts (*XWnt-5a, XWnt-7b, XWnt-8b, XWnt-11*) are not required for this dorsal β-catenin signal. The dorsalizing activity of Wnt ligands, however, is lost at or shortly after the midblastula transition (MBT) around 7–8 h of development. Soon afterward, during gastrulation, Wnt signaling is thought to play roles in nervous system patterning and notochord-somite boundary formation, and perhaps in suppressing dorsal axis formation on the ventral side.

The components of canonical Wnt pathway play different roles in the body axis formation of *Xenopus*. In embryos, ectopic expression of Wnts such as Wnt1 or Wnt8a, can induce the formation of a secondary body axis. However, XWnt-3a plays a major role in anterior–posterior patterning of the neuroectoderm and mesoderm. The β-catenin is required for axis formation and enriched dorsally by the two-cell stage in a manner dependent on cortical rotation. XTcf-3 is required for early Wnt signaling to establish the dorsal embryonic axis and closely related Xlef-1 is required for Wnt signaling to pattern the mesoderm after the onset of zygotic transcription. A number of studies have indicated that CKII has a critical role in the establishment of the dorsal embryonic axis. Dvl has been shown recently to be enriched dorsally in one-cell embryos, and ectopic GFP-tagged Dvl is transported along the microtubule array during cortical rotation. The activity of GSK-3 plays dual roles in *Xenopus* axis formation depending on its distribution and association with two GSK-3 binding proteins, GBP and Axin.

3.2.1.2 The development of zebrafish body axes

In zebrafish, maternally Wnt/β-catenin signaling is essential for the formation of organizer (also known as "shield"). The zygotic Wnt/β-catenin signaling is activated by Wnt ligands after MBT to antagonize the organizer and be involved in anterior-posterior patterning of the neural axis. In the zebrafish embryo, β-catenin accumulates specifically in nuclei of dorsal margin blastomeres at as early as the 128-cell stage. This asymmetric nuclear localization of β-catenin is an early marker of the dorsoventral axis. Soon after the MBT, β-catenin activates the expression of a number of zygotic genes, including *bozozok, chordin, Dkk1, squint* (*sqt*) and FGF signals. These β-catenin targets act to inhibit the action of ventralizing factors or, in the case of Sqt, induce mesendodermal fates at the dorsal margin. However, genetic studies in zebrafish have shown that Wnt8 signals are essential for the establishment of ventral and posterior fates. During gastrulation, Wnt8 mRNA and strong activity of a Wnt/β-catenin responsive reporter are evident at the ventrolateral margin. Simultaneous reduction of Wnt3a and Wnt8 activities results in a stronger expansion of dorsoanterior fates, indicating that these two Wnts have overlapping functions. Wnt inhibitors, such as Cerberus, Frzb1 and Dkk1, can function as head inducers. The Wnt antagonist Dkk1 is expressed early in the dorsal margin and dorsal yolk syncytial layer and during gastrulation in the developing prechordal plate, where it could function to counteract the ventralizing and posteriorizing effects of canonical Wnt signaling. Another Wnt antagonist Caveolin-1 (Cav-1) can maternally regulate dorsoventral patterning by limiting nuclear translocation of active β-catenin in zebrafish (Mo et al, 2010).

3.2.1.3 The fate of mouse body axis

Wnt/β-catenin signaling also plays multiple roles in the production and patterning of the mouse primary axes similar to that in frog and fish. The Wnt/β-catenin signaling precedes primitive streak formation and is present in epiblast cells that will go on to form the primitive streak. The N-terminally nonphosphorylated form of β-catenin as well as Wnt/β-catenin signaling is first detectable in the extraembryonic visceral endoderm in day-5.5 embryos. Before the initiation of gastrulation at day 6.0, Wnt/β-catenin signaling is asymmetrically distributed within the epiblast and is localized to a small group of cells adjacent to the embryonic–extraembryonic junction. At day 6.5 and onward, Wnt/β-catenin signaling was detected in the primitive streak and mature node. The expression of Wnt3, high levels of β-catenin and TCF-responsive promoter activity are detected at the site of primitive streak formation in the embryo posterior; conversely, the Wnt inhibitor *Dkk1* was expressed in anterior visceral endoderm. Extensive studies have indicated that *Wnt3* and *β-catenin* knockout mice fail to form the primitive streak, whereas knockout of the Wnt inhibitor Dkk1 results in an anterior truncation. In this way, the role for Wnt in early head-tail development within the mouse embryo could be viewed as similar to that for A-P patterning in frogs (Marikawa, 2006). In the mouse embryo, Axin is a maternal protein present throughout development and *Axin* mutations lead to axis duplication, similar to the effects of ectopic Wnt8 expression.

3.2.2 Embryonic stem cell (ESC)

Canonical Wnt signaling has been implicated in the control of various types of stem cells and may act as a niche factor to maintain stem cells in a self-renewing state. The stem cells contain tissue-specific somatic stem cells, tumor (or cancer) stem cells and ESC (Reya & Clevers, 2005; Nusse, 2008; Valkenburg et al, 2011), and the details of the former two types of stem cells are showed in Section 3.2.3 and 4.1, respectively. Mammalian ESCs provides an excellent model system for studying cell fate determination in early development of mouse and human. Studies have shown that activation of Wnt/β-catenin signaling in human and mouse ES cells enhance the expression of pluripotency genes and may facilitate the self-renewal of stem cells. For example, in ESCs, overexpression of Wnt1 or stabilized β-catenin or lack of APC results in the inhibition of neural differentiation and in the activation of downstream targets of Wnt signaling, including cyclins and c-myc.

Most of Wnt signaling components are involved in the control of ESC differentiation. For example, ESCs cultured in Wnt3a-conditioned medium undergo mesendoderm differentiation. Under the condition of elevated β-catenin activity, cultured mouse ESCs at high density embark on neural differentiation. Inhibition of GSK-3β transiently enhances the maintenance of ESCs. In addition, in mouse ESCs, loss of Tcf3 function promotes self-renewal in the absence of leukemia inhibitory factor (LIF), but these cells cannot form embryoid bodies. Canonical Wnt/β-catenin signal is reported to regulate nuclear orphan receptor Nr5a2 (also known as liver receptor homologue-1, Lrh-1) expression. β-catenin and Tcf3 are targeted to Nr5a2 and Nr5a2 and in turn directly activate the expression of Tbx3, Nanog, and Oct3/4, which are components of the core pluripotency network. Based on these findings, a model has been proposed for the effects of canonical Wnt signaling pathway on the ESCs (Tanaka et al, 2011). Moreover, an elevated level of Wnt signaling activity can promote the maintenance of pluripotency, but the normal level of Wnt/ β-catenin signaling has no apparent impact on ESCs.

Reseaches identified Wnt ligands expressed in human ESCs or pluripotent stem cells. For instance, *Wnt3, 5a* and *10b* mRNAs are expressed in undifferentiated human ES cells; *Wnt5a* and *8b* mRNAs in embryoid body; *Wnt6, 8b* and *10b* mRNAs in ESC-derived endoderm precursor cells; *Wnt4, 5a, 6, 7a, 7b* and *10a* mRNAs in ES cells-derived neural precursor cells. The expression patterns of Wnt ligands indicate that canonical Wnt signaling plays important roles in maintenance and differentiation of human ESCs. However, it appears that roles of Wnt signaling in the maintenance and differentiation of human and mouse ESCs are controversial. For example, human ESCs cannot be maintained by supplementation of Wnt3a in the absence of feeder cells, raising the possibility that feeder cells produce factors that synergize with Wnt signals to support the self-renewal of ESCs.

3.2.3 Organogenesis and development

Single molecules in canonical Wnt pathway are important regulators in animal development and implicated in tissue homeostasis of adult organisms. In adult animals, there are tissue-specific somatic stem cells (SCs) niches in adults have been found in mesenchymal, hematopoietic, neural, epidermal and gastrointestinal tissues. It is well known that many signaling pathways and their signaling networks, including Wnt, FGF, Notch, Hedgehog, and TGFβ/BMP, are essential for animal development. In this section, we mainly discuss the roles and molecular mechanisms of canonical Wnt pathway in the control of animal organgenesis and in the fate determination of somatic stem cells.

3.2.3.1 Cardiovascular system development

1. Cardiomyocytes differentiation

The Wnt/β-catenin signaling is essential for cardiac differentiation (Cohen et al, 2008). Canonical signaling through Wnt1 and Wnt3a expression in the anterior mesoderm inhibits the expression of early cardiac genes in the cardiac crescent of chick and frog embryos, including Nkx2.5 and GATA4. However, conditional deletion of β-catenin1 by cytokeratin 19 (Krt19)-Cre results in formation of ectopic heart tissues in the endoderm, suggesting that downregulation of β-catenin activity promotes cardiac differentiation. Although lots of Wnts are expressed during cardiac specification of mouse embryo, but their molecular mechanism remains unclear. It has been shown that a bi-phasic regulation of Wnt/β-catenin signaling is existed in mouse cardiac differentiation: activation of Wnt/β-catenin signaling pathway in the early phase; inhibition of this pathway and activation of the noncanonical pathway in later phases. The biphasic role for this pathway is also found in zebrafish cardiac differentiation. However, Wnt11, a non-canonical Wnt signaling ligand that can activate the caspase 3/8 to degrade β-catenin and thereby inhibits canonical Wnt signaling, is required at later stages of cardiac differentiation. These data suggest that Wnt/β-catenin signaling mainly plays a suppressive role in the cardiogenesis.

2. Vascular development and remodeling

Wnt/β-catenin signaling has been shown to play important roles in vascular development and remodeling (Tian et al, 2010; van de Schans et al, 2008). Loss of β-catenin also leads to defective endocardial cushion/cardiac valve development through defective endothelial-mesenchymal transformation. Several Wnt ligands, such as Wnt2a, Fzd5, have been implicated in regulating EC development and associated with abnormal placental vascular development. Inhibition of canonical Wnt signaling often results in decreased vascular smooth muscle cells (VSMCs) proliferation and *cyclin D1* expression.

3.2.3.2 Hematopoietic system development

1. Hematopoiesis

Hematopoietic stem cells (HSCs) have the ability to generate all lineages of blood cells, including red blood cells, platelets, lymphocytes, monocytes, and macrophages. Wnt2b is a key factor for hematopoietic stem or progenitor cells. Purified Wnt3a proteins promote the self-renewal of HSCs derived from Bcl2-transgenic mice. Therefore, the self-renewal of HSCs is likely promoted by the canonical Wnt signaling activation and Wnt signals can provide signals for HSC fate determination in the stem cell niche (Staal & Luis, 2010). However, some studies have shown that constitutive activation of β-catenin impairs multilineage differentiation and causes exhaustion of the HSC pool. The controversial results may be resulted from: (i) different levels of Wnt/β-catenin signaling activation; (ii) dosage responses of Wnt signaling required; (iii) the interference by other signals in the context of Wnt activation; and (iiii) Wnt proteins in various blood cell types.

2. Lymphopoiesis

The canonical Wnt signaling plays a crucial role in Lymphopoiesis, such as T cell and B cell development. The canonical Wnt signaling is aasociated with most immature stages of T cell development. Overexpression of cell autonomous inhibitors of β-catenin and Tcf (ICAT) blocks the development of earliest stage T cells in the thymus. Similarly, the secreted Wnt inhibitor DKK1 can inhibit the thymocyte differentiation at the most immature stages. On the contrary, overexpressing activated forms of β-catenin leads to the generation of more thymocytes and activates proliferation-associated genes in immature thymocytes. The canonical Wnt signaling can regulate B cell development. *Lef1*-deficient mice have a mild block of B lymphopoiesis in fetal but not in adult, and show defects in B cell proliferation. Depletion of Fz9 leds to pronounced splenomegaly, thymic atrophy, and lymphadenopathy with age, with accumulation of plasma cells in lymph nodes during mouse development. In addition, treatment of human B cell progenitors with Wnt3a in the stromal cell co-culture assays negatively regulates the cell proliferation.

3.2.3.3 Nervous system development

1. Neural crest stem cells (NCSCs)

Wnt/β-catenin can induce sensory neurogenesis by acting instructively on embryonic neural crest stem cell (NCSCs) (Toledo et al, 2008). In the central nervous system (CNS), the activation of β-catenin leads to the amplification of the neural progenitor pool. Constitutive expression of β-catenin in neural stem/progenitor cells results in the expansion of the entire neural tube. In addition, Wnt ligands, such as Wnt3a, promote the differentiation of neural SCs in the neocortex at E11.5 at the expense of neural SC expansion. Continuous neurogenesis in adult happens only in two specialized niches of the adult CNS, subventricular zone (SVZ) and subgranular zone (SGZ).

2. Neural crest formation

Canonical Wnt signaling has been found in early stages of neural crest development, such as neural crest induction and melanocyte formation. For example, ablation of β-catenin results in a decrease of tissue mass in the spinal cord and brain, and the neuronal precursor population, and a lack of melanocytes and sensory neural cells in dorsal root ganglia.

3. Neuronal differentiation

Numerous components of canonical Wnt signaling have been shown to regulate the precise patternings of developmenting neural tissue. Wnt1 acts as a mid-hindbrain organizer and the ablation of Wnt-1 causes severe deficiencies during mid–hindbrain formation in mice; Wnt-3, -3a, -7b and -8b, can participate in the development of the forebrain (gives rise to hippocampus). The functions of Wnts in neuronal differentiation depend on signals with temp-spatial distribution, triggering the differentiation of precursor cells to neurons.

4. The development of dopaminergic (DA) neurons

DA precursors can respond to canonical Wnts. For example, before the appearance of DA neurons, the expression of Wnt-1 and Wnt-3a is detected in the developing ventral midbrain (VM). In addition, the GSK-3β-specific inhibitor kenpaullone increases the DA differentiation through stabilizing β-catenin in ventral mesencephalic precursors. There are 13 Wnt ligands, all 10 Fzds receptors, and several intracellular Wnt signaling modulators are identified to developmentally regulate the development of midbrain and the DA precursors respond to Wnts in a very specific/temporal manner.

5. Synapses

The function of Wnt signaling pathway in synapses has been characterized during neuronal development. Wnts play roles in the formation of the sensory–motor connections in mouse spinal cord. Wnt-3 and 7a can promote synaptogenesis inducing the clustering of synapsin I, a presynaptic protein involved in synapse formation and function. This effect is controlled by the canonical pathway and can be mimicked by the GSK-3β inhibition induced by lithium. Interestingly, the Dvl-1 is found to present in synaptosomes of adult mice and it also co-localized with the presynaptic markers synaptophysin, bassoon and VAMP-2.

6. Sympathetic nervous system development

A recent study has shown that Fz3 acts at early developmental stages to maintain a pool of dividing sympathetic precursors, likely via activation of β-catenin, and Fz3 functions at later stages to promote innervation of final peripheral targets by post-mitotic sympathetic neurons.

7. Canonical Wnt signaling in brain

It is known that the expression of specific Wnt ligands occurs in distinct regions of developing human brain (Malaterre et al, 2007). The major role of Wnt1 is to regulate the proliferation of precursor populations in the developing mid-/hindbrain region; Wnt7b is expressed in cerebral cortical and diencephalic progenitor cells during early human development; Wnt3a appears to have a very specific role in the development of the hippocampus, a structure involved in integrating many of the higher order tasks, such as memory and learning. β-catenin in the E9.5 telencephalon is highly enriched at the apical end of the neural precursor cells and colocalized with N-cadherin at adherens junctions, implying that the main role of β-catenin at this stage of telencephalic specification is to promote neuroepithelial adhesion. Other canonical Wnt pathway-related factors are also implicated in a number of aspects of brain development. GSK-3β and β-catenin transcriptional partners LEF1 and TCF4 are expressed during brain development in mouse. These results suggested that brain developent respond to canonica Wnt signaling pathway in a very specific and temporal manner.

3.2.3.4 Reproductive system development

1. Gonadal development

Many Wnt genes are expressed in gonads. Wnt1, 3 and 7a are specifically expressed in the testis; Wnt5a, Wnt6 and Wnt9a are specifically expressed in the ovary; Wnt4 is expressed in mouse gonads in both sexes at embryonic day 9.5 (E9.5) and becomes ovary-specific at the time of sex determination around E11.5. These expression patterns of multiple Wnt genes in the gonads suggest that canonical Wnt signaling pathway is essential for gonadal development. Activation of Wnt/β-catenin signaling is required for female differentiation (Liu et al, 2009). Although β-catenin is present in gonads of both sexes, it is necessary for ovarian differentiation but dispensable for testis development. Lacking β-catenin, defects in ovaries are strikingly similar to those found in the R-spondin1 (Rspo1) and Wnt4 knockout mouse ovaries, including formation of testis-specific coelomic vessel, appearance of androgen-producing adrenal-like cells and loss of female germ cells. Studie have found that activation of β-catenin in otherwise normal XY mice effectively disrupts the male program and results in male-to-female sex-reversal.

The expression of sex determining gene Sry (sex-determining region Y) within the initially bipotential gonad is sufficient to induce the male developmental program. Both human *SRY* and mouse *Sry* are capable of repressing the Rspo1/Wnt/β-catenin signaling, thereby switching on testis determination. Interestingly, the HMG box of human SRY can bind directly to β-catenin while the mouse Sry binds to β-catenin *via* its HMG box and glutamine-rich domain.

2. Mammary stem cells and Mammary gland development

Several lines of evidence suggest that canonical Wnt signaling is involved in the maintenance of the stem/progenitor pool in the mammary gland. The stem/progenitor fraction is increased in the hyperplastic mammary glands of MMTV–Wnt-1 and MMTV–ΔNβ-catenin transgenic mice and in primary cultures of mammary epithelial cells treated with Wnt-3a. In addition, Lrp5 is expressed in the basal epithelium and cells with high expression have a 200-fold greater ability to regenerate a mammary tree when transplanted into cleared mammary fatpads. Embryos overexpressing the Wnt antagonist Dkk1, as well as animals deficient for Lrp6 or Lef-1, fail to form mammary placodes. These findings validate the importance of Wnt/β-catenin in mediating the activity of mammary stem cells.

The canonical Wnt signaling is essential for specification and morphogenesis of the mammary gland. Numerous components of the Wnt signaling cascade are expressed during embryonic mammary morphogenesis, including Wnt ligands (*i.e.*, Wnt1, 2, 3, 3a, 5a, 5b, 6, 7b, 10a, 10b, 11), receptors (*i.e.*, Fzd1-9, LRP5, LRP6), and downstream DNA-binding proteins (*i.e.*, Tcf1, 3, and 4 and Lef1). Wnt2, Wnt5a and Wnt7b are enriched in the terminal end bud microenvironment. Targeting other positive acting elements of the Wnt pathway, such as Lrp6, Lrp5, Lef1 and Pygo2, can result in placodal impairments, ranging from loss to reduced size and degeneration, while stimulating β-catenin signaling produces the converse effect - acceleration, expansion and induction of placodes and placodal markers. During mammary development, Wnt5a is considered to negatively regulate the Wnt/β-catenin pathway. Constitutive expression of the canonical Wnt4 leads to more highly branched ducts in virgin females, similar to what occurs during early pregnancy.

3. Prostate stem cells (PSCs) and Prostate gland development

Evidence of canonical Wnt signaling involvement in prostate stem cells is based on limited studies. A few findings suggest that Wnt signaling regulates the terminal differentiation of basal cells into luminal cells by controlling the proliferation and/or maintenance of epithelial progenitor cells. For example, more p63 (basal cell marker) positivity is seen in the ductal region of Wnt3a-treated cultures while fewer p63 positive cells are present in Dkk1-treated cultures. These results are supported by the CK8 (luminal cell marker) immunostaining. The expression of many Wnt signaling molecules such as Fzd6 and Wnt2 is increased in both fetal and adult PSC. This result means that adult PSCs acquire characteristics of self-renewing primitive fetal prostate stem cells, which in turn might also be characteristic of oncogenesis.

The canonical Wnt pathway has been implicated in prostate development (Kharaishvili et al, 2011). Wnt antagonist sFRP2 is highly expressed early in prostate development and down-regulated at later time points. It is indicated that both enhancement and reduction of canonical Wnt signaling can adversely affect branching morphogenesis in the developing rat prostate model. Treated with Wnt3a, rat ventral prostate cultures at postnatal day 2 (P2) show blunted and enlarged ductal tips at 7th day, while Dkk-treated prostates exhibit poor epithelial branching. The highest level of Axin2 is detected on P2, consistent with a higher progenitor cell population; while the level declines over time according to prostate maturation when the majority of the epithelial cells are terminally differentiated luminal cells. Other Wnts and components including three canonical Wnts (Wnt2, Wnt2b and Wnt7b), Fzd2 and 4 and Dvl are also highly expressed on P3 in ventral lobes. Except for

Wnt7b, all of them show a high expression at birth with levels declining during and after the completion of morphogenesis. Those results suggest that the canonical Wnt signaling is temporally regulated during prostate development.

3.2.3.5 Skeletal development

1. Mesenchymal stem cells (MSCs)

The MSCs can differentiate into mesoderm-derived chondrocytes, osteocytes, adipocytes, fibroblasts, myocytes as well as nonmesoderm-derived hepatocytes, and neurons. Canonical Wnt signals are required for maintenance of undifferentiated MSCs, inhibition of adipocyte maturation, dedifferentiation of adipocytes, and inhibition of osteoblastic differentiation (Ling et al, 2009). MSCs express a number of Wnt ligands including Wnt2, Wnt4, Wnt5a, Wnt11 and Wnt16, and several Wnt receptors including FZD2, 3, 4, 5 and 6, as well as various coreceptors and Wnt inhibitors. Exogenous application of Wnt3a to cell cultures expands the multipotential population of MSCs by up-regulation of cyclin D1 and c-Myc. Moreover, the overexpression of LRP5 can increase proliferation of MSCs. Dkk1 is required for the arrested hMSC to re-enter into cell cycle and subsequent proliferation. Interestingly, studies have revealed that canonical Wnt signaling stimulates hMSC proliferation at low dose while inhibits it at high dose. This dual effect of Wnt signaling suggests the intensity of Wnt signals can lead to different or even opposite biological functions.

2. Cartilage development

Cartilage development is initiated by chondrogenesis, which requires mesenchymal condensation and cartilage nodule formation. A variety of different Wnt signaling components positively or negatively regulate different stages of chondrogenesis and cartilage development (Chun et al, 2008). Chondrogenesis is inhibited by Wnt-3a via a β-catenin-dependent mechanism; Wnt-1 and -7a also inhibit chondrogenesis without significant effects on early condensation. Chondrocyte maturation and mineralization are also blocked or delayed by the forced expression of FrzB, Fzd-1, or Fzd-7. In contrast to the inhibition of chondrocyte maturation, constitutively active form of β-catenin promotes growth plate chondrocyte terminal differentiation and overexpression of Wnt-8c and -9a in chick sternal chondrocytes enhance hypertrophic maturation by upregulating type X collagen and Runx2.

3. Osteoblastogenesis and bone formation

Canonical Wnt signaling plays an important role in osteoblastogenesis and bone formation. Wnt activity in bone marrow varies throughout stages of development and has important contributions from several Wnts. Wnt7b is induced during osteoblastogenesis; Wnt10b is expressed in bone marrow; Wnt1, 4, and 14 are expressed in calvarial tissue and osteoblast cultures; Wnt1 and Wnt3a are induced by BMP2 in a mesenchymal precursor cell line. Wnt/β-catenin signaling promotes the bone formation via stimulation of the development of osteoblasts. Inhibition of GSK3 enzymatic activity with lithium chloride (LiCl) or small molecules (e.g. Chir99021 and LY603281-31-8) stimulates mesenchymal precursors to differentiate into osteoblasts. This result is supported by observations with Wnt3a, Wnt1 and Wnt10b, which activate signaling through β-catenin and stimulate osteoblastogenesis. However, Dkk1 can reduce osteoblastogenesis by inhibiting the activity of this pathway. Studies suggest that activation of Wnt/β-catenin signaling inhibits adipogenesis of mesenchymal precursors, which may have clinical importance due to the positive correlation reported between marrow adipose content and bone fractures.

3.2.3.6 Eye development

The canonical Wnt signaling pathway has been shown to be required at multiple points in development of the eye, from specification of the eye field to differentiation of the retina and determination of retinal polarity (de Iongh et al, 2006). Here, we mainly discuss the important roles in the eye development in vertebrates.

1. Eye specification

Most of the studies on eye specification have been carried out in *Xenopus* and zebrafish embryos. During zebrafish mid-late gastrulation, canonical Wnts (Wnt1, 8b, 10b and 11) and Fzds (Fzd3, 5, 8a) are detected in the anterior neural plate (ANP). Wnt1, 8b and 10b are expressed in domains caudal to the eye field (delineated by *Rx3*, eye marker). Fzd8a expression domain overlaps the expression of several anterior neural ectoderm markers including Six3, which is expressed in the presumptive eye fields. Fzd5 expression domain appears to completely overlap the eye field delineated by Rx3. Zebrafish mutants (*masterblind* and *headless*) with mutations of *axin* and *tcf3* exhibit defects in eye formation. In addition, inhibition of GSK-3β results in eye reduction or loss. Dkk1 induces complete heads with two-well formed eyes in larger eyes. Overexpression of Wnt8b or treatment with LiCl to activate the canonical Wnt signaling, results in the loss of anterior structures (including eyes) and the loss of *six3* and *rx1* expression. These results indicate that canonical Wnt signaling inhibits eye formation. Recent inverstigations suggest that activation of Dkk2 by PITX2 can locally suppress the canonical Wnt signaling activity in eye development.

2. Lens development

Recent studies have documented the involvement of various components of the Wnt signaling pathway in lens morphogenesis and differentiation. Expression of various Wnts (Wnt2b, 7a, 7b, 8a, and 8b), Fzd, Dkk and Lef/Tcf, has been identified in the developing eye of various species. Expression of these Wnt components is restricted to the lens epithelium and down-regulated as cells exit the cell cycle and initiate differentiation into lens fiber cells. However, Wnt7b continues to be expressed in the cortical fibers of the lens undergoing terminal differentiation. The expression pattern of Wnt components in the lens placode and effects of deleting β-catenin in the ocular ectoderm indicate that Wnt signals play an important role during lens induction and early morphogenesis. Analysis of the *Tcf/Lef-LacZ* mice shows that there is transient activation of Wnt signaling in the anterior lens epithelium between E13.5 and E14.5 after closure of the lens vesicle. Several lines of evidence indicate that Wnt signals also play key roles in the differentiation of the lens fibers. The active (non-phosphorylated) form of β-catenin and inactivated GSK-3β can be found in lens fiber as well as epithelial cells.

3. Retinal development

Wnt1, -3, -5a, -5b, -7b and -13 (Wnt2b) are found in embryonic and fetal retinae, and Wnt5a, -5b, -10a and -13 in the adult retinal. In the embryonic mouse retina at E12.5, Wnt receptors Fzd3, Fzd4, Fzd6 and Fzd7 are expressed throughout the optic cup and Fzd4 is detected in the RPE (optic cup, optic stalk). The expression patterns of *sfrps* are variable during early morphogenesis. The dynamic expression patterns of Wnt, Fzd and Sfrp genes in the developing retina suggest the involvement of canonical Wnt signaling pathway.

3.2.3.7 Liver development

Canonical Wnt pathway also is essential for liver development (Nejak-Bowen & Monga, 2008). 15 Wnts and 9 Fzs are identified in an adult mouse liver, and the Wnts expressed in various cell types of liver (Table.2). These findings suggest that distinct Wnt signals in various cell types might be associated with their different functions.

Cell type of mouse liver	Wnt ligands
Hepatocytes	1, 2, 4, 5a, 5b, 9a, 9b, 11
Biliary epithelial cells	2, 2b, 3, 4, 5a, 5b, 8b, 9a, 9b, 10a, 10b, 11
Sinusoidal endothelial cells	2, 2b, 3, 4, 5a, 5b, 8b, 9a, 9b, 10a, 11
Stellate and Kuffer cells	2, 2b, 3, 4, 5a, 5b, 6, 7a, 8b, 9a, 9b, 10a, 10b,11, 16

Table 2. Wnt genes expressed in various cell types within liver (Thompson & Monga, 2007).

In hepatocytes, Active β-catenin is detectable immediately prior to gastrulation at E5.5 in the extra- embryonic visceral endoderm and in a narrow region of cells in the epiblast at E6. Two associations with β-catenin are important in hepatocytes: One association is the connection between β-catenin and E-cadherin at the hepatocyte membrane and the other association is that of β-catenin with the hepatocyte growth factor (HGF) and receptor c-Met.

Several lines of evidence have identified that the regulation of Wnt/β-catenin signaling is a requirement for postnatal liver development. It is well known that liver derivation from the foregut endoderm occurs around somite stages 5 to 6 as a result of signaling from mesoderm in the form of FGFs and BMP4, both of which are incidentally downstream targets of the Wnt pathway. Wnt ligands such as Wnt2b, is expressed at these stages and positively regulates the induction and specification of zebrafish liver. In mouse, temporal expression of β-catenin during mouse prenatal liver development indicates its important role in hepatocyte expansion during early liver development (Lade & Monga, 2011). sFRP5 is expressed in the ventral foregut endoderm that gives rise to the liver at mouse E8.5 and can modulate Wnt activity by delineating borders between organs in the developing gut.

Canonical Wnt signaling is also important in normal liver growth and regeneration. The expression level of β-catenin is increased during postnatal development and can promote hepatic growth in mouse. In adult resting liver, the Wnt/β-catenin pathway is quiescent. When liver is not being challenged by chemical, metabolic or dietary stress, β-catenin is not required for normal physiologic function. However, if liver is injured, proliferation of the normally quiescent hepatocytes and cholangiocytes, followed by proliferation of the hepatic stellate cells and endothelial cells, quickly restores the liver to its original mass. During this regeneration process, levels of β-catenin are dramatically increased in the partial hepatectomy (PHx) model.

3.2.3.8 Kidney development

A number of Wnt family members are expressed in the mouse embryonic kidney (Merkel et al, 2007; Pulkkinen et al, 2008): Wnt-2b, -4, -5b, -6, -7b, -9b and -11 are expressed during kidney ontogeny; Wnt-6, -7b, -9b and 11 are expressed in the branching ureteric bud (UB) during the early stages of organogenesis; while Wnt-2b and -4 are detected in the kidney mesenchymal cells. In wild type mice, UB-produced Wnt9b is necessary for tubule formation, at least in part through its activation of Wnt4 expression in the adjacent mesenchyme. However, the precise mechanism for Wnt function in tubule formation remains to be defined.

3.2.3.9 Other organgenesis

1. Epithelial stem cells

Epithelial stem cells present in many tissues, including skin, intestine, lung, kidney, and so on. The canonical Wnt signaling pathway is shown to play important roles in two leading epithelial stem cell models (Gu et al, 2010): the intestine and hair follicle. The canonical Wnt signaling is required for the normal homeostasis of epithelial stem cells. Depletion of TCF4 or overexpression of Wnt inhibitor Dkk1 in intestinal stem cells (ISCs) results in a dramatic reduction in proliferation of crypt cells. Inhibition of the Wnt pathway by conditional ablation of β-catenin or by ectopic expression of Dkk1 specifically in epithelia, blocks hair follicle formation during embryogenesis and causes a loss of the postnatal HFSC niche. Conversely, constitutive activation of Wnt pathway results in massive proliferation of epithelial stem/progenitor cells.

2. Lung development

Canonical Wnt signaling is known to regulate epithelial and mesenchymal cell biology in an autocrine and paracrine fashion (Pongracz & Stockley, 2006). Several Wnt ligands, receptors, and components of the canonical pathway are expressed in a highly cell-specific fashion in the developing lung. For instance, Wnt2 is highly expressed in the distal mesenchyme, whereas Wnt7b is expressed predominantly in the epithelium. However, transgenic deletion of Wnt2 does not result in any detectable defects of lung development and function, probably due to functional redundancy of Wnt2 proteins. β-catenin-dependent signaling is central to the formation of the peripheral airways of the lungs and responsible for conducting gas exchange, but is dispensable for the formation of the proximal airways. Apart from β-catenin and Wnts, mRNA of Fz-1, -2 and -7 and several intracellular signaling molecules including Tcf-1, -3, -4, Lef1, and secreted Fz related proteins (sFRP-1, -2 and -4) have been found to be expressed in the developing lung in specific and spatio-temporal patterns. The canonical Wnt signaling appears to be able to fulfill their roles in maintenance of adult lung structure: the components of canonical Wnt pathway such as Wnt-3, -4, -5a, -7a, -7b, -10b, and -11 as well as Fz-3, -6 and -7, Dvl, and Dkk are expressed in primary lung tissue and cell lines derived from adult lung tissue.

3. Intestinal development

Intestinal crypts constitute a niche in which epithelial progenitors replicate and prepare to differentiate in response to Wnt signals. After appearance of villi, canonical Wnt signaling was first detected. However, intervillus cells lacking signs of canonical Wnt signaling proliferate actively during villus morphogenesis. In late gestation and briefly thereafter, conspicuous Wnt activity is evident in differentiated, postmitotic villus epithelium. Further investigations indicate that neither Tcf4 nor candidate Wnt targets CD44 and cyclinD1 are expressed in late fetal villus cells with a high Wnt activity. Instead, these cells express the related factor Tcf3 and a different Wnt target, c-Myc. Premature and downregulated β-catenin activity can cause severe villus dysmorphogenesis in transgenic mice. Lrp5 and Lrp6 are recently found to play redundant roles in intestinal epithelium development and might regulate intestinal stem/precursor cell maintenance by regulating the canonical Wnt signaling.

4. Pancreatic development

Previous studies have demonstrated the importance of canonical Wnt signaling in pancreatic development (Wells et al, 2007). The expression of Wnt1 under control of the pdx-1 promoter is associated with murine pancreatic agenesis. Other components of Wnt pathway are detectable during pancreatic organogenesis, including Wnt2, 2b, 3, 4, 5a, 5b, 7a, 7b, 14 and 15. All of ten Fzs proteins are found to express in pancreas, with the strongest expression of Fz1, 2, 4, 5, and 6 and colocalized expression of Frz 1-7 in the islets of Langerhans. Dkk 1, 3, and 4 as well as sFRP 1, 4, and 5 are expressed in the exocrine fraction, while sFRP 2 and 3 are detectable at low levels. The effects of β-catenin on mouse pancreatic development show somewhat conflicting findings (Murtaugh, 2008). The loss of β-catenin/Wnt signaling in the developing mouse results in transient pancreatitis, but exocrine pancreas has eventually recovered. In addition, a significant role of the Wnt pathway in endocrine lineage development using β-catenin knockout mice is identified. However, other studies indicate that β-catenin/Wnt signaling is essential for development of exocrine pancreas, but plays no role in endocrine development. Therefore, mechanisms underlying the regulation of pancreatic development by canonical Wnt signaling require further investigations.

5. Hair follicle and skin development

The hair follicle is an appendant miniorgan of skin. Canonical Wnt signals play an important role in hair follicle development. β-catenin inhibition or Dkk1 overexpression specifically blocks hair follicle formation during embryogenesis, and the former results in a loss of the postnatal hair follicle stem cells (HFSC) niche. Wnt10b may promote hair-follicle growth by inducing the switch from telogen to anagen. Several Wnts such as Wnt4, 10a and 10b, are expressed in the skin. Alteration of the levels and timing of LEF-1 expression during skin embryogenesis in transgenic mice disrupts the positioning and orientation of hair follicles, confirming a central role for LEF-1 in hair patterning and morphogenesis. Wnt3 or Dvl2 overexpression in transgenic mouse skin causes a short-hair phenotype owing to altered differentiation of hair shaft precursor cells and hair shaft structural defects.

3.3 Reprogramming

Reprogramming of nuclei allows the dedifferentiation of differentiated cells. Cell-cell fusion is a way to force the fate of a cell, and in the case of fusion with ESCs, this mechanism induces cellular reprogramming, that is, dedifferentiation of somatic cells. For example, ESCs treated for 24 hours with Wnt3a or with the GSK3 inhibitor, 6-bromoindirubin-30-oxime (BIO), can reprogram somatic cells after polyethylene glycol (PEG)-mediated fusion. Recent studies demonstrate that fusion-mediated reprograming of a somatic cell is greatly enhanced by dose-dependent activation of the Wnt/β-catenin signaling pathway. ESCs expressing whatever amount of β-catenin can fuse, but normally the fate of the resulting hybrids is to undergo apoptosis, unless low levels of nuclear β-catenin allow them to undergo reprogramming instead (Lluis et al, 2010). Further studies using genetic knockout

ESC models suggest that the canonical Wnt signaling pathway play important roles in reprogramming. It is known that the maintainance of mouse ESC (mESC) self-renewal requires the growth factor leukemia inhibitory factor (LIF), which stimulates two parallel pathways: Stat3/Klf4/Sox2 and PI3K/Tbx3/Nanog. In mouse ESCs, β-catenin promotes pluripotency gene expression, including Oct4, Nanog and Tbx3, depending on the regulation of Lrh-1.

4. Canonical Wnt signaling in human diseases

Abnormal expression of components in canonical Wnt signaling pathway is often associated with human diseases including almost of all human cancers (Fig.4). In addition to β-catenin, APC, GSK-3β, and Caveolin-1 are considered as key molecules in oncogenic cellular transformation, hyperplasia and metastasis owing their abilities to modulate many signaling pathways in tumor cells. Some components of this pathway such as β-catenin and Caveolin-1 are also nvolved in tumor multi-drug resistance (MDR). Additionally, the abnormal activity of canonical Wnt signaling has been shown to function in the development and progression of cardiovascular diseases, fibrosis, regeneration, wound healing, obesity, schizophrenia, osteoarthritis (OA) and diabetes.

4.1 The activity of canonical Wnt pathway in cancers and therapy

4.1.1 Tumorigenesis and cancer stem cells (CSCs)

Genetic predisposition, environmental factor, and aging are risk factors of human cancers. Dysregulation of canonical Wnt signaling always results in development of various tumors (Fig.4). Down-regulated canonical Wnt signaling inhibitors caused by epigenetic silencing and genetic alteration often cause the carcinogenesis, such as colon cancer, prostate cancer and Esophageal Squamous Cell Carcinoma.

Cancer stem cells (CSCs) are closely associated with tumorgenesis. CSCs are characterized by their tumorigenic properties, the ability to self-renew and formation of differentiated progeny. Similar to normal stem cells, CSCs express some specific surface markers (CD133, CD44 and others). CSCs contain many of active signaling pathways that are found in normal stem cells, such as Wnt, Notch, and Hedgehog (Hh). A number of studies have demonstrated that the Wnt/β-catenin pathway is crucial in the maintenance of CSCs from lung, leukemia, breast, melanoma, colon, liver and cutaneous cancers.

4.1.1.1 Colorectal cancer and intestinal cancer stem cells (ICSCs)

1. Colorectal cancer (CRC)

The majority of CRC is caused by mutations in key components of the canonical Wnt signaling pathway. In colon cancer, nearly 90% of these tumors harbor mutations that result in β-catenin mutation. Germline loss-of-function mutations in the APC gene were originally identified to be associated with familial adenomatous polyposis (FAP), about 1% of which progress to CRC. Furthermore, 85% of cases of sporadic intestinal neoplasia have mutations in APC, while activating mutations in β-catenin are found in approximately 50% of CRC tumors lacking APC mutations. Recently, investigatons suggest that β-catenin stabilization and C-terminal binding protein 1 (CtBP1) following APC inactivation contribute to adenoma initiation as the first step, and that KRAS activation and β-catenin nuclear localization act synergistically to promote adenoma progression to carcinoma. The promoter of sFRPs is often hypermethylated in CRCs, suggesting that reintroduction of sFRP can reverse the Wnt signaling in CRCs. Moreover, when DACT3 (a member of the Dpr/Frodo family) expression is restored by the inhibition of histone methylation and deacetylation, the Wnt signaling is ihhibited and CRC cell apoptosis is induced.

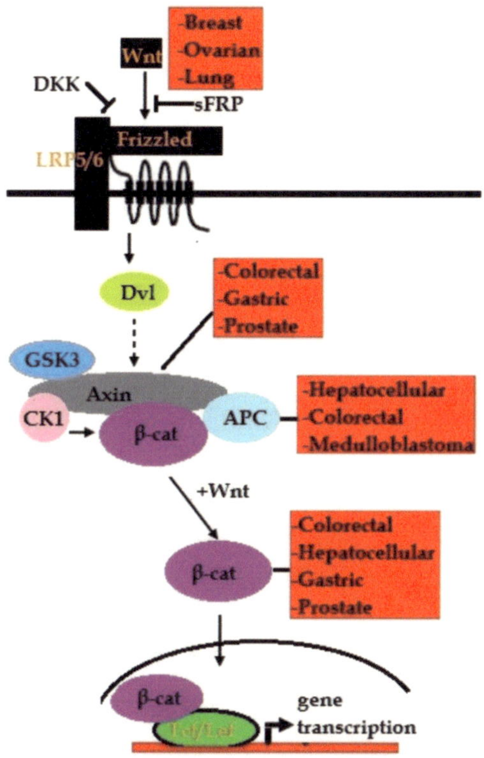

Fig. 4. Canonical Wnt signaling and dysregulation in cancers.The Wnt signaling pathway is comprised of extracellular, cytoplasmic and nuclear signaling events that are amenable to therapeutic intervention. Dysregulation at these stages are common in numerous cancers, captured in the white boxes. (Curtin & Lorenzi, 2010)

2. Intestinal cancer stem cells (ICSCs)

Extensive researches have been performed to find out which cell type is required for the cancer-initiating mutation. A critical work has shown that APC inactivation in Lgr5-positive stem cells at the crypt bottom leads to transformation within days. In contrast, APC inactivation in progenitors or differentiated cells does not cause tumor formation even after 30 weeks. These studies indicate that the cellular origin of CRC initiation might be within normal stem cells of the intestine, rather than progenitors or differentiated cells. Another study has demonstrated that severe polyposis in Apc loss-of-function mutant (Apc1322T) mice is associated with increased expression of the stem cell marker Lgr5 and other stem cell markers (Musashi1, Bmi1, and the Wnt target CD44). Furthermore, the Wnt target gene CD44 has been identified as a marker for colorectal cancer stem cells, and deletion of CD44 in APCMin/+ (heterozygous APC) mice attenuates intestinal tumorigenesis. Overall, these studies support a cancer stem cell model that Wnt signaling plays a key role in the regression of intestinal tumorigenesis.

4.1.1.2 Breast cancer and cancer stem cells (BCSCs)

1. Breast cancer

Studies in both mouse models and human breast cancers have revealed that canonical Wnt signaling is critical to mammary tumorigenesis. The mouse mammary tumor virus (MMTV) is found to integrate into the *Int-1* (*Wnt1*) locus and overexpression of Wnt1 induces mammary tumorigenesis. In human breast cancer, numerous reports have identified that the canonical Wnt pathway is dysregulated. Aberrant β-catenin expression is associated with basal and triple-negative breast cancers and poor clinical outcome. In addition, overexpression of Lrp5 correlates with basal breast cancers. Down-regulation of the sFRPs is observed in breast cancers. Although strong evidence has shown the dysregulation of Wnt pathway in human breast cancer, there are conflicting studies that fail to find an association of this pathway with metastasis or clinical outcome.

2. Breast cancer stem cells (BCSCs)

Studies in breast cancer demonstrate that stem cell populations are more resistant to radiation treatment and Wnt/β-catenin signaling mediates the resistance. These CSCs populations exhibit altered DNA repair in response to radiation and increased AKT (a serine-threonine protein kinase) and β-catenin activities. Blocking the AKT and β-catenin activation by inhibitor perifosine sensitizes the cells to radiation. These studies have underscored the importance of Wnt signaling in breast cancer and the targets for effective therapeutics.

4.1.1.3 Canonical Wnt signaling in prostate cancer and cancer stem cells (PCSCs)

1. Prostate cancer

Canonical Wnt pathway has been widely studied in prostate cancer (Kharaishvili et al, 2011). Wnt ligands are up-regulated in prostate cancer, and their expression often correlates with aggressiveness and metastasis. It is shown that elevated levels of Wnt1, Wnt5a, Wnt7b, and Wnt11 are closely associated with prostate cancer aggressiveness. In addition, Dkk1 expression increases during prostate cancer initiation but decreases during metastasis. Other Wnt pathway members such as Fz4 and Wif1 are found to be dysregulated in prostate cancer.Furthermore, in many cases of prostate cancer, APC is mutated and hypermethylated to a silent form and β-catenin is frequently mutated to an active form.

2. Prostate cancer stem cells (PCSCs)

Several lines of evidence have identified that Wnt signaling can induce prostate cancer initiation, EMT and metastasis, suggesting that canonical Wnts may play a role in the regulation of PCSCs (Bisson et al, 2009). Treatment of PCSCs with Wnt inhibitors can reduce prostasphere size and self-renewal. In contrast, the addition of Wnt3a causes increased prostasphere size and self-renewal. This process is associated with a significant increase in nuclear β-catenin, CD133 and CD44 expression. Moreover, Wnt3a treatment increases the self-renewal of putative PCSCs independent of androgen signaling.

4.1.1.4 Hepatocellular tumors and liver cancer stem cells

1. Hepatoblastoma

Hepatoblastoma is the most common malignant liver tumor. Nuclear and cytoplasmic localization of β-catenin are reported in 90% to 100% of all hepatoblastomas, familial and sporadic due to mutations in APC, CTNNB1, Axin1 and Axin2.

2. Hyperplasia and hepatic Adenoma, Hepatocellular carcinoma (HCC)

The Wnt/β-catenin pathway has been examined in several rare benign liver neoplasms and the analysis demonstrates that abnormal cytoplasmic or nuclear localization of β-catenin in 30% of hepatic adenomas from patients. A more recent analysis indicates mutation of β-catenin in only 12% of adenomas, but 46% of these adenomas progressed to HCC. This finding suggests that development of aberrant activity in the Wnt/β-catenin pathway is an important step toward progression to HCC.

The Wnt/β-catenin pathway is also an important player in the progression of hepatic adenoma and HCC. Studies have found that 20% to 90% of HCCs display activated β-catenin because of diverse mechanisms including mutation in genes encoding for *CTNNB1, Axin-1* and *Axin-2,* as well as fz7 upregulation and GSK-3β inactivation. However, the status of Wnts in HCC remains to be examined. Liver-specific deletion of APC can induce β-catenin stabilization and increased HCC. In addition, transgenic mouse models overexpressing c-myc or TGF-β result in mutation and/or nuclear translocation of β-catenin in liver tumors. Interestingly, simultaneous mutation of β-catenin and H-ras leads to 100% incidence of HCC in mice. These findings suggest that β-catenin activation is likely an initiating or contributory factor in a significant subset of HCCs. Several studies have shown that dyregulations of β-catenin in HCC are associated with hepatitis virus, such as hepatitis B virus (HBV) and hepatitis C virus (HCV). In addition, mutations in the Axin and Axin2 genes result in truncated proteins that are detected in about 10% of HCCs.

It is found that mutations in the β-catenin gene are evident only in a small subset of cholangiocarcinomas. Although the role of canonical Wnt signaling in biliary development is beginning to be understood, further investigations are needed.

3. Liver cancer stem cells

Wnt/β-catenin signaling plays an important role in the maintainance of liver CSCs. For example, elevated expression of Wnt and its downstream mediators are shown in EpCAM+ liver CSCs. It has been demonstrated that murine hepatic stem/progenitor cells transduced with mutant β-catenin can acquire excessive self-renewal capability and tumorigenicity.

4.1.1.5 Leukaemia and leukemia stem cells (LSCs)

1. Leukemia stem cells (LSCs)

Similar to HSCs, LSCs engage in complex bidirectional signals within the hematopoietic microenvironment. Two different stages of leukemia progression called "pre-LSCs" and established leukemia (LSCs) are identified in a syngeneic retroviral model of MLL-AF9 induced acute myeloid leukemia (AML). The homing and microlocalization of pre-LSCs is most similar to long-term HSCs and dependent on cell-intrinsic Wnt signaling. In contrast, the homing of established LSCs is most similar to that of committed myeloid progenitors and distinct from HSCs. In addition, Dkk1 can impair HSC function, while does not affect pre-LSCs, LSC homing, or AML development. Moreover, cell-intrinsic Wnt activation is observed in human and murine AML samples. For example, Wnt3a can affect the self-renewal of AML and T-lymphoblastic leukemia (T-ALL) cells.

2. LSCs associated with AML, CML and MLL

Acute myelogenous leukemia (AML) is the most common acute leukemia in adults. Only small subsets of AML cells (called LSCs) are capable of extensive proliferation and self-renewal, with several markers similar to HSCs. Recent studies have demonstrated that Wnt/β-catenin signaling is required for self-renewal of LSCs derived from either HSC or more differentiated granulocyte macrophage progenitors (GMP). As discussed before, the Wnt/β-catenin pathway is normally active in HSCs, but not in GMP. In addition, β-catenin is not absolutely required for self-renewal of adult HSCs, while β-catenin is required for LSC development and maintenance in AML (Wang et al, 2010). Thus, targeting the Wnt/β-catenin pathway may represent a new therapeutic opportunity in AML.

A conditional β-catenin knockout model has identified the Wnt/β-catenin pathway as being essential for the self-renewal of normal and chronic myelogenous leukemia (CML) stem cells: the impairment of HSC self-renewal in β-catenin$^{-/-}$ mice pre-empted the subversion of this property for the generation of CML LSCs (Deshpande & Buske C, 2007).

Previous studies have found that β-catenin is activated during development of mixed lineage leukaemia (MLL) leukemic stem cells (LSCs) (Yeung et al, 2010). Suppression of β-catenin can reverse LSCs to a pre-LSC-like stage and significantly reduce the growth of human MLL leukemic cells. Conditional deletion of β-catenin can completely abolish the oncogenic potential of MLL-transformed cells. In addition, established MLL LSCs that have acquired resistance against GSK3 inhibitors are resensitized by suppression of β-catenin expression. These results unveil previously unrecognized multiple functions of β-catenin in the establishment and drug-resistant properties of MLL stem cells, highlighting it as a potential therapeutic target for an important subset of AMLs.

4.1.1.6 Other cancers

1. Lung cancer

The canonical Wnt pathway is important for the development of human lung cancer. Although increased levels of β-catenin have been reported in different types of lung cancers, mutations of APC and β-catenin are rare in lung cancers. Dysregulations of specific Wnt molecules (e.g. Wnt1, Wnt2 and Wnt7a) leading to oncogenic signaling are detected in lung cancer. Other components of canonical Wnt pathway are found to be associated with lung cancer. Overexpression of Dvl has been reported in 75% of non-small cell lung cancer samples compared with autologous matched normal lung tissue controls. Downregulation of Wnt pathway antagonists like Dkk3, Wif, Caveolin-1 and sFRP have been reported in various types of lung cancers.

2. Esophageal carcinoma

The roles of canonical Wnt signaling in esophageal carcinoma remain not well understood. Some components, including APC, β-catenin, Dkk1 and Caveolin-1, are found to express in esophageal carcinoma. The expression of Dkk1 is upregulated on both mRNA and protein levels in esophageal carcinoma tissues compared with the adjacent normal esophageal tissues. The positive rates of APC and E-cadherin in esophageal carcinoma are lower than those in the normal group and the abnormal expression rates of β-catenin and cyclin D1 in esophageal carcinoma are higher than those in the normal group.

3. Ovarian cancer

Endometrioid ovarian carcinoma (EOC) frequently exhibit constitutive activation of canonical Wnt signaling, usually as a result of oncogenic mutations that stabilize and dysregulate the β-catenin protein. For example, the majority of low-grade endometrioid ovarian carcinomas often display nuclear immunoreactivity for β-catenin (70% of cases), and these cases often harbour mutations in the β-catenin gene at codons for residues phosphorylated by GSK-3β (54% of cases). However, high-grade endometrioid ovarian carcinomas do not display nuclear β-catenin immunoreactivity and progression is not associated with β-catenin mutations. Moreover, nuclear β-catenin in low-grade endometrioid EOC is also associated with squamous differentiation and correlates with good prognosis and lack of relapse. The EOC also shows constitutive activation of the canonical Wnt signaling pathway, usually as a result of oncogenic mutations in the APC and Axin tumor suppressor proteins. However, some studies have indicated that mutations in Axin are existed in cell lines of endometrioid EOC, while a study from other group has found that no mutations in either APC or Axin in human endometrioid EOC.

Mechanisms for activation of canonical Wnt signaling in ovarian carcinoma exhibit histotype dependence. EOC is strongly associated with active mutations in β-catenin. In contrast with endometrioid EOC, ovarian carcinomas of serous, clear-cell and mucinous histotypes have rarely been associated with activating mutations in the key proteins of the Wnt signaling pathway. Recent studies have shown that both GSK-3β and Axin2 are overexpressed in serous ovarian cancer. These findings implicate activation of Wnt/β-catenin signaling in serous EOC in the absence of activating mutations in either APC, Axin or β-catenin (Barbolina et al, 2011).

4.1.2 Potential roles in cancer therapy

As discussed before, canonical Wnt signaling is active in most of cancers and involed in the self-renewal and differentiation of cancer stem cells. Thus, inhibition of Wnt signaling activity represents a valuable strategy for cancer therapy. Several classes of drugs targeting the Wnt pathway are under development or on the market. These drugs belong to non-steroidal anti-inflammatory drugs (NSAIDs), vitamin D derivatives, antibody-based treatments, small molecule inhibitors, and so on (Table 3).

4.2 Cardiovascular diseases

4.2.1 Cardiac hypertrophy

Cardiomyocytes are terminally differentiated cells existing in heart and the abnormal increase in their individual sizes often leads cardiac hypertrophy. The canonical Wnt signaling pathway has been found to induce physiological and pathological hypertrophies. Cardiomyocyte-specific overexpression of GSK-3β in transgenic mice negatively regulates physiologic concentric hypertrophy (normal growth) of ventricular cardiomyocytes, leading to a smaller heart with depressed contractility. In addition, Fz2 expression is upregulated during hypertrophic development in the rat heart. Using the model of mice lacking the Dvl-1 gene, an attenuated hypertrophic response upon pressure overload induced by aortic constriction, an increased GSK-3β and Akt activities and reduced β-catenin protein levels are observed in these mice. Moreover, it is interesting that β-catenin levels are found to be relatively high in the embryonic heart compared with the adult heart, whereas in hypertrophic hearts an increase in β-catenin content is observed. It is also found that β-catenin is stabilized by hypertrophic stimuli, and that overexpression of β-catenin can induce hypertrophic growth of cardiomyocyte. Cardiomyocyte-specific deletion of β-catenin is shown to attenuate the hypertrophic response upon aortic constriction *in vivo*.

Inhibitors	Subcategory	Therapeutic	Pathway target	Development stage
Small molecules	NSAIDs	Aspirin	β-catenin	Clinical
Existing drugs and natural compounds		Sulindac,	β-catenin	Clinical
		Celecoxib	TCF	Clinical
	Vitamins	retinoids	β-catenin	Clinical
		1α25,-dihydroxy-VitaminD3	β-catenin	Clinical
	Polyphenols	Querucetin	Unknown	Preclinical
		EGCG	Unknown	Preclinical
		Curcumin	Unknown	Preclinical
		Resveratrol	Unknown	Phase II
		DIF	GSK-3β	Preclinical
Molecular targeted drugs		PNU 74654	β-catenin/TCF	Discovery
		2,4-diamino-quinazoline	β-catenin/TCF	Preclinical
		ICG-001-related analogs	CBP	Phase I(2010)
		NSC668036	Dvl	Discovery
		FJ9	Dvl	Discovery
		3289-8625	Dvl	Discovery
		IWR	Axin	Discovery
		IWP	Porcupine	Discovery
		XAV939	Tankyrase1&2	Discovery
Biologics		Antibodies	Wnt proteins	Preclinical
		Recombinant proteins	WIF1 and SFRPs	Preclinical
		RNA interference	Wnt proteins	Preclinical

Table 3. A summary of various Wnt therapeutics (Curtin & Lorenzi, 2010; Takahashi-Yanaga & Kahn, 2010)

4.2.2 Heart failure

In the failing heart, the abnormal expression of sFRPs is identidfied. sFRP3 and 4 are elevated in failing ventricles compared to donor hearts, which is not the case for sFRP1 and 2, and a reduced Wnt/β-catenin signaling is observed. Although these observations have indicated the abnormal activity of canonical Wnt signaling is associated with heart failture in human, the mechanisms underlying this association remain to be further investigated.

4.2.3 Myocardial infarction (MI) and infarct healing

MI is associated with hypertrophy and directly caused by an acute occlusion of a coronary artery. Similar to that during hypertrophic development, Fz2 expression is found to be gradually upregulated in the first 10 days after myocardial infarction in the rat. The upregulation of Wnt-10b and Fzd-1, -2, -5 and -10 and the downregulation of Wnt-7b are also observed in the infarct area at 1 week after infarction in the mouse. It is worth noting that *Fz2* mRNA is detected in the border zone of the infarct area at 1 week after infarction, whereas at 2 weeks after MI, the expression is migrated into the centre of the infarct area. Dvl, directly downstream of Fz, shows high levels of expression exclusively at 4 days after MI and remains upregulated during the first week after MI. The expression patterns of both Fz2 and Dvl closely resemble the location of myofibroblasts in the infarct area. These results indicate the myofibroblasts are the Fz2 and Dvl expressing cells and may be involved in infarct healing. This conclusion is supported by overexpressing FrzA (a homologue of sFRP1) to block Wnt signaling. This intervention shows a profound effect on infarct healing: the infarct size is reduced by more than 50% at 15 days post-MI and a concomitant improvement of cardiac function is observed in the FrzA-overexpressing mice compared to wildtype controls. This effect could be attributed to reduced cardiomyocyte apoptosis, limiting the scar area. Reduced infarct size and improved function can be induced by adenoviral overexpression of β-catenin in the border zone of the infarcted rat heart, suggesting an important role of Wnt/β-catenin signaling in infarct healing.

4.2.4 Aging

Aging is the main risk factor for cardiovascular diseases, but the molecular mechanisms are poorly understood. In human mammary arteries, the expression of Fz4 and several targets of Wnt/β-catenin signaling pathway such as the Wnt-inducible secreted protein 1 (WISP1), versican, osteopontin (SPP1), insulin-like growth factor binding protein 2 (IGFBP-2), and p21, are modified with age, suggesting an activation of the Wnt /β-catenin pathway in the aging process. In aging mammary arteries, the increase in β-catenin-activating phosphorylation at position Ser675 is found. Wnt3a or Wnt1 treatment of human vascular smooth muscle cells (VSMCs) induces β-catenin phosphorylation at Ser675 and the expression of WISP1, SPP1, and IGFBP-2. These findings suggest that the activation of Wnt pathway occurs in aging human mammary artery cells, but fails to induce the proliferation of aging vascular cells (Marchand et al, 2011).

4.2.5 Other vascular diseases

Canonical Wnt pathway regulates endothelial dysfunction and vascular smooth muscle cell (VSMC) proliferation and migration and thereby intimal thickening. Moreover, the pathway has the capacity to regulate inflammation and foam cell formation, pathological angiogenesis and calcification, which are crucial processes in plaque formation and stability. Furthermore, it is apparent that altered expression of a handful of Wnt pathway proteins occurs in or regulates atherogenesis. All of those findings indicate that canonical Wnt pathway acts as an important regulator of vascular diseases, such as atherosclerosis, coronary artery disease and hypertension (van de Schans et al, 2008; Tsaousi et al, 2011).

4.3 Nervous system diseases

4.3.1 Neural tube defects (NTD)

Various components of the Wnt signaling pathway have been implicated in NTD. For example, *Dvl2* null mutants have thoracic spina bifida, and *Dvl1/2* double mutants produce even more severe NTD. Mutations of axin, a Wnt pathway inhibitor, can result in incomplete closure of the neural tube or malformation of the head folds. Alterations (hypoactivity, hyperactivity and missense mutations) to LRP6 can cause NTD.

4.3.2 Primitive neuroectodermal tumors (PNETS)

Activation of canonical Wnt pathway can lead to PNETS. In some cerebellar and cerebral PNETS, mutations that lead to nuclear accumulation of β-catenin are present. Interestingly, stabilized β-catenin is not sufficient to cause the development of brain tumors, while stabilized β-catenin together with forced expression of c-Myc, a downstream target of the Wnt signaling pathway, can lead to increased tumors.

4.3.3 Alzheimer's disease (AD)

Alzheimer's disease (AD) is a neurodegenerative disorder associated with aging and characterized by fibrillar deposits of Aβ in subcortical brain regions. The main proteinaceous component of the amyloid deposited in AD is the amyloid-β-peptide (Aβ peptide), a 40- to 42-residue peptide that has been isolated from senile plaque cores. As discussed before, canonical Wnt signaling pathway is involved in neural induction and patterning during nervous system development. Thus, abnormal activity of this pathway is associated with neurodegenerative disorders, such as AD. Apparently, Aβ can bind with the extracellular cysteine-rich domain (CRD) of the Fz to inhibit Wnt/β-catenin signaling. Studies have indicated the exposure of rat hippocampal neurons to Aβ results in three hallmarks related with Wnt signaling: (i) destabilization of endogenous levels of β-catenin; (ii) an increase in GSK-3β activity; and (iii) a decrease in Wnt target gene transcription. In fact, relationship between Aβ-induced neurotoxicity and a decrease in the cytoplasmic levels of β-catenin has been observed. Inhibition of GSK-3β by lithium is shown to protect rat hippocampal neurons from Aβ-induced damage. Moreover, the conditioned media containing Wnt-3a and Wnt-7a are able to overcome the neurotoxic consequences induced by Aβ. In addition, LRP5/6 is also associated with AD.

4.3.4 Parkinson's disease (PD)

Parkinson's disease (PD) is caused by degeneration of the dopaminergic (DA) neurons of the substantia nigra. The canonical Wnt signaling has a role in promoting adult DA neurogenesis (Inestrosa & Arenas, 2009). Parkin, an E3 ubiquitin ligase linked to familial PD, can directly interact with β-catenin and regulates β-catenin levels *in vivo*. The stabilization of β-catenin in differentiated primary ventral midbrain neurons results in increased levels of cyclin E and proliferation, followed by increased levels of cleaved PARP and loss of DA neurons. In addition, Wnt3a signaling also causes death of post-mitotic DA neurons in parkin null animals, suggesting that both increased stabilization and decreased degradation of β-catenin can result in DA cell death.

4.3.5 Schizophrenia

Schizophrenia is a psychiatric disorder characterized by "positive" symptoms such as delusions, hallucinations, and disorganized speech and "negative" symptoms such as lack of emotional affect and motivation. The canonical Wnt signaling pathway is a candidate for dysregulating brain development, which cause neuroanatomical defects associated with schizophrenia (Okerlund & Cheyette, 2011). Studies have shown that Wnt1 is upregulated in schizophrenic brains, and some genes associated with susceptibility to the disease are core components of the Wnt signaling pathway, such as TCF4, Dkk proteins (especially Dkk1 and Dkk3), GSK-3β, Fz3, sFRP1 and Dvl3. Taken together, the genetic and pharmacological data suggest a potential connection between canonical Wnt signaling and the pathogenesis and therapeutics of schizophrenia.

4.4 Polycystic kidney disease

Cystic kidney disease is the most common genetic cause of end-stage renal failure. These diseases are characterized by the progressive development of cysts in the nephron and collecting ducts, and patients often require dialysis and kidney transplantation. One class cystic kidney disease is polycystic kidney disease (PKD), which contains two types of autosomal dominant (ADPKD) and autosomal recessive PKD (ARPKD). ADPKD typically arises during adulthood, whereas ARPKD arises during childhood and is much more severe. A second class of cystic nephropathy is characterized as glomerulocystic kidney disease, including medullary cystic kidney disease (MCKD) and nephronophthisis (NPHP). NPHP is inherited in a recessive fashion and like ARPKD. Two genes have been identified for the development of ADPKD: polycystic kidney disease gene 1 (*PKD1*) and *PKD2* that encode polycystin-1 (PC1) and polycystin-2 (PC2), respectively. However, 11 candidate genes are identified in the NPHP and NPHP-like disorders.

The canonical Wnt signaling is suggested to affect the cystogenesis. For example, the C-terminus of PC1 can facilitate the nuclear accumulation of β-catenin and the downstream transcription is decreased by overexpression of the C-terminus *in vitro*. In kidney, PC1 expression is increased in cystic epithelium of patients with PKD. Cysts arise in animal models of PKD with complete or partial loss of protein (as in, *Pkd1-/-*, *Pkd1+/-* and hypomorphic mice) and with overexpression of PC1 protein, suggesting the kidney is especially sensitive to gene dosage. These studies indicate that PC1 expression seems to be tightly regulated in the kidney, and canonical Wnt signaling might also require similar fine tuning. Other canonical Wnt components are also associated with cystic renal disease. For example, APC inactivation leads to cystic renal phenotypes in mice. Further evidence for a role of canonical Wnt signaling in renal cyst disease comes from work with NPHP animal models. Nphp2 and Nphp3 both negatively regulate the canonical Wnt cascade through regulation of Dvl, both *in vitro* and *in vivo* in *Xenopus laevis* embryos. Canonical Wnt activity is also affected in a mammalian model of NPHP: knockout mice for *Ahi1*, a gene mutated in the ciliopathy Joubert syndrome (JS), have decreased the canonical Wnt signaling in the kidney compared to wild-type mice.

4.5 Fibrosis

4.5.1 Kidney fibrosis

The Wnt/β-catenin signaling is involved in the pathogenesis of renal fibrosis (He et al, 2009). It has been identified that the majority of 19 different Wnts and 10 frizzled receptor genes are expressed at various levels in the normal mouse kidney. All members of the Wnt family except Wnt5b, Wnt8b, and Wnt9b are upregulated in the fibrotic kidney with distinct dynamics after unilateral ureteral obstruction. In addition, the expression of most Fzd receptors and Wnt antagonists is also induced. Furthermore, obstructive injury leads to a dramatic accumulation of β-catenin in the cytoplasm and nuclei of renal tubular epithelial cells, indicating activation of the canonical Wnt signaling. Numerous Wnt/β-catenin target genes (c-Myc, Twist, lymphoid enhancer-binding factor 1, and fibronectin) are also induced and their expression is closely correlated with renal β-catenin abundance. Wnt antagonist Dkk1 can inhibit myofibroblast activation, suppress expression of fibroblast-specific protein 1, type I collagen, and fibronectin, and reduce total collagen content in the model of obstructive nephropathy. In summary, these results suggest that Wnt/β-catenin signaling is involved in the promotion of renal fibrosis.

4.5.2 Lung fibrosis

The canonical Wnt signaling pathway is associated with pulmonary fibrosis based on studies in animal models and human diseases. Idiopathic pulmonary fibrosis (IPF) is the most common form of lung fibrosis. Studies have revealed the overexpression of Wnt genes, including Wnt-2 and -5a, the receptors Fz7 and -10, and Wnt regulators, such as sFRP1 and -2, in IPF lungs compared with normal lungs or those with other interstitial lung diseases. In addition, several Wnt target genes, such as matrix metalloproteinase 7, osteopontin, or Wnt1-inducible signaling protein (WISP) 1, are recently identified in experimental and idiopathic lung fibrosis. Furthermore, the nuclear localization of β-catenin is found in alveolar epithelial type II (ATII) cells and interstitial fibroblasts in IPF lungs. These results suggest the existence of an activated canonical Wnt signaling in IPF. Morover, abnormal activities of other canonical Wnt signaling components, such as GSK-3β, are observed in ATII cells. The increased activity of the Wnt pathway in IPF is confirmed by increased phosphorylation of LRP6 and GSK-3.

4.5.3 Liver fibrosis

Liver fibrosis represents chronic wound repair and is causally associated with persistent hepatic stellate cell (HSC) activation. Expression of Wnt and Fz genes is induced in HSC isolated from experimental cholestatic liver fibrosis, and Dkk-1 expression ameliorates this form of liver fibrosis in mice. These results suggest canonical Wnt signaling plays a role in liver fibrosis through activating HSC (Cheng et al, 2008). Moreover, both Wnt1 and Wnt10b potently suppress adipocyte differentiation via its inhibition of the adipogenic transcription factors CCAAT/enhanced binding protein family (C/EBP) and peroxisome proliferator-activated receptor-γ (PPARγ). The activated rat HSCs are shown to express higher levels of Wnt4, Wnt5, and Fz2 in culture and experimental liver fibrosis model .

4.6 Other diseases

4.6.1 Diabetes

It is known that the canonical Wnt pathway is involved in the development and genesis of mouse pancreatic islets, pancreatic beta cell growth. The canonnial Wnt signaling is also associated with diabetes (Jin, 2008). Several components of this pathway play important roles in normal cholesterol metabolism and glucose-induced insulin secretion and the production of the incretin hormone glucagon-like peptide-1 (GLP-1). For example, polymorphisms in *TCF7L2,* also known as TCF-4, have by far the biggest effect on the risk of type 2 diabetes. The human LRP5 gene is mapped to within the IDDM4 region, which is linked to type 1 diabetes on chromosome 11q13, and polymorphisms in LRP5 have shown to be associated with obesity phenotypes, and missense mutations in LRP6 are shown to be associated with the risk of bone loss, early coronary disease and the metabolic syndrome. In addition, forkhead box transcription factor subgroup O (FOXO) and TCF proteins are able to compete for the limited pool of β-catenin, and ageing will lead to increased FOXO-mediated gene transcription and reduce TCF-mediated gene transcription. Thus, these findings indicate that type 2 diabetes is an age-dependent disease.

4.6.2 Obesity

Obesity is linked to major adverse health outcomes such as insulin resistance and type 2 diabetes. With obesity, adipose tissue mass expands and adipocyte (fat cell) size increases. As previously discussed, canonical Wnt signaling pathway is essential for adipogenesis and type 2 diabetes. Thus, canonical Wnt signaling plays an important role in the genesis of obesity.

4.6.3 Osteoporosis and Osteoarthritis (OA)

Osteoporosis and osteoarthritis (OA) cause significant morbidity in the middle-age and elderly population. Bone tissue and chondrogenesis are involved in the pathogenesis of OA, which is characterized with subchondral sclerosis and the formation of osteophytic new bone. It is well known that the canonical Wnt pathway has emerged as an important regulator of chondrogenesis, bone development and remodeling. Thus, it is indicated that this Wnt pathway may be involved in the pathogenesis of OA (Velasco et al., 2010). For example, loss-of-function mutations of the LRP5 gene can result in osteoporosis, whereas activating mutations are associated with increased bone mass. It is reported that targeted deletion of the FrzB gene can increase the injury-associated loss of articular cartilage in mice, in association with increased cortical bone thickness and density. Recent work has found that expression of seven genes (BCL9, Fz5, Dvl2, EP300, FrzB, LRP5, and TCF7L1) is consistently upregulated both in tissue samples and in cell cultures from patients with knee osteoarthritis. These studies also demonstrate that three SNPs of the LRP5 gene and one in the LRP6 gene show marginally significant differences in allelic frequencies across the patient groups.

5. Conclusion and prospection

The canonical Wnt signaling is widely known as one of the key pathways that are essential for the embryogenesis of vertebrates. In recent years, increasing lines of evidence have demonstrated that abnormal activivation of this pathway is closely associated with the development and progression of human diseases such as various tumors. Although investigations have provided new insights into the molecular mechanism underlying the roles and regulation of canonical Wnt signaling in animal models and patients, many critical questions remain to be answered. For example, it is largely unclear how the expression of components in this pathway is spatiotemporally controlled and secreted during embryonic development, what mechanisms are involved in the control of Wnt/β-catenin activity by newly identified proteins, and what factors control the nuclear import of β-catenin that is necessary for the expression of downstream genes. Since the functions of canonical Wnt signaling in the formation of animal organs such as liver and the development of some of human diseases are not well understood, it will be of great interest to investigate its effects on activity and regulation of key signaling molecules in developmental and pathological contexts. We firmly believe that a better understanding of canonical Wnt signaling regulation will have a broad impact on biology and medicine.

6. Acknowledgements

In this chaper, we have cited many findings in previous publications and the origins of many results in the text are not mentioned due to the limitiation of reference numbers. Therefore, we would like to take this opportunity to express our sincere gratitude to all authors whose works are cited in this chapter.

7. References

Andersson, E. R.; Sandberg, R. & Lendahl, U. (2011). Notch signaling: simplicity in design, versatility in function. *Development* 138, 3593-612, ISSN (Print):0950-1991; (Online):1477-9129

Aoki, K. & Taketo, M. M. (2007). Adenomatous polyposis coli (APC): a multi-functional tumor suppressor gene. *J Cell Sci* 120, 3327-35, ISSN (Print): 0021-9533 ISSN (Online): 1477-9137

Arce, L.; Yokoyama, N. N. & Waterman, M. L. (2006). Diversity of LEF/TCF action in development and disease. *Oncogene* 25, 7492-504, ISSN: 0950-9232

Barbolina, M. V.; Burkhalter, R. J. & Stack, M. S. (2011). Diverse mechanisms for activation of Wnt signalling in the ovarian tumour microenvironment. *Biochem J* 437, 1-12, ISSN: 0264-6021

Bejsovec, A. (2005). Wnt pathway activation: new relations and locations. *Cell* 120, 11-4, ISSN: 0092-8674

Bisson, I. & Prowse, D. M. (2009). WNT signaling regulates self-renewal and differentiation of prostate cancer cells with stem cell characteristics. *Cell Res* 19, 683-97, ISSN: 1001-0602

Callow, M. G.; Tran, H.; Phu, L.; Lau, T.; Lee, J.; Sandoval, W. N.; Liu, P. S.; Bheddah, S.; Tao, J.; Lill, J. R. et al. (2011). Ubiquitin ligase RNF146 regulates tankyrase and Axin to promote Wnt signaling. *PLoS One* 6, e22595, ISSN: 1932-6203

Cheng, J. H.; She, H.; Han, Y. P.; Wang, J.; Xiong, S.; Asahina, K. & Tsukamoto, H. (2008). Wnt antagonism inhibits hepatic stellate cell activation and liver fibrosis. *Am J Physiol Gastrointest Liver Physiol* 294, G39-49, ISSN: 0193-1857

Cheong, J. K. & Virshup, D. M. (2011). Casein kinase 1: Complexity in the family. *Int J Biochem Cell Biol* 43, 465-9, ISSN: 1357-2725

Chun, J. S.; Oh, H.; Yang, S. & Park, M. (2008). Wnt signaling in cartilage development and degeneration. *BMB Rep* 41, 485-94, ISSN: 1976-6696

Cohen, E. D.; Tian, Y. & Morrisey, E. E. (2008). Wnt signaling: an essential regulator of cardiovascular differentiation, morphogenesis and progenitor self-renewal. *Development* 135, 789-98, ISSN (Print):0950-1991; (Online):1477-9129

Curtin, J. C. & Lorenzi, M. V. (2010). Drug discovery approaches to target Wnt signaling in cancer stem cells. *Oncotarget* 1, 563-77, ISSN: 1178-6930

de Iongh, R. U.; Abud, H. E. & Hime, G. R. (2006). WNT/Frizzled signaling in eye development and disease. *Front Biosci* 11, 2442-64, ISSN: 1093-9946

Deshpande, A. J. & Buske, C. (2007). Knocking the Wnt out of the sails of leukemia stem cell development. *Cell Stem Cell* 1, 597-8, ISSN: 1934-5909

Grumolato, L.; Liu, G.; Mong, P. & Aaronson, S. (2010). Canonical and noncanonical Wnts use a common mechanism to activate completely unrelated coreceptors. *Genes Dev* 24, 2517-2530, ISSN (printed): 0890-9369 (electronic): 1549-5477

Gu, B.; Watanabe, K. & Dai, X. (2010). Epithelial stem cells: an epigenetic and Wnt-centric perspective. *J Cell Biochem* 110, 1279-87, ISSN: 0730-2312

Guder, C.; Philipp, I.; Lengfeld, T.; Watanabe, H.; Hobmayer, B. & Holstein, T. W. (2006). The Wnt code: cnidarians signal the way. *Oncogene* 25, 7450-60, ISSN: 0950-9232

Habas, R. & Dawid, I.B. (2005). Dishevelled and Wnt signaling. Is the nucleus the final frontier? *J Bio* 4, 2, ISSN: 1741-7007

He, W.; Dai, C.; Li, Y.; Zeng, G.; Monga, S. P. & Liu, Y. (2009). Wnt/beta-catenin signaling promotes renal interstitial fibrosis. *J Am Soc Nephrol* 20, 765-76, ISSN: 1046-6673

Huang, H. C. & Klein, P. S. (2004). The Frizzled family: receptors for multiple signal transduction pathways. *Genome Biol* 5, 234, ISSN: 1474-760X

Inestrosa, N. C. & Arenas, E. (2009). Emerging roles of Wnts in the adult nervous system. *Nat Rev Neurosci* 11, 77-86, ISSN: 1471-0048

Itasaki, N. & Hoppler, S. (2010). Crosstalk between Wnt and bone morphogenic protein signaling: a turbulent relationship. *Dev Dyn* 239, 16-33, ISSN: 1058-8388

Jin, T. (2008). The WNT signalling pathway and diabetes mellitus. *Diabetologia* 51, 1771-80, ISSN: 0012-186X

Kharaishvili, G.; Simkova, D.; Makharoblidze, E.; Trtkova, K.; Kolar, Z. & Bouchal, J. (2011). Wnt signaling in prostate development and carcinogenesis. *Biomed Pap Med Fac Univ Palacky Olomouc Czech Repub* 155, 11-8, ISSN: 1673-2588

Kim, K. A.; Wagle, M.; Tran, K.; Zhan, X.; Dixon, M. A.; Liu, S.; Gros, D.; Korver, W.; Yonkovich, S.; Tomasevic, N. et al. (2008). R-Spondin family members regulate the Wnt pathway by a common mechanism. *Mol Biol Cell* 19, 2588-96, ISSN: 1059-1524

Lade, A. G. & Monga, S. P. (2011). Beta-catenin signaling in hepatic development and progenitors: which way does the WNT blow? *Dev Dyn* 240, 486-500, , ISNN: 1058-8388

Li, J.; Sutter, C.; Parker, D. S.; Blauwkamp, T.; Fang, M. & Cadigan, K. M. (2007). CBP/p300 are bimodal regulators of Wnt signaling. *Embo J* 26, 2284-94, ISSN: 0261-4189

Li, Y.; Li, Q.; Long, Y. & Cui, Z. (2011). LZTS2 regulates embryonic cell movements and dorsoventral patterning through interaction with and the export of nuclear β-Catenin in zebrafish. *J Biol Chem*, doi: 10.1074/jbc.M111.267328 jbc.M111.267328

Ling, L.; Nurcombe, V. & Cool, S. M. (2009). Wnt signaling controls the fate of mesenchymal stem cells. *Gene* 433, 1-7, ISSN: 0378-1119

Liu, C. F.; Bingham, N.; Parker, K. & Yao, H. H. (2009). Sex-specific roles of beta-catenin in mouse gonadal development. *Hum Mol Genet* 18, 405-17, ISSN: 0964-6906

Lluis, F.; Pedone, E.; Pepe, S. & Cosma, M. P. (2010). The Wnt/beta-catenin signaling pathway tips the balance between apoptosis and reprograming of cell fusion hybrids. *Stem Cells* 28, 1940-1949, ISSN: 1066-5099

MacDonald, B. T.; Tamai, K. & He, X. (2009). Wnt/beta-catenin signaling: components, mechanisms, and diseases. *Dev Cell* 17, 9-26, ISSN: 1534-5807

Malaterre, J.; Ramsay, R. G. & Mantamadiotis, T. (2007). Wnt-Frizzled signalling and the many paths to neural development and adult brain homeostasis. *Front Biosci* 12, 492-506, ISSN: 1093-9946

Marchand, A.; Atassi, F.; Gaaya, A.; Leprince, P.; Le Feuvre, C.; Soubrier, F.; Lompré, A. M. & Nadaud, S. (2011). The Wnt/beta-catenin pathway is activated during advanced arterial aging in humans. *Aging cell* 10, 220-232, ISSN: 1474-9718

Marikawa, Y. (2006). Wnt/beta-catenin signaling and body plan formation in mouse embryos. *Semin Cell Dev Biol* 17, 175-84, ISSN: 1084-9521

Masckauchan, T. N. & Kitajewski, J. (2006). Wnt/Frizzled signaling in the vasculature: new angiogenic factors in sight. *Physiology (Bethesda)* 21, 181-8, ISSN: 1548-9213

Merkel, C. E.; Karner, C. M. & Carroll, T. J. (2007). Molecular regulation of kidney development: is the answer blowing in the Wnt? *Pediatr Nephrol* 22, 1825-38, ISSN: 0931-041X

Mo, S.; Wang, L.; Li, Q.; Li, J.; Li, Y.; Thannickal, V. J. & Cui, Z. (2010). Caveolin-1 regulates dorsoventral patterning through direct interaction with beta-catenin in zebrafish. *Dev Biol* 344, 210-23, ISSN: 0012-1606

Murtaugh, L. C. (2008). The what, where, when and how of Wnt/beta-catenin signaling in pancreas development. *Organogenesis* 4, 81-86, ISSN: 1547-6278

Nejak-Bowen, K. & Monga, S. P. (2008). Wnt/beta-catenin signaling in hepatic organogenesis. *Organogenesis* 4, 92-9, ISSN: 1547-6278

Nusse, R. (1999). WNT targets. Repression and activation. *Trends Genet* 15, 1-3, ISSN: 0168-9525

Nusse, R. (2008). Wnt signaling and stem cell control. *Cell Res* 18, 523-7, ISSN: 1001-0602

Okerlund, N. D. & Cheyette, B. N. (2011). Synaptic Wnt signaling-a contributor to major psychiatric disorders? *J Neurodev Disord* 3, 162-74, ISSN: 1866-1947

Pongracz, J. E. & Stockley, R. A. (2006). Wnt signalling in lung development and diseases. *Respir Res* 7, 15, ISSN: 1465-9921

Pulkkinen, K.; Murugan, S. & Vainio, S. (2008). Wnt signaling in kidney development and disease. *Organogenesis* 4, 55-9, ISSN: 1547-6278

Rao, T. P. & Kuhl, M. (2011). An updated overview on Wnt signaling pathways: a prelude for more. *Circ Res* 106, 1798-806, ISSN: 0009-7330

Reya, T. & Clevers, H. (2005). Wnt signalling in stem cells and cancer. *Nature* 434, 843-50, ISSN: 0028-0836

Rubin, J. S.; Barshishat-Kupper, M.; Feroze-Merzoug, F. & Xi, Z. F. (2006). Secreted WNT antagonists as tumor suppressors: pro and con. *Front Biosci* 11, 2093-2105, ISSN: 1093-9946

Schulte, G. (2010). International Union of Basic and Clinical Pharmacology. LXXX. The class Frizzled receptors. *Pharmacol Rev* 62, 632-67, ISSN: 0031-6997

Schulte, G.; Schambony, A. & Bryja, V. (2010). beta-Arrestins - scaffolds and signalling elements essential for WNT/Frizzled signalling pathways? *Br J Pharmacol* 159, 1051-8, ISSN: 0007-1188

Staal, F. J. & Luis, T. C. (2010). Wnt signaling in hematopoiesis: crucial factors for self-renewal, proliferation, and cell fate decisions. *J Cell Biochem* 109, 844-9, , ISSN: 0730-2312

Takahashi-Yanaga, F. & Kahn, M. (2010). Targeting Wnt signaling: can we safely eradicate cancer stem cells? *Clin Cancer Res* 16, 3153-3162, ISSN: 1078-0432

Tanaka, S. S.; Kojima, Y.; Yamaguchi, Y. L.; Nishinakamura, R. & Tam, P. P. (2011). Impact of WNT signaling on tissue lineage differentiation in the early mouse embryo. *Dev Growth Differ* 53, 843-56, ISSN: 0012-1592

Teo, J. L. & Kahn, M. (2010). The Wnt signaling pathway in cellular proliferation and differentiation: A tale of two coactivators. *Adv Drug Deliv Rev* 62, 1149-55, ISSN: 0169-409X

Thompson, M. D. & Monga, S. P. (2007). WNT/beta-catenin signaling in liver health and disease. *Hepatology* 45, 1298-305, ISSN: 0270-9139

Tian, Y.; Cohen, E. D. & Morrisey, E. E. (2010). The importance of Wnt signaling in cardiovascular development. *Pediatr Cardiol* 31, 342-8, ISSN: 0172-0643

Toledo, E. M.; Colombres, M. & Inestrosa, N. C. (2008). Wnt signaling in neuroprotection and stem cell differentiation. *Prog Neurobiol* 86, 281-96, ISSN: 0301-0082

Tsaousi, A.; Mill, C. & George, S. J. (2011). The Wnt pathways in vascular disease: lessons from vascular development. *Curr Opin Lipidol* 22, 350-7, ISSN: 0957-9672

Valkenburg, K.; Graveel, G.; Zylstra-Diegel, C.; Zhong, Z. & Williams, B. (2011). Wnt/β-catenin Signaling in Normal and Cancer Stem Cells. *Cancers* 3, 2050-2079, ISSN: 2072-6694

van Amerongen, R. & Nusse, R. (2009). Towards an integrated view of Wnt signaling in development. *Development* 136, 3205-14, ISSN (Print):0950-1991; (Online):1477-9129

van de Schans, V. A.; Smits, J. F. & Blankesteijn, W. M. (2008). The Wnt/frizzled pathway in cardiovascular development and disease: friend or foe? *Eur J Pharmacol* 585, 338-45, ISSN: 0014-2999

Velasco, J.; Zarrabeitia, M. T.; Prieto, J. R.; Perez-Castrillon, J. L.; Perez-Aguilar, M. D.; Perez-Nunez, M. I.; Sanudo, C.; Hernandez-Elena, J.; Calvo, I.; Ortiz, F. et al. (2010). Wnt pathway genes in osteoporosis and osteoarthritis: differential expression and genetic association study. *Osteoporos Int* 21, 109-18, ISSN (printed): 0937-941X (electronic): 1433-2965

Wang, Y.; Krivtsov, A. V.; Sinha, A. U.; North, T. E.; Goessling, W.; Feng, Z.; Zon, L. I. & Armstrong, S. A. (2010). The Wnt/beta-catenin pathway is required for the development of leukemia stem cells in AML. *Science* 327, 1650-1653, ISSN: 0036-8075

Wells, J. M.; Esni, F.; Boivin, G. P.; Aronow, B. J.; Stuart, W.; Combs, C.; Sklenka, A.; Leach, S. D. & Lowy, A. M. (2007). Wnt/beta-catenin signaling is required for development of the exocrine pancreas. *BMC Dev Biol* 7, 4, ISSN: 1471-213X

Wodarz, A. & Nusse, R. (1998). Mechanisms of Wnt signaling in development. *Annu Rev Cell Dev Biol* 14, 59-88, ISSN: 1081-0706

Yeung, J.; Esposito, M. T.; Gandillet, A.; Zeisig, B. B.; Griessinger, E.; Bonnet, D. & So, C. W. (2010). beta-Catenin mediates the establishment and drug resistance of MLL leukemic stem cells. *Cancer Cell* 18, 606-18, ISSN: 1535-6108

Ying, Y. & Tao, Q. (2009). Epigenetic disruption of the WNT/beta-catenin signaling pathway in human cancers. *Epigenetics* 4, 307-12, ISSN: 1559-2294

5

Congenital Anomalies of Thoracic Systemic and Pulmonary Veins Visualized with Computed Tomography

Elżbieta Czekajska-Chehab, Sebastian Uhlig,
Grzegorz Staśkiewicz and Andrzej Drop
Ist Department of Radiology, Medical University of Lublin
Poland

1. Introduction

Introduction of multidetector computed tomography (MDCT) into daily clinical use has been a breakthrough in the thoracic imaging. It allowed one breathhold scanning of the entire chest, and thin sections made multiplanar and volumetric reconstructions easily available. Initially, the main interest focused on the abdominal aorta and its branches, however, it turned out, that MDCT allows for an excellent visualization and assessment of thoracic veins, including their anatomical variants and thrombosis. Thin collimation combined with secondary reconstructions allows preliminary diagnosis of vascular anomalies even in precontrast scanning. Secondary reconstructions in oblique or curved planes, three-dimensional reconstructions and ECG-gating allow clear identification of venous pathologies.

2. Embryology of thoracic veins

Formation of blood vessels occurs around the day 17 of the fetal development, and occurs within the splanchnopleuric mesoderm of the yolk sac. At about day 21, blood islands within the yolk sac may be observed. Central parts of the islands host hemoblasts, while the outer layers form the blood vessels. Developing veins form three main systems, which carry blood into the sinus venosus (Dudek & Fix, 2004):

- vitelline veins, which form part of part of inferior vena cava (IVC), hepatic veins and sinusoids, ductus venosus, portal vein and its tributaries (superior and inferior mesenteric veins – SMV and IMV, splenic vein); this venous system collects the blood from the fetal GI tract;
- umbilical veins, which carry blood from placenta - both contribute to the hepatic sinusoids, left one forms ligamentum teres
- cardinal veins, which collect the blood from the body:
    - anterior, which form superior vena cava (SVC), internal jugular veins (IJV);
    - posterior, which form part of IVC, common iliac veins;
    - subcardinal, which form part of IVC, renal and gonadal veins;
    - supracardinal, which form part of IVC, intercostal veins, azygos and hemiazygos veins.

The systemic veins are derived from cardinal veins (CVs), which apart from umbilical and vitelline vessels are one of three main elements of foetal venous system. CVs in the form of paired structures located symmetrically on both sides of embryo's body appear in 4th week of gestation. System of CVs is comprised of anterior cardinal veins (ACVs) draining cranial parts of the body and posterior cardinal veins (PCVs) providing drainage from caudal parts. ACV and PCV join together into common cardinal vein - CCV (Cuvier ducts), entering the sinus venosus of early heart eventually.

At 8th week of fetal life left brachiocephalic vein is being formed connecting the left and right ACVs. As a consequence the portion of left ACV below this connection partially obliterates forming the „ligament of Marshall" and the remaining, distal section of left ACV forms coronary sinus and oblique vein of the heart. Right ACV remains patent and together with right CCV becomes the precursor of superior vena cava system (Fasouliotis et al., 2002; Ratliff et al., 2006).

Most of PCVs undergo atrophy and their patent remnants form renal segment of inferior vena cava (IVC) and common iliac veins. Simultaneously, subcardinal and supracardinal veins are being formed. Both subcardinal and supracardinal veins (SVs) are involved in development of IVC, also SVs give the origin to the azygos system of veins. Usually SVs develop anastomosis at the level of thoracic spine. Right SV becomes azygos vein (AV), however according to data in literature its arch may be delivered from the upper segment of the right PCV (Demos et al., 2004). The left one below anastomosis transforms into hemiazygos vein (HV) and above the anastomosis obliterates. In some cases only the cranial section of left SV remains patent as accessory HV (Fasouliotis et al., 2002; Arslan et al., 2000).

3. Multidetector computed tomography of thoracic vascular system- optimization of scanning protocol, imaging pitfalls, collateral circulation

3.1 Optimization of the scanning protocol and imaging pitfalls

Optimal MDCT imaging of thoracic veins may be difficult, as there is no possibility of concomitant optimal enhancement of systemic, pulmonary and cardiac veins, because of different contrast inflow rate into particular vessels, asymmetrical enhancement of right and left sides of the thorax, dependent on the side of intravenous contrast administration, as well as artifacts and collateral circulation.

MDCT assessment of thoracic venous anomalies usually occurs in two situations: a more typical one involves incidental diagnosis of venous pathology in patients diagnosed for unrelated conditions, e.g. suspected neoplasm or coronary disease. In such cases, the examination is reviewed by radiologist after the scanning is over, and modification of the protocol is not possible. In cases of the precontrast scanning, preliminary assessment is possible, and appropriate modifications can be applied, including early postcontrast scanning (23-30s) for pulmonary veins evaluations, and late phase (60-120s) for systemic veins. Furthermore, ECG-gating utilization can be considered.

Less frequent setting is an examination performed for assessment of particular venous anomaly, e.g. before ablation or resynchronization therapy, as well as confirmation of anomalies suggested by echocardiography or chest x-ray. Such setting allows for optimal modification of the scanning protocol, like reduction of field of view (FOV), ECG-gating or bolus tracking for optimized visualization of pulmonary veins, cardiac veins or coronary sinus.

Technical features of MDCT allow for correct diagnosis of any thoracic venous pathology. Potential pitfalls are caused by limited knowledge of venous physiology and vascular anomalies and variants, focusing on arteries and pulmonary parenchyma, as well as lack of preliminary assessment of the precontrast scans. In our opinion, the most significant cause is insufficient awareness and interest in this type of pathology.

3.2 Thoracic collateral venous circulation pathways

Collateral circulation is particularly important in patients with obstruction of SVC, which may be caused by benign, malignant or iatrogenic conditions.

Four main groups of collateral thoracic veins include: azygos system of veins - communication between SVC and ascending lumbar vein; subfascial system of epigastric veins - collateral circulation between brachiocephalic vein and external femoral vein; subcutaneous system of superficial epigastric vein and vertebral veins. Less frequently, systemic-pulmonary or intramuscular pathways are involved.

Azygos system of veins provides communication between SVC and ascending lumbar veins, which receive lumbar veins, forming anastomosis with IVC. Azygos system consists of veins of posterior wall of the trunk, which receive multiple tributaries, particularly within their course through the mediastinum (Figure 1, Figure 2). Azygos system forms the best developed anastomosis between vena cava systems, with its tributaries arising from both parietal, as well as visceral (in particular mediastinal and bronchial) veins.

Subcutaneous veins of the trunk connect axillary and femoral veins (Figure 3). Superficial system anastomoses with the subfascial system by means of perforating veins, which carry blood from medial aspect of breasts and sternal branches of internal thoracic veins.

Subfascial veins connect external iliac vein and subclavian vein via internal thoracic and inferior epigastric veins. Internal thoracic veins (ITV) are tributaries of brachiocephalic veins. They are formed by junction of musculophrenic veins and superior epigastric veins. Internal thoracic veins anastomose at the posterior surface of sternum. Parietal tributaries of ITV are anterior intercostal veins, which provide anastomosis with the azygos sysem, by means of posterior intercostals. Additional tributaries of brachiocephalic veins, frequently widened in patients with SVC syndrome, are pericardiophrenic veins.

Vertebral plexuses form two vascular rings located outside the vertebrae: anterior and posterior external vertebral plexus, as well as inner, internal vertebral plexuses located within the vertebral canal. In the cervical region, anterior external plexus anastomoses with vertebral veins, in thoracic region with posterior intercostal veins, in lumbar - lumbar veins. At the anterior aspect of sacral bone it anastomoses with median and lateral sacral veins. Posterior external plexus is best developed in the cervical region, anastomosing with occipital, vertebral and deep cervical veins.

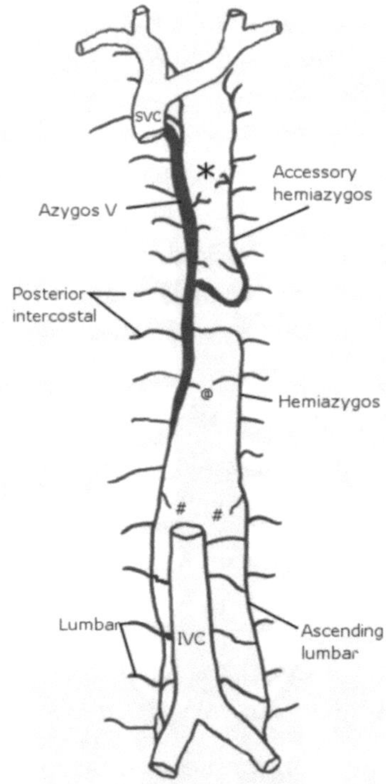

Fig. 1. Azygos system of veins. Multiple anastomoses of this system include parietal veins (lumbar, ascending lumbar, intercostal, @-superior phrenic) as well as visceral (#-renal, *-mediastinal, including: bronchial, esopahgeal, pericardiac) veins.

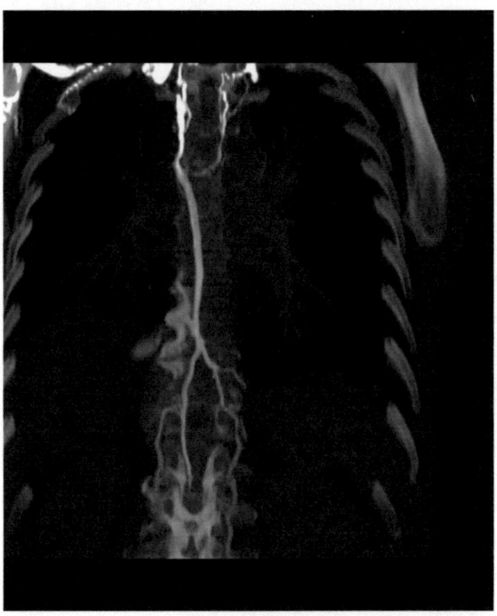

Fig. 2. Curved multiplanar reformation. Widening of azygos sytem of veins in a patient with left-sided SVC syndrome.

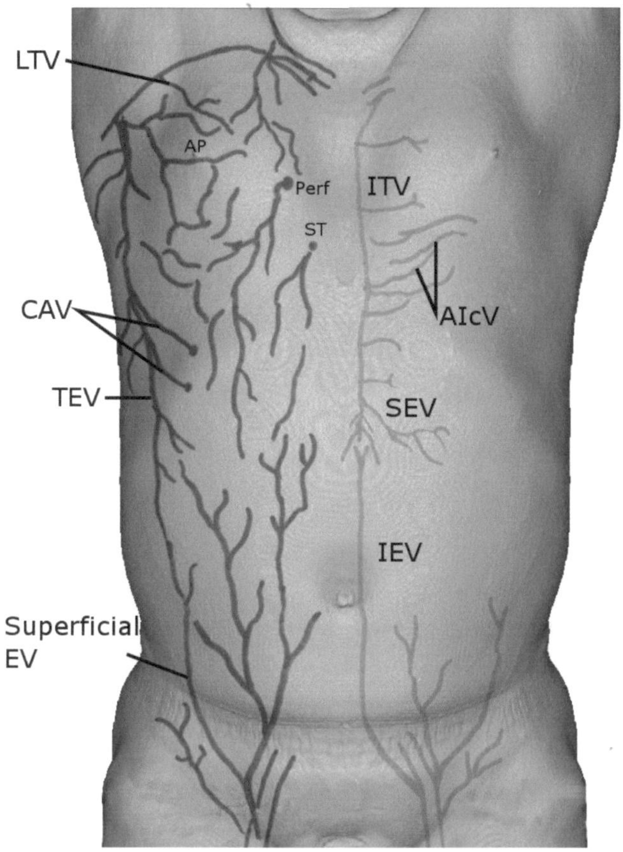

Fig. 3. Superficial and subfascial systems of veins. Superifical veins: Superificial EV - superficial epigastric vein, TEV - thoracoepigastric veins, CAV - costoaxillary veins, LTV - lateral thoracic vein, AP - areolar plexus. ST - sternal branches of internal thoracic vein, Perf - perforating branches.

4. Thoracic veins anomalies

4.1 Anomalies of the superior vena cava (SVC)

4.1.1 Persistent left superior vena cava

Persistent left superior vena cava (PLSVC) results from disturbances in process of obliteration of left ACV what leads to its patency. The defect occurs in 0,3 - 0,5% of the general population, usually in bilateral configuration with the right sided superior vena cava (Biffi et al., 2001; Tak et al., 2002) - Figure 4, Figure 5. Its prevalance is significantly higher when it is combined with other congenital heart defects, heterotaxy syndromes or some genetical disorders (Anagnostopoulos et al., 2009; Ho et al., 2004).

Solitary PLSVC is less common finding with an incidence reaching 33% among the individuals with this anomaly (Fang et al., 2007), Figure 6. PLSVC both in unilateral or bilateral configuration reaches the right atrium through the coronary sinus typically, Figure 7. Very seldom it is connected with the left atrium (Ardilouze et al., 2009).

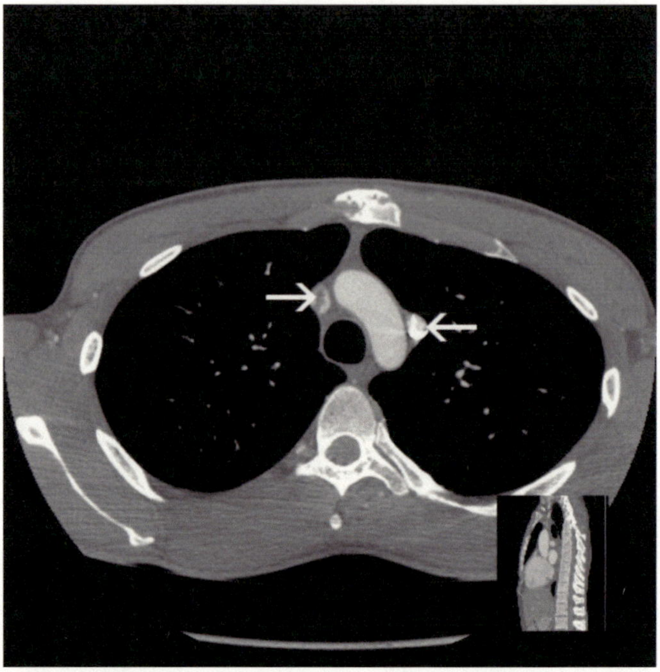

Fig. 4. Axial CT image presents bilateral superior venae cavae (arrows).

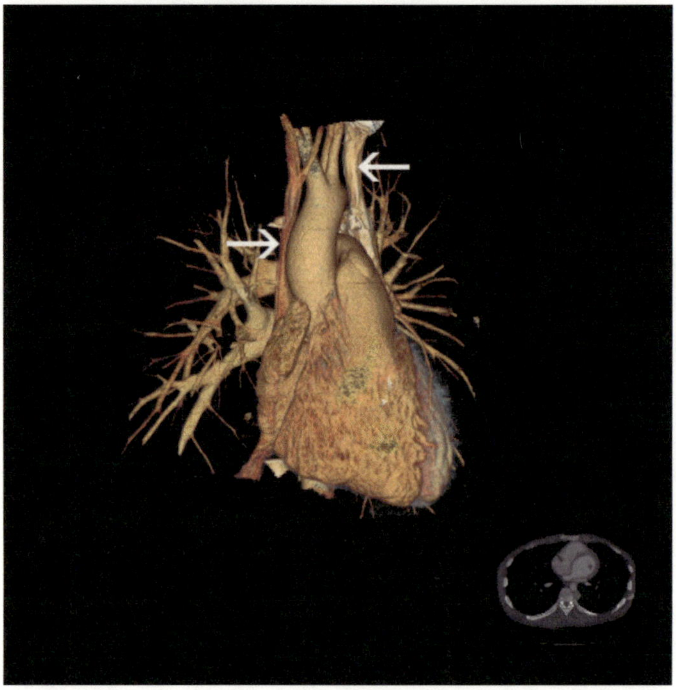

Fig. 5. Volumetric reconstruction presents bilateral superior venae cavae (arrows).

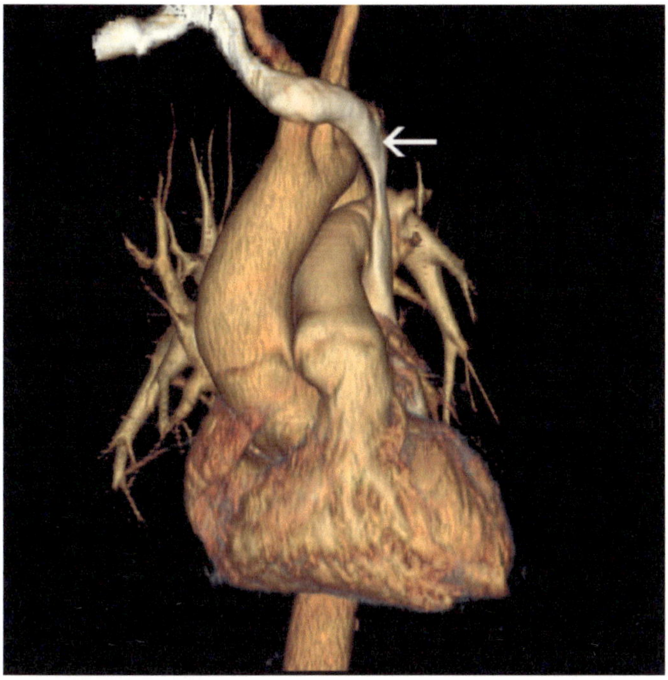

Fig. 6. Volumetric reconstruction presents single left-sided SCV (arrow).

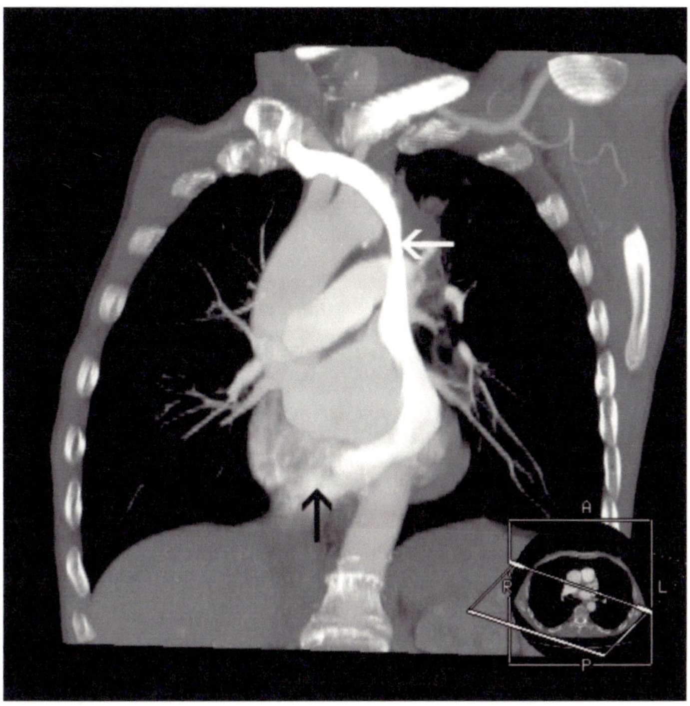

Fig. 7. Maximum intensity projection shows single left-sided SVC (white arrow), with a typical opening into widened coronary sinus (black arrow).

In the majority of cases, when PLSVC is not associated with other congenital heart defects, it remains hemodynamically asymptomatic. However, the anomaly may predispose to cardiac arrhythmias and simultaneously, the most important clinical implications of PLSVC are difficulties in placing pacemaker or in ablation procedure (Biffi et al.,2001; Horlitz et al., 2006; Morgan et al., 2002). Usually during this procedure the PLSVC is revealed most frequently as an incidental finding (Figure 8, Figure 9).

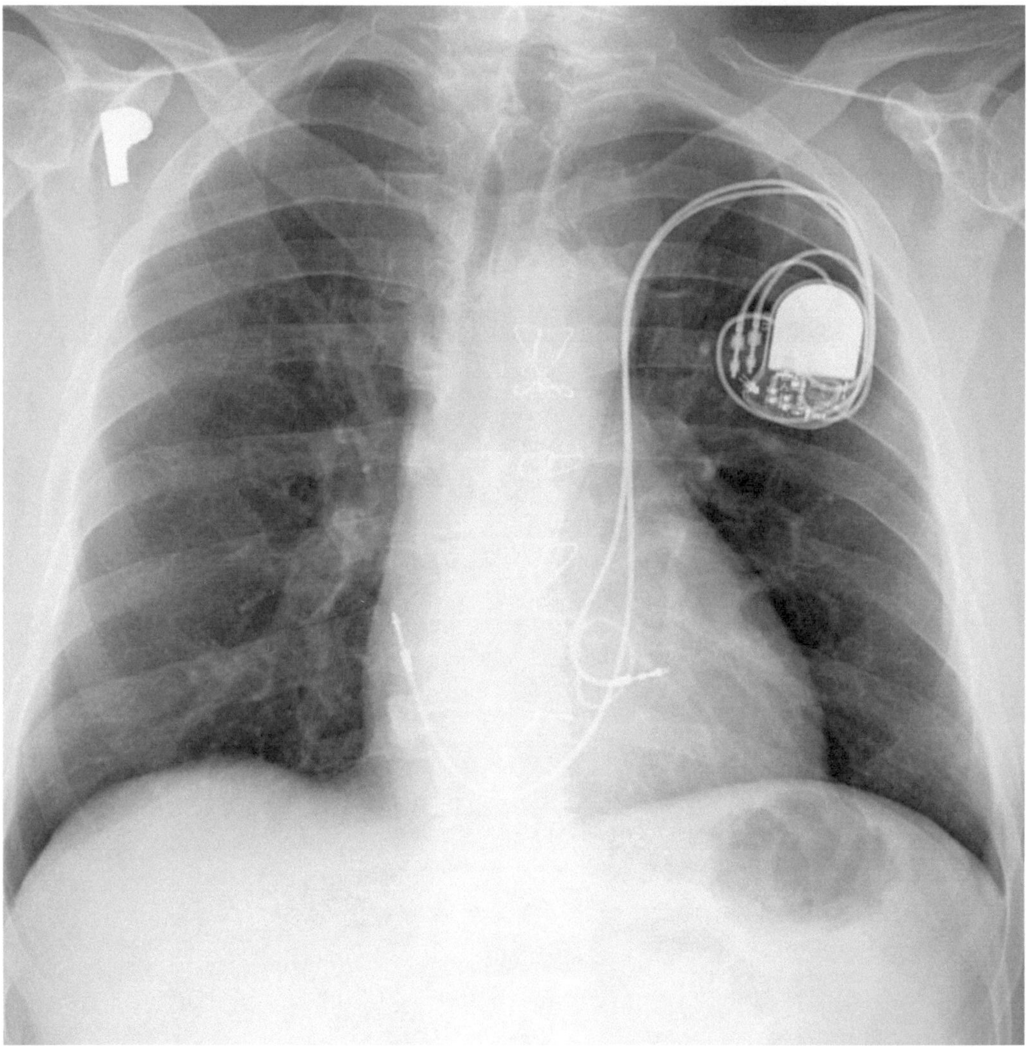

Fig. 8. Anteroposterior chest radiograph. Pacemaker electrodes passing through left-sided SVC, entering distal coronary sinus.

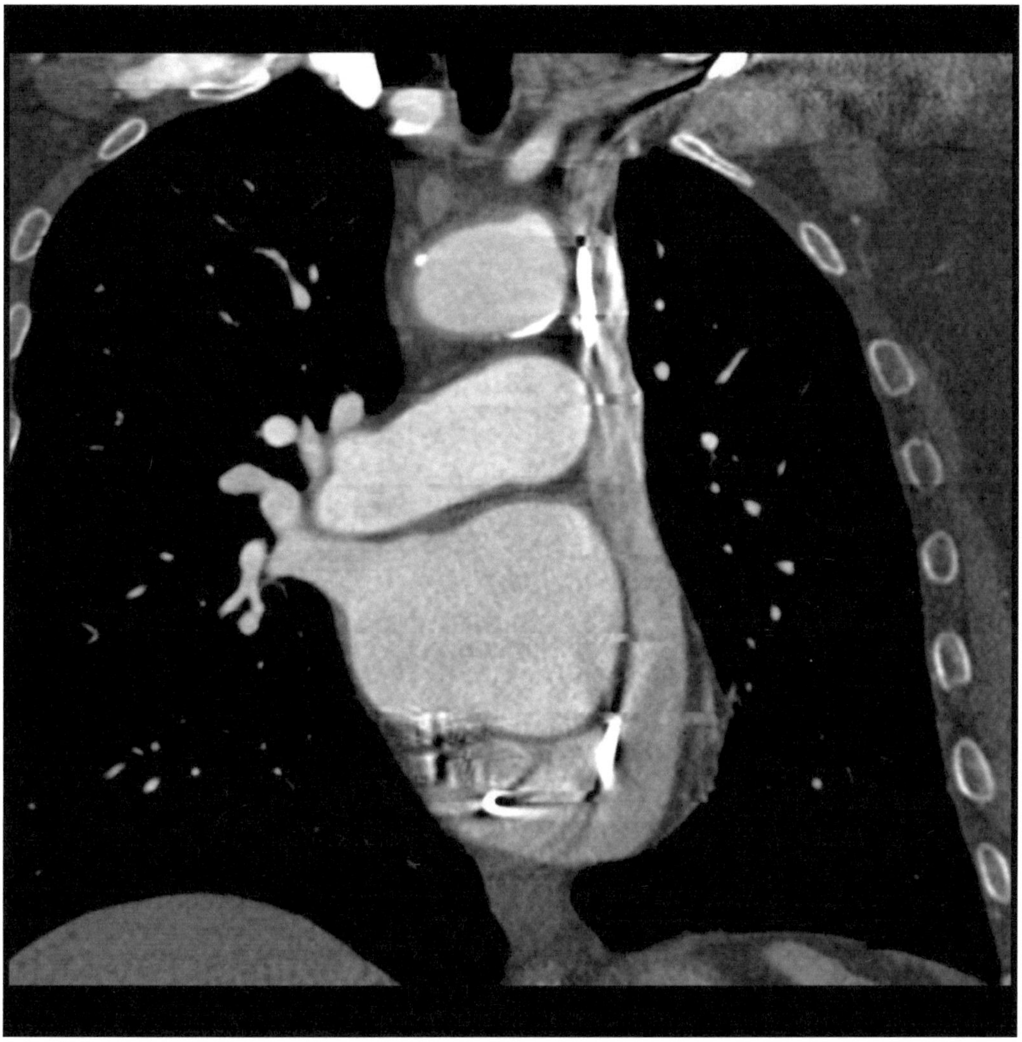

Fig. 9. Curved multiplanar reformation, CT. Pacemaker electrodes passing through single PLSVC into coronary sinus.

4.1.2 Aneurysm of SVC

In contrary to PLSVC, aneurysms of thoracic veins including SVC are extremely rare with merely about 30 cases reported in the literature (Varma et al., 2003). Both congenital and acquired causes of the pathology are possible. It may be fusiform or saccular and in the latter form can reach enormous size being unusual cause of mediastinal „mass" (Figure 10). Basing on few case reports it can induce complications, such as pulmonary embolism or be the source of intrathoracic bleeding after rupture. Saccular aneurysms are usually treated surgically (Enright & Kanne, 2010).

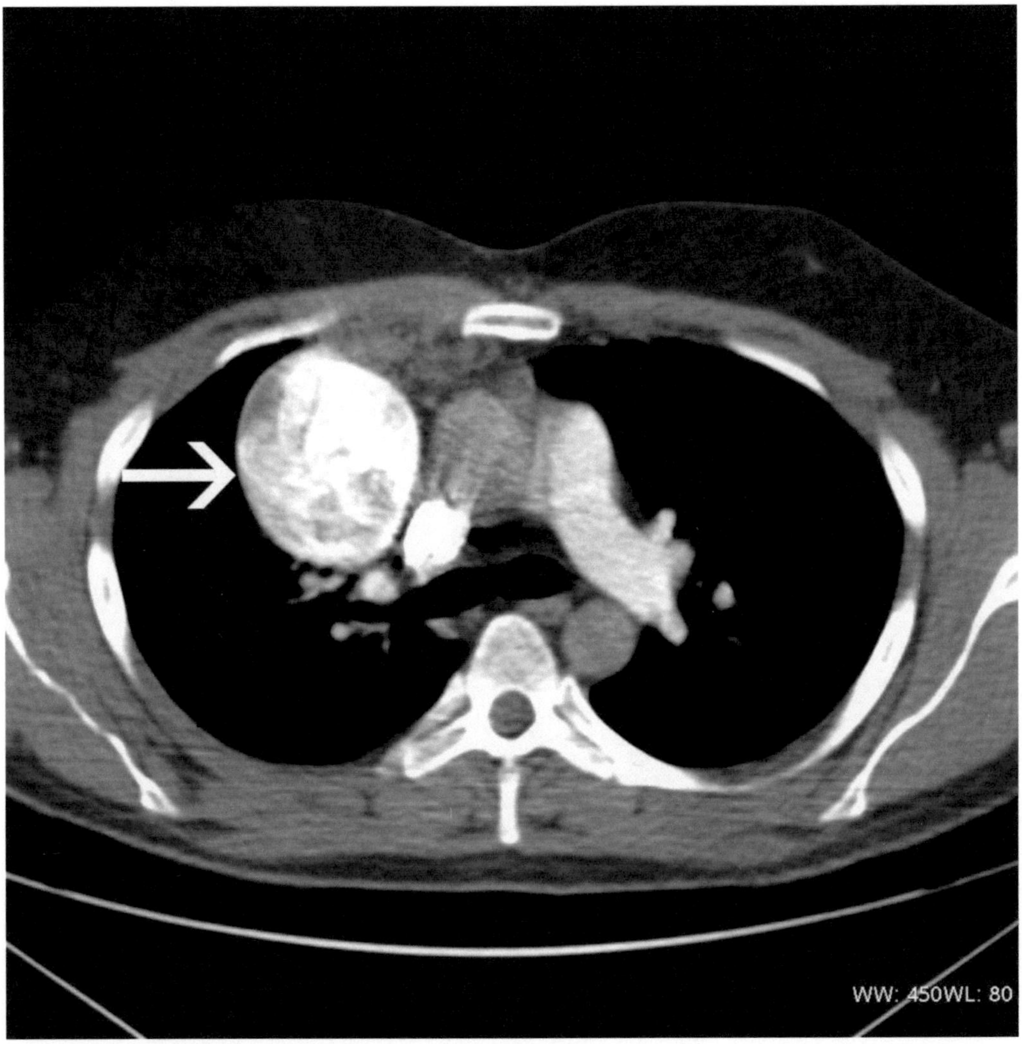

Fig. 10. Axial scan, CT. Saccular aneurysm of SVC (arrow)

4.2 Anomalies of the Azygos Veins (AV)

Azygos lobe: The most common variant of azygos system of veins is azygos lobe. It appears in about 1% of population and its appearance is attributed to incorrect migration of proximal section of right PCV, which is considered to be precursor of azygos arch. Instead of locating over the right lung's apex it penetrates its parenchyma pulling either visceral or parietal layers of pleura. In consequence azygos fissure composed of four layers of pleura is formed. Less frequently hemiazygos lobe may develop. Since azygos and hemiazygos lobes are asymptomatic, they are usually detected incidentally on x-rays (Figure 11) or CT examinations (Caceres et al., 1998; Demos et al., 2004).

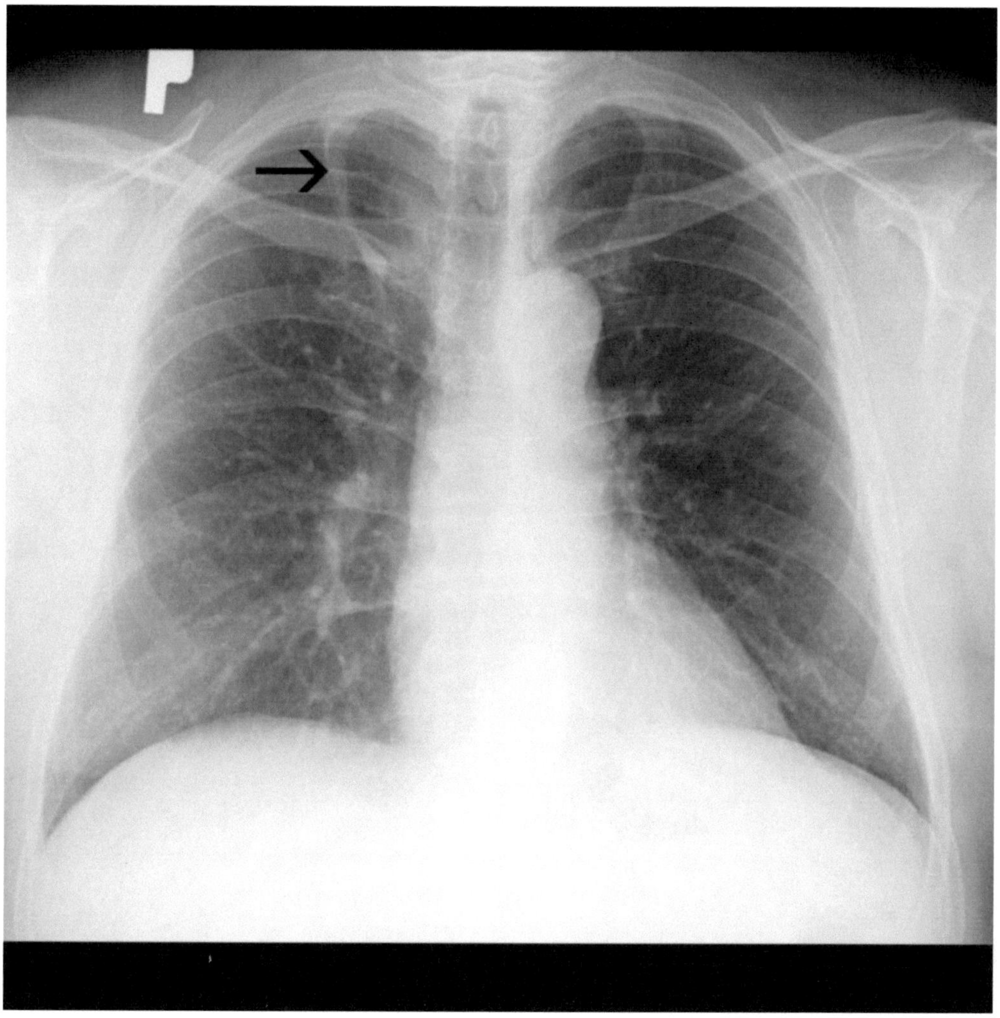

Fig. 11. Anteroposterior chest radiograph. Azygos lobe in the upper right lung field as an incidental finding, black arrow indicates accessory fissure.

Azygos and hemiazygos continuation of IVC: Azygos continuation of IVC results from disturbances in development of hepatic segment of IVC leading to interruption of the vessel. The drainage of caudal parts of the body is continued through the AV, with an exception of hepatic veins which empty to the right atrium directly, usually through one, common vessel. AV becomes widened and drains to SVC through prominent azygos arch.

Hemiazygos continuation is related to left sided IVC. Usually it drains directly to AV through anastomosis at the level of thoracic spine and the blood flow is continued through AV. However, other routes are possible including direct drainage to the coexistent PLSVC or through accessory HV (Demos et al., 2004)], furthermore, in absence of confluence of brachiocephalic veins, isolated drainage of left and right sides of the upper body may exist, with right brachiocephalic vein forming SVC, and left brachiocephalic vein opening into accessory hemiazygos vein (Figure 12).

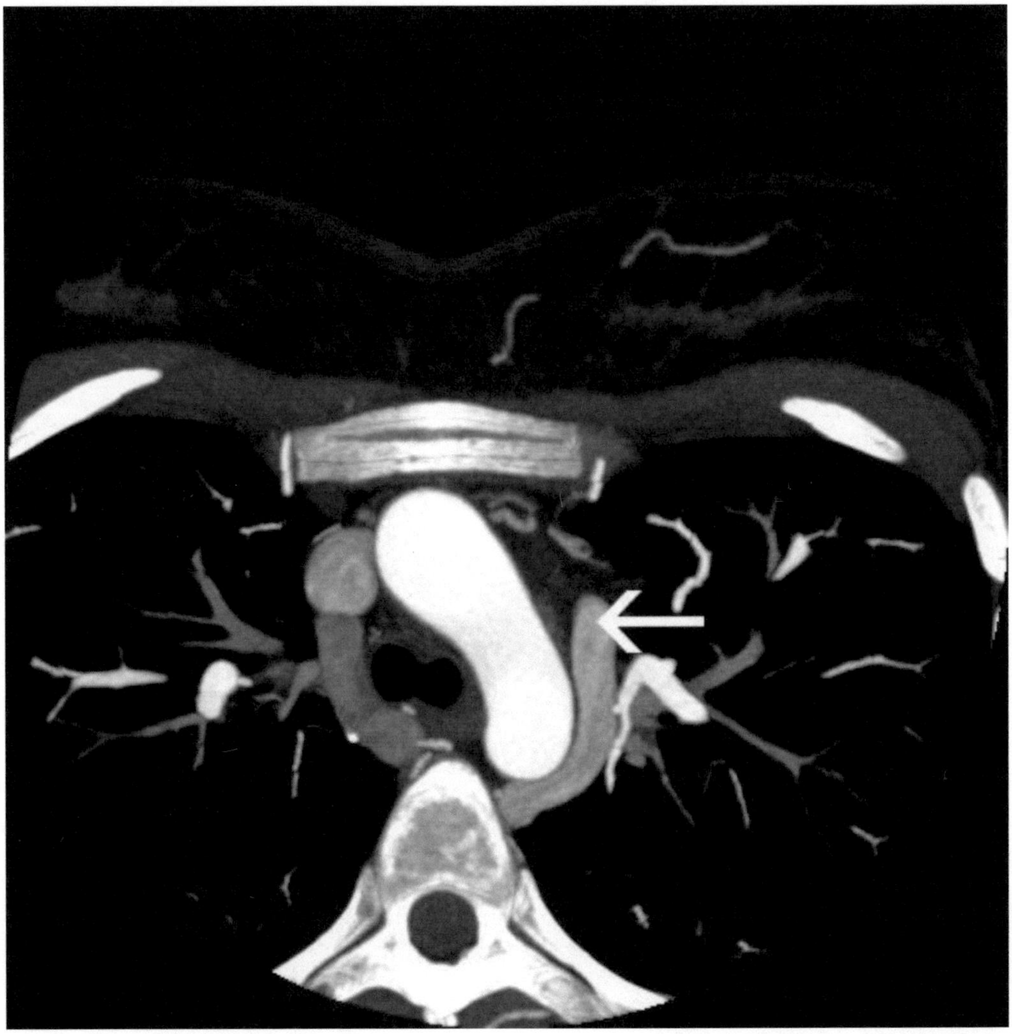

Fig. 12. Axial MIP reconstruction presents widening of accessory hemiazygos vein in a patients with absence of confluence of brachioceplaic trunks. Arrow indicates anomalous connection of left brahiocephalic trunk with accessory hemiazygos vein.

Both anomalies may be isolated and their frequency in general population is less then 0,3%. More often they are concomitant to other cardiovascular defects appearing up to 2% of these individuals. Typically, they are related with polysplenia-heterotaxy syndrome (Bronshtein et al., 2010), Figure 13.

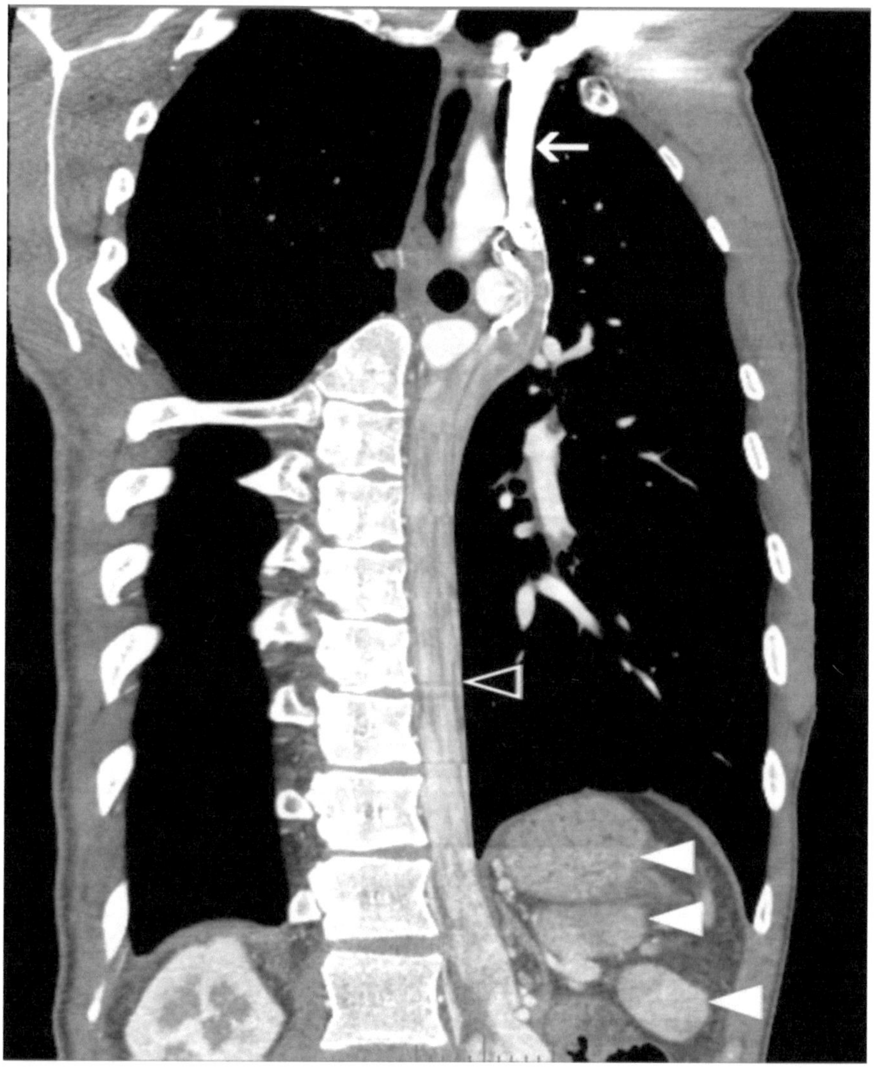

Fig. 13. Multiplanar curved line reformation of thoracic CT examination in a patient with heterotaxy-polysplenia syndrome. Arrow - PLSVC, blank arrowhead - hemiazygos vein, arrowheads - multiple spleens.

4.3 Coronary sinus anomalies and coronary veins variants

Three systems of cardiac veins should be distinguished (von Lüdinghausen, 1987): tributaries of the coronary sinus, anterior cardiac veins and atrial cardiac veins. In morphological study of 350 dissected human hearts (von Lüdinghausen, 1987), it was observed, that in over a half of cases, coronary sinus collects blood from cardiac veins except for anterior cardiac veins, including small cardiac vein, which drain into the right atrium independent of the coronary sinus. In 21% of cases, all veins of the cardiac ventricles open into the right atrium via coronary sinus. Ostial valve of the coronary sinus (Thebesian valve) was observed by von Lüdinghausen in 80% of specimens, and almost in half of the cases it was large. Such arrangement should be considered as a possible cause of problems with catheterization of the coronary sinus. In patients with narrowing or hypotrophy of coronary sinus ostium (Figure 14), accessory communications of cardiac veins can be visualized.

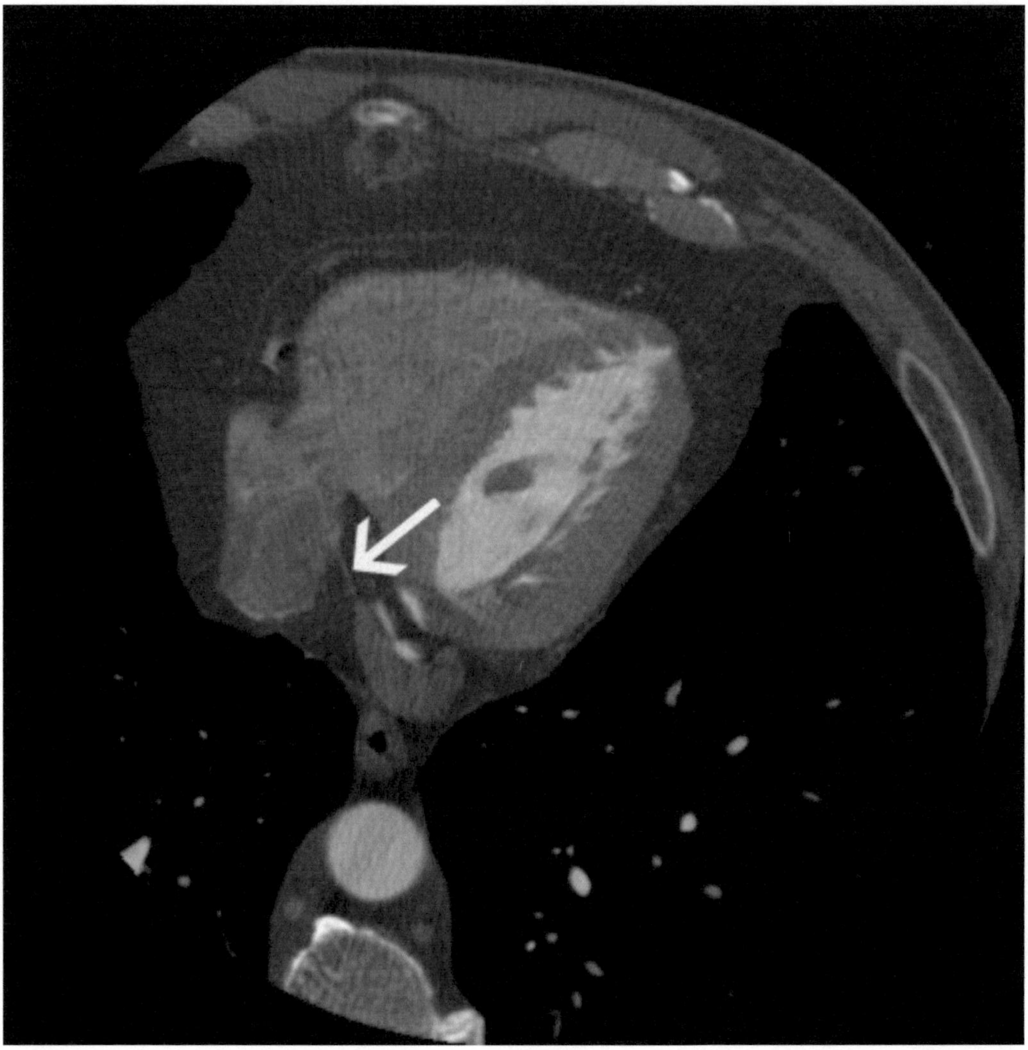

Fig. 14. Axial scan, CT. Narrowing of coronary sinus (arrow) ostium.

Figure 15 presents opening of great cardiac vein into SVC. Occasionally, anomalous communications of cardiac veins are seen, with L-R shunt between great cardiac vein and pulmonary veins (Figure 16).

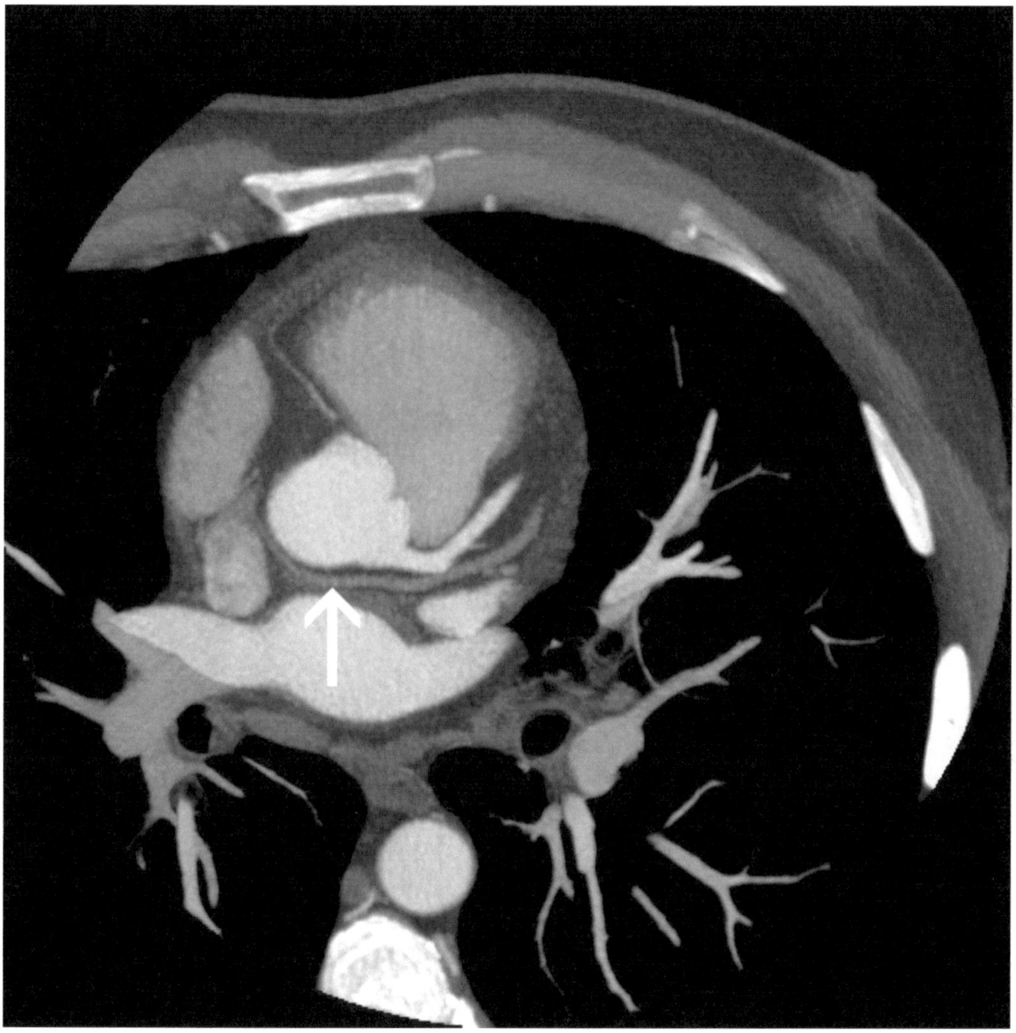

Fig. 15. Axial scan, maximum intensity projection. Anomalous course of great cardiac vein (arrow) with its opening into SVC.

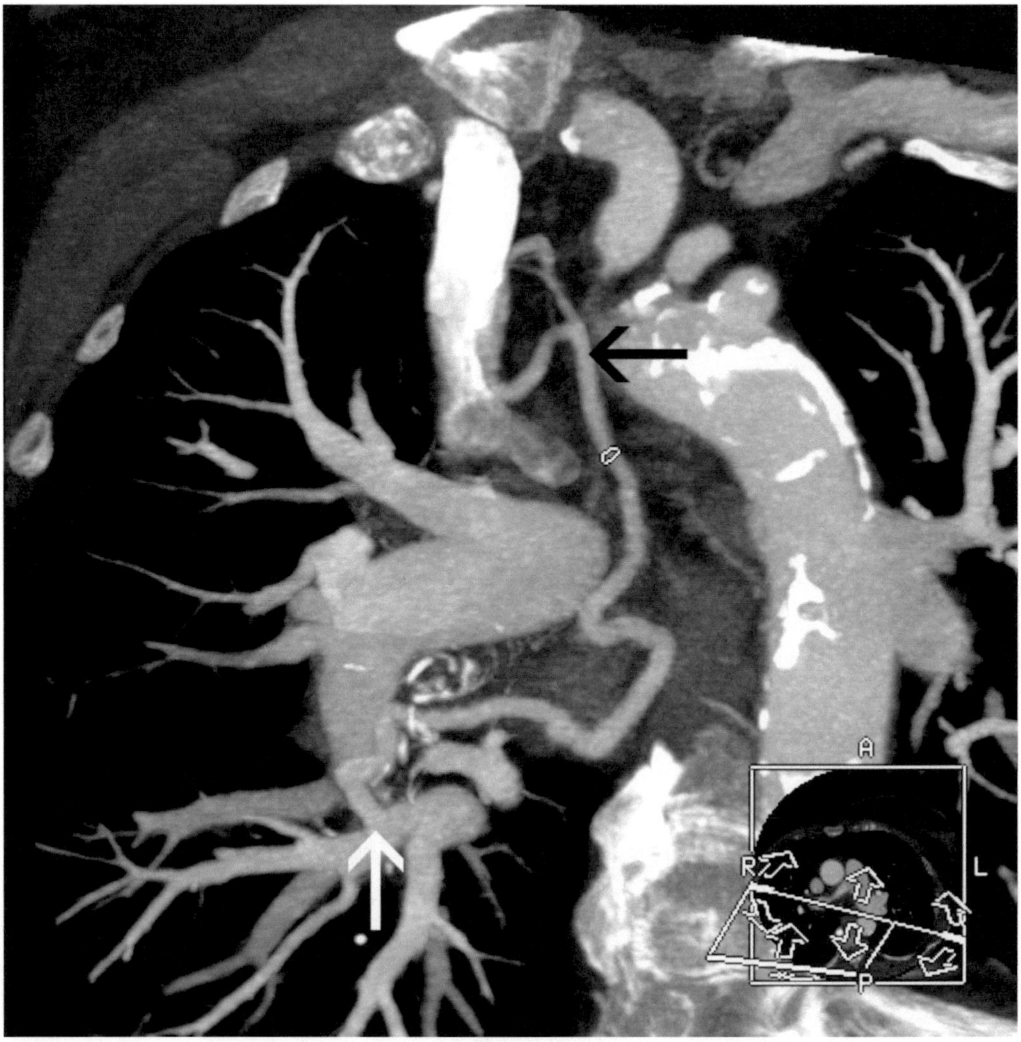

Fig. 16. Curved multiplanar reformation. L-R shunt between right inferior pulmonary vein (white arrow) and SVC via cardiac veins (black arrow)

4.4 Pulmonary veins anomalies

As lungs are initially drained by a vascular plexus with multiple connections with cardinal veins, persistence of these connections may produce a persistent communication with systemic veins and formation of anomalous pulmonary venous return (APVR) (Moore, 1973). Typical formation of the left atrium involves formation of four separate pulmonary veins, however, disturbed regression of primitive pulmonary vein may produce accessory pulmonary veins, Figure 17, Figure 18.

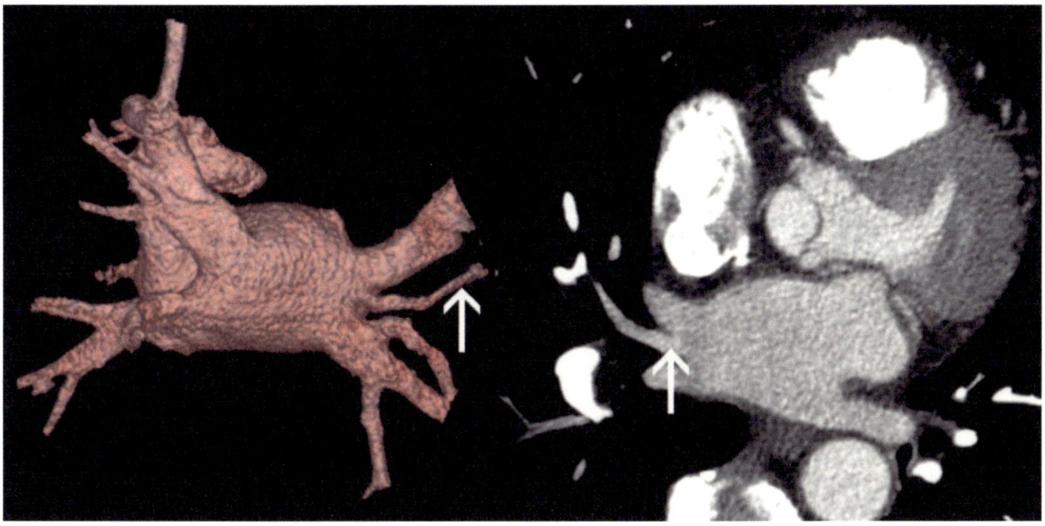

Fig. 17. Accessory middle right pulmonary vein (arrow) seen at volumetric reconstruction and axial scan.

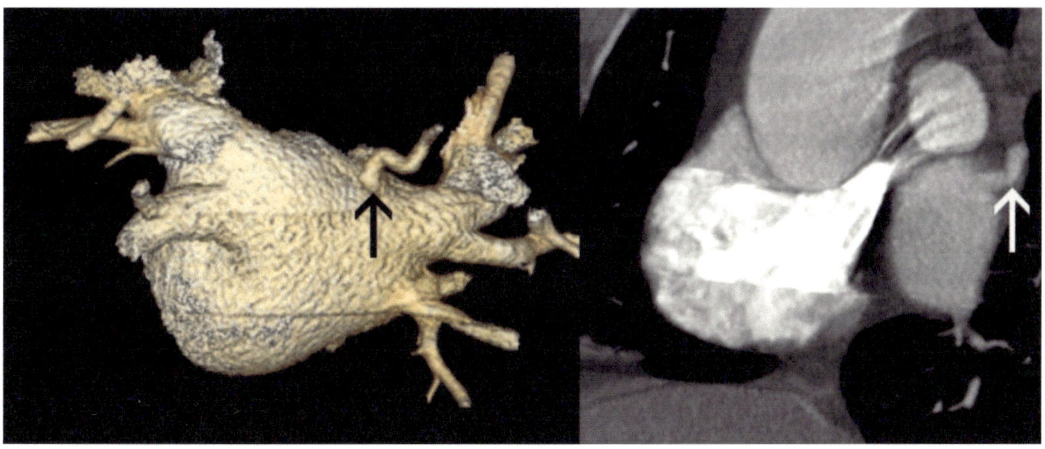

Fig. 18. Accessory posterior right pulmonary vein (arrow) seen at volumetric reconstruction and sagittal view.

Single pulmonary veins are a rare anomaly. Rey et al. (1986) reported group of patients with anomalous unilateral single pulmonary vein, which most frequently occurred on the right side, as in presented case (Figure 19). Bilateral single pulmonary veins are rarely reported, e.g. by Hidvegi and Lapin (1998).

Anomalous pulmonary venous return (APVR) may occur in the total or partial forms. Total anomalous pulmonary venous return is a more severe form of this anomaly, where all pulmonary veins drain outside of the left atrium, and are directed into right atrium via anomalous connections. TAPVR may produce severe symptoms, including cyanosis, difficulty breathing, low blood pressure and acidosis. Signs and symptoms are less severe in partial anomalous pulmonary venous return (PAPVR), which is an anomalous connection of some of pulmonary veins into systemic circulation. PAPVR constitutes for about 1-2% of congenital heart malformations. It occurs in almost all cases of sinus venosus type of ASD and about 15% of ASD II.

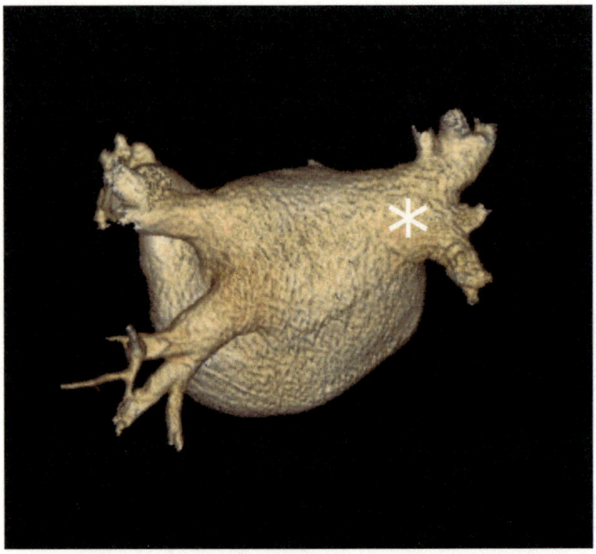

Fig. 19. Single pulmonary vein. Volumetric reconstruction, posterior view.

In right-sided PAPVR, anomalous drainage may carry blood from the right pulmonary vein into SVC, right atrium, inferior vena cava or infradiaphragmatic veins. When accompanied by hypoplastic right lung, it produces typical „scimitar syndrome". Left sided PAPVR involves drainage via persistent vertical vein. In our retrospective review of 1840 cardiac CT examinations, we observed PAPVR in 23 cases. Right-sided PAPVR produced communication with SVC in 13 cases (Figure 20), right atrium - 3 cases (Figure 21) and into IVC (scimitar syndrome) in 1 case (Figure 22). Left-sided PAPVR involved 5 cases of pulmonary drainage into left brachiocephalic vein via vertical vein.

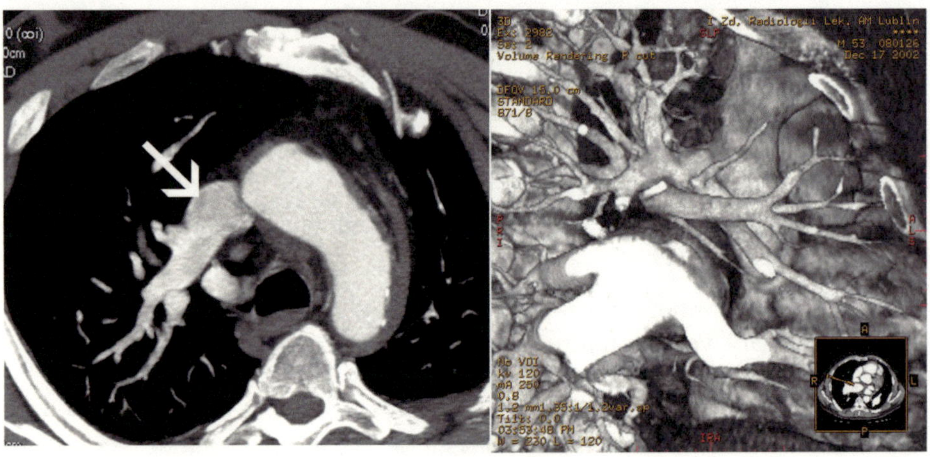

Fig. 20. PAPVR. Arrow indicates opening of pulmonary vein into SVC.

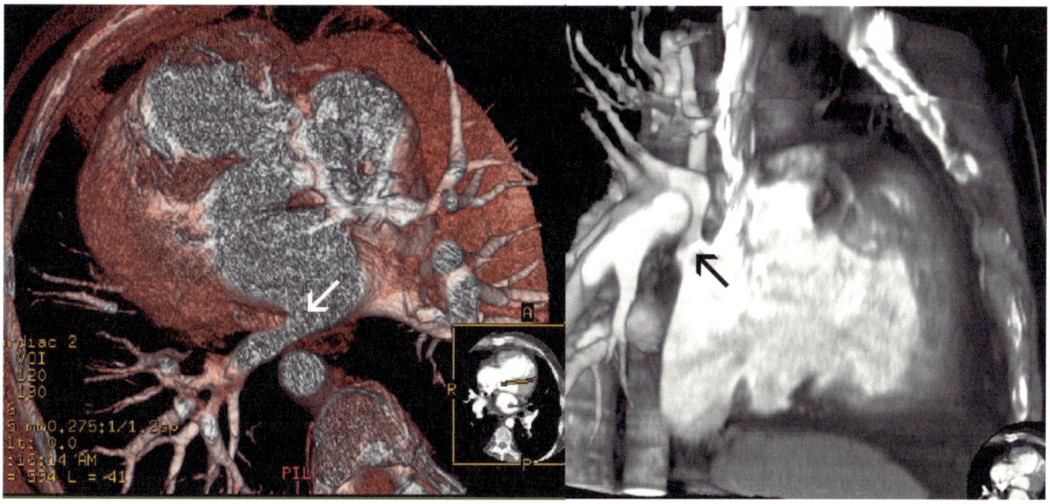

Fig. 21. PAPVR. Arrows indicate opening of pulmonary vein into right atrium

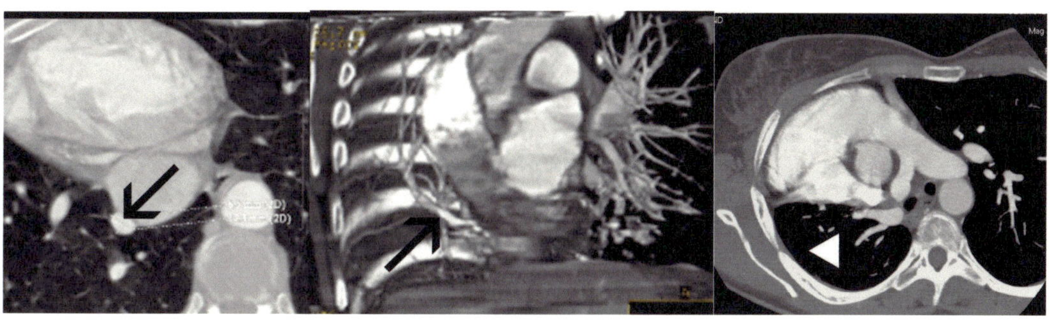

Fig. 22. Scimitar syndrome. Arrows indicate pulmonary vein draining hypoplastic right lung (arrowhead) into IVC.

5. References

Anagnostopoulos P.V., Pearl J.M., Octave C., Cohen M., Gruessner A., Wintering E., Teodori M.F. (2009) Improved current era outcomes in patients with heterotaxy syndromes. *Eur J Cardiothorac Surg*; 35: 871-7; discussion 877-8.

Ardilouze P., Bricot V., Maurel C., Christiaens L. (2009) A rare case of left superior vena cava draining into left atrium demonstrated by MDCT. *Int J Cardiol*; 131: e65-6.

Arslan G., Cubuk M., Ozkaynak C., Sindel T., Luleci E. (2000) Absence of the azygos vein. *Clin Imaging*; 24: 157-158.

Biffi M., Boriani G., Frabetti L., Bronzetti G., Branzi A. (2001) Left superior vena cava persistence in patients undergoing pacemaker or cardioverter-defibrillator implantation: a 10-year experience. *Chest*; 120: 139-144.

Bronshtein M., Khatib N., Blumenfeld Z. (2010) Prenatal diagnosis and outcome of isolated interrupted inferior vena cava. *Am J Obstet Gynecol*; 202: 398.e1-398.e4.

Caceres J., Mata J.M., Andreu J. (1998) The azygos lobe: normal variants that may simulate disease. *Eur J Radiol*; 27: 15-20.

Demos T.C., Posniak H.V., Pierce K.L., Olson M.C., Muscato M. (2004) Venous anomalies of the thorax. *AJR Am J Roentgenol*; 182: 1139-1150.
Dudek R.W., Fix J.D. (2004) Embryology, Lippincott Williams & Wilkins
Enright T.R., Kanne J.P. (2010) Saccular superior vena cava aneurysm - incidental diagnosis by MDCT. *Clin Radiol*; 65: 421-422.
Fang C.C., Jao Y.T., Han S.C., Wang S.P. (2007) Persistent left superior vena cava: multi-slice CT images and report of a case. *Int J Cardiol*; 121: 112-114.
Fasouliotis S.J., Achiron R., Kivilevitch Z., Yagel S. (2002) The human fetal venous system: normal embryologic, anatomic, and physiologic characteristics and developmental abnormalities. *J Ultrasound Med*; 21: 1145-1158.
Hidvegi R.S., Lapin J. (1998) Anomalous bilateral single pulmonary vein demonstrated by 3-dimensional reconstruction of helical computed tomographic angiography: case report. *Can Assoc Radiol J*;49:262 -265.
Ho V.B., Bakalov V.K., Cooley M., Van P.L., Hood M.N., Burklow T.R., Bondy C.A. (2004) Major vascular anomalies in Turner syndrome: prevalence and magnetic resonance angiographic features. *Circulation*; 110: 1694-1700.
Horlitz M., Schley P., Thiel A., Shin D.I., Müller M., Klein R.M., Gülker H. (2006) Wolff-Parkinson-White syndrome associated with persistent left superior vena cava. *Clin Res Cardiol*; 95: 133-135.
von Lüdinghausen M. (1987) Clinical anatomy of cardiac veins, Vv. cardiacae. *Surg Radiol Anat*;9(2):159-68.
Moore K.L. (1973) The developing human (clinically oriented embryology). Philadelphia, Pa: Saunders.
Morgan D.R., Hanratty C.G., Dixon L.J., Trimble M., O'Keeffe D.B. (2002) Anomalies of cardiac venous drainage associated with abnormalities of cardiac conduction system. *Europace*; 4: 281-287.
Ratliff H.L., Yousufuddin M., Lieving W.R., Watson B.E., Malas A., Rosencrance G, McCowan RJ. (2006) Persistent left superior vena cava: case reports and clinical implications. *Int J Cardiol*; 113: 242-246.
Rey C., Vaksmann G., Francart C. (1986) Anomalous unilateral single pulmonary vein mimicking partial anomalous pulmonary venous return. *Cathet Cardiovasc Diagn*; 12:330 -333
Tak T., Crouch E., Drake G.B. (2002) Persistent left superior vena cava: incidence, significance and clinical correlates. *Int J Cardiol*; 82: 91-93.
Varma P.K., Dharan B.S., Ramachandran P., Neelakandhan K.S. (2003) Superior vena caval aneurysm. *Interact Cardiovasc Thorac Surg*; 2: 331-333.

6

Hox Genes: Master Regulators of the Animal Bodyplan

A.J. Durston
Institute of Biology, Sylvius Laboratory, Wassenaarseweg, Leiden, The Netherlands

1. Introduction

Typical vertebrates- like dogs and cats and fish - usually have their head-tail body axis parallel to the ground. The head is at the front end and the tail at the back. All limbs (legs or fins) are used for locomotion. In this configuration, we know the head- tail axis as the anteroposterior (main) axis. The upper side of the animal is called its dorsal side and the lower side its ventral side. In humans, the anteroposterior axis is held upright. Only the hind limbs are used for walking. Your front is your ventral side and your back your dorsal side. We use the terminology for a typical vertebrate in the sections that follow.

During embryonic development, a developing animal is built by a hierarchy of genes. These include effector genes, encoding building blocks of the embryo- like muscle actin and keratin. They also include developmental control genes, which control the expression or action of other genes. These can be genes encoding proteins controlling the genesis, secretion or transduction of intercellular signals or genes encoding proteins controlling transcription or translation or protein action. Such developmental control genes regulate each other and may be organised in very large hierarchies. Hox genes are developmental control genes.

2. Discovery and cloning of the *Hox* genes, their role and regulation in *Drosophila*

Hox genes were first discovered as homeotic genes in the fruitfly *Drosophila*. They are sometimes referred to as: homeotic selector genes or: *HOMC* genes. They are characterised by the fact that a gain or loss of function mutation in a typical *Hox* gene can result in conversion of one large or small part of the main body axis to another. These are clearly developmental control genes acting high up in the hierarchy. In the case of the *Hox* genes, the conversions take place between different parts of the anteroposterior axis. One famous example is: *Bithorax*, discovered by Nobel prize winner Ed Lewis, which makes a four winged fly in its loss of function format. *Drosophila* normally has only two wings, on the mid thorax. The posterior thorax has vestigial 'halteres' . *Bithorax* is a gene for posterior thorax which converts this to mid thorax by loss of function (Lewis, 1978, 1995). In another equally famous example, discovered by Walter Gehring, *Antennapedia*, a gene for mid thorax converts part of the fly's head to mid thorax and therefore antennae to legs by misregulated gain of function (Carrasco et al., 1984) Vertebrate *Hox* genes similarly have drastic phenotypes but loss of function phenotypes are more difficult to visualise because each vertebrate *Hox* function is mediated by multiple *Hox* genes and these must all be knocked out. See Fig. 1.

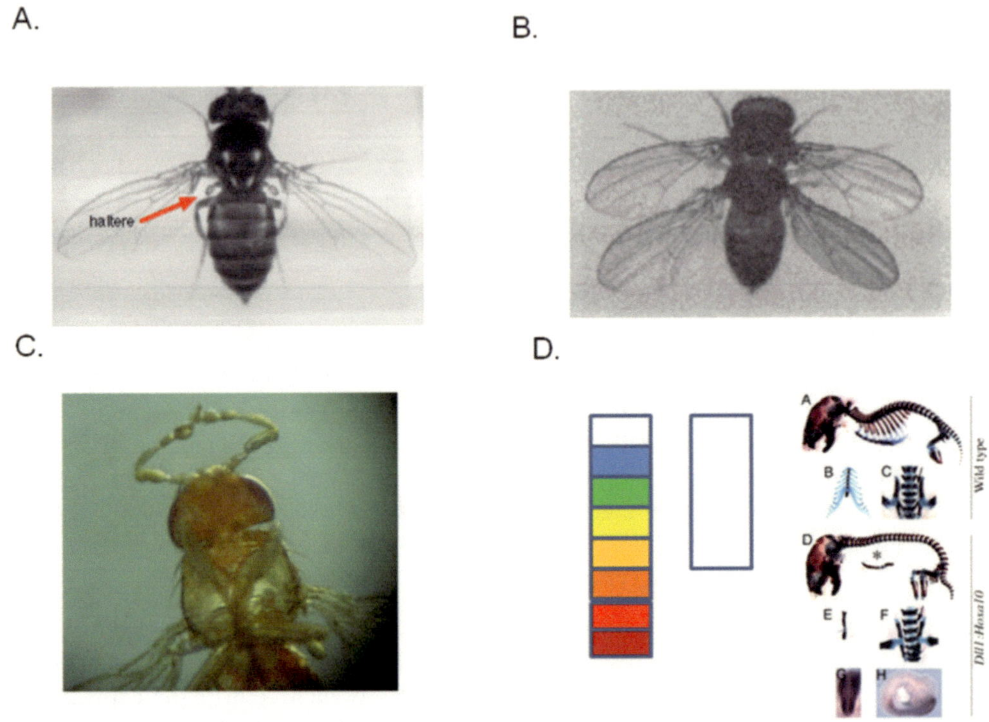

Fig. 1. **Hox gene phenotypes**
The function of Hox genes is indicated by gain and loss of function phenotypes. The figure shows this in Drosophila and vertebrates. A. A wild type Drosophila fly This has two wings on the anterior thorax and two halteres (red arrow) on the posterior thorax. B. A four winged fly, caused by a loss of function mutation in ultrabithorax, a gene for posterior thorax (Lewis, 1995). The halteres are transformed to wings. C Antennapedia mutation: anterior thoracic legs replace antennae on the head, due to a misregulated gain of function mutation for the gene Antennapedia (a gene for anterior thorax), leading to its expression in the head segments (Gehring, 1987). D. In vertebrates, mouse genetics has been bedevilled by the fact that there are 4 Hox clusters, with parallel functions. This once led to the erroneous idea that vertebrate Hox loss of function mutations have mild phenotypes. In fact, if you knock out all of the paralogues of a particular Hox paralogue group (pg), or ectopically express a Hox gene this can give a dramatic phenotype. Left: wild type Xenopus hindbrain. This has 8 segments (rhombomeres) 2-8 each express a different combination of Hox genes and so have different identities, indicated by the different colours. 1 (white) expresses no Hox genes. Its identity is determined by the gene Gbx2. Middle: hindbrain in Xenopus where Hox pg1 has been knocked down using morpholinos. The hindbrain is drastically anteriorised to the identity of r1. It is also shorter (redrawn from McNulty et al., 2005). Right: Skeletons of two mice. Above: wild type. Below, a mouse ectopically expressing HoxC10. The HoxC10 mouse is drastically different. For example, it lacks ribs (Carapuco et al., 2005). The thoracic vertebrae are posteriorised to abdominal identity. This is because Hox pg10 controls the transition from tthorax to abdomen, in the vertebral column.

These genes typically determine the identity of individual *Drosophila* body segments or groups of adjacent segments. In the early 80's strategies were developed for cloning developmental control genes. The first genes cloned were the *hox* genes *Bithorax-* by Hogness and his colleagues (Bender et al., 1983) (and *Antennapedia-* by the Gehring group (Carrasco et al., 1984). This was possible because these transcription factor genes contain a large highly conserved region- the homeobox- which encodes a 60 amino acid DNA binding domain and can be picked up by homology screening. It has, in fact emerged that *Hox* genes encode a subfamily of transcription factors and that the homeobox and another conserved region, the haxapeptide, are important in determining their specificity.

3. *Hox* clustering and colinearity: The key property

A key property of *Hox* genes is that they are often clustered in complexes. *Hox* complexes are among the most remarkable regions of the genome.. A *Hox* complex usually consists of up to 9-13 closely related Hox genes arranged in tandem . These genes specify patterning along body axes in all bilateria (Gehring *et al.*, 2009, Duboule, 2007). Invertebrates have a single *Hox* complex, or dispersed *Hox* genes, but tetrapod vertebrates typically possess four similar *Hox* complexes (*HoxA–D*), located on different chromosomes (Duboule, 2007). (Fig. 2) The *Hox* complexes also contain 5 micro RNA (*miRNA*) genes intercalated at homologous positions (Pearson et al., 2005; Yekta *et al.*, 2004, 2008; Woltering and Durston, 2007; Ronshaugen et al., 2005).

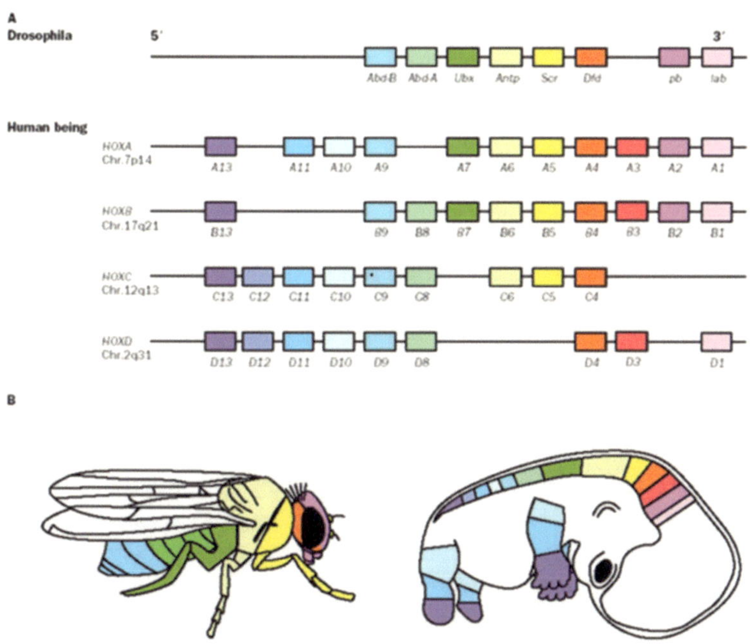

Fig. 2. **Hox Spatial and Functional Collinearity**
The four human and one Drosophila Hox complexes are homologues. The colour coding in Panels A and B shows the correspondence between the genomic order of Hox genes in the Hox complexes (A) and their spatial sequence of expression and action zones along the main body axis in Drosophila and human (B). From Goodman, 2003.

The 3′ to 5′ order of *Hox* genes along a chromosome corresponds to the order in which they act along body axes; this collinear property links clustering to function, emphasizing that *Hox* complexes are functional units or meta genes No one *Hox* gene can pattern an axis but a whole *Hox* cluster can. (Mainguy *et al.*, 2007, Duboule 2007). Hox collinearity is crucial in embryogenesis and includes 3 important and interrelated properties: functional colinearity describes the spatial order in which *Hox* genes act along a body axis; spatial colinearity refers to the spatial order in which the *Hox* genes are expressed, and temporal colinearity is the time sequence in which they are expressed (**Text Box 1**). The organization of *Hox* complexes is highly conserved, and *Hox* and *mir* genes not only have remained clustered through bilaterian evolution but are also in close proximity to each other despite their very complex and dynamic expression patterns. Individual *Hox* genes are also very highly conserved in Evolution.

Text box 1: ***Collinearity***

Collinearity describes the sequential expression of a genomic cluster of Hox genes along an embryonic axis and associated properties.

There are three important forms of collinearity: Spatial collinearity is the sequential 3′ to 5′ expression of Hox genes along a body axis. This occurs from anterior to posterior along the main body axis and also in other axes, for example from proximal to distal in developing limbs. Spatial colinearity can be associated with time dependence. The most 3′ gene is expressed first and more 5′ genes are expressed sequentially later. This is defined as temporal collinearity and, in early vertebrate development, spatial collinearity is generated from pre-existing temporal collinearity by time space translation. The gastrula's organiser interacts with Hox expressing non organiser mesoderm to translate a temporal sequence of Hox codes to a spatially collinear pattern. We also define a third property, functional collinearity- – which is the capacity of Hox genes to collinearly define region-specific structures along an axis.

Hox collinearity and the organisation of the *Hox* complexes are phenomena that have long fascinated developmental, molecular and evolutionary biologists. These phenomena represent an important example of genomic regulation. Understanding the structure and function of *Hox* genes is crucially important, because they are implicated in a growing number of diseases, including important cancers (Grier *et al.*, 2005). See also below.

Research and thinking on *Hox* collinearity has concentrated on three aspects. First, there is the question of how collinearity evolved, which is clearly one of the keys to understanding this phenomenon. Second, there are three mechanistic ideas. The first is that Hox spatial colinearity is secondary and due to an upstream hierarchy of spatially ordered genes. Hox collinearity is thus not utilised. The second is that collinearity is based on transcriptional regulation, and specifically that it is limited by the progressive 3′ to 5′ opening of *Hox* cluster chromatin and/or mediated by global control regions. The third model is that collinearity depends on interactions among the *Hox* genes themselves. These interactions include 'posterior prevalence', - a negative interaction among Hox proteins that clearly relates to functional collinearity in *Drosophila* (and possibly also to spatial and temporal collinearity; see **Text Box 1**).

In this article, we review the basis of *Hox* evolution and of the three longstanding mechanistic hypotheses to explain *Hox* gene collinearity. But we also propose a new explanation. Based on evidence from *Amphibian* and other vertebrate embryos, we reason that synchronised temporally collinear expression of the *Hox* complexes in early vertebrate embryos involves *trans*-acting factors and intercellular interactions. We review data implicating activating as well as repressive interactions among the *Hox* genes themselves, and timed signals from the somitogensis clock. This model provides a mechanistic link between the different aspects of collinearity. A review of potential collinearity mechanisms is now opportune because new data that have never been reviewed in the literature are now available and because the existing, entrenched models are limiting in the sense that they direct research in the same direction- that of chromatin opening and transcriptional control- and that they do not explain all of the facts (below). This has spurred us to interpret the data in a different light. The field gains a new perspective from this new synthesis of the data.

4. The evolution of *Hox* genes in different taxa, including vertebrates

Hox genes are available in all metazoans that have been studied. In all bilateria where there is information, they are concerned with patterning the main body axis. Invertebrates have one *Hox* gene complex: vertebrates have 4 or 8. The 4 *Hox* gene complexes typically present in most tetrapod vertebrates arose through 2 rounds of genome duplication during evolution. *Xenopus laevis* and teleost fishes have 8 *Hox* complexes because of 3 genome duplications. Even the individual *Hox* genes are strongly conserved in evolution throughout the animal kingdom (Carrasco et al., 1984; Gehring *et al.* 2009; Duboule 2007, DeRobertis, 2008) and are recognisable by having distinct conserved sequences. The *Hox* genes corresponding to the same position in each of the different vertebrate *Hox* complexes are conserved. They have very similar homeoboxes and hexapeptides and are called a paralogue group. *Hox* genes in invertebrates may be clustered and show collinearity or they may be scattered in the genome to various extents. Different extents of fragmentation, from atomised to fully clustered have been identified. The clustered format is thought to be ancestral.

Text box 2: ***An evolutionary explanation of collinearity***

It has been proposed that colinearity evolved by repeated tandem duplication of an ancestral ur-Hox gene and sequential evolutionary modifications of the duplicates, leading to generation of an organised gene array from an evolutionary ground state . This idea can conceivably explain how a genomic sequence could relate to a spatial or temporal sequence of gene expression. Please note that, if this is the explanation of collinearity, it is the explanation and obviates the need for an explicit collinearity mechanism involving interactions between or clustering of the Hox genes. The upstream mechanism for Hox expression will be whatever it evolved to be in order to regulate the spatially collinear localised expression of the individual Hox genes- as with the segmentation gene hierarchy in Drosophila. The spatially collinear axial expression pattern of the Drosophila Hox genes is thus secondary and determined by the spatially ordered expression patterns of the gap genes. Nonetheless, we think that explicit collinearity mechanisms evolved- see main text.

Evolution of *Hox* collinearity is particularly important because it can potentially offer an explanation of how collinear properties connect to *Hox* complex structure. The only other potential explanation for this comes from the chromatin opening model (below). It should be noted that whereas clustered *Hox* genes in organisms having *Hox* clusters show the normal spatially collinear sequence of *Hox* gene expression, so do *Hox* genes in fragmented clusters, from the split cluster seen in *Drosophila* to atomised *Hox* genes in organisms having no clustering- like *Oikopleura* (Duboule 2007, Seo *et.al.* 2004). These show 'trans collinearity' where the spatial sequence of expression of the Hox genes corresponds with their 3′ to 5′ genomic sequence in the ancestral cluster. It is thus clear that the spatial ordering of *Hox* gene expression does not rely soley on clustering. Presumably, *Hox* spatial collinearity evolved in an ancestral organism with clustered *Hox* genes and and persisted after cluster disintegration during evolution. This already demonstrates that *Hox* collinearity properties can persist in the absence *Hox* clustering and therefore of progressive chromatin opening. It has been proposed that a *Ho*x complex, whose function is to pattern an axis, acts as a meta gene or functional unit, where no one *Hox* gene can execute the whole function but the whole complex does (Mainguy *et al.*, 2007, Duboule, 2007). It has also been proposed that spatial collinearity has been a selective pressure that drives *Hox* clustering rather than vice versa. (Duboule 2007).

It has been proposed that *Hox* colinearity evolved by repeated tandem duplication of an ancestral ur-*Hox* gene and stepwise sequential evolutionary modifications of the duplicates, leading to generation of an organised gene array from an evolutionary ground state (Lewis 1978 1995; Gehring *et al.*,2009) (**Text Box 2, Fig.3A**). Lewis proposed that the modifications arose by unequal recombination between adjacent *Hox* genes. This idea can conceivably explain how a genomic sequence could generate ordered properties like spatial or temporal sequences of gene expression. Please note that, if this is the explanation of collinearity, it obviates any need for a dedicated collinearity mechanism. The upstream mechanism for *Hox* expression will be whatever it evolved to be in order to regulate the correctly localised expression of the individual *Hox* genes. This is the case with the gap-segmentation gene hierarchy in *Drosophila,* (see below). Nonetheless, we think that dedicated collinearity mechanisms evolved. Lewis showed that 5′ posterior drosophila *Hox* genes are epistatic to the *Hox* gene *Antennapedia.* If they are ectopically expressed in the normal *Antennapedia* domain, the most posterior *Hox* gene expressed dominates. If the most posterior *Hox* gene is deleted, the phenotype obtained is that of the most posterior *Hox* gene still expressed. And so on. This interaction was called posterior prevalence (below) and was thought by Lewis to reflect the fact that *Antennapedia* represents an ancestral ground state, while posterior *Hox* genes are derived from the ground state by tandem duplication and stepwise sequential modification (as above). It has been reported relatively recently by Gehring *et al.,* (2009) that the anterior *Drosophila Hox* genes have also evolved from the *Antennapedia* ancestral ground state and that these have developed anterior prevalence.

5. The mechanism of *Hox* collinearity

There are various ideas about this (Fig. 3).

1. In the section above, we have described the idea that collinear *Ho*x complexes arose by tandem duplication and sequential modification of an ancestral *ur-Hox* gene. In this case, no special mechanism is required to generate spatial collinearity. The

upstream mechanism for *Hox* expression will be whatever it evolved to be in order to regulate the correctly localised expression of the individual *Hox* genes. This is the case with the gap-segmentation gene hierarchy in *Drosophila* (Nuesslein- Volhard, 1995), where the spatial ordering of the *Hox* genes is secondary. The spatially expressed gap genes are the primary determinats of the spatially ordered *Hox* gene expression pattern (Kehle et al., 1998, Mito et al., 2006) . Later on, other genes, including the *Hox* genes themselves, the cofactor *teashirt*, polycomb group genes and segmentation genes play a role (Gebelein and Mann, 2007, Rusch and Kaufman, 2000 Mito et al., 2006) (Fig 3A, 3B).

2. The idea has developed in the mouse that temporal collinearity is due to progressive opening of *Hox* complex chromatin, from 3′ to 5′ (Fig 3C). (. This idea has become rather popular. There is some evidence for this (Soshnikova and Duboule 2009, Cambeyron and Bickmore, 2004, Van der Hoeven et al, 1996, Kmita et al., 2000) but the idea has limited application. It can not apply in animals with dispersed *Hox* genes that behave colinearly. It is not even the whole story in vertebrates, presumably including the mouse. Synchronised temporal colinearity between the different *Hox* complexes during gastrulation (Wacker et al., 2004, Durston et al., 2010, 2011) indicates the importance of trans acting factors and intercellular signals for temporal collinearity.
3. There is evidence that interactions between *Hox* genes are important. These can obviously not account for the relation between *Hox* complex structure and collinear properties but they are part of the story. Working in *D. melanogaster*, E. B. Lewis showed that loss-of-function mutations in posterior *Hox* genes drive the segmental phenotype towards that of the more anterior thoracic segment T2, which is determined by the *Hox* gene *Antennapedia* (Lewis, 1978, 1995). Struhl used *esc-Drosophila* embryos, which show constitutive activation of gene expression, in combination with *Hox* loss of function mutations to elucidate the functional hierarchy of *Drosophila Hox* genes (Struhl, 1983). All *Drosophila* segments were transformed to the phenotype of the most posterior functional *Hox* gene expressed. Posterior prevalence in *Drosophila* has been thought to underly functional collinearity only, not spatial collinearity. Experimentally derived ubiquitous expression of *Hox* genes under promoters that are known to be transcriptionally irrepressible leads to transformations only in regions anterior to the functional domain of the gene. For example, the thoracic *Antennapedia*, when ubiquitously expressed, suppresses Hox genes of the head, resulting in posterior transformation of head segments towards a thoracic identity while not affecting the abdomen – here, the effect of *Antp* is phenotypically suppressed by *bithorax*-complex genes such as *Ubx* (Gonzalez-Reyes *et al.*, 1990 Gibson and Gehring, 1988). However, posterior prevalence occurs not only postranslationally (Plaza et al., 2008) but also at the levels of transcription (Beachy et al., 1988, Hafen et al., 1984, Appel and Sakonju, 1993, Struhl and White, 1985) and posttranscriptional regulation of mRNA abundance (Yekta et al., 2004, 2008, Woltering and Durston, 2007, Ronshaugen et al.,2005) (Text box 3). It can thus also potentially regulate the mRNA expression of *Hox* genes. Namely, spatial and temporal collinearity. *Hox* interactions also occur during vertebrate gastrulation. These include posterior prevalence (Hooiveld et al, 1999, Woltering and Durston, 2007) but also 3′ to 5′ activation of *Hox* gene expression (McNulty et al, 2006, Hooiveld et al., 1999) See Fig. 3E, Fig. 5.

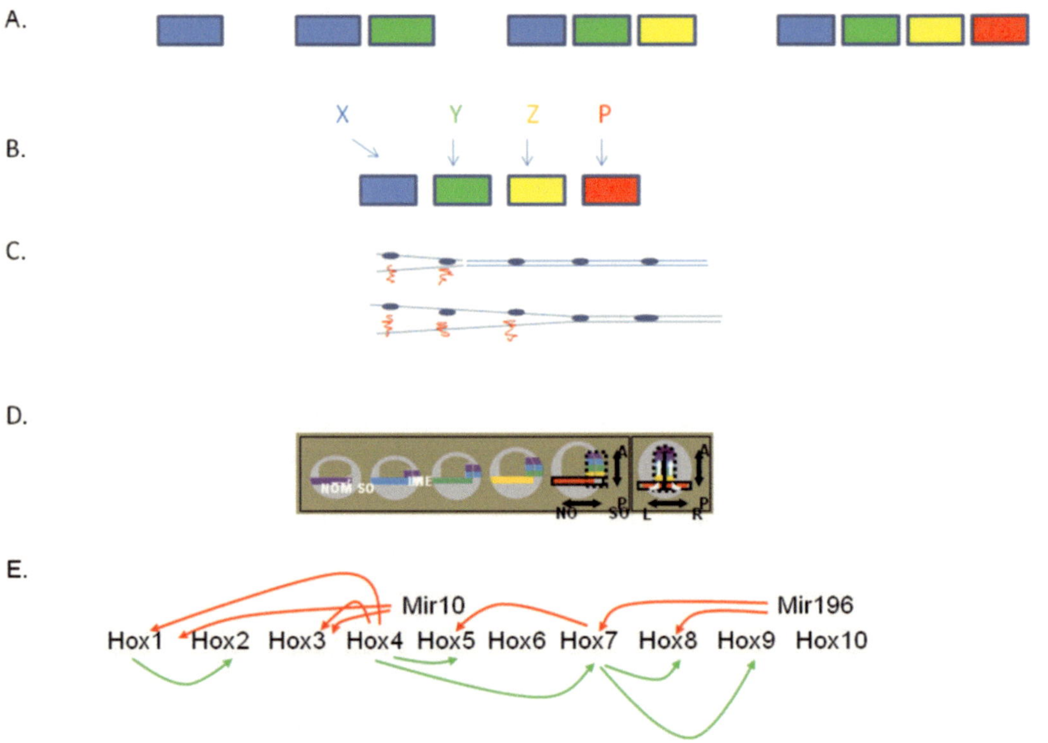

Fig. 3. **Some facts and ideas about Hox colinearity**
A. Tandem duplication and sequential modification. Clustered Hox genes are thought to have evolved by tandem duplication of an ancestral Ur-Hox gene. The duplicates are then thought to have been progressively modified, so they become more and more different from each other. The figure shows tandem duplication and progressive modification towards the right. The ur- Hox gene (left, blue) duplicates and the right hand daughter is modified (green). The green Hox gene duplicates again and its right hand daughter is modified (yellow). The yellow Hox gene duplicates again and its right hand daughter is modified (red). This type of mechanism can give collinear properties.
B. The associated upstream mechanism needed to generate spatial collinearity. If such a Hox cluster is to generate spatial colinearity without an explicit colinearity mechanism, an individual input is needed to turn on each Hox gene to ensure it is expressed at exactly the right axial position. The inputs concerned are going to need an axial pattern themselves. This kind of mechanism is used in Drosophila, where the gap genes provide the inputs. Gap genes specify the primary axial positions where the Hox genes are expressed and segmentation genes, the Hox genes themselves, polycomb group genes and cofactors like teashirt refine this information, restricting Hox expression by specific segment boundaries. In this situation, the Hox genes thus do not provide the primary axial patterning information. They are secondary. It is likely that this kind of mechanism is general in invertebrates, which probably have no temporal colinearity or colinearity mechanism and have had to evolve an ad hoc mechanism to generate spatial collinearity. Something like this may also occur in the vertebrate hindbrain, where the gastrula's colinearity mechanism is presumably the primary patterning mechanism and hindbrain genes confirm or alter the patterning information.
C. Progressive chromatin opening: the basic idea. This is an idea proposed by Duboule and colleagues to account for vertebrate temporal collinearity. The Hox complex chromatin opens from 3′ to 5′. This opening progressively permits Hox gene transcription, from 3′ to 5′.

D. Time- space translation. Vertebrates show early Hox collinearity. There is a temporally collinear sequence of Hox gene expression in the gastrula. This is used to generate a spatially collinear axial sequence of Hox gene expression. For details, see Fig. 4.
E. Hox interactions.What regulates vertebrate temporal collinearity? Not just chromatin opening, as proposed by Duboule. The different vertebrate Hox clusters are expressed with synchronous temporal collinearity. What may be involved are interactions between different Hox genes. The figure shows some interactions between Hox genes in the vertebrate gastrula.

Text box 3: ***The Level Of Action***

All effects above on activation or repression of Hox genes during gastrulation result in more or less Hox mRNA.but not all act on transcription. Recent evidence shows that Hox complex mRNA availability is strongly regulated posttranscriptionally, involving such phenomena as polycistronic transcripts, sense/ antisense transcript interactions and alternative splicing. At least one early vertebrate Hox interaction; downregulation of more 3′ Hox mRNA's by Hoxb4 is micro RNA mediated (posttranscriptional). We note that the important parameter for colinearity is the sum total of the (activating and repressing) inputs on each Hox gene (there may be many). We think it very significant that posterior prevalence (pp) acts at 3 different levels. If a Hox gene is activated transcriptionally, its mRNA can still be destabilised by pp miR action. If the Hox protein is made, it can still be inactivated by pp protein-protein interactions. We think that pp is the most important Hox-Hox colinearity interaction and that it needs to be dominant, to ensure the 3′ to 5′ directionality of colinearity

6. *Hox* function in vertebrates

Hox genes have several different roles in development

Vertebrates are unique in being the only type of metazoan animals in which the ancestral *Hox* cluster has been duplicated due to genome duplications. In most tetrapod vertebrates, there are four *Hox* clusters, on different chromosomes, presumably due to 2 genome duplications. Teleost fish have 8 clusters, due to 3 genome duplications.

6.1 *Hox* genes in the developing CNS and hindbrain

There is much evidence that *Hox* genes are important in early anteroposterior patterning of the vertebrate central nervous system. There is an approximately spatially collinear sequence of *Hox* expression in the early neural plate and neural tube. Anterior boundaries for expression of different *Hox* genes distinguish between different parts of the developing CNS- for example, some boundaries distinguish between the different segments in the hindbrain. Much work has been done to characterise the regulatory gene networks that regulate *Hox* expression and *Hox* function in the developing CNS, particularly those that pattern the developing hindbrain: a segmented structure. These networks do not appear to contain any mechanism that mediates collinearity, which is presumably set up earlier in the mesoderm and transferred to the developing CNS. (see below). The hindbrain regulators seem to maintain this early pattern or alter it. They have an ad hoc nature, as do the upstream regulators in *Drosophila*. They do not necessarily maintain spatial collinearity. For example, the primary *Hoxb1* expression domain is at a non collinear position. This work has been reviewed extensively in recent review articles (Wright, 1993, Krumlauf, 1994, Tumpel et al., 2009, Schneider-Manoury et al., 1998) and will not be discussed further here. The role of *Hox* genes in patterning the developing vertebrate CNS is limited to the hindbrain and spinal cord. The fore- and mid- brain are patterned by other regulators, including the *Otx* and *Emx* gene families (Cecchi et al., 2000) . The patterning of the anterior CNS by these gene families is actually conserved in *Drosophila,* but the anterior CNS region where they act here is very small, compared with the vertebrate forebrain.

6.2 *Hox* genes in axial mesoderm

Besides specifying A-P levels early on, in the developing central nervous system, *Hox* genes specify A-P levels in mesoderm. We are talking here about the axial and paraxial mesoderm. *Hox* genes are expressed in and specify A-P levels in, the presomitic and somitic mesoderm and the lateral plate mesoderm. *Hox* genes are not expressed in and do not specify A-P levels in the early notochord, which is derived from the *Hox*-negative organiser mesoderm in the gastrula. *Hox* patterning of axial mesoderm is covered by excellent recent reviews (Carapuco et al.,2005, Burke et al., 1995). We will not discuss it further here, except for one aspect (below).

The expression of *Hox* genes in the presomitic and somitic mesoderm is interesting because it correlates with the process of somitogenesis, the primary process of segmentation in the early vertebrate embryo, which occurs in this mesoderm. Vertebrate somitogenesis (segmentation of axial mesoderm) works via a mechanism where an oscillating system of gene expression generates a spatial pattern by time–space translation, just as in genesis of the vertebrate axial *Hox* pattern (see below and text box 1). The temporal oscillation in gene expression (somitogenesis clock) generates spatially periodic segments in the axial mesoderm: the somites (Palmeirim *et al.*, 1997). This is closely linked to collinear *Hox* expression. *Hox* spatial expression boundaries coincide with somite/segment boundaries and several vertebrate somitogenesis genes are known to regulate *Hox* expression (Peres *et al.,* 2006; Dubrulle *et al.*, 2001, Dubrulle and Pourquie, 2004, Zakany *et al.*, 2001).

6.3 *Hox* genes in gastrulation

Hox genes are expressed earlier in development than in the developing central nervous system and axial mesoderm. This is interesting because the *Hox* genes set up the primary axial pattern during these early stages. The *Hox* genes are already expressed during gastrulation. For example, in the non-organiser mesoderm (NOM) of the *Xenopus laevis* gastrula, where *Hox* genes are first expressed in the embryo and are expressed with temporal colinearity (Fig.4a). This mesoderm manifests a sharply timed temporally collinear sequence of *Hox* gene expression that is translated in time and space by interactions with the Spemann organiser (SO) to to generate a spatially collinear pattern of *Hox* gene expression along the main body axis of the organism (Wacker et al., 2004a; Durston et al., 2010, 2011) The mechanism for this is shown in Figure 4b. .In short, the temporal sequence of *Hox* gene expression in the mesoderm is sequentially frozen, from anterior to posterior and is transferred to the developing neural plate, which overlies the internalising mesoderm, in the gastrula. (Text Box 1, Fig. 4a,b).

A.

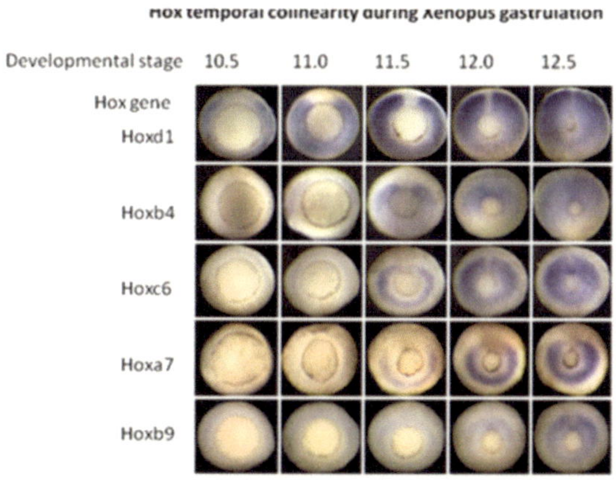

B.

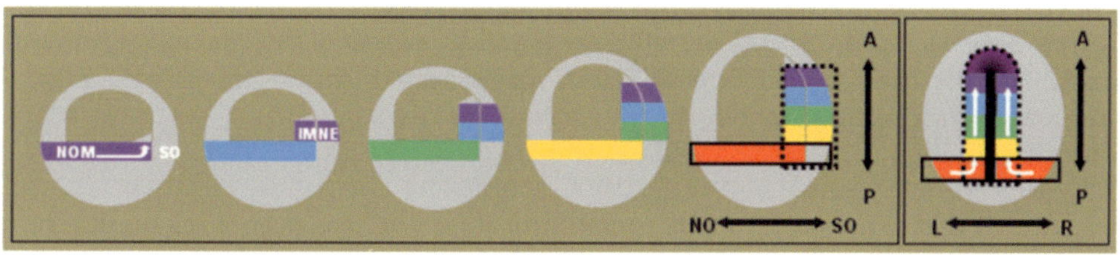

Fig. 4. **Temporal Collinearity AndTime space translation.**

A. Temporal Collinearity In the Xenopus Gastrula

The figure shows Hox expression patterns at sequential stages during gastrulation in Xenopus. From Wacker et al., 2004. The embryos are seen from underneath, where a ring (the blastopore) shows the position where mesoderm tissue invaginates during gastrulation. This ring gets smaller as gastrulation proceeds and the upper tissues in the embryo spread out and cover the lower part of the embryo (epiboly).The expression of several different Hox genes, seen as blue colour by in situ hybridisation, is in each case initially in the gastrula mesoderm in the zone above (outside) the ring. Hox expression is thus seen as a blue ring, and since it is initially only in part of the mesoderm (non organiser nesoderm), the ring is initially broken. This ring of Hox expression gets smaller as the blatopore ring gets smaller and mesoderm invaginates into the embryo.The figure shows expression of a sequence of Hox genes with different paralogue numbers, from 1 to 9. It will be seen that the Hox gene with the lowest paralogue number starts expression first and later numbers start sequentially later. It will also be seen that the Hox genes in this time sequence include members of all of the 4 primary vertebrate paralogue groups (a,b,c,d).

B. Time-space translation

Timed interactions between the Hox expressing non-organiser mesoderm and the Spemann organiser generate positional information during vertebrate gastrulation (Wacker et al., 2004). The drawings show simplified 2-dimensional representations of Xenopus gastrulae. The first 5 drawings show parasagittal (ventral to dorsal) two dimensional representations of gastrula profiles, starting at the beginning of gastrulation and then at sequential stages till the end. The last (6th.) drawing shows the end of gastrulation, from the dorsal side (profile at the level of the dorsal axial mesoderm). Hox expressing tissue (NOM (NO and I) and, late in gastrulation neurectoderm (N)) is represented by different colours, each of which represents a different hox code. Initially, the coloured bar represents the broken ring of NOM in the wall of the embryo. The later internal coloured blocks at the dorsal side of the embryo represent the involuted NOM mesoderm. The coloured blocks next to them in the wall of the embryo represent the overlying neurectoderm, which also comes to express hox genes. Hox expression is copied from the gastrula mesoderm to the neurectoderm. The SO is shown only in the last drawing, as the heavy median black line. By this stage, it has become the notochord and a head mesodermal portion. The first 5 drawings represent paraxial profiles, where the organiser is not available. The black dotted line in the last drawing depicts the sphere of influence of the SO. N: neurectoderm, NO: non-organiser mesoderm; S,: Spemann organiser; A: Anterior; P: Posterior; L: Left; R: Right. N nonorganiser; S Spemann organiser. The white arrows reflect directions of cell movement flow. To dorsal, anterior and internal(drawings 1 and 6). -There is a collinear time sequence of hox expression in non involuted non-organiser mesoderm (NOM) in the gastrula (depicted by the spectral sequence of colours). -During gastrulation involution movements continuously bring cells from the NOM into the inside of the embryo See stack of blocks of different colours, reflecting a history of the collinear hox mesodermal time sequence, in the internal involuted mesoderm. -Stable (ectodermal) Hox expression is induced by a combination of signals from the SO and the Hox expressing NOM. See corresponding blocks of sequential spectral colours in the gastrula's mesoderm and outer layer, reflecting a vertical transfer of the Hox codes from involuted mesoderm to overlying neurectoderm. A "Hox stripe" as part of the anterior–posterior Hox pattern is thus formed at the dorsal side.

A striking feature of the *Xenopus* gastrula mesoderm's temporally collinear *Hox* expression sequence is that expression of *Hox* genes from different *Hox* complexes occurs in the same perfectly temporally collinear sequence (Fig. 4A). The temporal collinearity of the different *Hox* complexes is therefore synchronised (Wacker et al., 2004a; Durston et al., 2010, 2011) . The different *Hox* paralogues (ie the different copies of each different Hox gene type, produced by the vertebrate genome duplications) in the different complexes are on different chromosomes, ruling out that *Hox* colinearity simply reflects cis-localised progressive opening of *Hox* complex chromatin for transcription. Trans acting signals are clearly needed to synchronise the different *Hox* complexes and, since we are dealing with a cell mass rather than a single cell, intercellular signals are also required. We note that these *trans*-acting factors and intercellular signals must be very sharply timed to enable synchronisation of the different *Hox* complexes and are probably timed to trigger expression of different *Hox* genes at different times. This conclusion was not a complete surprise. It is known that trans acting factors must mediate collinearity in organisms with dispersed Hox genes. This is, however, the first evidence that vertebrate temporal collinearity is also mediated by trans acting factors.

The involvement of trans acting factors and intercellular signals has been investigated and three sectors of the regulatory gene hierarchy have become interesting.

1. There is evidence that the *Hox* genes themselves are involved, via *Hox-Hox* interactions including posterior prevalence and via interactions involving micro RNA's. These interactions drive initiation of *H*ox complex expression as well as progression of temporally collinear expression through the *Hox* complexes (Hooiveld et al., 1999, Woltering and Durston, 2008, McNulty et al., 2005) (Fig. 5A). There is much evidence that *Hox* genes in vertebrates and *Drosophila* show activating as well as repressive interactions, including posterior prevalence McNulty *et al.*, 2006; Hooiveld *et al.*, 1999;

Woltering and Durston, 2008; Le Pabic *et al.*, 2010; Lobe. 1995, Maconochie *et al.*, 1997; Gould *et al.*, 1997; Bergson and McGinnis,1990 ; Miller *et al.*, 2001, Wellik and Capecchi, 2003) and that they drive conventional intercellular signalling pathways(eg. Graba *et al.* 1995, Bruhl 2004, Manak *et al*1994, Michaut *et al.*, 2011, Morsi el Kadi *et al.*, 2002, Pearson *et al.*, 2005) as well as acting as signalling molecules themselves (Bloch-Gallego *et al.*, 1993, Chatelin *et al.*, 1996).

2. There is evidence that the signalling factor *Wnt 8* acts as a signal to initiate synchronous expression of the different Hox complexes. (In der Rieden et al., 2010)
3. There is evidence that the somitogenesis clock is involved (Fig. 5B). Vertebrate somitogenesis (segmentation of axial mesoderm) works via a mechanism where an oscillating system of gene expression generates a spatial pattern by time-space translation, just as in genesis of the vertebrate axial *Hox* pattern (see above and text box 1). This dynamic process is known to start during gastrulation in chicken and *Xenopus* (Peres *et al,* 2006; Jouve *et al.*, 2002) and it drives activation of Hox gene expression. *Xdelta2* is a *Xenopus* oscillating somitogenesis gene (Jen *et al.*, 1997, 1999). It is already expressed during gastrulation and then generates presomitic stripes so its expression is already oscillatory. It regulates expression of *Hox* genes during gastrulation (Peres *et al.*, 2006). This gene could help to drive synchronised temporally collinear expression of the *Hox* complexes. It could do so either by regulating only initiation of expression of *Hox* complexes (via *labial Hox* genes) or by driving initiation and 3′ to 5′ progression, (repeatedly inducing expression of different *Hox* genes). We note that *XDelta2* drives expression of at least 3 different *Hox* paralog groups including *labial*). If *delta* drives progression as well as initiation, a repeated periodic pulsatile signal is required. The idea that the somitogenesis clock drives *Hox* temporal collinearity is very attractive because both of these timers are known to operate already in the gastrula and because of the evidence linking *Hox* patterning and segmentation (above). Such a signalling pathway might act separately from the *Hox* genes or be downstream of them. *XDelta 2* is indeed downstream of Hox genes as well as upstream. There is a positive feedback loop (McNulty *et al.*, 2006, Peres *et al.*, 2006). *XDelta 2* may thus mediate *Hox* induced signalling. These findings indicate that the axial segmentation mechanism may help to drive Hox expression in vertebrates, just as in *Drosophila.*

The *X. laevis* example was chosen because the data are most complete for this system; however, the conclusions are strongly supported by many findings in other vertebrates (zebrafish, chicken and mouse) (Gaunt and Strachan, 1996, Alexandre *et al.* 1996, Deschamps *et al.*, 1999). This example illustrates that *Hox* colinearity cannot depend solely on the collinear opening of chromatin. Because the *Hox* complexes are synchronised, *trans*-actingfactors and intercellular signals must be involved – *trans*-acting factors would be necessary for coordinating the sequential 3′ to 5′ activation of *Hox* genes in and between *Hox* clusters, and intercellular signals would enable the coordinated activation of *Hox* gene expression between cells in a tissue. An alternative explanation is that only the most 3′ *Hox* genes (*Hox1*) transactivate, and the remaining timing is provided by synchronised opening of the *Hox* complexes. The different structures of the 4 primary vertebrate *Hox* complexes (with different *Hox* paralogues missing from each) would, however, make it difficult for progressive opening of different *Hox* complexes to stay synchronous. Since the gastrula mesoderm is a cell mass, not a single cell, trans-activation needs to be accompanied by intercellular signalling.

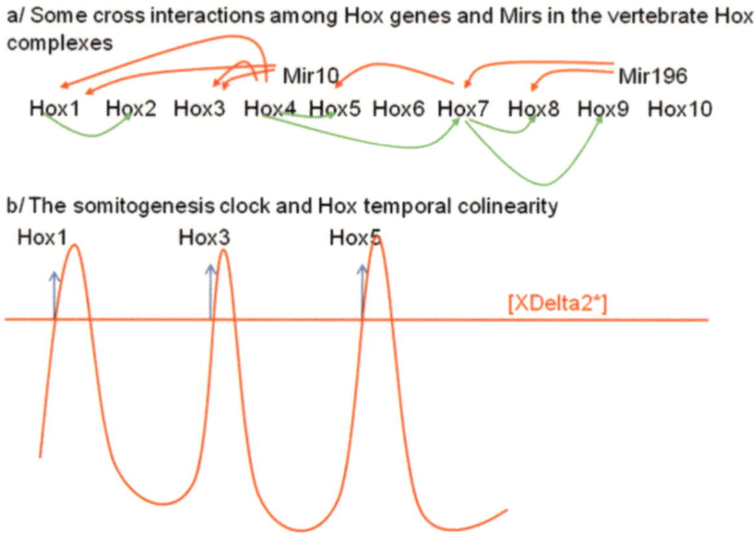

Fig. 5. **Regulators of vertebrate Hox temporal colinearity: Hox-Hox interactions and Somitogenesis oscillations**

A. some cross interactions between Hox genes and Mirs in the vertebrate Hox complexes during vertebrate gastrulation. Red: repression. Green: activation

B. The somitogenesis clock and Hox temporal collinearity. We show an oscillating concentration of XDelta2. Sequential peaks of XDelta2 activate expression of different Hox genes. [XDelta2]; The threshold concentration of XDelta2 at which Hox expression is activated.*

6.4 *Hox* genes in later development and in. limbs, hairs, haematopoiesis, the pancreas, etc

Vertebrate *Hox* genes have many other functions than specifying levels in the main body axis, in the central nervous system and in axial mesoderm. They regulate the axial patterning of limbs (Zakany and Duboule, 2007). They mediate patterning and differentiation in hairs (Awgulevich, 2003), the gut (Kawazoe et al., 2002), the pancreas (Gray et al., 2011), the blood (Magli et al.,. See articles for details. These other functions will not be discussed further here. Many of these *Hox* functions have been elucidated by gain and loss of function expts. In general, loss of function mutation in a single vertebrate *Hox* gene delivers a deceptively mild phenotype. This has bedevilled the analysis of *Hox* function using mouse genetics. It is because each vertebrate *Hox* gene is a member of a paralogue group of at up to 4 or 8 *Hox* genes which have parallel and shared functions. Where measures have been takn to knock out a whole paralogue group, a suitably dramatic phenotype is obtained. See Fig. 1.

6.5 Modified use of *Hox* genes in elongated vertebrates: Snakes and Caecilians

The elongated, snake-like skeleton, as it has convergently evolved in numerous reptilian and amphibian clades, is from a developmental biologist's point of view amongst the most fascinating anatomical peculiarities in the animal kingdom. This kind of body plan is characterized by a greatly increased number of vertebrae, a reduction of skeletal regionalization along the primary body axis and loss of the limbs. Recent studies conducted in both mouse and snakes now hint at how changes in gene regulatory circuitries of the *Hox* genes and the somitogenesis clock could underlie these striking departures from standard tetrapod morphology. These studies show that particular snake Hox genes have changed their specificities by mutations in the homeobox. This leads to their failing to specify the expected axial boundaries and enables particular body regions, especially the thorax, to become drastically extended (Woltering et al., 2009, Di Poi et al., 2010).

7. Conclusions

Hox genes are upstream regulators in the developmental hierarchy that are of great importance for the bodyplan. They specify and differentiate between different zones along the main body axis. These genes show collinearity- clustering associated with acquisition of ordered properties within the gene cluster- a spectacular phenomenon that has attracted much interest. A *Hox* cluster is actually a metagene. It, but not an individual *Hox* gene, can fulfil a developmental function- patterning the body axis. In Drosophila, and probably in all other invertebrates- the full potential of the *Hox* genes is not realised. The expression of each individual *Hox* gene is regulated by other spatially regulated genes and so *Hox* collinearity is not used to pattern the main body axis. In vertebrates, temporal collinearity has been developed and this is used to pattern the main body axis and develop spatial collinearity, by time-space translation. It is presently generally assumed that the mechanism of temporal collinearity is progressive 3′ to 5′ opening for transcription of *Hox* complexes. This may be important. However, we develop a different mechanistic hypothesis: that collinearity is partly mediated by *Hox* gene interactions. This idea was already indicated by earlier investigations of posterior prevalence. We review new evidence that trans-acting factors and intercellular signals mediate vertebrate *Hox* collinearity; that these include interactions among *Hox* genes, including posterior prevalence, as well as somitogenesis signals. We propose that these *Hox* interactions have a role in generating *Hox* temporal and spatial collinearity as well as functional collinearity. We note also that an evolutionary explanation for collinearity actually probably obviates any requirement for a dedicated collinearity mechanism. Our conclusions open new perspectives for research into the mechanisms underlying collinearity. Testing this model will require a much more extensive investigation and description of early vertebrate *Hox* temporal collinearity.

8. Acknowledgements

We thank Dr. Moises Mallo and 'Genes and Development' for permission to reproduce a figure from [10] in Fig. 1e. We thank Dr. Frances Goodman and 'The Lancet' for permission to reproduce Fig. 6 from [79] in Fig 2. We also thank 'Developmental Biology' for permission to reproduce our own material from [69] in Figs 4 A and B. We also acknowledge that the idea that the somitogenesis oscillation could drive Hox gene expression (as indicated in Fig.5) was first published 30 years ago by H. Meinhardt [78]

9. References

Alexandre D, Clarke JD, Otoxby E, Yan YL, Jowett T, Holder N. (1996)Ectopic expression of *Hoxa-1* in the zebrafish alters the fate of the mandibular arch neural crest and phenocopies a retinoic acid-induced phenotype. *Development.*;122(3):735-746.

Appel B, Sakonju S, (1993) Cell-type-specific mechanisms of transcriptional repression by the homeotic gene products *UBX* and *ABD-A* in *Drosophila* embryos. *EMBO J.* 12(3): 1099–1109.

Awgulewitsch A. Hox in hair growth and development. Naturwissenschaften. 2003 May;90(5):193-211. Epub 2003 Apr 26.

Beachy PA, Krasnow MA, Gavis ER, Hogness DS.(1988) An *Ultrabithorax* protein binds sequences near its own and the *Antennapedia* P1 promoters. *Cell.* 1988;55(6):1069-1081.

Bender W, Spierer P, Hogness DS Chromosomal walking and jumping to isolate DNA from the Ace and rosy loci and the bithorax complex in Drosophila melanogaster. *J Mol Biol.* 1983 Jul 25;168(1):17-33.

Bergson C, and McGinnis W, (1990) An autoregulatory enhancer element of the *Drosophila* homeotic gene *Deformed EMBO Journal* 9,.13.4287-4297,

Bloch- Gallego E, Le Roux I, Joliot AH, Volovitch M, Henderson CE, Prochiantz A. (1993) *Antennapedia* homeobox peptide enhances growth and branching of embryonic chicken motoneurons in vitro. *J Cell Bio*l. 120(2):485-492.

Bruhl, T. et al. (2004) Homeobox *A9* transcriptionally regulates the *EphB4* receptor to modulate endothelial cell migration and tube formation. *Circ. Res.* 94, 743–751

Burke AC, Nelson CE, Morgan BA, Tabin C. Hox genes and the evolution of vertebrate axial morphology. Development. 1995 Feb;121(2):333-46.

Cambeyron S, Bickmore WA, (2004) Chromatin decondensation and nuclear reorganization of the *HoxB* locus upon induction of transcription. Genes Dev. 18(10): 1119–1130.

Carapuco M, Novoa A, Bobola N, Mallo M (2005) *Hox* genes specify vertebral types in the presomitic mesoderm. *Genes Dev.*;19(18):2116-2121

Carrasco AE, McGinnis W, Gehring WJ, De Robertis EM, (1984) Cloning of an X. laevis gene expressed during early embryogenesis coding for a peptide region homologous to Drosophila homeotic genes. *Cell.*;37(2):409-414.

Cecchi C, Mallamaci A, Boncinelli E. Otx and Emx homeobox genes in brain development. Int J Dev Biol. 2000;44(6):663-8.

Changes in Hox genes' structure and function during the evolution of the squamate body plan. Nature. 2010 Mar 4;464(7285):99-103.

Chatelin J, Volovitch M, Joliot AH, Perez F, Prochiantz A. (1996) Transcription factor *hoxa-5* is taken up by cells in culture and conveyed to their nuclei. *Mech Dev.* 55(2):111-117.

De Robertis EM, (2008) Evo-devo: variations on ancestral themes. *Cell.* 132(2):185-195.

Deschamps J, Van den Akker E, Forlani S, De Graaff W, Oosterveen T, Roelen B, Roelofsma J. (1999) Initiation, establishment and maintenance of Hox gene expression patterns in the mouse. *Int J Dev Biol.* 43(7):635-650.

Di-Poï N, Montoya-Burgos JI, Miller H, Pourquié O, Milinkovitch MC, Duboule D.

dMi-2, a hunchback-interacting protein that functions in polycomb repression. Science. 1998 Dec 4;282(5395):1897-900.

Duboule D, (1994).Temporal colinearity and the phylotypic progression: a basis for the stability of a vertebrate Bauplan and the evolution of morphologies through heterochrony. *Dev Suppl.* 135-42

Duboule D,(2007) The rise and fall of *Hox* gene clusters. *Development* 134(14): 2549-2460.

Dubrulle J, Pourquie O. (2004) Coupling segmentation to axis formation. *Development.*;131(23):5783-5793

Dubrulle J.,. McGrew MJ, Pourquié O, (2001).*Cell* 106, 219

Durston A, Jansen H, and Wacker S, (2011) Time-Space Translation: A Developmental Principle. The Scientific World In Press.

Durston A., Jansen HJ Wacker SA,.(2010) Review: Time-Space Translation Regulates Trunk Axial Patterning In The Early Vertebrate Embryo. *Genomics* 95, 250-255.

Gaunt SJ, Strachan L. (1996) Temporal colinearity in expression of anterior *Hox* genes in developing chick embryos. *Dev Dyn.*;207(3):270-280

Gebelein B, Mann RS Compartmental modulation of abdominal Hox expression by engrailed and sloppy-paired patterns the fly ectoderm. Dev Biol. 2007 Aug 15;308(2):593-605. Epub 2007 May 24.

Gehring WJ, Kloter U, and Suga H, (2009). Evolution of the *Hox* Gene Complex from an Evolutionary Ground State. *Current Topics in Developmental Biology* 88: 35-61

Gibson G, Gehring W. (1988) Head and thoracic transformations caused by ectopic expression of *Antennapedia* during *Drosophila* development. *Development* , 102, 657-675.

Gomez C, Ozbudak EM, Wunderlich J, Baumann D, Lewis J, Pourquié O. Control of segment number in vertebrate embryos. Nature. 2008 Jul 17;454(7202):335-9. Epub 2008 Jun 18.

Gonzalez Reyes G, Urquia N, Gehring WJ, Struhl G Morata G, (1990), Are cross-regulatory interactions between homoeotic genes functionally significant?, *Nature* 344 78–80.

Goodman FR. Congenital abnormalities of body patterning: embryology revisited. Lancet 2003 23, 362(9384),651-62.

Gould A, Morrison A, Sproat G, White RA, Krumlauf R. (1997) Positive cross-regulation and enhancer sharing: two mechanisms for specifying overlapping *Hox* expression patterns. *Genes Dev.* 11(7):900-13.

Graba Y. et al. (1995) DWnt-4, a novel Drosophila *Wnt* gene acts downstream of homeotic complex genes in the visceral mesoderm. *Development* 121, 209–218.

Gray S, Pandha HS, Michael A, Middleton G, Morgan R. HOX genes in pancreatic development and cancer. JOP. 2011 May 6;12(3):216-9.

Grier DG, Thompson A, Kwasniewska A, McGonigle GJ, Halliday HL, (2005) The pathophysiology of *HOX* genes and their role in cancer. *J. Pathol* 205(2): 154–71.

Hafen E, Levine M, Gehring WJ.(1984) Regulation of *Antennapedia* transcript distribution by the *bithorax* complex in Drosophila. *Nature.*;307(5948):287-289.

Hooiveld M, Morgan R, In Der Rieden P, Houtzager E, Pannese M,, Damen K, Boncinelli E, Durston A, (1999) Novel colinear interactions between vertebrate *Hox* genes. *Int. J. Dev. Biol.* 43:665-674

In Der Rieden PMJ, Lloret Vilaspasa F, Durston AJ, (2010). *Xwnt8* directly initiates expression of *labial Hox* genes. *Dev. Dynamics* 29: 226-239

Jen WC, Gawantka V, Pollet N, Niehrs C, Kintner C. (1999) Periodic repression of *Notch* pathway genes governs the segmentation of Xenopus embryos. *Genes Dev.*;13(11):1486-1499

Jen WC, Wettstein D, Turner D, Chitnis A, Kintner C. (1997) The *Notch* ligand, *X-Delta-2*, mediates segmentation of the paraxial mesoderm in Xenopus embryos. *Development*. 1997;124(6):1169-1178.

Jouve C, Iimura T, Pourquie O.(2002) Onset of the segmentation clock in the chick embryo: evidence for oscillations in the somite precursors in the primitive streak. *Development*.;129(5):1107-1111

Kawazoe Y, Sekimoto T, Araki M, Takagi K, Araki K, Yamamura K.

Kehle J, Beuchle D, Treuheit S, Christen B, Kennison JA, Bienz M, Müller J.

Kmitam M., et al., (2000) Mechanisms of *Hox* gene colinearity: transposition of the anterior *Hoxb1* gene into the posterior *HoxD* complex. *Genes Dev.* 14(2):198-211..

Krumlauf R, (1994) *Hox* genes in vertebrate development *Cell* 78, 2, 191-201

Krüppel acts as a gap gene regulating expression of hunchback and even-skipped in the intermediate germ cricket Gryllus bimaculatus. Dev Biol. 2006 Jun 15;294(2):471-81. Epub 2006 Apr 17.

Le Pabic P, Scemama JL, Stellwag EJ. (2010) Role of *Hox PG2* genes in Nile tilapia pharyngeal arch specification: implications for gnathostome pharyngeal arch evolution. 12(1):45-60.

Lewis EB, (1978) A Gene Complex Controlling Segmentation in Drosophila *Nature* 276: 565-568

Lewis EB, Nobel lecture, December 8, 1995. The *bithorax* complex: The first fifty years. In: H. Lifshitz, Editor, *Genes, Development and Cancer. The Life and Work of Edward B. Lewis, Kluwer Academic Publishers, Norwell, MA*

Lobe CG, (1995) Activation of *Hox* gene expression by *Hoxa-5*. *DNA Cell Biol.*;14(10):817-23.

Maconochie MK, et al, (1997) Cross-regulation in the mouse *HoxB* complex: the expression of *Hoxb2* in rhombomere 4 is regulated by *Hoxb1*. Genes Dev. 11, 1885–1895.

Magli MC, Largman C, Lawrence HJ. Effects of HOX homeobox genes in blood cell differentiation. J Cell Physiol. 1997 Nov;173(2):168-77.

Mainguy G, Koster J, Woltering J, Jansen H, Durston A, (2007).Extensive polycistronism and antisense transcription in the Mammalian *Hox* clusters. *PLoS ONE* 2(4):e356.

Manak JR, Mathies LD, Scott MP (1994) Regulation of a *decapentaplegic* midgut enhancer by homeotic proteins. *Development* 120, 3605–3612

McNulty C, Peres J, Van Den Akker W, Bardine N, Durston A. (2005) A Knockdown of the complete *Hox* paralogous group *1* leads to dramatic hindbrain and neural crest defects. *Development*.;132(12):2861-2871

Meinhardt H. Models For Biological Pattern Formation. Academic Press. (1982)

Michaut L, Jansen H, Bardine N, Durston A, Gehring WJ, (2011) Analysing the function of a *hox* gene: an evolutionary approach. *Evolution and Development* under review

Miller DF, Rogers BT, Kalkenbrenner A, Hamilton B, Holtzman SL, Kaufman T.(2001) Cross-regulation of *Hox* genes in the *Drosophila melanogaster* embryo. *Mech Dev*.102(1-2):3-16.

Mito T, Okamoto H, Shinahara W, Shinmyo Y, Miyawaki K, Ohuchi H, Noji S.

Morsi El Kadi A, In Der Rieden P, Durston A, Morgan R, (2002). The small GTPase *Rap-1* is an immediate downstream target for *Hoxb4* transcriptional regulation. Mech. Dev.*113*, 131-139

Nuesslein- Volhard (1995) *Nobel lecture*

Palmeirim I, Henrique D, Ish Horowicz D, Pourquie O, (1997) Avian *hairy* gene expression identifies a molecular clock linked to vertebrate segmentation and somitogenesis. *Cell.*;91(5):639-48.

Pearson JC, Lemons D, McGinnis W, (2005) Modulating *Hox* Gene Functions During Animal Body Patterning. *Nature Reviews Genetics* 6, 893,

Peres J, McNulty C, Durston A. (2006) Interaction between *X-Delta-2* and *Hox* genes regulates segmentation and patterning of the anteroposterior axis. *Mech Dev.*;123(4):321-333.

Plaza S, Prince F, Adachi Y, Punzo C, Cribbs DL, Gehring WJ. (2008) Cross-regulatory protein-protein interactions between *Hox* and *Pax* transcription factors. *Proc Natl Acad Sci U S A.*;105(36):13439-13444.

Region-specific gastrointestinal Hox code during murine embryonal gut development. Dev Growth Differ. 2002 Feb;44(1):77-84.

Ronshaugen M, Biemar F, Piel J, Levine M, Lai EC,, (2005).The Drosophila microRNA *iab-4* causes a dominant homeotic transformation of halteres to wings. *Genes Dev.*;19(24):2947-2952.

Rusch DB, Kaufman TC.Regulation of proboscipedia in Drosophila by homeotic selector genes.Genetics. 2000 Sep;156(1):183-94.

Schneider-Maunoury S, Gilardi-Hebenstreit P, Charnay P. How to build a vertebrate hindbrain. Lessons from genetics. C R Acad Sci III. 1998 Oct;321(10):819-34.

Seo HC, Edvardsen RB, Maeland A D, Bjordal M, Jensen MF, Hansen A, Flaat M, Weissenbach J, Lehrach H, Wincker P, (2004). *Hox* cluster disintegration with persistent anteroposterior order of expression in *Oikopleura dioica. Nature* 431: 67 - 71.

Soshnikova N, Duboule D, (2009) Epigenetic Temporal Control of Mouse *Hox* Genes in Vivo *Science* 324, 1320-1323.

Struhl G, White RA. Regulation of the *Ultrabithorax* gene of *Drosophila* by other *bithorax* complex genes. *Cell.* 1985;43(2 Pt 1):507-519.

Struhl, (1983) Role of the *esc*+ gene product in ensuring the selective expression of segment-specific homeotic genes in *Drosophila. J. Embryol. Exp. Morphol.* 76:, 297–331

Tümpel S, Wiedemann LM, Krumlauf R.Hox genes and segmentation of the vertebrate hindbrain. Curr Top Dev Biol. 2009;88:103-37

Van Der Hoeven F, Zakany J, Duboule D, (1996) Transpositions in the *HoxD* complex reveal a hierarchy of regulatory controls. *Cell.*;85(7):1025-1035.

Wacker SA, Jansen HJ, McNulty CL, Houtzager E, Durston AJ. (2004a). Timed interactions between the *Hox* expressing non-organiser mesoderm and the Spemann organiser generate positional information during vertebrate gastrulation. *Dev Biol.* ;268(1):207-219

Wellik DM, Capecchi MR, (2003) *Hox10* and *Hox11* genes are required to globally pattern the mammalian skeleton, *Science* 301 363–367.

Woltering JM, and Durston A, (2008) *MiR10* represses *HoxB1*a and *HoxB3a* in Zebrafish. *PLoS ONE.*;3(1):e1396.

Woltering Joost M., Freek J. Vonk, Hendrik Müller[3], Nabila Bardine, Merijn A.G. de Bakker, Antony J. Durston & Michael K. Richardson (2009) Molecular regionalisation of the snake and caecilian body plan. Dev Bio. 332(1):82-9.

Wright CV. (1993) Hox genes and the hindbrain. Curr Biol. 1993 Sep 1;3(9):618-21.

Yekta S, Tabin CJ, Bartel DP (2008) MicroRNAs in the Hox network: an apparent link to posterior prevalence *Nat Rev Genet.* 9(10): 789–796.

Yekta S, Shih H, Bartel DP (2004) MicroRNA-directed cleavage of *HOXB8* mRNA. *Science* 304(5670): 594–596.

Zakany J, Duboule D. The role of Hox genes during vertebrate limb development. Curr Opin Genet Dev. 2007 Aug;17(4):359-66. Epub 2007 Jul 20.

Zakany J, Kmita M, Alarcon P, De La Pompa L, Duboule D (2001) Localized and transient transcription of *Hox* genes suggests a link between patterning and the segmentation clock. *Cell.*;106(2):207-217.

7

In Vitro Organogenesis of *Protea cynaroides* L. Shoot-Buds Cultured Under Red and Blue Light-Emitting Diodes

How-Chiun Wu[1] and Elsa S. du Toit[2]
[1]*Department of Natural Biotechnology, Nanhua University, Dalin Township, Chiayi*
[2]*Department of Plant Production and Soil Science, University of Pretoria, Pretoria*
[1]*Taiwan R.O.C*
[2]*South Africa*

1. Introduction

Protea cynaroides L. (King Protea), which belongs to the Proteaceae family, is a slow-growing, semi-hardwood shrub. The *Protea* genus has the widest distribution area of all the southern Africa Proteaceae, ranging from the predominantly winter or all-year round rainfall area of the Cape in South Africa to the subtropical and tropical areas of southern Africa (Paterson-Jones, 2007). They occupy a variety of habitats from sea level to up to 1500 metres. *P. cynaroides* species vary widely in colour, shape and flowering time (Matthews, 1993). Its growth habits vary from dwarf variants to dense, bushy forms reaching heights of 2 m, which are commonly used in cultivation. The most characteristic feature of its blossom is its flowerhead, which typically consists of hundreds of flowers (Rebelo, 2000). Its flowerhead shape ranges from small, narrow, goblet-shapes to large, wide, flat types. Their colours range from greenish-white to deep pink and red (Matthews, 1993). Due to their wide variability, flowers can be seen throughout the year, depending on the variety. In their natural habitat, *P. cynaroides* are found in well-drained, acidic, nutrient-deficient soils. Their ability to thrive in soil with low nutrients is assisted by the growth of proteoid roots, which are specialized roots that look like very fine bottlebrushes, and are very efficient at absorbing nutrients. The King Protea is a well-known cut flower in many parts of the world, and is a highly sought after commodity in the international flower market due to its attractive flowerhead and long vase life. The demand for the King Protea has remained consistent on the international market and its market price has remained relatively high over the years. Current important production areas include: Australia, South Africa, California, Portugal, Israel, Zimbabwe, Hawaii, Chile, New Zealand, and Ecuador (Dorrington, 2008). Due to its popularity, production areas are expanding in Europe, with new plantations being established in Portugal and Spain (Leonardt, 2008).

King Proteas are plants that are difficult to grow and fertilize (Littlejohn et al., 2003). The major factors identified for successful cultivation are well-drained, sandy acidic soils with low phosphor content and pH ranging from 3.5 to 5.8 (Silber, et al., 2001). Although higher pH levels can be tolerated, these plants have low mineral requirements and are therefore not tolerant to salt concentrations that would appear normal to other plants (Montarone & Allemand, 1995). Stem cuttings are commonly used to vegetatively propagate *P. cynaroides*, however, root formation usually needs several months to take place, and typically have low success rates. *In vitro* propagation techniques are widely used to propagate numerous economically important plants. Under *in vitro* conditions, growers are able to mass-produce plants in a relatively short period of time. In addition, *in vitro* propagation is also used to overcome problems that are found in traditional vegetative propagation, such as poor root formation of cuttings, slow growth rates, and susceptibility of cuttings to diseases. In traditional sexual propagation, problems such as seed dormancy and low germination rate are often overcome via *in vitro* propagation. The significant successes in this field have been extensively reported, which in most cases have dramatically changed the way plants are propagated.

Over the years, very few studies investigating the *in vitro* propagation of *P. cynaroides* have been reported. According to Tal et al. (1992), recurrent difficulties encountered in the propagation of proteas *in vitro* include phenolic oxidation and necrosis of clonal explants. These factors have resulted in limited success and prevented progress in this area of research. The first attempt to propagate *P. cynaroides in vitro* was carried out by Ben-Jaacov & Jacobs (1986). In their study, growth of axillary buds was successful through the establishment of nodal stem segments. More recently, advances were made in the *in vitro* establishment of *P. cynaroides* nodal explants by treating shoot segments with antioxidants (ascorbic acid and citric acid) after surface sterilization to reduce oxidative browning and increase axillary bud growth (Wu & du Toit, 2004). In another study, *P. cynaroides* apical buds were used as explants and successfully establishment *in vitro* by Thillerot et al. (2006). Proliferation of buds were subsequently achieved in the multiplication stage, however, it was reported that bud growth was slow, possibly due to apical dominance. Most importantly, *in vitro* rooting *of P. cynaroides* explants in the studies described above was never achieved. Moreover, growth of *P. cynaroides* shoots *in vitro* remains to be slow and inconsistent. With the aim to produce complete plantlets more efficiently, somatic embryogenesis of *P. cynaroides* was studied. Results showed that somatic embryos were able to form directly on mature zygotic embryos and cotyledons (Wu et al., 2007b), and germinate into plantlets. While studying the induction of somatic embryos in *P. cynaroides* cotyledons, it was discovered that the cotyledonary nodes possessed a high organogenic potential to produce shoot-buds. However, the growth rates of the axillary buds and shoot-buds were slow, and subsequent attempts to multiply these explants were not successful. The slow growth rate of these buds may be attributed to the absence of a root system, since the growth rate of *P. cynaroides* somatic embryos, which possessed a root system, was relatively high. It is likely that the uptake of nutrients by rootless *P. cynaroides* buds were highly inefficient. Therefore, in order to increase the growth rates of axillary buds and shoot-buds in the multiplication stage, induction of adventitious roots is required. The use of growth regulators to promote rooting of buds has been ineffective (Wu et al., 2007b).

Light is an important stimulus for plant development. It is also widely known that spectral quality is a key factor in plant morphogenesis (Okamoto et al., 1997). Conventional fluorescent lamps, which have a wide range of wavelengths from 350 to 750 nm, are the most commonly used light source in plant tissue culture (Economou & Read, 1987). Due to the difficulty in controlling the light quality of fluorescent lamps, and with technological advances in recent years, the use of light emitting diodes (LEDs) as an alternative light source for explants cultured *in vitro* has attracted considerable interest. The advantages that LEDs have over fluorescent lamps are their wavelength specificity, light intensity adjustability, low thermal energy output, small mass, and long life (Bula et al., 1991; Brown et al., 1995; Okamoto et al., 1997). Numerous studies have been conducted to investigate the effectiveness of specific light qualities emitted by LEDs in promoting growth and morphogenesis of different plants. An overview of the available literature shows that red LEDs (620-680 nm), blue LEDs (420-480), a combination of red and blue LEDs, and LEDs emitting far-red light (735 nm), at various wavelengths and intensities are commonly used as light sources in research studies.

Light quality studies have been carried out on important agricultural crops such as banana (Nhut et al., 2002), lettuce (Okamoto et al., 1996), pepper (Brown et al., 1995), potato (Jao & Fang, 2004), spinach (Yanagi & Okamoto, 1997) and wheat (Goins et al., 1997) In addition, floral plants such as anthurium (Budiarto, 2010), calla lily (Chang et al., 2003; Jao et al., 2005), gerbera (Wang et al., 2011), *Lilium* (Lian et al., 2002; Lin et al., 2008) and *Pelargonium* (Appelgren, 1991) amongst others, have also been studied. Results from different studies have shown that red and blue lights in particular, have a significant influence on plant photomorphogenesis. However, the responses of plants to different light qualities vary widely. Studies showed that culturing *Lilium* explants under a combination of red and blue LEDs produced larger bulblets, and a higher number of roots (Lian et al., 2002). Findings by Appelgren (1991) revealed that growing *Pelargonium* plantlets *in vitro* under red light significantly stimulated stem elongation, while inhibition of stem elongation was found under blue light. In a recent study, red and blue LEDs were found to induce root formation in anthuriums (Budiarto, 2010). Similarly, a higher rooting percentage and higher root numbers of grape explants were obtained when cultured under red LEDs (Poudel et al., 2008).

From the literature described above, it is clear that LEDs have numerous advantages over conventional fluorescent lamps, and that light emitted by LEDs are highly beneficial to the growth and morphogenesis in a wide range of plant species. In order for *in vitro* propagation to become an alternative method of propagation for *P. cynaroides*, stimulating adventitious root formation and promoting vegetative growth of *P. cynaroides* explants *in vitro* must be achieved. Adventitious root formation in *P. cynaroides* explants has never been reported before. The use of LEDs as a light source is ideal to study the effects of specific wavelengths on organogenesis, particularly adventitious root formation, in difficult-to-grow plants such as *P. cynaroides*. Therefore, the aim of this study was to investigate the effects of light quality emitted by light-emitting diodes (LEDs) on the induction of adventitious roots and bud growth of *P. cynaroides* shoot-buds.

2. Materials and methods

2.1 Embryo excision and culture conditions

P. cynaroides seedlings were established using mature embryos excised from seeds. Surface-sterilization of the seeds and excision of the embryos was done according to Wu et al. (2007a) with modifications. Hairs on *P. cynaroides* seeds were first removed by hand and only plump-looking, healthy seeds were selected for germination. For surface sterilization, the seeds were placed in 99% sulphuric acid (H_2SO_4) for 30 seconds. The seeds were then immediately transferred to sterilized distilled water and rinsed for 5 mins to remove traces of sulphuric acid. This was repeated twice. Afterwards, the embryo was removed from the seed by carefully cutting open the seed coat with a scalpel. After excision, the embryos were placed into the growth medium in an upright position. Only the bottom half of the embryo was in direct contact with the growth medium. Half-strength Murashige and Skoog medium (Murashige & Skoog, 1962) supplemented with 30 g L^{-1} sucrose and 9 g L^{-1} agar was used for germinating the embryos. Ten mL of growth medium were dispensed into glass test tubes (25 mm x 150 mm^2). The pH of the medium was adjusted to 5.8 prior to adding agar. The medium was autoclaved for 20 min at 121°C and 104 KPa. Embryos in the test tubes (one embryo/tube) were placed in a growth chamber with a 16-h photoperiod. An alternating temperature regime of 21°C/12°C (light/dark) was used throughout the germination period. Cool white fluorescent tubes provided 50 µmol m^{-2} sec^{-1} photosynthetically active radiation (PAR). The PAR was measured at plant height with a light meter (LI-1800, LI-COR Inc.). Separation of the two cotyledons was observed after approximately 10 days (Fig. 1A). Growth and greening of the cotyledons occurred after 20 days (Fig. 1B). After 40 days, germinated embryos (Fig. 1C), which consisted of two cotyledons and a radicle, were subcultured to fresh medium for the induction of adventitious bud formation.

2.2 Induction of adventitious bud formation

Germinated seedlings were transferred to half-strength MS medium media containing 2 mg L^{-1} benzyladenine (BA) and 0.5 mg L^{-1} naphthalene acetic acid (NAA) to induce the formation of shoot-buds. Glass culture vessels (100 mm x 150 mm^2) containing 50 mL of growth medium were used. The pH of the growth medium was adjusted to 5.8 before autoclaving. Each glass vessel contained five explants. The cultures were placed in a growth room with the temperature adjusted to 25±2°C. Cool white fluorescent tubes provided 50 µmol m^{-2} sec^{-1} PAR with a 16-h photoperiod. Direct formation of shoot-buds on the cotyledons was observed after approximately 40 days (Fig. 1D). Almost identical shoot-buds were selected, removed and transferred to fresh medium for the light quality experiment.

2.3 Light quality treatments and culture conditions

After each shoot-bud was removed from the cotyledons, they were weighed under sterile conditions. Shoot-buds with similar weights (10 mg) were selected for this experiment. The shoot-buds were grown in glass test tubes placed in customized LED lighting systems. The explants were exposed to the following light treatments: red LEDs (660 nm), blue LEDs (450 nm), and total darkness. Conventional cool white fluorescent lamps were used as the control. The LEDs were purchased from Ryh Dah Inc. (Taiwan). The lighting systems were constructed with aluminum boxes (50 cm (L) x 50 cm (W) x 25 cm (H)), and equipped with three hundred red or blue LEDs spaced 2 cm apart, on the cover of the box. A temperature sensor, timer and two fans were also installed on each lighting system. The LED lighting systems were placed in a growth room throughout the entire duration of the experiment. In all treatments, the PAR, photoperiod and temperature were adjusted to 50 µmol m^{-2} sec^{-1}, 16 h, and 25±2°C, respectively. The wavelengths of the light sources were measured with a spectroradiometer (International Light Technologies, ILT900). The spectral distributions of red, blue LEDs and fluorescent lights are shown in Fig. 2. Shoot-buds were cultured in 10 mL of growth medium in test tubes (1 shoot-bud/tube) containing half-strength MS media supplemented with 0.1 mg L^{-1} NAA, 30 g L^{-1} sucrose and 9 g L^{-1} agar.

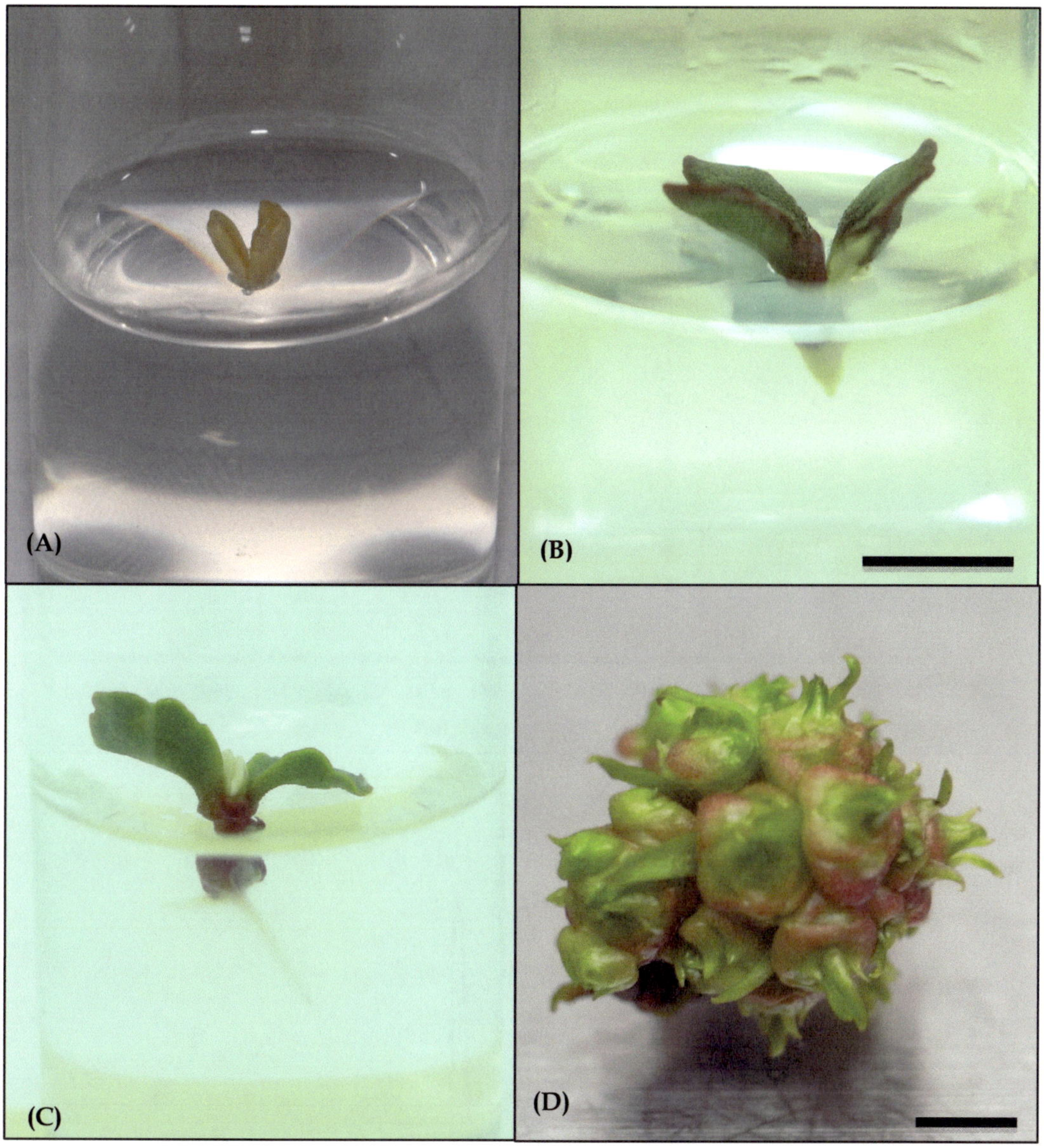

Fig. 1. Germination of *P. cynaroides* zygotic embryo after **(A)** 10 days, **(B)** 20 days, and **(C)** 40 days. **(D)** Direct shoot-bud formation on cotyledonary node 40 days after subculturing to half-strength MS medium with 2 mg L^{-1} BA and 0.5 mg L^{-1} NAA (Bar = 0.5 cm).

2.4 Statistical analysis

A completely randomized design was used in all treatments. Eight replications per treatment were used. Data for rooting percentage, number of roots, root length, root fresh weight, number of leaves, and bud fresh weight were recorded after 45 days in culture. The experiment was repeated twice. Data were analyzed using Duncan's Multiple Range test to compare treatment means. Differences were considered significant when $P<0.001$. Statistical analyses were done using the Statistical Analysis System (SAS) program (SAS Institute Inc., 1996).

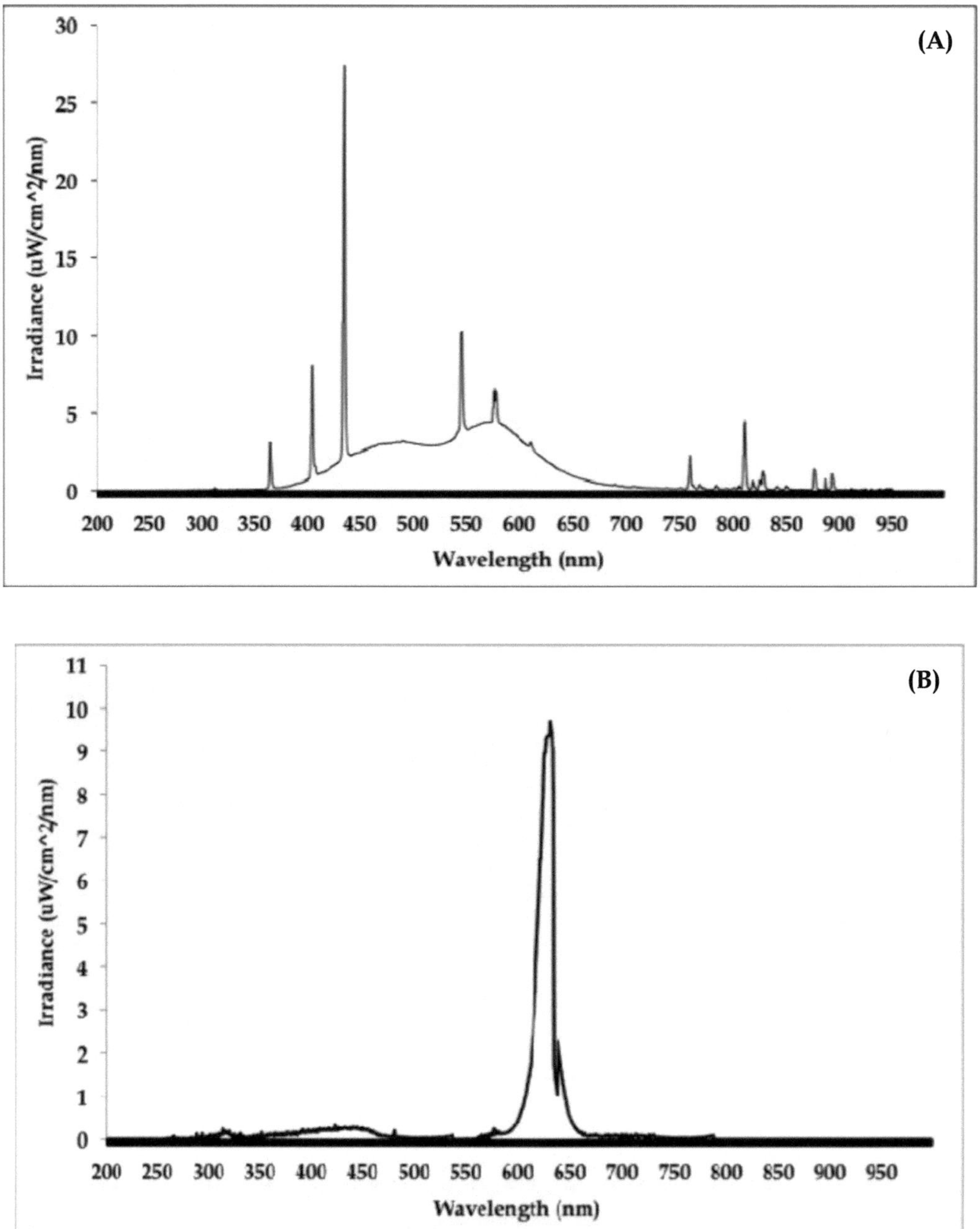

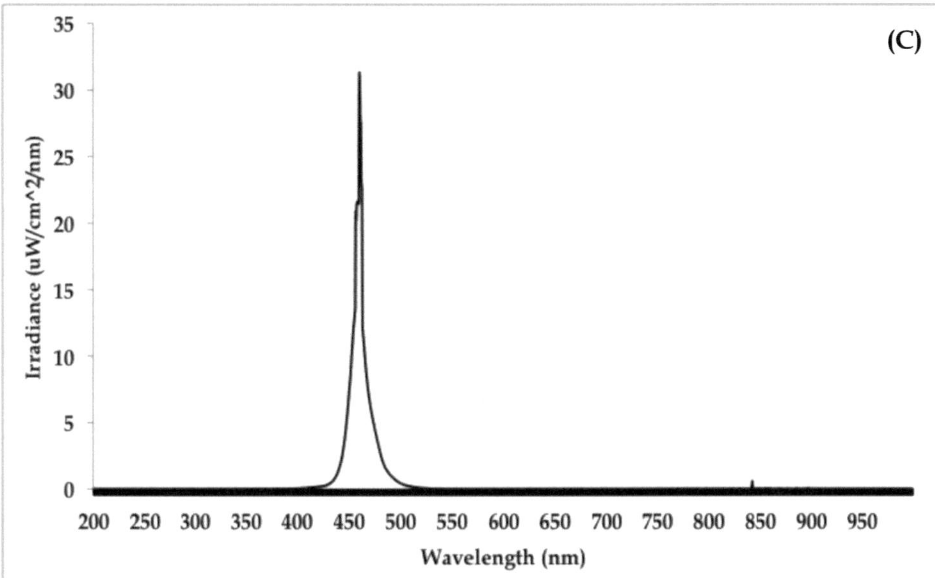

Fig. 2. Spectral distribution of **(A)** fluorescent lamp, **(B)** red LED, and **(C)** blue LED.

3. Results

Results of the study are shown in Fig. 3 and Fig. 4. Vegetative growth of explants in all treatments was very slow. As Fig. 3 shows, elongation of the shoot-buds did not take place. However, root formation, growth of new leaves and increase in bud weight occurred after 30 days in culture. From a visual observation of the buds, browning of the leaves and bud tissues of explants cultured under conventional white fluorescent light (control) were clearly evident (Fig. 3A). On the other hand, very little to no browning of the leaves or tissues was observed on explants grown under red LEDs, blue LEDs or in the dark (Fig. 3B, 3C, 3D). In addition, adventitious buds exposed to blue light seemed to possess the greenest leaves (Fig. 3C), while those grown in the dark exhibited light green leaves and tissues (Fig. 3D). In terms of root formation, adventitious roots were found on explants cultured under red LEDs after 30 days (Fig. 3B), while root formation on explants grown under the other light conditions were only evident towards the end of the study at day 45 (Fig. 4A).

Results of the analyses of the different growth parameters after 45 days in culture are shown in Fig. 4. A significantly higher rooting percentage was observed in adventitious buds cultured under red LEDs (Fig. 4A). Furthermore, the rooting percentage of explants irradiated by white fluorescent light and those grown in the dark were similar. In contrast, the rooting percentage of buds cultured under blue LEDs was significantly lower than all the other light treatments. In terms of the number of roots formed on explants, results showed a similar trend to that of rooting percentage (Fig. 4B). Adventitious buds irradiated by red LEDs produced the highest mean number of roots, while those exposed to light emitted by blue LEDs produced a significantly lower number of roots. No significant differences were observed between the number of roots formed by explants under white fluorescent lights and in the dark (Fig. 4B). In addition, results showed that although red LEDs induced the highest rooting percentage and root numbers, the lengths of these roots were comparable to those formed in the dark (Fig. 4C). Moreover, the roots formed on buds irradiated by white fluorescent light and blue LEDs were similar in length.

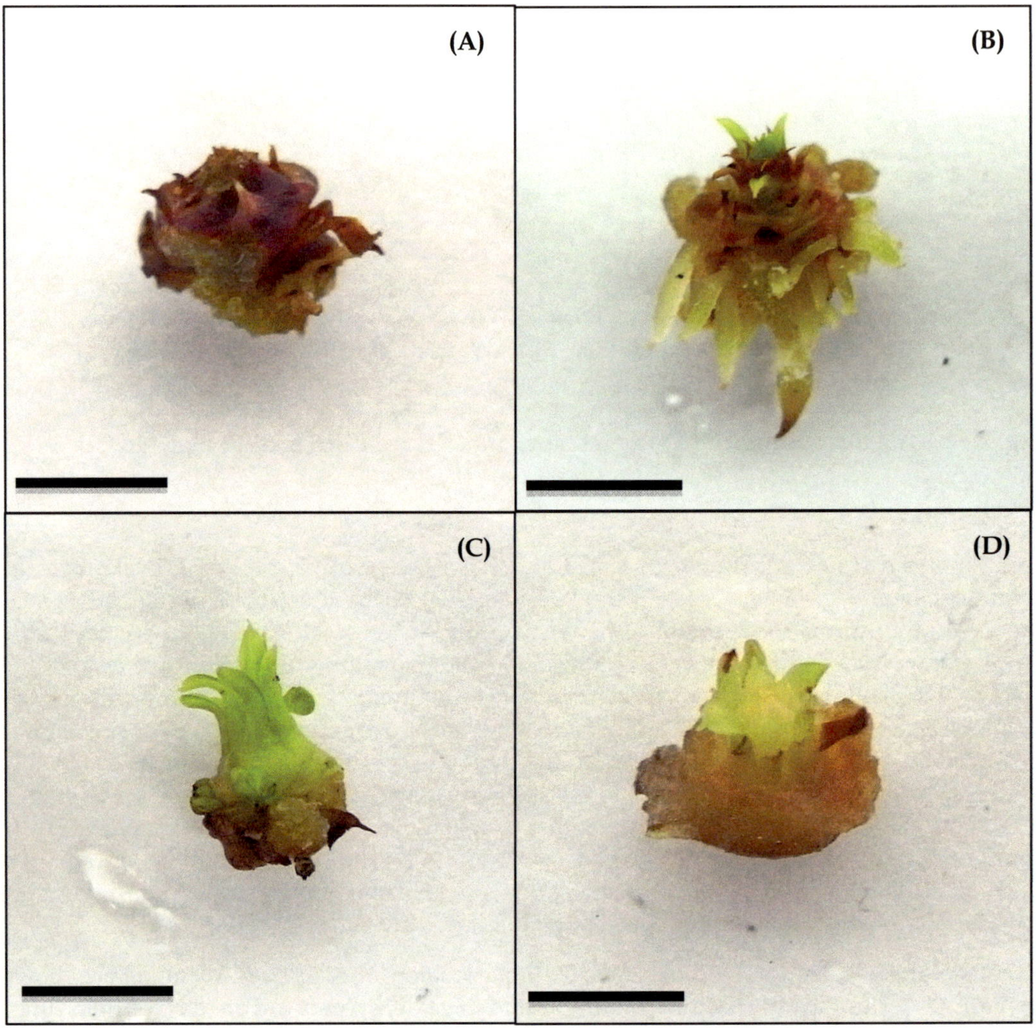

Fig. 3. Response of explants to **(A)** white fluorescent light, **(B)** red LED light, **(C)** blue LED light, **(D)** total darkness, after 30 days in culture (Bar = 0.5 cm).

As a result of the similar root lengths found between explants grown under red LEDs and those grown in the dark, the root fresh weight (per root) of these two treatments were not significantly different (Fig. 4D). Furthermore, the root fresh weight of buds exposed to light emitted by white fluorescent lamps and blue LEDs were similar, and were significantly lower than those cultured under red LEDs and in the dark. Results of this study showed that red LEDs also induced the formation of the highest number of new leaves on the buds (Fig. 4E). However, compared to those cultured under blue LEDs and in the dark, the leaf numbers were not significantly different. Surprisingly, buds cultured under conventional white fluorescent light produced the least number of new leaves, which were significantly lower than those exposed to red LEDs, blue LEDs or those grown in the dark. The fresh weight of buds was found to be the highest when irradiated by red LEDs or grown in the dark (Fig. 4F). The lowest bud fresh weight was found in explants cultured under either white fluorescent light or blue LEDs.

4. Discussion

Overall results of this study demonstrated the difficulties in propagating *P. cynaroides* explants *in vitro*. Besides the direct formation of a high number of adventitious buds without an intervening callus phase on cotyledons (Fig. 1D), the subsequent vegetative growth of these buds were limited. Although the rate and severity of phenolic oxidation of the adventitious shoot-buds were not analysed, phenolic oxidation of explants were visually evident in buds cultured under conventional fluorescent lamps, while those irradiated by light emitted by LEDs or grown in the dark were less pronounced (Fig. 3). Phenolic oxidation has been previously reported to be one of the recurrent difficulties faced by researchers attempting to propagate *Protea* species *in vitro* (Tal et al., 1992; Thillerot et. al., 2006). An important finding of this study is the poor overall performance of conventional white fluorescent lamps compared to monochromatic light or growing explants in the dark. Although it is commonly known that growing plants in the absence of light reduces phenolic oxidation (Sivaci et al., 2007), it is morphogenetically and physiologically disadvantageous for explants to be exposed to total darkness for a prolonged period of time. Based on visual observation of the buds in this study, it seems that individual light quality plays an important role in oxidation process of *P. cynaroides* explants. Results of these observations indicate that monochromatic light may be the answer to reducing phenolic oxidation, which has so often been described by other authors as a barrier to successful propagation of the *Protea* species. A detailed study on the influences of individual light quality on phenolic oxidation is needed.

With regard to the organogenic growth and development of *P. cynaroides* adventitious shoot-buds, overall findings from this study showed that the buds responded positively to light emitted by red LEDs. On the other hand, buds cultured under white fluorescent lamps, which are commonly used as a light source for explants, showed poor growth in all parameters measured (Fig. 4). In the initial stages of the experiment, new vegetative growths were evident in these explants, however, as time progressed and browning of the buds took place, further growth of leaves and buds were severely limited (data not shown). A comparison of the overall root growth of *P. cynaroides* buds between red and blue LEDs showed a clear beneficial effect of red LEDs over blue LEDs in all root growth parameters. In literature, wide-ranging responses to different light qualities by various plant species have been reported. For example, no differences were found in rooting percentage, root number and root length between red and blue LEDs in two of the three grape cultivars tested (Poudel et al., 2008). Similarly, findings by Wang et al. (2011) showed that no significant differences in root number and root length were observed between *Gerbera* plantlets cultured under red LEDs and blue LEDs.

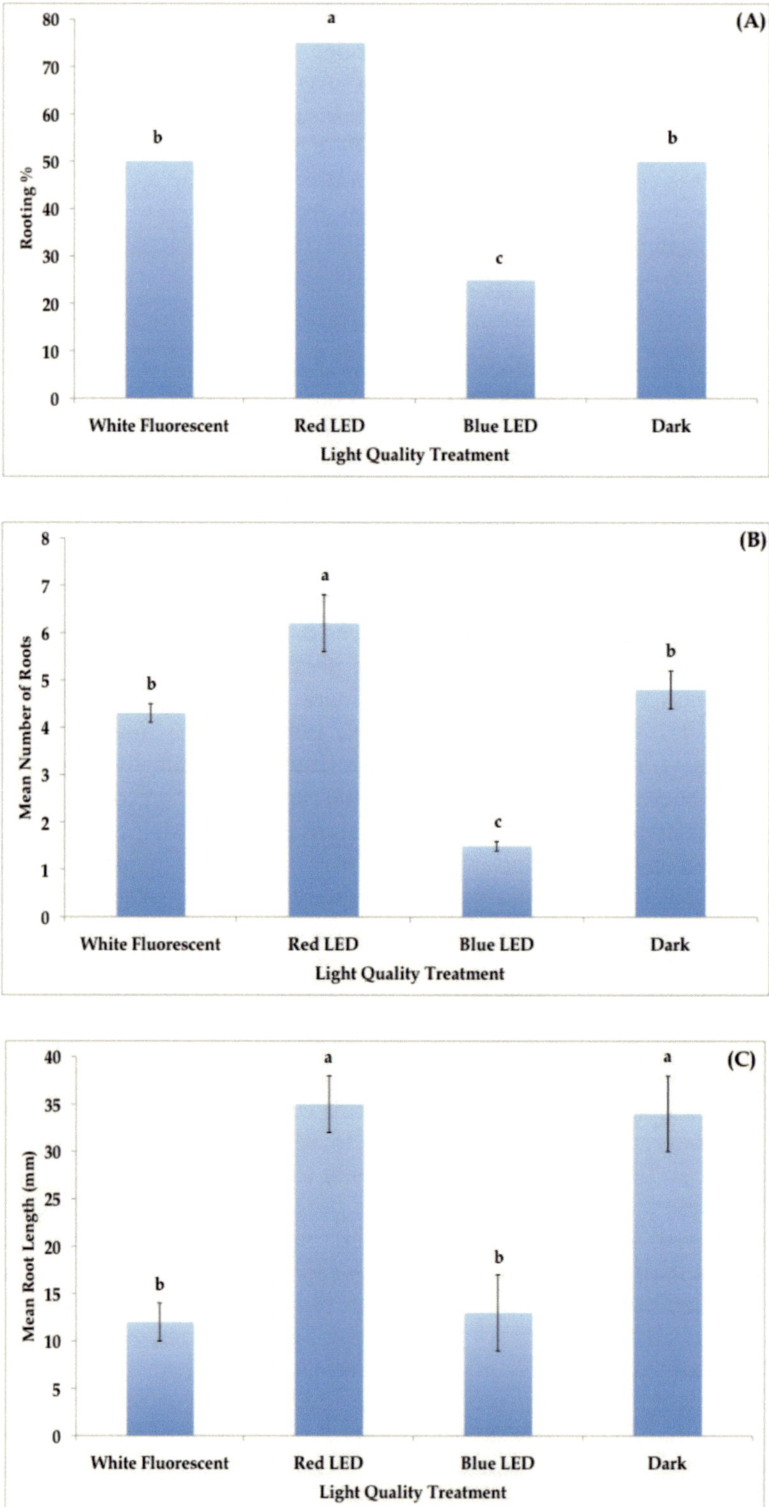
(A)
Rooting %
0
10
20
30
40
50
60
70
80
b
a
c
b
White Fluorescent
Red LED
Blue LED
Dark
Light Quality Treatment
(B)
Mean Number of Roots
0
1
2
3
4
5
6
7
8
b
a
c
b
White Fluorescent
Red LED
Blue LED
Dark
Light Quality Treatment
(C)
Mean Root Length (mm)
0
5
10
15
20
25
30
35
40
b
a
b
a
White Fluorescent
Red LED
Blue LED
Dark
Light Quality Treatment

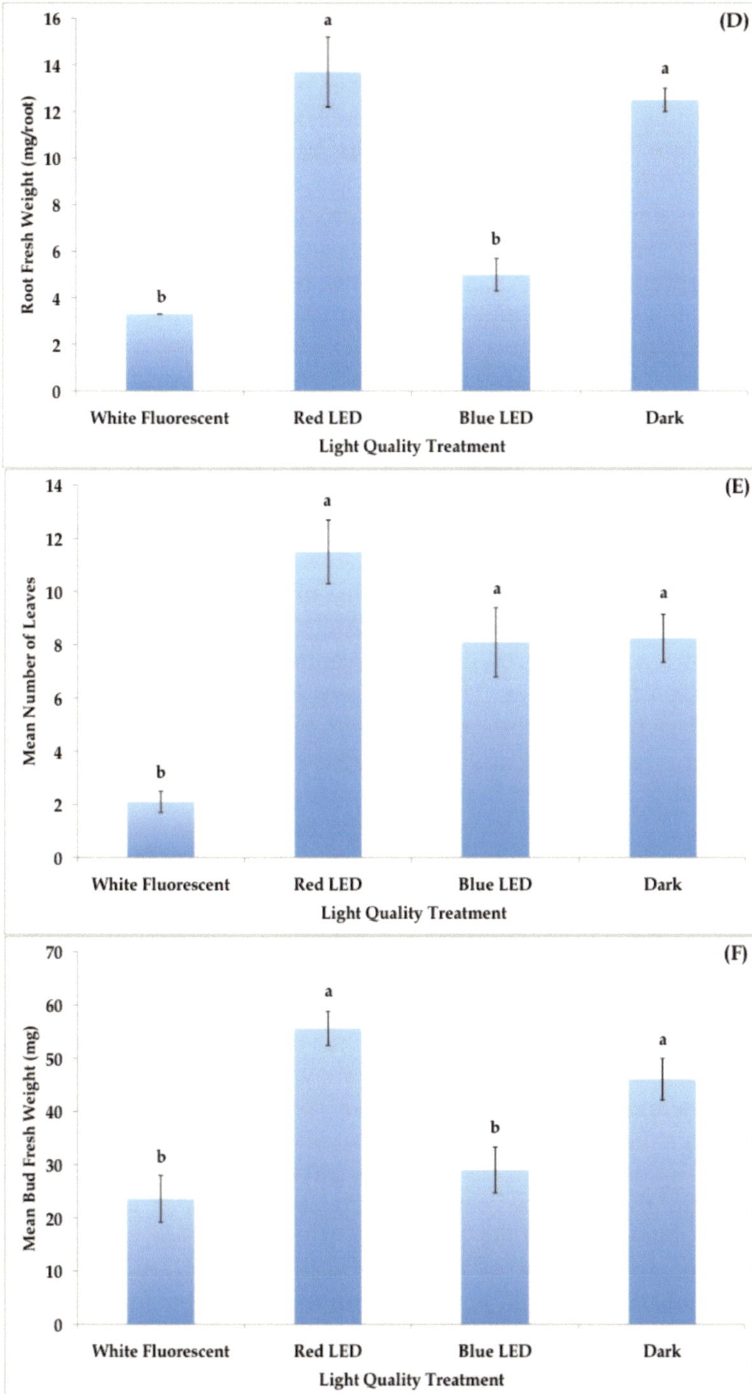

Fig. 4. Response of adventitious buds to light quality treatments after 45 days in culture. **(A)** Rooting percentage; **(B)** Root number; **(C)** Root length; **(D)** Root fresh weight; (per root) **(E)** Leaf number; **(F)** Bud fresh weight.

On the other hand, red light was found to be inhibitory toward the formation of roots in *Cattleya* microcuttings (Cybularz-Urban et al., 2007). In their study, the number of roots and root length produced by the microcuttings under red light were significantly lower than those exposed to blue light. Similar results were also found in cherry plantlets where, compared to red light, irradiation by blue lights significantly increased the root numbers (Iacona & Muleo, 2010). Nevertheless, an overview of literature seems to indicate that red light in general are stimulatory to root formation. The positive effects of red LEDs in the present study are in agreement with this trend. For example, the number of roots formed in *Dieffenbachia* explants significantly increased under red light, while root growth of explants cultured under blue light were similar to those irradiated by conventional white fluorescent tubes, which were found to produce significantly lower number of roots (Gabarkiewicz et al., 1997). Red light was also found to stimulate root formation in anthurium (Budiarto, 2010), cotton (Li et al., 2010) and strawberry (Nhut et al., 2003) explants.

In terms of leaf growth, results of the present study seem to be in agreement with those reported in other plant species. Poudel et al. (2008) reported that in their *in vitro* propagation of three grape cultivars, no significant differences were found in the number of leaves formed by shoots cultured under red and blue LEDs. Similar findings were also reported in *Gerbera jamesonii* where an almost identical number of leaves was found in plantlets cultured under red LEDs and blue LEDs (Wang et al. (2011). However, according to Nhut & Nam (2010), red LEDs promote leaf growth, but the amount of chlorophyll decreases, thereby reducing the quality of the leaves. This statement is supported by results of a study by Chang et al. (2003) where the chlorophyll content of calla lily leaves were found to be significantly higher when grown under blue lights compared to those cultured under red lights. This however, is in contrast to results of a study by Kim et al. (2004), who found the chlorophyll content (SPAD value) to be similar between chrysanthemum plantlets cultured under red LEDs and blue LEDs. It is almost certain that, in terms of chlorophyll content, the response of different plant species to red and blue LEDs varies widely. Further studies are needed to analyse the leaves of *P. cynaroides* explants to clarify the relationship between light quality and chlorophyll content.

The poor leaf growth of *P. cynaroides* buds under conventional fluorescent lamps was, to a certain extent, expected. As mentioned above, phenolic browning is a problem that has not been totally resolved. The results of this study showed the severity of this problem in the browning of leaves and tissues (Fig. 3A). When compared to explants in the other light treatments, the negative effects of browning is clearly evident in explants grown under white fluorescent lights, and analyses of the growth parameters further illustrates its negative influence on the overall growth of the shoot-buds. The lack of elongated growth of *P. cynaroides* shoot-buds in the LED treatments is an issue that needs to be resolved. A possible explanation for the lack of shoot-bud elongation could be due monochromatic lights causing an imbalance of light energy distribution available for photosystems I and II, which inhibits shoot growth (Kim et al., 2004). However, this does not explain the lack of elongation of shoot-buds cultured in the dark, which were less affected by phenolic browning, and is known to induce cell elongation. It is therefore probable that different growth regulator concentrations in the medium are needed to promote cell elongation in *P. cynaroides*. Growth regulators alone, or in combination with light quality could improve the growth of *P. cynaroides* explants.

Results of this study indicate that the significantly higher bud weight of shoot-buds cultured under different light conditions (Fig. 4F) is related to their overall root growth (Fig. 4A-C). As suggested earlier, the formation of roots is vital for the efficient absorption of nutrients, and thus is directly related to explant growth. Results showed that dark-grown buds and those irradiated by red LEDs produced the most roots, which in turn resulted in the highest bud weight. In contrast, poor root growth of buds cultured under blue LEDs resulted in lower bud weight. Under white fluorescent lamps, although rooting percentage and the number of roots were similar to those grown in the dark, however, due to phenolic browning, growth and development of the shoot-buds were severely inhibited.

5. Conclusion

The induction of adventitious root formation on *P. cynaroides* buds was achieved for the first time. In sharp contrast to blue LEDs, red LEDs were found to be the most suitable light source for root induction. Phenolic browning of shoot-buds cultured under conventional white fluorescent lamps resulted in poor overall vegetative growth, as are commonly reported. Of particular interest was that phenolic browning of *P. cynaroides* shoot-buds does not seem to occur under monochromatic red or blue lights. This finding could be an important break through in reducing browning of *P. cynaroides* explants *in vitro*. In addition, the results of this study suggest that the light quality emitted by red and blue LEDs were both beneficial to the vegetative growth of *P cynaroides* shoot-buds *in vitro*. Successful induction of adventitious roots on this difficult-to-grow plant has provided a step closer to the realization of micropropagation as an alternative means for propagating *P. cynaroides*. However, further studies are needed to investigate the effects of red and blue LED combinations at different ratios on the growth and development of *P. cynaroides* explants. In addition, the induction of shoot elongation and development through the use of growth regulators is required. Further analysis of the relationship between light quality and phenolic browning, is needed.

6. Acknowledgement

Financial support in the form of a research grant (NSC 98-2313-B-343-001) from the National Science Council of Taiwan (R.O.C) is gratefully acknowledged.

7. References

Appelgren, M. (1991). Effects of light quality on stem elongation of *Pelargonium in vitro*. *Scientia Horticulturae*, Vol.45, pp. 345-351, ISSN 0304-4238

Ben-Jaacov, J. & Jacobs, G. (1986). Establishing *Protea, Leucospermum* and *Serruria in vitro*. *Acta Hor*ticulturae, Vol.185, pp. 39-52, ISSN 0567-7572

Brown, C. S.; Schurger, A. C. & Sager, J.C. (1995). Growth and photomorphogenesis of pepper plants under red light-emitting diodes with supplemental blue or far-red lighting. *Journal of the American Society for Horticultural Sciences*, Vol.120, No.4, pp. 808-813

Budiarto, K. (2010). Spectral quality affects morphogenesis on Anthurium plantlet during *in vitro* culture. *Agrivita*, Vol. 32, No.3, pp. 234-240, ISSN 0126-0537

Bula, R.J.; Morrow, R.C.; Tibbitts, T.W.; Barta, D.J.; Ingnatius, R.W. & Martin, T.S. (1991). Light-emitting diodes as a radiation source for plants. *HortScience*, Vol.26, pp. 203-205, ISSN 1432-1904

Chang, H.S.; Chakrabarty, E.J.; Hahn, E.J., & Paek, K.Y. (2003). Micropropagation of Calla Lily (*Zantedeschia albomaculata*) via *in vitro* shoot tip proliferation. *In Vitro Cellular and Developmental Biology – Plant*, Vol.39, pp. 129-134, ISSN 1054-5476

Cybularz-Urban, T.; Hanus-Fajerska, E. & Swiderski, A. (2007). Effect of light wavelength on *in vitro* organogenesis of a *Cattleya* hybrid. *Acta Biologica Cracoviensia*, Vol.49, No.1, pp. 113-118, ISSN 0001-5296

Dorrington, P. (2008). Proceedings of the 13th International Protea Association Conference. *Protea Newsletter International*, Vol.1, No.1, pp. 1-19, Stellenbosch, South Africa, September 3-6, 2008

Economou, A.S. & Read, P.E. (1987). Light treatments to improve efficiency of *in vitro* propagation systems. *HortScience*, Vol.22, pp. 751-754, ISSN 0018-5345

Gabarkiewicz, B.; Gabryszewska, E.; Rudnicki, R. & Goszczynska, D. (1997). Effects of light quality on *in vitro* growing of *Dieffenbachia* cv. Compacta. *Acta Horticulturae*, Vol.418, pp. 159-162, ISSN 0567-7572

Galen, C.; Rabenold, J.J. & Liscum, E. (2007). Functional ecology of a blue light receptor: effects of phototropin-1 on root growth enhance drought tolerance in *Arabidopsis thaliana*. *New Phytologist*. Vol.173, No.1, pp. 91–99, ISSN 1469-8137

Goins, G.D.; Yorio, N.C.; Sanwo, M.M. & Brown, C.S. (1997). Photomorphogenesis, photosynthesis, and seed yield of wheat plants grown under light emitting diodes (LEDs) with or without supplemental blue lighting. *Journal of Experimental Botany*, Vol.48, No.7, pp. 1407-1413. ISSN 1460- 2431

Iacona, C. & Muleo, R. (2010). Light Quality affects *in vitro* adventitious rooting and *ex vitro* performance of cherry rootstock Colt. *Scientia Horticulturae*, Vol.125, pp. 630-636, ISSN 0304-4238

Jao, R.C. & Fang, W. (2004). Effects of frequency and duty ratio on the growth of potato plantlets *in vitro* using light emitting diodes. *HortScience*, Vol.39, No.2, pp. 375-379, ISSN 0018-5345

Jao, R.C; Lai, C.C.; Fang, W. & Chang, S.F. (2005). Effects of red light on the growth of Zantedeschia plantlets *in vitro* and tuber formation using light-emitting diodes. *HortScience*, Vol.40, No.2, pp. 436-438, ISSN 0018-5345

Kim, S.; Hahn, E.; Heo, J. & Paek, K. (2004). Effects of LEDs on net photosynthetic rate, growth and leaf stomata of chrysanthemum plantlets *in vitro*. *Scientia Horticulturae*, Vol.101, pp. 143-151, ISSN 0304-4238

Leonardt, K. (2008). Regional grower reports. *Protea Newsletter International*, Vol.1, No.1, pp. 8-12

Li, H.; Xu, Z. & Tang, C. (2010). Effect of light-emitting diodes on growth and morphogenesis of upland cotton (*Gossypium hirutum* L.) plantlets *in vitro*, *Plant, Cell, Tissue and Organ Culture*, Vol.103, No.2, pp. 155-163, ISSN 1573-5044

Lian, M.L; Murthy, H.N. & Paek, K.Y. (2002). Effects of light emitting diodes (LEDs) on the *in vitro* induction and growth of bulblets of *Lilium* oriental hybrid 'Pesaro'. *Scientia Horticulturae*, Vol.94, pp. 365-370, ISSN 0304-4238

Lin, B.; Tai, T. & Chung, J. (2008). Effects of six types of LED radiation on scale multiplication, leaf formation and rooting of *Lilium* Oriental Hybrid 'Casa Blanca' *in vitro*. *Journal of the Taiwan Society for Horticultural Science*, Vol.54, No.3, pp. 223-230, ISSN 1819-8317

Littlejohn, G.M.; van den Berg, G.C. & Matlhoahela, P. (2003). Within plant distribution of macronutrients in Protea 'Cardinal'. *Acta Horticulturae*, Vol.602, pp. 93-98, ISSN 0567-7572

Matthews, L. (1993). *The Protea growers handbook*, Trade Winds Press, ISBN 0731803256, South Africa

Montarone, M. & Allemand, P. (1995). Growing Proteaceae soilless under shelter. *Acta Horticulturae*, Vol.387, pp. 73-84, ISSN 0567-7572

Murashige, T. & Skoog, F. (1962). A revised medium for rapid growth and bioassays with tobacco tissue cultures. *Physiologia Plantarum*, Vol.15, 473-497, ISSN 1399-3054

Nhut, D.T.; Hong, L.T.A.; Watanabe, H.; Goi, M. & Tanaka, M. (2002). Growth of banana plantlets cultured *in vitro* under red and blue light-emitting diode (LED) irradiation source. *Acta Horticulturae*, Vol.575, pp. 117-124, ISSN 0567-7572

Nhut, D.T.; Takamura, T.; Watanabe, H.; Okamoto, K. & Tanaka, M. (2003). Responses of strawberry plantlets cultured *in vitro* under superbright red and blue light-emitting diodes (LEDs). *Plant, Cell, Tissue and Organ Culture*, Vol.73, No.1, pp. 43-52, ISSN 1573-5044

Nhut, D.T. & Nam, N.B. (2010). Light-emitting diodes (LEDs): An artificial lighting source for biological studies. *Proceedings of the International Federation for Medical and Biological Engineering (IFMBE)*, Vol.27, pp. 134-139. ISSN 1680-0737

Okamoto, K.; Yanagi, T. & Kondo, S. (1997). Growth and morphogenesis of lettuce seedlings raised under different combinations of red and blue light. *Acta Horticulturae*, Vol.435, pp. 149-157, ISSN 0567-7572

Okamoto, K.; Yanagi, T. & Takita, S. (1996). Development of plant growth apparatus using blue and red LED as artificial light source. *Acta Horticulturae*, Vol.440, pp. 111-116, ISSN 0567-7572

Paterson-Jones, C. (2007). *Protea*. Struik Publishers, ISBN 1770075240, Cape Town, South Africa

Poudel, P.; Kataoko, I. & Mochioka, R. (2008). Effect of red- and blue-light-emitting diode on growth and morphogenesis of grapes. *Plant, Cell, Tissue and Organ Culture*, Vol.92, No2. pp. 147-153, ISSN 1573-5044

Quail, P.H. (2002). Phytochrome photosensory signalling networks. *Nature Reviews Molecular Cell Biology*, Vol.3, pp. 85–93, ISSN 1471-0080

Robelo, T. (2000). *Field guide to the Proteas of the Cape Peninsula*, National Botanical Institute, Cape Town, South Africa

SAS Institute Inc. (1996). The SAS system for Windows. *SAS Institute Inc.*, Cary, North Carolina, USA

Silber, A.; Mitchnick, B. & Ben-Jaacov, J. (2001). Phosphorous nutrition and rhizosphere pH in *Leucadendron* Safari Sunset'. *Acta Horticulturae*, Vol.545, pp. 135-143, ISSN 0567-7572

Sivaci, A.; Sokmen, M. & Gunes, T. (2007). Biochemical changes in green and etiolated stems of MM106 apple rootstock. *Asian Journal of Plant Sciences*, Vol.6, No.5, pp. 839-843, ISSN 1682-3974

Tal, E.; Solomon, H.; Ben-Jaacov, J. & Watad, A.A. (1992). Micropropagation of selected *Leucospermum cordifolium*: Effect of antibiotics and GA_3. *Acta Horticulturae*, Vol.316, pp. 55-58, ISSN 0567-7572

Thillerot, F.; Choix, A.; Poupet, M. & Montarone. (2006). Micropropagation of *Leucospermum* 'High Gold' and three cultivars of Protea. *Acta Horticulturae*, Vol.716, pp. 17-24, ISSN 0567-7572

Wang, Z.; Li, G.; He, S.; Teixeira da Silva, J.A. & Tanaka, M. (2011). Effect of cold cathode fluorescent lamps on growth of *Gerbera jamesonii* plantlets *in vitro*. *Scientia Horticulturae*, Vol. 130, pp. 482-484 ISSN 0304-4238

Wu, H.C. & du Toit, E.S. (2004). Reducing oxidative browning during *in vitro* establishment of *Protea cynaroides*. *Scientia Horticulturae*, Vol.100, pp. 355-358, ISSN 0304-4238

Wu, H.C.; du Toit, E.S. & Reinhardt, C.F. (2007a). Micrografting of *Protea cynaroides*. *Plant, Cell, Tissue and Organ Culture*, Vol.89, No.1, pp. 23-28, ISSN 1573-5044

Wu, H.C.; du Toit, E.S. & Reinhardt, C.F. (2007b). A protocol for direct somatic embryogenesis of *Protea cynaroides* L. using zygotic embryos and cotyledon tissues. *Plant, Cell, Tissue and Organ Culture*, Vol.89, No.2, pp. 217-224, ISSN 1573-5044

Yanagi, T. & Okamoto, K. (1997). Utilization of super-bright light emitting diodes as an artificial light source for plant growth. *Acta Horticulturae*, Vol.418, pp. 223-228, ISSN 0567-7572

8

Development of the Site of Articulation Between the Two Human Hemimandibles (Symphysis Menti)

Ahmed F. El Fouhil
College of Medicine, King Saud University
Saudi Arabia

1. Introduction

Symphysis menti was long ago considered as an axial midline symphysis present between the two halves of the fetal mandible and continues until the end of the first postnatal year when synostosis occurs (Bannister et al., 1995).

Previous studies have been focused on the development of the human symphysis menti in the first half of the fetal period (Kjaer, 1975). However, further development of this region till the occurrence of the complete fusion had not been fully investigated. Moreover, most studies on Meckel's cartilage had clarified its role in the development of mandible (O'Rahilly and Gardner, 1972). However, the role of such cartilage in the formation of the symphysis menti had received sporadic attention.

The aim of the present work was to study the different developmental stages of the human symphysis menti throughout the whole fetal period and postnatally till the occurrence of occlusion.

2. Material and methods

Thirty-two human specimens of different ages covering the fetal period and the first year of postnatal life were legally obtained from the Gynecology and Obstetrics, and Pathology Departments, Faculty of Medicine, Ain Shams University, Cairo, Egypt. According to their ages, the specimens were divided into eight groups (Table 1).

The mandible of all ages were scanned, using a General Electric 9800 Computarized Tomography (C.T.) scanner at 1.5 mm section thickness (512 x 512 matrix size 9.6 – 15.0 cm DF OV), using an edge enhancement (bone) algorithm in the axial and coronal scan planes. Three-dimensional (3 D) C.T. reconstructions were performed by an experienced operator on a CEMAX VIP 3 D work station for all two-dimensional C.T. data sets. Three-dimensional images were generated for each specimen.

In all abortions, the lower jaw was taken as a whole. In postmortem specimens, the body of the mandible was separated from the two rami and obtained as a single unit. The specimens were fixed in 10% formalin solution for one week. After fixation, specimens were decalcified by using neutral EDTA decalcifying solution for a period ranging from five to fifteen days according to each specimen. Decalcified specimens were processed for light microscopic study. They were dehydrated, cleared and embedded in paraffin blocks. Serial sections (4 - 5 micron thick) were obtained from each block and mounted on clean glass slides. The slides were deparaffinized and rehydrated. The sections were stained with Haematoxylin and Eosin and Masson's trichrome stains.

Group	Age	Number of specimens
First	9 weeks, intrauterine	3 abortions
Second	12 weeks, intrauterine	4 abortions
Third	28 weeks, intrauterine	8 postmortem
Fourth	40 weeks, intrauterine	5 postmortem
Fifth	One month, postnatal	3 postmortem
Sixth	Two months, postnatal	4 postmortem
Seventh	Five months, postnatal	3 postmortem
Eighth	One year, postnatal	2 postmortem

Table 1. Number of specimens for each age group.

3. Results

3.1 First group (nine weeks, intrauterine)

3.1.1 Histology

The symphyseal region consisted of mesenchymal tissue bounded labially and orally by trabeculae of immature bone formed of irregularly arranged collagen fibers with increased number of osteocytes. Such tabeculae were separated by spaces filled with newly formed bone marrow. Orally, the symphyseal region was also bounded by Meckel's cartilage that appeared as two symmetrical rod-like, cartilaginous structures. Rostrally, the two rods were separated by a thin rim of mesenchymal tissue (Fig. 1). While caudally, such rim was markedly thickened (Fig. 2). The medial portion of each rod showed signs of endochondral ossification (Fig. 1). Ossification proceeded in a latero-medial direction.

3.1.2 Three-dimensional C.T. scanning

The mandible appeared as two bilateral bony structures separated from each other, in the median plane, by a defect.

3.2 Second group (twelve weeks, intrauterine)

3.2.1 Histology

The mesenchymal tissue in the caudal portion of the symphyseal region showed two well defined, rounded to oval cartilaginous structures appearing do novo, unrelated and completely separated from Meckel's cartilage (Fig. 3). Such structures showed a marked hypercellularity and hypertrophy in their central region.

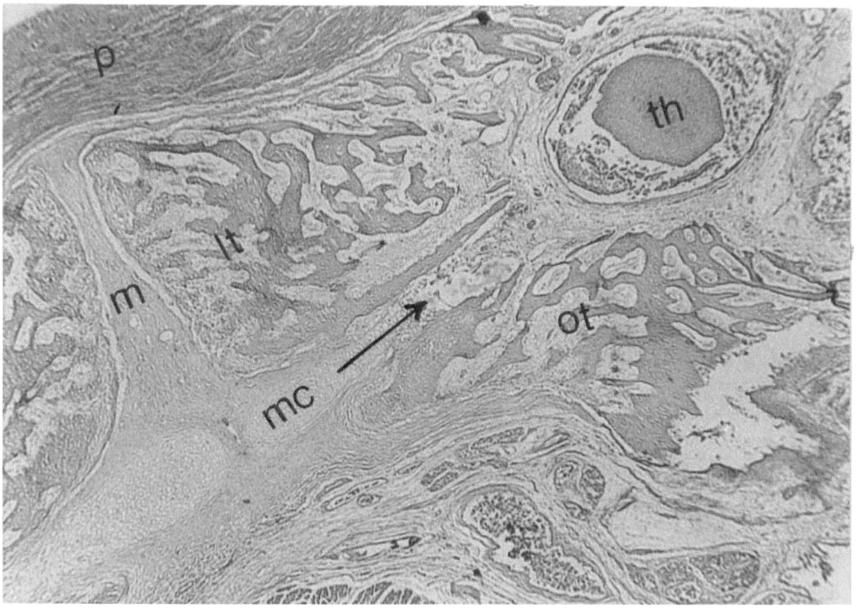

Fig. 1. A photomicrograph in the rostral portion of a nine-week old fetal mandible, showing the mesenchymal tissue in the midline (m), bounded by labial bony trabeculae (lt). Notice the closeness of the bilateral portions of Meckel's cartilage (mc). Oral bony trabeculae could be identified (ot). th = tooth premordium; p = lip; arrow = endochondral ossification in Meckel's cartilage. (Haematoxylin and Eosin x 20).

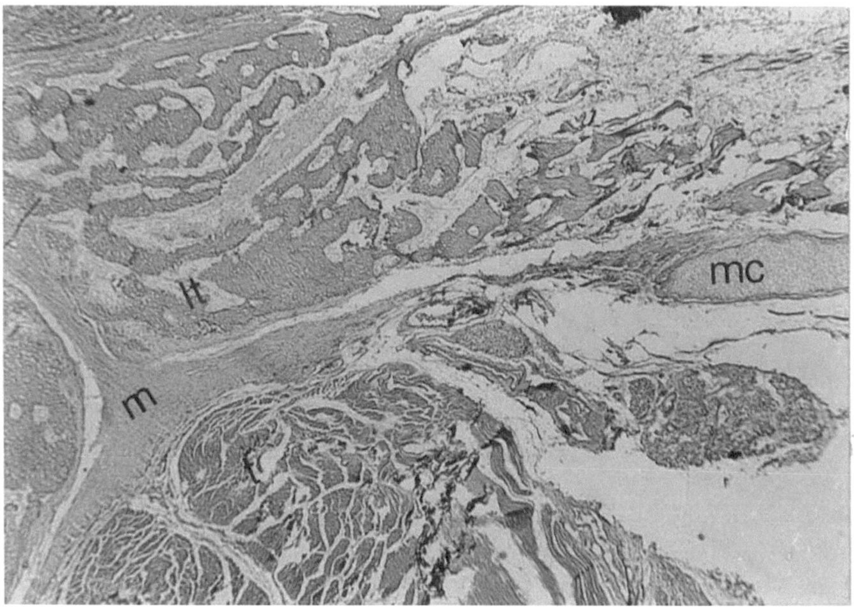

Fig. 2. A photomicrograph in the caudal portion of a nine-week old fetal mandible. Notice the wide separation of Meckel's cartilage (mc) from the mesenchymal tissue in the midline (m). t = tongue; lt = labial bony trabeculae. (Haematoxylin and Eosin x 20).

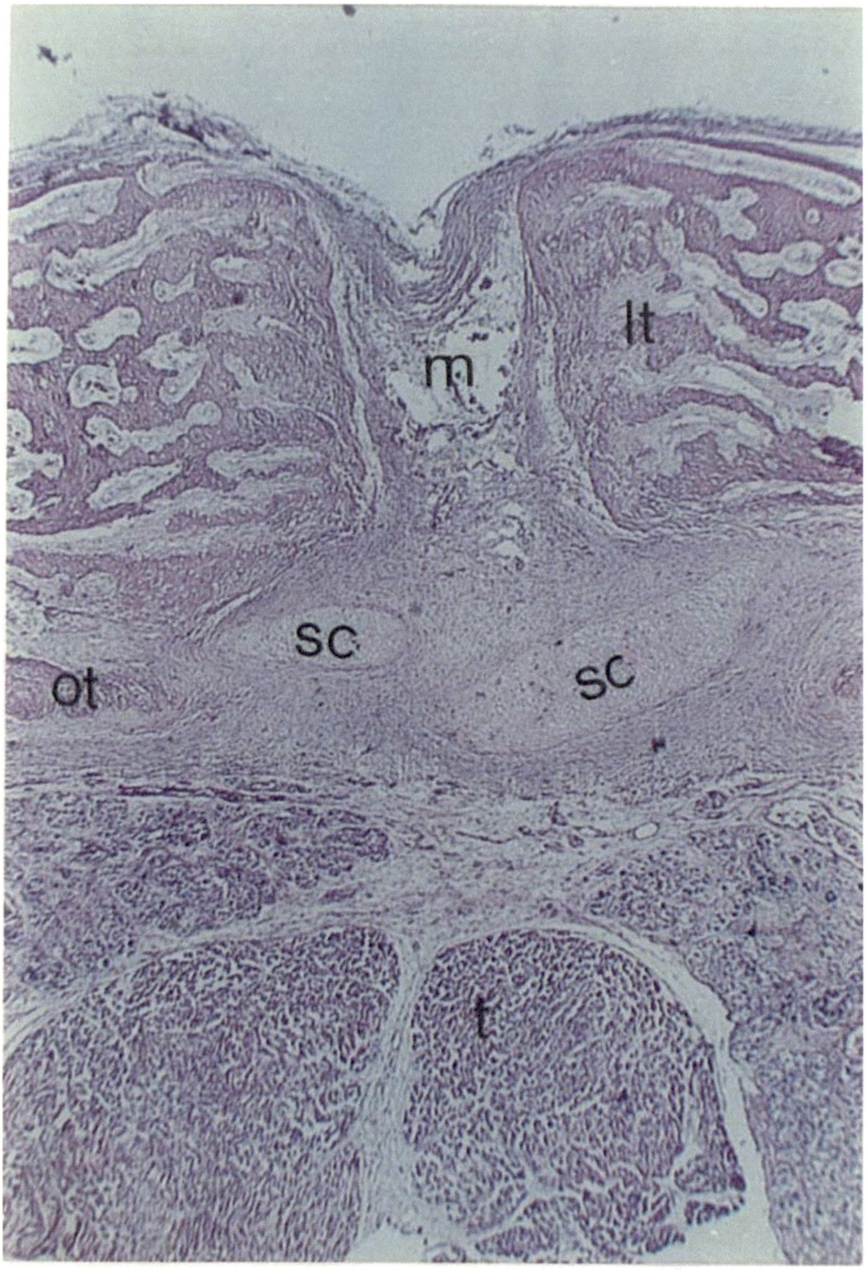

Fig. 3. A photomicrograph of a twelve-week old fetal mandible, showing mesenchymal tissue in the midline (m). Two secondary cartilages (sc) could be identified in the caudal portion of such mesenchyme. lt = labial bony trabeculae; ot = oral bony trabeculae; t = tongue. (Haematoxylin and Eosin x 20).

3.2.2 Three-dimensional C.T. scanning

The defect between the hemimandibles was still observed (Fig. 4).

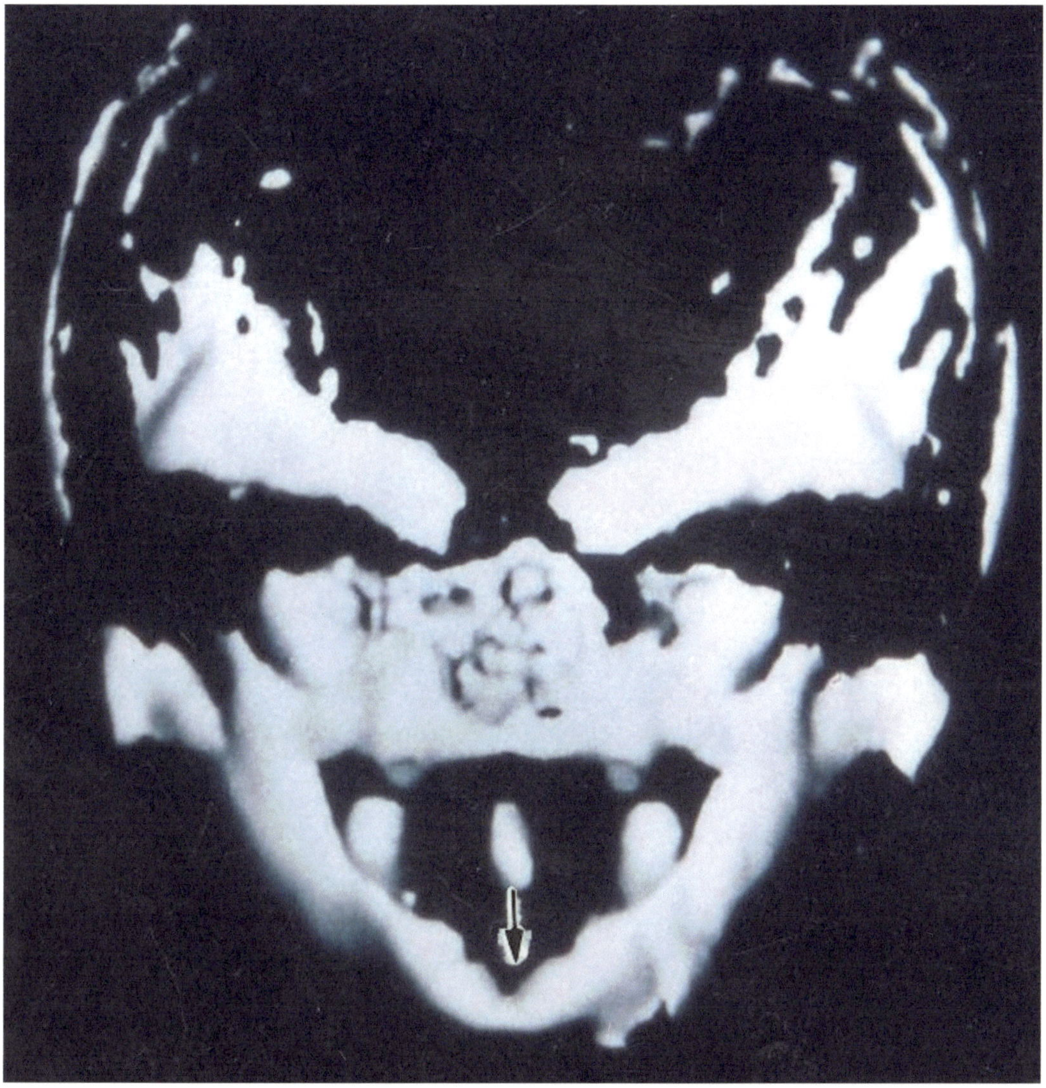

Fig. 4. A photograph of a three-dimensional C.T. scan of a twelve-week old fetal skull, with a top view of the mandible. Notice the triangular defect between the hemimandibles (arrow).

3.3 Third group (twenty-eight weeks, intrauterine)

3.3.1 Histology

A centrifugal pattern of matrix calcification had been observed in the symphyseal secondary cartilaginous structures (Fig. 5).

3.3.2 Three-dimensional C.T. scanning

The defect between the hemimandibles became narrower in its rostral portion (Fig. 6).

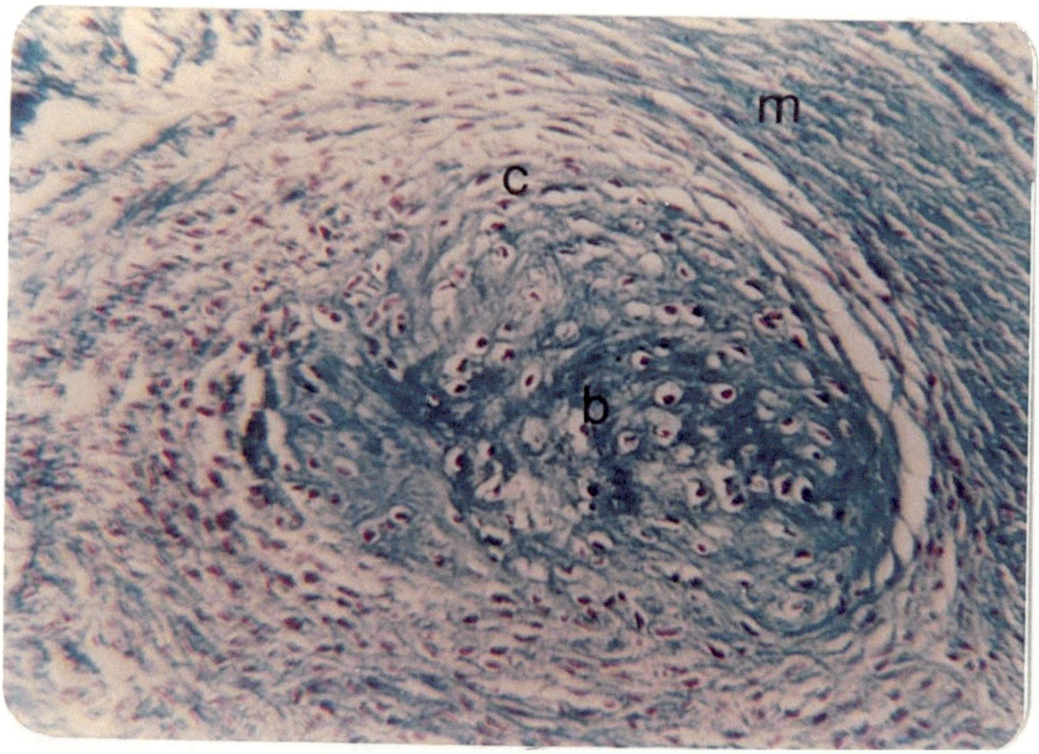

Fig. 5. A photomicrograph of a twenty-eight-week old fetal mandible, showing the symphyseal secondary cartilage. Notice the centrifugal ossification in the secondary cartilage. b = bone; c = cartilage; m = symphyseal mesenchymal tissue. (Masson's trichrome x 200).

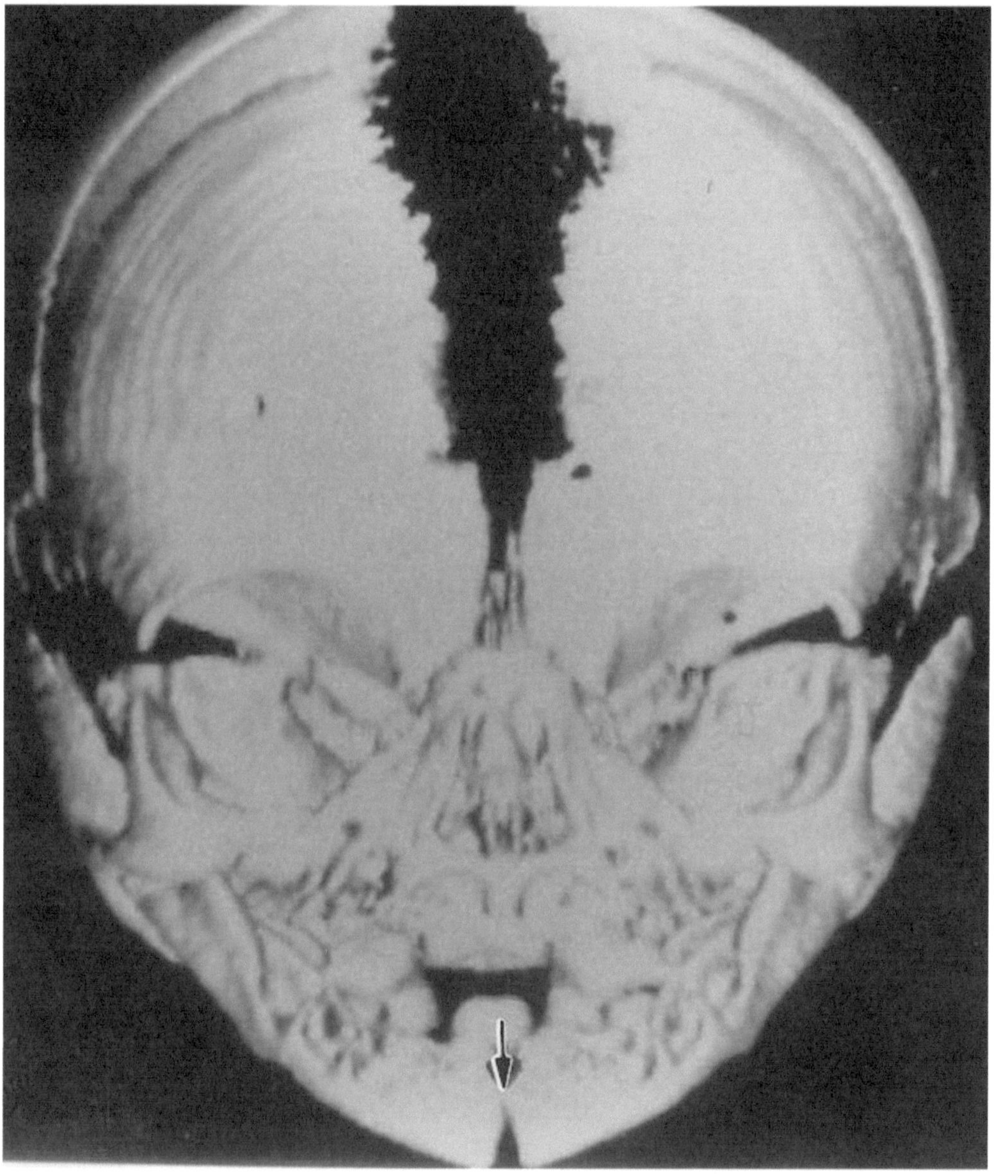

Fig. 6. A photograph of a three-dimensional C.T. scan of a twenty-eight-week old fetal skull, frontal orientation. Notice the triangular defect between the hemimandibles (arrow).

3.4 Fourth group (forty weeks, intrauterine)

3.4.1 Histology

The ossification process in the symphyseal secondary cartilages had completed leading to the formation of a single mental ossicle. The symphyseal region had decreased considerably in size and was bounded by bony trabeculae with very few remains of Meckel's cartilage in the form of ill-defined patches of cartilage (Figs 7, 8).

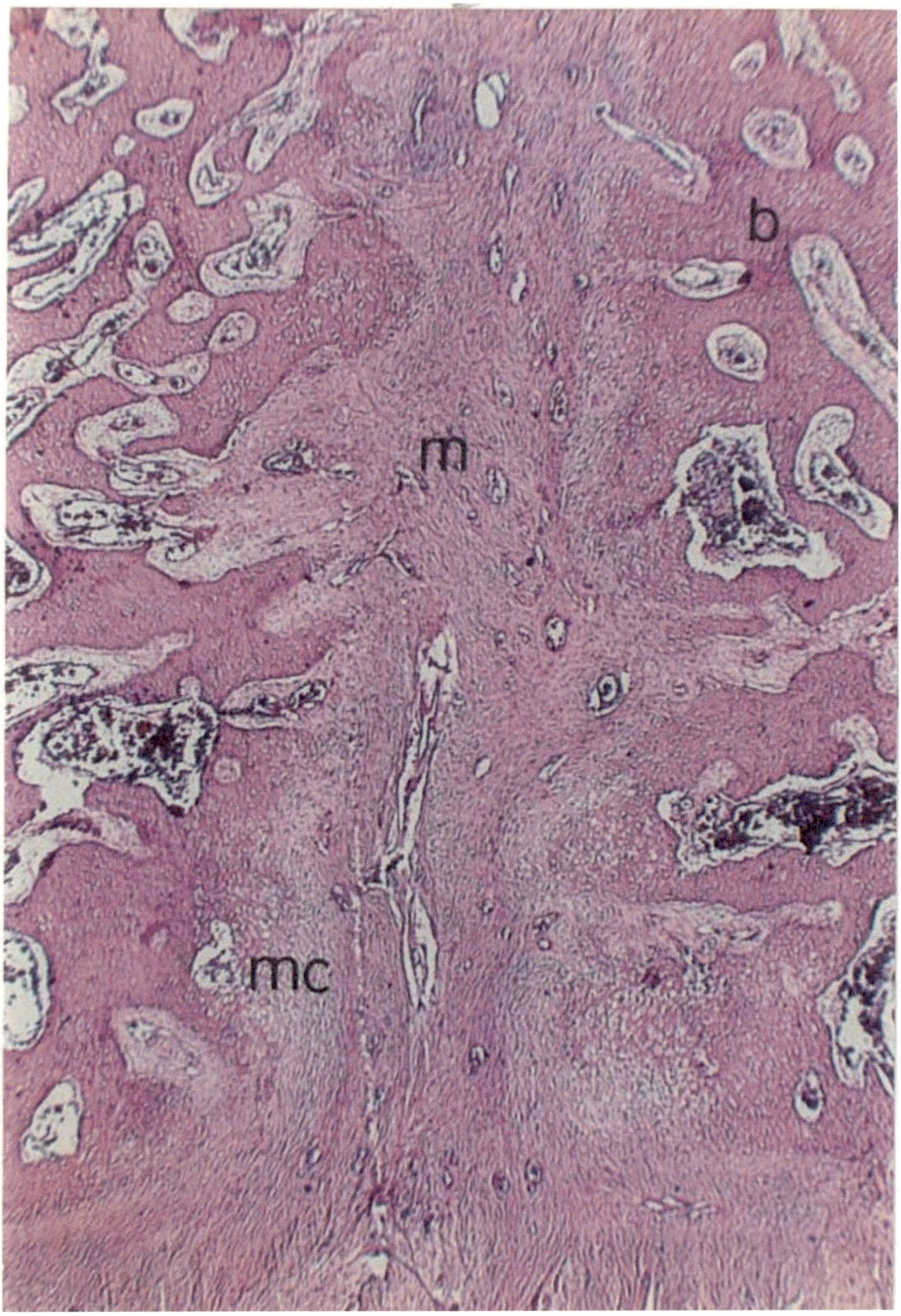

Fig. 7. A photomicrograph in the rostral portion of a forty-week old fetal mandible, showing the mesenchymal tissue in the midline (m), bounded on either side by bony trabeculae (b). Notice the remains of Meckel's cartilage (mc) in the caudal portion. (Haematoxylin and Eosin x 20).

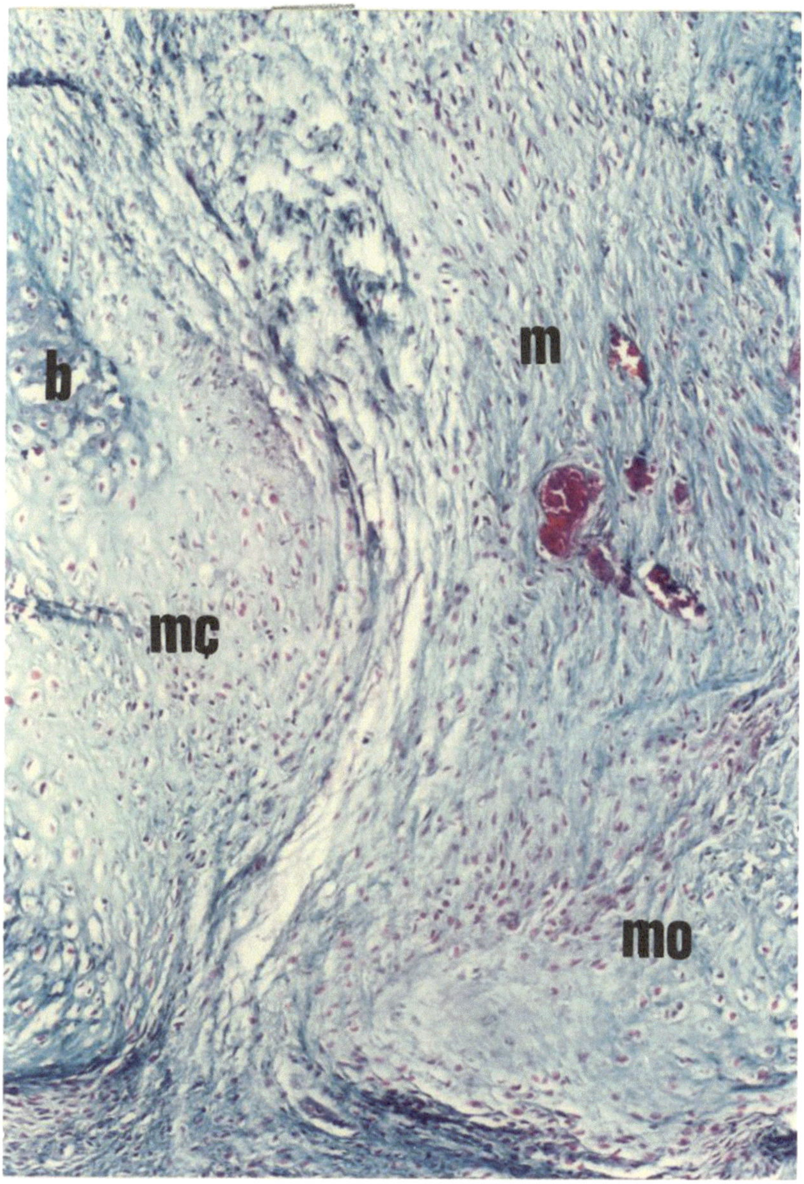

Fig. 8. A photomicrograph in the caudal portion of a forty-week old fetal mandible, showing the mesenchymal tissue (m). A mental ossicle (mo) is present in the caudal portion of the mesenchyme. mc = remains of Meckel's cartilage; b = bone of the hemimandible. (Masson's trichrome x 100).

3.4.2 Three-dimensional C.T. scanning

In serial caudo-rostral axial cuts in the symphyseal region (Fig. 9), a mental ossicle, completely separated from the hemimandibles, was only detected in the caudal cuts. Such ossicle was decreasing in size rostrally, denoting its conical shape.

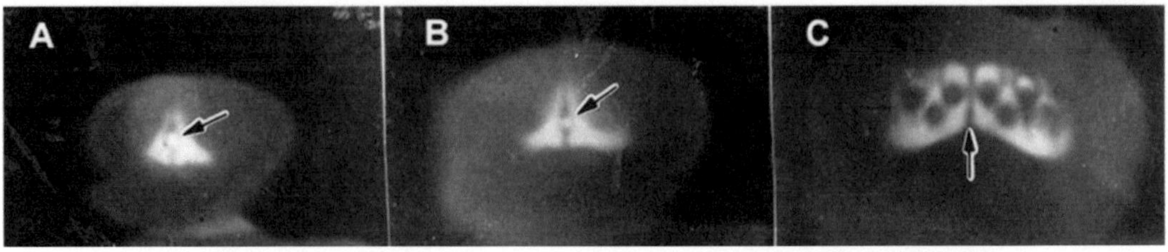

Fig. 9. A photograph of a three-dimensional C.T. scan, showing serial caudo-rostral cuts in a forty-week old fetal mandible:

a. A caudal cut shows a rounded mental ossicle (arrow) completely separated from the hemimandibles by a defect.
b. A more rostral cut shows a decrease in the size of the mental ossicle (arrow), denoting its conical shape.
c. The most rostral cut shows a midline defect (arrow) between the hemimandibles. The mental ossicle is not observed at this level.

3.5 Fifth group (one month, postnatal)

3.5.1 Histology

The mental ossicle appeared as a triangular structure, completely surrounded with symphyseal mesenchymal tissue (Fig. 10). Bony trabeculae forming the hemimandibles were growing towards the symphyseal region. No remains of Meckel's cartilage could be identified.

3.5.2 Three-dimensional C.T. scanning

The cone-shaped mental ossicle had increased in size, minimizing the gap between it and the hemimandibles. Rostral to the ossicle, the two hemimandibles were separated by a small midline defect (Fig. 11).

3.6 Sixth group (two months, postnatal)

3.6.1 Histology

The caudal portion of the mental ossicle appeared to fuse with both hemimandibles, while its rostral portion was still separated from them by mesenchymal tissue (Fig. 12).

3.6.2 Three-dimensional C.T. scanning

The mental ossicle had completely fused with the caudal portions of the hemimandibles, while a thin defect existed between the hemimandibles, rostral to the mental ossicle (Fig. 13).

3.7 Seventh group (five months, postnatal)

3.7.1 Histology

The mental ossicle had completely fused with both hemimandibles. A rim of symphyseal mesenchymal tissue was still separating the two hemimandibles, rostral to the mental ossicle (Fig. 14).

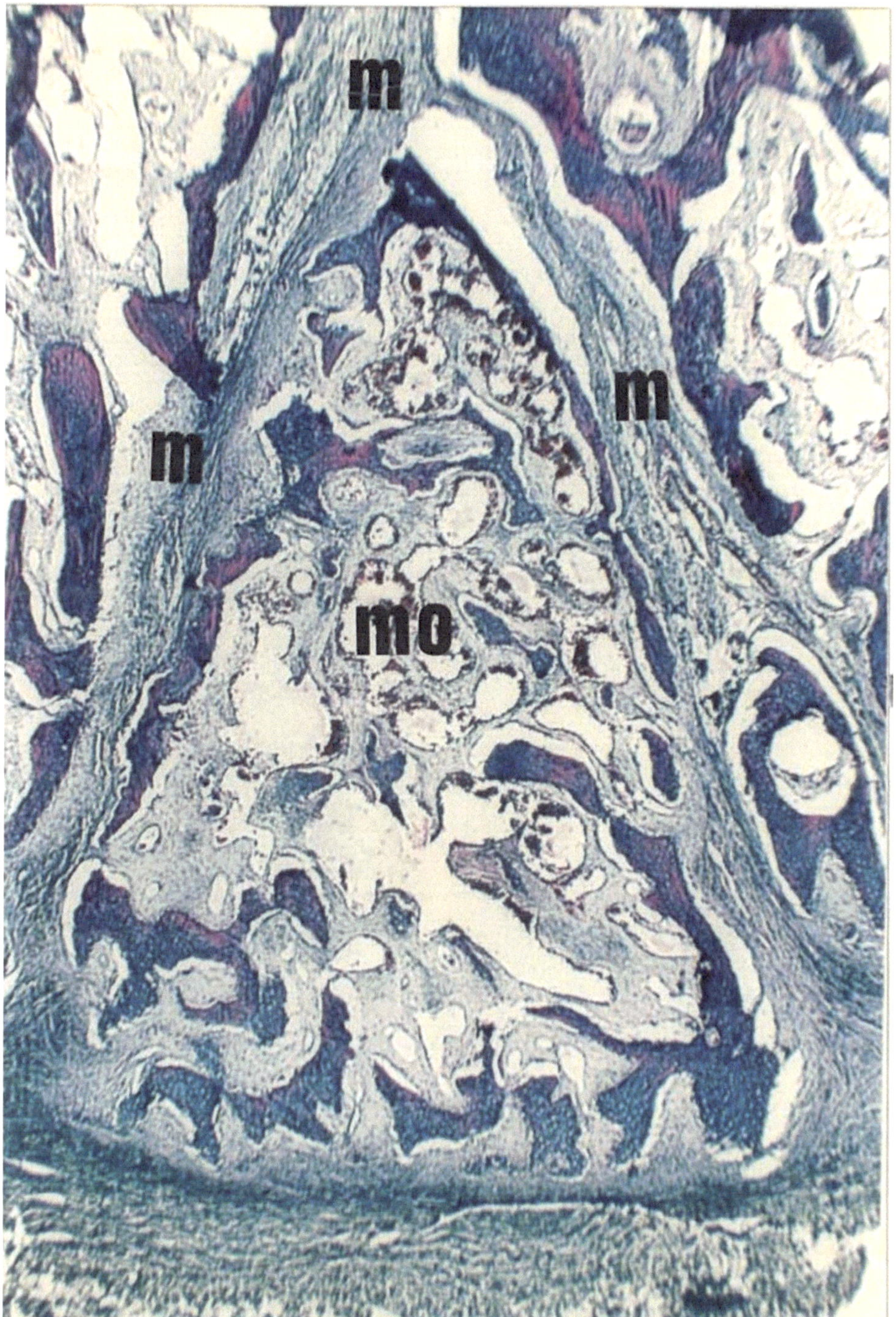

Fig. 10. A photomicrograph in the caudal portion of a one-month old infant mandible, showing a triangular mental ossicle (mo) present in the caudal portion of the symphyseal mesenchymal tissue (m). (Masson's trichrome x 200).

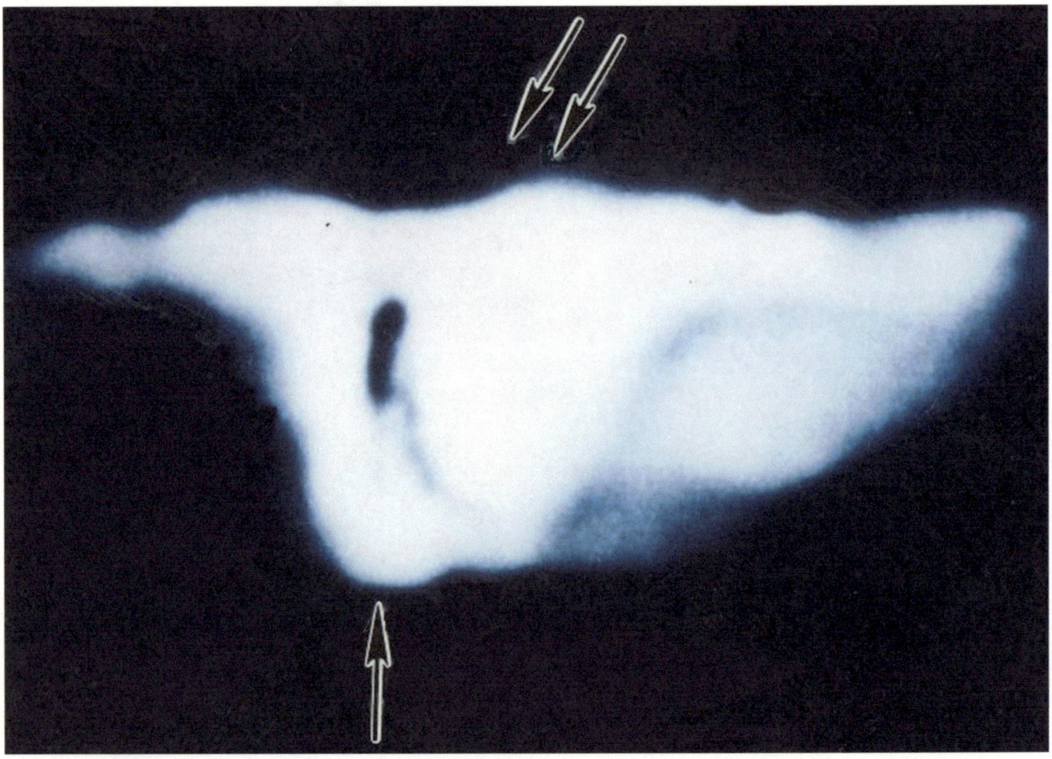

Fig. 11. A photograph of a three-dimensional C.T. scan of a one-month old infant mandible. Notice the mental ossicle (arrow) and the midline defect (double arrows) between the hemimandibles, rostral to the mental ossicle.

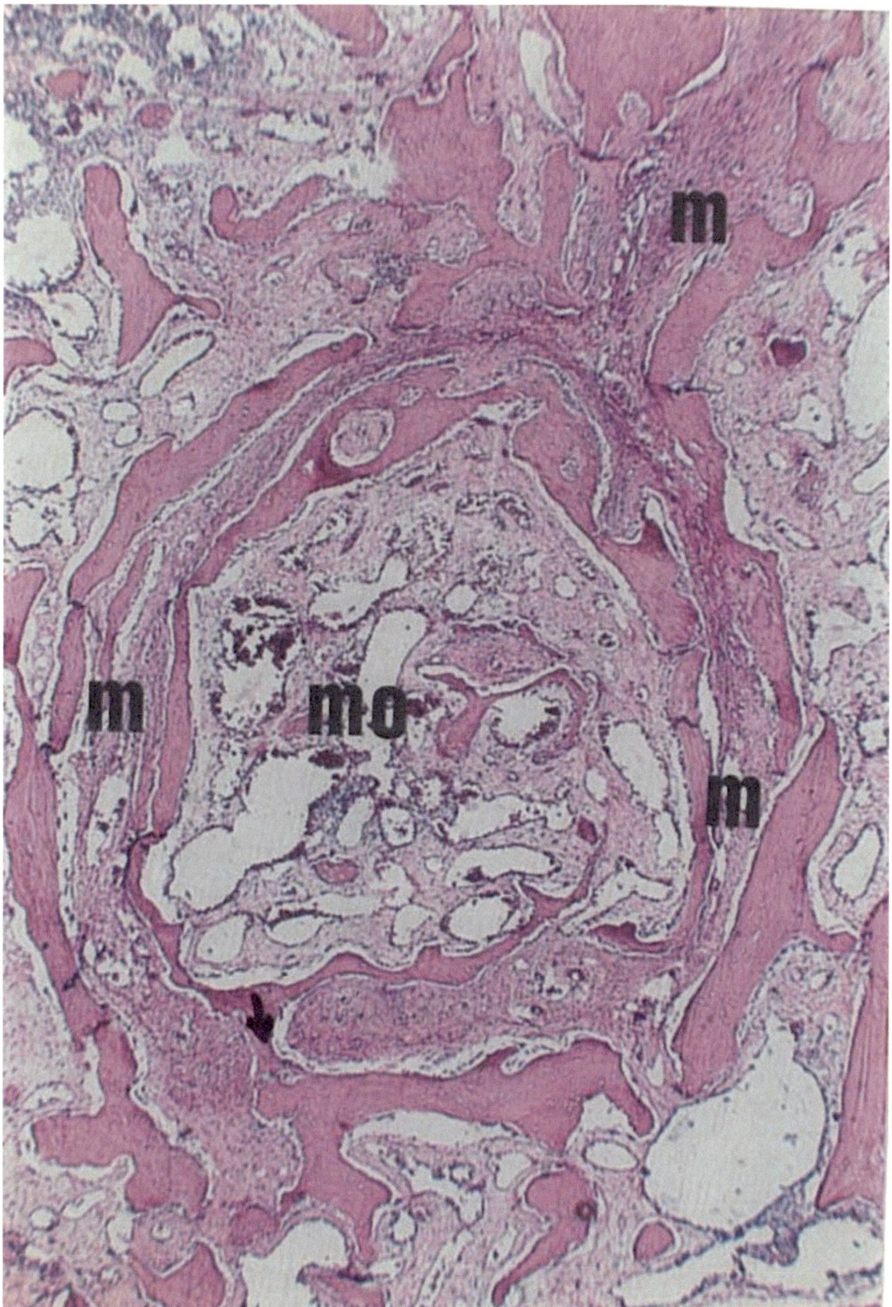

Fig. 12. A photomicrograph of a two-month old infant mandible. Notice that the caudal portion of the mental ossicle (mo) had started to fuse with both hemimandibles (arrow), while its rostral portion was still separated from the hemimandibles by a rim of mesenchymal tissue continuous with the midline mesenchyme (m). (Haematoxylin and Eosin x 20).

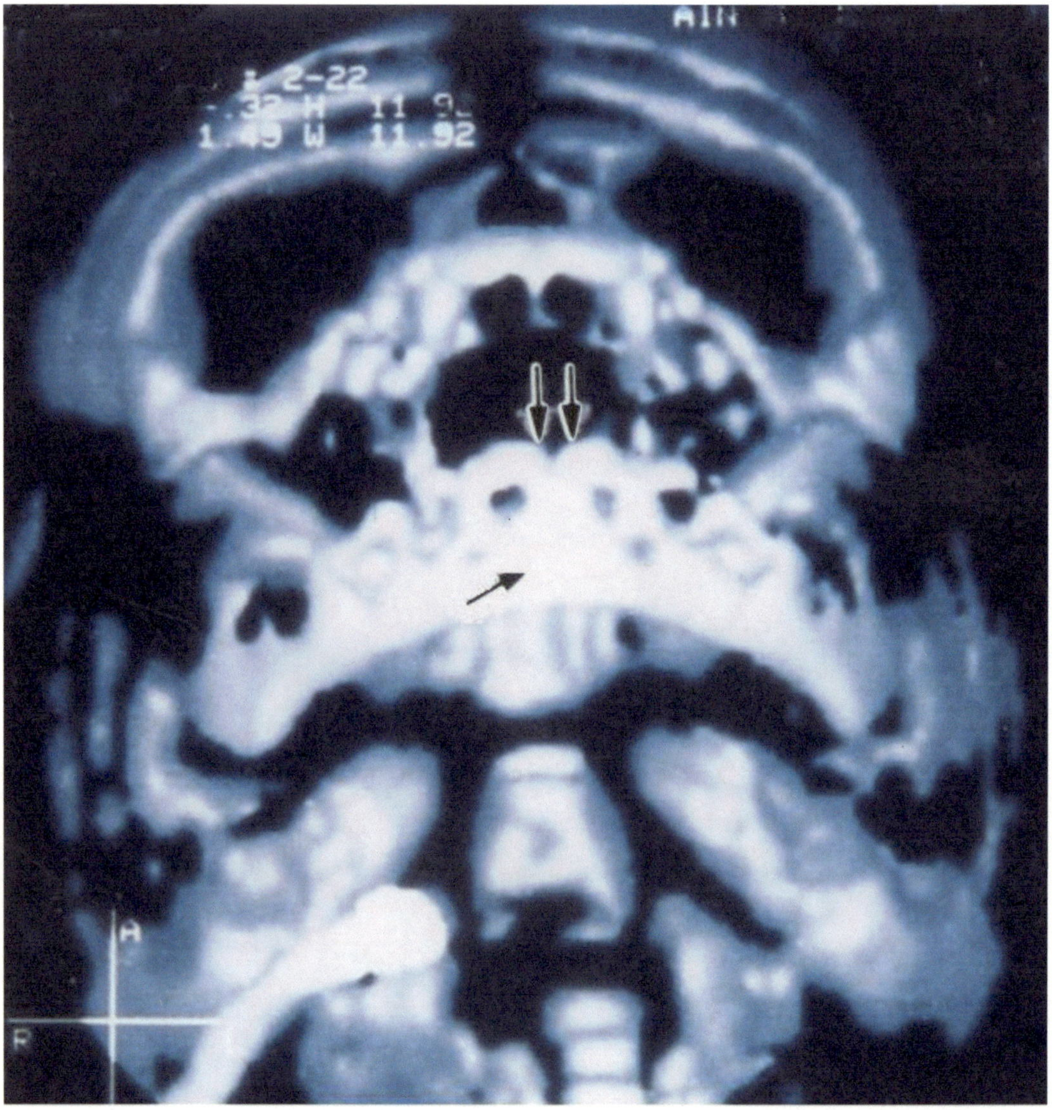

Fig. 13. A photograph of a three-dimensional C.T. scan of a two-month old infant skull, showing the fusion of the mental ossicle (arrow) with the hemimandibles. Notice the midline defect (double arrows) between the hemimandibles, rostral to the mental ossicle.

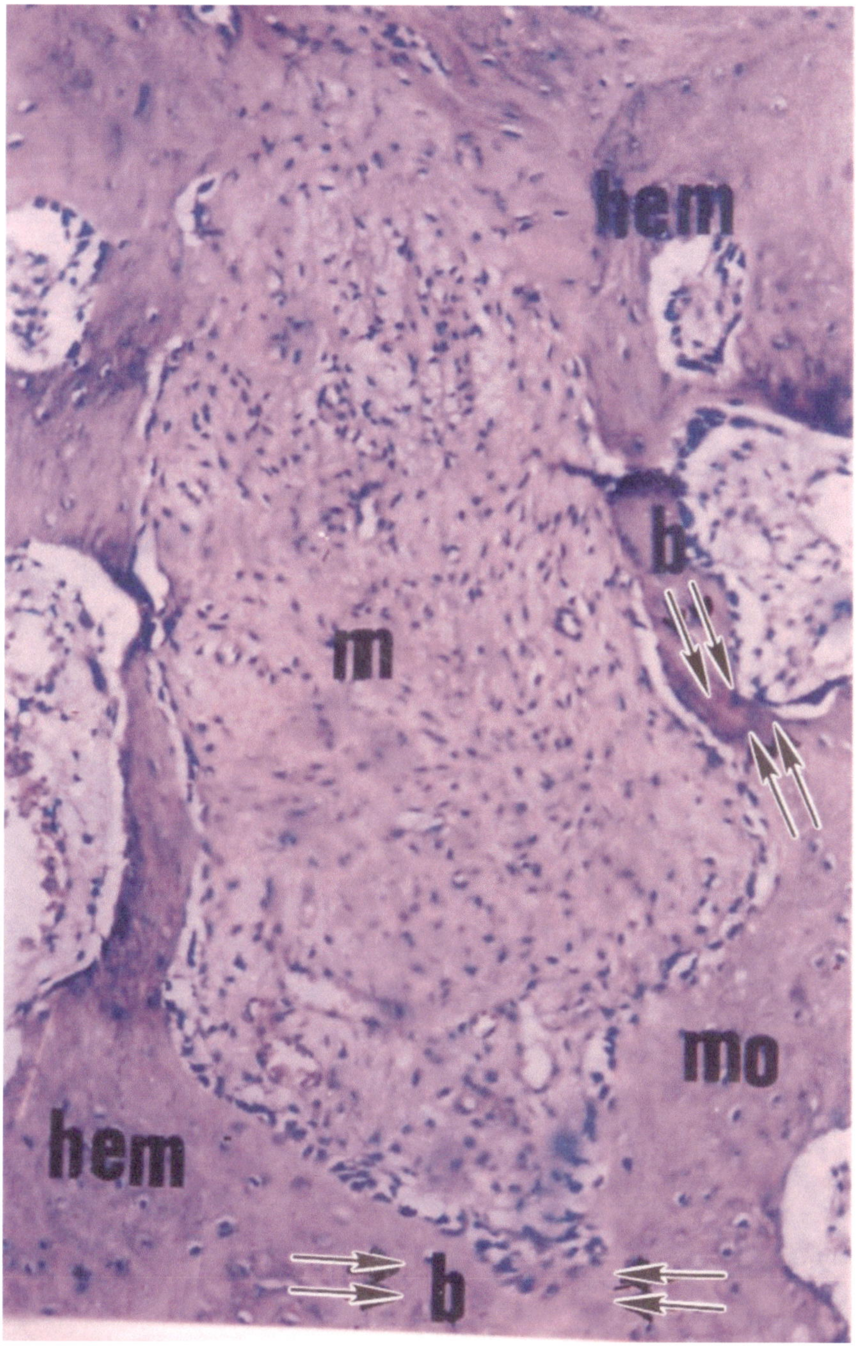

Fig. 14. A photomicrograph of a five-month old infant mandible, showing the complete fusion of the mental ossicle (mo) with the hemimandibles (hem) forming a single bony trabecula (b). Rostrally, remains of the symphyseal tissue (m) still separate the hemimandibles. The arrows show the direction of fusion between the mental ossicle and each hemimandible. (Haematoxylin and Eosin x 100).

3.7.2 Three-dimensional C.T. scanning

The rostral portion of the symphyseal region appeared fused from the inside. Its outer aspect showed a narrow midline defect between the two hemimandibles (Fig. 15).

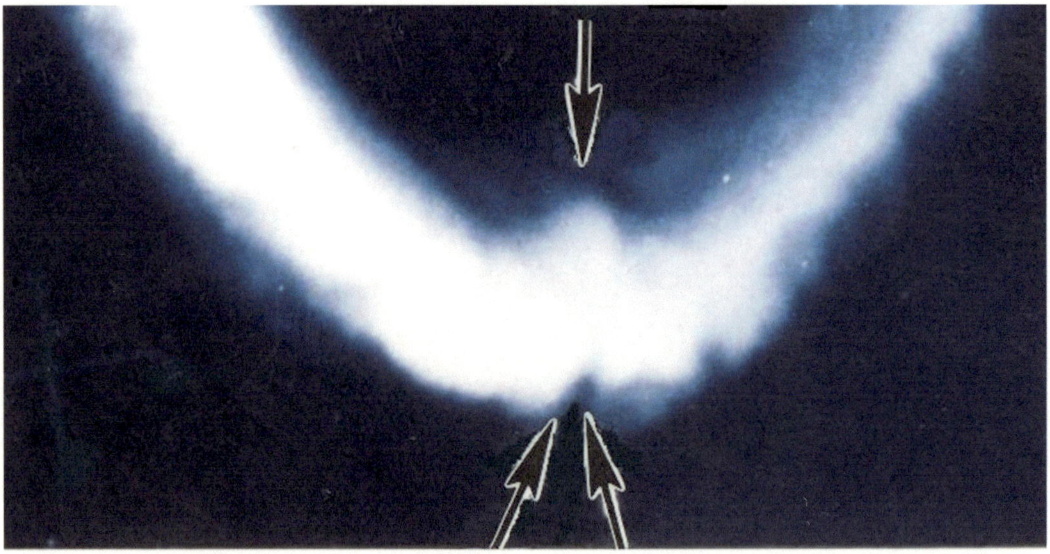

Fig. 15. A photograph of a three-dimensional C.T. scan of a five-month old infant mandible, top view. Notice the complete inward fusion (arrow), while a small midline defect still exists outward (double arrows).

3.8 Eighth group (one year, postnatal)

3.8.1 Histology

The symphyseal region was completely obliterated. The bony trabeculae became continuous across the midline (Fig. 16).

3.8.2 Three-dimensional C.T. scanning

The mandible appeared as a single bone (Fig. 17).

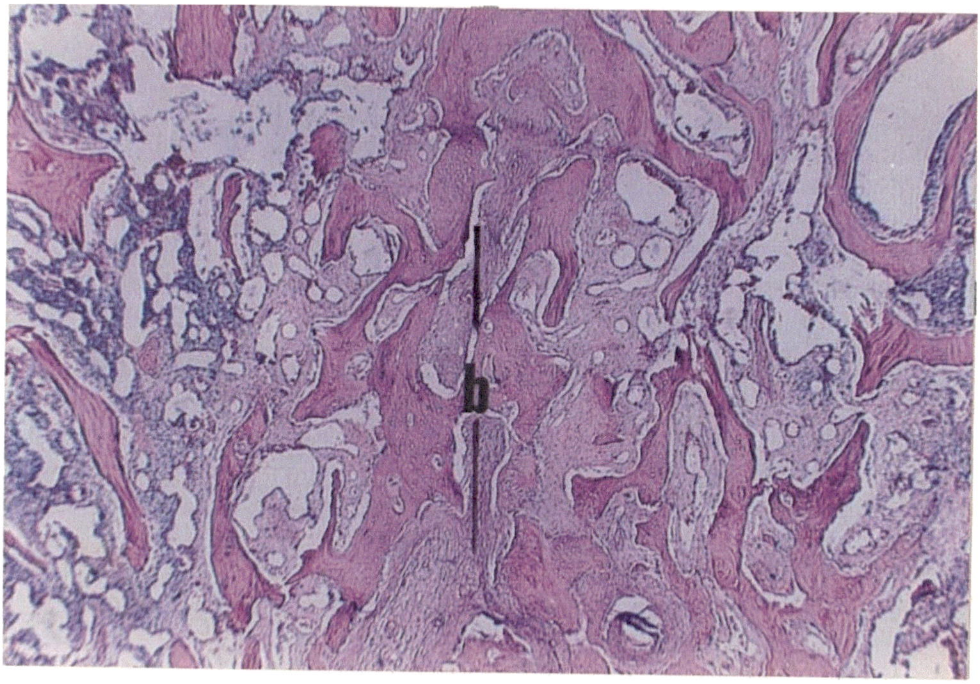

Fig. 16. A photomicrograph of a one-year old infant mandible, showing a complete closure of the symphysis menti resulting in a single mandible. Notice the complete midline encroachment (line) by bony trabeculae (b). (Haematoxylin and Eosin x 20).

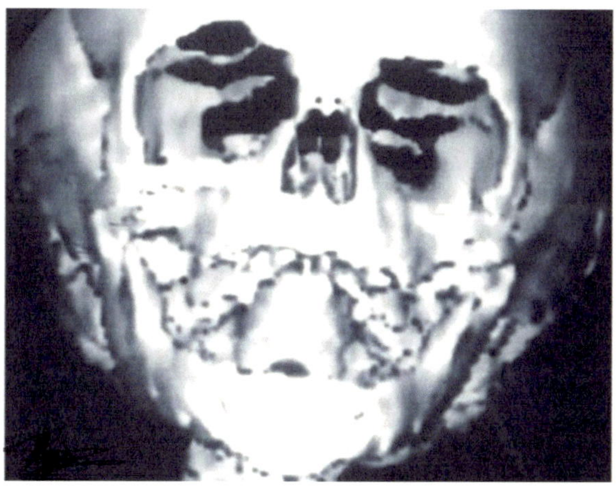

Fig. 17. A photograph of a three-dimensional C.T. scan of a one-year old infant skull, showing a complete obliteration of the symphyseal region. The mandible appears as a single bone.

4. Discussion

The role of Meckel's cartilage in the formation of the human mandible remained for a long time a subject of debate. Callender (1869) and Dieulafe and Herpin (1906) stated that

Meckel's cartilage was the origin of the whole mandible. On the other hand, Magitot and Robin (1862) denied any role for Meckel's cartilage in the development of the mandible. Stieda (1875) suggested that Meckel's cartilage directed mandibular ossification without taking part in that process. The present study had clarified the active role of Meckel's cartilage in the development of the medial portions of the hemimandibles. By the ninth week in utero, signs of endochondral ossification were observed, in the medial portions of the two rods of Meckel's cartilage, proceeding towards the midline and leading to the ossification of the most medial ends of the hemimandibles. Such findings were in agreement with those of Friant (1957) who stated that a small fraction of Meckel's cartilage, extending from the mental foramen almost to the site of the future symphysis probably became ossified. The present study showed no evidence of contribution of Meckel's cartilage in the development of the rest of the body of the mandible. The mandibular body consisted of irregular bony trabeculae in between spaces filled with mesenchymal tissue denoting its membranous origin. Meckel's cartilage completely disappeared in the lateral portions of the hemimandibles. These findings were in agreement with reports of Bannister et al. (1995). In their studies on the human mandible, Dieulafe and Herpin (1906) as well as Kjaer (1975) observed a temporary fusion of the bilateral portions of Meckel's cartilage across the midline. The present study showed no evidence of any fusion of the two portions of Meckel's cartilage. Such fusion was only confirmed in rodents (Bhaskar, 1986; Bareggi et al., 1994).

The present study revealed the presence of two well defined, rounded to oval cartilaginous structures in the caudal portion of the symphyseal mesenchyme. Previous studies had described similar structures. Sperber and Tobias (1981), Osburn (1981) and Bareggi et al. (1994) termed these structures "secondary cartilages". The term "secondary cartilage" is used to describe cartilage developing in association with membrane bones of the skull to provide them with articular cartilage (Cormack, 1987). On the other hand, Kjaer (1975) and Hamilton (1976) used the term "accessory cartilages" being, according to them, derived from the rostral connection of the bilateral portions of Meckel's cartilage. The present study demonstrated that there was a difference in the time of appearance between Meckel's cartilage that appeared as early as the ninth week in utero and the two cartilaginous structures not detected before the twelfth week in utero. Furthermore, in all serial sections examined, a distance always exists between both structures. The difference in ossification, regarding its time of occurrence (earlier in Meckel's cartilage) and its pattern (latero-medial in Meckel's cartilage and centrifugal in the two cartilaginous structures) would confirm the absence of any relationship between Meckel's cartilage and the cartilaginous structures. Therefore, the present study found the term "secondary cartilages" more appropriate to describe these two cartilaginous structures. Many authors believe that the symphyseal secondary cartilages appear after Meckel's cartilage and always maintain their own individuality (Friant, 1960 and 1968; Bertolini et al., 1967; Durst-Zirkovic and Davila. 1974, Goret-Nicase and Dhem, 1982; Goret-Nicase and Pilet, 1983).

After their studies on the human mandible using plain X-ray, Lebourg and Champagne (1951), Sicher (1962) and Scott and Symons (1982) described several mental ossicles in the symphyseal region. However, the present study, using a more advanced technique, namely the three-dimensional C.T. scanning, revealed that endochondral ossification of the secondary cartilages led to the formation of a single mental ossicle, conical in shape. The

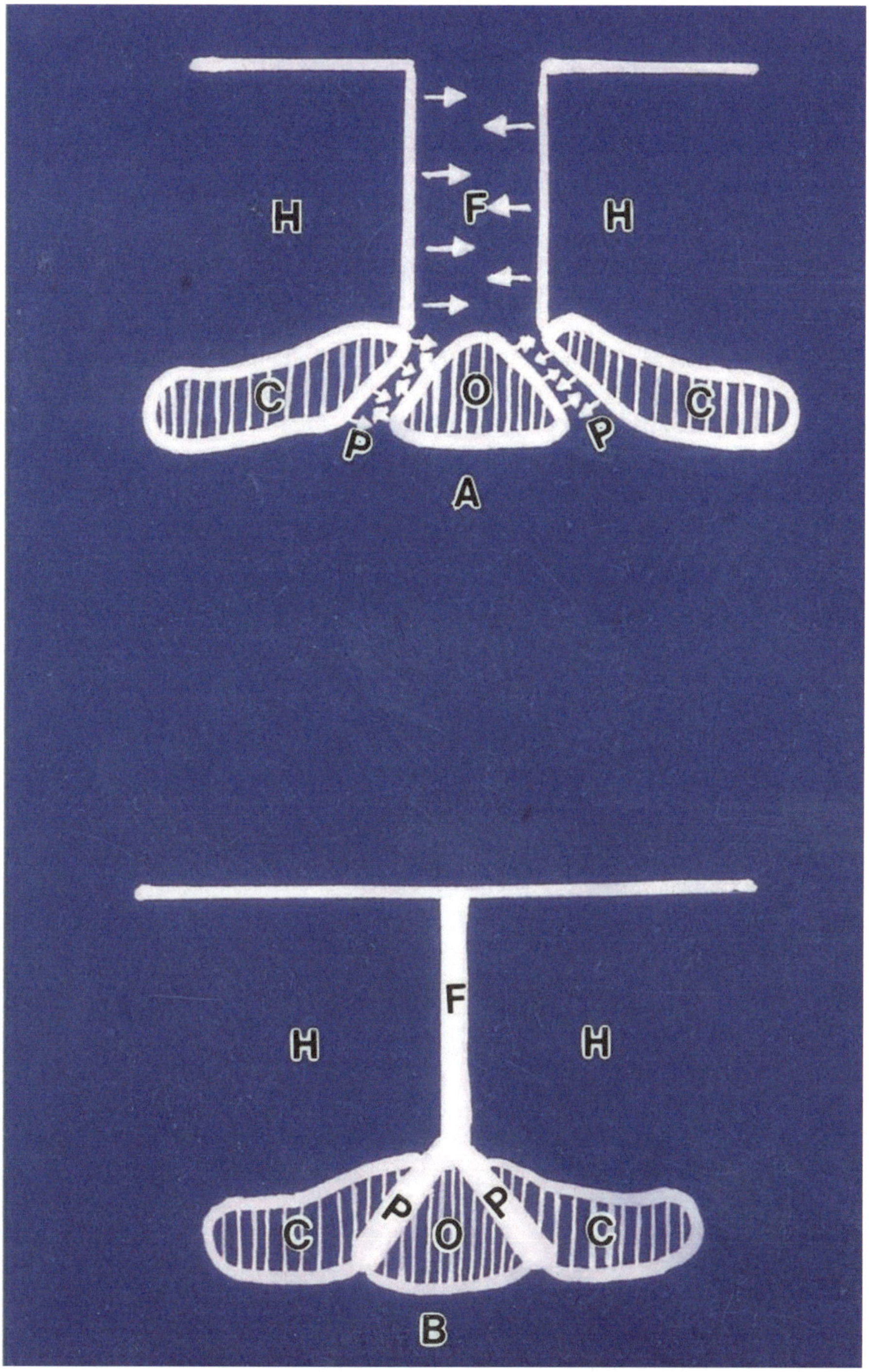

Fig. 18. A schematic presentation of the articulations between the two hemimandibles. A) Before fusion. B) After fusion. C = Meckel's cartilage; O = mental ossicle; H = hemimandible; F = fibrous joint; P = primary cartilaginous joint.

present study also studied the process of fusion of the mental ossicle with the hemimandibles. Such process proceeded in a caudo-rostral direction and led to the incorporation of the mental ossicle with the hemimandibles. Around the fifth month postnatally, fusion of the parts of the hemimandibles rostral to the mental ossicle, from an inward to an outward direction, followed the latter process. The mandible became a single bone before the end of the first postnatal year.

The nature and type of the human symphysis menti remained unsettled. Further, the details of fusion of this joint were uncertain. Kjaer (1975) stated that the symphysis menti might be compared to a suture. Sperber and Tobias (1981) considered the symphysis menti as a type of syndesmosis that was converted to synostosis. Bannister et al. (1995) mentioned that it is a fibrous joint. The present study had demonstrated that the rostral portion of the symphyseal region differed in architecture from the caudal portion. Rostrally, the symphyseal region was bounded on both sides by labial bony trabeculae, membranous in origin, separated in the midline by mesenchymal tissue. The bony trabeculae extended towards the midline, and by the end of the first postnatal year, a synostosis was well apparent. Caudally, the picture was different, due to the presence of two secondary hyaline cartilages in the symphyseal mesenchyme bounded on both sides by Meckel's cartilage. Both of them underwent endochondral ossification. Ossification in the secondary cartilages led to the formation of a mental ossicle that fused with the most medial ends of the hemimandibles derived from Meckel's cartilage. A synostosis was detected on both sides of the mental ossicle before the end of the first postnatal year. This picture simulated a primary cartilaginous joint (Fig. 18).

5. Summary

At the ninth week I.U., the symphysis menti was only formed of mesenchymal tissue bounded on either side by labial bony trabeculae, Meckel's cartilage and oral bony trabeculae. Rostrally, the bilateral rods of Meckel's cartilage approached each other but were separated by a rim of mesenchymal tissue. A triangular defect appeared between the two hemimandibles. By the twelfth week I.U., two secondary cartilaginous structures, completely separated from Meckel's cartilage, were observed in the caudal portion of the midline mesenchyme. By the twenty-eighth week I.U., signs of endochondral ossification appeared in the secondary cartilages and ended by the formation of a mental ossicle at the fortieth week I.U. The mental ossicle appeared conical in shape, and showed consistent gradual growth reaching its maximum by the age of first month P.N. Finally, complete fusion of the mental ossicle with the hemimandibles had occurred by the age of five months P.N., while the hemimandibles were still separated by a rim of mesenchymal tissue rostral to the mental ossicle. Fusion of the hemimandibles in that region proceeded from an inward to an outward direction. Thus, by the end of the first year P.N., the mandible became a single bone. The single mental ossicle is not an integral part of the symphyseal region, but is rather a contributor in the construction of the symphysis menti. Moreover, the symphysis menti is not simply a midline one as thought long ago. Instead, there are two different sites of articulations between the hemimandibles. The first one was located in the midline, between the rostral portions of the hemimandibles and simulated a fibrous joint. The second one was observed to lie on either side of the midline, between the mental ossicle and the caudal portion of each hemimandible, and simulated in structure a primary cartilaginous joint. Both articulations ended by synostosis, by the end of the first year P.N.

6. References

[1] Bannister LH, Berry MN, Collins P, Dyson M, Dussek JE and Ferguson MWJ (1995). Gray's Anatomy, 38th Ed., New York: Churchill Livingstone.

[2] Barreggi R; Narducci P; Grill V; Sandrucci MA and Bratina F (1994). On the presence of a secondary cartilage in the mental symphyseal region of human embryos and fetuses. Surg. Radiol. Anat., 16 (4): 379-384.

[3] Bertolini R; Wendler D and Hartmann E (1967). Die entwicklung der symphysis menti beim. Menschen Anat. Anz., 121: 55-71.

[4] Bhaskar SN (1986). Orban's Oral Histology and Embryology, 10th Ed., St louis: The CV Mosby Company.

[5] Callender GW (1869). The formation and early growth of the bones of the human face. Trans. Roy. Soc. (London), 159: 163-172.

[6] Cormack DH (1987). Histology, 9th Ed., Philadelphia: Lippincott Company.

[7] Dieulafe L and Herpin A (1906). Dévelopment de l'os maxillaire inférieur. J. Anat. Physiol. Paris, 42: 239-252.

[8] Durst-Zircovic B and Davila S (1974). Strukturelle veränderungen des Meckelschen Knorpels in laufe der Bildung des corpus mandibulae. Anat. Anz., 135: 12-23.

[9] Friant M (1957). Anatomie comparée. Le début de l'ossification du cartilage de Meckel. C. R. Acad.. Sci., 244: 1017-1073.

[10] Friant M (1960). L'évolution du cartilage de Meckel humain, jusqu'à la fin du sixième mois de la vie foetale. Acta Anat., 41: 228-239.

[11] Friant M (1968). Les transformations du cartilage de Meckel humain. Folia Morphol., 16: 215-225.

[12] Goret-Nicase M and Dhem A (1982). Presence of chondroid tissue in the symphyseal region of the growing human mandible. Acta Anat., 113: 189-195.

[13] Goret-Nicase M and Pilet D (1983). A few observations about Meckel's cartilage in the human. Anat. Embryol., 167: 363-370.

[14] Hamilton WJ (1976). Textbook of human anatomy, second Ed., London: The MacMillan Press Ltd.

[15] Kjaer I (1975). Histochemical investigations on the symphysis menti in the human fetus related to fetal skeletal maturation in the hand and foot. Acta Anat., 93: 606-633.

[16] Lebourg L and Champagne G (1951) A propos du dévelopment mandibulaire post-natal. Précisions sur la chronologie de la suture symphysaire. Stomatol. Chin. Maxillofac., 52: 891-897.

[17] Magitot E and Robin C (1862). Mémoire sur une organe transitoire de la vie foetale désignée sous the nom de Meckel. Ann. Sci. Nat. Zool., 18: 213- 241.

[18] O'Rahilly R and Gardner E (1972). The initial appearance of ossification in staged human embryos. Am J Anat., 134: 291-308.

[19] Osborn JW (1981). Dental Anatomy and Embryology, Vol. 1, Oxford: Blackwell Scientific Publications.

[20] Scott JH and Symons NB (1982). Introduction to Dental Anatomy, 9th Ed., New York: Churchill Livingstone.

[21] Sicher H (1962). Temporomandibular articulation concepts and misconcepts. J. Oral. Surg., 20: 281-284.

[22] Sperber GH and Tobias PV (1981). Cranifacial Embryology, 3rd Ed., London: Wright PSG.

[23] Stieda L (1875). Studien über die Entwicklung der Knocken und des Knochenge webes. Arch. F. Mikr. Anat., 11: 235-363.

9

Combinatorial Networks Regulating Seed Development and Seed Filling

Ming-Jun Gao[1], Gordon Gropp[1], Shu Wei[2],
Dwayne D. Hegedus[1] and Derek J. Lydiate[1]
[1]*Agriculture and Agri-Food Canada,*
Saskatoon Research Centre, Saskatoon, Saskatchewan,
[2]*School of Tea & Food Science, Anhui Agricultural University, Hefei,*
[1]*Canada*
[2]*China*

1. Introduction

Seeds offer plants a unique opportunity to suspend their life cycles in a desiccated state. This enables them to endure adverse environmental conditions and then resume growth by using endogenous storage products when more favorable conditions develop. Seed development is pivotal to the reproductive success of flowering plants (Angiosperms). It is initiated by the process of double fertilization that gives rise to the embryo and the endosperm. The embryo develops following fertilization of the haploid egg cell by one of the sperm cells leading to the formation of a diploid zygote. In contrast, the triploid endosperm results from the fertilization of the maternal homodiploid central cell of the ovule by another sperm cell (Weterings & Russell, 2004). The diploid embryo and the triploid endosperm develop concertedly inside the maternal ovule and are protected by a seed coat constituted of maternally derived inner and outer integuments. The seed coat provides an important interface between the embryo and the external environment (Haughn & Chaudhury, 2005). Thus, different genome combinations contribute to seed ontogeny.

Seed formation is an intricate genetically programmed process that is correlated with changes in metabolite levels and is regulated by a complex signaling network mediated by sugar and hormone levels (Wobus & Weber, 1999; Lohe & Chaudhury, 2002; Weber et al., 2005; Holdsworth et al., 2008; Sun et al., 2010). Most of the basic knowledge regarding cellular differentiation, growth regulation, imprinting and signal transduction pertaining to seed development comes from studies with *Arabidopsis thaliana* (Goldberg et al., 1989; Laux & Jürgens, 1997; Harada, 1999; Smeekens, 2000; Finkelstein et al., 2002; North et al., 2010; Bauer & Fischer, 2011). There is sufficient evidence to state that the fundamental regulatory mechanisms governing seed development and maturation are similar for all plant seeds (Weber et al., 2005). Seed development can be divided into two stages, embryo morphogenesis and maturation, the latter being characterized by storage compound accumulation, acquisition of desiccation tolerance, growth arrest and entry into a dormancy period that is broken upon germination (Harada, 1999). In addition to the diversity of shapes and sizes, a common element in plant seeds is the storage reserves that generally consist of starch, storage lipid triacylglycerols (TAGs) and specialized seed storage proteins (SSPs). Given the importance of seeds, such as those of legumes or cereals, in human and animal diets, much research has been devoted to improving qualitative and quantitative traits associated with seed components such as palatability and nutritional quality. As such, understanding the metabolism and development during seed filling has been a major focus of plant research. The recent development of a range of chemical, physiological, molecular genetics and post-genomics approaches has allowed rapid progress toward understanding the processes of early seed development, maturation, dormancy, after-ripening and germination, but has also provided opportunities to control and modify both the quality and quantity of seed products (Mazur et al., 1999; Hills, 2004 ; Baud et al., 2008; North et al., 2010). In recent years, much effort has been devoted to elucidating the intricate regulatory networks that control seed development and maturation, where hormone and sugar signaling together with a set of developmentally regulated transcription factors and chromatin remodeling proteins are involved. Here, we summarize the most recent advances in our understudying of this complex regulatory network and its role in the control of seed development and seed filling.

2. Genomic imprinting and early seed development

Genomic imprinting is a genetic phenomenon that occurs in the placenta of mammals and in the endosperm of angiosperms, in which a set of alleles that reside in the same nucleus and share the same DNA sequence is expressed in a parent-of-origin manner. Imprinting is an epigenetic process that is independent of classical Mendelian inheritance. According to the parental conflict theory (Haig & Wilczek, 2006), imprinting is described as a battle between the maternal and paternal genomes over limited maternal resources. The mother, which may carry progeny from several fathers, will attempt to distribute resources equally to all of her offspring. Conversely, the father will try to extract the maximum maternal resource for his progeny at the expense of others. Therefore, alleles that support the allocation of maternal resources for maximal growth of seeds are expressed paternally, whereas alleles that confine resource distribution from mother to seed are expressed maternally. Thus, the endosperm that is critical for embryo and seed development becomes a site where maternal and paternal genomes compete for resources via imprinting or parent-of-origin-specific gene expression.

Most imprinted genes known from flowering plants are preferentially expressed in the endosperm and some are known to be fundamental for proper early seed development (Table 1) (Gehring et al., 2004; Berger & Chaudhury, 2009; Bauer & Fischer, 2011). At least nineteen imprinted genes have been characterized in maize (*Zea mays)* (Table 2) and *Arabidopsis* (Berger & Chaudhury, 2009; Bauer & Fischer, 2011). The *R* gene was the first imprinted gene identified in maize (Kermicle, 1970) that promotes anthocyanin accumulation in the outer aleurone layer of the endosperm. All maize kernels have a fully red colored aleurone layer when a red *RR* female is crossed with a colorless *rr* male, whereas mottled aleurone pigmentation is produced by the reciprocal mating (Kermicle, 1970). Moreover, the mottled phenotype is present regardless of the number of paternal *R* alleles and maternally inherited *R* alleles are always associated with the solid red color. Other imprinted genes that are maternally expressed in the maize endosperm include the *MO17* allele of the *dzr1* locus (Chaudhuri & Messing, 1994), one of the *α-zein* alleles (Lund et al., 1995), maize enhancer of *Zeste1* gene (*Mez1*) (Haun et al., 2009) and fertilization independent endosperm1 (*Fie1*) (Danilevskaya et al., 2003). In *Arabidopsis*, several imprinted genes involved in early seed development have been identified and include the *FIS* (*FERTILIZATION INDEPENDENT SEED*) genes *MEDEA* (*MEA*) (Grossniklaus & Schneitz, 1998; Kiyosue et al., 1999), *FERTILIZATION INDEPENDENT ENDOSPERM* (*FIE*) (Ohad et al., 1996), *FIS2* (Luo et al., 1999), and *MULTI-COPY OF IRA1* (*MSI1*) (Köhler et al., 2003; Ingouff et al., 2007), the *MEA* homologs *CURLY LEAF* (*CLF*) or *SWINGER* (*SWN*) (Makarevich et al., 2006), and other maternally imprinted genes such as *MATERNALLY EXPRESSED PAB C-TERMINAL* (*MPC*) (Tiwari et al., 2008) and *FLOWERING WAGENINGEN* (*FWA*) (Kinoshita et al., 2004; Köhler & Hennig, 2010).

Protein	Protein complex	Protein domains	Expression pattern during seed development	Loss-of-function phenotypes	References
FIS2	FIS (FERTILIZATION INDEPENDENT SEED)	C2H2 Zn finger	Endosperm, embryo, female gametophyte	Initiation of seed development in the absence of fertilization; embryo lethality; endosperm cellularization	Luo et al., 1999
MEA	FIS	SET	Endosperm, female gametophyte	Embryo lethality; cellularized endosperm without pollination	Grossniklaus & Schneitz, 1998; Kiyosue et al., 1999
MSI1	FIS, VRN, EMF?	WD 40	Embryo, female gametophyte	Parthenogenetic development including proliferation of unfertilized endosperm and embryos	Ach et al., 1997
FIE	FIS, EMF, VRN	WD 40	Endosperm, embryo, female gametophyte	Initiation of endosperm development in the absence of fertilization; flowers formed in seedlings and non-reproductive organs	Ohad et al., 1999

Table 1. PcG proteins required for early seed development in *Arabidopsis*

Gene name	Acronym	Potential function	References
R-mottled allele *dzr1*	*R*	Transcription factor The allele in the MO17 ecotype is maternally imprinted and zein accumulation is regulated	Kermicle, 1970 Chaudhuri & Messing, 1994
Fertilization independent endosperm 1	*Fie1*	PcG complex	Danilevskaya et al., 2003; Gutiérrez-Marcos et al., 2006; Hermon et al., 2007
Fertilization independent endosperm 1	*Fie2*	PcG complex	Danilevskaya et al., 2003; Gutiérrez-Marcos et al., 2006
No-apical-meristem related protein 1	*Nrp1*	Unknown	Guo et al., 2003
Maize enhancer of Zeste 1	*Mez1*	PcG complex	Haun et al., 2009
Maternally expressed gene 1	*Meg1*	Cysteine-rich peptide	Gutiérrez-Marcos et al., 2004

Table 2. Imprinted genes and their function in maize

In plants and animals, homeotic genes encoding the polycomb group (PcG) and trithorax group (trxG) proteins are key players in maintaining repressive and active state of targets, respectively, and are crucial for developmental patterning and growth control (Simon & Tamkun, 2002). PcG and trxG proteins form higher order complexes that have intrinsic histone methyltransferase (HMTase) activity for various types of lysine methylation at the amino-terminus of core histone proteins. This property is conferred by the conserved 130-residue SET (Su(var), Enhancer of Zeste, Trithorax) domain (Cao & Zhang, 2004). The FIS proteins MEA, FIE, MSI1 and FIS2 interact and form a protein complex called MEA-FIE complex that is similar to the PRC2 (Polycomb Repressive Complex 2) in animals (Simon & Tamkun, 2002; Köhler & Makarevich, 2006; Baroux et al., 2007). Mutation of any FIS component, such as MEA, leads to the formation of seeds independent of fertilization. Moreover, *fis* mutants have a prominent maternally determined phenotype after fertilization. Seed that carries a maternally inherited *fis* allele eventually aborts with an embryo that has arrested at the late heart stage and a multinucleate endosperm that fails to cellularize (Ohad et al., 1996; Grossniklaus & Schneitz, 1998; Kiyosue et al., 1999; Luo et al., 1999; Köhler et al., 2003; Ingouff et al., 2007). This phenotype is in part owing to the derepression of the type I MADS-box gene *PHERES1* (*PHE1*). *PHE1* is a direct target gene of the MEA-FIE complex in the embryo at the globular stage and in the central domain of the endosperm (Köhler et al., 2003). Mutation of *MEA* results in elevated expression of the maternal *PHE1* allele through removal of the trimethylation marks from histone 3 lysine 27 (H3K27me3), whereas this has little effect on the activity of the paternal *PHE1* allele, suggesting targeting specificity of the MEA-FIE complex to the maternal *PHE1* allele (Köhler et al., 2005; Makarevich et al., 2006). In contrast to the action of MEA that is required for PcG target repression during gametophyte and early seed development, MEA homologs CLF/SWN have been demonstrated to repress *PHE1* expression by the action of H3K27me3 at later stages of sporophyte development (Makarevich et al., 2006). In maize, genome-wide analysis of transcriptome changes during early seed development identified transcripts of sixteen loci that were exclusively of maternal origin, suggesting a general mechanism for delayed paternal genome expression in plants (Grimanelli et al., 2005).

What are the underlying mechanisms that control genomic imprinting? DNA methylation was among the first recognized epigenetic modifications that affected early seed development (Finnegan et al., 1996). It has been demonstrated that methylation at CpG sites and plant-specific CpNpG and CpNpN was involved in embryo patterning (Xiao et al., 2006). METHYLTRANSFERASE1 (MET1) is the principal maintenance methyltransferase in *Arabidopsis* and is the homolog of mammalian Dnmt1 that maintains cytosine methylation at CG sites (Finnegan & Dennis, 1993; Kankel et al., 2003). *MET1* is expressed mainly in sperm cells (Jullien et al., 2008) and *met1* mutants display global reduction of CpG and CpNpG methylation and accompanied developmental abnormalities (Finnegan et al., 1996). Genetic and molecular studies have shown that MET1-conferred DNA methylation is involved in the imprinting of *FIS* genes (Xiao et al., 2003; Kinoshita et al., 2004; Jullien et al., 2006). The paternal MEA alleles in the endosperm are hypermethylated, whereas the maternal alleles are hypomethylated. MET1 targets methylation at CG sites in the MEA promoter and in the 3′ untranslated region (3′UTR) (Gehring et al., 2006). Recently, *MPC* and *FWA* were found to be inactivated throughout the plant life cycle until gametogenesis (Jullien et al., 2006; Tiwari et al., 2008). During male gametogenesis, these genes were repressed in sperm cells by the action of MET1 (Jullien et al., 2006; Tiwari et al., 2008). During endosperm development, the inherited paternal allele remains silenced by MET1, whereas the inherited maternal alleles are transcriptionally active (Gutiérrez-Marcos et al., 2006; Hermon et al., 2007; Tiwari et al., 2008). It was therefore suggested that the differential expression between the two parental alleles is established by the status of DNA methylation that has been epigenetically inherited from the gametes (Huh et al., 2007). This hypothesis is supported by the pattern of expression of the *PcG* genes *Fie1* and *Fie2* in maize (Danilevskaya et al., 2003). Maternally imprinted *Fie1* and *Fie2* were expressed solely during early endosperm development (Danilevskaya et al., 2003; Gutiérrez-Marcos et al., 2006). Imprinting of these two genes corresponded to the presence of differentially methylated regions at the parental alleles, which are inherited from the gametes, with high methylation in the sperm cells and none or little in the central cell, though *Fie2* did not display a DNA methylation status in the gametes as did *FIE1* (Gutiérrez-Marcos et al., 2006; Baroux et al., 2007). MET1-mediated DNA methylation is involved in the epigenetic control of seed size. During male gametogenesis, endosperm growth in *met1* mutants was inhibited and smaller seeds were produced (Luo et al., 2000; Garcia et al., 2005; Xiao et al., 2006; FitzGerald et al., 2008). This is probably due to the ectopic expression of imprinted paternal alleles of loci such as *FIS2* and *FWA*. Seeds derived from crosses between wild-type pollen and ovules from *MET1* antisense plants (*MET1a/s*) display increased seed size (Adams et al., 2000; Luo et al., 2000), owing to the loss of MET1 activity in the female gametes, the integuments, or both (Berger & Chaudhury, 2009). Similar results were obtained from crosses between wild-type pollen and homozygous *met1/met1* ovules, resulting in the formation of larger seeds, which is due to ovules with more cells and autonomous elongation (FitzGerald et al., 2008). Therefore, MET1 was proposed to play a role in inhibiting ovule proliferation and elongation and the effect of MET1 on seed size results mainly from the maternal controls (Berger & Chaudhury, 2009).

What are the mechanisms leading to the removal of DNA methylation marks from *FIS* genes in the central cell? DEMETER (DME) has been identified as a transcriptional activator that regulates *MEA*, *FIS2*, *FWA* and *MPC* expression in the central cells (Choi et al., 2002; Kinoshita et al., 2004; Gehring et al., 2006; Jullien et al., 2006; Morales-Ruiz et al., 2006; Tiwari et al., 2008; Bauer & Fischer, 2011). *DME* encodes a DNA glycosylase that removes methylated cytosine through its 5-methylcytosine DNA glycosylase activity at target loci (Choi et al., 2002; Kinoshita et al., 2004; Gehring et al., 2006; Jullien et al., 2006; Morales-Ruiz et al., 2006; Tiwari et al., 2008). *DME* is expressed predominantly in the central cell before fertilization where it activates target genes such as *MEA* (Choi et al., 2002). In *dem* mutant endosperm, the maternal *MEA* allele is not expressed due to hypermethylation and *dem* seeds eventually abort (Gehring et al., 2006). This finding suggests that DME removes DNA methylation marks at the maternal *MEA* allele in the central cell, resulting in hypomethylation and activation of *MEA* in the early endosperm, whereas the paternal imprinted *MEA* is methylated and transcriptionally silenced in the endosperm (Baroux et al., 2007; Huh et al., 2007). However, DME is not sufficient to remove all DNA methylation marks from targets such as *FIS2* as evidenced by the continued expression of *FIS2* and *MPC* in the *dme* mutant during female gametogenesis (Choi et al., 2002; Jullien et al., 2006). Recently, an additional mechanism was identified in which the Retinoblastoma pathway is involved in the regulation of maternal imprinting (Jullien et al., 2008). The *Arabidopsis* homolog RETINOBLASTOMA RELATED (RBR) directly silences *MET1* expression via interaction with MSI1 during the late stage of female gametogenesis. When the Retinoblastoma pathway is inactive, expression of *FIS2* and *FWA* in the central cell is completely repressed (Jullien et al., 2008; Berger & Chaudhury, 2009). Partial repression of *MET1* by the Retinoblastoma pathway results in DNA hemi-methylation, the preferred substrate for the 5-methylcytosine glycosylase DME (Jullien et al., 2008), and complete demethylation by DME at the promoter regions of target alleles such as *FIS2* and *FWA* leads to activation of these genes in the central cell. After fertilization, the active maternal allele inherits the demethylation marks, whereas the inactive paternal allele inherits the methylation marks (Berger & Chaudhury, 2009; Gehring et al., 2009) (Fig. 1). Deep sequencing of endosperm or embryo DNA immunoprecipited with antisera against methylcytosine demonstrated a global reduction in DNA methylation on CG sites in the endosperm. The global CG methylation level is reduced by 15-20% in the endosperm in comparison to the levels in vegetative tissues or embryos (Gehring et al., 2009; Hsieh et al., 2009). In maize, a reduction of maternal DNA methylation might also occur in the endosperm (Lauria et al., 2004). Additionally, large amounts of maternally inherited non-coding small RNAs might also affect the genome-wide DNA methylation in the endosperm and the embryos via their links to *de novo* DNA methyltransferases (Mosher et al., 2009). Recent genome-wide deep sequencing of cDNA libraries (Hsieh et al., 2011) or RNA derived from seeds of reciprocal intraspecific crosses (Gehring et al., 2011) has identified many genes that show imprinted gene expression in *Arabidopsis* endosperm. These genes include transcription factors, proteins involved in hormone signaling and regulators for histone modifications and chromatin remodeling (Gehring et al., 2011; Hsieh et al., 2011). These studies demonstrate that parent-of-origin effect on gene expression is a complex phenomenon and may affect multiple aspects of early seed development.

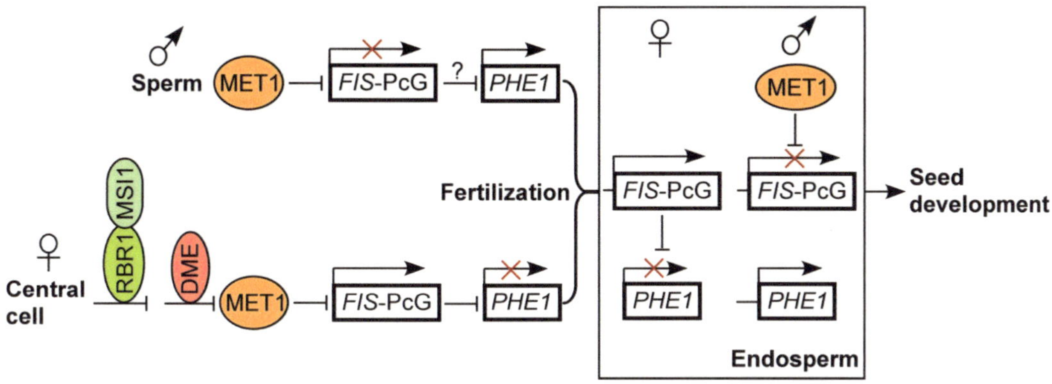

Fig. 1. A proposed model for the epigenetic control of early seed development. The FIS-PcG complex includes proteins encoded by *FIS* class genes such as *MEA* and *FIS2* (Simon & Tamkun, 2002; Köhler & Makarevich, 2006; Baroux et al., 2007). Both maternal and paternal alleles of these imprinted genes are repressed via DNA methylation from the activity of the DNA methyltransferase MET1 in the central cell and sperm (Gehring et al., 2006; Jullien et al., 2006; Huh et al., 2007). During female gametogenesis, MET1 activity is partially repressed by the Retinoblastoma pathway involving RBR1 and its interacting partner MSI1 through DNA hemi-methylation, the preferred substrate for the 5-methylcytosine glycosylase DME (Jullien et al., 2008). The complete demethylation on *MET1* in the mature central cell is mediated by DME, resulting in imprinted expression of the *FIS-PcG* genes (Jullien et al., 2008). During early endosperm development, the inherited paternal *FIS-PcG* alleles remain silenced by MET1, whereas the imprinted maternal alleles are active leading to the repression of target genes such as the maternal *PHE1* through lysine27 on histone H3 (H3K27) methylation. The mechanism underlying *PHE1* activation in sperm cell remains unknown. In contrast to the *FIS* genes *MEA* and *FIS2* that are proposed to play a role for the repression of endosperm proliferation (Kiyosue et al., 1999; Ingouff et al., 2007), paternal-specific expression of *PHE1* in the chalazal domain of the endosperm promotes endosperm development (Köhler et al., 2005).

In conjunction with DNA methylation, histone methylation also modulates genomic imprinting. Histone methylation mediated by the SET domain-containing PcG complex represses target genes by modifying the chromatin at or near target gene loci. This suppressive mechanism was proposed to regulate endosperm cell proliferation, as mutation of the target *FIS* class genes *MEA*, *FIS2* or *FIE* results in the autonomous central cell divisions (Ohad et al., 1996; Chaudhury et al., 1997; Grossniklaus & Schneitz, 1998; Kiyosue et al., 1999). As described above, the endosperm is the only site where imprinting is known to take place; however, seeds may also form when genomic imprinting mechanisms are bypassed (Nowack et al., 2007). When *CDKA;1* mutant pollen was crossed with the *FIS* gene mutants, *mea*, *fis2* and *fie*, viable single-fertilized seeds with homodiploid endosperm were produced despite smaller seed size than wild type (Nowack et al., 2007). *CDKA;1* encodes a cdc2/cdc28 homolog. Mutation of *CDKA;1* leads to the generation of pollen with only one sperm (Iwakawa et al., 2006; Nowack et al., 2006) that preferentially fertilizes the egg cell while the diploid central cell remains unfertilized. Embryos from egg cells pollinated with *cdka;1* mutant pollen abort at about 3 days after pollination and only a few divisions of the unfertilized central cell occur (Nowack et al., 2006). Furthermore, when repression exerted by the *FIS* genes such as *MEA* in the female gametophyte is disrupted, single-fertilized seeds form (Nowack et al., 2007). This suggests that functional endosperm can arise from the central cell in the female gametophyte without a paternal contribution and that genomic imprinting in the endosperm is not always essential for seed development. This hypothesis is supported by the demonstration that fertilization of the diploid central cell acts as a trigger that initiates proliferation of the multicellular endosperm (Nowack et al., 2007).

3. Seed maturation and seed filling

According to several models, seed development can be divided into two stages; morphogenesis and maturation. The maturation phase is initiated once the embryo and endosperm have completed the morphogenesis and patterning stages (Wobus & Weber, 1999). While early embryo morphogenesis is mainly maternally controlled, transition to the maturation phase requires a switch from maternal to filial control (Weber et al., 2005). After the switch is initiated, the embryo continues to grow for a short period of time until it matures; the seed then accumulates storage products, develops desiccation tolerance and produces a protective seed coat. Maturation ends with the completion of a desiccation phase after which seed growth arrests and it enters into dormancy, thus, the embryo enters into a quiescent state but retains the capacity to regenerate after imbibition (Harada, 1999). The spatial and temporal regulation of the maturation processes requires the concerted action of several signaling pathways that integrate information from genetic and epigenetic programs, and from both hormonal and metabolic signals (Wobus & Weber, 1999; Weber et al., 2005). Moreover, recent discoveries have led to a better understanding of ABA signaling and metabolic regulation in the maternal to filial switch leading to the maturation phase (Gutierrez et al., 2007; Cutler et al., 2010).

3.1 A regulatory network for seed maturation

Precise spatial and temporal regulation of gene expression is required for proper seed maturation. The expression of genes involved in the regulation of metabolism occurring during seed maturation is highly coordinated (Vicente-Carbajosa et al., 1998; Santos-Mendoza et al., 2005; Gutierrez et al., 2007; Holdsworth et al., 2008; Sun et al., 2010). The maize *Opaque2* (*O2*) was one of the first genes encoding a plant transcription factor to be characterized (Hartings et al., 1989; Schmidt et al., 1990). The *O2* orthologs, *SPA* from wheat (*Triticum aestivum*) and *BLZ2* from barley (*Hordeum vulgare*), were reported to have the same functions as *O2* in their corresponding species (Albani et al., 1997; Oñate et al., 1999). In *Arabidopsis*, three members of the B3 family of transcription factors, LEAFY COTYLEDON (LEC) 2, ABSCISIC ACID-INSENTITIVE 3 (ABI3) and FUSCA 3 (FUS3) and a fourth regulator, a HAP3 subunit of the CCAAT-box binding transcription factor (CBF) LEC1, are key regulators of seed maturation processes (Fig. 2). A redundant gene regulatory network linking these master regulators was elucidated by examining the expression of *ABI3*, *FUS3* and *LEC2* in *abi3*, *fus3*, *lec1* and *lec2* single, double and triple mutants (To et al., 2006). Using Affymetrix GeneChips to profile *Arabidopsis* genes active in seeds from fertilization to maturation, 289 seed-specific genes have been identified, including 48 transcription factors such as *LEC1*, *LEC2* and *FUS3* (Le et al., 2010). In combination with ABA, GA, auxin and sugar signaling, this regulatory network governs most seed-specific traits, such as accumulation of storage compounds, acquisition of desiccation tolerance and entry into quiescence, in a partially redundant manner (Harada, 1999; Brocard-Gifford et al., 2003; Gazzarrini et al., 2004; Kagaya et al., 2005b; To et al., 2006; Stone et al., 2008). *LEC1* and *LEC2* are expressed early in embryogenesis and ectopic expression of these two regulators is sufficient to confer embryonic traits to vegetative organs (Lotan et al., 1998; Stone et al., 2001; Santos-Mendoza et al., 2005). *ABI3* and *FUS3* expression occurs later in embryogenesis and their overexpression results in ectopic expression of some seed maturation genes, such as *At2S3* and *CRC*, in vegetative tissues in an ABA-dependent manner, demonstrating that the SSP gene expression is controlled by LEC1 through the regulation of *ABI3* and *FUS3* (Parcy et al., 1994; Kagaya et al., 2005b). Genetic and molecular studies have shown that ABI3, FUS3 and LEC2 regulate oleosin gene expression and lipid accumulation (Crowe et al., 2000; Santos-Mendoza et al., 2005; Baud et al., 2007). Loss of *ABI3* function alters accumulation of seed storage reserves and leads to loss of desiccation tolerance, dormancy, ABA sensitivity upon germination and chlorophyll degradation (Vicente-Carbajosa & Carbonero, 2005). In addition, the APETALA2 (AP2) protein, ABI4, and the bZIP domain factor, ABI5, are involved in many aspects of seed maturation through their interaction with the major regulators LEC2, ABI3 and FUS3 (Carles et al., 2002; Brocard-Gifford et al., 2003; Lara et al., 2003; Acevedo-Hernández et al., 2005). In addition to these complex genetic interactions, *ABI3* expression was found to be regulated by both post-transcriptional and post-translational mechanisms. After excision of the long 5′-untranslated region (UTR) of the *ABI3* transcript, *ABI3-GUS* expression level was markedly increased, suggesting that *ABI3* expression is negatively regulated by its own 5′-UTR (Ng et al., 2006). Moreover, *ABI3* levels are regulated by an ABI3-interacting protein, AIP2 an E3 ligase that targets ABI3 to the 26S proteasome for degradation (Zhang et al., 2005). The ectopic expression of the *ABI3* maize ortholog, Viviparous (*VP1*), in *Arabidopsis* leads to the expression of a subset of seed-specific genes in vegetative tissues, indicating that *VP1* is a key determinant for embryonic traits (Suzuki et al., 2003). This also suggests that ABI3-dependent regulatory mechanisms are conserved in both dicots and cereals.

Seed maturation-related genes, such as those governing SSP and lipid accumulation, are controlled by the interaction of transcriptional regulators with *cis*-acting elements in their promoters. The best characterized *cis*-elements include the RY repeat (CATGCA), ACGT-box (CACGTG) and AACA motif, that are recognized by B3, bZIP and MYB domain transcription factors, respectively. Functional analysis and *in vitro* protein-DNA interaction assays demonstrated binding of the B3 factors (LEC2, ABI3 and FUS3) to RY repeats (Reidt et al., 2000; Kroj et al., 2003; Mönke et al., 2004; Braybrook et al., 2006), and bZIP factors (ABI5, AtbZIP10, AtbZIP25 and bZIP53) to ACGT-boxes (Bensmihen et al., 2002; Lara et al., 2003; Alonso et al., 2009; Reeves et al., 2011). Moreover, ABI5 and its homolog EEL play antagonistic roles to influence the expression of the late embryogenesis abundant (LEA) gene, *AtEm1*, through competition for the same DNA binding site (Bensmihen et al., 2002). In addition to direct binding to DNA elements, the major regulators indirectly regulate the expression of seed maturation genes. Genetic and molecular studies have shown that LEC1 and LEC2 act upstream of ABI3 and FUS3 and control SSP gene expression through the regulation of *ABI3* and *FUS3* expression (Kagaya et al., 2005b; To et al., 2006). ABI3 functions as a seed-specific transcriptional co-activator that physically interacts with ABI5, AtZIP10 and AtZIP25 (Nakamura et al., 2001; Lara et al., 2003). Recently, another G-box binding group C bZIP factor, bZIP53, was shown to be a key regulator of seed maturation gene expression and enhanced expression by heterodimerization with bZIP10 or bZIP25 (Alonso et al., 2009). *FUS3* expression in the protoderm and its negative regulation of TRANSPARENT TESTA GLABRA1 (TTG1) are critical for embryogenesis (Tsuchiya et al., 2004). Moreover, *FUS3* was induced by auxin and indirectly influences the seed maturation process by positive and negative regulation of ABA and GA synthesis, respectively (Gazzarrini et al., 2004).

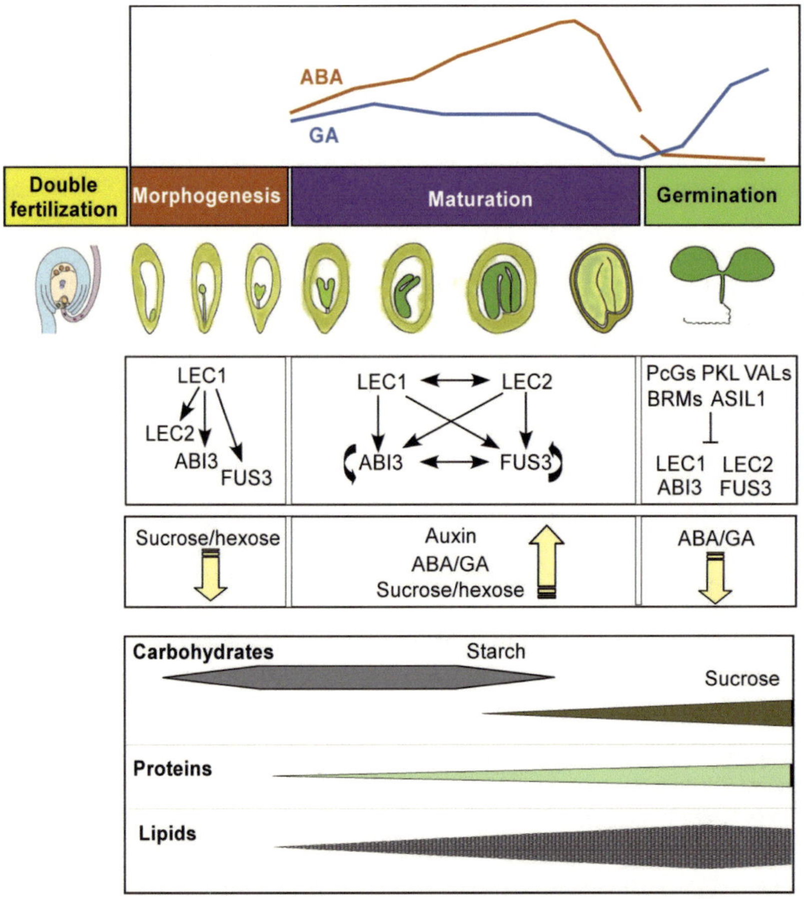

Fig. 2. Schematic representation of seed development in *Arabidopsis*. Embryogenesis after double fertilization in angiosperms involves two phases, morphogenesis and maturation. During the morphogenesis phase (approximately the first one third of the time of embryogenesis), the basic body plan is established and generates the different morphological domains of the embryo, the embryonic tissue and organ systems. After transition to the maturation phase, the embryo undergoes typical seed filling, growth arrest, acquisition of desiccation tolerance and entry into quiescence. Major reserves synthesized and accumulated during maturation phase include starch, storage proteins and lipids. Transition into the maturation phase is coordinated by the interactions of stage-specific developmental regulators such as the LEC regulators and the competing effects of sugars (sucrose-hexose ratio), hormones (ABA-GAs balance) and their synchronized interactions. The germination potential of seeds and seedling establishment are determined by the after-ripening process, hormones (GAs) and multiple embryonic repressors. Adapted from Refs. (Baud et al., 2002; Weber et al., 2005; Braybrook & Harada, 2008).

In monocots, the starchy endosperm is the prevalent storage domain, where carbohydrates and SSPs accumulate during maturation. Cereal SSP genes were among the first plant genes to be characterized. The AACA motif and the bipartite endosperm box (EB) encompassing the GCN4-like motif (GLM, ATGAGTCAT) and the prolamin box (PB, TGTAAAG) are the best characterized *cis*-elements affecting SSP gene expression (Forde et al., 1985; Wu et al., 2000). *In vitro* and *in vivo* protein-DNA interaction assays have identified direct targeting of the barley R2R3MYB factor HvGAMYB, wheat GAMYB and rice (*Oryza sativa)* OsMYB5 to the AACA motif. The Dof (DNA binding with one finger) proteins BPBF (prolamin box binding factor) and SAD (scutellum and aleurone-expressed DOF) bind to the PB box, while OPAQUE2 (O2)-like bZIP proteins, SPA (in wheat), BLZ1 and BLZ2 (in barley), bind to the GLM motif (Albani et al., 1997; Mena et al., 1998; Vicente-Carbajosa et al., 1998; Wu et al., 1998; Oñate et al., 1999; Díaz et al., 2002; Yanagisawa, 2002; Diaz et al., 2005). GAMYB was reported to activate expression of the endosperm-specific genes, such as *Itr1* which encodes the trypsin inhibitor BTI-CMe (Díaz et al., 2002). Dof proteins, BPBF and SAD, and the O2-like bZIP proteins, BLZ1 and BLZ2, activated expression of the B-hordein storage protein gene *Hor2* in barley (Mena et al., 1998; Vicente-Carbajosa et al., 1998; Oñate et al., 1999; Diaz et al., 2005). The maize Dof protein PBF was demonstrated to trans-activate the *γ-zein* gene (*γZ*) through the PB box (Marzábal et al., 2008). In addition, the R1MYB-SHA-QYF family proteins, HvMCB1 and HvMYBS3, were shown to regulate endosperm-specific gene expression through binding to the GATA motif (Rubio-Somoza et al., 2006a; 2006b). Recently, the barley FUSCA3 (HvFUS3) was demonstrated to bind to the RY-box present in the promoters of many endosperm genes (Moreno-Risueno et al., 2008). *HvFUS3* encodes a B3 domain protein that is expressed in the endosperm and embryo of developing seeds. *HvFUS3* expression peaks during the mid maturation phase and it participates in the transcriptional activation of the endosperm-specific genes *Hor2* and *Itr1* (Moreno-Risueno et al., 2008). Moreover, HvFUS3 was determined to trans-activate seed-specific genes *in planta* through interaction with the O2-like bZIP factor BLZ2 (Moreno-Risueno et al., 2008), indicating the involvement of both a B3 domain protein and a bZIP factor in the combinatorial regulation of endosperm-specific gene expression. In maize, O2 affects grain size and composition and is important in carbon allocation and amino acid biosynthesis during seed development (Hunter et al., 2002; Manicacci et al., 2009). In addition, two R1MYB transcription factor family proteins from wheat, MCB1 (MYB-related CAB promoter-binding protein) and MYBS3, were shown to interact with GARC (GA response complex) and to be involved in the regulation of SSP gene expression (Rubio-Somoza et al., 2006a; 2006b). Recent deep sequencing analysis of the transcriptome in developing rice seeds identified many differentially expressed novel transcripts and genes that are involved in the biosynthesis of starch and storage proteins. Hundreds of novel conserved patterns of *cis*-elements were found in the upregulated genes in the rice cultivars with high milling yield and good eating quality (Venu et al., 2011). Similar to the studies in *Arabidopsis* as described above, these discoveries indicate that complex combinatorial interactions of different transcription factors are pivotal for the regulation of the seed maturation program in cereals.

With the exception of those directly targeting SSP genes for which the regulatory elements in their promoters are well defined, little progress has been made in understanding the interactions between the master regulators and other target proteins, called secondary transcription factors (STF), that are also essential for the regulation of seed maturation processes. Nonetheless, part of the seed maturation program is regulated by indirect means mediated by STF. In rice, mutual interactions have been demonstrated between two transcriptional activators, a DOF–related rice prolamin box binding protein (RPBF) and a RISBZ1 bZIP factor (Yamamoto et al., 2006). In barley, the formation of binary or ternary complexes with PBF and DOF regulatory proteins are important for controlling SSP gene expression (Rubio-Somoza et al., 2006a; 2006b; Yamamoto et al., 2006). In *Arabidopsis*, mutation of LEC-type regulators (LEC1, LEC2 and FUS3) led to reduced accumulation of SSPs and major seed lipid TAGs, while ectopic expression in seedlings caused SSPs and TAGs to accumulate in vegetative tissues (Kagaya et al., 2005b; Santos-Mendoza et al., 2005; Braybrook et al., 2006; Wang et al., 2007). The master regulator LEC2 was also shown to control seed oil accumulation through regulation of WRINKLED1 (WRI1) (Baud et al., 2007) that directly targets fatty acid synthetic genes (Baud et al., 2009; Maeo et al., 2009). WRI1 is an AP2-type transcription factor with two AP2-binding domains (Cernac & Benning, 2004) and functions downstream of LEC1 ad LEC2. Ectopic expression of *WRI1* leads to the upregulation of fatty acid synthetic and glycolytic genes in seedlings (Baud et al., 2007; Mu et al., 2008). *In vitro* and *in vivo* analyses demonstrated that WRI1 was able to bind to the AW-box [CnTnG](n)$_7$[CG] of *BCCP2* (acetyl-CoA carboxylase) and *PI-PKβ1* (a subunit of pyruvate kinase) (Baud et al., 2009; Maeo et al., 2009). These studies provide insight into the understanding of the role of WRI1 in the regulation of oil synthesis during seed maturation. Some other downstream regulatory complexes have also been identified. For instance, biosynthesis of flavonoids, which are found in most seeds and grains and are major metabolites in the embryo and seed coat (Lepiniec et al., 2006), is regulated by a complex with six components including TRANSPARENT TESTA GLABRA1 (TTG1), the expression of which is repressed by FUS3 in the protoderm (Tsuchiya et al., 2004). Discovery of additional STFs and their interactions with the upstream master regulators will allow better exploration of the molecular mechanisms that control seed filling.

3.2 Hormonal signaling during seed maturation

The phytohormone ABA, an endogenous messenger derived from epoxycarotenoid, has a wide rage of functions in plant development, and in responses to biotic and abiotic stresses through its interaction with the Mg-chelatase H subunit (CHLH) and PYR1/RCAR1 (Shen et al., 2006; Ma et al., 2009; Park et al., 2009; Cutler et al., 2010). Many factors involved in ABA signaling have been characterized (Finkelstein, 2006; Razem et al., 2006; Adie et al., 2007; Hirayama & Shinozaki, 2007). ABA is the key hormone regulating several seed maturation processes including the initiation of the maturation phase, filling of seed reserves and entrance into dormancy (Nambara & Marion-Poll, 2003; Finch-Savage & Leubner-Metzger, 2006). ABA is initially synthesized in the maternal tissues and subsequently in the embryo (Nambara & Marion-Poll, 2003; Frey et al., 2004). Many genes for seed ABA biosynthesis have been identified including *ABA1* (*ABA DEFICIENT1*) encoding a zeaxanthin epoxidase that functions in first step of the ABA biosynthesis, NCEDs encoding 9-cis-epoxycarotenoid dioxygenases and *ABA2/GIN1* (*GLUCOSE INSENSITIVE1*)/*SDR1* (*SHORT-CHAIN DEHYDROGENASE REDUCTASE1*)/*SIS4* (*SUGAR-INSENSITIVE4*) encoding a cytosolic short-chain dehydrogenase/reductase involved in the conversion of xanthoxin to ABA-aldehyde during ABA biosynthesis (Nambara & Marion-Poll, 2003). A subset of ABA response mutants have been isolated and served as tools for dissecting the ABA singaling pathway (Kucera et al., 2005). For example, mutant analyses reveal that the ABA-activated protein kinases, PP2Cs (serine-threonine phosphatase type 2C) ABI1 and ABI2, and the transcriptional regulators ABI3, ABI4 and ABI5, are involved in the ABA signaling pathway and associated with seed dormancy (Finkelstein et al., 2002; Himmelbach et al., 2003). In *Arabidopsis*, ABA level is dynamically modulated and increases concurrent with the initiation of seed maturation phase, remains high throughout the maturation phase, declines at late maturation and is very low during germination and seedling establishment (Fig. 2) (Nambara & Marion-Poll, 2003; Seo et al., 2009). During seed maturation, ABA signaling is intimately associated with the actions of the master regulators LEC1, LEC2, ABI3 and FUS3 (Finkelstein et al., 2002; Gutierrez et al., 2007; Braybrook & Harada, 2008). For instance, *FUS3* expression leads to the elevation of ABA levels (Gazzarrini et al., 2004) and exogenous application of ABA enhances *FUS3* expression (Kagaya et al., 2005a; 2005b). As well, activation of embryonic gene (e.g. storage protein, LEA and oleosin genes) expression by LEC1, FUS3 and ABI3 is enhanced by ABA application (Parcy et al., 1994; Kagaya et al., 2005a; 2005b). A number of genes have been characterized that regulate ABA homeostasis. In *Arabidopsis*, CYP707A1 and CYP707A2 are major regulators for ABA degradation in the embryo at mid maturation and in both the embryo and the endosperm during late maturation (Okamoto et al., 2006). In barley and bean (*Phaseolus vulgaris*), the expression of *CYP707A* genes is the major mechanism controlling ABA catabolism in seeds (Millar et al., 2006; Yang et al., 2006). Moreover, *HvNCED2* was shown to upregulate ABA biosynthesis during grain development, whereas *HvCYP707A1* downregulated ABA levels during the subsequent seed maturation phase (Chono et al., 2006).

GA is also important in controlling seed maturation, germination and seedling growth (Seo et al., 2009). As shown in Fig. 2, GA levels are suppressed throughout the seed maturation phase until germination at which time GA levels elevate significantly. It was demonstrated that ABA interacts with GA during the maturation process (Seo et al., 2006). GA biosynthesis is suppressed by ABA in developing seeds through activation of *AtGA2ox6*. Seed maturation and germination are not determined by ABA alone, but instead by the ABA/GA ratio (Karssen et al., 1983; Giraudat et al., 1994; Dubreucq et al., 1996; Debeaujon & Koornneef, 2000; Finkelstein et al., 2002; Koornneef et al., 2002; Ogawa et al., 2003). At the beginning of the maturation phase, ABA levels increases in seeds and the resulting elevated ABA/GA ratio promotes maturation, induces dormancy and inhibits germination. Consistent with the lower ABA/GA ratio in the seeds of *lec2* and *fus3* mutants, and with the precocious cell differentiation and growth of mutant embryos, FUS3 and LEC2 were found to inhibit GA biosynthesis through the repression of GA biosynthetic genes (Curaba et al., 2004; Gazzarrini et al., 2004). However, reduced GA levels alone are not sufficient to confer desiccation tolerance during late maturation phase and SSP accumulation was defective in the *fus3* mutant in spite of the GA status (Gazzarrini et al., 2004). Additionally, *ABI3* and *FUS3* were shown to be regulated by ABA and/or GA at the post-translational level. AIP2 (ABI3-interacting protein 2), an E3 ligase controlled by ABA, can trigger the degradation of ABI3 (Zhang et al., 2005). Besides the importance of ABA/GA ratio for the regulation of seed maturation, the balance between ABA and other hormones is also important. For example, grain-filling rate in wheat was correlated with increases in the ABA/ethylene ratio (Yang et al., 2006).

Genetic and molecular studies have shown that auxin plays an essential role in embryogenesis and post-embryonic organ formation through its dynamic directional distribution (Tanaka et al., 2006). During embryogenesis, auxin accumulation is directed by PIN-FORMED (PIN)-mediated polar transportation from the apical cells to the hypophysis, the founder cell of the root stem-cell system (Tanaka et al., 2006). It has been suggested that auxin is required for the embryonic regulators FUS3, LEC1 and LEC2 to potentiate embryogenesis and seed maturation processes (Gazzarrini et al., 2004; Casson & Lindsey, 2006; Stone et al., 2008). ABI3 has been shown to be involved auxin signaling and lateral root development (Brady & McCourt, 2003). Auxin-responsive genes can be activated by the ectopic expression of *LEC2* (Braybrook & Harada, 2008) and *FUS3* expression was induced by auxin (Gazzarrini et al., 2004). ASIL1 (for *Arabidopsis* 6b-interacting protein 1-like 1), a trihelix transcriptional repressor of seed maturation genes in *Arabidopsis*, is not responsive to ABA, but is moderately induced by auxin (Gao et al., 2009). In dry or imbibed wild-type seeds, *LEC1* and *LEC2* transcripts were not observed, whereas expression was elevated in *asil1* mutants at 1 h after imbibition with this increase being enhanced by the application of auxin (Gao et al., 2009). Given the fact that somatic embryogenesis is induced by the synthetic auxin 2,4-D (2,4-dichlorophenoxyacetic acid) (Mordhorst et al., 1998) and that derepression of *LEC1* and *LEC2* in imbibed *asil1* mutant seeds was enhanced by auxin, similar to ABA, it was suggested to function as a signal for the activation of embryonic genes. Auxin accumulation is also dynamically changed during germination and vegetative growth. For example, auxin activity was highly localized in the radical tips of germinating and germinated seeds (Liu et al., 2007) and the initiation sites of organ primordia in roots and shoots correspond to regions with increased auxin levels (Tanaka et al., 2006). *ASIL1* expression also exhibited a modest response to auxin and the level of *ASIL1* transcript is elevated at 1h post-imbibition, therefore the rise in *ASIL1* transcript levels may correspond to the distribution of auxin in cells of germinating seeds (Gao et al., 2009). LEC1 and LEC2 function upstream of other embryonic and seed maturation genes (To et al., 2006) and their ectopic expression is sufficient to provoke the embryonic program in vegetative tissues (Lotan et al., 1998; Stone et al., 2001; Santos-Mendoza et al., 2005). Therefore, expression of these two major regulators of embryonic programming should be strictly prevented during germination and seedling development. Given the up-regulation of *ASIL1* by auxin and the derepression of embryonic genes in germinating *asil1* seeds as well as in 2-week-old *asil1* seedlings, ASIL1 may prevent ectopic expression of *LEC1* and *LEC2* in cells that encounter elevated auxin levels during germination and vegetative growth (Gao et al., 2009). Although significant progress has been made in understanding the connection between seed maturation and auxin signaling, the precise roles that auxin plays and its mode of action during the maturation phase remain to be established. Only minor auxin-related traits have been detected in *lec* mutants during early embryogenesis (Lotan et al., 1998; Stone et al., 2001). The *lec1* and *lec2* mutants have strongly reduced ability to generate somatic embryos (Gaj et al., 2005), whereas ectopic expression of *LEC1* and *LEC2* in seedlings induced the formation of embryonic traits (Lotan et al., 1998; Stone et al., 2001). Therefore, it has been proposed that LEC transcription factors seem to build an environment in somatic cells that prime them to respond to auxin and undergo somatic embryogenesis; this competence might be affected by the repression of GA synthesis by LEC regulators or influenced by ABA signaling alone or by the ABA/GA balance (Braybrook & Harada, 2008).

3.3 Sugar signaling and metabolic regulation

Sugars generated by photosynthesis play a key role in plant development as structural components, storage molecules, energy sources and as intermediates for the synthesis of other organic molecules. In addition, sugars may act as signaling molecules that regulate the expression of genes involved in photosynthesis and metabolism. High sugar levels lead to a negative feedback on photosynthesis while promoting starch biosynthesis. Conversely, low sugar levels increase photosynthetic gene expression and promote storage reserve mobilization while limiting the use of carbohydrates to metabolic processes (Wobus & Weber, 1999; Rook et al., 2006). For instance, many plant developmental processes, such as seed germination, seedling establishment, flowering and senescence, are influenced by glucose (Gibson, 2000; Smeekens, 2000; Gibson, 2005; Rolland et al., 2006). Gene expression can be regulated by sugar-induced signal transduction through diverse mechanisms at the transcriptional, post-transcriptional, translational and post-translational levels (Rolland et al., 2006). Many studies have determined that the initiation of seed maturation processes is triggered by sugar signaling, notably the sucrose/hexose ratio in the embryos (Fig. 2) (Weber et al., 2005). During endosperm or cotyledon differentiation, gradients in metabolite concentrations emerge and provide signals for the transition into the maturation phase (Weber et al., 2005). Glucose concentration is directly correlated with cell division. This is supported by the observation of higher levels of glucose in nondifferentiated premature regions and low levels in mature starch-accumulating regions (Borisjuk et al., 2003). Conversely, young embryos contain moderately low levels of sucrose and the highest concentration of sucrose occurs in the actively elongating and starch-accumulating cells during maturation, which is consistent with the expression of genes involved in the storage compound synthesis (Borisjuk et al., 2002). This alteration in sugar balance is correlated with the establishment of an epidermis-localized sucrose uptake system via the formation of transfer cells (Offler et al., 2003). A strong and transient increase in sucrose uptake occurs while free hexose levels decrease markedly in the embryo. Sucrose signaling subsequently controls storage filling and differentiation processes in seeds through the regulation of gene expression and metabolic enzyme activities (Gibson, 2005; Rolland et al., 2006). In *Arabidopsis*, mutation of the gene encoding sugar transporter SUC5 delayed the conversion of sugar to lipids and AtSUC5 plays a major role in the progression into maturation phase (Baud et al., 2005). More interestingly, seed mass was increased in an *ap2* (*apetala2*) mutant, which is characterized by an increase in embryo cell size and number. This phenotype is the consequence of a prolonged period of cell division regulated by elevation of hexose/sucrose ratio (Ohto et al., 2005). In *tps1* (*TREHALOSE-6-PHOSPHATE SYNTHASE1*) mutant embryos, starch instead of lipids accumulated due to the downregulation of genes involved in the starch-sucrose breakdown and the upregulation of genes responsible for the lipid mobilization for gluconeogenesis, demonstrating the importance of trehalose in the sugar signaling pathway regulating the maturation phase (Gómez et al., 2006). As such, sugar signaling was suggested to be a ubiquitous regulatory system involved in seed maturation (Gutierrez et al., 2007).

Seed storage metabolism involves the movement of intermediates between several distinct subcellular compartments including mitochondria, plastids and cytosol (Fait et al., 2006). In cells of heterotrophic embryos, ATP is mainly generated in bioenergetic organelles, the mitochondria, by respiration and is imported into plastids through ATP/ADP translocators in a rate-limiting manner (Tjaden et al., 1998; Rawsthorne, 2002). Studies in legumes, barley and maize have shown that ATP levels are associated with seed maturation processes. ATP levels are low in young cotyledons and increase toward maturation starting from the abaxial region. The active storage-accumulating regions contain high levels of ATP during maturation (Borisjuk et al., 2003; Rolletschek et al., 2004). The photoheterotrophic plastids in seed embryos are different from leaf chloroplasts with regard to morphology and physiology. These differences include elevated cyclic electron transport via photosystem II, but a low capacity for photosynthetic CO_2 fixation (Asokanthan et al., 1997). Seed photosynthesis plays a role in controlling biosynthetic fluxes through the production of ATP and O_2 by preventing hypoxic conditions inside the seed (Rolletschek et al., 2005a; Weber et al., 2005). The low O_2 levels in developing seeds affect enzymatic activity, gene expression patterns, mitochondrial ATP production, and metabolite fluxes. Hypoxia leads to energy depletion so that embryo cells are stressed and storage reserve accumulation is constrained (Borisjuk et al., 2003; Rolletschek et al., 2004; Rolletschek et al., 2005a; Weber et al., 2005; Borisjuk & Rolletschek, 2009). Therefore, photosynthesis in developing seeds is important for storage reserve synthesis and accumulation (Borisjuk et al., 2005; Rolletschek et al., 2005a; Fait et al., 2006). The energy status is also important for controlling the flux of substrates into different storage products (Rolletschek et al., 2005b). In general, energy demand is highest for lipids, followed by storage proteins, and lowest for starch (Weber et al., 2005). For instance, in *Brassica napus*, the developmental transfer from starch to lipid storage at mid maturation is accompanied by increased ATP/ADP ratios. Starch synthesis is saturated at lower ATP levels than is lipid synthesis (Vigeolas et al., 2003). Moreover, during seed maturation in oilseeds *B. napus* and soybean (*Glycine max*), the biosynthetic switch from starch to lipids is linked to the import of specific metabolites, suggesting that the relative fluxes into different storage products are not only energy dependant but also developmentally controlled (Eastmond & Rawsthorne, 2000; Weber et al., 2005).

Seed maturation is also influenced by nitrogen metabolism because storage protein accumulation depends on nitrogen uptake and availability (Golombek et al., 2001; Miranda et al., 2001; Rolletschek et al., 2005c). Asparagine is acquired from the phloem, metabolized and reconstructed in the seed coat and unloaded at later stages. In soybean, the level of asparagine in developing cotyledons plays a rate-limiting role in protein biosynthesis (Hernandez-Sebastia et al., 2005). Moreover, amino acid biosynthesis controls storage protein synthesis. For example, in soybean, pea (*Pisum sativum*), Fava bean (*Vicia faba*) and wheat, phosphoenolpyruvate carboxylase (PEPC), a ubiquitous and highly regulated enzyme, is as a determinant of SSP biosynthesis. Therefore, PEPC has become a promising target for increasing protein content of crop seeds. For example, overexpression of PEPC in bean seeds resulted in the accumulation of up to 20% more protein per gram seed dry weight due to the shift of metabolic fluxes from sugars/starch into organic acids and free amino acids during maturation; seed dry weight was higher by 20% - 30% possibly owing to elevated carbon fixation (Fait et al., 2006). A major metabolic switch has been identified that is associated with the transition from seed filling to the desiccation phase. Seed metabolism is fundamentally changed during this switch. Seed storage accumulation during maturation is associated with the reduction of most sugars, amino acids and organic acids. However, desiccation tolerance is associated with increases in the content of distinct sugars, organic acids, nitrogen-rich amino acids and shikimate-derived metabolites (Fait et al., 2006). Similarly, studies using gene profiling in *Medicago truncatula* seeds have demonstrated that lipids, starch and oligosaccharides are mobilized, consistent with the elevation in sucrose level during the early desiccation stage (Buitink et al., 2006). Protein phosphorylation was shown to be involved in the metabolic regulation during seed maturation as the storage-associated enzyme PEPC is activated by phosphorylation (Goldberg & Fischer, 1999). In legume seeds, SPS (sucrose-phosphate synthase) activity is inhibited by phosphorylation during the switch from high hexose to high sucrose levels (Weber et al., 2005). In rice seeds, a calcium-dependent protein kinase (CDPK) isoform was found to control storage reserve accumulation by phosphorylation of sucrose synthase (Asano et al., 2002). Overexpression of *CDPK2* in rice arrests seed development at an early stage (Morello et al., 2000). A large number of functionally diverse phosphoproteins were expressed during seed filling in *B. napus* (Agrawal & Thelen, 2006). *OsCPK23* is markedly upregulated in developing seeds in comparison to mature leaves (Ray et al., 2007). The 12S globulin cruciferin was found to be the major phosphorylated storage protein in *Arabidopsis* seeds (Wan et al., 2007) and protein tyrosine kinases and protein tyrosine phosphatases were shown to be involved in the storage protein accumulation and lipid reserve mobilization processes (Ghelis et al., 2008). Recently, the leucine-rich repeat receptor kinase encoded by *IKU2* (*HAIKU2*) was shown to directly target the positive seed regulator SHB1 (Zhou et al., 2009). Mutation of *IKU2* reduced seed size and affected embryo and endosperm development (Luo et al., 2005).

3.4 Sugar and ABA signal interaction

As described above, transition of embryo morphogenesis into the maturation phase is governed by sugars and ABA signaling and their coordinated interaction (Brocard-Gifford et al., 2003; Gibson, 2004). Genetic and molecular studies demonstrated that sugar signaling in higher plants is intimately associated with hormone signaling, in particular with ABA (Leon & Sheen, 2003; Rook et al., 2006; Dekkers et al., 2008). Four independent screens have been conducted to identify sugar response mutants: *sun* (sucrose uncoupled), *isi* (impaired sucrose induction), *gin* and *sis*. All four screens identified the ABA deficient mutants (*aba2*/*isi4*/*gin1*/*sis4* and *aba3*/*gin5*) and *ABA insensitive4* (i.e. *abi4*/*sun6*/*isi3*/*gin6*/*sis5*) (Arenas-Huertero et al., 2000; Huijser et al., 2000; Laby et al., 2000; Rook et al., 2001) suggesting genetic interactions between sugar and ABA signaling pathways. Furthermore, ABA biosynthetic and signaling genes were found to be regulated by glucose. Several sugar signaling mutants, such as *gin1*, *gin5*, *isi4* and *sis4*, exhibit lower endogenous ABA levels (Arenas-Huertero et al., 2000; Laby et al., 2000; Rook et al., 2001), which is consistent with the previously identified ABA deficient mutants *aba1*, *aba2* and *aba3* that show a *gin* phenotype (Arenas-Huertero et al., 2000; Huijser et al., 2000; Laby et al., 2000). Transcripts of several ABA biosynthetic genes, such as *ABA1*, *AAO3* and *ABA3*, are increased by low concentrations of glucose (2%) (Cheng et al., 2002), as well as by ABA itself (Xiong et al., 2001; Cheng et al., 2002; Seo & Koshiba, 2002). These observations suggest that ABA biosynthetic genes and ABA accumulation are directly regulated by glucose. ABI4 and ABI5 were shown to be involved in ABA signaling and play important roles during seed development (Finkelstein, 1994; Brocard et al., 2002). As indicated above, sugar response mutants, such as *sun6*, *isi3*, *gin6* and *sis5*, are allelic to *abi4*. The *abi4* mutant was isolated based on its ability to germinate in the presence of high levels of ABA (3 μM) (Finkelstein, 1994). Expression of *ABI4* was activated by 6% glucose in an ABA-dependent fashion, but had a limited response to ABA alone (Arenas-Huertero et al., 2000; Cheng et al., 2002). These investigations indicate that ABA biosynthetic and signaling genes can be regulated by both glucose and ABA. Besides *abi4* and *abi5, abi8* mutants also displayed a glucose insensitive phenotype, although this phenotype was not as obvious as that of the *abi4* mutant (Arenas-Huertero et al., 2000; Huijser et al., 2000; Laby et al., 2000; Brocard-Gifford et al., 2003). Similar to *ABI4, ABI5* expression is also induced by glucose in an ABA-dependent manner (Cheng et al., 2002) and overexpression of *ABI5* increased sensitivity to glucose (Brocard et al., 2002). Additionally, *ABI3* expression was also found to be induced by glucose in an ABA-dependent manner, although not as significant as *ABI4* and *ABI5* (Cheng et al., 2002). Overexpression of *ABI3* confers hypersensitivity to sugars (Finkelstein et al., 2002; Zeng & Kermode, 2004) and *abi3* mutants were insensitive to glucose in combination with ABA (Nambara & Marion-Poll, 2003). A similar sugar-ABA interaction was shown for the regulation of *ApL3* (ADP pyrophosphorylase large subunit) in starch biosynthesis in rice (Akihiro et al., 2005). These findings clearly connect sugar to ABA signaling; however, a number of genes are coregulated by sugar and ABA (Li et al., 2006). Additionally, *ABI1, ABI2* and *ABI3* appear not to have a major role in sugar signaling (Arenas-Huertero et al., 2000; Huijser et al., 2000; Laby et al., 2000). Taken together, genetic and molecular analyses of sugar signaling have uncovered complex and extensive interactions between sugar and ABA signaling pathways. Whether a direct molecular link exists between sugar and ABA signaling pathways remains unresolved, and more efforts might be devoted to the establishment of their connections in a more direct and specific way.

3.5 Epigenetic regulation of seed maturation

Accumulation of seed reserves is a major process during the seed maturation phase. The main storage products accumulated during seed filling are storage proteins, oil (often TAG) and carbohydrates (often starch). Recently, advances have been made toward understanding the regulatory, metabolic and developmental control of seed filling (Baud et al., 2008; Gallardo et al., 2008; Santos-Mendoza et al., 2008; North et al., 2010). The regulatory networks governing seed maturation in *Arabidopsis* are repressed prior to germination so that seed storage reserves are not accumulated during vegetative development (Fig. 2). Therefore, studies on the expression of seed maturation genes in non-seed tissues would facilitate understanding of the regulatory mechanisms underlying seed filling. Chromatin modification has been implicated in the repression of these regulatory networks. Phaseolin is the major SSP of bean. Phaseolin (*phas*) gene expression is temporally and spatially regulated and is completely inactive during the vegetative phase of plant development (Bustos et al., 1989; van Der Geest et al., 1995). Silencing of the *phas* gene in vegetative tissues was associated with the presence of a nucleosome positioned over the three phased TATA boxes present in the *phas* promoter (Kadosh & Struhl, 1998). Ectopic expression of the ABI3-like factor *ALF* potentiated the chromatin structure over the TATA region of the phas promoter and caused *phas* expression in vegetative tissues in an ABA-dependent manner (Goldberg & Fischer, 1999). In developing seeds, this repressive structure is remodeled concomitant with gene activation, leading to the disruption of condensed chromatin configuration and allowing transcription factors to access the *phas* promoter (Li & Hall, 1999). Chromatin immunoprecipitation assays demonstrated that histone acetylation and methylation-directed chromatin remodeling contributed to the regulation of *phas* expression (Ng et al., 2006). Acetylation and deacetylation of lysine residue in the amino-terminal tail were shown to be involved in the reversible modification of chromatin structure and had the opposite effect on transcriptional regulation (Berger,

2002). Acetylation is catalyzed by histone acetyltransferase (HAT) and results in transcriptional activation (Brownell & Allis, 1996; Kuo & Allis, 1998; Kuo et al., 2000). Deacetylation is catalyzed by histone decaetylase (HDAC) and is linked to transcriptional repression (Kadosh & Struhl, 1998; Rundlett et al., 1998). Inhibition of HDAC activity with trichostatin A during germination led to elevated expression of embryogenesis-related genes (Tanaka et al., 2008).

Several proteins have been identified that act as negative regulators of seed maturation gene expression (Table 3 and Fig. 2). PICKLE (PKL), a CHD3 chromatin remodeling factor belonging to the SWI/SNF class, acts in concert with GA to ensure that embryonic traits are not expressed after germination (Ogas et al., 1997; Ogas et al., 1999). *pkl* mutants expressed seed maturation genes in primary roots (Ogas et al., 1997; Ogas et al., 1999; Rider et al., 2003; Henderson et al., 2004; Li et al., 2005). The VP1/ABI3-LIKE (VAL) B3 proteins VAL1 and VAL2, also referred to as HSI2 and HSL1, respectively (Tsukagoshi et al., 2007), act together with sugar signaling to repress ectopic expression of seed maturation genes in seedlings and were necessary for the transition from seed maturation to active vegetative growth (Suzuki et al., 2007; Tsukagoshi et al., 2007). *VAL1* and *VAL2* encode B3 domain proteins with an ERF-associated amphiphilic repression (EAR) motif. Interestingly, a CW domain of unknown function and a putative plant homeodomain (PHD)-like zinc (Zn)-finger domain are frequently present in chromatin remodeling factors and were present in the VAL1 and VAL2 (Suzuki et al., 2007). It was revealed that VAL1/HSI2 functions as a repressor of a sugar-inducible reporter gene (Tsukagoshi et al., 2005). Most of the embryonic and seed maturation genes including *LEC1, ABI3, FUS3* and genes for seed storage compounds were derepressed in seedlings of a double mutant of *VAL1* and *VAL2* (Suzuki et al., 2007; Tsukagoshi et al., 2007). As noted above, PcG group proteins establish epigenetic inheritance of repressed gene expression states through histone methylation of H3K27 (Köhler & Grossniklaus, 2002). Genetic and molecular studies demonstrated that *FUS3* is regulated by the PcG proteins, for example, *FUS3* expression is derepressed in leaves of a double mutant of *CLF* and *SWN* and chromatin immunoprecipitation corroborated the direct targeting of *FUS3* by the PcG protein MEA (Makarevich et al., 2006). A member of BRAHMA (BRM)-containing SNF2 chromatin remodeling ATPase was also found to be involved in repression of some seed maturation genes in leaves. Mutation of *BRM* led to the accumulation of transcripts from *2S, FUS3* and some other embryogenesis-related genes in leaf tissues (Tang et al., 2008). Recently, a new embryonic repressor ASIL1 was isolated by its interaction with the *Arabidopsis* 2S albumin *At2S3* promoter (Gao et al., 2009). ASIL1 has domains conserved in the plant-specific trihelix family of DNA binding proteins and belongs to a subfamily of 6b-interacting protein 1-like factors. It is interesting that the trihelix domain of ASIL1 is highly similar to the SANT (Switching-defective protein 3 (Swi3), Adaptor 2 (Ada2), Nuclear receptor co-repressor (N-CoR), Transcription factor (TF)IIIB) domain that functions as a unique histone-interaction module in chromatin remodeling (Boyer et al., 2004). This structural feature suggests that ASIL1 may function as a gene-specific DNA-binding factor to regulate seed maturation genes by recruiting a chromatin remodeling complex. Identification of proteins that interact with ASIL1 will provide further insight into this possible regulatory mechanism. *asil1* seedlings exhibit a global shift in gene expression to a profile resembling late embryogenesis. *LEC1* and *LEC2* were markedly derepressed during early germination, as was a large subset of seed maturation genes, such as those encoding SSPs and oleosins, in seedlings of *asil1* mutants. Consistent with this, *asil1* seedlings accumulated 2S albumin and oil with a fatty acid composition similar to that of seed-derived lipid. Moreover, ASIL1 specifically binds to a GT element that overlaps the G-box and is in close proximity to the RY repeats of the *At2S* promoters. It was suggested that ASIL1 targets GT-box–containing embryonic genes by competing with the binding of transcriptional activators to this promoter region. Thus, ASIL1 represents a novel component of the regulatory framework that negatively controls expression of seed maturation genes during post-embroyonic growth (Gao et al., 2009). This finding supports the notion that embryonic traits are actively repressed during and after germination and are directly or indirectly regulated by epigenetic means (Fig. 2).

Gene	Acronym	Protein category	Protein domains	DNA-binding property	Potential function in embryonic gene repression	References
VP1/ABI3-LIKE	*VILs*	B3	B3, Zn finger	Yes	Repression of master regulators of seed maturation LEC1, ABI3 and FUS3, and many seed maturation genes	Suzuki et al., 2007; Tsukagoshi et al., 2007
ASIL1	*ASIL1*	Trihelix	Trihelix	Yes	Repression of master regulators of seed maturation LEC1, LEC2, ABI3 and FUS3, and many seed maturation genes	Gao et al., 2009
PICKLE	*PKL*	SNF2	SNF2, CHD3, PHD	No	Repression of master regulators of seed maturation LEC1, LEC2 and FUS3, and many seed maturation genes	Ogas et al., 1997; Rider et al., 2003; Henderson et al., 2004; Li et al., 2005
CURLY LEAF/ SWINGER	*CLF/ SWN*	PcG	SET	No	Repression of master regulators of seed maturation LEC1, LEC2 and FUS3, and many seed maturation genes	Makarevich et al., 2006
BRAHAM	*BRM*	SNF2	SNF2	No	Many seed maturation genes	Tang et al., 2008
HDA6/19	*HDA6/19*	HDAC	HDAC	No	Repression of master regulators of seed maturation LEC1, ABI3 and FUS3, and many seed maturation genes	Tanaka et al., 2008

Table 3. Genes involved in seed repression in *Arabidopsis* seedlings

4. Conclusion

Seeds are the key link between two sporophytic generations in the life cycle of flowering plants. Seed development is an intricate genetically programmed process that is correlated with changes in metabolite levels and regulated by a complex signaling network mediated by sugars and hormones. The coordinated expression of embryo and endosperm tissues is required for proper early seed development, which is primarily maternally controlled through epigenetic mechanisms such as histone- and DNA-methylation. The transition to the maturation phase requires a switch to filial control which is denoted by a distinct hormone and metabolite profile. Genetic, physiological and cytological approaches have been employed to dissect the molecular mechanisms underlying seed development. Such studies have elucidated the elaborate regulatory and metabolic pathways governing the onset of seed maturation, seed filling, acquisition of desiccation tolerance and after-ripening phases. Considering the importance of seeds for human food, animal feed and sustainable feedstocks for biofuel production, much effort has been devoted to the genetic and metabolic control of starch, protein and lipid deposition in cereal grains and oilseeds. Molecular, physiological and genetic approaches are being used in combination to identify the individual steps in the pathways leading to storage compound synthesis and the factors that regulate these processes. Currently, these tools and knowledge are being applied to engineer crop plants with altered seed compositions and metabolite profiles to improve seed yield, quality and utility.

5. References

Acevedo-Hernández; G.J., León, P. & Herrera-Estrella, L.R. (2005). Sugar and ABA responsiveness of a minimal RBCS light-responsive unit is mediated by direct binding of ABI4. *Plant Journal*, Vol.43, No.4, (August 2005), pp. 506-519, ISSN 0960-7412

Ach, R.A.; Taranto, P. & Gruissem, W. (1997). A conserved family of WD-40 proteins binds to the retinoblastoma protein in both plants and animals. *Plant Cell*, Vol.9, No.9, (September 1997), pp. 1595-1606, ISSN 1040-4651

Adams, S.; Vinkenoog, R.; Spielman, M.; Dickinson, H.G. & Scott, R.J. (2000). Parent-of-origin effects on seed development in *Arabidopsis thaliana* require DNA methylation. *Development*, Vol.127, No.11, (June 2000), pp. 2493-2502, ISSN 0950-1991

Adie, B.A.; Pérez-Pérez, J.; Pérez-Pérez, M.M.; Godoy, M.; Sánchez-Serrano, J.J.; Schmelz, E.A. & Solano, R. (2007). ABA is an essential signal for plant resistance to pathogens affecting JA biosynthesis and the activation of defenses in *Arabidopsis*. *Plant Cell*, Vol.19, No.5, (May 2007), pp. 1665-1681, ISSN 1040-4651

Agrawal, G.K. & Thelen, J.J. (2006). Large scale identification and quantitative profiling of phosphoproteins expressed during seed filling in oilseed rape. *Molecular & Cellular Proteomics*, Vol.5, No.11, (November 2006), pp. 2044-2059, ISSN 1535-9476

Akihiro, T.; Mizuno, K. & Fujimura, T. (2005). Gene expression of ADP-glucose pyrophosphorylase and starch contents in rice cultured cells are cooperatively regulated by sucrose and ABA. *Plant Cell Physiology*, Vol.46, No.6, (June 2005), pp. 937-946, ISSN 0032-0781

Albani, D.; Hammond-Kosack, M.C.U.; Smith, C., Conlan, S.; Colot, V., Holdsworth, M.J. & Bevan, M.W. (1997). The wheat transcriptional activator SPA: a seed-specific bZIP protein that recognizes the GCN4-like motif in the bifactorial endosperm box of prolamin genes. *Plant Cell*, Vol.9, No.2, (February 1997), pp. 171-184, ISSN 1040-4651

Alonso, R.; Oñate-Sánchez, L.; Weltmeier, F.; Ehlert, A.; Diaz, I.; Dietrich, K.; Vicente-Carbajosa, J. & Dröge-Laser, W. (2009). A pivotal role of the basic leucine zipper transcription factor bZIP53 in the regulation of Arabidopsis seed maturation gene expression based on heterodimerization and protein complex formation. *Plant Cell*, Vol.21, No.6, (June 2009), pp. 1747-1461, ISSN 1040-4651

Arenas-Huertero, F.; Arroyo, A.; Zhou, L.; Sheen, J. & León, P. (2000). Analysis of *Arabidopsis* glucose insensitive mutants, *gin5* and *gin6*, reveals a central role of the plant hormone ABA in the regulation of plant vegetative development by sugar. *Genes & Development*, Vol.14, No.16, (August 2000), pp. 2085-2096, ISSN 0890-9369

Asano, T.; Kunieda, N.; Omura, Y.; Ibe, H.; Kawasaki, T.; Takano, M.; Sato, M.; Furuhashi, H.; Mujin, T.; Takaiwa, F.; Wu, C.Y.; Tada, Y.; Satozawa, T.; Sakamoto, M. & Shimada, H. (2002). Rice SPK, a calmodulin-like domain protein kinase, is required for storage product accumulation during seed development: phosphorylation of sucrose synthase is a possible factor. *Plant Cell*, Vol.14, No.3, (March 2002), pp. 619-628, ISSN 1040-4651

Asokanthan, P.; Johnson, R.W.; Griffith, M. & Krol, M. (1997). The photosynthetic potential of canola embryos. *Physiologia Plantarum*, Vol.101, No.2, (October 1997), pp. 353-360, ISSN 0031-9317

Baroux, C.; Pecinka, A.; Fuchs, J.; Schubert, I. & Grossniklaus, U. (2007). The triploid endosperm genome of *Arabidopsis* adopts a peculiar, parental-dosage-dependent chromatin organization. *Plant Cell*, Vol.19, No.6, (June 2007), pp. 1782-1794, ISSN 1040-4651

Baud, S.; Boutin, J.-P.; Miquel, M.; Lepiniec, L. & Rochat, C. (2002). An integrated overview of seed development in *Arabidopsis thaliana* ecotype WS. *Plant Physiology and Biochemistry*, Vol.40, No.2, (February 2002), pp. 151-160, ISSN 0981-9428

Baud, S.; Dubreucq, B. ; Miquel, M. ; Rochat, C. & Lepiniec, L. (2008). Storage Reserve Accumulation in Arabidopsis: Metabolic and Developmental Control of Seed Filling. *The Arabidopsis Book*, Vol.6,.No.e0113, ISSN 1543-8120

Baud, S.; Wuillème, S.; To, A.; Rochat, C. & Lepiniec, L. (2009). Role of WRINKLED1 in the transcriptional regulation of glycolytic and fatty acid biosynthetic genes in *Arabidopsis*. *Plant Journal*, Vol.60, No.6, (December 2009), pp. 933-947, ISSN 0960-7412

Baud, S.; Mendoza, M.S.; To, A.; Harscoët, E.; Lepiniec, L. & Dubreucq, B. (2007). WRINKLED1 specifies the regulatory action of LEAFY COTYLEDON2 towards fatty acid metabolism during seed maturation in *Arabidopsis*. *Plant Journal*, Vol.50, No.5, (June 2007), pp. 825-838, ISSN 0960-7412

Baud, S.; Wuillème, S.; Lemoine, R.; Kronenberger, J.; Caboche, M.; Lepiniec, L. & Rochat, C. (2005). The AtSUC5 sucrose transporter specifically expressed in the endosperm is involved in early seed development in *Arabidopsis*. *Plant Journal*, Vol.43, No.6, (September 2005), pp. 824-836, ISSN 0960-7412

Bauer, M.J. & Fischer, R.L. (2011). Genome demethylation and imprinting in the endosperm. *Current Opinion in Plant Biology*, Vol.14, No.2, (April 2011), pp. 162-167, ISSN 1369-5266

Bensmihen, S.; Rippa, S.; Lambert, G.; Jublot, D.; Pautot, V.; Granier, F.; Giraudat, J. & Parcy, F. (2002). The homologous ABI5 and EEL transcription factors function antagonistically to fine-tune gene expression during late embryogenesis *Plant Cell*, Vol.14, No.6, (June 2002), pp. 1391-1403, ISSN 1040-4651

Berger, F. & Chaudhury, A. (2009). Parental memories shape seeds. *Trends in Plant Science*, Vol.14, No.10, (October 2009), pp. 550-556, ISSN 1360-1385

Berger, S.L. (2002). Histone modifications in transcription regulation. *Current Opinion in Genetics & Development*, Vol.12, No.2, (April 2002), pp. 142-148, ISSN 0959-437X

Borisjuk, L. & Rolletschek, H. (2009). The oxygen status of the developing seed. *New Phytologist*, Vol.182, No.1, (October 2009), pp. 17-30, ISSN 0028-646X

Borisjuk, L.; Rolletschek, H.; Wobus, U. & Weber, H. (2003). Differentiation of legume cotyledons as related to metabolic gradients and assimilate transport into seeds. *Journal of Experimental Botany*, Vol.54, No.382, (January 2003), pp. 503-512, ISSN 0022-0957

Borisjuk, L.; Walenta, S.; Rolletschek, H.; Mueller-Klieser, W.; Wobus, U. & Weber, H. (2002). Spatial analysis of plant development: sucrose imaging within Vicia faba cotyledons reveals specific developmental patterns. *Plant Journal*, Vol.29, No.4, (February 2002), pp. 521-530, ISSN 0960-7412

Borisjuk, L.; Nguyen, T.H.; Neuberger, T.; Rutten, T;, Tschiersch, H.; Claus, B.; Feussner, I.; Webb, A.G.; Jakob, P.; Weber, H.; Wobus, U. & Rolletschek, H. (2005). Gradients of lipid storage, photosynthesis and plastid differentiation in developing soybean seeds. *New Phytologist*, Vol.167, No.3, (September 2005), pp. 761-776, ISSN 0028-646X

Boyer, L.A.; Latek, R.R. & Peterson, C.L. (2004). The SANT domain: a unique histone-tail-binding module? *Nature Reviews Molecular Cell Biology*, Vol.5, No.2, (February 2004), pp. 158-163, ISSN 1471-0072

Brady, S.M. & McCourt, P. (2003). Hormone cross-talk in seed dormancy. *Journal of Plant Growth Regulation*, Vol.22, No.1, (July 2003), pp. 25-31, ISSN 0721-7595

Braybrook, S.A. & Harada, J.J. (2008). LECs go crazy in embryo development. *Trends in Plant Science*, Vol.13, No.12, (December 2008), pp. 624-630, ISSN 1360-1385

Braybrook, S.A.; Stone, S.L.; Park, S.; Bui, A.Q.; Le, B.H.; Fischer, R.L.; Goldberg, R.B. & Harada, J.J. (2006). Genes directly regulated by LEAFY COTYLEDON2 provide insight into the control of embryo maturation and somatic embryogenesis. *Proceedings of the National Academy of Sciences USA*, Vol.103, No.9, (February 2006), pp. 3468-3473, ISSN 0027-8424

Brocard-Gifford, I.M.; Lynch, T.J. & Finkelstein, R.R. (2003). Regulatory networks in seeds integrating developmental, abscisic acid, sugar, and light signaling. *Plant Physiology*, Vol.131, No.1, (January 2003), pp. 78-92, ISSN 0032-0889

Brocard, I.M.; Lynch, T.J. & Finkelstein, R.R. (2002). Regulation and role of the *Arabidopsis abscisic acid-insensitive 5* gene in abscisic acid, sugar, and stress response. *Plant Physiology*, Vol.129, No.4, (August 2002), pp. 1533-1543, ISSN 0032-0889

Brownell, J.E. & Allis, C.D. (1996). Special HATs for special occasions: linking histone acetylation to chromatin assembly and gene activation. *Current Opinion in Genetics & Development*, Vol.6, No.2, (April 1996), pp. 176-184, ISSN 0959-437X

Buitink, J.; Leger, J.J. ; Guisle, I. ; Vu, B.L. ; Wuillème, S. ; Lamirault, G. ; Le Bars, A. ; Le Meur, N. ; Becker, A. ; Küster, H. & Leprince, O. (2006). Transcriptome profiling uncovers metabolic and regulatory processes occurring during the transition from desiccation-sensitive to desiccation-tolerant stages in *Medicago truncatula* seeds. *Plant Journal*, Vol.47, No.5, (September 2006), pp. 735-750, ISSN 0960-7412

Bustos, M.M.; Guiltinan, M.J.; Jordano, J.; Begum, D.; Kalkan, F.A. & Hall, T.C. (1989). Regulation of beta-glucuronidase expression in transgenic tobacco plants by an A/T-rich, cis-acting sequence found upstream of a French bean beta phaseolin gene. *Plant Cell*, Vol.1, No.9, (September 1989), pp. 839-853, ISSN 1040-4651

Cao, R. & Zhang, Y. (2004). The functions of E(Z)/EZH2-mediated methylation of lysine 27 in histone H3. *Current Opinion in Genetics & Development*, Vol.14, No.2, (April 2004), pp. 155-164, ISSN 0959-437X

Carles, C.; Bies-Etheve, N.; Aspart, L.; Léon-Kloosterziel, K.M.; Koornneef, M.; Echeverria, M. & Delseny, M. (2002). Regulation of *Arabidopsis thaliana* Em genes: Role of ABI5. *Plant Journal*, Vol.30, No.3, (May 2002), pp. 373-383, ISSN 0960-7412

Casson, S.A. & Lindsey, K. (2006). The turnip mutant of *Arabidopsis* reveals that *LEAFY COTYLEDON1* expression mediates the effects of auxin and sugars to promote embryonic cell identity. *Plant Physiology*, Vol.142, No.2, (October 2006), pp. 526-541, ISSN 0032-0889

Cernac, A. & Benning, C. (2004). WRINKLED1 encodes an AP2/EREB domain protein involved in the control of storage compound biosynthesis in *Arabidopsis*. *Plant Journal*, Vol.40, No.4, (November 2004), pp. 575-585, ISSN 0960-7412

Chaudhuri, S. & Messing, J. (1994). Allele-specific parental imprinting of dzr1, a posttranscriptional regulator of zein accumulation. *Proceedings of the National Academy of Sciences USA*, Vol.91, No.11, (May 1994), pp. 4867-4871, ISSN 0027-8424

Chaudhury, A.M.; Ming, L.; Miller, C.; Craig, S.; Dennis, E.S. & Peacock, W.J. (1997). Fertilization-independent seed development in *Arabidopsis thaliana*. *Proceedings of the National Academy of Sciences USA*, Vol.94, No.8, (April 1997), pp. 4223-4228, ISSN 0027-8424

Cheng, W.H.; Endo, A.; Zhou, L.; Penney, J.; Chen, H.C.; Arroyo, A.; Leon, P.; Nambara, E.; Asami, T.; Seo, M.; Koshiba, T. & Sheen, J. (2002). A unique short-chain dehydrogenase/reductase in *Arabidopsis* glucose signaling and abscisic acid biosynthesis and functions. *Plant Cell*, Vol.14, No.11, (November 2002), pp. 2723-2743, ISSN 1040-4651

Choi, Y.; Gehring, M.; Johnson, L.; Hannon, M.; Harada, J.J.; Goldberg, R.B.; Jacobsen, S.E. & Fischer, R.L. (2002). DEMETER, a DNA glycosylase domain protein, is required for endosperm gene imprinting and seed viability in *Arabidopsis*. *Cell*, Vol.110, No.1, (July 2002), pp. 33-42, ISSN 0092-8674

Chono, M.; Honda, I.; Shinoda, S.; Kushiro, T.; Kamiya, Y.; Nambara, E.; Kawakami, N.; Kaneko, S. & Watanabe, Y. (2006). Field studies on the regulation of abscisic acid content and germinability during grain development of barley: molecular and chemical analysis of pre-harvest sprouting. *Journal of Experimental Botany*, Vol.57, No.10, (June 2006), pp. 2421-2434, ISSN 0022-0957

Crowe, A.J.; Abenes, M.; Plant, A. & Moloney, M.M. (2000). The seed-specific transactivator, ABI3, induces oleosin gene expression. *Plant Science*, Vol.151, No.2, (February 2000), pp. 171-181, ISSN 0168-9452

Curaba, J.; Moritz, T.; Blervaque, R.; Parcy, F.; Raz, V.; Herzog, M. & Vachon, G. (2004). *AtGA3ox2*, a key gene responsible for bioactive gibberellin biosynthesis, is regulated during embryogenesis by LEAFY COTYLEDON2 and FUSCA3 in *Arabidopsis*. *Plant Physiology*, Vol.136, No.3, (November 2004), pp. 3660-3669, ISSN 0032-0889

Cutler, S.R.; Rodriguez, P.L.; Finkelstein, R.R. & Abrams, S.R. (2010). Abscisic acid: emergence of a core signaling network. *Annual Review of Plant Biology*, Vol.61, pp. 651-679, ISSN 1543-5008

Danilevskaya, O.N.; Hermon, P.; Hantke, S.; Muszynski, M.G.; Kollipara, K. & Ananiev, E.V. (2003). Duplicated fie genes in maize: expression pattern and imprinting suggest distinct functions. *Plant Cell*, Vol.15, No.2, (February 2003), pp. 425-438, ISSN 1040-4651

Debeaujon, I. & Koornneef, M. (2000). Gibberellin requirement for *Arabidopsis* seed germination is determined both by testa characteristics and embryonic abscisic acid. *Plant Physiology*, Vol.122, No.2, (February 2000), pp. 415-424, ISSN 0032-0889

Dekkers, B.J.; Schuurmans, J.A. & Smeekens, S.C. (2008). Interaction between sugar and abscisic acid signalling during early seedling development in *Arabidopsis*. *Plant Molecular Biology*, Vol.67, No.1-2, (May 2008), pp. 151-167, ISSN 0167-4412

Diaz, I.; Martinez, M.; Isabel-LaMoneda, I.; Rubio-Somoza, I. & Carbonero, P. (2005). The DOF protein, SAD, interacts with GAMYB in plant nuclei and activates transcription of endosperm-specific genes during barley seed development. *Plant Journal*, Vol.42, No.5, (June 2005), pp. 652-662, ISSN 0960-7412

Díaz, I.; Vicente-Carbajosa, J.; Abraham, Z.; Martínez, M.; Isabel-LaMoneda, I. & Carbonero, P. (2002). The GAMYB protein from barley interacts with the DOF transcription factor BPBF and activates endosperm-specific genes during seed development. *Plant Journal*, Vol.29, No.4, (February 2002), pp. 453-464, ISSN 0960-7412

Dubreucq, B.; Grappin, P. & Caboche, M. (1996). A new method for the identification and isolation of genes essential for *Arabidopsis thaliana* seed germination. *Molecular Genetics and Genomics*, Vol.252, No.1-2, (August 1996), pp. 42-50, ISSN 1617-4623

Eastmond, P.J. & Rawsthorne, S. (2000). Coordinate changes in carbon partitioning and plastidial metabolism during the development of oilseed rape embryos. *Plant Physiology*, Vol.122, No.3, (March 2000), pp. 767-774, ISSN 0032-0889

Fait, A.; Angelovici, R.; Less, H.; Ohad, I.; Urbanczyk-Wochniak, E.; Fernie, A.R. & Galili, G. (2006). *Arabidopsis* seed development and germination is associated with temporally distinct metabolic switches. *Plant Physiology*, Vol.142, No.3, (November 2006), pp. 839-854, ISSN 0032-0889

Finch-Savage, W.E. & Leubner-Metzger, G. (2006). Seed dormancy and the control of germination. *New Phytologist*, Vol.171, No.3, pp. 501-523, ISSN 0028-646X

Finkelstein, R.R. (1994). Mutations at two new *Arabidopsis* ABA response loci are similar to the *abi3* mutations. *Plant Journal*, Vol.5, No.6, pp. 765-771, ISSN 0960-7412

Finkelstein, R.R. (2006). Studies of abscisic acid perception finally flower. *Plant Cell*, Vol.18, No.4, (April 2006), pp. 786-791, ISSN 1040-4651

Finkelstein, R.R.; Gampala, S.S.L. & Rock, C.D. (2002). Abscisic acid signaling in seeds and seedlings. *Plant Cell*, Vol.14 (Suppl), pp. S15-45, ISSN 1040-4651

Finnegan, E.J. & Dennis, E.S. (1993). Isolation and identification by sequence homology of a putative cytosine methyltransferase from *Arabidopsis thaliana. Nucleic Acids Research*, Vol.21, No.10, (May 1993), pp. 2383-2388, ISSN 0305-1048

Finnegan, E.J.; Peacock, W.J. & Dennis, E. (1996). Reduced DNA methylation in *Arabidopsis thaliana* results in abnormal plant development. *Proceedings of the National Academy of Sciences USA*, Vol.93, No.16, (August 1996), pp. 8449-8454, ISSN 0027-8424

FitzGerald, J.; Luo, M.; Chaudhury, A. & Berger, F. (2008). DNA methylation causes predominant maternal controls of plant embryo growth. *PLoS ONE*, Vol.3, No.e2298, ISSN 1932-6203

Forde, B.G.; Heyworth, A.; Pywell, J. & Kreis, M. (1985). Nucleotide sequence of a B1 hordein gene and the identification of possible upstream regulatory elements in endosperm storage protein genes from barley, wheat and maize. *Nucleic Acids Research*, Vol.13, No.20, (October 1985), pp. 7327-7339, ISSN 0305-1048

Frey, A.; Godin, B.; Bonnet, M.; Sotta, B. & Marion-Poll, A. (2004). Maternal synthesis of abscisic acid controls seed development and yield in *N. plumbaginifolia. Planta*, Vol.218, No.6, (April 2004), pp. 958-964, ISSN 0032-0935

Gaj, M.D.; Zhang, S.; Harada, J.J. & Lemaux, P.G. (2005). Leafy cotyledon genes are essential for induction of somatic embryogenesis of *Arabidopsis. Planta*, Vol.222, No.6, (December 2005), pp. 977-988, ISSN 0032-0935

Gallardo, K.; Thompson, R. & Burstin, J. (2008). Reserve accumulation in legume seeds. *Comptes Rendus Biologies*, Vol.331, No.10, (October 2008), pp. 755-762, ISSN 1631-0691

Gao, M.-J.; Lydiate, D.J.; Li, X.; Lui, H.; Gjetvaj, B.; Hegedus, D.D. and Rozwadowski, K. (2009). Repression of seed maturation genes by a trihelix transcriptional repressor in *Arabidopsis* seedlings. *Plant Cell*, Vol.21, No.1, (January 2009), pp. 54-71, ISSN 1040-4651

Garcia, D.; Gerald, J.N.F. & Berger, F. (2005). Maternal control of integument cell elongation and zygotic control of endosperm growth are coordinated to determine seed size in *Arabidopsis. Plan Cell*, Vol.17, No.1, (January 2005), pp. 52-60, ISSN 1040-4651

Gazzarrini, S.; Tsuchiya, Y.; Lumba, S.; Okamoto, M. & McCourt, P. (2004). The transcription factor FUSCA3 controls developmental timing in *Arabidopsis* through the hormones gibberellin and abscisic acid. *Developmental Cell*, Vol.7, No.3, (September 2004), pp. 373-385, ISSN 1534-5807

Gehring, M.; Choi, Y. & Fischer, R.L. (2004). Imprinting and seed development. *Plant Cell*, Vol.16 (suppl), (March 2004), pp. S203-S213, ISSN 1040-4651

Gehring, M.; Bubb, K.L. & Henikoff, S. (2009). Extensive demethylation of repetitive elements during seed development underlies gene imprinting. *Science*, Vol.324, No.5933, (June 2009), pp. 1447-1451, ISSN 0036-8075

Gehring, M.; Missirian, V. & Henikoff, S. (2011). Genomic analysis of parent-of-origin allelic expression in *Arabidopsis thaliana* seeds. *PLoS One*, Vol.6, (August 2011), No.e23687, ISSN 1932-6203

Gehring, M.; Huh, J.H.; Hsieh, T.F.; Penterman, J.; Choi, Y.; Harada, J.J.; Goldberg, R.B. & Fischer, R.L. (2006). Demeter DNA glycosylase establishes MEDEA polycomb gene self-imprinting by allele-specific demethylation. *Cell*, Vol.124, No.3, (February 2006), pp. 495-506, ISSN 0092-8674

Ghelis, T.; Bolbach, G.; Clodic, G.; Habricot, Y.; Miginiac, E.; Sotta, B. & Jeannette, E. (2008). Protein tyrosine kinases and protein tyrosine phosphatases are involved in abscisic acid-dependent processes in *Arabidopsis* seeds and suspension cells. *Plant Physiology*, Vol.148, No.3, (November 2008), pp. 1668-1680, ISSN 0032-0889

Gibson, S.I. (2000). Plant sugar-response pathways. Part of a complex regulatory web. *Plant Physiology*, Vol.124, No.4, (December 2000), pp. 1532-1539, ISSN 0032-0889

Gibson, S.I. (2004). Sugar and phytohormone response pathway: navigating a signalling network. *Journal of Experimental Botany*, Vol.55, No.395, (January 2004), pp. 253-264, ISSN 0022-0957

Gibson, S.I. (2005). Control of plant development and gene expression by sugar signalling. *Current Opinion in Plant Biology*, Vol.8, No.1, (February 2005), pp. 93-102, ISSN 1369-5266

Giraudat, J.; Parcy, F. ; Bertauche, N. ; Gosti, F. ; Leung, J. ; Morris, P.C. ; Bouvier-Durand, M. & Vartanian, N. (1994). Current advances in abscisic acid action and signalling. *Plant Molecular Biology*, Vol.26, No.5, (December 1994), pp. 1557-1577, ISSN 0167-4412

Goldberg, R.B. & Fischer, R.L. (1999). Mutations in *FIE*, a WD Polycomb group gene, allow endosperm development without fertilization. *Plant Cell*, Vol.11, No.3, (March 1999), pp. 407-415, ISSN 1040-4651

Goldberg, R.B.; Barker, S.J. & Perez-Grau, L. (1989). Regulation of gene expression during plant embryogenesis. *Cell*, Vol.56, No.2, (January 1989), pp. 149-160, ISSN 0092-8674

Golombek, S.; Rolletschek, H.; Wobus, U. & Weber, H. (2001). Control of storage protein accumulation during legume seed development. *Journal of Plant Physiology*, Vol.158, No.4, pp. 457-464, ISSN 0032-0889

Gómez, L.D.; Baud, S.; Gilday, A.; Li, Y. & Graham, I.A. (2006). Delayed embryo development in the *ARABIDOPSIS TREHALOSE-6-PHOSPHATE SYNTHASE 1* mutant is associated with altered cell wall structure, decreased cell division and starch accumulation. *Plant Journal*, Vol.46, No.1, (April 2006), pp. 69-84, ISSN 0960-7412

Grimanelli, D. ; Perotti, E. ; Ramirez, J. & Leblanc, O. (2005). Timing of the maternal-to-zygotic transition during early seed development in maize. *Plant Cell*, Vol.17, No.4, (April 2005), pp. 1061-1072, ISSN 1040-4651

Grossniklaus, U. & Schneitz, K. (1998). The molecular and genetic basis of ovule and megagametophyte development. *Seminars in Cell & Developmental Biology*, Vol.9, No.2, (April 1998), pp. 227-238, ISSN 1084-9521

Guo, M.; Rupe, M.A.; Danilevskaya, O.N.; Yang, X. & Hu, Z. (2003). Genome-wide mRNA profiling reveals heterochronic allelic variation and a new imprinted gene in hybrid maize endosperm. *Plant Journal*, Vol.36, No.1, (October 2003), pp. 30-44, ISSN 0960-7412

Gutiérrez-Marcos, J.F.; Costa, L.M.; Dal Prà, M.; Scholten, S.; Kranz, E.; Perez, P. & Dickinson, H.G. (2006). Epigenetic asymmetry of imprinted genes in plant gametes. *Nature Genetics*, Vol.38, No.8, (August 2006), pp. 876-878, ISSN 1061-4036

Gutiérrez-Marcos, J.F.; Costa, L.M.; Biderre-Petit, C.; Khbaya, B.; O'Sullivan, D.M.; Wormald, M.; Perez, P. & Dickinson, H.G. (2004). *Maternally expressed gene1* Is a novel maize endosperm transfer cell-specific gene with a maternal parent-of-origin pattern of expression. *Plant Cell*, Vol.16, No.5, (May 2004), pp. 1288-1301, ISSN 1040-4651

Gutierrez, L.; Van Wuytswinkel, O.; Castelain, M. & Bellini, C. (2007). Combined networks regulating seed maturation. *Trends in Plant Science*, Vol.12, No.7, (July 2007), pp. 294-300, ISSN 1360-1385

Haig, D. & Wilczek, A. (2006). Sexual conflict and the alternation of haploid and diploid generations. *Philosophical Transactions of the Royal Society B: Biological Sciences*, Vol.361, No.1466, (February 2006), pp. 335-343, ISSN 0962-8436

Harada, J.J. (1999). Signaling in plant embryogenesis. *Current Opinion in Plant Biology*, Vol.2, No.1, (February 1999), pp. 23-27, ISSN 1369-5266

Hartings, H.; Maddaloni, M.; Lazzaroni, N.; Di Fonzo, N.; Motto, M.; Salamini, F. & Thompson, R. (1989). The *O2* gene which regulates zein deposition in maize endosperm encodes a protein with structural homologies to transcriptional activators. *EMBO Journal*, Vol.8, No.10, (October 1989), pp. 2795-2801, ISSN 0261-4189

Haughn, G. & Chaudhury, A. (2005). Genetic analysis of seed coat development in *Arabidopsis*. *Trends in Plant Science*, Vol.10, No.10, (October 2005), pp. 472-477, ISSN 1360-1385

Haun, W.J.; Danilevskaya, O.N.; Meeley, R.B. & Springer, N.M. (2009). Disruption of imprinting by mutator transposon insertions in the 5' proximal regions of the *Zea mays Mez1* locus. *Genetics*, Vol.181, No.4, (April 2009), pp. 1229-1237, ISSN 0016-6731

Henderson, J.T.; Li, H.C.; Rider, S.D.; Mordhorst, A.P.; Romero-Severson, J.; Cheng, J.C.; Robey, J.; Sung, Z.R.; de Vries, S.C. & Ogas, J. (2004). *PICKLE* acts throughout the plant to repress expression of embryonic traits and may play a role in gibberellin-dependent responses. *Plant Physiology*, Vol.134, No.3, (March 2004), pp. 995-1005, ISSN 0032-0889

Hermon, P.; Srilunchang, K.O.; Zou, J.; Dresselhaus, T. & Danilevskaya, O.N. (2007). Activation of the imprinted Polycomb Group Fie1 gene in maize endosperm requires demethylation of the maternal allele. *Plant Molecular Biology*, Vol.64, No.4, (July 2007), pp. pp. 387-395, ISSN 0167-4412

Hernandez-Sebastia, C.; Marsolais, F., Saravitz, C.; Israel, D.; Dewey, R.E. & Huber, S.C. (2005). Free amino acid profiles suggest a possible role for asparagines in the control of storage-product accumulation in developing seeds of low- and high-protein soybean lines. *Journal of Experimental Botany*, Vol.56, No.417, (May 2005), pp. 1951-1963, ISSN 0022-0957

Hills, M.J. (2004). Control of storage-product synthesis in seeds. *Current Opinion in Plant Biology*, Vol.7, No.3, (June 2004), pp. 302-308, ISSN 1369-5266

Himmelbach, A.; Yang, Y. & Grill, E. (2003). Relay and control of abscisic acid signaling. *Current Opinion in Plant Biology*, Vol.6, No.5, (October 2003), pp. 470-479, ISSN 1369-5266

Hirayama, T. & Shinozaki, K. (2007). Perception and transduction of abscisic acid signals: keys to the function of the versatile plant hormone ABA. *Trends in Plant Science*, Vol.12, No.8, (July 2007), pp. 343-351, ISSN 1360-1385

Holdsworth, M.J.; Bentsink, L. & Soppe, W.J. (2008). Molecular networks regulating Arabidopsis seed maturation, after-ripening, dormancy and germination. *New Phytologist*, Vol.179, No.1, (April 2008), pp. 33-54, ISSN 0028-646X

Hsieh, T.F.; Ibarra, C.A.; Silva, P.; Zemach, A.; Eshed-Williams, L.; Fischer, R.L. & Zilberman, D. (2009). Genome-wide demethylation of *Arabidopsis* endosperm. *Science*, Vol.324, No.5933, (June 2009), pp. 1451-1454, ISSN 0036-8075

Hsieh, T.F.; Shin, J.; Uzawa, R.; Silva, P.; Cohen, S.; Bauer, M.J.; Hashimoto, M.; Kirkbride, R.C.; Harada, J.J.; Zilberman, D. & Fischer, R.L. (2011). Regulation of imprinted gene expression in *Arabidopsis* endosperm. *Proceedings of the National Academy of Sciences USA*, Vol.08, No.5, (February 2011), pp. 1755-1762, ISSN 0027-8424

Huh, J.H.; Bauer, M.J.; Hsieh, T.F. & Fischer, R. (2007). Endosperm gene imprinting and seed development. *Current Opinion in Genetics & Development*, Vol.17, No.6, (December 2007), pp. 480-485, ISSN 0959-437X

Huijser, C.; Kortstee, A.; Pego, J.; Weisbeek, P.; Wisman, E. & Smeekens, S. (2000). The *Arabidopsis SUCROSE UNCOUPLED-6* gene is identical to *ABSCISIC ACID INSENSITIVE-4*: involvement of abscisic acid in sugar responses. *Plant Journal*, 23, No.5, (September 2000), pp. 577-585, ISSN 0960-7412

Hunter, B.G.; Beatty, M.K.; Singletary, G.W.; Hamaker, B.R.; Dilkes, B.P.; Larkins, B.A. & Jung, R. (2002). Maize opaque endosperm mutations create extensive changes in patterns of gene expression. *Plant Cell*, 14, No.10, (October 2002), pp. 2591-2612, ISSN 1040-4651

Ingouff, M.; Hamamura, Y.; Gourgues, M.; Higashiyama, T. & Berger, F. (2007). Distinct dynamics of HISTONE3 variants between the two fertilization products in plants. *Current Biology*, Vol.17, No.12, (June 2007), pp. 1032-1037, ISSN 0960-9822

Iwakawa, H.; Shinmyo, A. & Sekine, M. (2006). *Arabidopsis* CDKA;1, a cdc2 homologue, controls proliferation of generative cells in male gametogenesis. *Plant Journal*, Vol.45, No.5, (March 2006), pp. 819-831, ISSN 0960-7412

Jullien, P.E.; Kinoshita, T.; Ohad, N. & Berger, F. (2006). Maintenance of DNA methylation during the *Arabidopsis* life cycle is essential for parental imprinting. *Plant Cell*, 18, No.6, (June 2006), pp. 1360-1372, ISSN 1040-4651

Jullien, P.E.; Mosquna, A.; Ingouff, M.; Sakata, T.; Ohad, N. & Berger, F. (2008). Retinoblastoma and its binding partner MSI1 control imprinting in *Arabidopsis*. *PLoS Biology*, Vol.6, (August 2008), No.e194, ISSN 1544-9173

Kadosh, D. & Struhl, K. (1998). Targeted recruitment of the Sin3-Rpd3 histone deacetylase complex generates a highly localized domain of repressed chromatin in vivo. *Molecular and Cellular Biology*, Vol.18, No.9, (September 1998), pp. 5121-5127, ISSN 0270-7306

Kagaya, Y.; Toyoshima, R.; Okuda, R.; Usui, H.; Yamamoto, A. & Hattori, T. (2005a). LEAFY COTYLEDON1 controls seed storage protein genes through its regulation of

FUSCA3 and *ABSCISIC ACID INSENSITIVE3*. *Plant Cell Physiology*, Vol.46, No.3, (March 2005), pp. 399-406, ISSN 0032-0781

Kagaya, Y.; Okuda, R.; Ban, A.; Toyoshima, R.; Tsutsumida, K.; Usui, H.; Yamamoto, A. & Hattori, T. (2005b). Indirect ABA-dependent regulation of seed storage protein genes by FUSCA3 transcription factor in *Arabidopsis*. *Plant Cell Physiology*, Vol.46, No.2, (February 2005), pp. 300-311, ISSN 0032-0781

Kankel, M.W.; Ramsey, D.E.; Stokes, T.L.; Flowers, S.K.; Haag, J.R.; Jeddeloh, J.A.; Riddle, N.C.; Verbsky, M.L. & Richards, E.J. (2003). *Arabidopsis* MET1 cytosine methyltransferase mutants. *Genetics*, Vol.163, No.3, (March 2003), pp. 1109-1122, ISSN 0016-6731

Karssen, C.M.; Brinkhorst Van der Swan, D.L.C.; Breekland, A.E. & Koornneef, M. (1983). Induction of dormancy during seed development by endogenous Abscisic-Acid - studies on Abscisic-Acid deficient genotypes of *Arabidopsis thaliana* (L.) Heynh. *Planta*, Vol.157, No.2, pp. 158-165, ISSN 0032-0935

Kermicle, J.L. (1970). Dependence of the R-mottled aleurone phenotype in maize on mode of sexual transmission. *Genetics*, Vol.66, No.1, (September 1970), pp. 69-85, ISSN 0016-6731

Kinoshita, T.; Miura, A.; Choi, Y.; Kinoshita, Y.; Cao, X.F.; Jacobsen, S.E.; Fischer, R.L. & Kakutani, T. (2004). One-way control of FWA imprinting in *Arabidopsis* endosperm by DNA methylation. *Science*, Vol.303, No.5657, (January 2004), pp. 521-523, ISSN 0036-8075

Kiyosue, T.; Ohad, N.; Yadegari, R.; Hannon, M.; Dinneny, J.; Wells, D.; Katz, A.; Margossian, L.; Harada, J.J.; Goldberg, R.B. & Fischer, R.L. (1999). Control of fertilization-independent endosperm development by the *MEDEA* polycomb gene in *Arabidopsis*. *Proceedings of the National Academy of Sciences USA*, 96, No.7, (March 1999), pp. 4186-4191, ISSN 0027-8424

Köhler, C. & Grossniklaus, U. (2002). Epigenetic inheritance of expression states in plant development: the role of Polycomb group proteins. *Current Opinion in Cell Biology*, Vol.14, No.6, (December 2002), pp. 773-779, ISSN 0955-0674

Köhler, C. & Makarevich, G. (2006). Epigenetic mechanisms governing seed development in plants. *EMBO Reports*, Vol.7, No.12, (December 2006), pp. 1223-1227, ISSN 1469-221X

Köhler, C. & Hennig, L. (2010). Regulation of cell identity by plant Polycomb and trithorax group proteins. *Current Opinion in Genetics & Development*, Vol.20, No.5, (October 2010), pp. 541-547, ISSN 0959-437X

Köhler, C.; Page, D.R.; Gagliardini, V. & Grossniklaus, U. (2005). The *Arabidopsis thaliana* MEDEA Polycomb group protein controls expression of PHERES1 by parental imprinting. *Nature Genetics*, 37, No.1, (January 2005), pp. 28-30, ISSN 1061-4036

Köhler, C.; Hennig, L.; Bouveret, R.; Gheyselinck, J.; Grossniklaus, U. & Gruissem, W. (2003). *Arabidopsis* MSI1 is a component of the MEA/FIE Polycomb group complex and required for seed development. *EMBO Journal*, Vol.22, No.18, (September 2003), pp. 4804-4814, ISSN 0261-4189

Koornneef, M.; Bentsink, L. & Hilhorst, H. (2002). Seed dormancy and germination. *Current Opinion in Plant Biology*, Vol.5, No.1, (February 2002), pp. 33-36, ISSN 1369-5266

Kroj, T.; Savino, G.; Valon, C.; Giraudat, J. & Parcy, F. (2003). Regulation of storage protein gene expression in *Arabidopsis. Development*, 130, No.24, (December 2003), pp. 6065-6073, ISSN 0950-1991

Kucera, B.; Cohn, M.A. & Leubner-Metzger, G. (2005). Plant hormone interactions during seed dormancy release and germination. *Seed Science Research*, Vol.15, No.4, pp. 281-307, ISSN 0960-2985

Kuo, M.H. & Allis, C.D. (1998). Roles of histone acetyltransferases and deacetylases in gene regulation. *Bioessays*, 20, No.8, (August 1998), pp. 615-626, ISSN 0265-9247

Kuo, M.H.; vom Baur, E.; Struhl, K. & Allis, C.D. (2000). Gcn4 activator targets Gcn5 histone acetyltransferase to specific promoters independently of transcription. *Molecular Cell*, Vol.6, No.6, (December 2000), pp. 1309-1320, ISSN 1907-2765

Laby, R.J.; Kincaid, M.S.; Kim, D. & Gibson, S.I. (2000). The *Arabidopsis* sugar-insensitive mutants *sis4* and *sis5* are defective in abscisic acid synthesis and response. *Plant Journal*, Vol.23, No.5, (September 2000), pp. 587-596, ISSN 0960-7412

Lara, P.; Onate-Sanchez, L.; Abraham, Z.; Ferrandiz, C.; Diaz, I.; Carbonero, P. & Vicente-Carbajosa, J. (2003). Synergistic activation of seed storage protein gene expression in *Arabidopsis* by ABI3 and two bZIPs related to OPAQUE2. *Journal of Biological Chemistry*, Vol.278, No.23, (June 2003), pp. 21003-21011, ISSN 0021-9258

Lauria, M.; Rupe, M.; Guo, M.; Kranz, E.; Pirona, R.; Viotti, A. & Lund, G. (2004). Extensive maternal DNA hypomethylation in the endosperm of *Zea mays*. *Plant Cell*, Vol.16, No.2, (February 2004), pp. 510-522, ISSN 1040-4651

Laux, T. & Jürgens, G. (1997). Embryogenesis: a new start in life. *Plant Cell*, Vol.9, No.7, (July 1997), pp.989-1000, ISSN 1040-4651

Le, B.H.; Cheng, C.; Bui, A.Q.; Wagmaister, J.A.; Henry, K.F.; Pelletier, J.; Kwong, L.W.; Belmonte, M.; Kirkbride, R.; Horvath, S.; Drews, G.N.; Fischer, R.L.; Okamuro, J.K.; Harada, J.J. & Goldberg, R. (2010). Global analysis of gene activity during *Arabidopsis* seed development and identification of seed-specific transcription factors. *Proceedings of the National Academy of Sciences USA*, Vol.107, No.18, (May 2010), pp. 8063-8070, ISSN 0027-8424

Leon, P. & Sheen, J. (2003). Sugar and hormone connections. *Trends in Plant Science*, Vol.8, No.3, (March 2003), pp. 110-116, ISSN 1360-1385

Lepiniec, L. ; Debeaujon, I. ; Routaboul, J.; Baudry, A. ; Pourcel, L. ; Nesi, N. & Caboche, M. (2006). Genetics and biochemistry of seed flavonoids. *Annual Review of Plant Biology*, Vol.57, pp. 405-430, ISSN 1543-5008

Li, G. & Hall, T.C. (1999). Footprinting in vivo reveals changing profiles of multiple factor interactions with the *ß-phaseolin* promoter during embryogenesis. *Plant Journal*, Vol.18, No.6, (June 1999), pp. 633-641, ISSN 0960-7412

Li, H.C.; Chuang, K.; Henderson, J.T.; Rider, S.D.J.; Bai, Y.; Zhang, H.; Fountain, M.; Gerber, J. & Ogas, J. (2005). *PICKLE* acts during germination to repress expression of embryonic traits. *Plant Journal*, Vol.44, No.6, (December 2005), pp. 1010-1022, ISSN 0960-7412

Li, Y.; Lee, K.K.; Smith, C.; Walsh, S.; Hadingham, S.A.; Sorefan, K.; Cawley, G. & Bevan, M.W. (2006). Establishing glucose- and ABA- regulated transcription networks in *Arabidopsis* by microarray analysis and promoter classification using a relevance vector machine. *Genome Research*, Vol.16, No.3, (March 2006), pp. 414-427, ISSN 1088-9051

Liu, P.P.; Montgomery, T.A.; Fahlgren, N.; Kasschau, K.D.; Nonogaki, H. & Carrington, J.C. (2007). Repression of AUXIN RESPONSE FACTOR10 by microRNA160 is critical for seed germination and post-germination stages. *Plant Journal*, Vol.52, No.1, (Octomber 2007), pp. 133-146, ISSN 0960-7412

Lohe, A.R. & Chaudhury, A. (2002). Genetic and epigenetic processes in seed development. *Current Opinion in Plant Biology*, Vol.5, No.1, (February 2002), pp. 19-25, ISSN 1369-5266

Lotan, T.; Ohto, M.; Yee, K.M.; West, M.A.; Lo, R.; Kwong, R.W.; Yamagishi, K.; Fischer, R.L.; Goldberg, R.B. & Harada, J.J. (1998). *Arabidopsis* LEAFY COTYLEDON1 is sufficient to induce embryo development in vegetative cells. *Cell*, Vol.93, No.7, (June 1998), pp. 1195-1205, ISSN 0092-8674

Lund, G.; Ciceri, P. & Viotti, A. (1995). Maternal-specific demethylation and expression of specific alleles of zein genes in the endosperm of *Zea mays* L. *Plant Journal*, Vol.8, No.4, (October 1995), pp. 571-581, ISSN 0960-7412

Luo, M.; Bilodeau, P.; Dennis, E.; Peacock, W.J. & Chaudhury, A.M. (2000). Expression and parent-of-origin effects for FIS2, MEA and FIE in the endosperm and embryo of developing *Arabidopsis* seeds. *Proceedings of the National Academy of Sciences USA*, Vol.97, No.19, (September 2000), pp. 10637-10642, ISSN 0027-8424

Luo, M.; Dennis, E.S.; Berger, F.; Peacock, W.J. & Chaudhury, A. (2005). *MINISEED3* (*MINI3*), a WRKY family gene, and *HAIKU2* (*IKU2*), a leucine-rich repeat (LRR) kinase gene, are regulators of seed size in *Arabidopsis*. *Proceedings of the National Academy of Sciences USA*, Vol.102, No.48, (November 2005), pp. 17531-17536, ISSN 0027-8424

Luo, M.; Bilodeau, P.; Koltunow, A.; Dennis, E.S.; Peacock, W.J. & Chaudhury, A.M. (1999). Genes controlling fertilization-independent seed development in *Arabidopsis thaliana*. *Proceedings of the National Academy of Sciences USA*, Vol.96, No.1, (January 1999), pp. 296-301, ISSN 0027-8424

Ma, Y.; Szostkiewicz, I.; Korte, A.; Moes, D.; Yang, Y.; Christmann, A. and Grill, E. (2009). Regulators of PP2C phosphatase activity function as abscisic acid sensors. *Science*, Vol.324, No.5930, (May 2009), pp. 1064-1068, ISSN 0036-8075

Maeo, K.; Tokuda, T.; Ayame, A.; Mitsui, N.; Kawai, T.; Tsukagoshi, H.; Ishiguro, S. & Nakamura, K. (2009). An AP2-type transcription factor, WRINKLED1, of Arabidopsis thaliana binds to the AW-box sequence conserved among proximal upstream regions of genes involved in fatty acid synthesis. *Plant Journal*, Vol.60, No.3, (July 2009), pp. 476-487, ISSN 0960-7412

Makarevich, G.; Leroy, O.; Akinci, U.; Schubert, D.; Clarenz, O.; Goodrich, J.; Grossniklaus, U. & Köhler, C. (2006). Different Polycomb group complexes regulate common target genes in *Arabidopsis*. *EMBO Reports*, Vol.7, No.9, (September 2006), pp. 947-952, ISSN 1469-221X

Manicacci, D.; Camus-Kulandaivelu, L.; Fourmann, M.; Arar, C.; Barrault, S.; Rousselet, A.; Feminias, N.; Consoli, L.; Francès, L.; Méchin, V.; Murigneux, A.; Prioul, J.L.; Charcosset, A. & Damerval, C. (2009). Epistatic interactions between Opaque2 transcriptional activator and its target gene CyPPDK1 control kernel trait variation in maize. *Plant Physiology*, Vol.150, No.1, (May 2009), pp. 506-520, ISSN 0032-0889

Marzábal, P.; Gas, E.; Fontanet, P.; Vicente-Carbajosa, J.; Torrent, M. & Ludevid, M.D. (2008). The maize Dof protein PBF activates transcription of gamma-zein during maize seed development. *Plant Molecular Biology*, Vol.67, No.5, (July 2008), pp. 441-454, ISSN 0167-4412

Mazur, B.; Krebbers, E. & Tingey, S. (1999). Gene discovery and product development for grain quality traits. *Science*, Vol.285, No.5426, (July 1999), pp. 372-375, ISSN 0036-8075

Mena, M.; Vicente-Carbajosa, J.; Schmidt, R.J. & Carbonero, P. (1998). An endosperm-specific DOF protein from barley, highly conserved in wheat, binds to and activates transcription from the prolamine-box of a native B-hordein promoter in barley endosperm. *Plant Journal*, Vol.16, No.1, (Octomber 1998), pp. 53-62, ISSN 0960-7412

Millar, A.A.; Jacobsen, J.V.; Ross, J.J.; Helliwell, C.A.; Poole, A.T.; Scofield, G.; Reid, J.B. & Gubler, F. (2006). Seed dormancy and ABA metabolism in Arabidopsis and barley: the role of ABA 8'-hydroxylase. *Plant Journal*, Vol.45, No.6, (March 2006), pp. 942-954, ISSN 0960-7412

Miranda, M.; Borisjuk, L.; Tewes, A.; Heim, U.; Sauer, N.; Wobus, U. & Weber, H. (2001). Amino acid permeases in developing seeds of *Vicia faba* L.: expression precedes storage protein synthesis and is regulated by amino acid supply. *Plant Journal*, Vol.28, No.1, (October 2001), pp. 61-72, ISSN 0960-7412

Mönke, G.; Altschmied, L.; Tewes, A.; Reidt, W.; Mock, H.P.; Bäumlein, H. & Conrad, U. (2004). Seed-specific transcription factors ABI3 and FUS3: molecular interaction with DNA. *Planta*, Vol.219, No.1, (May 2004), pp. 158-166, ISSN 0032-0935

Morales-Ruiz, T.; Ortega-Galisteo, A.P.; Ponferrada-Marín, M.I.; Martínez-Macías, M.I.; Ariza, R.R. & Roldán-Arjona, T. (2006). DEMETER and REPRESSOR OF SILENCING 1 encode 5-methylcytosine DNA glycosylases. *Proceedings of the National Academy of Sciences USA*, Vol.103, No.18, (May 2006), pp. 6853-6858, ISSN 0027-8424

Mordhorst, A.P.; Voerman, K.J.; Hartog, M.V.; Meijer, E.A.; van Went, J.; Koornneef, M. & de Vries, S.C. (1998). Somatic embryogenesis in *Arabidopsis thaliana* is facilitated by mutations in genes repressing meristematic cell divisions. *Genetics*, Vol.149, No.2, (June 1998), pp. 549-563, ISSN 0016-6731

Morello, L.; Frattini, M.; Gianì, S.; Christou, P. & Breviario, D. (2000). Overexpression of the calcium-dependent protein kinase *OsCDPK2* in transgenic rice is repressed by light in leaves and disrupts seed development. *Transgenic Research*, Vol.9, No.6, (December 2000), pp. 453-462, ISSN 0962-8819

Moreno-Risueno, M.A.; González, N.; Díaz, I.; Parcy, F.; Carbonero, P. & Vicente-Carbajosa, J. (2008). FUSCA3 from barley unveils a common transcriptional regulation of seed-specific genes between cereals and *Arabidopsis*. *Plant Journal*, Vol.53, No.6, (March 2008), pp. 882-894, ISSN 0960-7412

Mosher, R.A.; Melnyk, C.W.; Kelly, K.A.; Dunn, R.M.; Studholme, D.J. & Baulcombe, D.C. (2009). Uniparental expression of PolIV-dependent siRNAs in developing endosperm of *Arabidopsis*. *Nature*, Vol.460, No.7252, (July 2009), pp. 283-286, ISSN 0028-0836

Mu, J.; Tan, H.; Zheng, Q.; Fu, F.; Liang, Y.; Zhang, J.; Yang, X.; Wang, T.; Chong, K.; Wang, X. & Zuo, J. (2008). LEAFY COTYLEDON1 is a key regulator of fatty acid biosynthesis in *Arabidopsis*. *Plant Physiology*, Vol.148, No.2, (October 2008), pp. 1042-1054, ISSN 0032-0889

Nakamura, S.; Lynch, T.J. & Finkelstein, R.R. (2001). Physical interactions between ABA response loci of *Arabidopsis*. *Plant Journal*, Vol.26, No.6, (June 2001), pp. 627-635, ISSN 0960-7412

Nambara, E. & Marion-Poll, A. (2003). ABA action and interactions in seeds. *Trends in Plant Science*, Vol.8, No.5, (May 2003), pp. 213-217, ISSN 1360-1385

Ng, D.W.; Chandrasekharan, M.B. & Hall, T.C. (2006). Ordered histone modifications are associated with transcriptional poising and activation of the phaseolin promoter. *Plant Cell*, Vol.18, No.1, (January 2006), pp. 119-132, ISSN 1040-4651

North, H.; Baud, S.; Debeaujon, I.; Dubos, C.; Dubreucq, B.; Grappin, P.; Jullien, M.; Lepiniec, L.; Marion-Poll, A.; Miquel, M.; Rajjou, L.; Routaboul, J.M. & Caboche, M. (2010). Arabidopsis seed secrets unravelled after a decade of genetic and omics-driven research. *Plant Journal*, Vol.61, No.6, (March 2010), pp. 971-981, ISSN 0960-7412

Nowack, M.K.; Grini, P.E.; Jakoby, M.J.; Lafos, M.; Koncz, C. & Schnittger, A. (2006). A positive signal from the fertilization of the egg cell sets off endosperm proliferation in angiosperm embryogenesis. *Nature Genetics*, Vol.38, No.1, (January 2006), pp. 63-67, ISSN 1061-4036

Nowack, M.K.; Shirzadi, R.; Dissmeyer, N.; Dolf, A.; Endl, E.; Grini, P.E. & Schnittger, A. (2007). Bypassing genomic imprinting allows seed development. *Nature*, Vol.447, No.7142, (May 2007), pp. 312-315, ISSN 0028-0836

Offler, C.E.; McCurdy; D.W.; Patrick, J.W. & Talbot, M.J. (2003). Transfer cells: cells specialized for a special purpose. *Annual Review of Plant Biology*, Vol.54, pp. 431-454, ISSN 1543-5008

Ogas, J.; Cheng, J.C.; Sung, Z.R. & Somerville, C. (1997). Cellular differentiation regulated by gibberellin in the *Arabidopsis thaliana* pickle mutant. *Science*, Vol.277, No.5322, (July 1997). pp. 91-94, ISSN 0036-8075

Ogas, J.; Kaufmann, S.; Henderson, J. & Somerville, C. (1999). PICKLE is a CHD3 chromatin-remodeling factor that regulates the transition from embryonic to vegetative development in *Arabidopsis*. *Proceedings of the National Academy of Sciences USA*, Vol.96, No.24, (November 1999), pp. 13839-13844, ISSN 0027-8424

Ogawa, M.; Hanada, A.; Yamauchi, Y.; Kuwalhara, A.; Kamiya, Y. & Yamaguchi, S. (2003). Gibberellin biosynthesis and response during *Arabidopsis* seed germination. *Plant Cell*, Vol.15, No.7, (July 2003), pp. 1591-1604, ISSN 1040-4651

Ohad, N.; Margossian, L.; Hsu Yung, C.; Williams, C.; Repetti, P. & Fischer, R.L. (1996). A mutation that allows endosperm development without fertilization. *Proceedings of the National Academy of Sciences USA*, Vol.93, No.11, (May 1996), pp. 5319-5324, ISSN 0027-8424

Ohad, N.; Yadegari, R.; Margossian, L.; Hannon, M.; Michaeli, D.; Harada, J.J.; Goldberg, R.B. & Fischer, R.L. (1999). Mutations in FIE, a WD polycomb group gene, allow endosperm development without fertilization. *Plant Cell*, Vol.11, No.3, (March 1999), pp. 407-416, ISSN 1040-4651

Ohto, M.; Fischer, R.L.; Goldberg, R.B.; Nakamura, K. & Harada, J.J. (2005). Control of seed mass by APETALA2. *Proceedings of the National Academy of Sciences USA*, Vol.102, No.8, (Febryary 2005), pp. 3123-3128, ISSN 0027-8424

Okamoto, M.; Kuwahara, A.; Seo, M.; Kushiro, T.; Asami, T.; Hirai, N.; Kamiya, Y.; Koshiba, T. &Nambara, E. (2006). CYP707A1 and CYP707A2, which encode abscisic acid 8 ¢-hydroxylases, are indispensable for proper control of seed dormancy and germination in *Arabidopsis*. *Plant Physiology*, Vol.141, No.1, (May 2006), pp. 97-107, ISSN 0032-0889

Oñate, L. ; Vicente-Carbajosa, J.; Lara, P. ; Díaz, I. & Carbonero, P. (1999). Barley BLZ2, a seed-specific bZIP protein that interacts with BLZ1 in vivo and activates transcription from the GCN4-like motif of B-hordein promoters in barley endosperm. *Journal of Biological Chemistry*, Vol.274, No.14, (April 1999), pp. 9175-9182, ISSN 0021-9258

Parcy, F.; Valon, C.; Raynal, M.; Gaubier-Comella, P.; Delseny, M. & Giradaut, J. (1994). Regulation of gene expression program during *Arabidopsis* seed development: roles of the ABI3 locus and of endogenous abscisic acid. *Plant Cell*, Vol.6, No.11, pp. 1567-1582, ISSN 1040-4651

Park, S.-Y.; Fung, P.; Nishimura, N.; Jensen, D.R.; Fujii, H.; Zhao, Y.; Lumba, S.; Santiago, J.; Rodrigues, A.; Chow, T.F.; Alfred, S.E.; Bonetta, D.; Finkelstein, R.R.; Provart, N.J.; Desveaux, D.; Rodriguez, P.L.; McCourt, P.; Zhu, J.K.; Schroeder, J.I.; Volkman, B.F. & Cutler, S.R. (2009). Abscisic acid inhibits type 2C protein phosphatases via the PYR/PYL family of START proteins. *Science*, Vol.324, No.5930, (May 2009), pp. 1068-1071, ISSN 0036-8075

Rawsthorne, S. (2002). Carbon flux and fatty acid synthesis in plants. *Progress in Lipid Research*, Vol.41, No.2, (March 2002), pp. 182-196, ISSN 0163-7827

Ray, S.; Agarwal, P.; Arora, R.; Kapoor, S. & Tyagi, A.K. (2007). Expression analysis of calcium-dependent protein kinase gene family during reproductive development and abiotic stress conditions in rice (*Oryza sativa* L. ssp. indica). *Molecular Genetics and Genomics*, Vol.278, No.5, (November 2007), pp. 493-505, ISSN 1617-4623

Razem, F.A.; El-Kereamy, A.; Abrams, S.R. & Hill, R.D. (2006). The RNA-binding protein FCA is an abscisic acid receptor. *Nature*, Vol.439, No.7074, (January 2006), pp. 290-294, ISSN 0028-0836

Reeves, W.M.; Lynch, T.J.; Mobin, R. & Finkelstein, R.R. (2011). Direct targets of the transcription factors ABA-Insensitive(ABI)4 and ABI5 reveal synergistic action by ABI4 and several bZIP ABA response factors. *Plant Molecular Biology*, Vol. 75, No.4-5, (March 2011), pp. 347-363, ISSN 0167-4412

Reidt, W.; Wohlfarth, T.; Ellerstrom, M.; Czihal, A.; Tewes, A.; Ezcurra, I.; Rask, L. & Bäumlein, H. (2000). Gene regulation during late embryogenesis: the RY motif of maturation-specific gene promoters is a direct target of the *FUS3* gene product. *Plant Journal*, Vol.21, No.5, (March 2000), pp. 401-408, ISSN 0960-7412

Rider, S.D.; Henderson, J.T.; Jerome, R.E.; Edenberg, H.J.; Romero-Severson, J. & Ogas, J. (2003). Coordinate repression of regulators of embryonic identity by PICKLE during germination in *Arabidopsis*. *Plant Journal*, Vol.35, No.1, (July 2003), pp. 33-43, ISSN 0960-7412

Rolland, F.; Baena-Gonzalez, E. & Sheen, J. (2006). Sugar sensing and signaling in plants: conserved and novel mechanisms. *Annual Review of Plant Biology*, Vol.57, pp. 675-709, ISSN 1543-5008

Rolletschek, H.; Koch, K.; Wobus, U. & Borisjuk, L. (2005a). Positional cues for the starch/lipid balance in maize kernels and resource partitioning to the embryo. *Plant Journal*, Vol.42, No.1, (April 2005), pp. 69-83, ISSN 0960-7412

Rolletschek, H.; Radchuk, R.; Klukas, C.; Schreiber, F.; Wobus, U. & Borisjuk, L. (2005b). Evidence of a key role for photosynthetic oxygen release in oil storage in developing soybean seeds. *New Phytologist*, Vol.167, No.3, (September 2005), pp. 777-786, ISSN 0028-646X

Rolletschek, H.; Borisjuk, L.; Radchuk, R.; Miranda, M.; Heim, U.; Wobus, U. & Weber, H. (2004). Seed-specific expression of a bacterial phosphoenolpyruvate carboxylase in *Vicia* narbonensis increases protein content and improves carbon economy. *Plant Biotechnology Journal*, Vol.2, No.3, (May 2004), pp. 211-219, ISSN 1467-7644

Rolletschek, H.; Hosein, F.; Miranda, M.; Heim, U.; Götz, K.P.; Schlereth, A.; Borisjuk, L.; Saalbach, I.; Wobus, U. & Weber, H. (2005c). Ectopic expression of an amino acid transporter (VfAAP1) in seeds of Vicia narbonensis and pea increases storage proteins. *Plant Physiology*, Vol.137, No.4, (April 2005), pp. 1236-1249, ISSN 0032-0889

Rook, F.; Hadingham, S.A.; Li, Y. & Bevan, M.W. (2006). Sugar and ABA response pathways and the control of gene expression. *Plant, Cell & Environment*, Vol.29, No.3, (March 2006), pp. 426-434, ISSN 0140-7791

Rook, F.; Corke, F.; Card, R.; Munz, G.; Smith, C. & Bevan, M.W. (2001). Impaired sucrose-induction mutants reveal the modulation of sugar-induced starch biosynthetic gene expression by abscisic acid signalling. *Plant Journal*, Vol.26, No.4, (May 2001), pp. 421-433, ISSN 0960-7412

Rubio-Somoza, I.; Martinez, M.; Diaz, I. & Carbonero, P. (2006a). HvMCB1, a R1MYB transcription factor from barley with antagonistic regulatory functions during seed development and germination. *Plant Journal*, Vol.45, No.1, (January 2006), pp. 17-30, ISSN 0960-7412

Rubio-Somoza, I.; Martinez, M.; Abraham, Z.; Diaz, I. & Carbonero, P. (2006b). Ternary complex formation between HvMYBS3 and other factors involved in transcriptional control in barley seeds. *Plant Journal*, Vol.47, No.2, (July 2006), pp. 269-281, ISSN 0960-7412

Rundlett, S.E.; Carmen, A.A.; Suka, N.; Turner, B.M. & Grunstein, M. (1998). Transcription repression by UME6 involves deacetylation of lysine 5 of histone H4 by RPD3. *Nature*, Vol.392, No.6678, (April 1998), pp. 831-835, ISSN 0028-0836

Santos-Mendoza, M. ; Dubreucq, B. ; Miquel, M. ; Caboche, M. & Lepiniec, L. (2005). LEAFY COTYLEDON 2 activation is sufficient to trigger the accumulation of oil and seed specific mRNAs in *Arabidopsis* leaves. *FEBS Letter*, Vol.579, No.21, (August 2005), pp. 4666-4670, ISSN 0014-5793

Santos-Mendoza, M. ; Dubreucq, B. ; Baud, S. ; Parcy, F. ; Caboche, M. & Lepiniec, L. (2008). Deciphering gene regulatory networks that control seed development and maturation in Arabidopsis. *Plant Journal*, Vol.54, No.4, (May 2008), pp. 608-620, ISSN 0960-7412

Schmidt, R.J.; Burr, F.A.; Aukerman, M.J. & Burr, B. (1990). Maize regulatory gene opaque-2 encodes a protein with a "leucine-zipper" motif that binds to zein DNA. *Proceedings of the National Academy of Sciences USA*, Vol.87, No.1, (January 1990), pp. 46-50, ISSN 0027-8424

Seo, M. & Koshiba, T. (2002). The complex regulation of ABA biosynthesis in plants. *Trends in Plant Science*, Vol.7, No.1, (January 2002), pp. 41-48, ISSN 1360-1385

Seo, M. ; Nambara, E. ; Choi, G. & Yamaguchi, S. (2009). Interaction of light and hormone signals in germinating seeds. *Plant Molecular Biology, Vol.*69, No.4, (March 2009), pp. 463-472, ISSN 0167-4412

Seo, M.; Hanada, A.; Kuwahara, A.; Endo, A.; Okamoto, M.; Yamauchi, Y.; North, H.; Marion-Poll, A.; Sun, T.P.; Koshiba, T.; Kamiya, Y.; Yamaguchi, S. & Nambara, E. (2006). Regulation of hormone metabolism in Arabidopsis seeds: phytochrome regulation of abscisic acid metabolism and abscisic acid regulation of gibberellin metabolism. *Plant Journal*, Vol.48, No.3, (November 2006), pp. 354-366, ISSN 0960-7412

Shen, Y.Y.; Wang, X.F.; Wu, F.Q.; Du, S.Y.; Cao, Z.; Shang, Y.; Wang, X.L.; Peng, C.C.; Yu, X.C.; Zhu, S.Y.; Fan, R.C.; Xu, Y.H. & Zhang, D.P. (2006). The Mg-chelatase H subunit is an abscisic acid receptor. *Nature*, Vol.443, No.7113, (October 2006), pp. 823-826, ISSN 0028-0836

Simon, J.A. & Tamkun, J.W. (2002). Programming off and on states in chromatin: mechanisms of Polycomb and trithorax group complexes. *Current Opinion in Genetics & Development*, Vol.12, No.2, (April 2002), pp. 210-218, ISSN 0959-437X

Smeekens, S. (2000). Sugar-induced signal transduction in plants. *Annual Review of Plant Physiology and Plant Molecular Biology*, Vol.51, (June 2000), pp. 49-81, ISSN 0167-4412

Stone, S.L.; Kwong, L.W.; Yee, K.M.; Pelletier, J.; Lepiniec, L.; Fischer, R.L.; Goldberg, R.B. & Harada, J.J. (2001). LEAFY COTYLEDON2 encodes a B3 domain transcription factor that induces embryo development. *Proceedings of the National Academy of Sciences USA*, Vol.98, No.20, (September 2001), pp. 11806-11811, ISSN 0027-8424

Stone, S.L.; Braybrook, S.A.; Paula, S.L.; Kwong, L.W.; Meuser, J.; Pelletier, J.; Hsieh, T.F.; Fischer, R.L.; Goldberg, R.B. & Harada, J.J. (2008). *Arabidopsis* LEAFY COTYLEDON2 induces maturation traits and auxin activity: Implications for somatic embryogenesis. *Proceedings of the National Academy of Sciences USA*, Vol.105, No.8, (February 2008), pp. 3151-3156, ISSN 0027-8424

Sun, X.; Shantharaj, D.; Kang, X. & Ni, M. (2010). Transcriptional and hormonal signaling control of Arabidopsis seed development. *Current Opinion in Plant Biology*, Vol.13, No.5, (October 2010), pp. 611-620, ISSN 1369-5266

Suzuki, M.; Wang, H.H. & McCarty, D.R. (2007). Repression of the LEAFY COTYLEDON 1/B3 regulatory network in plant embryo development by VP1/ABSCISIC ACID INSENSITIVE 3-LIKE B3 genes. *Plant Physiology*, Vol.143, No.2, (February 2007), pp. 902-911, ISSN 0032-0889

Suzuki, M.; Ketterling, M.G.; Li, Q.B. & McCarty, D.R. (2003). Viviparous1 alters global gene expression patterns through regulation of abscisic acid signalling. *Plant Physiology*, Vol.132, No.3, (July 2003), pp. 1664-1677, ISSN 0032-0889

Tanaka, H.; Dhonukshe, P.; Brewer, P.B. & Friml, J. (2006). Spatiotemporal asymmetric auxin distribution: A means to coordinate plant development. *Cellular and Molecular Life Sciences*, Vol.63, No.23, (December 2006), pp. 2738-2754.

Tanaka, M.; Kikuchi, A. & Kamada, H. (2008). The *Arabidopsis* histone deacetylases HDA6 and HDA19 contribute to the repression of embryonic properties after germination. *Plant Physiology*, Vol.146, No.1, (January 2008), pp. 149-161, ISSN 0032-0889

Tang, X.; Hou, A.; Babu, M.; Nguyen, V.; Hurtado, L.; Lu, Q.; Reyes, J.C.; Wang, A.; Keller, W.A.; Harada, J.J.; Tsang, E.W. & Cui, Y. (2008). The *Arabidopsis* BRAHMA chromatin remodelling ATPase is involved in repression of seed maturation genes in leaves. *Plant Physiology*, Vol.147, No.3, (July 2008), pp. 1143-1157, ISSN 0032-0889

Tiwari, S.; Schulz, R.; Ikeda, Y.; Dytham, L.; Bravo, J.; Mathers, L.; Spielman, M.; Guzmán, P.; Oakey, R.J.; Kinoshita, T. & Scott, R.J. (2008). MATERNALLY EXPRESSED PAB C-TERMINAL, a novel imprinted gene in *Arabidopsis*, encodes the conserved C-terminal domain of polyadenylate binding proteins. *Plant Cell*, Vol.20, No.9, (September 2008), pp. 2387-2398, ISSN 1040-4651

Tjaden, J.; Möhlmann, T.; Kampfenkel, K.; Henrichs, G. & Neuhaus, H.E. (1998). Altered plastidic ATP/ADP-transporter activity influences potato (*Solanum tuberosum* L.) tuber morphology, yield and composition of starch. *Plant Journal*, Vol.16, No.5, pp. 531-540, ISSN 0960-7412

To, A.; Valon, C.; Savino, G.; Guilleminot, J.; Devic, M.; Giraudat, J. & Parcy, F. (2006). A network of local and redundant gene regulation governs *Arabidopsis* seed maturation. *Plant Cell*, Vol.18, No.7, (July 2006), pp. 1642-1651, ISSN 1040-4651

Tsuchiya, Y.; Nambara, E.; Naito, S. & McCourt, P. (2004). The FUS3 transcription factor functions through the epidermal regulator TTG1 during embryogenesis in *Arabidopsis*. *Plant Journal*, Vol.37, No.1, (January 2004), pp. 73-81, ISSN 0960-7412

Tsukagoshi, H.; Morikami, A. & Nakamura, K. (2007). Two B3 domain transcriptional repressors prevent sugar-inducible expression of seed maturation genes in *Arabidopsis* seedlings. *Proceedings of the National Academy of Sciences USA*, Vol.104, No.7, (February 2007), pp. 2543-2547, ISSN 0027-8424

Tsukagoshi, H.; Saijo, T.; Shibata, D.; Morikami, A. & Nakamura, K. (2005). Analysis of a sugar response mutant of *Arabidopsis* identified a novel B3 domain protein that functions as an active transcriptional repressor. *Plant Physiology*, Vol.138, No.2, (June 2005), pp. 675-685, ISSN 0032-0889

van Der Geest, A.; Frisch, D.A.; Kemp, J.D. & Hall, T.C. (1995). Cell ablation reveals that expression from the phaseolin promoter Is confined to embryogenesis and microsporogenesis. *Plant Physiology*, Vol.109, No.4, (December 1995), pp. 1151-1158, ISSN 0032-0889

Venu, R.; Sreerekha, M.; Nobuta, K.; Beló, A.; Ning, Y.; An, G.; Meyers, B.C. & Wang, G.L. (2011). Deep sequencing reveals the complex and coordinated transcriptional regulation of genes related to grain quality in rice cultivars. *BMC Genomics*, Vol.12, pp. 190, ISSN 1471-2164

Vicente-Carbajosa, J. & Carbonero, P. (2005). Seed maturation: developing an intrusive phase to accomplish a quiescent state. *International Journal of Developmental Biology*, Vol.49, No.5-6, pp. 645-651, ISSN 0214-6282

Vicente-Carbajosa, J.; Oñate, L.; Lara, P.; Diaz, I. & Carbonero, P. (1998). Barley BLZ1: a bZIP transcriptional activator that interacts with endosperm-specific gene promoters. *Plant Journal*, Vol.13, No.5, (March 1998), pp. 629-640, ISSN 0960-7412

Vigeolas, H.; van Dongen, J.T.; Waldeck, P.; Hühn, D. & Geigenberger, P. (2003). Lipid storage metabolism is limited by the prevailing low oxygen concentrations within developing seeds of oilseed rape. *Plant Physiology*, Vol.133, No.4, (December 2003), pp. 2048-2060, ISSN 0032-0889

Wan, L.; Ross, A.R.; Yang, J.; Hegedus, D.D. & Kermode, A.R. (2007). Phosphorylation of the 12 S globulin cruciferin in wild-type and abi1-1 mutant *Arabidopsis thaliana* (thale cress) seeds. *Biochemical Journal*, Vol.404, No.2, (June 2007), pp. 247-256, ISSN 0264-6021

Wang, H.; Guo, J.; Lambert, K.N. & Lin, Y. (2007). Developmental control of Arabidopsis seed oil biosynthesis. *Planta*, Vol.226, No.3, (August 2007), pp. 773-783, ISSN 0032-0935

Weber, H.; Borisjuk, L. & Wobus, U. (2005). Molecular physiology of legume seed development. *Annual Review of Plant Biology*, Vol.56, pp. 253-279, ISSN 1543-5008

Weterings, K. & Russell, S.D. (2004). Experimental analysis of the fertilization process. *Plant Cell*, Vol.16 (suppl), pp. S107-S118, ISSN 1040-4651

Wobus, U. & Weber, H. (1999). Seed maturation: genetic programmes and control signals. *Current Opinion in Plant Biology*, Vol.2, No.1, (February 1999), pp. 33-38, ISSN 1369-5266

Wu, C.Y.; Suzuki, A.; Washida, H. & Takaiwa, F. (1998). The GCN4 motif in a rice glutelin gene is essential for endosperm-specific gene expression and is activated by Opaque-2 in transgenic rice plant. *Plant Journal*, Vol.14, No.6, (June 1998), pp. 673-683, ISSN 0960-7412

Wu, C.Y.; Washida, H.; Onodera, Y.; Harada, K. & Takaiwa, F. (2000). Quantitative nature of the prolamin-box, ACGT and AACA motifs in a rice glutelin gene promoter: minimal cis-element requirements for endosperm-specific gene expression. *Plant Journal*, Vol.23, No.3, (August 2000), pp. 415-421, ISSN 0960-7412

Xiao, W.; Custard, K.D.; Brown, R.C.; Lemmon, B.E.; Harada, J.J.; Goldberg, R.B. & Fischer, R.L. (2006). DNA methylation is critical for *Arabidopsis* embryogenesis and seed viability. *Plant Cell*, Vol.18, No.4, (April 2006), pp. 805-814, ISSN 1040-4651

Xiao, W.; Gehring, M.; Choi, Y.; Margossian, L.; Pu, H.; Harada, J.J.; Goldberg, R.B.; Pennell, R.I. & Fischer, R.L. (2003). Imprinting of the MEA Polycomb gene is controlled by antagonism between MET1 methyltransferase and DME glycosylase. *Developmental Cell*, Vol.5, No.6, (December 2003), pp. 891-901, ISSN 1534-5807

Xiong, L.M.; Gong, Z.Z.; Rock, C.D.; Subramanian, S.; Guo, Y.; Xu, W.Y.; Galbraith, D. & Zhu, J.K. (2001). Modulation of abscisic acid signal transduction and biosynthesis by an Sm-like protein in *Arabidopsis*. *Developmental Cell*, Vol.1, No.6, (December 2001), pp. 771-781, ISSN 1534-5807

Yamamoto, M.P.; Onodera, Y.; Touno, S.M. & Takaiwa, F. (2006). Synergism between RPBF Dof and RISBZ1 bZIP activators in the regulation of rice seed expression genes. *Plant Physiology*, Vol.141, No.4, (June 2006), pp. 1694-1707, ISSN 0032-0889

Yanagisawa, S. (2002). The Dof family of plant transcription factors. *Trends in Plant Science*, Vol.7, No.12, (December 2002), pp. 555-560, ISSN 1360-1385

Yang, J.; Zhang, J.; Liu, K.; Wang, Z. & Liu, L. (2006). Abscisic acid and ethylene interact in wheat grains in response to soil drying during grain filling. *New Phytologist*, Vol.171, No.2, pp. 293-303, ISSN 0028-646X

Zeng, Y. & Kermode, A.R. (2004). A gymnosperm *ABI3* gene functions in a severe abscisic acid-insensitive mutant of *Arabidopsis* (*abi3-6*) to restore the wild-type phenotype and demonstrates a strong synergistic effect with sugar in the inhibition of post-germinative growth. *Plant Molecular Biology*, Vol.56, No.5, (November 2004), pp. 731-746, ISSN 0167-4412

Zhang, X.R. ; Garreton, V. & Chua, N.H. (2005). The AIP2 E3 ligase acts as a novel negative regulator of ABA signaling by promoting ABI3 degradation. *Genes & Development*, Vol.19, No.13, (July 2005), pp. 1532-1543, ISSN 0890-9369

Zhou, Y.; Zhang, X.; Kang, X.; Zhao, X.; Zhang, X. & Ni, M. (2009). SHORT HYPOCOTYL UNDER BLUE1 associates with MINISEED3 and HAIKU2 promoters in vivo to regulate *Arabidopsis* seed development. *Plant Cell*, Vol.21, No.1, (January 2009), pp. 106-117, ISSN 1040-4651

10

Plant Somatic Embryogenesis: Some Useful Considerations

Antonia Gutiérrez-Mora, Alejandra Guillermina González-Gutiérrez, Benjamín Rodríguez-Garay, Azucena Ascencio-Cabral and Lin Li-Wei
Centro de Investigación y Asistencia en Tecnología y Diseño del Estado de Jalisco, Unidad de Biotecnología Vegetal, Guadalajara, Jalisco, México

1. Introduction

This review chapter discusses basic clues of plant somatic embryogenesis. Firstly, the similarities between zygotic and somatic embryogenesis will be compared, starting from the polarity of the egg cell inside the embryo sac and ending with the mature embryo inside a seed.

The rest of the chapter will review and discuss the most important factors needed for the conversion of a somatic cell into an embryo and finally into a whole plant.

2. Zygotic embryogenesis *versus* somatic embryogenesis

2.1 Zygotic embryogenesis

In order to understand the formation and production of plant somatic embryos it is important to briefly look at the process of zygotic embryogenesis given their high similarity. Double fertilization is one of the main characteristics of angiosperms where one male gamete fertilizes the egg cell and a second male gamete fertilizes the central cell of the embryo sac (Russell, 1993).

Embryogenesis has evolved as a successful reproductive strategy in higher plants. The life cycle of angiosperm plants (flowering plants) is divided into two phases: the diploid sporophytic phase and the haploid gametophytic phase (Fan et al., 2008). The functions of the gametophyte are short lived and less complex than those of the sporophyte and are only devoted to produce haploid male and female gametes (Fan et al., 2008; Reiser & Fischer, 1993; Yadegari & Drews, 2004). Male gametes or microgametophytes (pollen grains) are developed inside the anthers and are formed from a pollen mother cell which undergoes a meiotic process that gives rise to a tetrad of haploid cells called microspores. During the maturation towards the pollen formation, the microspore suffers an asymmetric mitotic division giving rise to a two new cells: the vegetative and the generative cells. The generative cell undergoes a second mitotic division producing two sperms, while the vegetative cell remains undivided and bears the capacity of producing the polen tube which will grow in the female tissue of the carpel serving as the sperm carrier (Mc Cormick, 2004) (Figure 1).

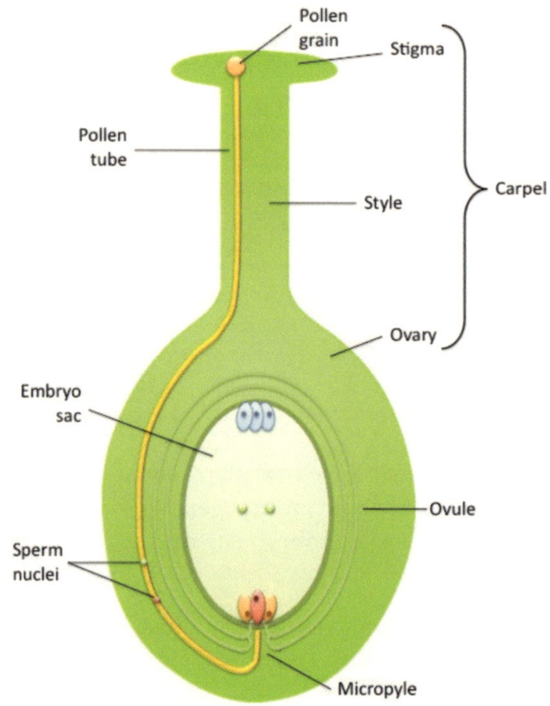

Fig. 1. Ideogram of an angiosperm female apparatus in the flower and the path of the pollen tube toward the embryo sac.

The female gametophyte called **embryo sac** is developed inside the carpel, which consists of three elements: the ovary, the style and the pollen grain receptacle called stigma. The ovary may hold one or several ovules which bear the female gametophyte or embryo sac. An ovule is formed by three layers of cells surrounding the embryo sac, the nucellus and the inner and outer integuments. The integuments do not join at the tip of the ovule leaving an opening called micropyle, which is the "door" for the penetration of the pollen tube into the embryo sac (Figures 1 and 2).

The female gametophyte, megagametophyte or embryo sac is developed inside the ovule. Each ovule contains one megaspore mother cell, which after two rounds of meiotic cell divisions gives rise to a strand of four haploid megaspores. In the majority of angiosperm plant species three of these cells degenerate, but the closest to the chalaza survives as the functional megaspore, enlarges and undergoes three mitotic divisions to form the embryo sac. The embryo sac may follow different patterns of development in different species, however the most common consists of four types of cells, arranged as follows: Three antipodal cells (at the chalazal end), one central cell containing two polar haploid nuclei (that generally migrate towards the center of the embryo sac), two synergid cells flanking the egg cell (all three positioned at the micropylar end) (Maheshwari, 1937; Yang et al., 2010) (Figure 2).

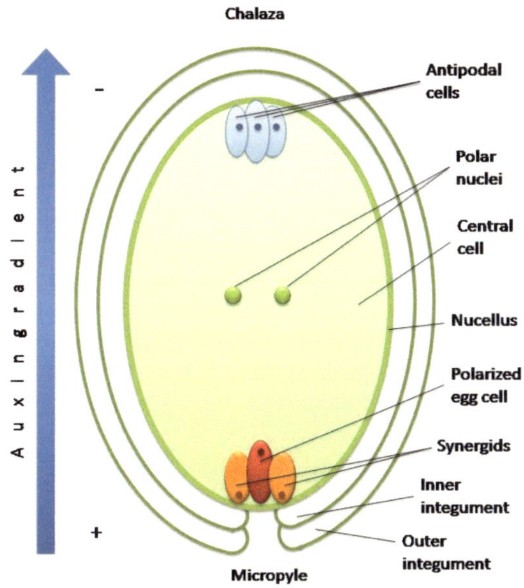

Fig. 2. Ideogram of the female angiosperm gametophyte showing the polarity of the embryo sac and the egg cell given mainly by an endogenous auxin gradient (blue arrow to the left). Modified from Pagnussat et al. (2009).

In the sexual reproduction of angiosperms, the pollen grain is transferred from the anther to the stigma where it germinates and forms the pollen tube (Yadegari & Drews, 2004) which travels long distances directed first by sporophytic signals and then by the female gametophyte (Wetering & Russell, 2004). Afterwards, the pollen tube reaches the micropyle where it is guided by signals generated by the synergid cells through high calcium concentrations (Tian & Russell, 1997). Then the spermatic cells are discharged into one of the synergids through the filiform apparatus (Yadegari & Drews, 2004). Double fertilization takes place when one spermatic nucleus fuses with the egg cell forming the zygote (diploid), while the second sperm fuses with the polar nuclei of the central cell to initiate the endosperm (generally triploid) (Russell, 1993).

The observed polarity of zygotic embryos starts with the formation of the embryo sac. This polarity in the embryo sac is due to a gradient of the natural auxin indole-acetic acid along the micropyle-chalaza axis whose expression starts at the micropylar region outside of the embryo sac. In the same manner and following this pattern, the haploid egg cell which after its fertilization produces the embryo, is also highly polarized with its nucleus located at the chalazal pole (Pagnussat et al., 2009). Pagnussat et al. (2009) reported that it is possible that auxin does not regulate the position of the nuclei during the embryo sac formation, however it participates in the regulation of cell fate at cellularization. After fertilization, the resulting diploid zygote remains highly polarized, while the other male gamete fuses with the central cell of the embryo sac which then develops into the triploid endosperm, acting as a nutritive and protective element for the embryo. In the majority of the plant species, the somatic embryogenesis process follows the above pattern. In the case of somatic embryogenesis being the initial somatic embryogenic cell equivalent to the zygote, and the *in vitro* culture medium being equivalent to the nutritive and protective endosperm (Figure 3).

In angiosperms, the first division of the zygote is highly asymmetric. Actin governs the migration of the premitotic nucleus into the future division plane and the placement of the preprophase band in these asymmetrically dividing cells (Rasmussen et al., 2011). Once fertilized, the zygote elongates and divides asymmetrically, with the smaller apical cell generating most of the embryo and the larger basal cell giving rise mainly to the extra embryonic suspensor. Subsequent divisions of the large basal cell give rise to the suspensor and at its tip the hypophyseal region where the radicle will be formed and finally giving the symmetry to the whole plant (Toonen & de Vries, 1996; Gutiérrez-Mora et al., 2004). The single-celled zygote soon acquires the potential to develop into an embryo undergoing a series of complex cellular and morphological processes that finally produce the sporophyte or plant (Rao, 1996). Further information in these topics can be found in Russell (1992); Rotman et al. (2003); Gutiérrez-Marcos et al. (2006); He et al. (2007) and Capron et al. (2008), among many others.

2.2 Somatic embryogenesis

Somatic embryogenesis is the maximum expression of cell **totipotency** in plant cells. In short, totipotency is the hability of a plant cell to undergo a series of complex metabolic and morphological coordinated steps to produce a complete and normal plant or sporophyte without the participation of the sexual processes. Thus, somatic embryogenesis is the developmental process by which theoretically any somatic cell develops into a zygotic like structure that finally forms a plant (Rao, 1996; Jiménez, 2005). Like their zygotic counterparts, somatic embryos have a single cell origin (Rao, 1996). The single cell origin of somatic embryos has been elegantly reported by several authors, in particular, this unicellular origin of somatic embryos has been reported in *Agave tequilana* (Gutiérrez-Mora et al., 2004; Portillo et al., 2007).

Usually, the somatic embryogenic process consists of two main steps, the induction of the process and the expression of the resultant embryos (Rodríguez-Garay et al., 2000; Gutiérrez-Mora et al., 2004; Jiménez, 2005). The process is initiated with somatic cells theoretically from any part of the plant, however, substantial differences in competence are found in practice. The cells which are more competent for somatic embryogenesis are generally those coming from young tissues, immature zygotic embryos among them. However, stems, roots and leaves may be useful as well. Usually, somatic embryos are induced by simple manipulation of the cultural *in vitro* conditions. One of the main elements in the culture medium are the growth regulator substances (GRS) such as auxins, cytokinins, abscisic acid and gibberellins among other components. Also, it is important to mention that the hormonal endogenous substances play important roles in the somatic embryogenic process. Out of the above mentioned GRS, auxins are the most important components in the induction of the process (Dodeman et al., 1997; Jiménez, 2005; Jiménez & Thomas, 2006; Rao, 1996; Feher, 2006). Somatic cells need the signal for the cell polarization and the asymmetric division given by auxins as it happens in their zygotic counterparts (Gutiérrez-Mora et al., 2004; Pagnussat et al., 2009). The participation of the other GRS is important in the balance of hormonal constituents needed to achieve somatic embryogenesis.

With regard to the initial steps of the development of a somatic embryo, the induction process is generally initiated by the action of a selected auxin (the most used auxin for most species is 2,4-Dichlorophenoxiacetic acid (2,4-D)) (Nomura & Komamine, 1986; Jiménez,

2005). In this revision the cellular process is illustrated by the formation of a somatic embryo of *Agave tequilana* Weber cultivar Azul (Gutiérrez-Mora et al., 2004; Portillo et al., 2007).

The initial induced somatic cell emulates its sexual counterpart "the zygote". This is a highly polarized cell with its nucleus positioned to an extreme of the cell, leaving the other extreme highly vacuolated (Figure 3a and a'). The first transversal cell division is asymmetrical giving rise to a small apical cell and a highly vacuolated basal cell (Figure 3b and b'). A second division of the apical cell gives rise to the embryo proper or two-celled proembryo and the highly vacuolated cell which is putatively the first cell of the suspensor (Figure 3c and c'). A third round of cell division produces a four-celled embryo head, and the first suspensor cell has suffered a second division. Observed subsequent cell divisions of the suspensor cells give rise to the putative hypophyseal region where the plant radicle will be formed. After this round of cell divisions, subsequent and well coordinated divisions will

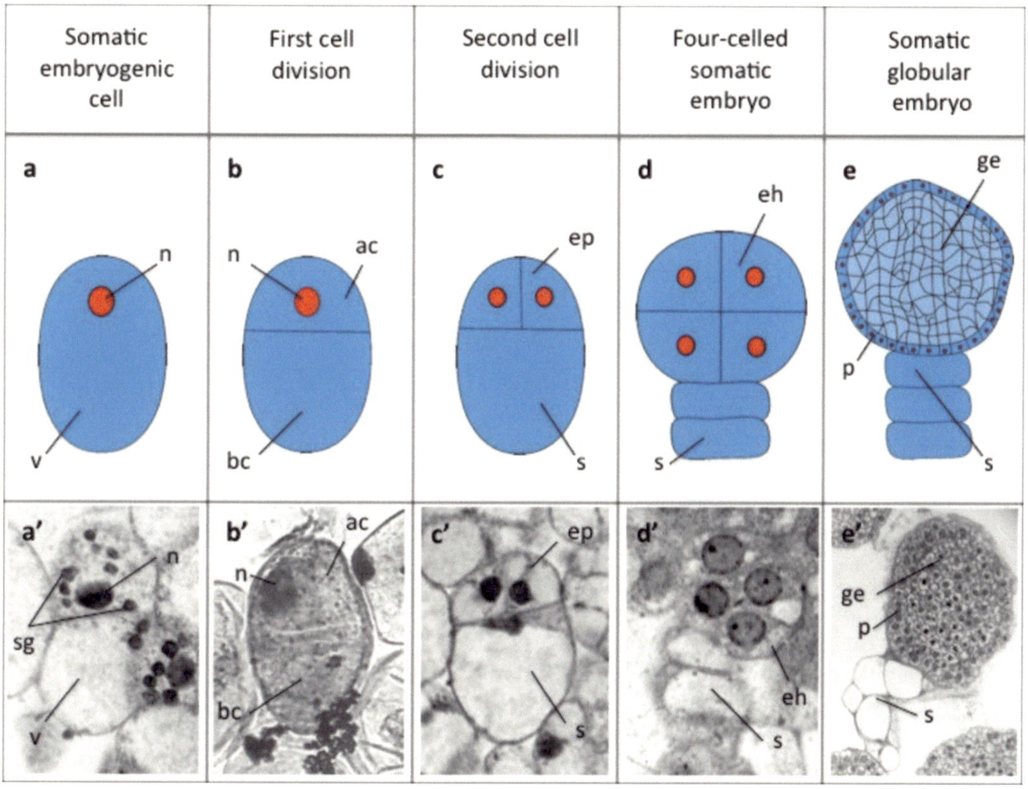

Fig. 3. Early cell divisions in the somatic embryogenesis of the monocotyledonous species *Agave tequilana* Weber var. Azul. **a) - e)**. Ideogram of the somatic embryogenic process, which represents the real somatic embryogenic process **a') - e')**. **n** – nucleus, **v** - vacuole, **sg** - starch granules, **ac** – apical cell, **bc** – basal cell, **ep** – embryo proper, **s** – suspensor, **eh** – embryo head, **p** – protoderm, **ge** – globular embryo. Figures 3a', 3c' and 3d' are from Portillo, L., et al. Somatic embryogenesis in *Agave tequilana* Weber cultivar azul. In Vitro Cellular and Developmental Biology – Plant, 2007, Vol. 43, pp. 569-575. Copyright© 2007 by the Society for In Vitro Biology, formerly the Tissue Culture Association. Reproduced with permission of the copyright owner.

form the globular stage of the somatic embryo (Figure 3e and e'). It is important to mention that at this globular stage the somatic embryos of most of the species are very similar having protoderm. Also, it is important to mention that in many species the suspensor is not observed because it does not remain and does not divide. However, this cellular and morphological point of the somatic embryo is important for the formation of the radicle and the final symmetry of the whole plant (Gutiérrez-Mora et al., 2004; Yeung et al., 1996; Supena et al., 2008).

Moreover, after the globular stage of the somatic embryos, the fate of their morphology follows their genetic lineage: monocotyledonous or dicotyledonous as it can be observed in Figure 4. A distinctive characteristic of the dicotyledonous species is the formation the cotyledon primordium (cp) which gives to the classical heart form to somatic embryos, similar to their zygotic counterparts. On the other hand, somatic embryos of monocotyledonous species show the classical torpedo shape which is disrupted at germination.

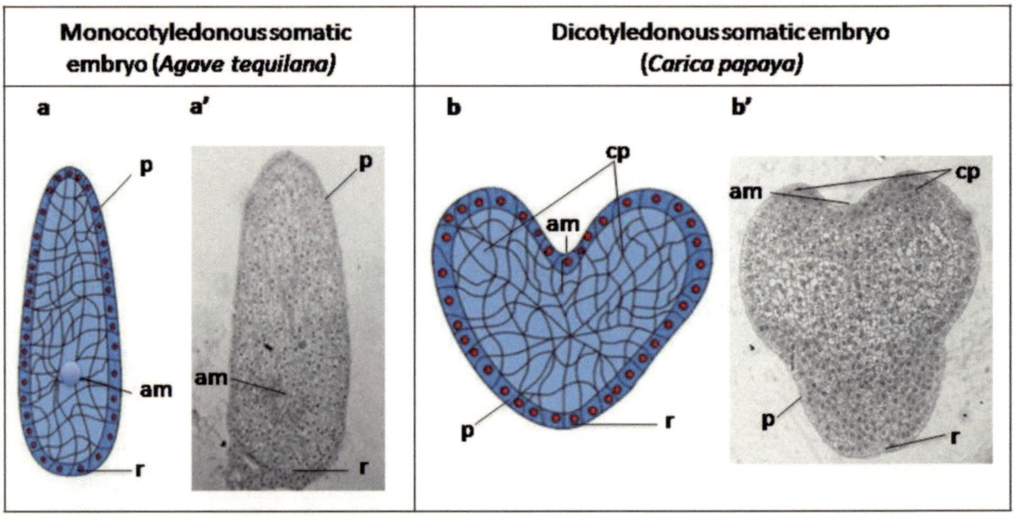

Fig. 4. Differential morphology between monocotyledonous and dicotyledonous somatic embryos after the globular stage. a) and a') Ideogram and real *Agave tequilana* (monocotyledonous) somatic embryo, respectively. b) and b') Ideogram and real *Carica papaya* (dicotyledonous) somatic embryo, respectively. **r** - radicle, **am** - apical meristem, **p** - protoderm, **cp** - cotyledonar primordium.

3. The role of phytohormones

Plants are sessile organisms which have endogenous signals (hormonal compounds) to cope biotic and abiotic challenges (Gilroy & Trewavas, 2001). Phytohormones are chemical cues which are produced at relatively low concentrations and move around the plant triggering diverse responses in tissues and cells. Some of the most important characteristics of endogenous hormonal elements are (Öpik & Rolfe, 2005):

They work at low concentrations, in general between 10^{-6} a 10^{-9} M at the site of action. High concentrations inhibit their action. A medium for hormonal transport is needed if the site of its synthesis is different from that for its action. Hormones are mainly transported through the vascular system of the plant. This is not always true as is the case for ethylene. It is necessary that the target site has the capacity to respond. Plant hormones are produced endogenously by the plant itself. Plant growth regulators (PGR) are synthetic compounds with hormone-like activity which are given to the plant under *in vitro* or *ex vitro* conditions. There exist several groups of these compounds according to their physiological action:

Auxins.- The original endogenous hormone is the Indole-3-acetic acid (IAA). Some of the most used synthetic PGR with auxin activity are indole-3-butyric acid (IBA), naphthaleneacetic acid (NAA), 2,4-dichlorophenoxyacetic acid (2,4-D), etc.

Cytokinins.- In whole plants the natural cytokinins are zeatin and zeatin riboside. Some of the most used synthetic compounds are kinetin, thidiazuron (TDZ), benzyladenine (BA), among others.

Gibberellins (GA).- In nature, plants produce more than 110 different kinds of GA, however the most used compounds are GA_1, GA_3, GA_4 and GA_7

Abscisic acid(ABA).- This is a natural compound which is used in both *in vitro* and *ex vitro* conditions.

The process of somatic embryogenesis requires different concentrations and combinations at its different stages in order to finally produce an embryo. The two most important stages, the induction and the expression of embryos may require different medium composition with regard to nutrients and growth regulators.

In nature, auxins are produced in apical and root meristems, young leaves, seeds and developing fruits, and their main functions are cell elongation and expansion, suppression of lateral buds, etc. (Öpik & Rolfe, 2005). In somatic embryogenesis this is considered one of the most important elements producing cell polarity and asymmetrical cell division. In general, relatively high auxin concentrations (2,4-D, IAA, etc.) favor callus formation and the induction process (cell polarity). Afterwards, when the induction stage has been achieved, it is necessary to reduce or eliminate the auxins in order to initiate the bilateral symmetry and the expression of the somatic embryos.

On the other hand, in nature, cytokinins are an important factor for cell division, and stimulate the formation and development of lateral or axilar buds, retard senecense and inhibit root formation. In *in vitro* somatic embryogenesis, cytokinins are utilized in combination with auxins and play an important role in cell proliferation. In the production of somatic embryos of some plants such as pea and soybean, the adition of cytokinins to the culture medium inhibits the induction effect of auxins (Lakshmanan & Taji, 2000). However, in other species such as *Zoysia japonica* (Asano et al., 1996), *Begonia gracilis* (Castillo & Smith, 1997) and *Oncidium sp.* (Chen & Chang, 2001), the use of cytokinins favours the induction of somatic embryos.

With regard to gibberellins (GA), in whole plants, these hormonal compounds are mainly produced in the apical zone, fruits and seeds. They stimulate stem growth and are responsible for the distances between nodes by stimulating cell elongation, also, they regulate the transition from the juvenile stage to the adult stage of the plant and promote seed germination by regulating the rupture of the embryo dormancy. In *in vitro* embryogenic cultures, the addition of GA promotes the regeneration process and the germination of somatic embryos (Li & Qu, 2002).

Finally, another important hormonal factor (but not the last) is the abscisic acid (ABA). This compound is produced mainly in chloroplasts. Its main functions are stomata closure, seed dormancy and the inhibition of axillary buds growth. The addition of ABA to *in vitro* embryogenic cultures inhibits the early embryo germination and stimulates the coordinated maturation of the somatic embryo. However, prolonged exposition to ABA, this element suppresses growth of the formed *in vitro* plants (Bozhkov et al., 2002).

Plant growth regulators are critical in determining the pathway of the plant cells. The effects of growth regulators in somatic embryogenesis have been studied in a variety of plant species. The potential of 2,4 D has been reported as the most efficient growth regulator in *Eleutherococcus sessiliflorus, Gymnema silvester, Holestemma ada-kodien, Paspalum scrobiculatum, Andrographis paniculata* (Choi et al., 2002; Kumar et al., 2002; Martin, 2004). Similarly, Malabadi et al. (2005) developed an effective protocol for inducing somatic embryogenesis in conifers using triacontanol (TRIA) as growth regulator. Moreover, adding Picloram (PIC), 6-benzylaminopurine (BAP) and naphthaleneacetic acid (NAA) was reported to influence plant regeneration via somatic embryogenesis in *Arachis pintoi* and *Arachis glabrata* (Rey & Mroginski, 2006; Vidoz et al., 2004). On the other hand, high-frequency regeneration via somatic embryogenesis of recalcitrant cotton (*Gossypium hirsutum L.*) was possible in medium containing kinentin and 2,4 dichlorophenoxyacetic acid fortified with B5 vitamins and the addition of zeatin (Khan et al., 2010). Carbenicillin, a well-known antibiotic in the culture media showed a growth regulator activity in somatic embryogenic callus induction (Shehata et al., 2010). The effects of 2,4-D, kinetin and 6-benzylaminopurine in the micropropagation of *Anthurium andreanum* 'Tera' through somatic embryogenesis were reported by Beyramizade et al. (2008). Germination of somatic embryos was possible in Pigeonpea *(Cajanus* L. Mills.), *Arachis pintoi and Pennisetum glaucum (L.) R. Br and Phalaenopsis* in MS medium supplemented with BA (Mohan & Krishnamurthy, 2002; Rey & Mroginski, 2006; Jha et al., 2009; Gow et al., 2010). Furthermore, it has been reported that the oxidative stress induced by specific grow regulators is associated with callus regeneration (Szechyńska et al., 2007). Exogenously supplying polyamines during the multiplication stage has been reported as being deleterious at successive stages of somatic embryo formation of *Panax ginseng*. Nevertheless, adding spermidine at the initiation stage enhanced the effect of the synthetic auxin 3-(benzo[b]selenyl) acetic acid (BSAA) (Kevers et al., 2002).

4. *In vitro* environmental factors

Plant regeneration through somatic embryogenesis has been reported in several studies. However, developing regeneration methods that meet the physical and chemical demands of the plant cells is still a largely empirical process. Identifying ideal *in vitro* culture conditions can be extremely difficult due to the wide number of factors that contribute to the induction, development and conversion of the somatic embryo into a plant. With the aim to overcome difficulties and determine optimum conditions for *in vitro* propagation via somatic embryogenesis, the effects of these factors have been studied in a significant number of plant species.

4.1 Culture medium

Culture medium is one of most important factors to be considered for *in vitro* plant cell culture and it can be used in either solid or liquid state. Also, it must supply the essential minerals required for growth and development. The most common medium used in in vitro plant cultures is that developed by Murashige and Skoog (1962) which has been reported to be used in plant regeneration of several species (Ascencio-Cabral et al., 2008; Castillo & Smith, 1997; Fitch et al., 1993; Mohan & Krishnamurthy, 2002; Kevers et al., 2002; Konieczny et al., 2008, among many others). Alternatively, B5 medium has been used for the *in vitro* regeneration of *Arabidopsis thaliana* (Gaj, 2001). Furthermore, Thuzar et al. (2011) revealed that using N6 medium in *in vitro* cultures promoted somatic embryogenesis and plant regeneration of *Elaeis guineensis* Jacq. As well as these, somatic embryogenesis of *Agave tequilana* has been reported when cultured on Schenk and Hildelbrant (SH) medium (Rodríguez-Sahagún et al., 2011).

4.2 Gelling agents

When plant cells or tissues are to be cultured on the surface of the medium, it must be solidified. Even though agar is the most frequent type of gelling agent used in culture media, the water potential of a medium solidified with gel is more negative than that of liquid medium, due to their matric potential (Amador & Stewart, 1987, as cited by George et al., 2008). Nevertheless, Ascencio-Cabral et al. (2008), reported a significant effect on plant regeneration from somatic embryos of *Carica papaya L* when media was solidified with Difco® Bacto Agar. Results showed that the gelling agent not only had a strong effect by itself but also it interacted positively with other factors such as light and the presence of the glucoside phloridzin, producing a high rate of healthy plantlets. Apart from this, the addition of phenolic glycosides into the growth medium have been reported to help reduce the occurrence of hyperhydricity and plant regeneration was improved (Ascencio-Cabral et al., 2008; Witrzens et al., 1988). Another example of the use of a gelling agent is Phytagel or Gellan gum. Complete plants were produced after somatic embryo germination. Cultures were transferred to the same basal medium without growth regulators, and solidified with 5g/l of the agar substitute Phytagel. After 16 weeks, somatic embryos started to germinate and developed typical plantlet morphology (Torres-Muñoz & Rodríguez-Garay, 1996).

4.3 Carbon source

Carbon sources have been reported to have a significant effect in *in vitro* plant regeneration. In general, sucrose is the carbohydrate of choice as carbon source, probably because it is the most common carbohydrate in the plant phloem (Murashige & Skoog, 1962; Thorpe, 1982; Lemos & Baker, 1998; Fuentes et al., 2000, as cited by Ahmad et al., 2007). Fitch et al. (1993) reported the effect on frequency of somatic embryos in cultures of *Carica papaya* L. when the culture medium was supplied with different concentrations of sucrose. Results showed that tissue in medium containing 7% of sucrose was able to enhance somatic embryogenesis (Fitch, 1993). In addition, Rybczyński et al. (2007) reported that supplementing 0.2-0.4% sucrose to culture media boost the efficiency of the photosynthetic apparatus of somatic embryos of *Gentiana kurroo*. However, other carbohydrates can also be suitable and in special conditions may be better than sucrose (Slater et al., 2003). Furthermore, somatic embryogenesis of *Citrus deliciosa* was promoted by supplementing the culture media with galactose (Cabasson et al., 1995). Selecting the suitable source of carbohydrates and the concentration has been reported to induce high-efficiency somatic embryogenesis in cell cultures of *Phalaenopsis and Prunus incisa* (Tokuhara & Mii, 2003; Cheong & Pooler, 2004).

4.4 Amino acids

Moreover, studies have been conducted to optimize different types and concentrations of amino acids on the induction of somatic embryogenesis in strawberry (*Fragaria x ananassa* Duch.) cultivars. Results revealed that stimulation of embryogenesis and embryo development was strictly dependent on the type and concentration of amino acid in the medium. Proline was much more effective than glutamine and alanine on induction and development of somatic embryogenesis (Gerdakaneh et al., 2011).

4.5 Environmental factors

Moreover, physical factors such as light, photoperiod, temperature, gaseous environment and osmotic pressure have to be controlled when cultured *in vitro*. In order to find the most suitable environmental conditions to produce somatic embryos several works have been conducted.

4.6 Temperature

Applying a heat-shock encouraged somatic embryogenesis in cultures of *Avena sativa* (Kiviharju & Pehu, 1998), *Zea mays, Triticum aestivum* L. and rye (Fu et al., 2008). Alternatively, a cold pre-treatment doubled the embryogenic response in *in vitro* maize cultures (Pescitelli et al., 1990). Thermal shock (cold and heat) and incubation in mannitol, cultures of *Dianthus chinensis* (Fu et al., 2008) showed a strong interaction between the genotype and culture conditions for the production of somatic embryos. Aslam et al. (2011) evaluated the effect of freezing and non-freezing temperature on somatic embryogenesis in *Catharanthus roseus* (L.), their results showed that somatic embryo development (production, maturation and germination) was sensitive to temperature variations.

4.7 Light

In addition, light has a significant effect in plant development. The importance of light in plant regeneration of wheat cultures has been reported in several studies (Liang et al., 1987; Jaramillo & Summers, 1991). Somatic embryogenesis in quince was reported as positively regulated by phytochrome (D'Onofrio et al., 1998). Furthermore, research conducted by Torné et al. (2001) demonstrated that somatic embryogenesis in *Araujia sericifera* was promoted by light provided by gro-lux lamps. Alternatively, light or dark treatments have been reported to induce embryogenesis in cultures of *Prunus incisa Thunb.* cv. (Cheong & Pooler, 2004). In contrast, the expression and the maturation of embryos of *Agave tequilana* Weber were successfully achieved when embryos were exposed to red light for 15 days in LOG medium at λ= 630 nm (Rodríguez-Sahagún et al., 2011). Germanà et al. (2005) evaluated the effect of light quality in a culture of *Citrus clementina* Hort. ex Tan., cultivar Nules; as a result embryogenic callus was produced only under photoperiodic conditions of white light. Ascencio-Cabral et al. (2008), reported a significant effect of light quality on germination and plant length from somatic embryos of *Carica papaya* L. In this study, embryos exposed to gro-lux and wide-spectrum light germinated healthier and developed regular roots. However, Gow et al. (2009) reported negative effects on direct somatic embryogenesis of *Phalaenopsis* orchids in cultures exposed to light; in addition, light induced embryo necrosis and low plantlet regeneration. Furthermore, varying the culture period effectively enhanced somatic embryogenesis when culture conditions were 60 days for induction in darkness and 45 days for subculture in light (Gow et al., 2010).

4.8 Ethylene biosynthesis

Another factor affecting somatic embryogenesis is ethylene biosynthesis which has been reported to inhibit regeneration (Giridhar et al., 2004), it has been reported that by blocking its synthesis plant regeneration increased. Giridhar et al. (2004) reported that by adding silver nitrate at different stages of the plant regeneration through somatic embryogenesis of *Coffea arabica* L. and *Coffea canephora* was good for the production of somatic embryos. Recent research conducted by Kępczyńska & Zielińska (2011) focused on the effects ethylene inhibitors binding to receptors at different phases of somatic embryogenesis in *Medicago sativa* L.; the findings showed that ethylene biosynthesis and its action influenced individual phases of somatic embryogenesis. Moreover, alterations of these processes affected adversely the activity of the production of somatic embryos.

5. A new whole plant

A great number of *in vitro* produced plants do not survive the transfer from the *in vitro* to the *ex vitro* environment under greenhouse or field conditions. Due to their anatomical and physiological characteristics, these kinds of plants need a gradual adaptation or acclimatization to *ex vitro* environments in order to survive and be productive. The greenhouse and field have substantially lower relative humidity, higher light level and septic environment that are stressful to micropropagated plants compared to *in vitro* conditions (Hazarika, 2003, Hazarika & Bora, 2010). Plantlets were developed within the culture vessels under low level of light, aseptic conditions, on a medium containing ample sugar and nutrients to allow for heterotrophic growth and in an atmosphere with a high level of humidity. These contribute a culture-induced phenotype that cannot survive the environmental conditions when directly placed in a greenhouse or field. The physiological and anatomical characteristics of micropropagated plantlets necessitate that they should be gradually acclimatized to the environment of the greenhouse or field (Kozai, 1991).

Abnormalities in morphology, anatomy and physiology of plantlets cultivated *in vitro* can be repaired after transfer to *ex vitro* conditions. However, many plant species need gradual changes in environmental conditions to avoid desiccation and photoinhibition. During acclimatization to *ex vitro* conditions, leaf thickness generally increases, leaf mesophyll progresses in differentiation into palisade and spongy parenchyma, stomatal density decreases and the stomatal shape changes from circular to an elliptical one. The most important changes include development of cuticle, epicuticular waxes, and effective stomatal regulation of transpiration leading to stabilization of water status. For photosynthetic parameters it seems very important at which conditions *in vitro* plantlets have been grown. According to this, transfer can be accompanied with a transient decrease in photosynthetic parameters. Further, an increase in chlorophyll content, maximum photochemical efficiency, actual quantum yield of photosystem II, and net photosynthetic rate is usually observed in dependence on the environmental conditions during acclimatization. Acclimatization can be speed up by hardening of plantlets *in vitro* or after transplantation by decreasing the transpiration rate by antitranspirants including ABA, or by increasing the photosynthetic rate by elevated CO_2 concentration (Pospíšilová et al., 1999).

Hyperhydricity is a factor which is considered as a physiological disorder that can be induced by diverse stress conditions. Previous research about hyperhydricity, report that the observed anatomical and physiological problems are the result of several altered or disrupted metabolic pathways, such as changes in the synthesis of proteins that negatively affect enzymes involved in the photosynthetic apparatus (Rubisco), also, the disruption in the synthesis of cellulose and lignin (PAL, glucan synthase) and the alteration of processes associated to ethylene synthesis (peroxidases). Changes in the synthesis of proteins affect enzymes which are linked to interconnected metabolic pathways. Low protein levels have been found in hyperhydric leaves as compared to normal leaves and a 30 kD protein has been found only in anomalous leaves (Van Huystee, 1987); and also other proteins (30-32 kD) associated to lignin synthesis (Kevers et al., 1984).

On the other hand, stems exhibit hypertrophy of cortical and pith parenchyma, large intercellular spaces, hypolignification of the vascular system (Kevers et al., 1985), and a reduced and/or abnormal vascular system (Letouzé & Daguin, 1987). Jausoro et al., (2010) reported disorganized cortex, epidermal holes, epidermal discontinuity, collapsed cells, and other structural characteristics were observed in hyperhydric shoots of *Handroanthus impetiginosus*.

Hyperhydricity is the expression of several phases with diverse degrees of abnormalities in affected plants. These plants are not able to survive the stress imposed by the transfer of the *in vitro* to the *ex vitro* environment. In order to have success in this transfer process, it is necessary that the plants to undergo through a gradual change to aquire their normal anatomical stage for a succesful aclimatization process (Debergh et al., 1992).

In order to overcome hyperhydricity, several strategies have been proposed, basically related to environmental issues that help to control relative humidity and water availability through the manipulation of solutes in de growth medium (Maene & Debergh, 1987). Plantlets with well developed leaves under low humidity and high irradiance show a photosynthetic and metabolic normal activity.

In *in vitro* cultures, the photosynthetic activity is scarce, for which the adaptation of the foliar system toward an active photosynthesis is necessary. For the above mentioned adaptation, several strategies have been proposed: elimination of carbon sources, mechanical defoliation of plantlets, induction of storage organs (Ziv & Lilien-Kipnis, 1990), use of growth retardants to inhibit foliar growth in order to improve the proliferation rate, meristems growth, and the enrichment of CO_2 under high luminic intensity (Ziv, 1989). Shoot hyperhydricity, resulting in failure to root and/or survive transplanting is a frequent problem in sunflower (Baker et al., 1999). Hyperhydricity can be controlled in various ways including improved vessel aeration (Rossetto et al., 1992), reducing cytokinin levels (Williams & Taji, 1991), increasing agar concentration (Brand, 1993) and changing the concentration of medium constituents (Ziv, 1989). Losses up to 60% of cultured shoots or explants have been reported due to hyperhydricity in commercial plant micropropagation

(Piqueras et al., 2002). On the other hand stems exhibit hypertrophy of cortical and pith parenchyma, large intercellular spaces, hypolignification of vascular system (Kevers et al., 1985), and a reduced and/or abnormal vascular system (Letouzé & Daguin, 1987).

6. Conclusion

Zygotic embryogenesis is a key process in flowering plants, and it is a well coordinated series of developmental events governed from the very beginning by cell polarity and asymmetric cell division in which male and female cells participate.

Somatic embryogenesis is almost a mirror copy of the above process, but without the participation of sexual organs and cells. Single somatic cells are programmed to follow similar developmental steps by the manipulation of *in vitro* environmental factors such as culture medium which includes several components: a gelling agent (when necessary), a carbon source, several nutrient elements and most importantly hormonal-like factors. Also, the somatic embryogenic processes need special physical environmental factors for the incubation of cell and tissue cultures, such as temperature and light among others.

The practical uses of somatic embryos include the massive propagation of plants of high commercial value and more importantly their use in basic research and in plant breeding programs where biotechnological tools are used.

7. Acknowledgments

This work was financially supported in part by SNICS-SAGARPA-México grant BEI-AGA-10-8. The authors wish to thank J. Aldana-Padilla for the artwork of figures 1 to 4 and to A. Valdivia-Ugalde for the photograph of figure 3b'. L. Li-Wei is a graduate student at PICYT-CIATEJ and financially supported by CONACyT-México. A.G. González-Gutiérrez is an undergraduate student at CUCBA-Universidad de Guadalajara. A. Ascencio-Cabral was a M.S. graduate student financially supported by CONACyT-México.

8. References

Ahmad, T.; Abbasi, N.K.; Hafiz, I.A. & Ali, A. (2007). Comparison of sucrose and sorbitol as main carbon sources in micropropagation of peach rootstock GF-677. *Pakistan Journal of Botany*, Vol.39, No.4, (August 2007), pp. 1269-1275, ISSN 2070-3368

Asano, Y.; Katsumoto, H.; Inokuma, C.; Kaneko, S.; Ito, Y. & Fujiie, A. (1996). Cytokinin and thiamine requirements and stimulative effects of riboflavin and *a*-ketoglutaric acid on embryogenic callus induction from the seeds of *Zoysiajaponica* Steud. *Journal of Plant Physiology*, Vol.149, No.3-4, pp. 413–417, ISSN 0176-1617

Ascencio-Cabral A.; Gutiérrez-Pulido, H.; Rodríguez-Garay, B. & Gutiérrez-Mora, A. (2008). Plant regeneration of *Carica papaya* L. through somatic embryogenesis in response to light quality, gelling agent and phloridzin. *Scientia Horticuturae*, Vol.2, No.118, (September 2008), pp. 155-160, ISSN 0304-4238

Aslam, J.; Mujib, A. & Sharma, M.P. (2011). Influence of freezing and non-freezing temperature on somatic embryogenesis and vinblastine production in *Catharanthus roseus* (L.) G. Don. *Acta Physiologiae Plantarum*, Vol.33, No.2, (March 2011), pp. 473-480, ISSN 1861-1664

Baker, C.M.; Muñoz-Fernandez, N. & Carter, C.D. (1999). Improved shoot development and rooting from mature cotyledons of sunflower. *Plant Cell, Tissue and Organ Culture,* Vol.58, No.1, (July 1999), pp. 39-49, ISSN 1573-5044

Beyramizade, E.; Azadi, P. &Mii, M. (2008). Optimization of factors affecting organogenesis and somatic embryogenesis of *Anthurium andreanum* Lind. 'Tera'. *Propagation of Ornamental Plants,* Vol.8, No.4, (December 2008), pp. 198-203, ISSN 1311-9109

Brand, M.H. (1993). Agar and ammonium nitrate influence hyperhydricity, tissue nitrate and total nitrogen content of service berry (*Amelanchier arborea*) shoots *in vitro. Plant Cell, Tissue and Organ Culture,* Vol.35, No.3, (December 1993), pp. 203-209, ISSN 1573-5044

Bozhkov, P.V.; Filonova, L.H. & von Arnold, S. (2002). A key developmental switch during Norway Spruce somatic embryogenesis is induced by withdrawal of growth regulators and is associated with cell death and extracellular acidification. *Biotechnology and Bioengineering,* Vol.77, No.6, (January 2002), pp 658–667, ISSN 1097-0290

Cabasson, C.; Ollitrault, P.; Côte, F.X.; Michaux-Ferrière, N.; Dambier, D.; Dalnic, R. & Teisson, C. (1995). Characteristics of *Citrus* cell culture during undifferentiated growth on sucrose and somatic embryogenesis on galactose. *Physiologia Plantarum,* Vol.93, No.3, (April 1995), pp. 464-470, ISSN 0031-9317

Capron, A.; Gourgues, M.; Neiva, L.S.; Faure, J.E.; Berger, F.; Pagnussat, G.; Krishnan, A.; Alvarez-Mejia, C.; Vielle-Calzada, J.P.; Lee, Y.R.; Liu, B. & Sundaresan, V. (2008) Maternal control of male-gamete delivery in *Arabidopsis* involves a putative GPI-anchored protein encoded by the *LORELEI* gene. *The Plant Cell,* Vol.20, No.11, (November 2008), pp. 3038-3049, ISSN 1532-298X

Castillo, B. & Smith, M.A.L. (1997). Direct somatic embryogenesis from *Begonia gracilis* explants. *Plant Cell Reports,* Vol.16, No.6, (March 1997), pp. 385–388, ISSN 1432-203X

Chen, J.T. & Chang, W.C. (2001). Effects of auxins and cytokinins on direct somatic embryogenesis on leaf explants of *Oncidium* 'Gower Ramsey'. *Plant Growth Regulation,* Vol.34, No.2, (June 2001), pp.229–232, ISSN 1435-8107

Cheong, E.J. & Pooler M.R. (2004). Factors affecting somatic embryogenesis in *Prunus incisa* cv. February Pink. *Plant Cell Reports,* Vol.22, No.11, (March 2004), pp. 810-815, ISSN 1432-203X

Choi, Y.E.; Ko, S.K.; Lee, K.S. & Yoon, E.S. (2002). Production of plantlets of *Eleutherococcus sessiliflorus* via somatic embryogenesis and successful transfer to soil. *Plant Cell, Tissue and Organ Culture,* Vol.69, No.2, (May 2002), pp. 201-204, ISSN 1573-5044

Debergh, P.; Aitken-Christie, J.; Cohen, D.; Grout, B.; von Arnold, S.; Zimmerman, R. & Ziv, M. (1992). Reconsideration of the term 'vitrification' as used in micropropagation. *Plant Cell, Tissue and Organ Culture,* Vol.30, No.2 (August 1992), pp. 135-140, ISSN 1573-5044

Dodeman, V.L.; Ducreux, G. & Kreis, M. (1997). Zygotic embryogenesis *versus* somatic embryogenesis. *Journal of Experimental Botany,* Vol.48, No.313, (August 1997), pp. 1493-1509, ISSN 1460 2431

D'Onofrio C.; Morini, S. & Bellocchi G. (1998).Effect of light quality on somatic embryogenesis of quince leaves. *Plant Cell, Tissue and Organ Culture,* Vol.53, No.2, (May 1998), pp. 91-98, ISSN 1573-5044

Fan, Y.F.; Jiang, L.; Gong, H.Q. & Liu, C.M. (2008). Sexual reproduction in higher plants I: Fertilization and the initiation of zygotic program. *Journal of Integrative Plant Biology,* Vol.50, No.7 (July 2008), pp. 860-867, ISSN 1744-7909

Feher, A. (2006). Why somatic plant cells start to form embryos?, In: *Plant Cell Monographs,* Vol. 2, Mujib, A. & Samaj, J. (Eds.), pp. 85-101, Springer-Verlag Berlin Heidelberg, Retrieved from http://www.springerlink.com/content/978-3-540-28717-9/#section=539745&page=1

Fitch, M.M. (1993). High frequency somatic embryogenesis and plant regeneration from papaya hypocotyls callus. *Plant Cell, Tissue and Organ Culture,* Vol.32, No.2, (February 2003), pp. 205-212, ISSN 1573-5044

Fitch, M.M.M.; Manshardt, R.M.; Gonsalves, D. & Slightom, J.L. (1993). Transgenic papaya plants from *Agrobacterium*-mediated transformation of somatic embryos. *Plant Cell Reports,* Vol.12, No.5, (March 1993), pp. 245-249, ISSN 0721-7714

Fu, X.P.; Yang, S.H. & Bao, M.Z. (2008). Factors affecting somatic embryogenesis in anther cultures of Chinese pink (*Dianthus chinensis*L.). *In Vitro Cellular & Developmental Biology-Plant,* Vol.44, No.3, (April 2008), pp. 194–202, ISSN 1054-5476

Gaj, M.D. (2001). Direct somatic embryogenesis as a rapid and efficient system for *in vitro* regeneration of *Arabidopsis thaliana. Plant Cell, Tissue and Organ Culture,* Vol.64, No.1, (October 2004), pp. 39-46, ISSN 1573-5044

George, E.F.; Hall, M.A. & De Klerk, G.J. (2008). *Plant Propagation by Tissue Culture* (Third Edition), AA Dordrecht, ISBN 978-1-4020-5004-6, The Netherlands

Gerdakaneh, M.A.A.; Sioseh-Mardah, A. & Sarabi, B. (2011). Effects of different amino acids on somatic embryogenesis of strawberry (*Fragaria* x *ananassa*Duch). *Acta Physiologiae Plantarum,* Vol.33, No.5, (February 2011), pp. 1847–1852, ISSN 1861-1664

Germanà, M.A.; Benedetta, C.; Calogero, I. & Rosario, M. (2005). The effect of light quality on anther culture of *Citrus clementina* Hort. ex Tan. *Acta Physiologiae Plantarum,* Vol.27, No.4, (June 2007), pp. 717-721, ISSN 1861-1664

Gilroy, S. & Trewavas, A. (2001). Signal processing and transduction in plant cells: the end of the beginning?. *Nature Reviews Molecular Cell Biology,* Vol.2, No.4, (April, 2001), pp. 307-314, ISSN 1471-0072

Giridhar, P.; Indu, E.P.; Vinod, K.; Chandrashekar, A.; Ravishankar, G.A. & Castellanos-Hernández, O.A. (2004). Direct somatic embryogenesis from *Coffea arabica* L. and *Coffea canephora* P. ex Fr. under the influence of ethylene action inhibitor-silver nitrate. *Acta Physiologiae Plantarum,* Vol.26, No.3, (September 2004), pp. 299-305, ISSN 1861-1664

Gow, W.P.; Chen, J.T. & Chang, W.C. (2009). Effects of genotype, light regime, explant position and orientation on direct somatic embryogenesis from leaf explants. *Acta Physiologiae Plantarum,* Vol.3, No.2, (November 2008), pp. 363-369, ISSN 1861-1664

Gow, W.P.; Chen, J.T. & Chang, W.C. (2010). Enhancement of direct somatic embryogenesis and plantlet growth from leaf explants of *Phalaenopsis* by adjusting culture period and explant length. *Acta Physiologiae Plantarum,* Vol.32, No.4, (December 2009), pp. 621-627, ISSN 1861-1664

Gutiérrez-Mora, A.; Ruvalcaba-Ruíz, D.; Rodríguez-Domínguez, J.M.; Loera-Quezada, M.M. & Rodríguez-Garay, B. (2004). Recent advances in the biotechnology of Agave: A cell approach, In: *Recent Research Developments in Cell Biology,* S.G. Pandalai, (Ed.), Vol.2, pp. 12-26, Transworld Research Network, ISBN 81-7895-142-8, Kerala, India.

Gutiérrez-Marcos, J.F.; Costa, L.M. & Evans, M.M.S. (2006). Maternal gametophytic baseless is required for development of the central cell and early endosperm patterning in maize (*Zea mays*). *Genetics,* Vol.174, No.1, (September 2006), pp. 317-329, ISSN 1943-2631

Hazarika, B.N. (2003). Acclimatization of tissue-cultured plants. *Current Science,* Vol.85, No.12, (December 2003) pp. 1704-1712, ISSN 0011-3891

Hazarika, B.N. & Bora, A. (2010). Hyperhydricity- A bottleneck to micropropagation of plants. *Acta Horticulturae,* Vol.865, pp. 95-101, ISBN 978-90-66053-96-0, Bangalore, India, June 30 2010

He, Y.C.; He, Y.Q.; Qu, L.H.; Sun, M.X. & Yang, H.Y. (2007). Tobacco zygotic embryogenesis in vitro: the original cell wall of the zygote is essential for maintenance of cell polarity, the apical-basal axis and typical suspensor formation. *The Plant Journal,* Vol.49, No.3, (February 2007), pp. 515-527, ISSN 1365-313X

Jausoro, V.; Lorente, B.E. & Apostolo, N.M. (2010). Structural differences between hyperhydric and normal *in vitro* shoots of *Handroanthus impetiginosus* (Mart. ex DC) Mattos (*Bignoniaceae*). *Plant Cell, Tissue and Organ Culture,* Vol.101, No.2, (May 2010), pp. 183-191, ISSN 1573-5044

Jaramillo, J. & Summers, W. (1991). Dark-light treatments influence induction of tomato anther callus. *HortScience.* Vol. 26, No.7, (July 1991), pp. 915-916, ISSN 0018-5345

Jha P.; Yadav, C.B.; Anjaiah, V. & Bhat, V. (2009). *In vitro* plant regeneration through somatic embryogenesis and direct shoot organogenesis in *Pennisetum glaucum* (L.) R. Br. *In vitro Cellular & Developmental Biology-Plant,* Vol.45, No.2, pp. 145-154, (April 2009), ISSN 1054-5476

Jiménez, V.M. (2005). Involvement of plant hormones and plant growth regulators on *in vitro* somatic embryogenesis. *Plant Growth Regulation,* Vol.47, No.2-3, (November 2005), pp. 91-110, ISSN 1573-5087

Jiménez, V.M. & Thomas, C. (2006). Participation of plant hormones in determination and progression of somatic embryogenesis, In: *Plant Cell Monographs,* Vol. 2, Mujib, A. & Samaj, J. (Eds.), pp. 103-118, Springer-Verlag Berlin Heidelberg, Retrieved from http://www.springerlink.com/content/978-3-540-28717-9/#section=539745&page=1

Kevers, C.; Coumans, M.C.; Coumans-Gillès, M.F. & Caspar, T.H. (1984). Physiological and biochemical events leading to vitrification of plants cultured *in vitro. Physiologia Plantarum,* Vol.61, No.1, (May 1984), pp. 69-74, ISSN 1399-3054

Kevers, C.; Gaspar, T.H. & Crevecoeur, M. (1985). Nature et teneur des polyamines de cals normaux et habitues de betterave sucriere. Effet des regulateurs de croissance du milieu de culture. *Botanica Helvetica,* Vol.95, pp. 117- 120, ISSN 0253-1453

Kevers, C.; Gaspar, T. & Dommes, J. (2002). The beneficial role of different auxins and polyamines at successive stages of somatic embryo formation and development of *Panax ginseng in vitro. Plant cell, Tissue and Organ Culture,* Vol.70, No.2, pp. 181-188, (August 2002), ISSN 0167-6857

Kępczyńska E. & Zielińska, S. (2011). Disturbance of ethylene biosynthesis and perception during somatic embryogenesis in *Medicago sativa* L. reduces embryos ability to regenerate. *Acta Physiologiae Plantarum*, Vol.33, No.5, (April 2011), pp. 1969-1980, ISSN 1861-1664

Khan, T.; Reddy, V.S. & Leelavathi, S. (2010). High-frequency regeneration via somatic embryogenesis of an elite recalcitrant cotton genotype (*Gossypium hirsutum* L.) and efficient *Agrobacterium*-mediated transformation. *Plant Cell, Tissue and Organ Culture*, Vol.101, No.3, (February 2010), ISSN 1573-5044

Kiviharju, E. & Pehu, E. (1998). The effect of cold and heat pretreatments on anther culture response of *Avena sativa* and *A. sterilis*. *Plant Cell, Tissue and Organ Culture*, Vol.54, No.2, (August 1998), pp. 97-104, ISSN 1573-5044

Konieczny, R.; Libik, M.; Tuleja, M.; Niewiadomska, E. & Miszalski, Z. (2008). Oxidative events during *in vitro* regeneration of sunflower. *Acta Physiologiae Plantarum*, Vol.30, No.27, (August 2007), pp. 71–79, ISSN 1861-1664

Kozai, T. (1991). Micropropagation under photoautotrophic conditions. In: *Micropropagation. Technology and Application*, Debergh, P.C., Zimmerman, R.H. (eds.), pp. 447-469, Kluwer Academic Publishers, ISBN 9780792308188, Dordrecht - Boston - London

Kumar, H.G.A.; Murthy, H.N. & Paek, K.Y. (2002). Somatic embryogenesis and plant regeneration in *Gymnema sylvestre*. *Plant Cell, Tissue and Organ Culture*, Vol.71, No.1, (October 2002), pp. 85–88, ISSN 1573-5044

Lakshmanan, P. & Taji, A. (2000). Somatic embryogenesis in leguminous plants. *Plant Biology*, Vol.2, No.2, (March 2000), pp.136–148, ISSN 1438- 8667

Letouzé, R. & Daguin, F. (1987). Control of vitrification and hypolignification process in *Salix babylonica* cultured *in vitro*. *Acta Horticulturae*, Vol.212, pp. 185-191, ISBN 978-90-66050-43-3, Gembloux, Belgium, September 1 1987

Li, L. & Qu, R. (2002). *In vitro* somatic embryogenesis in turf-type Bermuda grass: roles of abscisic acid and gibberellic acid, and occurrence of secondary somatic embryogenesis. *Plant Breeding*, Vol.121, No.2, (April 2002) pp. 155–158, ISSN 0179-9541

Liang, G.H., Xu, A. & Tang, H. (1987). Direct generation of wheat haploids via anther culture. *Crop Science*. Vol.27, No.2, (March-April 1987), pp. 336–339, ISSN 1435-0653

Lemos, E.E.P. & Baker, D.A. (1998). Shoot regeneration in response to carbon source on internodal explants of *Annona muricata* L. *Plant Growth Regulation*, Vol.25, No.2, (July 1998), pp.105–112, ISSN 1573-5087

Maene, L. & Debergh, P.C. (1987). Optimization of the transfer of tissue cultured shoots to *in vivo* conditions. *Acta Horticulturae*, Vol.12, pp. 335-348, ISBN 978-90-66050-43-3, Gembloux, Belgium, September 1 1987

Maheshwari, P. (1937). A critical review of the types of embryo sacs in angiosperms. *The New Phytologist*, Vol.36, No.5, (December 1937), pp. 359-417, ISSN 1469-8137

Malabadi, R.B.; Gangadhar, M.G.S. & Nataraja, K. (2005). *Plant* regeneration via somatic embryogenesis in *Pinus kesiya* (Royle ex. Gord.) influenced by triacontanol. *Acta Physiologiae Plantarum*, Vol.27. No.4, (August 2005), pp. 531-537, ISSN 1861-1664

Martin, K.P. (2004). Plant regeneration protocol of medicinal important *Andrographics paniculata* (Burm. F.) Wallich ex Nees via somatic embryogenesis. *In Vitro Cellular & Developmental Biology-Plant*, Vol.40. No.2, (March 2004), pp.204-209, ISSN 1054-5476

Mc Cormick, S. (2004). Control of male gametophyte development. *The Plant Cell*, Vol.16, No.1 (January 2004), pp. S142-S153, ISSN 1532-298X

Mohan, M.L. & Krishnamurthy, K.V. (2002). Somatic embryogenesis and plant regeneration in pigeon pea. *Biologia Plantarum*, Vol.45, No.1, (April, 2002), pp. 19-25, ISSN 0006-3134

Murashige, T. & Skoog. F. (1962). A revised medium for rapid growth and bio assays with tobacco cultures. *Physiologia Plantarum,* Vol.15, No.3, (July 1962), pp. 473-497, ISSN 1399-3054

Nomura, K. & Komamine, A. (1986). Somatic embryogenesis in cultured carrot cells. *Development, Growth & Differentiation*, Vol.28, No.6, (November 1986), pp. 511-517, ISSN 1440-169

Öpik, H. & Rolfe, S. (2005). Plant growth hormones In: The physiology of flowering plants. 4thedition. Willis A. J. pp.177 - 202, CAMBRIDGE, ISBN 978-0-521-66485-1, New York, USA

Pagnussat, G.C.; Alandete-Saez, M.; Bowman, J.L. & Sundaresan, V. (2009). Auxin-dependent patterning and gamete specification in the *Arabidopsis* female gametophyte. *Science*, Vol.324, No.5935 (June 2009), pp. 1684-1689, ISSN 1095-9203

Pescitelli, S. M.; Johnson, C. D. & Petolino, J. F. (1990). Isolated microspore culture of maize: effect of isolation technique, reduced temperature and sucrose level. *Plant Cell Reports,* Vol.8, No.10 (March 1990), pp.628-631, ISSN 1432-203X

Piqueras, A.; Cortian, M.; Serna, M.D. & Casa, J.L. (2002). Polyamines and hyperhydricity in micropropagated carnation plants. *Plant Science,* Vol.162, No.5, (May 2002), pp. 671-678, ISSN 0168-9452

Portillo, L.; Santacruz-Ruvalcaba, F.; Gutiérrez-Mora, A. & Rodríguez-Garay, B. (2007). Somatic embryogenesis in *Agave tequilana* Weber cultivar azul. *In Vitro Cellular and Developmental Biology - Plant*, Vol.43, No.6, (December 2007), pp. 569-575, ISSN 1054-5476

Pospíšilová, J.; Tichá, I.; Kadleček, P.; Haisel, D. & Plzáková, Š. (1999). Acclimatization of micropropagated plants to *ex vitro* conditions. *Biologia Plantarum*, Vol.42, No.4, (December 1999), pp. 481-497, ISSN 0006-3134

Rao, K.S. (1996). Embryogenesis in flowering plants: recent approaches and prospects. *Journal of Biosciences*, Vol.21, No.6, (December 1996), pp. 827-841, ISSN 0973-7138

Rasmussen, C.G.; Humphries, J.A. & Smith, L.G. (2011). Determination of symmetric and asymmetric division planes in plant cells. *Annual Review of Plant Biology,* Vol. 62, pp. 387-409, ISSN 1543-5008

Reiser, L. & Fischer, R.L. (1993). The ovule and the embryo sac. *The Plant Cell,* Vol.5, No.10, (October 1993), pp. 1291-1301, ISSN 1532-298X

Rey, H.Y. & Mgroginski, L.A. (2006). Somatic embryogenesis and plant regeneration in diploid and triploid *Arachis pintoi*. *Biologia Plantarum*, Vol.50, No.1, (December 2005), pp. 152-155, ISSN 0006-3134

Rodríguez-Garay, B.; Santacruz-Ruvalcaba, F.; Loera-Quezada, M.M. & Gutiérrez-Mora, A. (2000). Embriogénesis sexual y somática en plantas. *Horticultura Mexicana,* Vol.8, No.1 (January 2000), pp. 104-113, ISSN 0188-9761

Rodríguez-Sahagún, A.; Acevedo-Hernández, G.; Rodríguez-Domínguez, J.M.; Rodríguez-Garay, B.; Cervantes-Martínez, J. & Castellanos-Hernández, O.A. (2011). Effect of light quality and culture medium on somatic embryogenesis of *Agave tequilana* Weber var. azul. *Plant Cell, Tissue and Organ Culture*, Vol.104, No.2, (August 2010), pp. 271-275, ISSN 1573-5044

Rossetto, M.; Dixon, K.W. & Bunn, E. (1992). Aeration: a simple method to control vitrification and improve *in vitro* culture of rare Australian plants. *In Vitro Cellular & Developmental Biology-Plant*, Vol.28, No.4 (October 1994), pp. 192–196, ISSN 1054-5476

Rotman, N.; Rozier, F.; Boavida, L., Dumas, C.; Beger, F. & Faure, J.E. (2003). Female control of male gamete delivery during fertilization in *Arabidopsis thaliana*. *Current Biology*, Vol.13, No.6, (March 2003), pp. 432-436, ISSN 0960-9822

Russell, S.D. (1992). Double fertilization. *International Review of Cytology*, Vol.140, pp. 357-388, ISSN 0074-7696

Russell, S.D. (1993). The egg cell: Development and role in fertilization and early embryogenesis. *The Plant Cell*, Vol.5, No.10, (October 1993), pp. 1349-1359, ISSN 1532-298X

Rybczyński, J.J.; Borkowska, B.; Fiuk, A.; Gawrońska, H.; Śliwińska E. & Mikuła, A. (2007). Effect of sucrose concentration on photosynthetic activity of *in vitro* cultures *Gentiana kurroo* (Royle) germlings. *Acta Physiologiae Plantarum*, Vol.29, No.5, (October 2007), pp. 445-453, ISSN 1861-1664

Shehata, A.M.; Wannarat, W.; Skirvin, R.M. & Norton, M.A. (2010). The dual role of carbenicillin in shoot regeneration and somatic embryogenesis of horse radish (*Armoracia rusticana*) *in vitro*. *Plant Cell, Tissue and Organ Culture*, Vol.102, No.3, (March 2010), pp. 397–402, ISSN 1573-5044

Slater, A.; Scott, N. & Fowler, M. (2003). *Plant biotechnology: the genetic manipulation of plants*, (2nd Edition) Oxford Press University, ISBN 0199282617, Oxford, United Kingdom.

Supena, E.D.J.; Winarto, B.; Riksen, T.; Dubas, E.; van Lammeren, A.; Offringa, R.; Boutilier, K. & Custers, J. (2008). Regeneration of zygotic-like microspore-derived embryos suggests an important role for the suspensor in early embryo patterning. *Journal of Experimental Botany*, Vol.59, No.4, (March 2008), pp. 803-814, ISSN 1460-2431

Szechyńska-Hebda, M.; Skrzypek, E.; Dąbrowska, G.; Biesaga-Kościelniak, J.; Filek, M. & Wędzony, M. (2007). The role of oxidative stress induced by growth regulators in the regeneration process of wheat. *Acta Physiologiae Plantarum*, Vol.29, No.4, (April 2007), pp. 327–337, ISSN 1861-1664

Thuzar, M.; Vanavichit, A.; Tragoonrung, S. & Jantasuriyarat, C. (2011). Efficient and rapid plant regeneration of oil palm zygotic embryos cv. 'Tenera' through somatic embryogenesis. *Acta Physiologiae Plantarum*, Vol.33, No.1, (May 2010), pp. 123–128, ISSN 1861-1664

Tian, H.Q. & Russell, S.D. (1997). Calcium distribution in fertilized and unfertilized ovules and embryo sacs of *Nicotiana tabacum L. Planta*, Vol.202, No.1, (April 1997), pp. 93-105, ISSN 1432-2048

Tokuhara, K. & Mii, M. (2003). High efficient somatic embryogenesis from cell suspension cultures of *Phalaenopsis* orchids by adjusting carbohydrate sources. *In vitro Cellular & Developmental Biology-Plant*, Vol.39, No.6, (December 2006), pp. 635–639, ISSN 1054-5476

Toonen, M.A.J. & de Vries, S.C. (1996). Initiation of somatic embryos from single cells. *In:* Embryogenesis: the generation of a plant, T.L. Wang, & A. Cuming, (Eds.), pp. 173-189, Bios Scientific Oxford, ISBN 1-8599-6065-0, Oxford, United Kingdom.

Torné, J.M.; Moysset, L.; Santos, M. & Simón E. (2001). Effects of light quality on somatic embryogenesis in *Araujia sericifera*. *Physiologia Plantarum*, Vol.111, No.3, (March 2011), pp. 405-411, ISSN 1399-3054

Torres-Muñoz, L., and B. Rodríguez-Garay. (1996). Somatic embryogenesis in the threatened cactus *Turbinicarpus pseudomacrochele* (Buxbaum & Backerberg). *Journal of professional Association for Cactus Development*, Vol.1, pp. 36-38, ISSN 1938-6648

Van Huystee, R.B. (1987). Some molecular aspects of plants peroxidase biosynthetics studies. *Annual Review of Plant Physiology*, Vol.38, (June 1987), pp. 205-219, ISSN 1543-5008

Vidoz, M.L.; Rey, H.R.; Gonzalez, A.M. & Mroginski, L.A. (2004).Somatic embryogenesis and plant regeneration through leaf culture in *Arachis glabrata* (Leguminose). *Acta Physiologiae Plantarum*, Vol.26, No.1. (October 2003), pp. 59-66, ISSN 1861-1664

Wetering, K. & Russell, S.D. (2004). Experimental analysis of the fertilization process. *The Plant Cell*, Vol.16, No.1, (January 2004), pp. S107-S118, ISSN 1532-298X

Williams, R.R. & Taji, A.M. (1991). Effects of temperature, gel concentration and cytokynins on vitrification of *Olearia microdisca* (J.M. Black) *in vitro* shoots cultures. *Plant Cell, Tissue and Organ Culture*, Vol.26, No.1, (July 1991), pp. 1-6, ISSN 1573-5044

Witrzens, B.; Scowcroft, W.R; Downes, R.W. & Larkin, P.J. (1988). Tissue culture and plant regeneration from sunflower (*Helianthus annus*) and interspecific hybrids (*H. tuberosus*X *H. annus*). *Plant Cell, Tissue and Organ Culture*, Vol.13, No.1, pp. 61-76, ISSN 1573-5044

Yadegari, R. & Drews, G.N. (2004). Female gametophyte development. *The Plant Cell*, Vo.16, No.1, (January 2004), pp. S133-S141, ISSN 1532-298X

Yang, W.C.; Shi, D.Q. & Chen, Y.H. (2010). Female gametophyte development in flowering plants. *Annual Review of Plant Biology*, Vol.61, (April 2010), pp. 89-108, ISSN 1543-5008

Yeung, E.C.; Rahman, M.H. & Thorpe, T.A. (1996). Comparative development of zygotic and microspore-derived embryos in *Brassica nap*us L. cv. Topas. I. Histodifferentiation. *International Journal of Plant Sciences*, Vol.157, No.1, (January 1996), pp. 27-39, ISSN 1537 5315

Ziv, M. (1989). Enhanced shoot and cormlet proliferation in liquid cultured *Gladiolus* buds by growth retardants. *Plant Cell, Tissue and Organ Culture*, Vol.17, No.2-3, (January 1989), pp. 101-110, ISSN 183-191

Ziv, M. & Lilien- Kipnis, H. (1990). Gladiolus, In: *Handbook of Plant Cell Culture*, D.A. Evans, W.R. Shark Y.P.S. Bajaj & P.A. Ammirato (Eds.), Vol.5, pp. 461-478, McGraw Hill Publishing Co. New York, ISBN 0029490111, New York

11

Gene Expression in Embryonic Neural Development and Stem Cell Differentiation

C. Y. Irene Yan[1], Felipe M. Vieceli[1], Tatiane Y. Kanno[1],
José Antonio O. Turri[1] and Mirian A. F. Hayashi[2]
[1]*Departamento de Biologia Celular e do Desenvolvimento,*
Universidade de São Paulo (USP)
[2]*Departamento de Farmacologia,*
Universidade Federal de São Paulo (UNIFESP)
Brazil

1. Introduction

Since all cells ultimately are derived from a single cell - the fertilized egg - a complete overview on the neuron development should peruse through initial steps of neural induction in the ectoderm of the blastula embryo, and the sequential activation of the neurogenic program in the neural tube through neurite outgrowth during final differentiation step.

The concept of neural induction, i.e. the definition of the neural plate domain in the ectoderm, was first proposed by Spemman and Mangold after the classic experiment in which transplantation of the frog embryo's dorsal blastopore lip induced a complete neural axis from the acceptor embryo's ectoderm. Since then, much effort has been made aimed at identify the signals that confer the neural bias to the ectoderm. The resulting picture clearly indicates that neural induction is a multi-step process that requires the interplay of various pathways. The result of neural induction is the definition of a neural plate composed by proliferating neuroepithelial cells expressing pan-neural genes.

However, acquisition of neural bias is not sufficient to propel the neuroepithelial cell towards terminal neural differentiation path. However, acquisition of neural bias is not sufficient to propel the neuroepithelial cell towards A terminal neural differentiation path. Cell fate plasticity remains high and demands continuous reinforcement to proceed towards a specific differentiation path. The transition from proliferating precursor cell to post-mitotic state is also a highly regulated step. Thus, proneural genes have an important role, regulating both cell cycle arrest and initiation of neural differentiation.

In recent years, the potential and promise held by embryonic stem cells as a source for new cell-reposition therapies have attracted the attention of the scientific and lay community. Stem cells are, by definition, self-propagating cells that are extremely plastic and can potentially differentiate into multiple types of cells. However, the same plasticity that holds the promise of generation of multiple tissues from a single cell line is also the characteristic that makes stem cell differentiation difficult to control. This has led to intense research aimed at understanding the process of cell differentiation. More often than not, stem cell biologists have approached differentiation from a developmental biology perspective. After all, the newly-fertilized egg is a single cell at its most undifferentiated and uncommitted state, and is exposed to all the signalling events necessary for generating all the differentiated tissues of a complete organism.

In support of this, several of the embryonic proneural genes and signalling pathways are also present during induction of ES-cell neural differentiation. An example of a protein that is active both in normal development and ES-cell differentiation is Ndel1. Ndel1 is a microtubule associated neuronal protein, which has been shown to be essential for neuronal differentiation and cell migration during the central nervous system development. Albeit the abundant literature on its functional role, expression modulation and protein positioning during the neuronal differentiation process, marginal attention has been paid for its localization and function in early neuronal development step. More recently, we have also demonstrated that its enzymatic activity plays an essential role in neurite outgrowth in differentiating PC12 cells. The Ndel1 gene expression modulation during the neuronal differentiation has been intensively studied and its expression in pluripotent ES cells undergoing neuronal differentiation has also been explored. Taken together, all these data strongly suggests that Ndel1 is a relevant component in the embryogenesis of the nervous system and in the differentiation of cells to neuronal phenotype.

2. Embryonic neural induction

The neural lineage derives from the ectodermal germ layer, which in turn originates through gastrulation from the epiblast. The ectoderm also gives rise to the epidermal lineage, and one of the first events that define the neural lineage is the choice between these two cell fates: neural or epidermal. Both lineages must be delimited both molecularly and anatomically. The earliest time point when we can detect this segregation is at the pre-gastrula epiblast. The epiblast receives signals that will generate a neural bias. Thereafter, this bias is progressively stabilized during neural specification and finally, the neural region is patterned in the three axes. Thus, neural induction can be subdivided into the response of the epiblast to neuralizing signals by adopting a neural bias at its central region, and the progressive stabilization of this bias through additional signals. Much of what we have learned about these events was gathered from experiments in the chick and amphibian embryo.

The precise stage at which the epiblast first demonstrates that it is competent to follow neural fate has been progressively pushed back as more molecular markers have become available. For instance, the early neural marker Sox3 and late marker Sox2 have been used as standard indicators of neural bias and specification (Fernandez-Garre et al., 2002; Rex et al., 1997; Streit et al., 2000, 1997; Uchikawa, 2003; Wood & Episkopou, 1999). These two genes have slightly different temporal expression pattern with an overlap at the neural induction stage. Sox3 is detected throughout the epiblast before neural induction in pre-gastrula embryos and becomes restricted to the future neuroepithelium as development progresses. Sox2 is first detected around the time when neural induction is believed to occur and thereafter its expression is limited to the neuroepithelium (Muhr et al., 1999; Rex et al., 1997).

The induction of neural fate in the ectoderm for a long time was claimed to be the 'default' fate, where the absence of additional extracellular signals is sufficient to drive towards neural bias. This model was mainly sustained on data obtained from dissociated amphibian ectodermal cell cultures (Wilson & Hemmati-Brivanlou, 1995). The mainstay of this model was that activation of ectodermal BMP signalling pathway conferred an epidermal bias. Thus, neural bias could be promoted by the absence signalling; i.e. inhibition of BMP signalling either through the addition of extracellular BMP inhibitors (e.g. Chordin, Noggin) or decrease of extracellular BMP concentration through dilution (Wilson & Hemmati-Brivanlou, 1995; reviewed in Almeida et al., 2010).

Lately, the default model has been modified by experiments done in whole avian and amphibian embryos. The current model sustains that ectopic expression of Sox2 and Sox3 and other neural bias markers is achieved when there is concomitant inhibition of BMP and stimulation of FGF signalling (Linker & Stern, 2004). In this revised model, FGF is an early neural inducer that acts by counteracting BMP signalling in the epiblast (Pera et al., 2003; Streit et al., 2000; Wilson et al., 2000, 2001). Thereafter, the presence of extracellular BMP inhibitors such as Chordin is required to maintain and stabilize the neuroepithelium's neural bias during gastrulation (Streit et al., 1998).

3. Cell cycle exit and neurogenic differentiation

The vertebrate neuroepithelium starts with a relatively small number of proliferative progenitor cells. At early developmental stages, progenitor cells proliferate rapidly through symmetric division and give rise only to additional progenitor cells, thus increasing the population of progenitor cells. Vertebrate neurons are generated in the ventricular zone, an epithelial layer that delimits the ventricles. Proliferation at the ventricular zone occurs in an unsynchronized fashion and is characterized by the process known as the interkinetic nuclear migration (Hayes & Nowakowski, 2000). This movement spans the apical-basal cell axis and positions the nucleus at the basal side during the G1 and S phase of mitosis and at the apical side during G2 and M phases (reviewed in Latasa et al. 2009). Once a certain critical mass is attained, the neuroepithelium produces neurons through asymmetric neurogenic divisions. In this scenario, one daughter cell remains proliferative and maintains the neuroblast pool, while the other arrests from the cell cycle and proceeds towards neurogenic differentiation to populate the central nervous system. The difference in fate is given by unequal distribution of proteins amongst the daughter cells, which will direct towards self-renewal or differentiation. The mechanism that controls this asymmetric distribution is still being investigated.

One of the hypotheses is that the choice between symmetric and asymmetric segregation depends on the position of the mitotic spindle. This proposal derives from results obtained in the ferret cortex. In this model system, asymmetrical cell division is determined by the position of the mitotic spindle relative to the apical surface of the neuroepithelium (Chenn & McConnell, 1995). When the cleavage plane is perpendicular, both daughter cells inherit equal portions of apical and basal membrane, thus generating proliferating progenitor cells symmetrically. Conversely, when the mitotic spindle is parallel, the unequal distribution of apical and basal membranes amongst the daughter cells leads to the birth of an apically-located proliferating progenitor and a basally-located postmitotic progenitor (Chenn & McConnell, 1995). However, in other vertebrates, the role of mitotic spindle positioning in determining the balance between asymmetric and symmetric division has been controversial (Konno et al., 2008; reviewed in Shioi et al., 2009; Zigman et al., 2005). The discrepancies observed in the various reports could be attributed to technical difficulties in imaging the apical domain of the pseudostratified neuroepithelial cells of the mammalian embryo. Irrespective of the role of mitotic spindle in the control of symmetric and asymmetric cell division, it is a consensus that the distinct cell fates arise from the asymmetric distribution of cellular components. As such, the PAR polarity proteins have been recently associated with unequal segregation of the progenitor cell components (Bultje et al., 2009; Ossipova et al., 2009; Tabler et al., 2010).

Naturally, the question arises about the nature of the proteins that direct towards self-renewal or differentiation of the neural progenitor cells. The cell-surface transmembrane Notch receptor has an evolutionary conserved role in determining cell-fate specification (reviewed in Pierfelice et al., 2011). Overwhelming evidence has indicated that Notch signalling is one of the main players in regulating the choice between proliferation and differentiation in the vertebrate nervous system. Activation of the Notch pathway is regulated by cell-cell signalling. In brief, Notch receptors are activated by Delta-like or Jagged proteins expressed on the membranes of neighbouring cells. Receptor activation results in the cleavage of the intracellular domain of Notch, its translocation to the nucleus and transcription of target genes. Of these, the Hes family of basic helix-loop-helix (bHLH) transcription factors has been consistently associated with the repression of proneural transcription factors expression, and consequently of neural differentiation. Thus, cells whose Notch pathway is triggered will remain in mitosis at the ventricular zone (Akai et al., 2005; Hammerle & Tejedor, 2007; Kawaguchi et al., 2008; Latasa et al., 2009; Le Roux et al., 2003). Conversely, inhibition of Notch signalling removes progenitor cells from mitosis (Hammerle & Tejedor, 2007). In other words, the Notch signalling pathway is intimately related to the binary cell fate choice between proliferation and differentiation. Although inhibition of Notch signalling is required for cell cycle arrest (Kawaguchi et al., 2008), it is insufficient to drive differentiation. Overexpression of the truncated form of the Delta ligand or of the Notch receptor induces cell cycle arrest, but does not increase the proportion of cells expressing differentiation markers (Akai et al., 2005; Hammerle & Tejedor, 2007).

4. The neurogenic transcriptional cascade

The transition from proliferative to postmitotic neuron is a highly-regulated multi-stepped process. Initiation of neurogenic differentiation requires expression of proneural bHLH transcription factors such as Neurogenin 1 and 2, which trigger a transcriptional cascade that culminates in the expression of terminal differentiation genes (Bertrand et al., 2002). Several of the vertebrate proneural genes were identified through homology with Drosophila achaete-scute (asc) and atonal (ato) family of genes. Overexpression of the orthologues of the asc (Xash1; Talikka et al., 2002) or ato (XNgnr1; Ma et al., 1996) induces ectopic neurogenesis and expression of downstream neurogenic bHLH transcription factors (Lin et al., 2004; Ma et al., 1996).

However, instead of generating multiple neural lineages, the overexpression of a single vertebrate proneural gene affects only specific neural subsets. For instance, Mash1-/- mice display severe defects in neurogenesis in the ventral telencephalon and the olfactory sensory epithelium (Casarosa et al., 1999; Horton et al., 1999). Similarly, Neurogenin1 (Ngn1) or

Neurogenin2 (Ngn2) single-mutant mice lack cranial sensory ganglia while Ngn1/2 double mutants also lack components of the peripheral nervous system (Fode et al., 1998; Ma et al., 1998, 1999). The complexity of the phenotypes generated confirm the diversity of existing genetic programs underlying the development of each neuronal subtype and implies that the importance of a single bHLH factor depends on the neural cell lineage (Powell & Jarman, 2008). This emphasizes the importance of using a wide array of marker genes to identify progression of neural differentiation, as a single proneural gene might not be involved in the differentiation of the neural lineage under investigation. Furthermore, it has important implications for experimental approaches that aim to direct the *in vitro* differentiation of stem cell lines.

Vertebrate proneural genes are first expressed, while precursor cells are still at the ventricular zone. Indeed, several of the above-mentioned proneural genes expression is regulated by the Delta-Notch pathway (Kageyama et al., 2008; Ma et al., 1996). However, neural differentiation does not occur in the ventricular zone. Rather, postmitotic neural precursors undergo migration towards outer layers of the neural tube. Proneural bHLH proteins are also involved in this migratory behaviour. Overexpression of Neurogenin1, Neurogenin2, NeuroD and Mash1 increases progenitor cell migration in the mouse cortex and regulates the expression of the cytoskeleton-regulating GTPases RhoA (Ge et al., 2006).

An anatomical consequence of this migratory behaviour coupled to differentiation is the organization of neural tube in distinct cell layers, compartmentalizing differentiation stages progressively in concentric layers, where internal layers harbour younger, more undifferentiated precursors and more external layers contain more mature neurons. This spatial organization facilitates the positioning of marker genes in the neurogenic programs hierarchy. For instance, Notch pathway receptor and ligand genes are expressed in the ventricular zone (Fig. 1; Le Roux et al., 2003; Myat et al., 1996) In contrast, consistent with

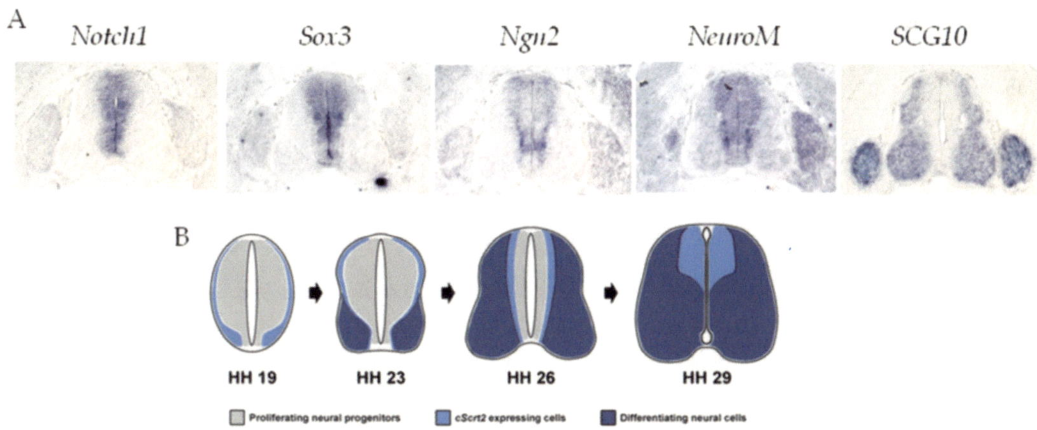

Fig. 1. Progression of neural differentiation is associated with more external layers of the neural tube. A) *In situ* hybridization for markers for proliferation (Notch1), transition between proliferation and cell cycle arrest (Sox3 and Ngn2), postmitotic differentiation (NeuroM) and late differentiation (SCG10) in chick HH26 truncal neural tube. B) Diagram summarizing the anatomical changes in the different differentiation compartments.

their role in initiating differentiation, Sox3 and Neurogenin1 are expressed at the ventricular layer and slightly beyond the proliferative zone as well (Fig. 1; Bylund et al., 2003). Ath3/NeuroM is mainly expressed by post-mitotic neural precursors, and the expression domain borders the external perimeter of Neurogenin1 and Sox3 (Fig. 1; Roztocil et al., 1997). This domain is also known as the intermediate layer and contains neural progenitors in the early stages of differentiation. Other markers for this stage include the RNA-binding protein Hu and the RNA splicing factor NeuN/Fox3 (Dent et al., 2010; Kim et al., 2009; Wakamatsu & Weston, 1997). Finally, the late differentiation marker SCG10 is expressed by cells at the outer border (mantle layer) of the neural tube (Fig. 1; Stein et al., 1988).

SCG10 encodes a membrane-associated protein associated with the growth cones of developing neurons (Stein et al., 1988). Its presence in the developing neural tube correlates with the onset of late differentiation events such as neuritogenesis. An additional marker that is widely used to characterize post-mitotic differentiating neurons is beta III tubulin (recognized by the monoclonal antibody Tuj1; Lewis & Cowan, 1988; Lee et al., 1990; Menezes and Luskin, 1994).

In the chick embryo truncal neural tube, beta III tubulin presence is particularly strong at the developing ventral root, corresponding to axons emitted by the motor neurons in the ventral lateral regions of the tube (Fig. 2). Thereafter, its presence becomes increasingly prevalent and can be detected in the outer mantle layer and in the developing dorsal root ganglions (Fig. 2). Beta III tubulin has been associated with the emergence of stable microtubule cytoskeletal scaffolds in axons and dendrite, suggesting that beta III tubulin is required for neurite maintenance (Ferreira and Caceres, 1992). Indeed, neurons with decreased levels of beta III tubulin have shorter neurites (Tucker et al., 2008). However, Tuj-1 immunoreactivity is not limited to neurons undergoing neuritogenesis. Beta III tubulin is also present in cells that are migrating from the ventricular and subventricular zone (O´Rourke et al., 1997).

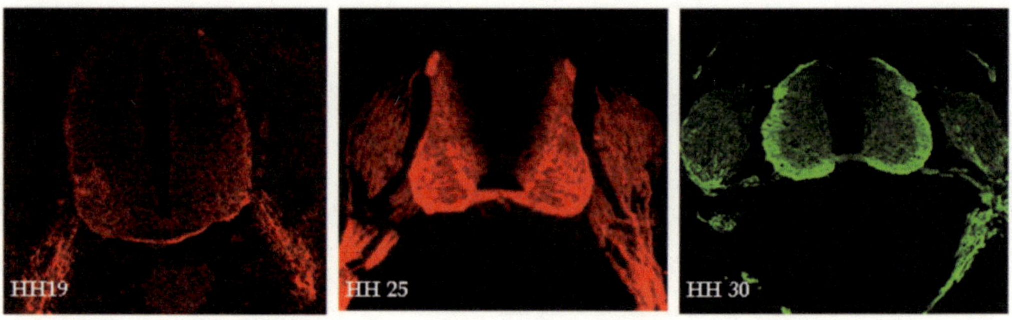

Fig. 2. Evolution of beta III tubulin expression in the chick truncal neural tube. Beta III tubulin was detected by immunohistochemistry with the monoclonal antibody Tuj1. The above staining shows that beta III tubulin is first detected in the motorneurons neurites that comprise the ventral root (HH19) and in some outer peripheral neurites. Thereafter, expression progresses so as to expand towards inner layers as well. At HH25, a strong immunofluorescent signal can be seen at the ventral motorneuron domain, ventral root and dorsal root ganglion. At HH30, beta III tubulin is clearly present in the axons of the outer mantle layer and is only excluded from the innermost layer that borders the ventricular region.

Consistent with the importance of microtubule cytoskeleton in the latter stages of neural differentiation, several microtubule-associated proteins such as MAP2 and Tau are also up-regulated. MAP2 and MAP1B double knockout mice have fiber tract malformations and retarded neuronal migration. Additionally, primary neuronal cultures derived from these mice display reduced neurite outgrowth (Teng et al., 2001).

5. Stem cell neural differentiation recapitulates embryogenesis

In vitro differentiation of embryonic stem cells into neural lineages aims to recapitulate the multistep process - from induction to terminal differentiation - of neural embryogenesis described above. Indeed as in embryonic epiblast induction, some cell lines, neural induction is more efficiently induced by the combination of fibroblast growth factor (FGF) signalling and bone morphogenetic protein (BMP) inhibition (LaVaute et al., 2009; Tropepe et al., 2001; Ying et al., 2003). In these reports, the endogenous production of BMP inhibitors was sufficient to avoid epidermal fate. However, conservation of embryogenic signalling is not a rule for all cell lines. Some iPSCs (induced Pluripotent Stem Cells) do not improve their neural differentiation rate with FGF signalling and/or BMP inhibition (Hu et al., 2010). Thus, the extent of recall of embryogenesis in these experimental paradigms is still an open question and begs for future analysis.

There are multiple protocols for *in vitro* neural induction and the depth of analysis regarding similarity with embryogenesis varies. Some groups provide a detailed comparison with embryogenesis. For instance, Abranches and collaborators report expression of Sox genes during the early phases of induced differentiation, interkinetic nuclear migration and Notch-signalling and subsequent expression of the postmitotic neural (Hu) and glial markers (GFAP) (Abranches et al., 2009). However, most reports concentrate on the detection of late developmental neural markers such as MAP2, Tau, NeuN and beta III tubulin, which have been generally accepted in the community as indication for stem cell neuronal differentiation (Tropepe et al., 2001).

For instance, Kerkis and collaborators detected the presence microtubule-associated proteins (MAPs), such as Lis1 and Ndel1, as neural markers at early stages of *in vitro* model for neuronal differentiation from pluripotent stem cells (Kerkis et al., 2011).

6. Lis1 and Ndel1: Microtubule associated proteins involved in neural development

The microtubule associated proteins (MAPs), Lis1 and Ndel1 are involved in neuronal differentiation and cell migration during the CNS development.

Lis1, also known as platelet-activating factor acetylhydrolase (PAF-AH), regulates microtubule function and is essential for proper neuronal migration during cortical development (Arai, 2002). Mutations in Lis1 gene have been associated with neuronal migration defects and abnormal layering of the cortex (Reiner et al., 1995; Saillour et al., 2009; Youn et al., 2009). For instance, haploinsufficiency of Lis1 alone causes congenital malformation of brain folds and grooves, i.e. lissencephaly. Lis 1 microdeletion is also part of the genetic causes of Miller-Dieker syndrome (MDS; Miller, 1963; Dieker et al., 1969; Reiner et al., 1993). Besides lissencephaly, MDS patients also present hypoplasic corpus callosum. Together, these data underscore the importance of Lis1 in proper neuronal migration and axon formation.

In support of the importance of Lis1 in neural development, Lis1-binding protein Ndel1 (Nuclear-distribution Element like-1) also plays a relevant role in the proper establishment of the nervous system. Lis1 and Ndel1 co-localize predominantly in the centrosome in early neuroblasts, and later, redistribute to axons during neuronal development (Shu et al., 2004; Guo et al., 2006; Bradshaw et al., 2008; Hayashi et al., 2010). The direct association of Lis1 with the Ndel1 fungal homologue was first shown in 2000 (Kitagawa et al., 2000), and soon after the interaction with the mammalian homologue was also demonstrated (Sweeney et al., 2001).

Ndel1 is also known as endooligopeptidase A or EOPA and was first isolated due to its ability to inactivate bioactive peptides. Ndel1/EOPA, is a thiol-sensitive enzyme inactivates physiologically important peptides such as bradykinin and neurotensin, and also converts opioid oligopeptides into enkephalins (Camargo et al., 1973, 1983, 1987; Gomes et al., 1993; Hayashi et al., 2000, 2005). The contribution of bradykinin and neurotensin neuropeptides in neurite outgrowth was also previously described (Zhao et al., 2003; Tischler et al., 1991; Robson and Burgoyne, 1989; Tischler et al., 1984).

In normal cortical development Ndel1 is involved in microtubule organization, nuclear translocation and neuronal positioning (Shu et al., 2004; Youn et al., 2009; Bradshaw et al., 2011). Knockdown or ablation of cortical Ndel1 function also results in impaired migration of neocortical projection neurons (Sasaki et al., 2005; Youn et al., 2009). Deletion of Ndel1 by RNAi leads to deficits in neuronal positioning and uncouples the centrosome from the nucleus, resulting in aberrant neuronal migration (Shu et al., 2004). Ndel1 homozygous knockout mice have similar deficits in neuronal positioning (Sasaki et al., 2005; Youn et al., 2009).

7. Expression of Ndel1 in the developing CNS and ES cells

Consistent with its importance in the development of the nervous system and its association with the microtubule cytoskeleton, Ndel1 domain of expression in the developing embryonic neural tube coincides with that of beta III tubulin in the outer mantle zone (Fig. 3). As mentioned in previous sections, the expression of beta III tubulin in post-mitotic cells is associated with neurons that are migrating or emmiting neurites. Thus, the co-localization shown here suggests that Ndel1 is involved in these processes as well in the chick developing neural tube.

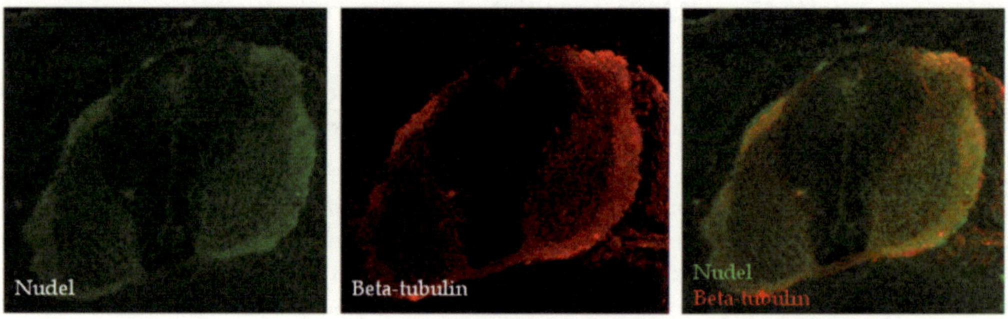

Fig. 3. Ndel1 expression co-localizes with beta III tubulin in the mantle zone of the embryonic neural tube. Immunofluorescence of adjacent slices of HH 30 embryos truncal neural tube with monoclonal anti-Ndel1 and anti beta III tubulin (Tuj1) antibodies. The overlay at the rightmost figure is provided for comparative purposes only.

Likewise, the dynamics of Ndel1 localization in stem cells during neural differentiation suggests that it is recruited for neurite extension. In undifferentiated ES cells, both Lis1 and Ndel1 show a perinuclear co-localization (Hayashi et al., 2011). In contrast, after the onset of neuronal differentiation, Lis1 presents a cytoplasmic and Ndel1 a perinuclear localization. Following differentiation, both Lis1 and Ndel1 co-localize in the outgrowing neurites (Kerkis et al., 2011).

The presence of Ndel1 persists in adult brains. Northern blot analysis confirmed its preferential expression in the rabbit and rodent CNS (Hayashi et al., 1996; 2000), although this could not be confirmed for humans (Guerreiro et al., 2005). Later, the presence of Ndel1 in the adult brain was confirmed by *in situ* hybridization studies, with higher expression in some regions, such as the hippocampus, cerebellum, and basal nucleus of Meynert (Hayashi et al., 2001). This study provided a basis for phenotypic identification of Ndel1-expressing neurons throughout the rat brain and showed a correlation between the distribution of Ndel1 neurons and systems responsible for motor, sensory, endocrine, and possibly for other functions. Together, these expression patterns argue in favour of a role for Ndel1 in neurite growth and maintenance.

8. *In vitro* assays for Ndel1 cellular function

As mentioned previously, clinical correlation data suggested strongly that Lis1 and Ndel1 are involved in neuronal migration during cortical layer formation. Lis1 and Ndel1 participate in nuclear and centrosomal transport in migrating neurons (Shu et al., 2004; Tsai et al., 2005). Additionally, they influence centrosome positioning in migrating non-neuronal cells (Dujardin et al., 2003; Stehman et al., 2007; Shen et al., 2008). Moreover, dominant negative overexpression of either the enzymatic active form of Ndel1 or its orthologue mNudE disrupted CNS lamination in *Xenopus laevis* embryos (Hayashi et al., 2004; Feng et al., 2000).

In an attempt to elucidate the exact role of Lis1 and Ndel1 in neuronal migration during cortical layer formation, we have used long-term adherent neurosphere cultures to mimic the development of cortical layers *in vitro* (Hayashi et al., 2011). In this experimental model, the neuropsheres grow for two weeks without splitting and the resulting aggregates present an inner core that would correspond to the inner cortical layer where migrating neurons originate from, and an outer layer that harbors neurons that finished their migration. In this experimental paradigm, a significant variation in spatial distribution of Lis1 and Ndel1 proteins was observed (Kerkis et al., 2011). Lis1, but not Ndel1, was detected in the rosette cells localized at the inner part of the cellular aggregates. In contrast, co-localization of both Lis1 and Ndel1 was observed in the cells at the peripheral layer of the cellular aggregates (Kerkis et al., 2011). Although further analysis with other MAPs would provide a better picture of the role of Lis1 and Ndel1 in neuronal migration during establishment of cortical layers, these data nonetheless indicate that these two proteins play a differential role in the establishment and maintenance of neuronal layers.

The role of Ndel1 in neurite outgrowth has been better characterized. Knockdown of Ndel1 expression in rat pheochromocytoma PC12 cell line inhibits neurite outgrowth. This inhibition can be rescued by wild-type Ndel1 ($Ndel1_{WT}$), but not by a mutant ($Ndel1_{mut273}$), which does not have enzymatic activity (Hayashi et al., 2010). This result indicates that

Ndel1 enzymatic activity plays a crucial role in neurite outgrowth. In support to this, a significant increase of Ndel1 promoter activity during the period of maximal neurite outgrowth was observed (Hayashi et al., 2010).

Clearly, the expression of Ndel1 shows strong correlation with the onset of various aspects of embryonic neural development and ES cells and PC12 cells neural differentiation. Thus, we directed our attention towards cis-regulatory elements that could regulate neuro-specific Ndel1 expression in a variety of experimental models.

9. Control of Ndel1 expression

The promoter of both rabbit and human Ndel1 gene was analyzed by the group in cultured cell lines. Interestingly, the Ndel1 promoter activity was shown to be very different in neuronal and non-neuronal cells, with a stronger activity in NH15 neuronal compared to C6 glial cells for the rabbit full-length promoter, thus confirming the preferential neuronal expression of. However, such difference was not observed for the human full-length promoter under the same conditions (Guerreiro et al., 2005).

We've isolated the rabbit promoter fragment -888/-744 as the region responsible for determining the neuronal-specific expression. This DNA segment contains potential binding motifs for the CP2 and SRY (sex-determining region Y) transcription factors. SRY is the founding member of the Sox (Sry-related HMG box) gene family (Sekido, 2010). Moreover, strong negative regulator elements were found within positions -755/-450 and -314/-245 in both human and rabbit promoters. Of these, at least one common negative cis-regulating region seems to be acting in the control Ndel1 expression in both species (Guerreiro et al., 2005). During neural development, these elements may restrict Ndel1 promoter activity to a neuronal subtype or a specific period of differentiation.

In the human Ndel1 promoter, the critical regulatory domain lies between -314/-245. Within this region we also found a single putative binding site for a member of the Sox transcription factor family. It is tempting to speculate on the identity of members of the Sox family, which now number more than 20, that regulate Ndel1 expression (Lefebvre et al., 2007). There are certain members of the Sox family, which we could speculatively nominate as candidates to mediate the increased expression of Ndel1. For instance, accumulated evidence has shown that Sox 11 is relevant for neurite outgrowth. As Neuro2a cells undergo retinoic acid-induced neuronal differentiation, Sox 11 levels increase significantly. Conversely, RNAi knockdown of Sox 11 inhibits axon outgrowth in Neuro2a cells, Dorsal Root Ganglion neurons and regeneration in nerve injury models (Jankowski et al., 2006; Jankowski et al., 2009).

10. Conclusion

Microtubule-associated proteins (MAPs) are essential for neuronal differentiation and cell migration during the central nervous system (CNS) development and also in the adult nervous system. In particular the distribution and role of lissencephaly (Lis1) and nuclear distribution element-like (Ndel1) allows the comparison between neural differentiation in stem cells and during embryo development. They are very powerful tools not only due to their putative role as expression markers of the differentiation process, but also due to their confirmed role in the cell maturation and migration processes. Furthermore, the study of cis-regulatory regions that confer neural-specificity to Ndel1 expression can increase our understanding of gene expression control during neural differentiation.

11. Acknowledgment

The authors are grateful for the continuous support by Fundação de Amparo à Pesquisa do Estado de São Paulo (FAPESP) and Conselho Nacional de Desenvolvimento Científico e Tecnológico (CNPq).

12. References

Abranches, E.; Silva, M.; Pradier, L.; Schulz, H.; Hummel, O.; Henrique, D. & Bekman, E. (2009). Neural differentiation of embryonic stem cells in vitro: a road map to neurogenesis in the embryo. *PLoS One*, Vol. 4(7), e6286.

Akai, J.; Halley, P.A. & Storey, K.G. (2005). FGF-dependent Notch signaling maintains the spinal cord stem zone. *Genes & Development*, Vol. 19(23), pp. 2877-2887.

Arai H. (2002). Platelet-activating factor acetylhydrolase. *Prostaglandins Other Lipid Mediat.*, Vol. 68-69, pp 83-94. Review.

Almeida, K.L.; Abreu, J.G. & Yan, C.Y.I. (2010). Neural Induction. In: *Perspectives of Stem Cells-From Tools for Studying Mechanisms of Neuronal Differentiation towards Therapy*, H. Ulrich, (Org.), Dordresch: Springer, ISBN 978-90-481-3374-1.

Bertrand, N.; Castro, D.S. & Guillemot, F. (2002). Proneural genes and the specification of neural cell types. *Nature Reviews Neuroscience*, Vol. 3(7), pp. 517-530.

Bradshaw, N.J.; Ogawa, F.; Antolin-Fontes, B.; Chubb, J.E.; Carlyle, B.C.; Christie, S.; Claessens, A.; Porteous, D.J. & Millar, J.K. (2008). DISC1, PDE4B, and NDE1 at the centrosome and synapse. *Biochemical and Biophysical Research Communications*, Vol. 377(4), pp. 1091-1096. Erratum in: *Biochemical and Biophysical Research Communications*, Vol. 384(3), pp. 400 (2009).

Bradshaw, N.J.; Soares, D.C.; Carlyle, B.C.; Ogawa, F.; Davidson-Smith, H.; Christie, S.; Mackie, S.; Thomson, P.A.; Porteous, D.J. & Millar, J.K. (2011). PKA phosphorylation of NDE1 is DISC1/PDE4 dependent and modulates its interaction with LIS1 and NDEL1. *J Neurosci*. Vol. 31(24), pp. 9043-54.

Brandon, N.J.; Handford, E.J.; Schurov, I.; Rain, J.C.; Pelling, M.; Duran-Jimeniz, B.; Camargo, L.M.; Oliver, K.R.; Beher, D.; Shearman, M.S. & Whiting, P.J. (2004). Disrupted in Schizophrenia 1 and Nudel form a neurodevelopmentally regulated protein complex: implications for schizophrenia and other major neurological disorders. *Molecular and Cellular Neurosciences*, Vol. 25(1), pp. 42-55.

Bultje, R.S.; Castaneda-Castellanos, D.R.; Jan, L.Y.; Jan, Y.N.; Kriegstein, A.R. & Shi, S.H. (2009). Mammalian Par3 regulates progenitor cell asymmetric division via notch signaling in the developing neocortex. *Neuron*, Vol. 63(2), pp. 189-202.

Burdick, K.E.; Kamiya, A.; Hodgkinson, C.A.; Lencz, T.; DeRosse, P.; Ishizuka, K.; Elashvili, S.; Arai, H.; Goldman, D.; Sawa, A. & Malhotra, A.K. (2008). Elucidating the relationship between DISC1, NDEL1 and NDE1 and the risk for schizophrenia:

evidence of epistasis and competitive binding. *Hum. Mol. Genet.*, Vol. 17, pp. 2462–2473.

Bylund, M.; Andersson, E.; Novitch, B.G. & Muhr, J. (2003). Vertebrate neurogenesis is counteracted by Sox1-3 activity. *Nature Neuroscience*, Vol. 6(11), pp. 1162-1168.

Camargo, A.C.; Shapanka, R. & Greene, L.J. (1973). Preparation, assay, and partial characterization of a neutral endopeptidase from rabbit brain. *Biochemistry*, Vol. 12(9), pp. 1838-1844.

Camargo, A.C.; Caldo, H. & Emson, P.C. (1983). Degradation of neurotensin by rabbit brain endo-oligopeptidase A and endo-oligopeptidase B (proline-endopeptidase). *Biochemical and Biophysical Research Communications*, Vol. 116(3), pp. 1151-1159.

Camargo, A.C.; Oliveira, E.B.; Toffoletto, O.; Metters, K.M. & Rossier, J. (1987). Brain endo-oligopeptidase A, a putative enkephalin converting enzyme. *Journal of Neurochemistry*, Vol. 48(4), pp. 1258-1263.

Casarosa, S.; Fode, C. & Guillemot, F. (1999). Mash1 regulates neurogenesis in the ventral telencephalon. *Development*, Vol.126(3), pp. 525-534.

Chenn, A. & McConnell, S.K. (1995). Cleavage orientation and the asymmetric inheritance of Notch1 immunoreactivity in mammalian neurogenesis. *Cell*, Vol. 82(4), pp. 631-641.

Dent, M.A.; Segura-Anaya, E.; Alva-Medina, J. & Aranda-Anzaldo, A. (2010). NeuN/Fox-3 is an intrinsic component of the neuronal nuclear matrix. *FEBS Letters*, Vol. 584(13), pp. 2767-2771.

Dieker, H.; Edwards, R.H.; Zurhein, G.; Chou, S.M.; Hartman, H.A. & Optiz, J.M. (1969). The lissencephaly syndrome. *Birth Defects*, Vol. 5, pp. 53-64.

Dobyns, W.B.; Stratton, R.F. & Greenberg, F. (1984). Syndromes with lissencephaly. I: Miller-Dieker and Norman-Roberts syndromes and isolated lissencephaly. *Am J Med Genet.*, Vol. 18(3), pp. 509-26.

Duan, X.; Chang, J.H.; Ge, S.; Faulkner, R.L.; Kim, J.Y.; Kitabatake, Y.; Liu, X.B.; Yang, C.H.; Jordan, J.D.; Ma, D.K.; Liu, C.Y.; Ganesan, S.; Cheng, H.J.; Ming, G.L.; Lu, B. & Song, H. (2007). Disrupted-In-Schizophrenia 1 regulates integration of newly generated neurons in the adult brain. *Cell*, Vol. 130(6), pp. 1146-58.

Dujardin, D.L.; Barnhart, L.E.; Stehman, S.A.; Gomes, E.R.; Gundersen, G.G. & Vallee, R.B. (2003). A role for cytoplasmic dynein and LIS1 in directed cell movement. *J Cell Biol.*, Vol. 163(6), pp. 1205-11.

Faulkner, N.E.; Dujardin, D.L.; Tai, C.Y.; Vaughan, K.T.; O'Connell, C.B.; Wang, Y. & Vallee, R.B. (2000). A role for the lissencephaly gene LIS1 in mitosis and cytoplasmic dynein function. *Nat Cell Biol.*, Vol. 2(11), pp. 784-91.

Feng, Y.; Olson, E.C.; Stukenberg, P.T.; Flanagan, L.A.; Kirschner, M.W. & Walsh, C.A. (2000). LIS1 regulates CNS lamination by interacting with mNudE, a central component of the centrosome. *Neuron*, Vol. 28(3), pp. 665-79.

Fernández-Garre, P.; Rodríguez-Gallardo, L.; Gallego-Díaz, V.; Alvarez, I.S. & Puelles, L. (2002). Fate map of the chicken neural plate at stage 4. *Development*, Vol. 129(12), pp. 2807-2822.

Fode, C.; Gradwohl, G.; Morin, X.; Dierich, A.; LeMeur, M.; Goridis, C. & Guillemot, F. (1998). The bHLH protein NEUROGENIN 2 is a determination factor for epibranchial placode-derived sensory neurons. *Neuron*, Vol. 20(3), pp. 483-494.

Ge, W.; He, F.; Kim, K.J.; Blanchi, B.; Coskun, V.; Nguyen, L.; Wu, X.; Zhao, J.; Heng, J.I.; Martinowich, K.; Tao, J.; Wu, H.; Castro, D.; Sobeih, M.M.; Corfas, G.; Gleeson, J.G.; Greenberg, M.E.; Guillemot, F. & Sun, Y.E. (2006). Coupling of cell migration with neurogenesis by proneural bHLH factors. *PNAS*, Vol. 103(5), pp. 1319-1324.

Gomes, M.D.; Juliano, L.; Ferro, E.S.; Matsueda, R.; Camargo, A.C. (1993). Dynorphin-derived peptides reveal the presence of a critical cysteine for the activity of brain endo-oligopeptidase A. *Biochem. Biophys. Res. Commun.* Vol. 197(2), pp. 501-507.

Guerreiro, J.R.; Winnischofer, S.M.; Bastos, M.F.; Portaro, F.C.; Sogayar, M.C.; de Camargo, A.C. & Hayashi, M.A. (2005). Cloning and characterization of the human and rabbit NUDEL-oligopeptidase promoters and their negative regulation. *Biochimica et Biophysica Acta*, Vol. 1730(1), pp. 77-84.

Guo, J.; Yang, Z.; Song, W.; Chen, Q.; Wang, F.; Zhang, Q. & Zhu, X. (2006). Nudel contributes to microtubule anchoring at the mother centriole and is involved in both dynein-dependent and -independent centrosomal protein assembly. *Molecular Biology of the Cell*, Vol. 17(2), pp. 680-689.

Hämmerle, B. & Tejedor, F.J. (2007). A novel function of DELTA-NOTCH signalling mediates the transition from proliferation to neurogenesis in neural progenitor cells. *PLoS One*, Vol. 2(11), e1169.

Hattori, M.; Adachi, H.; Tsujimoto, M.; Arai, H. & Inoue, K. (1994). Miller-Dieker lissencephaly gene encodes a subunit of brain platelet-activating factor acetylhydrolase [corrected]. *Nature*, Vol. 370(6486), pp. 216-8. Erratum in: *Nature*, Vol. 370(6488), pp. 391.

Hayashi, M.A.; Gomes, M.D.; Rebouças, N.A.; Fernandes, B.L.; Ferro, E.S. & de Camargo, A.C. (1996). Species specificity of thimet oligopeptidase (EC 3.4.24.15). *Biological Chemistry Hoppe-Seyler*, Vol. 377(5), pp. 283-291.

Hayashi, M.A.; Portaro, F.C.; Tambourgi, D.V.; Sucupira, M.; Yamane, T.; Fernandes, B.L.; Ferro, E.S.; Rebouças, N.A. & de Camargo, A.C. (2000). Molecular and immunochemical evidences demonstrate that endooligopeptidase A is the predominant cytosolic oligopeptidase of rabbit brain. *Biochemical and Biophysical Research Communications*, Vol. 269(1), pp. 7-13. Erratum in: *Biochemical and Biophysical Research Communications*, Vol. 272(1), pp. 309 (2000).

Hayashi, M.A.; Pires, R.S.; Rebouças, N.A.; Britto, L.R. & Camargo, A.C. (2001). Expression of endo-oligopeptidase A in the rat central nervous system: a non-radioactive in situ hybridization study. *Brain Research. Molecular Brain Research*, Vol. 89(1-2), pp. 86-93.

Hayashi, M.A.; Portaro, F.C.; Bastos, M.F.; Guerreiro, J.R.; Oliveira, V.; Gorrão, S.S.; Tambourgi, D.V.; Sant'Anna, O.A.; Whiting, P.J.; Camargo, L.M.; Konno, K.; Brandon, N.J. & Camargo, A.C. (2005). Inhibition of NUDEL (nuclear distribution element-like)-oligopeptidase activity by disrupted-in-schizophrenia 1. *PNAS*, Vol. 102(10), pp. 3828-3833.

Hayashi, M.A.F.; Guerreiro, J.R.; Charych, E.; Kamiya, A.; Barbos, R.L.; Machado, M.F.; Campeiro, J.D.; Oliveira, V.; Sawa, A.; Camargo, A.C. and Brandon, N.J. (2010) Assessing the role of endooligopeptidase activity of Ndel1 (nuclear-distribution gene E homolog like-1) in neurite outgrowth. *Mol Cell Neurosci*. Vol. 44(4), pp. 353-61.

Hayashi, M.A.F.; Lizier, N.F.; Pereira, L. & Kerkis, A. (2011). Pluripotent stem cells as an in vitro model of neuronal differentiation. *Embryonic Stem Cells – Differentiation and Pluripotent Alternatives*, Book 3, Vol. 4, pp. 81-98.

Hayashi, M.A.F.; Portaro, F.C.V. & Camargo, A.C.M. (2005). Cytosolic oligopeptidases: features and possible physiopathological roles in the immune and nervous systems. *Current Medicinal Chemistry* (Hilversum), Vol. 4, pp. 269-277.

Hayes, N.L. & Nowakowski, R.S. (2000). Exploiting the dynamics of S-phase tracers in developing brain: interkinetic nuclear migration for cells entering versus leaving the S-phase. *Developmental Neuroscience*, Vol. 22(1-2), pp. 44-55.

Horton, S.; Meredith, A.; Richardson, J.A. & Johnson, J.E. (1999). Correct coordination of neuronal differentiation events in ventral forebrain requires the bHLH factor MASH1. *Molecular and Cellular Neurosciences*, Vol. 14(4-5), pp. 355-369.

Hu, B.Y.; Weick, J.P.; Yu, J.; Ma, L.X.; Zhang, X.Q.; Thomson, J.A. & Zhang, S.C. (2010). Neural differentiation of human induced pluripotent stem cells follows developmental principles but with variable potency. *PNAS*, Vol. 107(9), pp. 4335-4340.

Jaaro-Peled, H.; Hayashi-Takagi, A.; Seshadri, S.; Kamiya, A.; Brandon, N.J. & Sawa, A. (2009). Neurodevelopmental mechanisms of schizophrenia: understanding disturbed postnatal brain maturation through neuregulin-1-ErbB4 and DISC1. *Trends Neurosci.*, Vol. 32(9), pp. 485-95.

Jankowski, M.P.; Cornuet, P.K.; McIlwrath, S.; Koerber, H.R. & Albers, K.M. (2006). SRY-box containing gene 11 (Sox11) transcription factor is required for neuron survival and neurite growth. *Neuroscience*, Vol. 143(2), pp. 501-14.

Jankowski, M.P.; McIlwrath, S.L.; Jing, X.; Cornuet, P.K.; Salerno, K.M.; Koerber, H.R. & Albers, K.M. (2009). Sox11 transcription factor modulates peripheral nerve regeneration in adult mice. *Brain Res.*, Vol. 1256, pp. 43-54.

Kageyama, R.; Ohtsuka, T.; Shimojo, H. and Imayoshi, I. (2008). Dynamic Notch signaling in neural progenitor cells and a revised view of lateral inhibition. *Nature Neuroscience*, Vol. 11(11), pp. 1247-1251.

Kamiya, A.; Tomoda, T.; Chang, J.; Takaki, M.; Zhan, C.; Morita, M.; Cascio, M.B.; Elashvili, S.; Koizumi, H.; Takanezawa, Y.; Dickerson, F.; Yolken, R.; Arai, H. & Sawa, A. (2006). DISC1–NDEL1/NUDEL protein interaction, an essential component for neurite outgrowth, is modulated by genetic variations of DISC1. *Hum. Mol. Genet.*, Vol. 15, pp. 3313–3323.

Kamiya, A.; Kubo, K.; Tomoda, T.; Takaki, M.; Youn, R.; Ozeki, Y.; Sawamura, N.; Park, U.; Kudo, C.; Okawa, M.; Ross, C.A.; Hatten, M.E.; Nakajima, K. & Sawa, A. (2005). A schizophrenia-associated mutation of DISC1 perturbs cerebral cortex development. *Nat Cell Biol.*, Vol. 7(12), pp. 1167-78. Erratum in: *Nat Cell Biol.*, 2006 Vol. 8(1), pp. 100.

Kawaguchi, D.; Yoshimatsu, T.; Hozumi, K. & Gotoh, Y. (2008). Selection of differentiating cells by different levels of delta-like 1 among neural precursor cells in the developing mouse telencephalon. *Development*, Vol. 135(23), pp. 3849-3858.

Kerkis, I.; Hayashi, M.A.F.; Lizier, N.F.; Cassola, A.C.; Pereira, L.V. & Kerkis, A. (2011). Pluripotent Stem Cells as an *In Vitro* Model of Neuronal Differentiation, InTech, ISBN 978-953-307-632-4, Vienna, Austria.

Kim, K.K.; Adelstein, R.S. & Kawamoto, S. (2009). Identification of neuronal nuclei (NeuN) as Fox-3, a new member of the Fox-1 gene family of splicing factors. *The Journal of Biological Chemistry*. Vol. 284(45), pp. 31052-31061.

Kitagawa, M.; Umezu, M.; Aoki, J.; Koizumi, H.; Arai, H. & Inoue, K. (2000). Direct association of LIS1, the lissencephaly gene product, with a mammalian homologue of a fungal nuclear distribution protein, rNUDE. *FEBS Lett.*, Vol. 479(1-2), pp. 57-62.

Konno, D.; Shioi, G.; Shitamukai, A.; Mori, A.; Kiyonari, H.; Miyata, T. & Matsuzaki, F. (2008). Neuroepithelial progenitors undergo LGN-dependent planar divisions to maintain self-renewability during mammalian neurogenesis. *Nature Cell Biology*, Vol. 10(1), pp. 93-101.

Latasa, M.J.; Cisneros, E. & Frade, J.M. (2009). Cell cycle control of Notch signaling and the functional regionalization of the neuroepithelium during vertebrate neurogenesis. *The International Journal of Developmental Biology*, Vol.53(7), pp. 895-908.

LaVaute, T.M.; Yoo, Y.D.; Pankratz, M.T.; Weick, J.P.; Gerstner, J.R. & Zhang, S.C. (2009). Regulation of neural specification from human embryonic stem cells by BMP and FGF. *Stem Cells*, Vol. 27(8), pp. 1741-1749.

Lefebvre, V.; Dumitriu, B.; Penzo-Méndez, A.; Han, Y. & Pallavi, B. (2007). Control of cell fate and differentiation by Sry-related high-mobility-group box (Sox) transcription factors. *Int J Biochem Cell Biol.*, Vol. 39(12), pp. 2195-214.

le Roux, I.; Lewis, J. and Ish-Horowicz, D. (2003). Notch activity is required to maintain floorplate identity and to control neurogenesis in the chick hindbrain and spinal cord. *The International Journal of Developmental Biology*, Vol. 47(4), pp. 263-272.

Lee, M.K.; Tuttle, J.B.; Rebhun, L.I., Cleveland, D.W. and Frankfuter, A. (1990) The expression and posttranslational modification of a neuron-specific beta-tubulin isotype during chick embryogenesis. *Cell Mot Cytosk*, Vol. 17: 118-132

Lewis, S.A. & Cowan, N.J. (1988). Complex regulation and functional versatility of mammalian alpha- and beta-tubulin isotypes during the differentiation of testis and muscle cells. *The Journal of Cell Biology*, Vol. 106(6), pp. 2023-2033.

Liang, Y.; Yu, W.; Li, Y.; Yu, L.; Zhang, Q.; Wang, F.; Yang, Z.; Du, J.; Huang, Q.; Yao, X. & Zhu, X. (2007). Nudel modulates kinetochore association and function of cytoplasmic dynein in M phase. *Mol Biol Cell*, Vol. 18(7), pp. 2656-66.

Lin, C.H.; Stoeck, J.; Ravanpay, A.C.; Guillemot, F.; Tapscott, S.J. & Olson, J.M. (2004). Regulation of neuroD2 expression in mouse brain. *Developmental Biology*, Vol. 265(1), pp. 234-245.

Linker, C. & Stern, C.D. (2004). Neural induction requires BMP inhibition only as a late step, and involves signals other than FGF and Wnt antagonists. *Development*, Vol. 131(22), pp. 5671-5681.

Ma, Q.; Kintner, C. & Anderson, D.J. (1996). Identification of neurogenin, a vertebrate neuronal determination gene. *Cell*, Vol. 87(1),pp. 43-52.

Ma, Q.; Sommer, L.; Cserjesi, P. & Anderson, D.J. (1997). Mash1 and neurogenin1 expression patterns define complementary domains of neuroepithelium in the developing

CNS and are correlated with regions expressing notch ligands. *The Journal of Neuroscience*, Vol. 17(10), pp. 3644-3652.

Ma, Q.; Chen, Z.; del Barco Barrantes, I.; de la Pompa, J.L. & Anderson, D.J. (1998). neurogenin1 is essential for the determination of neuronal precursors for proximal cranial sensory ganglia. *Neuron*, Vol. 20(3), pp. 469-482.

Ma, Q.; Fode, C.; Guillemot, F. & Anderson, DJ. (1999). Neurogenin1 and neurogenin2 control two distinct waves of neurogenesis in developing dorsal root ganglia. *Genes & Development*, Vol. 13(13), pp. 1717-1728.

McKenney, R.J.; Vershinin, M.; Kunwar, A.; Vallee, R.B. & Gross, S.P. (2010). LIS1 and NudE induce a persistent dynein force-producing state. *Cell*, Vol. 141(2), pp. 304-14.

Menezes, J.R.L. and Luskin, M.B. (1994). Expression of neuron-specific tubulin defines a novel population in the proliferative layers of the developing telencephalon. *J. Neurosci.* 14(9): 5399-5416.

Millar, J.K.; Wilson-Annan, J.C.; Anderson, S.; Christie. S.; Taylor, M.S.; Semple, C.A.; Devon, R.S.; St Clair, D.M.; Muir, W.J.; Blackwood, D.H. & Porteous, D.J. (2000). Disruption of two novel genes by a translocation co-segregating with schizophrenia. *Hum Mol Genet.*, Vol. 9(9), pp. 1415-23.

Miller, J.Q. (1963). Lissencephaly in two siblings. *Neurology*, Vol. 13, pp. 841-850.

Mori, D.; Yamada, M.; Mimori-Kiyosue, Y.; Shirai, Y.; Suzuki, A.; Ohno, S.; Saya, H.; Wynshaw-Boris, A. & Hirotsune, S.(2009). An essential role of the aPKC-Aurora A-NDEL1 pathway in neurite elongation by modulation of microtubule dynamics. *Nat Cell Biol.*, Vol. 11(9), pp. 1057-68.

Muhr, J.; Graziano, E.; Wilson, S.; Jessell, T.M. & Edlund, T. (1999). Convergent inductive signals specify midbrain, hindbrain, and spinal cord identity in gastrula stage chick embryos. *Neuron*, Vol. 23(4), pp. 689-702.

Myat, A.; Henrique, D.; Ish-Horowicz, D. & Lewis, J. (1996). A chick homologue of Serrate and its relationship with Notch and Delta homologues during central neurogenesis. *Developmental Biology*, Vol. 174(2), pp. 233-247.

Nguyen, M.D.; Shu, T.; Sanada, K.; Larivière, R.C.; Tseng, H.C.; Park, S.K.; Julien, J.P. & Tsai L.H. (2004). A NUDEL-dependent mechanism of neurofilament assembly regulates the integrity of CNS neurons. *Nat Cell Biol.*, Vol. 6(7), pp. 595-608.

Nicodemus, K.K.; Callicott, J.H.; Higier, R.G.; Luna, A.; Nixon, D.C.; Lipska, B.K.; Vakkalanka, R.; Giegling, I.; Rujescu, D.; Clair, D.S.; Muglia, P.; Shugart, Y.Y. & Weinberger, D.R. (2010). Evidence of statistical epistasis between DISC1, CIT and NDEL1 impacting risk for schizophrenia: biological validation with functional neuroimaging. *Hum. Genet.*, Vol. 127 (4), pp. 453-454.

O´Rourke, N.A.; Chenn, A. And McConnell, S.K. (1997) Postmitotic neurons migrate tangentially in the cortical ventricular zone. *Development*, 124: 997-1005.

Ossipova, O.; Ezan, J. & Sokol, S.Y. (2009). PAR-1 phosphorylates Mind bomb to promote vertebrate neurogenesis. *Developmental Cell*, Vol. 17(2), pp. 222-233.

Pera, E.M.; Ikeda, A.; Eivers, E. & De Robertis, E.M. (2003). Integration of IGF, FGF, and anti-BMP signals via Smad1 phosphorylation in neural induction. *Genes & Development*, Vol. 17(24), pp. 3023-3028.

Pierfelice, T.; Alberi, L. & Gaiano, N. (2011). Notch in the vertebrate nervous system: an old dog with new tricks. *Neuron*, Vol. 69(5), pp. 840-855.

Powell, L.M. & Jarman, A.P. (2008). Context dependence of proneural bHLH proteins. *Current Opinion in Genetics & Development*, Vol. 18(5), pp. 411-417.

Reiner, O.; Carrozzo, R.; Shen, Y.; Wehnert, M.; Faustinella, F.; Dobyns, W.B.; Caskey, C.T. & Ledbetter, D.H. (1993). Isolation of a Miller-Dieker lissencephaly gene containing G protein beta-subunit-like repeats. *Nature*, Vol. 364(6439), pp. 717-721.

Reiner, O.; Albrecht, U.; Gordon, M.; Chianese, K.A.; Wong, C.; Gal-Gerber, O.; Sapir, T.; Siracusa, L.D.; Buchberg, A.M.; Caskey, C.T. & Eichele, G. (1995) Lissencephaly gene (LIS1) expression in the CNS suggests a role in neuronal migration. *J Neurosci.*, Vol. 15(5 Pt 2), pp. 3730-8.

Reiner, O.; Sapoznik, S. & Sapir, T. (2006). Lissencephaly 1 linking to multiple diseases: mental retardation, neurodegeneration, schizophrenia, male sterility, and more. *Neuromolecular Med.*, Vol. 8(4), pp. 547-65

Rex, M.; Orme, A.; Uwanogho, D.; Tointon, K.; Wigmore, P.M.; Sharpe, P.T. & Scotting, P.J. (1997). Dynamic expression of chicken Sox2 and Sox3 genes in ectoderm induced to form neural tissue. *Developmental Dynamics*, Vol. 209(3), pp. 323-332.

Robson, S.J. & Burgoyne, R.D. (1989). L-type calcium channels in the regulation of neurite outgrowth from rat dorsal root ganglion neurons in culture. *Neurosci Lett*, Vol. 104(1-2), pp. 110-4.

Roztocil, T.; Matter-Sadzinski, L.; Alliod, C.; Ballivet, M. & Matter, J.M. (1997). NeuroM, a neural helix-loop-helix transcription factor, defines a new transition stage in neurogenesis. *Development*, vol. 124(17), pp. 3263-3672.

Saillour, Y.; Carion, N.; Quelin, C.; Leger, P.L.; Boddaert, N.; Elie, C.; Toutain, A.; Mercier, S.; Barthez, M.A.; Milh, M.; Joriot, S.; des Portes, V.; Philip, N.; Broglin, D.; Roubertie, A.; Pitelet, G.; Moutard, M.L.; Pinard, J.M.; Cances, C.; Kaminska, A.; Chelly, J.; Beldjord, C. & Bahi-Buisson, N. (2009). LIS1-related isolated lissencephaly: spectrum of mutations and relationships with malformation severity. *Archives of Neurology*, Vol. 66(8), pp. 1007-1015.

Sasaki, S.; Mori, D.; Toyo-oka, K.; Chen, A.; Garrett-Beal, L.; Muramatsu, M.; Miyagawa, S.; Hiraiwa, N.; Yoshiki, A.; Wynshaw-Boris, A. & Hirotsune, S. (2005). Complete loss of Ndel1 results in neuronal migration defects and early embryonic lethality. *Molecular and Cellular Biology*, Vol. 25(17), pp. 7812-7827.

Sekido, R. (2010). SRY: A transcriptional activator of mammalian testis determination. *Int J Biochem Cell Biol.*, Vol. 42(3), pp. 417-20.

Shen, Y.; Li, N.; Wu, S.; Zhou, Y.; Shan, Y.; Zhang, Q.; Ding, C.; Yuan, Q.; Zhao, F.; Zeng, R. & Zhu, X. (2008). Nudel binds Cdc42GAP to modulate Cdc42 activity at the leading edge of migrating cells. *Dev Cell*, Vol. 14(3), pp. 342-53.

Shim, S.Y.; Samuels, B.A.; Wang, J.; Neumayer, G.; Belzil, C.; Ayala, R.; Shi, Y.; Shi, Y.; Tsai, L.H. & Nguyen, M.D. (2008). Ndel1 controls the dynein-mediated transport of vimentin during neurite outgrowth. *J Biol Chem.*, Vol. 283(18), pp. 12232-40

Shioi, G.; Konno, D.; Shitamukai, A. & Matsuzaki, F. (2009). Structural basis for self-renewal of neural progenitors in cortical neurogenesis. *Cerebral Cortex*, Vol. 19, pp. i55-61.

Shu, T.; Ayala, R.; Nguyen, M.D.; Xie, Z.; Gleeson, J.G. & Tsai, L.H. (2004). Ndel1 operates in a common pathway with LIS1 and cytoplasmic dynein to regulate cortical neuronal positioning. *Neuron*, Vol. 44(2), pp. 263-277.

Siller, K.H.; Serr, M.; Steward, R.; Hays, T.S. & Doe, C.Q. (2005). Live imaging of Drosophila brain neuroblasts reveals a role for Lis1/dynactin in spindle assembly and mitotic checkpoint control. *Mol Biol Cell* Vol. 16(11), pp. 5127-40.

St Clair, D.; Blackwood, D.; Muir, W.; Carothers, A.; Walker, M.; Spowart, G.; Gosden, C. & Evans, H.J. (1990). Association within a family of a balanced autosomal translocation with major mental-illness. *Lancet*, Vol. 336, pp. 13–16.

Stein, R.; Mori, N.; Matthews, K.; Lo, L.C. & Anderson, D.J. (1988). The NGF-inducible SCG10 mRNA encodes a novel membrane-bound protein present in growth cones and abundant in developing neurons. *Neuron*, Vol. 1(6), pp. 463-476.

Stehman, S.A.; Chen, Y.; McKenney, R.J. & Vallee, R.B. (2007). NudE and NudEL are required for mitotic progression and are involved in dynein recruitment to kinetochores. *J Cell Biol.*, Vol. 178(4), pp. 583-94.

Streit, A.; Sockanathan, S.; Pérez, L.; Rex, M.; Scotting, P.J.; Sharpe, P.T.; Lovell-Badge, R. & Stern C.D. (1997). Preventing the loss of competence for neural induction: HGF/SF, L5 and Sox-2. *Development*, Vol. 124(6), pp. 1191-1202.

Streit, A.; Lee, K.J.; Woo, I.; Roberts, C.; Jessell, T.M. & Stern, C.D. (1998). Chordin regulates primitive streak development and the stability of induced neural cells, but is not sufficient for neural induction in the chick embryo. *Development*, Vol. 125(3), pp. 507-519.

Streit, A.; Berliner, A.J.; Papanayotou, C.; Sirulnik, A. & Stern, C.D. (2000). Initiation of neural induction by FGF signalling before gastrulation. *Nature*, Vol. 406(6791), pp. 74-78.

Sweeney, K.J.; Prokscha, A. & Eichele, G. (2001). NudE-L, a novel Lis1-interacting protein, belongs to a family of vertebrate coiled-coil proteins. *Mech Dev.*, Vol. 101(1-2), pp. 21-33.

Tabler, J.M.; Yamanaka, H. & Green, J.B. (2010). PAR-1 promotes primary neurogenesis and asymmetric cell divisions via control of spindle orientation. *Development*, Vol. 137(15), pp. 2501-2505.

Talikka, M.; Perez, S.E. & Zimmerman, K. (2002). Distinct patterns of downstream target activation are specified by the helix-loop-helix domain of proneural basic helix-loop-helix transcription factors. *Developmental Biology*, Vol. 247(1), pp. 137-148.

Tarricone, C.; Perrina, F.; Monzani, S.; Massimiliano, L.; Kim, M.H.; Derewenda, Z.S.; Knapp, S.; Tsai, L.H. & Musacchio, A. (2004). Coupling PAF signaling to dynein regulation: structure of LIS1 in complex with PAF-acetylhydrolase. *Neuron*, Vol. 44(5), pp. 809-21.

Taya, S.; Shinoda, T.; Tsuboi, D.; Asaki, J.; Nagai, K.; Hikita, T.; Kuroda, S.; Kuroda, K.; Shimizu, M.; Hirotsune, S.; Iwamatsu, A. & Kaibuchi, K. (2007). DISC1 regulates the transport of the NUDEL/LIS1/14-3-3epsilon complex through kinesin-1. *J Neurosci.*, Vol. 27(1), pp. 15-26.

Teng, J.; Takei, Y.; Harada, A.; Nakata, T.; Chen. J. & Hirokawa, N. (2001). Synergistic effects of MAP2 and MAP1B knockout in neuronal migration, dendritic outgrowth, and microtubule organization. *The Journal of Cell Biology*, Vol. 155(1), pp. 65-76.

Tischler, A.S.; Lee, Y.C.; Perlman, R.L.; Costopoulos, D.; Slayton, V.W.; Bloom, S.R. (1984). Production of "ectopic" vasoactive intestinal peptide-like and neurotensin-like immunoreactivity in human pheochromocytoma cell cultures. *J Neurosci*, Vol. 4(5), pp. 1398-404.

Tischler, A.S.; Ruzicka, A.; Dobner, P.R. (1991). A protein kinase inhibitor, staurosporine, mimics nerve growth factor induction of neurotensin/neuromedin N gene expression. *J Biol Chem*, Vol. 266(2), pp. 1141-6.

Toth, C.; Shim, S.Y.; Wang, J.; Jiang, Y.; Neumayer, G.; Belzil, C.; Liu, W.Q.; Martinez, J.; Zochodne, D. & Nguyen, M.D. (2008). Ndel1 promotes axon regeneration via intermediate filaments. *PLoS One*, Vol. 3(4), pp. e2014.

Tropepe, V.; Hitoshi, S.; Sirard, C.; Mak, T.W.; Rossant, J. & van der Kooy, D. (2001). Direct neural fate specification from embryonic stem cells: a primitive mammalian neural stem cell stage acquired through a default mechanism. *Neuron*, Vol. 30(1), pp. 65-78.

Tsai, J.W.; Chen, Y.; Kriegstein, A.R. & Vallee, R.B. (2005). LIS1 RNA interference blocks neural stem cell division, morphogenesis, and motility at multiple stages. *J Cell Biol.*, Vol. 170(6), pp. 935-45.

Tucker, R.P.; Tran, H; Gong, Q (2008) Neurogenesis and neurite outgrowth in the spical cord of chicken embryos and in primary cultures of spinal neurons following knockdown of Class III beta tubulin with antisense morpholinos. *Protoplasma* 234: 97-101.

Uchikawa, M.; Ishida, Y.; Takemoto, T.; Kamachi, Y. & Kondoh H. (2003). Functional analysis of chicken Sox2 enhancers highlights an array of diverse regulatory elements that are conserved in mammals. *Developmental Cell*, Vol. 4(4), pp. 509-519.

Vergnolle, M.A. & Taylor, S.S. (2007). Cenp-F links kinetochores to Ndel1/Nde1/Lis1/dynein microtubule motor complexes. *Curr Biol.*, Vol. 17(13), pp. 1173-9.

Wakamatsu, Y. & Weston, J.A. (1997). Sequential expression and role of Hu RNA-binding proteins during neurogenesis. *Development*, Vol. 124(17), pp. 3449-3460.

Wilson, P.A. & Hemmati-Brivanlou, A. (1995). Induction of epidermis and inhibition of neural fate by Bmp-4. *Nature*, Vol. 376(6538), pp. 331-333.

Wilson, S.I.; Graziano, E.; Harland, R.; Jessell, T.M. & Edlund, T. (2000). An early requirement for FGF signalling in the acquisition of neural cell fate in the chick embryo. *Current Biology*, Vol. 10(8), pp. 421-429.

Wilson, S.I.; Rydström, A.; Trimborn, T.; Willert, K.; Nusse, R.; Jessell, T.M. & Edlund, T. (2001). The status of Wnt signalling regulates neural and epidermal fates in the chick embryo. *Nature*, Vol. 411(6835), pp. 325-330.

Wood, H.B. & Episkopou, V. (1999). Comparative expression of the mouse Sox1, Sox2 and Sox3 genes from pre-gastrulation to early somite stages. *Mechanisms of Development*, Vol. 86(1-2), pp. 197-201.

Ying, Q.L.; Stavridis, M.; Griffiths, D.; Li, M. & Smith, A. (2003). Conversion of embryonic stem cells into neuroectodermal precursors in adherent monoculture. *Nature Biotechnology*, Vol. 21(2), pp. 183-186.

Youn, Y.H.; Pramparo, T.; Hirotsune, S. & Wynshaw-Boris, A. (2009). Distinct dose-dependent cortical neuronal migration and neurite extension defects in Lis1 and Ndel1 mutant mice. *The Journal of Neuroscience*, Vol. 29(49), pp. 15520-15530.

Zhao, Y.; Biermann, T., Luther C, Unger T, Culman J, Gohlke P. (2003) Contribution of bradykinin and nitric oxide to AT2 receptor-mediated differentiation in PC12 W cells. *J Neurochem*, Vol. 85(3), pp. 759-67.

Zigman, M.; Cayouette, M.; Charalambous, C.; Schleiffer, A.; Hoeller, O.; Dunican, D.; McCudden, C.R.; Firnberg, N.; Barres, B.A.; Siderovski, D.P. & Knoblich, J.A. (2005). Mammalian inscuteable regulates spindle orientation and cell fate in the developing retina. *Neuron*, Vol. 48(4), pp. 539-545.

12

Recent Advances of *In Vitro* Embryogenesis of Monocotyledon and Dicotyledon

Sun Yan-Lin[1,2] and Hong Soon-Kwan[2,3]
[1]*School of Life Sciences, Ludong University, Yantai, Shandong*
[2]*Department of Bio-Health Technology, College of Biomedical Science, Kangwon National University, Chuncheon, Kangwon-Do,*
[3]*Institute of Bioscience and Biotechnology, Kangwon National University, Chuncheon, Kangwon-Do,*
[1]*China*
[2,3]*Korea*

1. Introduction

Plant tissue and cell culture is a rapid way of achieving plant breeding through the protoplast fusion and regeneration novel hybrid, the production of large numbers of identical individuals and disease and/or pest resistant varieties, thus indirectly increasing the crop yield. Particularly for some plant species, they cannot be improved by conventional breeding because of poor seed germination, frequency of seedling death, or/and environmental challenges such as habitat destruction and illegal and indiscriminate collection. Based on the plasticity and totipotency of plants, plant tissue and cell culture techniques offer a viable tool for mass multiplication and germplasm conservation of some plants, especially those rare and endangered medicinal plants while at the same time facilitating pharmaceutical and other commercial needs (Sahoo & Chand, 1998; Anis & Faisal, 2005). Owing to these useful applications, plant tissue culture technology has now become a remarkably important, useful tool in experimental studies.

The concept of *in vitro* plant cell culture was firstly developed by Gottlieb Haberlandt, a German scientist in 1902. He isolated single fully differentiated individual plant cells from different plant species and cultured them in a nutrient medium containing glucose, peptone, and Knop's salt solution. However, Haberlandt did not succeed to induce plant cells to divide. Later, Hanning (1904) initiated a new line of investigation involving the culture of embryogenic tissue. He excised embryogenic tissues like mature embryos from *Raphanus sativus*, *R. landra*, *R. caudatus*, and *Cochlearia donica* to culture them to maturity on mineral salts and sugar solution. Until in 1934, Gautheret (1934) found successful results on *in vitro* culture of plants. In the following few years, single somatic cells of some green plants have been induced to develop into entire individuals and eventually produce flowers and fruits (Vasil & Hilderbrandt, 1965). In addition, studies of plant tissue culture in monocotyledons were a bit later than that in dicotyledons: Loo (1945) firstly performed stem cultures *in vitro* from apical meristems of monocotyledonous *Asparagus officinalis*; until in 1951, Morel &

Wetmore (1951) successfully obtained the proliferation *in vitro* from tuber of monocotydelonous *Amorphophallus rivieri*. Based on one hundred years' investigation, plant tissue culture technologies have achieved a great progress in many aspects including the effects of plant growth regulators, auxins, and cytokinins, genotype-dependence, callus type-dependence and so on. However, plant tissue and cell cultures in medicinal plants and recalcitrant crops, especially monocotyledonous species and grass species are still deficient. In this chapter, recent advances of *in vitro* embryogenesis of monocotyledon, the halophyte *Leymus chinensis* (Trin.) Tzvel (=*Aneurolepidium chinensis* Trin. Kitag, Poaceae, LC, thereafter) and dicotyledon, the medicinal plant, *Eleutherococcus senticosus* (Rupr. et Maxim.) Harms (=*Acanthopanax senticosus*, Araliaceae, ES, thereafter) will be presented.

LC, a perennial rhizomatous grass belonging to the tribe Poaceae (Czerepanov, 2007), is widely distributed through Northern China, Mongolia and Siberia (Liu et al., 2002a). Due to its intrinsic adaptation to highly alkaline-sodic soil conditions (Jin et al., 2006), this plant species has been used to protect soil and water from loss in arid areas of Northwest of China. Combined with its fine agronomic properties such as rich productivity, high protein content, and palatable to cattle, this plant species has become a major candidate in artificial grassland construction and grassland ecological environment improvement (Jia, 1987). Despite the LC population is common in distinctive regions of China, especially in Songnen Steppe, LC grasslands are being seriously ruined owing to deteriorating environmental conditions, animal destroy, and human destructive activities (Wang et al., 2005). Moreover, the protandry in LC, which limits pollination within flowering shoots, results in self-incompatible and then causes the propagation problem in low seed-set and fecundity (Huang et al., 2004; Wang et al., 2005). Plant breeding or trait improvement in this plant species becomes important and urgently needed.

For *in vitro* embryogenesis of LC, the first report was performed by Gao (1982), using rhizome as explants resulting in about 20% callus induction frequency and 24.2% plant regeneration frequency. Later in 1990, Cui et al. (1990) investigated young rhizome and mature seeds as explants to induce callus induction, and referred to the relationship with callus status and plant regeneration in LC for the first time. However, their callus induction and plant regeneration frequencies were still not very high. In the following few years, many scientists continued to attempt the optimal tissue culture conditions and explants for *in vitro* tissue culture of LC (Liu et al., 2002b; Liu et al., 2004; Sun & Hong 2009, 2010a, 2010b). Induction of embryogenic calli, considered as the most critical step for the success in plant regeneration, is influenced by genotype, explants type, and medium composition as well as by their interaction (Rachmawati & Anzai, 2006). In this chapter, we will summarize the factors influencing LC callus induction, embryogenesis, and plant regeneration efficiency, and focus their interaction.

ES, called Siberian ginseng, Ciwujia in Chinese and Gasiogalpi in Korean, is a woody medicinal plant, distributed in southeast Russia, northeast China, Korea, and Japan (Lee, 1979; Hahn et al., 1985). The cortical root and stem tissues of this species have long been used for medicinal properties (Umeyama et al., 1992; Davydov & Krikorian, 2000). Main active compounds such as triterpene saponins isolated from ES possess important pharmacological activities, including inhibiting histamine release, improving immune system, fighting cancer and aging, and improving adrenal function (Umeyama et al., 1992; Gaffney et al., 2001). However, the poor and/or even failed seed setting, seed dormancy and over-exploitation always puzzle this species (Yu et al., 2003). Thus, improving its propagation efficiency on enhancing yield and quality to achieve efficient farm cultivation and considerable economic benefits has become an important issue. To achieve this goal, many investigations have been reported, including conventional propagations, habitat conditions, molecular classification, and mass production through *in vitro* tissue cultures.

Conventional propagations of ES have two means: seed propagation and stem cutting propagation. However, until now, two propagations are still considered difficult because of long-term stratification prior to the maturation of the zygotic embryos in mature seeds or difficultly rooting induction from stem cuts (Isoda & Shoji, 1994). Based on this situation, plant cell culture techniques have been applied as a new means for propagation of this species (Choi et al., 1999a, b). Compared with the rise and development of tissue culture in LC, the tissue culture studies in ES initiate relatively late. The first callus induction attempt was done in 1991, and this work reported plant regeneration could be successfully achieved through direct secondary somatic embryogenesis from immature zygotic embryos (Gui et al., 1991). Later, somatic embryos were produced directly from the surface of zygotic embryos of this species without forming an intervening callus (Choi & Soh, 1993). In this report, two kinds of somatic embryos were induced from various explants, including hypocotyls, cotyledon, radicle: one was single embryos with closed radicle mainly formed on cotyledon and radicle, the other was polyembryos mainly formed on hypocotyls. To improve the *in vitro* tissue culture conditions, Yu et al. (1997a, b) attempted to induce embryogenic callus from immature embryos, and obtained high callus formation of 83% on modified SH medium and 100% on B5 medium with 2,4-D addition. Plant regeneration capability of embryogenic callus was different depending on the mature degree of the explants, immature embryos. Choi et al. (1999a) established a high frequency of plant production *via* somatic embryogenesis from callus with cultured on MS medium with 1.0 mg/l 2,4-D for somatic embryo induction and then MS medium lacking 2,4-D before plant regeneration. In the following report by Choi et al. (1999b), various explants such as cotyledon, hypocotyl and root were investigated in plant regeneration *via* direct somatic embryogenesis, of which hypocotyls segments showed the highest somatic embryo formation frequency (75%). This report obtained the highest germination rate of 93% from somatic embryos, and thus established an efficient means for mass propagation though somatic embryogenesis of ES. As known that the somatic embryogenesis and plant regeneration in plants were genotype-specific and explants-specific (Liu et al., 2004; Sun & Hong, 2010), Li & Yu (2002) investigated somatic embryogenesis from various explants including young leaf, stem, node, petiole, peduncle, flower and root using three different genotypes of ES accession Korea, Russia, and Japan. In this report, the highest callus formation frequency was obtained from flower explants, and normal plantlets were produced from somatic embryos when transferred to 1/4 MS medium.

To achieve *in vitro* mass propagation of ES, cell suspension cultures using hypocotyls-derived callus have been firstly conducted by Choi et al. (1999a). However, the somatic embryo formation capacity of suspension cultured cells was significantly lower compared to that from callus cultures. Later, improved cell suspension cultures were observed that 35 g dotyledonary embryos (about 12,000) were converted to 567 g fresh mass of plantlets with initially culture in 500-ml flask, followed by culture in 10-l plastic tank, and then low-strength MS medium (Choi et al., 2002). This report established an efficient protocol for the mass production of ES plantlet from tank culture of somatic embryos. In the year 2003, the *in vitro* mass propagation conditions were further improved by shortening the maturation time from immature zygotic embryos to somatic embryos within one month (Han & Choi, 2003). Based on the above results, it indicated that *in vitro* mass propagation could be practically applicable for systematic procedure of plant production of ES, and the *in vitro* plantlets could be satisfied as a source of medicinal raw materials, just like *Panax ginseng* (Furuya et al., 1983). Due to no comprehensive review of *in vitro* embryogenesis and plant regeneration on ES to date, we here, summarize the currently available scientific information on ES, aiming to provide the basis of further understanding this species.

2. *In vitro* embryogenesis of monocotyledon

The halophyte forage grass, LC was used as the model monocotyledonous plant for understanding embryogenic callus induction and plant regeneration. The factors affecting embryogenic callus induction efficiency and plant regeneration potential would be summarized as follow:

2.1 Explants type

Plant tissue culture of LC has been investigated using nearly all readily available explants such as mature embryos (Liu et al., 2002b; Kim et al., 2005), mature seeds (Cui et al., 1990; Qu et al., 2004; Kim et al., 2005; Wei et al., 2005; Kong et al., 2008; Sun & Hong, 2009, 2010a), leaf base segments (Liu et al., 2002b; Kim et al., 2005; Sun & Hong, 2009, 2010a), rhizoma (Gao, 1982; Lu et al., 2009), immature inflorescence (Liu et al., 2004), immature spikes (Liu et al., 2002b; Zhang et al., 2007), and root segments (Sun & Hong, 2009), shown in Table 1. In our previous studies (Sun & Hong, 2009; 2010a), mature seed is considered as the optimal explants to induce embryogenic callus, with 56.4 ~ 88.3% of callus induction frequencies. Similar results have been observed in reports of Cui et al. (1990) and Kim et al. (2005) that found mature seeds could produced the highest callus induction frequencies among young rhizome, embryos and leaves as explants, respectively. Using mature seeds as explants to induce callus, it is not only due to the highest callus induction efficiency, but also several advantages such as convenient acquisition and easy conservation in bulk quantities. Except using mature seeds as explants, Liu et al. (2002) suggested that immature stacys were the optimal explants for callus induction with compared to mature embryos and leaf sections, and only calli from immature stacys could regenerate plants. Lu et al. (2009) investigated roots, rhizoma and leaves as explants to induce callus, and found rhizoma are the optimal explants among these three explants. Sun & Hong (2009) have further attempted root segments as explants for callus induction, and increased callus induction frequencies to 71.0 ~ 75.0 %, respectively. However, because the status of calli derived from root segments was less efficient to regenerate shoots or plantlets than that from mature seeds followed by that from leaf base segments, root segments did not use as the optimal explants in further experiments. And in later studies, Sun & Hong (2010a) continued to use mature seeds as the optimal explants and obtained high callus induction frequencies, and authors have also successfully transformed some genes into this grass using this system (data not published).

Plant species	Isolate	Explants	Reference
Aneurolepidium chinensis	---	Rhizoma	Gao 1982
Aneurolepidium chinensis (Trin.) Kitag	Wild-type collected from Jilin, China	Young rhizoma	Cui et al. (1990)
	Wild-type collected from Nei Mongolia, China	Mature seeds	
Leymus chinensis (Trin.) Tzvel.	NM-1	Immature stacys	Liu et al. (2002)
		Mature embryos	
		Leaf sections	
Leymus chinensis (Trin.)	Wild-type collected from Jilin, China in 2001	Mature seeds	Qu et al. (2004)
Leymus chinensis	Nongmu 1	Immature inflorescence	Liu et al. (2004)
	Jisheng 1		
	C-5		
	C-4		
	C-3		
	W4		
	C-2		
	C-6		
Leymus chinensis	Wild-type collected from Jilin, China in 2002	Mature seeds	Qu et al. (2005)
Leymus chinensis (Trin.)	Wild-type collected from Anda, Heilongjiang, China in 2003	Embryos	Kim et al. (2005)
		Seeds	
		Leaves	
Aneurolepidium chinensis (Trin.) Kitag	A (grey-green leaf) collected from Daqing, Heilongjiang, China	Mature seeds	Wei et al. (2005)
	B (yellow-green leaf) collected from Daqing, Heilongjiang, China		
	C (grey leaf) collected from Daqing, Heilongjiang, China		
Leymus chinensis	Zaipei-3	Young spikes	Zhang et al. (2007)
Leymus chinensis	Wild-type collected from Daan, China in July, 2004	Mature seeds	Kong et al. (2008)
Leymus chinensis	---	Roots	Lu et al. (2009)
		Rhizoma	
		Leaves	
Leymus chinensis (Trin.) Tzvel.	WT, wild-type collected from Siping, Jilin, China	Mature seeds	Sun & Hong (2009)
		Leaf base segments	
		Root segments	
	JS, a new variety collected from Jisheng Wildrye Excellent Seed Station, Changchun, Jilin, China	Mature seeds	
		Leaf base segments	
		Root segments	
Leymus chinensis (Trin.)	WT, wild-type collected from Siping, Jilin, China	Mature seeds	Sun & Hong (2010a)
		Leaf base segments	
	JS, a new variety collected from Jisheng Wildrye Excellent Seed Station, Changchun, Jilin, China	Mature seeds	
		Leaf base segments	

Table 1. Summary of different isolates and explants of *Leymus chinensis* (Trin.) Tzvel. or *Aneurolepidium chinensis* (Trin.) Kitag., used in different tissue culture systems. --- means undefined in the relevant reference

2.2 Genotypes

Tissue culture capacities are estimated by callus induction and plant regeneration efficiency. For LC, the tissue culture capacities according to different genotypes are shown in Table 2. Cui et al. (1990) only could induce 29.05% of explants into calli and 23.68% of calli into shoots or plantlets using wild-type collected from Inner Mongolia of China, while in the following few years, Liu et al. (2002) have obtained nearly 3 times of callus induction frequency (88%) using NM-1 collected from Inner Mongolia of China compared to that in the study of Cui et al. (1990). In the report of Liu et al. (2002), they suggested that only embryogenic calli derived from immature stacys could be used for plant regeneration, but not other explants; NM-1 had the highest plant regeneration frequency (38%) among all ten genotypes such as WZMQY, SL, and JIS-1. Of them, WZMQY could only induce 3% of embryogenic calli into shoots or plantlets, YHT-w had obtained just 20% of plant regeneration frequency, and JIS-1 as a new variety from Jisheng Chinese Wildrye Excellent Seed Station, Jilin, China, had only resulted in 5% of plant regeneration frequency. Liu et al. (2004) optimized further the tissue culture systems of this grass, suggested that all eight genotypes including Nongmu 1 [the same as NM-1 in Liu et al. (2002)], C-2 ~ 6 (populations derived from Nongmu 1), Jisheng 1 [the same as JIS-1 in Liu et al. (2002)] and W4, had relatively high callus induction frequencies and plant regeneration frequencies, especially in Nongmu 1 and Jisheng 1. Nongmu 1 showed 90.29% of callus induction frequency, and C-6, one of its populations showed 93.21% of callus induction frequency, while the plant regeneration frequencies of Nongmu 1 and C-6 reached 43.66% and 9.46%, respectively. Qu et al. (2004) investigated mature seeds of wild-type collected in Jilin of China as explants and obtained 24% of callus induction frequency and 26.67% of plant regeneration frequency. Kim et al. (2005) used various explants of wild-type collected from Heilongjiang of China and found seeds as the optimal explants for callus induction had 68% of callus induction frequency and 36% of plant regeneration frequency; Wei et al. (2005) used mature seeds of wild-type plants collected from Heilongjiang of China and obtained relatively low callus induction and plant regeneration frequencies, of which A with grey-green leaves had the highest callus induction frequency (20%), but relatively low plant regeneration frequency (2%), B with yellow-green leaves had the lowest callus induction frequency (6%), but the highest plant regeneration frequency (4%). Kong et al. (2008) optimized the tissue culture conditions using mature seeds of wild-type collected from Heilongjiang of China as explants, and obtained 48.3% of callus induction frequency. In the study of Sun & Hong (2009), they used both genotypes, WT (wild-type) and JS [a new variety, same as JIS-1 in the report of Liu et al. (2002) and Jisheng 1 in the report of Liu et al. (2004)], collected from Jilin of China, suggesting that WT had slightly higher callus induction and plant frequency frequencies than JS which had been improved to 88.3% and 70.8 %, respectively. In another study of Sun & Hong (2010a), they also used WT and JS as explants and had 75.6% and 71.0% of callus induction and plant regeneration frequencies, respectively. In this report, WT also showed higher callus induction and plant regeneration potential than JS.

Isolate	Collection origin and year	Explants	Callus induction frequency (%)	Plant regeneration frequency (%)	Reference
w	Inner Mongolia, China	Mature seeds	29.05	23.68	Cui et al. (1990)
w	Jilin, China	Young rhizoma	22.50	14.80	

Isolate	Collection origin and year	Explants	Callus induction frequency (%)	Plant regeneration frequency (%)	Reference
NM-1	Ximeng, Inner Mongolia, China	Immature stacys	88	38	Liu et al. (2002)
NM-1	Ximeng, Inner Mongolia, China	Leaf sections	60	0	
NM-1	Ximeng, Inner Mongolia, China	Mature embryos	45	0	
WZMQY	Hailaer, Inner Mongolia, China	Immature stacys	---	3	
SL	Shuangliao, Jilin, China	Immature stacys	---	11	
GLT	Gaolintun, Inner Mongolia, China	Immature stacys	---	21	
YHT-w	Yihuta, Inner Mongolia, China	Immature stacys	---	20	
CL-w	Changling, Jilin, China	Immature stacys	---	8	
HUIG	Changlin, Jilin, China	Immature stacys	---	8	
CHC-01	Changchun, Jilin, China	Immature stacys	---	10	
JIS-1	Changchun, Jilin, China	Immature stacys	---	6	
JIS-4	Changchun, Jilin, China	Immature stacys	---	12	
Nongmu 1	Inner Mongolia, China	Immature inflorescence	90.29	43.66	Liu et al. (2004)
C-2	Inner Mongolia, China	Immature inflorescence	54.23	7.69	
C-3	Inner Mongolia, China	Immature inflorescence	90.72	6.67	
C-4	Inner Mongolia, China	Immature inflorescence	87.12	5.71	
C-5	Inner Mongolia, China	Immature inflorescence	87.79	12.82	
C-6	Inner Mongolia, China	Immature inflorescence	93.21	9.46	
Jisheng 1	Jilin, China	Immature inflorescence	33.35	10.34	
W4	Inner Mongolia, China	Immature inflorescence	64.95	4.71	
w	Jilin, China in 2001	Mature seeds	24	26.67	Qu et al. (2004)
w	Anda, Heilongjiang, China in 2003	Seeds	68	36	Kim et al. (2005)
w	Anda, Heilongjiang, China in 2003	Leaves	51	36	
w	Anda, Heilongjiang,	Embryos	39	36	

Isolate	Collection origin and year	Explants	Callus induction frequency (%)	Plant regeneration frequency (%)	Reference
	China in 2003				
A (grey-green leaf)	Daqing, Heilongjiang, China	Mature seeds	20	2	Wei et al. (2005)
B (yellow-green leaf)	Daqing, Heilongjiang, China	Mature seeds	6	4	
C (grey leaf)	Daqing, Heilongjiang, China	Mature seeds	12	2	
w	Daqing, Heilongjiang, China	Mature seeds	48.3	---	Kong et al. (2008)
WT	Siping, Jilin, China	Mature seeds	88.3	70.8	Sun & Hong (2009)
WT	Siping, Jilin, China	Root segments	71.0	70.8	
WT	Siping, Jilin, China	Leaf base segments	66.7	70.8	
JS	Changchun, Jilin, China	Mature seeds	83.3	68.1	
JS	Changchun, Jilin, China	Root segments	75.0	68.1	
JS	Changchun, Jilin, China	Leaf base segments	74.7	68.1	
WT	Siping, Jilin, China	Mature seeds	75.6	71.0	Sun & Hong (2010a)
WT	Siping, Jilin, China	Leaf base segments	30.0	71.0	
JS	Changchun, Jilin, China	Mature seeds	56.4	69.2	
JS	Changchun, Jilin, China	Leaf base segments	28.9	69.2	

Table 2. Summary of callus induction and plant regeneration frequencies in tissue culture systems using different genotypes. --- means undefined or unverified in the relevant reference. w means wild-type plants in its collection origin

2.3 Medium compositions

2.3.1 Culture media for callus induction

Except effects of explants type and genotypes, the effect of medium compositions in each stage of LC tissue culture is also important and never neglected (Table 3). Gao (1982) has conducted three culture media to induce callus using rhizoma, but could only induce 20% of explants into callus, which also had not high potential of plant regeneration. To improve callus induction conditions, Cui et al. (1990) attempted Murashige and Skoog (MS, Murashige & Skoog, 1962), B5 and 8114 containing 1 ~ 4 mg/l 2,4-dichlorophenoxyacetic acid (2,4-D) to induce callus, suggesting that B5 or MS with 4 mg/l 2,4-D is the most appropriate for callus induction of this grass. Despite there is no a great increase in callus induction frequencies, with about 22%, the study of Cui et al. (1990) is the first report talking about the importance of callus type for regeneration and optimization method of callus types with cultured on B5 or MS with 1 mg/l 2,4-D before shoot organogenesis. Later, Liu et al. (2002) detected effect of various 2,4-D concentrations (0.5 ~ 2.5 mg/l) on callus induction frequency, suggesting that 2.0 mg/l 2,4-D could induce the highest callus induction frequency, but the callus induction frequencies depend on different plant genotypes. Qu et al. (2004) talked effects of various culture medium types (MS, B5, N6 and MSB) and 2,4-D concentrations (0 ~ 4.0 mg/l) on callus induction frequency, and showed that 2.5 mg/l 2,4-D when added into MS culture medium, induce relatively higher callus compared to other 2,4-D concentrations and there was no significant change on callus induction frequencies among MS, B5, N6 and MSB media all supplemented with 2.0 mg/l 2,4-D. Liu et al. (2004) firstly attempted N6 medium in LC, that is more appropriate for tissue culture of gramineous plants due to lower concentrations of inorganic salts, and some components such as glutamine, proline, and casein hydrolytes that might act as nitrogen supplier also helped enhancement of callus induction. Kim et al. (2005) increased the concentrations of thiamine·HCl (VB1), glycine, and inositol in MS basic salts with additional application of 1.0 mg/l, 2.0 mg/l, and 100 mg/l, respectively. With the addition of 1.5 mg/l 2,4-D, it could cause the highest callus induction frequency. Lower and higher 2,4-D concentrations did not satisfy the demands of high callus induction frequency. However, Wei et al. (2005) suggested that effect of 1.0 mg/l 2,4-D on callus induction is remarkable, and the effect on callus induction is inversely proportionate to the 2,4-D concentration. In this study, compact embryogenic callus could be translated from soft and watery callus with 1 ~ 2 times of subculture on the same medium used for callus induction. Zhang et al. (2007) continued to use 2.0 mg/l 2,4-D as the optimal 2,4-D concentration for callus induction of LC according to the report of Liu et al. (2004). The difference was that there was a process of callus status regulation with transferring callus onto MS medium supplemented with 1.0 mg/l abscisic acid (ABA), 100 mg/l casein hydrolytes, 300 ~ 500 mg/l glutamine, 500 mg/l proline and 2.0 mg/l 2,4-D from MS medium only containing 2.0 mg/l 2,4-D. Newly formed callus appeared white, translucent, watery, and nearly ropy with slow growth, that could not be used for plant regeneration (Zhang et al., 2007; Sun & Hong, 2010a). In Zhang et al. (2007) study, they also investigated N6/MS medium alternation to stimulate the formation of embryogenic callus and the proliferation, and make embryogenic callus compact. Compared to MS medium that is in favor of the embryogenesis of callus and the proliferation of embryogenic callus, N6 medium contains higher nitrate-nitrogen concentrations that results in the formation of compact structure of embryogenic callus, the maintenance of the embryogenesis. In the studies of Kong et al. (2008) and Lu et al. (2009), they all applied only 2,4-D to induce callus production, however, the former suggested 2.0 mg/l 2.4-D is the optimal concentration, while the later suggested moderate low 2,4-D concentration (0.5 mg/l) is more suitable in callus induction from rhizoma than high concentration (1.0 mg/l) and low concentration (0.1 mg/l). To optimize the tissue culture conditions further, Sun & Hong (2009) investigated effects of plant hormone 2,4-D, nitrogen supplier and high osmosis maker, glycine and proline, nitrate-nitrogen enhancer, KNO_3 on callus induction by $L_9(3^4)$ orthogonal test, suggesting that using mature seeds as explants demands higher 2,4-D concentration, the optimal medium compositions varies in different explants and genotypes. In our following study, Sun & Hong (2010a) added freshly 5.0 mg/l L-glutamic acid combined with 2.0 mg/l 2,4-D in MS medium, suggesting that the inclusion could significantly promote primary callus induction. Culturing on the same medium for 1 ~ 2 months was essential for the embryogenic callus maturation and the optimization of callus status.

Isolate	Optimal components in media	plant regeneration	Reference
w	B5 or MS + 2,4-D 4 mg/l	MS + 0.5 mg/l BA	Cui et al. (1990)
NM-1	MS + 2 mg/l 2,4-D	MS + 1.0 mg/l KT, 0.5 mg/l NAA	Liu et al. (2002)
WZMQY		MS + 1.0 mg/l KT, 0.5 ~ 1.0 mg/l NAA	
SL		MS + 1.0 mg/l KT, 0.5 mg/l NAA	
GLT		MS + 1.0 mg/l KT, 0.5 mg/l NAA	
YHT-w		MS + 1.0 mg/l KT, 0.5 mg/l NAA	
CL-w		MS + 1.0 mg/l KT, 1.5 mg/l NAA	
HUIG		MS + 1.0 mg/l KT, 0.5 ~ 1.0 mg/l NAA	
CHC-01		MS + 1.0 mg/l KT, 0.5 mg/l NAA	
JIS-1		MS + 1.0 mg/l KT, 1.0 mg/l NAA	
JIS-4		MS + 1.0 mg/l KT, 0.6 mg/l NAA	
w	MS + 2.5 mg/l 2,4-D	MS + 0.5 mg/l BA	Qu et al. (2004)
Nongmu 1	N6 + 5.0 mg/l Glutamine, 500 mg/l Proline, 500 mg/l Casein hydrolytes, 2.0 mg/l 2,4-D	N6 + 1.0 mg/l KT, 1.0 mg/l BA	Liu et al. (2004)
Jisheng 1			
C-5			
C-4			
C-3			
W4			
C-2			
C-6			
w	MS + 1.5 mg/l 2,4-D, 1.0 mg/l Thiamine·HCl, 2.0 mg/l Glycine, 100 mg/l Myo-inositol	MS + 2.0 mg/l KT, 0.5 mg/l NAA	Kim et al. (2005)
A (grey-green leaf)	MS + 1.0 mg/l 2,4-D	1/2 MS + 0.5 ~ 1.5 mg/l NAA	Wei et al. (2005)
B (yellow-green leaf)	MS + 2.0 mg/l 2,4-D		
C (grey leaf)	MS + 1.0 mg/l 2,4-D		
Zaipei-3	MS + 2.0 mg/l 2,4-D	MS/N6 + 2.0 mg/l 2,4-D, 1.0 mg/l ABA, 100 mg/l Casein hydrolytes, 300 ~ 500 mg/l Glutamine, 500 mg/l Proline	Zhang et al. (2007)
w	MS + 2.0 mg/l 2,4-D	---	Kong et al. (2008)
---	MS + 0.5 mg/l 2,4-D	---	Lu et al. (2009)

Isolate	Optimal components in media	plant regeneration	Reference
WT	MS + 1.0 mg/l 2,4-D, 4.0 mg/l Glycine, 0.3 g/l Proline, 1.0 g/l KNO3	MS + 0.2 mg/l NAA, 2.0 mg/l KT, 2.0 g/l casamino acid	Sun & Hong (2009)
	MS + 1.0 mg/l 2,4-D, 4.0 mg/l Glycine, 0.3 g/l Proline, 1.0 g/l KNO3		
	MS + 0.5 mg/l 2,4-D, 2.0 mg/l Glycine, 0.5 g/l Proline, 1.0 g/l KNO3		
JS	MS + 2.0 mg/l 2,4-D, 1.0 mg/l Glycine, 1.0 g/l Proline, 1.0 g/l KNO3		
	MS + 0.5 mg/l 2,4-D, 2.0 mg/l Glycine, 0.5 g/l Proline, 1.0 g/l KNO3		
	MS + 1.0 mg/l 2,4-D, 1.0 mg/l Glycine, 0.5 g/l Proline, 2.0 g/l KNO3		
WT	MS + 2.0 mg/l 2,4-D, 5.0 mg/l L-glutamic acid	MS + 0.2 mg/l NAA, 2.0 mg/l KT, 2.0 g/l casamino acid	Sun & Hong (2010a)
JS		MS + 0.5 mg/l NAA, 2.0 mg/l KT, 2.0 g/l casamino acid	

Table 3. Summary of the optimal medium compositions in callus induction and plant regeneration stages. --- means undefined or unverified in the relevant reference. w means wild-type plants in its collection origin

2.3.2 Culture media for plant regeneration

The final aim of plant tissue culture is still plant regeneration, of which the appropriate concentration combination of medium compositions in plant regeneration media plays an important role (Table 3). From 1982, Gao (1982) has been able to regenerate whole plants from rhizoma, just with low plant regeneration frequency (24.2%). Later in 1990, Cui et al. (1990) performed plant regeneration on MS medium containing 0.5 mg/l 6-benzyladenine (BA), but this still did not largely enhance plant regeneration frequency (14.8 ~ 23.68%). Qu et al. (2004) also investigated plant regeneration on MS medium containing 0.5 mg/l BA, and similar results were obtained, with 26.67% of the plant regeneration frequency. Liu et al. (2002) attempted kinetin (KT) and α-naphthalene acetic acid (NAA) to induce shoot organogenesis in plant regeneration stage, and obtained 38% of the highest plant regeneration frequency using NM-1 genotype. In 2004, Liu et al. (2004) further optimized plant regeneration medium compositions using N6 medium supplemented with 1.0 mg/l KT and 1.0 mg/l BA, and increased plant regeneration frequency (43.66%) once again using Nongmu 1 genotype. In this study, plant regeneration efficiencies varying according to different genotypes are obvious that C-4 and W4 showed only 5.71 ~ 4.71% of plant regeneration frequency. In following study of Liu et al. (2006), it was reported that N6 medium supplemented with 0.3 ~ 2.5 mg/l BA and 0.3 ~ 2.5 mg/l KT could efficiently regulate callus status and thus induce high plant regeneration frequency. Kim et al. (2005) also detected effects of NAA and KT on plant regeneration frequency and found 0.5 mg/l

NAA the most suitable for plant regeneration of wild-type plants collected from Heilongjiang, China when combined with 2.0 mg/l KT in MS medium. Wei et al. (2005) reported that embryogenic callus induction and shoot organogenesis could be accomplished one-step on consistent culture media. Zhang et al. (2007) found ABA, casein hydrolytes, glutamine and proline combined with alternately culture on MS/N6 medium could efficiently improve callus status, and stimulate plant regeneration. Summarized previous studies, Sun & Hong (2009, 2010a) freshly added 2.0 g/l casamino acid combined with 2.0 mg/l KT and low concentrations of NAA (0.2 ~ 0.5 mg/l) in MS medium to increase plant regeneration efficiency, and resulted in relatively high frequencies (54.0 ~ 71.0%).

2.4 Other effects on callus induction

2.4.1 Temperature

Optimal temperature is mainly considered as the requirement of plant growth, however, temperature as one influence factor in plant tissue culture is rarely reported. For LC, most tissue culture systems have been performed under 22 ~ 28℃ without special explanation (Table 4). Until in 2008, Kong et al. (2008) firstly brought forward that variable temperature results in high callus induction and proliferation frequencies through improving the callus status. Callus induction frequency under variable 16℃/26℃ was twice higher compared to that under invariable 26℃, that was explained that alternating temperature could break seed dormancy and thus induce callus induction.

Isolate	Explants	Temperature (°C)	Objection and Remarks	Reference
---	Rhizoma	---	Plant regeneration	Gao 1982
Wild-type collected from Jilin, China	Young rhizoma	---	Regulation of callus status and plant regeneration	Cui et al. (1990)
Wild-type collected from Nei Mongolia, China	Mature seeds			
NM-1	Immature stacys	25	Plant regeneration	Liu et al. (2002)
	Mature embryos		Non regenerated plants	
	Leaf sections		Non regenerated plants	
Wild-type collected from Jilin, China in 2001	Mature seeds	26	Plant regeneration	Qu et al. (2004)
Nongmu 1	Immature inflorescence	25	Plant regeneration	Liu et al. (2004)
Jisheng 1				
C-5				
C-4				
C-3				
W4				
C-2				
C-6				
Wild-type collected from Jilin, China in 2002	Mature seeds	---	Research on salt-tolerance of callus	Qu et al. (2005)
Wild-type collected from Anda, Heilongjiang, China in 2003	Embryos	24 ± 2	Plant regeneration	Kim et al. (2005)
	Seeds			
	Leaves			

Isolate	Explants	Temperature (°C)	Objection and Remarks	Reference
A (grey-green leaf) collected from Daqing, Heilongjiang, China	Mature seeds	25 ± 2	*In vitro* 12 plants regenerated from this system	Wei et al. (2005)
B (yellow-green leaf) collected from Daqing, Heilongjiang, China				
C (grey leaf) collected from Daqing, Heilongjiang, China				
Zaipei-3	Young spikes	22-26	Regulation of callus status	Zhang et al. (2007)
Wild-type collected from Daan, China in July, 2004	Mature seeds	16/26	Research on the relationship between variable cultivating temperature and seed dormancy and callus induction frequency	Kong et al. (2008)
---	Roots	---	Optimation of callus induction	Lu et al. (2009)
	Rhizoma			
	Leaves			
WT, wild-type collected from Siping, Jilin, China	Mature seeds	28 ± 2	Plant regeneration and optimization of callus induction medium by four-factor-thee-level $[L_9(3^4)]$ orthogonal test	Sun & Hong (2009)
	Leaf base segments			
	Root segments			
JS, a new variety collected from Jisheng Wildrye Excellent Seed Station, Changchun, Jilin, China	Mature seeds			
	Leaf base segments			
	Root segments			
WT, wild-type collected from Siping, Jilin, China	Mature seeds	28 ± 2	Optimization of callus induction and plant regeneration media by the addition of growth regulators and plant regeneration	Sun & Hong (2010a)
	Leaf base segments			
JS, a new variety collected from Jisheng Wildrye Excellent Seed Station, Changchun, Jilin, China	Mature seeds			
	Leaf base segments			

Table 4. Summary of temperature used for callus induction and plant regeneration of *L. chinensis*. --- means undefined or unverified in the relevant reference

2.4.2 Seed dormancy

Seed dormancy of LC is the key factor in the inhibition of germination rate that is considered as the main connection with callus induction frequency (Cui et al., 1990), thus, breaking dormancy becomes the sticking point of increasing germination rate and subsequent enhancing callus induction frequency. Ma et al. (2005) has reported that dormancy style of LC belongs to inhibitor-induced physiological dormancy, and one of the key inhibitors is ABA. However, Zhang et al. (2007) reported that low concentration of ABA helps the callus embryogenesis and maintenance of callus compact structure. Zhang et al.

(2007) also suggested that low concentration of ABA creates high-osmotic and dry conditions to stimulate cell growth, while high concentration inhibits the callus embryogenesis regulation and even cause callus browning. Except the variable temperature applied by Kong et al. (2008), many methods including polyethylene glycol (PEG) treatment, exogenous hormone addition and saturation in flowing cold water have also been investigated by scientists (Ma et al., 2005).

2.4.3 Nitrogen source

High ammonium-nitrogen MS medium is reported to be able to stimulate the callus embryogenesis, while low ammonium-nitrogen B5 medium is more suitable for tissue and suspension cell culture of some plant species than MS medium (Table 5). Early in 1990, Cui et al. (1990) have investigated callus induction of LC on B5 medium, but have not obtained significant results compared to that on MS medium. Later, the results of Qu et al. (2004) suggested further B5 did not cause significantly high callus induction frequency in tissue culture of LC. Except B5 medium, high nitrate-nitrogen N6 medium is reported to favor in the formation of callus compact structure and maintenance of callus embryogenesis (Table 5). From the year of 2004, Qu et al. (2004) and Liu et al. (2004) have chosen N6 as basic salts in optimal tissue culture media. However, Qu et al. (2004) found that using N6 and even MSB medium for callus induction did not have remarkable changes compared to using MS medium. Until in 2007, Zhang et al. (2007) further investigated MS/N6 alternating medium to meet needs of callus induction, embryogenesis and maintenance. To improve the callus status and maintain the embryogenesis, many scientists also added some organic nitrogen

Component	MS	N6	B5	MSB
	Concentration (mg/l)	Concentration (mg/l)	Concentration (mg/l)	Concentration (mg/l)
KNO_3	1900	2830	2500	1900
NH_4NO_3	1650	463		1650
KH_2PO4	170	400		170
$MgSO_4 \cdot 7H_2O$	370	185	250	370
$CaCl_2 \cdot 2H_2O$	440	165	150	440
KI	0.83	0.80	0.75	0.83
H_3BO_3	6.2	1.6	3.0	6.2
$MnSO_4 \cdot 4H_2O$	22.3	4.4	10	22.3
$(NH_4)_2SO_4$			134	
$ZnSO_4 \cdot 7H_2O$	8.6	1.5	2.0	8.6
$Na_2MoO_4 \cdot 2H_2O$	0.25		0.025	0.25
$CuSO_4 \cdot 5H_2O$	0.025		0.025	0.025
$CoCl_2 \cdot 6H_2O$	0.025		0.025	0.025
Na_2-EDTA	37.3	37.3	37.3	37.3
$FeSO_4 \cdot 7H_2O$	27.8	27.8	27.8	27.8
Inositol	100		100	100
Glycine	2.0	2.0		2.0
Nicotinic acid	0.5	0.5	1.0	1.0
VB1	0.1	1.0	10	10
VB6	0.5	0.5	1.0	1.0

Table 5. Components of common culture media including MS, N6, B5 and MSB

sources, such as glutamine, proline, casein hydrolytes, glycine and casamino acids (Liu et al., 2004; Zhang et al., 2007; Sun & Hong 2009, 2010a), and many evidence suggested that these accessions of organic nitrogen sources, or even additional nitrate-nitrogen sources like KNO_3 (Sun & Hong 2009), have greatly improved the callus status and enhanced the callus embryogenesis and maintenance.

2.4.4 Others

Pre-culture on medium with lower 2,4-D concentrations than medium used for primary callus induction before transferring onto plant regeneration medium results in efficient and rapid plant regeneration (Liu et al., 2002b). Cui et al. (1990) firstly attempted this method in improvement of callus status, suggesting that removing 2,4-D and adding inositol and casein hydrolytes could regulate callus status to increase plant regeneration frequency. Later, this method continued to be used in many studies (Liu et al., 2002b; Qu et al., 2004; Kim et al., 2005; Wang et al., 2006; Kong et al., 2008), as well as suggesting that lower 2,4-D concentration could help the following plant regeneration. In addition, to quicken the production of embryogenic callus and *in vitro* regenerated plants of LC, a novel plant regeneration system from suspension-derived callus has been established by Sun & Hong (2010). This cell suspension culture system makes significantly greater increment of callus biomass and more stable culture conditions than the conventional tissue culture system.

3. *In vitro* embryogenesis of dicotyledon

The medicinal plant, ES was used as the model dicotyledonous plant for understanding the embryogenic callus induction and plant regeneration. The factors affecting embryogenic callus induction efficiency and plant regeneration potential would be presented here.

3.1 General introduction of ES

ES is a woody medicinal plant that grows only in cold regions of Asia (Lee, 1979). Due to the over-exploitation of ES, combined with poor seed setting and/or failure to set seed (Yu et al., 2003), this plant has become an endangered species in several countries, and even classified as rare, protected plants by the Environmental Ministry in Korea (Jung et al., 2004). To develop the farm cultivation of ES, many investigations are involved in the natural growth conditions of habitats. As known that the region, Hokkaida in Japan is the location adapting to the natural growth and seed production of ES, Park et al. (1995) therefore compared the natural condition factors such as local temperature and sunshine duration of Hokkaida in Japan with several locations in Korea to select a proper seed production site in Korea. This investigation suggested that Daegwanryeong in Korea is the most suitable for ES cultivation from seed propagation, because its climate characteristics are mostly similar to those of Hokkaido. In the further investigation, Park et al. (1996) mentioned Mountain Deokyu situated at 127°45′E, 35°52′N, is one of main habitats of ES in Korea. To understand more habitat information to instruct farm cultivation of ES in Korea, Park et al. (1996) surveyed the local climate, soil components, and symbiotic plant species as information inferences. To optimize the cultivation conditions of ES, Han et al. (2001) investigated the effect of shading treatments on the growth of ES, and suggested that 50% shading net treatment was most effective for yield. Kim et al. (2003) deemed that shading treatments could increase not only apparent quantum yield, but carboxylation efficiency and re-phosphorylation.

Since long-term stratification during afterripening period is required to induce maturation of the zygotic embryos in mature seeds (Isoda & Shoji, 1994), Park et al. (1997) studied the characteristics of embryo elongation after stratification and the dehiscence rate during afterripening period, which would help improve seed propagation of this species.

In addition, seed dormancy also entangles germination and propagation of this species. ES is known to have double dormancy: morphological rudimentary dormancy influenced by surrounding endosperm, and physiological dormancy after post-maturation of zygotic embryos (You et al., 2005). To date, several studies have been attempted to break seed dormancy in order to promote the seed germination, but most studies only focus on its physiological dormancy. For example, Li et al. (2003a) investigated a method for breaking the physiological dormancy of dehisced ES seeds, and suggested that storage at 5℃ for 85 d could most effectively increase germination rates up to more than 90%. In the report by Li et al. (2003b), they performed cold stratification before sowing, combined with gibberellic acid (GA_3) soak. This result showed 10 d-cold stratification at 4℃ following afterripening, and soaking in 500 ppm GA_3 for 3 d could also effectively promote germination. As the effective influence of GA_3 soak on germination, Lim et al. (2008) also applied this method as pretreatment of ES seeds, however, due to the different experimental materials and specific sensitivity to GA_3 soak, they elucidated the optimal GA_3 concentration was 300 mg/l for promoting the seed afterripening. And Toros sterilization was synchronously performed in ES seeds, showing positive effect on reducing dehiscent rates and suppressing fungi actions. To break another dormancy of ES, You et al. (2005) applied endosperm removal during *in vitro* culture of excised seeds and plant regeneration, and the removal of endosperm tissue not only broke the morphological rudimentary dormancy but markedly stimulated the growth of rudimentary zygotic embryos. To improve the efficiency of dormancy breaking, GA_3 treatment in 2.0 mg/l was together used in the *in vitro* culture of excised seeds.

Except of seed propagation, stem cutting propagation is widely used for propagation of ES, however, difficult rooting is a major problem to resolve. Park et al. (1994) suggested that rooting could be successfully induced from cut of stems after 3 ~ 12 d-culture, and the season for cutting propagation is also important, the late September being the best cutting season in Korea. Han et al. (2001) indicated that up-ground 30 cm-length cutting was the most effective for branching stem length, plant height and yield.

Despite a great process has been achieved on conventional propagation, this propagation pattern is known limited by some disadvantages, such as requiring enormous time and labor, and particularly long-term stratification for ES (Choi & Jeong, 2002). Thus, the establishment of more efficient propagation methods is urgently needed. Decently, *in vitro* callus induction and plant regeneration through embryogenesis has become rapid, efficient propagation means.

3.2 *In vitro* plant regeneration

Based on the plasticity and totipotency of plants, tissue culture technology has now become a remarkably useful tool in experimental studies, such as rapidly achievement of plant breeding and mass propagation. Based on one hundred years' investigation, plant tissue culture technologies have achieved a great progress in many aspects including the effects of plant growth regulators, auxins, and cytokinins, genotype-dependence, and callus type-dependence.

3.2.1 Effect of 2,4-D

In general, 2,4-D is an important inducer for somatic embryogenesis, and this inducer has also been used for the induction of somatic embryos of ES in many investigations (Gui et al., 1991; Han & Choi, 2003). And the importance of 2,4-D has been early affirmed by Gui et al. (1991) that 0.5 mg/l 2,4-D could produce mature embryos developed somatic embryos directly from swollen cotyledon and embryo axes, but most embryos only germinated on the above medium without 2,4-D. In the following investigations, the most optimal callus induction media were mainly composed with 2,4-D alone or combined with the addition of another growth inducer, thidiazuron (TDZ). For instance, Choi & Soh (1993) suggested that 1.0 mg/l 2,4-D could induce more calli from various explants of ES, and successfully achieve the transference from callus induction to plant regeneration on the same medium. Yu et al. (1997b) suggested that treatment with 2,4-D had better efficiency in callus induction than treatment of TDZ, however the plant regeneration was reversed. Yu et al. (1997a) have investigated the effects of 2,4-D and TDZ on callus formation and plant regeneration, suggesting that treatment of 2,4-D induced more calli than treatment of TDZ alone, and treatment of 2,4-D combined with TDZ had higher callus formation than treatment of 2,4-D alone. In addition, Yu et al. (1997a) also attempted various basic salts as main medium, such as WPM and SH, among which SH medium containing 1.0 mg/l 2,4-D showed 83% of callus induction frequency. Yu et al. (1997a) suggested that plant regeneration differed depending on the mature degree of immature embryo. Choi et al. (1999a) induced directly embryogenic callus without intervening callus formation on MS medium containing 1.0 mg/l 2,4-D, but the embryogenic callus formation frequency was not very high. However, embryogenic calli were transferred to MS medium lacking 2,4-D to induce somatic embryo development, and amounts of somatic embryos were produced. Li & Yu (2002) attempted to induce callus from various explants, different genotypes, and both 2,4-D concentrations (2.0 mg/l and 4.0 mg/l), and suggested that MS medium containing 2.0 mg/l 2,4-D combined with 2.0 mg/l TDZ, or 4.0 mg/l 2,4-D and 1.0 mg/l TDZ had the highest efficiency in callus formation. According to callus induction of ES, the most optimal 2,4-D concentrations were reported to be arranged between 0.5 mg/l and 4.0 mg/l (Table 6). Generally, the concentrations of alone 2,4-D were relatively low, arranging between 0.5 mg/l and 1.0 mg/l, while the concentrations of 2,4-D combined with TDZ showed higher than those with alone 2,4-D addition, arranging between 1.0 mg/l and 4.0 mg/l.

From our summary, it was obvious that 2,4-D is critical for callus initiation and embryogenic callus formation in ES, particularly when combined with the supplement of TDZ.

3.2.2 Effects of other callus inducers

Except the important growth inducer, 2,4-D, other many growth inducers also played important roles in callus induction, somatic embryo maturity, and even plant regeneration (Table 7). In the early report of Gui et al. (1991), BA and NAA were also used for callus induction and embryogenesis. Medium supplemented BA combined with NAA or 2,4-D only caused embryos enlarge, swell, callus, but did not produce somatic embryos or adventitious buds or shoots. This suggested that BA or NAA was not more efficient than 2,4-D in embryogenesis of ES. However, 0.5 mg/l 2,4-D or 1.0 ~ 3.0 mg/l indole-3-acetic acid (IAA) or 0.5 mg/l zeatin or 0.2 mg/l NAA was suggested to be favored in somatic embryo development and maturity by Gui et al. (1991). Later, TDZ that has both auxin- and cytokinin-like activity and can be substituted for auxins or combinations of auxins and cytokinins (Shen et al., 2007; Singh et al., 2003), was used to improve the callus induction conditions of ES (Yu et al., 1997a). It was suggested that alone TDZ, IAA, NAA, or BA with different concentrations was investigated to induce callus induction (Yu et al., 1997a), only alone BA could induce callus successfully. The callus induction frequency caused by alone BA was very low, reaching only 20%. However, if optimal concentration of TDZ (0.7 mg/l) mixed with the addition of 2,4-D, the callus induction frequency was largely increased, having 4-5-fold increase (Yu et al., 1997a). For plant regeneration, Yu et al. (1997a) suggested that the combination of growth inducers did not had better regeneration efficiency than single addition of growth inducer, and lower concentration of TDZ showed the highest plant regeneration frequency in MS, MSB5, and B5 medium. In the following study by Yu et al. (1997b), the optimal concentration of TDZ showed closed relationships with the basic salts in callus induction medium, suggesting that alone 2,4-D without the addition of TDZ produced high callus induction frequency using SH medium as the basic salts, while higher concentration of TDZ was required to be combined with 2,4-D when using WPM medium as the basic salts (Table 6). In addition, Li & Yu (2002) firstly attempted to use indole-3-butyric acid (IBA), combined with TDZ to induce callus, however, the callus induction frequencies of different ES genotypes were generally lower than those with the treatment of 2,4-D combined with TDZ.

Growth inducers	Concentration (mg/l)	Remarks	References
2.4-D	0.5		Gui et al. (1991)
	1		Choi & Soh (1993)
	2	Combined with the addition of 0.7 mg/l TDZ	Yu et al. (1997a)
	1	Using SH medium as the basic salts	Yu et al. (1997b)
	1	Combined with the addition of 3.0 mg/l TDZ, using WPM medium as the basic salts	
	1		Choi et al. (1999a)
	1		Choi et al. (1999b)
	2	Combined with the addition of 2.0 mg/l TDZ	Li & Yu (2002)
	4	Combined with the addition of 1.0 mg/l TDZ	

Table 6. The most optimal concentrations of 2,4-D in callus induction

Growth inducers	Concentration (mg/l)	Treatment for somatic embryo development	References
BA	0.5 ~ 2.0	2,4-D 0.5 mg/l, or IAA 1.0 ~ 3.0 mg/l, or zeatin 0.5 mg/l, or NAA 0.2 mg/l	Gui et al. (1991)
NAA	0.5		
TDZ	0.7	2,4-D 1.0 ~ 4.0 mg/l, or TDZ 0.02 ~ 2.2 mg/l, or IAA 1.0 ~ 2.0 mg/l, or NAA 1.0 ~ 2.0 mg/l, or BA 1.0 mg/l	Yu et al. (1997a)
TDZ	3.0	Combination of 2,4-D 0.1 ~ 2.0 mg/l and TDZ 0.1~3.0 mg/l	Yu et al. (1997b)
TDZ	0.07 ~ 10	Combination of the addition of TDZ with 2,4-D or IBA, and culture in MS free liquid medium	Li & Yu (2002)
IBA	10		

Table 7. Other growth inducers during callus induction stage and treatment for somatic embryo development

3.2.3 Explant type

Explant type is another important factor affecting callus initiation efficiency. Generally, younger, more rapidly growing tissue is most effective. There have been many evidences indicating that plant regeneration potentials in many plant species have a direct correlation with the developmental stage of the explants tissue, such as in rice (Sahrawat & Chand, 2001), wheat (Wernicke & Milkovits, 1984), oat (Chen et al., 1995). For the monocotyledonon LC, mature seed has been reported to be the optimal explant for callus initiation according to the description of Part 2.1. For the dicotyledon ES, the investigations and attempts about appropriate explants have also been much studied (Table 8).

First, swollen cotyledon and embryo axes were used to induce callus, and they develop somatic embryos from the epidermal or subepidermal layer of the cotyledons or embryonic axes (Gui et al., 1991). The precedence of both explants, though, was not discussed, the somatic embryos rapidly developed into globular or heart-shaped structures, and germinated normally. Choi & Soh (1993) attempted various explants to initiate callus induction, including cotyledon, hypocotyl, radicle, and intact embryo and wounded embryo, of which wounded embryo produced the highest somatic embryo formation (77.8%). With 6 week-culture, wounded embryo-derived callus appeared torpedo shape and even cotyledonary embryo, while other calli derived from intact embryo, cotyledon, hypocotyl, or radicle appeared globular, heart shape, few torpedo shape, but no cotyledonary embryo. Later, immature embryo was firstly used as explant by Yu et al. (1997a, b), and produced high somatic embryo formation.

Embryogenic cells treated as artificial seeds for obtaining plants directly have been reported for several crops of agricultural interest (Kitto & Janick, 1985; Redenbaugh et al., 1986; Choi & Jeong, 2002). To achieve ES embryogenic cells as artificial seeds, Choi et al. (1999a, b) investigated different explants to attempt to initiate callus induction in a simple and efficient way. Among cotyledon, hypocotyl, and root of zygotic embryos, hypocotyl was considered as the most optimal explant of ES, and had the highest frequency of somatic embryo formation. Using hypocotyl-derived embryogenic cells from this system, mass production through large-scale tank culture were successfully obtained, with approximately 27-fold increment of fresh weight of somatic embryo after 4 week-culture (Choi et al., 2002). In addition, mass production through cell suspension culture was also done by comparing the somatic embryo formation from cotyledon, hypocotyl, and radicle-derived embryogenic cells (Han & Choi, 2003). In this study, embryogenic cells derived from hypocotyl of zygotic embryos showed the highest growth rate and somatic embryo formation of 89%. Based on the above suggestions, it is indicated that even mass production of plant cell through large-scale suspension culture has been successfully obtained, ES plantlets produced from this system could be more convenient to be used as a source of medicinal raw materials. However, due to direct sowing of artificial seeds in the field for practical use, low soil survival becomes a major problem (Redenbaugh et al., 1986). Herein, Choi & Jeong (2002) overcame the problem of low soil survival, and reported firstly encapsulated somatic embryos as ES artificial seeds to achieve all development status from artificial seeds to whole plants. Later, Jung et al. (2004) further improved this system with the addition of carbon sources to the encapsulation matric, and obtained that 96% of the encapsulated embryos converted to plantlets with well-elongated epicotyls.

Explants used in the study	The most optimal explant	Somatic embryo formation (%)	References
Swollen cotyledon	---	83.3	Gui et al. (1991)
Embryo axes			
Hypocotyl	Wounded embryo	77.8±9.6	Choi & Soh (1993)
Cotyledon			
Radicle			
Embryo (intact and wounded)			
Immature embryos	Immature embryos	86.7	Yu et al. (1997a)
Immature embryos	Immature embryos	83.3	Yu et al. (1997b)
Hypocotyl	Hypocotyl	---	Choi et al. (1999a)
Cotyledon	Hypocotyl	75	Choi et al. (1999b)
Hypocotyl			
Root			
Young leaf	Petiole	3.0	Li & Yu (2002)
Stem			
Node			
Petiole			
Penduncle			
Flower			
Root			
Cotyledon from zygotic embryo, seedling, and plant	Hypocotyl from zygotic embryo	89±7.2	Han & Choi (2003)
Hypocotyl from zygotic embryo, seedling, and plant			
Radicle from zygotic embryo, seedling, and plant			

Table 8. Explants of callus initiation and somatic embryo formation. --- means undefined in the relevant reference

3.2.4 Other effects on embryogenesis and plant regeneration

As known that seed dehydration accompanied by the maturation of zygotic embryos results in the dormancy of zygotic embryos (Gray et al., 1987), thus, the desiccation of somatic embryos not detrimental to survival is very efficient in the long-term conservation of somatic embryos. In light of these theories, Choi & Jeong (2002) investigated the dormancy characteristics of ES somatic embryos and induced encapsulated somatic embryos maintain in the dormancy status by a high sucrose treatment. Moreover, maintaining ES somatic embryos from cell suspension cultures under low temperature (4°C) was also considered to be able to achieve long-term animatingly conservation (Li et al., 2004). These treatments help a long-term conservation of artificial seeds and an enhanced resistance to dehydration of somatic embryos. You et al. (2005) carried out that removal of endosperm from seeds could markedly stimulate the growth of rudimentary zygotic embryos to induce more rapid germination of rudimentary zygotic embryos by *in vitro* culture of excised seeds. And in their later investigation (You et al., 2006), the roles of plasmolyzing pretreatment for zygotic embryos were evaluated on the induction of somatic embryos, suggesting that this pretreatment could result in sharply increased callose concentration in ES zygotic embryos, and callose accumulation could then stimulate the reprogramming of epidermal cells into embryogenically competent cells and finally induce somatic-embryo development from single cells. The further and detailed mechanism of enhanced somatic embryo formation through plasmolysis treatment was revealed that the expression level of callose synthase gene increased with response to 2,4-D, sucrose, and mannitol, and the callose played an important role in separating cell in epidermis from neighboring cells and consequently developing into embryogenic potential cells (Xilin et al., 2010).

3.3 Application for biochemical and biological events

Somatic embryogenesis has been studied as a model system for understanding the physiological, biochemical, and molecular biological events occurring during plant embryo development (Zimmerman, 1993). Among them, production of secondary metabolites through cell culture, particularly in medical plant, has long been used for commercial purposes (Roberts, 2007). To improve the culture conditions and then increase the production efficiency, many scientists have been investigated many factors affecting growth of culture materials and *in vivo* accumulation of active compounds. Ahn et al. (2003) investigated the effect of inorganic nitrogen sources such as KNO_3 and NH_4NO_3 on cell growth and production of chlorogenic acid and eleutheroside E derivative. In another investigation by Ahn et al. (2007), the effect of NO_3^- and NH_4^+ on the adventitious root growth of ES and production of eleutheroside derivatives were investigated, and eleutheroside B (249 µg/g), E (788 µg/g), and E1 (43 µg/g) were increased at the highest levels by 40, 120, and 40 mM total nitrogen source, respectively. These results suggested that production of secondary metabolites through *in vitro* cultured cells could be manipulated by controlling the total concentration of nitrogen sources and the concentration ratio of NO_3^- and NH_4^+ in the culture medium.

Except of nitrogen sources, light is another important factor affecting growth and organogenesis, but a factor stressing plants to consequently regulate the secretion mechanism of secondary products (Shohael et al., 2006a). Higher H_2O_2 content, malondialdehyde content and lipoxygenase activities were observed in cultured embryos under red light compared dark grown embryos, as well as activities of some antioxidant enzymes such as catalase, superoxide dismutase, glutathione *S* transferase, and ascorbate peroxidase were also stimulated in red light irradiated embryos. Of course, the contents of eleutheroside E and E1 were synchronously accumulated 51% and 21% higher than control under red light irradiation. Jeong et al. (2009) compared the effects of red, blue, and far-red light by irradiation of light emitting diodes (LEDs) with white fluorescent lamp, on growth, morphogenesis and eleutheroside contents of *in vitro* cultured ES. The results indicated that *in vitro* cultured plantlets under the red/blue LEDs were taller than control, and those under blue LED showed greater leaf area, root length, and fresh weight than other light sources. Contents of eleuthroside B and E in plantlets were higher under blue LED, while content of eleuthroside E1 was the highest under fluorescent lamps.

Ahn et al. (2007, 2010) investigated the impacts of jasmonic acid (JA) on adventitious root culture of ES and eleutherosides accumulation, suggesting that JA inhibited the root growth but increased eleutherosides accumulation, as well as total phenolic contents and antioxidant activity. The highest levels of accumulation of eleutheroside B (359.9 μg/g), E (798.1 μg/g), and E1 (197 μg/g) were found under 40, 10, and 10 μM of methyl jasmonate addition, respectively.

Effects of temperature on secondary metabolite production such as eleutheroside B, E, E1, total phenolics, flavonoids, and chlorogenic acid and antioxidant enzyme activities were investigated by Shohael et al. (2006b), suggesting that culture at 24°C caused the highest production efficiency of secondary metabolites, and either lower or higher temperature could cause severe oxidative stress to form a cellular damage. Based on above results, the production of secondary metabolites, one side, was considered as the consequent result of cultured cell metabolism, the other side, as the outcome stimulated by some stress treatments. Therefore, to control the balance between reactive oxygen species (ROS) formation derived by stress treatments and consumption correlated with an array of antioxidant enzymes and redox metabolites becomes required and important. Shohael et al. (2007) further examined the ascorbate-glutathione cycle enzymes and other enzymes metabolism during somatic embryogenesis of ES, and suggested that the alterations of the glutathione redox systems play a significant role in somatic embryo development.

Genetic improvement of another application of plant tissue culture, and a good approach to improve plant physiological traits and augment the drug-yielding capacity of medicinal plants (Tejavathi & Shailaja, 1999). To authors' knowledge, only two transformation events through *Agrobacterium*-mediated transformation occurred in ES. Jo et al. (2005) transformed the human lactoferrin (*hLf*) gene into ES cells, and these transgenic ES cultured cells could produce *hLf* protein as cell growth increasing proportionally. As lactoferrin is an iron-binding glycoprotein with many biological roles, including the protection against microbial and virus infection and stimulation of the immune system, *hLf* transgenic ES plants could be used as a medicinal raw material for production of secondary metabolites. Another successful transformation event of ES was obtained in the report by Seo et al. (2005) that a squalene synthass-encoding gene derived from *Panax ginseng* (*PgSS1*) was successfully introduced into ES plants through *Agrobacterium*-mediated transformation. The transgenic plants showed up to 3-fold of squalene synthase enzyme activity higher than that of wild-type plants. Moreover, the introduced *PgSS1* gene in transgenic plants enhanced the metabolisms of phytosterol and triterpenoides, with 2.0 ~ 2.5-fold increments of their levels. These results indicated that transgenic ES cultured cells would be biotechnologically useful for the commercial production of medicinal plant cell cultures.

4. Conclusions

All biotechnological approaches like genetic engineering, haploid induction, or somaclonal variation to improve traits strongly depend on an efficient *in vitro* plant regeneration system. Since LC as a monocotyledonous grass species and also a halophyte and ES as a dicotyledonous medicinal plant species, have increasingly great ecological and economic significant, this review would help efficiently improve traits through genetically modification.

5. Acknowledgment

This work was supported by Nutraceutical Bio Brain Korea 21 Project Group.

6. References

Ahn, J.K.; Lee, W.Y. & Park, E.J. (2010). Effect of methyl jasmonate on the root growth and the eleutheroside accumulation in the adventitious root culture of *Eleutherococcus senticosus*. *Journal of Korean Forest Society*, Vol.99, No.3, (June 2010), pp. 331-336, ISSN 0445-4650

Ahn, J.K.; Lee, W.Y. & Park, S.Y. (2003). Effect of nitrogen source on the cell growth and production of secondary metabolites in bioreactor cultures of *Eleutherococcus senticosus*. *Korean Journal of Plant Biotechnology*, Vol.30, No.3, pp. 301-305, ISSN 1598-6365

Ahn, J.K.; Park, Y.K.; Lee, W.Y. & Park, S.Y. (2007). Increment of eleutherosides and antioxidant activity in *Eleutherococcus senticosus* adventitious root by jasmonic acid. *Journal of Korean Forest Society*, Vol.96, No.5, pp. 539-542, ISSN 0445-4650

Anis, M. & Faisal, M. (2005). *In Vitro* regeneration and mass multiplication of *Psoralea corylifolia*–An endangered medicinal plant. *Indian Journal of Biotechnology*, Vol.4, No.2, (April 2005), pp. 261-264, ISSN 0972-5849

Chen, H.C.; Xu, G.J.; Loschke, D.C.; Tomaska, L. & Rolfe, B.G. (1995). Efficient callus formation and plant regeneration from leaves of oats (*Avena sativa* L.). *Plant Cell Reports*, Vol.14, No.6, pp. 393-397, doi:10.1007/BF00238604, ISSN 0721-7714

Choi, Y.E. & Jeong, J.H. (2002). Dormancy induction of somatic embryos of Siberian ginseng by high sucrose concentrations enhances the conservation of hydrated artificial seeds and dehydration resistance. *Plant Cell Reports*, Vol.20, No., pp. 1112-1116, ISSN 0721-7714. doi:10.1007/s00299-002-0455-y

Choi, Y.E. & Soh, W.Y. (1993). Structural aspects of somatic embryos derived from cultured zygotic embryos in *Acanthopanax senticosus* L. *Korean Journal of Plant Tissue Culture*, Vol.20, No.5, pp. 261-266, ISSN 1015-5880

Choi, Y.E.; Kim, J.W. & Yoon, E.S. (1999a). High frequency of plant production *via* somatic embryogenesis from callus or cell suspension cultures in *Eleutherococcus senticosus*. *Annals of Botany*, Vol.83, No.3, pp. 309-314, ISSN 0305-7364

Choi, Y.E.; Lee, K.S.; Kim, E.Y.; Kim, Y.S.; Han, J.Y.; Kim, H.S.; Jeong, J.H. & Ko, S.K. (2002). Mass production of Siberian ginseng plantlets through large-scale tank culture of somatic embryos. *Plant Cell Reports*, Vol.21, No.1, pp. 24-28, ISSN 0721-7714. doi:10.1007/s00299-002-0470-z

Choi, Y.E.; Yang, D.C. & Yoon, E.S. (1999b). Rapid propagation of *Eleutherococcus senticosus via* direct somatic embryogenesis from explants of seedlings. *Plant Cell, Tissue and Organ Culture*, Vol.58, No.2, pp. 93-97, ISSN 0167-6857

Cui, Q.H.; Zhang, Y.Z.; Piao, T.F.; Gu, D.F.; Zhang, W.Q.; Xu, Y.K.; Sun, Z.L. & Liu, H.X. (1990). Embryogenic callus and plant regeneration of *Aneurolepidium chinensis* (Trin.) Kitag. *Journal of Jilin Agricultural University*, Vol.12, pp. 1-5 ISSN 1000-5684

Czerepanov, S.K. (2007). *Vascular plants of Russia and adjacent states (the former USSR)*, Cambridge University Press, pp. 377-378, ISBN 0-521-45006-3, Cambridge, UK

Davydov, M. & Krikorian, A.D. (2000). *Eleutherococcus senticosus* (Rupr. and Maxim.) Maxim. (Araliaceae) as an adaptogen: a closer look. *Journal of Ethnopharmacology,* Vol.72, No.2000, pp. 345-393, ISSN 0378-8741

Fowler, M.W. (1983). Commercial applications and economic aspects of mass plant cell culture, In: *Plant biotechnology,* S.H. Mantell & H. Smith, (Ed.), 3-37, Cambridge University Press, Cambridge, UK

Furuya, T.; Yoshikawa, T.; Orihara, Y. & Oda, H. (1983). Saponin production in cell suspension cultures of *Panax ginseng*. *Planta Medica,* Vol.48, No.2, (June 1983), pp. 83-87, ISSN 0032-0943

Gaffney, B.T.; Hügel, H.M. & Rich, P.A. (2001). The effects of *Eleutherococcus senticosus* and *Panax ginseng* on steroidal hormone indices of stress and lymphocyte subset numbers in endurance athletes. *Life Sciences,* Vol.70, No.4, (December 2001), pp. 431-442, ISSN 0024-3205

Gao, T.S. (1982). Induction of callus and regeneration of plantlets from the rhizome explants of *Aneurolepidium chinensis. Acta Botanica Sinica,* Vol.24, pp. 182-185, ISSN 1672-6650

Gautheret, R.J. (1934). Culture du tissus cambial. *Comptes Rendus Hebdomadaires des Séances de l'Académie des Sciences,* Vol.198, pp. 2195-2196, ISSN 0001-4036

Gray, D.J.; Conger, B.V. & Songstad, D.D. (1987). Desiccated quiescent somatic embryos of orchardgrass for use as synthetic seeds. *In Vitro Cellular & Developmental Biology,* Vol.23, No.1, (January 1987), pp. 29-33, ISSN 0883-8364

Gui, Y.; Guo, Z.; Ke, S. & Skirvin, R.H. (1991). Somatic embryogenesis and plant regeneration in *Acanthopanax senticosus. Plant Cell Reports,* Vol.9, No.9, pp. 514-516, ISSN 0721-7714

Hahn, D.R.; Kim, C.J. & Kim, J.H. (1985). A study on chemical constituents of *Acanthopanax koreanum* Nakai and its pharmaco-biological activities. *Yakhak Hoeji,* Vol.29, pp. 357-361, ISSN 0377-9556

Han, J.S.; Kim, S.K.; Kim, S.W. & Kim, Y.J. (2001). Effects of shading treatments and harvesting methods on the growth of *Eleutherococcus senticosus* Maxim. *Korean Journal of Medicinal Crop Science,* Vol.9, No.1, pp. 1-7, ISSN 1225-9306

Han, J.Y. & Choi, Y.E. (2003). Mass production of *Eleutherococcus senticosus* plants through *in vitro* cell culture. *Korean Journal of Plant Biotechnology,* Vol.30, No.2, pp. 167-172, ISSN 1598-6365

Hanning, E. (1904). Zur Physiologie pflanzlicher Embryonen. I. Über die Kultur von cruciferen Embryonen ausserhalb des Embryosacks. *Botanische Zeitung,* Vol.62, pp. 45-80

Huang, Z.; Zhu, J.; Mu, X. & Lin, J. (2004). Pollen dispersion, pollen viability and pistil receptivity in *Leymus chinensis*. *Annals of Botany,* Vol.93, No.3, (January 2004), pp. 295-301, ISSN 0305-7364

Isoda, S. & Shoji, J. (1994). Studies on the cultivation of *Eleutherococcus senticosus* Maxim. II. On the germination and raising of seedling. *Nature Medicine,* Vol.48, pp. 75-81, ISSN 1078-8956

Jeong, J.H.; Kim, Y.S.; Moon, H.K.; Hwang, S.J. & Choi, Y.E. (2009). Effects of LED on growth, morphogenesis and eleutheroside contents of *in vitro* cultured plantlets of *Eleutherococcus senticosus* Maxim. *Korean Journal of Medicinal Crop Science,* Vol.17, No.1, pp. 39-45, ISSN 1225-9306

Jia, S.X. (1987). *Forage floras of China,* Agricultural Press, pp. 19-35, ISBN 978-1-930723-59-7, Beijing, China

Jin, H.; Plaha, P.; Park, J.Y.; Hong, C.P.; Lee, I.S.; Yang, Z.H.; Jiang, G.B.; Kwak, S.S.; Liu, S.K.; Lee, J.S.; Kim, Y.A. & Lim, Y.P. (2006). Comparative EST profiles of leaf and root of *Leymus chinensis*, a xerophilous grass adapted to high pH sodic soil. *Plant Science,* Vol.170, No.6, (June 2006), pp. 1081-1086, ISSN 0168-9452

Jo, S.H.; Kwon, S.Y.; Kim, J.W.; Lee, K.T.; Kwak, S.S. & Lee, H.S. (2005). Transgenic Siberian ginseng cultured cells that produce high levels of human lactoferrin. *Korean Journal of Plant Biotechnology,* Vol.32, No.3, pp. 209-215, ISSN 1598-6365

Jung, S.J.; Yoon, E.S.; Jeong, J.H. & Choi, Y.E. (2004). Enhanced post-germinative growth of encapsulated somatic embryos of Siberian ginseng by carbohydrate addition to the encapsulation matrix. *Plant Cell Reports,* Vol.23, No.6, (November 2004), pp. 365-370, doi:10.1007/s00299-004-0821-z, ISSN 0721-7714

Kim, M.D.; Jin, H.; Park, E.J.; Kwon, S.Y.; Lee, H.S. & Kwak, S.S. (2005). Plant regeneration through somatic embryogenesis of *Leymus chinensis* Trin. *Korean Journal Plant Biotechnology,* Vol.32, No.1, pp. 51-55, ISSN 1598-6365 (in Korean with English abstract)

Kim, P.G.; Lee, K.Y.; Hur, S.D.; Kim, S.H. & Lee, E.J. (2003). Effects of shading treatment on photosynthetic activity of *Acanthopanax senticosus. Korean Journal of Ecology,* Vol.26, No.6, pp. 321-326, ISSN 1225-0317

Kitto, S. & Janick, J. (1985). Production of synthetic seeds by encapsulating asexual embryos of carrot. *Journal of the American Society for Horticultural Science,* Vol.110, pp. 277-282, ISSN 0003-1062

Kong, X.J.; Liang, Z.W.; Ma, H.Y. & Liu, M. (2008). Effect of variable cultivating temperature on frequency of embryogenic callus inducting from *Leymus chinensis. Biotechnology,* Vol.18, No.5, pp. 60-62, ISSN 1004-311X (in Chinese with English abstract)

Lee, W.T. (1979). Distribution of *Acanthopanax* plants in Korea. *Korean Journal of Pharmacognosy,* Vol.10, No.3, pp. 103-107, ISSN 0253-3073

Li, C.H. & Yu, C.Y. (2002). Effect of genotype and explant on somatic embryogenesis and acclimatization of *Acanthopanax senticosus. Korean Journal of Medicinal Crop Science,* Vol.10, No.3, pp. 217-221, ISSN 1225-9306

Li, C.H.; Lim, J.D.; Heo, K.; Kim, M.J.; Lee, C.O.; Lee, J.G.; Cui, X.S. & Yu, C.Y. (2004). Long-term cold storage and plant regeneration of suspension cultured somatic embryos of *Eleutherococcus senticosus* Maxim. *Korean Journal of Medicinal Crop Science,* Vol.12, No.6, (December 2004), pp. 494-499, ISSN 1225-9306

Li, C.H.; Lim, J.D.; Kim, M.J. & Yu, C.Y. (2003b). Effects of GA_3 on seed germination and seedling survival rate of *Acanthopanax senticosus* Maxim. *Korean Journal of Medicinal Crop Science,* Vol.11, No.3, pp. 207-211, ISSN 1225-9306

Li, C.H.; Lim, J.D.; Kim, M.J.; Heo, K. & Yu, C.Y. (2003a). Dehisced seed germination and seedling growth affected by chilling period in *Eleutherococcus senticosus* Maxim. *Korean Journal of Medicinal Crop Science,* Vol.11, No.5, pp. 347-351, ISSN 1225-9306

Lim, S.H.; Jeong, H.N.; Kang, A.S. & Jeon, M.S. (2008). Influence of GA_3 soak and seed dressing with Toros (Tolclofos methyl) wp. on the dehiscence of *Eleutherococcus senticosus* Maxim seeds. *Korean Journal of Medicinal Crop Science,* Vol.16, No.2, pp. 106-111, ISSN 1225-9306

Liu, G.S.; Li, X.F.; Su, M. & Qi, D.M. (2006). *A protocol for enhancing plant regeneration frequency of Leymus chinensis and the appropriative tissue culture media,* State

Intellectual Property Office of the People's Republic of China, Institute of Botany of the Chinese Academy of Science, No.200610078404

Liu, G.S.; Liu, J.S.; Qi, D.M.; Chu, C.C. & Li, H.J. (2004). Factors affecting plant regeneration from tissue cultures of Chinese leymus (*Leymus chinensis*). *Plant Cell Tissue & Organ Culture,* Vol.76, No.2, (February 2004) pp. 175-178, doi:10.1023/B:TICU.0000007251.96785.18, ISSN 0167-6857

Liu, G.S.; Wang, E.H.; Liu, J.; Qi, D.M. & Li, F.F. (2002b). Plant regeneration of *Leymus chinensis* via *in vitro* culture. *Acta Agrestia Sinica,* Vol.10, No.3, pp. 198-202, ISSN 1007-0435

Liu, J.; Zhu, Z.Q.; Liu, G.S.; Qi, D.M. & Li, F.F. (2002a). AFLP variation analysis on the germplasm resources of *Leymus chiensis*. *Acta Botanica Sinica,* Vol.44, No.7, pp. 845-851, ISSN 1672-9072

Loo, S.W. (1945). Cultivation of excised stem tips of *Asparagus in vitro*. *American Journal of Botany,* Vol.32, pp. 13-17, ISSN 0002-9122

Lu, X.Y.; Li, X.Z.; Zhou, H.X.; Xia, H.Z.; Li, Z.Y. & Wang, Y.M. (2009). Callus induction of *Leymus chinensis*. *Beijing Agriculture,* Vol.15, No., pp. 18-20, ISSN 1000-6966 (in Chinese with English abstract)

Ma, H.Y.; Liang, Z.W. & Chen, Y. (2005). Research progress on improving germination rate of *Leymus chinensis*. *Chinese Journal of Grassland,* Vol.27, No.4, pp. 64-68, ISSN 1673-5021 (in Chinese with English abstract)

Morel, G. & Wetmore, R.H. (1951). Tissue culture of monocotyledons. *American Journal Botany,* Vol.38, pp. 18-140, ISSN 0002-9122

Murashige, T. & Skoog, F. (1962). A revised medium for rapid growth and bio assays with tobacco tissue cultures. *Physiologia Plantarum,* Vol.15, No.3, pp. 473-497, ISSN 0031-9317, doi:10.1111/j.1399-3.54.1962.tb08052.x

Park, H.K.; Park, M.S.; Kim, T.S.; Choi, I.L.; Jang, Y.S. & Kim, G.S. (1994). Cutting propagation of *Eleutherococcus senticosus* MAXIM. *Korean Journal of Medicinal Crop Science,* Vol.2, No.2, pp. 133-139, ISSN 1225-9306

Park, H.K.; Park, M.S.; Kim, T.S.; Kim, S.; Choi, K.G. & Park, K.H. (1997). Characteristics of embryo growth and dehiscence during the after-ripening period in *Eleutherococcus senticosus*. *Korean Journal of Crop Science,* Vol.42, No.6, pp. 673-677, ISSN 0252-9777

Park, M.S.; Kim, Y.J.; Park, H.K.; Chang, Y.S. & Lee, J.H. (1995). Using air temperature and sunshine duration data to select seed production site for *Eleutherococcus senticosus* Max. *Korean Journal of Crop Science,* Vol.40, No.4, pp. 444-450, ISSN 0252-9777

Park, M.S.; Kim, Y.J.; Park, H.K.; Kim, S.; Kim, G.S. & Chang, Y.S. (1996). Habitat environment of *Eleutherococcus senticosus* Max. at Mt. Deokyu. *Korean Journal of Crop Science,* Vol.41, No.6, pp. 710-717, ISSN 0252-9777

Qu, T.B.; Wang, P.W.; Guan, S.Y. & Liu, L.Z. (2004). Establishment of regeneration system of *Leymus chinensis* culture. *Acta Prataculturral Science,* Vol.13, No.5, pp. 91-94, ISSN 1004-5759 (in Chinese with English abstract)

Rachmawati, D. & Anzai, H. (2006). Studies on callus induction, plant regeneration and transformation of Javanica rice cultivars. *Plant Biotechnology,* Vol.23, No.5, pp. 521-524, ISSN 1342-4580

Redenbaugh, K.; Paasch, B.D.; Nichol, J.W.; Kossler, M.E.; Viss, P.R. & Walker, K.A. (1986). Somatic seeds: encapsulation of asexual plant embryos. *Nature Biotechnology,* Vol.4, pp. 797-801, ISSN 1087-0156. doi:10.1038/nbt0986-797

Roberts, S.C. (2007). Production and engineering of terpenoids in plant cell culture. *Nature Chemical Biology*, Vol.3, (June 2007), pp. 387-395, ISSN 1552-4469. doi:10.1038/nchembio.2007.8

Sahoo, Y.& Chand, P.K. (1998). Micropropagation of *Vitex negundo* L., a woody aromatic medicinal shrub, through high-frequency axillary shoot proliferation. *Plant Cell Reports*, Vol.18, No.3, (July 1998), pp. 301-307, doi:10.1007/s002990050576, ISSN 0721-7714

Sahrawat, A.K. & Chand S. (2001). High-frequency plant regeneration from coleoptiles tissue of indica rice (*Oryza sativa* L.). *In Vitro Cellular & Developmental Biology. Plant*, Vol.37, No.1, (January 2001), pp. 55-61, doi:10.1079/IVP2000114, ISSN 1054-5476

Seo, J.W.; Jeong, J.H.; Shin, C.G.; Lo, S.C.; Han, S.S.; Yu, K.W.; Harada, E.; Han, J.Y. & Choi, Y.E. (2005). Overexpression of squalene synthase in *Eleutherococcus senticosus* increases phytosterol and triterpene accumulation. *Phytochemistry*, Vol.66, No.8, (February 2005), pp. 869-877, ISSN 0031-9422. doi:10.1016/j.phytochem.2005.02.016

Shen, X.L.; Chen, J.J. & Kane, M.E. (2007). Indirect shoot organogenesis from leaves of *Dieffenbachia* cv. Camouflage. *Plant Cell Tissue & Organ Culture*, Vol.89, No.2-3, (February 2007), pp. 83-90, doi:10.1007/s11240-007-9214-7, ISSN 0167-6857

Shohael, A.M.; Ali, M.B.; Hahn, E.J. & Paek, K.Y. (2007). Glutathione metabolism and antioxidant responses during *Eleutherococcus senticosus* somatic embryo development in a bioreactor. *Plant Cell Tissue & Organ Culture*, Vol.89, No.2-3, (May 2007), pp. 121-129, doi:10.1007/s11240-9220-9, ISSN 0167-6857

Shohael, A.M.; Ali, M.B.; Yu, K.W.; Hahn, E.J. & Paek, K.Y. (2006b). Effect of temperature on secondary metabolites production and antioxidant enzyme activities in *Eleutherococcus senticosus* somatic embryos. *Plant Cell Tissue & Organ Culture*, Vol.85, No.2, pp. 219-228, ISSN 0167-6857. doi:10.1007/s11240-005-9075-x

Shohael, A.M.; Ali, M.B.; Yu, K.W.; Hahn, E.J.; Islam, R. & Park, K.Y. (2006a). Effect of light on oxidative stress, secondary metabolites and induction of antioxidant enzymes in *Eleutherococcus senticosus* somatic embryos in bioreactor. *Process Biochemistry*, Vol.41, pp. 1179-1185, ISSN 1359-5113. doi:10.1016/j.procbio.2005.12.015

Singh, N.D.; Sahoo, L.; Sarin, N.B. & Jaiwal, P.K. (2003). The effect of TDZ on organogenesis and somatic embryogenesis in pigeonpea (*Cajanus cajan* L. Millsp). Plant Science Vol.164, No.3, (March 2003), pp. 341-347, doi:10.1016/S0168-9452(02)00418-1, ISSN 0168-9452

Sun, Y.L. & Hong, S.K. (2009). Somatic embryogenesis and *in vitro* plant regeneration from various explants of the halophyte *Leymus chinensis* (Trin.). *Journal of Plant Biotechnology*, 36, No.3, pp. 236-243, ISSN 1598-6365

Sun, Y.L. & Hong, S.K. (2010a). Effects of plant growth regulators and L-glutamic acid on shoot organogenesis in the halophyte *Leymus chinensis* (Trin.). *Plant Cell Tissue & Organ Culture*, Vol.100, No.3, (December 2009), pp. 317-328, doi:10.1007/s11240-009-9653-4, ISSN 0167-6857

Sun, Y.L. & Hong, S.K. (2010b). Establishment of a novel plant regeneration system from suspension-derived callus in the halophytic *Leymus chinensis* (Trin.). *Journal of Plant Biotechnology*, Vol.27, No.2, (June 2010), pp. 228-235, ISSN 1598-6365

Tejavathi, D.H. & Shailaja, K.S. (1999). Regeneration of plants from the cultures of *Bacopa monnieri* (L.) Pennell. *Phytomorphology*, Vol.49, No.4, pp. 447-452, ISSN 0031-9449

Umeyama, A.; Shoji, N.; Takei, M.; Endo, K. & Arihara, S. (1992). Ciwujianosides D1 and C1: powerful inhibitors of histamine release induced by anti-immunoglobulin E from rat peritoneal mast cells. *Journal of Pharmaceutical Sciences,* Vol.81, No.7, (July 1992), pp. 661-662, ISSN 0022-3549

Vasil, V. & Hildebrandt, A.C. (1965). Differentiation of tobacco plants from single, isolated cells in microcultures. *Science,* Vol.150, No.3698, (November 1965), pp. 889-892, doi:10.1126/science.150.3698.889, ISSN 0036-8075

Wang, P.W.; Qu, T.B.; Guan, S.Y. & Qu, J. (2006). *Selection of salt-tolerant mutants of Leymus chinensis.* State Intellectual Property Office of the People's Republic of China, Jilin Agriculture University, No.200610163263

Wang, Y.S.; Zhao, L.M.; Wang, H.; Wang, J.; Huang, D.M.; Hong, R.M.; Teng, X.H. & Miki, N. (2005). Molecular genetic variation in a clonal plant population of *Leymus chinensis* (Trin.) Tzvel. *Journal of Integrative Plant Biology,* Vol.47, No.9, pp. 1055-1064, ISSN 1672-9072

Wei, Q.; Hu, G.F.; Li, F.L. & Hu, B.Z. (2005). Study on callus inducement and plant regeneration in seeds of *Aneurolepidium chinensis* (Trin.) Kitag.. Journal of Northeast Agricultural University, Vol.36, No.1, pp. 41-44, ISSN 1005-9369 (in Chinese with English abstract)

Wernicke, W. & Milkovits, L. (1984). Developmental gradients in wheat leaves – Response of leaf segments in different genotypes cultured *in vitro*. *Journal of Plant Physiology,* Vol.115, pp. 49-58, ISSN 0176-1617

Xilin, H.; An, Y.; Xia, D.A. & You, X.L. (2010). Plasmolysis treatment enhances the expression of callose synthase gene in zygotic embryos of *Eleutherococcus senticosus*. *Journal of Forestry Research,* Vol.21, No.2, pp. 189-192, ISSN 1993-0607. doi:10.1007/s11676-010-0030-2

You, X.L.; Choi, Y.E. & Yi, J.S. (2005). Rapid *in vitro* germination of zygotic embryos *via* endosperm removal in *Eleutherococcus senticosus*. *Journal of Plant Biotechnology,* Vol.7, No.1, pp. 75-80, ISSN 1598-6365

You, X.L.; Yi, J.S. & Choi, Y.E. (2006). Cellular change and callose accumulation in zygotic embryos of *Eleutherococcus senticosus* caused by plasmolyzing pretreatment result in high frequency of single-cell-derived somatic embryogenesis. *Protoplasma,* Vol.227, pp. 105-112, doi:10.1007/s00709-006-0419-3, ISSN 1615-6102

Yu, C.Y.; Kim, J.K. & Ahn, S.D. (1997a). Callus formation and plant regeneration from immature embryos of *Eleutherococcus senticosus*. *Korean Journal of Medicinal Crop Science,* Vol.5, No.1, pp. 49-55, ISSN 1225-9306

Yu, C.Y.; Kim, S.H.; Lim, J.D.; Kim, M.J. & Chung, I.M. (2003). Intraspecific relationship analysis by DNA markers and in vitro cytotoxic and antioxidant activity in *Eleutherococcus senticosus*. *Toxicology in Vitro,* Vol.17, No.2, (April 2003), pp. 229-236, doi:10.1016/S0887-2333(03)00008-0, ISSN 0887-2333

Yu, C.Y.; Lim, J.D.; Seong, E.S. & Kim, J.K. (1997b). Effect of embryo maturity and medium on callus formation regeneration from immature embryos of *Eleutherococcus senticosus*. *Korean Journal of Plant Resources,* Vol.10, No.2, pp. 122-127, ISSN 1226-3591

Zhang, Y.; Li, X.F.; Liu, G.S. & Chen, Y.F. (2007). Regulation of callus status of *Leymus chinensis*. *Journal of Northwest Sci-Tech University of Agriculture and Forestry (Natural Science Edition),* Vol.35, No.5, pp. 111-114, ISSN 1671-9387 (in Chinese with English abstract)

Zimmerman, J.L. (1993). Somatic embryogenesis: a model for early development in higher plants. *The Plant Cell,* Vol.5, No.10, (October 1993), pp. 1411-1423, ISSN 1040-4651

13

Induced Androgenic Embryogenesis in Cereals

Danial Kahrizi[1] and Maryam Mirzaei[2]
[1]*Agronomy and Plant Breeding Department, Faculty of Agriculture, Razi University, Kermanshah,*
[2]*Department of Plant Breeding, Islamic Azad University, Kermanshah Branch, Kermanshah, Iran*

1. Introduction

Plant breeding, a system of gene pooling through generations of phenotypic selection has long been the only method available for crop improvement. For many years *in vitro* plant breeding has been used in many plants for different traits improvement.

The method of *in vitro* plant breeding has been used for improving different traits in many crops. Gamethophytic embryogenesis is one of the methods for production of haploid plants.

Androgenesis is defined as culture of female gametophytic cells/tissues on a plant tissue culture medium in sterile conditions. Androgenesis can be used as anther culture or isolated microspore culture (IMC).

The production of haploids and doubled haploids (DHs) through androgenic embryogenesis allows a single-step development of complete homozygous lines from heterozygous stuck plants, reduction the time required to produce homozygous plants in comparison with the conventional breeding methods that employ several generations of autogamy.

Androgenic embryogenesis is one the different methods of embryogenesis present in the plant kingdom, and it consists in the capacity of male (microspore or anther) to permanently switch from their gametophytic pathway of development towards a sporophytic one. Differently from somatic embryogenesis, which provides the clonal propagation of the genotype (unless the somaclonal variation), androgenic embryogenesis results in haploid plants (unless spontaneous or induced chromosome duplication occurs), because such plants are derived from the regeneration of male gametes, products of meiotic segregation.

Androgenic embryogenesis (also referred to as androgenesis) is regarded as one of the most striking examples of cellular totipotency, but also as a form of atavism. It is an important survival adaptation mechanism in the plant kingdom that is expressed only under certain circumstances and as a consequence of an environmental stress. In comparison to conventional breeding methods, androgenic embryogenesis makes the production of homozygous lines feasible and shortens the time required to produce such lines, allowing the single-step development of completely homozygous lines from the heterozygous parents. Conventional methods performed to achieve homozygosity consist of carrying out several backcrosses or selfing; as such, they are time-consuming and labour-intensive procedures.

2. Isolated microspore technique

The technique of isolated microspore culture, performed by removing somatic anther wall, requires better equipment and more skills compared to anther culture, although the earlier provides the better method for investigating cellular, physiological, biochemical and molecular processes involved in androgenic embryogenesis.

The isolated microspore culture is as a powerful tool of *in vitro* plant breeding for haploid and doubled haploid plant production. This technique may allow faster production of new varieties than using conventional breeding methods and has been successfully employed in many crop plants. The microspore is at the centre of a variety of topics in modern plant science and breeding. High frequency regeneration of fertile plants (doubled haploids) from isolated microspores is an important tool for different plant breeding and biotechnological applications.

Microspore culture is a form of androgenesis in which the developing immature pollen grain is stressed into switching pathways to become a sporophytic cell with the potential to regenerate into a green plant. Microspores can be isolated in large numbers providing a relatively uniform population of haploid, single cells capable of developing directly into embryos and plants. Thus, they provide excellent tools for studying embryogenesis, *in vitro* selection in culture and cell cycles relative to transformation.

Successful microspore tissue culture systems require a responsive genotype and a healthy homogenous population of donor plants producing physiologically healthy material. The genotype of the donor material can affect ethylene production, endogenous auxin and cytokinin activity, androgenic embryogenesis, plant regeneration and albinism.

The regeneration potential of the culture is dependent upon donor plants, staging, pre-treatment, isolation and culture media. Haploid plants must be chromosome doubled to restore fertility for use in plant breeding. Chromosome doubling of microspore-derived from plantlets and calli is a critical step in haploid breeding programs.

In a research an experiment was conducted to determine the responses of five barley genotypes to androgenic embryogenesis and spontaneous chromosome doubling (Kahrizi and Mohammadi, 2009). For study on effect of genotype upon androgenesis, after microspore culture, the number of embryos per 100 used anthers was measured. Results showed that genotype significantly affected the embryoid formation . This result is in agreement with the results of Castillo et al. (2000) but is in disagreement with Li and Devaux, (2003) and Kasha *et al.* (2004) that reported there was no significant difference in embryo induction among genotypes.

3. Chromosome doubling

Chromosome doubling to induce polyploidy has been widely used in plant breeding programs to restore fertility in sterile genotypes and to overcome crossing barriers.

The doubled haploids represent useful tools for applied breeding and genetic analysis.

For androgenesis experiments, colchicine is used in doubling the chromosomes. It has been applied to regenerated plants after transfer to soil or *in vitro* either initially in the microspore culture substrate. Colchicines however, is toxic carcinogenic and expensive.

For androgenesis experiments, colchicine, (S)-N-(5,6,7,9-tetrahydro-1,2,3,10-tetramethoxy-9-oxobenzo[a]heptalen-7-yl) acetamide, is the most commonly used antimitotic agent in doubling the chromosomes of seedling from such experiments (Inagaki, 1985), or *in vitro* either initially in the microspore culture substrate (Hansen and Anderson, 1998a). Colchicine, however, has a relatively low efficiency for plant microtubules and has carcinogenic effects for human and is expensive (Hansen & Anderson, 1998b).

In cytogenetic section of Kahrizi and Mohammadi (2009) research focused on chromosome doubling of haploids without applying any antimitotic agent as well as effect of genotype upon chromosome doubling was studied.

Spontaneous chromosome doubling rates among microspore-derived from wheat plants are 15-25%. It has been revealed that spontaneous chromosome doubling in barley constituted 70-80% of regenerated population and only 15-20% plantlets were haploids.

Barley is important as a global crop and as a leading mode plant for isolated microspore culture and cereal transformation studies.

The utility of doubled haploid lines in barley breeding programs have been demonstrated, and a number of cultivars have been developed using this system. Microspore culture in barley has been improved more than in other cereals and thus is preferred for investigations such as microspore transformation.

4. Factors influencing androgenic embryogenesis

The success of androgenic embryogenesis is influenced with numerous factors such as: (Bajaj, 1990)

1. The growth and development of stock (donor) plants. Including:
   1.1 Photo period
   1.2 Light quality and intensity
   1.3 Temperature
   1.4 Nutrition and fertilizers
   1.5 CO_2 concentration
   1.6 Biotic and abiotic stresses

   The variation in androgenetic response is dependent upon the donor plants' growth environment. This has been reported in many of crops, including wheat (Picard & De Buyer 1975), rice (Chaleff & Stolarz 1981) and maize (Genovesi, 1990). The donor plants' physiology and vigor were found to greatly influence androgenic response frequency (Nitsch et al. 1982). Genovesi (1990) approved that anthers of weak donor plants produced only a few embryos or calli *in vitro*. This is probably indicative of the importance of endogenous factors for androgenic response. He also mentioned the importance of environmental factors, such as the influence of photoperiod, light intensity and quality, temperature and nutrition on the donor plant vigor. Field grown donor plants gave better embryo induction frequencies (Dieu & Beckert 1986). Nitsch *et al.* (1982) suggested that the stock plants be grown under optimal conditions and that pesticide treatment be avoided. androgenesis also respond differentially to incubation conditions such as temperature, light quality and quantity, CO_2 concentration. Abiotic stresses play a very important role in androgenic induction.

2. Microspore developmental stage

   Many investigators, who have reported success in maize anther culture, agreed that the uninucleate microspore is the most responsive stage for culture. However, some have shown a preference for the mid-uninuleate stage, while others preferred the late-uninuleate stage.

   The best time for harvesting wheat spikes is when the majority of microspores are at the mid- to late-uninucleate stage. During this period, microspores are most susceptible to androgenic induction treatment.

3. Microspore density

   Various microspore densities ranging from 2×10^4 to 2×10^5 / ml had been reported effective for embryo induction, a high density is not necessary for success. In fact, a density of 7–8 × 10^3 / ml is quite effective for embryoid development (Zheng et al., 2002b). The effective density ranges from 5 × 10^3 to 2 × 10^4 / ml. Relatively low but adequate microspore density eases the competition for nutrients, oxygen, and space for cell divisions and embryoid formation, hence improves both the number and quality of embryoids. The co-culture of microspores with ovaries and/or ovary-conditioned medium (OVCM) makes it possible to employ a lower density. In addition, microspores of high purity in culture also contribute to the success of using lower microspore densities.

4. Pretreatments. It may be treat on stock plant, spike, anther or microspores that including:
   4.1 Cold pretreatment
   4.2 Warm pretreatment
   4.3 Chemical pretreatment

Low or high temperature shocks are applied as a pre-treatment or at the early stages of induction in most protocols developed for both, mono and dicotyledonous plants. Temperature pretreatments are believed to improve androgenesis by diverting normal gametophytic development into a sporophytic pathway leading to the production of haploid embryo like structure (Nitsch et al. 1982). Genovesi (1990) reported highly significant effects of post-treatment with high temperature on embryoid formation. The role of temperature in androgenic induction is now better understood. It is described as one of many stress factors influencing microspore transition from gametophytic to sporophytic development.

Osmotic and starvation stress are nowadays frequently applied to cereals in combination with a relatively short, 3–5 day treatment with low temperature.

Different stress pretreatments including cold shock (Gustafson et al., 1995; Hu and Kasha, 1999), sugar starvation alone and in combination with cold shock or heat shock (Mejza et al., 1993; Touraev et al., 1996; Hu and Kasha, 1997, 1999) and inducer chemicals alone or in combination with heat shock (Zheng et al., 2001; Liu et al., 2002).

5. Inductive media for embryogenesis

   Improvements in the formulation of culture media have also contributed to the progress of androgenic methods. The composition of basic salts and micro-elements is wide and varied. The most often modified components are: (1) the source of organic nitrogen, (2) carbohydrates, and (3) growth regulators. Several media are applied for androgenic embryogenesis in different cereal plants that is shown in table 1.

6. Compositions of Media

Improvements in the composition of culture media have also contributed to the progress of androgenic methods. The composition of basic salts and micro-elements is wide and varied. The most often modified components are: (1) the source of organic nitrogen, (2) carbohydrates, and (3) growth regulators.

The first significant step towards better efficiency in barley androgenesis was achieved by lowering the ammonium nitrate content and enriching the glutamine level as a source of organic nitrogen.

Carbohydrates provide as a source of energy, building material and a component that regulates the osmotic properties of the culture media. The most spectacular success in protocols efficiency was achieved by the replacement of sucrose by maltose in numerous versions of induction media. In wheat, triticale, rye and rice the concentration of maltose ranges from 60 to 90 g/l of induction media.

In the examples cited above for cereals, the concentration of sucrose in the regeneration media is in the order of 20–30 g/l, which is a standard amount in many other protocols. Sucrose and maltose are the main sugar components of the media throughout the literature with few examples of other carbohydrates tested.

Several substances are active as growth regulators *in vitro*, many of them are synthetic analogous of plant hormones. The kind of substance, its concentration and the proportions in which several components are composed remain of substantial importance in regulating cell division and morphogenesis. In many protocols for isolated microspore culture, growth regulators are omitted in the induction medium.

In barley androgenic cultures, BAP, IAA, NAA and PAA are added to the induction media alone or in combination at various concentrations. The improved protocol contains 1 mg/l of BAP with 10 mg/l of PAA. On the other hand, in anther culture of wheat, triticale and rye 2, 4-D and kinetin are used in the induction media and NAA with kinetin to stimulate regeneration. Abscisic acid (ABA) was applied to improve regeneration of induced embryos.

Microspore suspensions are often cultured without the addition of growth regulators although the most successful media are conditioned with ovaries. Conditioning with an actively growing suspension culture was also successfully applied to induce in vitro development of isolated zygotes. It can be presumed that the ovaries provide a source of active ingredients, phytohormones or other signaling molecules important for androgenic induction or embryo maturation. However, the data from detailed analysis of conditioned media have not yet been published.

Maize microspore culture was used recently as a model to study androgenic processes. Among others, the latter authors showed that arabinogalactan proteins added to the medium improved regeneration in low responsive genotypes. This discovery opens up new possibilities in improving the regeneration process, and may have beneficial effects for other species. It is probable, that other molecules that play regulatory role are secreted into the conditioned media however, to prove this hypothesis more detail studies of media during culture are required.

7. Microspore separation method, releasing and purifying microspores

   At least seven different approaches exist for isolating microspores include mechanical separation, blending, maceration, stirring, vortexing, sonication and floating.

   Shedding is a technique first developed by Sunderland and Roberts (1977) in which cultured tobacco anthers shed their microspores into a liquid medium. These microspores were then collected and cultured for callus development and plant regeneration. The shedding technique was later adopted in wheat. More recently, a 6-7 day pretreatment in 0.3 M mannitol plus macronutrients was recommended for shedding microspores or for a step preceding mechanical isolation of microspores (Kasha et al., 1990). Magnetic-bar stirring is a derivative of shedding in that a stirring force is added to help release the microspores still enclosed within the anther wall. In effect, magneticbar stirring serves to increase microspore yields from the natural shedding. The shedding and stirring procedures, however, are not effective means in wheat microspore cultures due to the low yields of microspores and plants subsequently recovered.

8. Genotype of stock plants.

   The androgenic embryogenesis is highly dependent to stock plant genotype. It may be as intraspecies or interspecies variations (Table 2).

Media	References
N6	Chu, 1978
Yu-Pei (YP)	Ku et al., 1981
MS	Murashige and Skoog, 1962
FHG	Hunter, 1988
CHB-2	Chu et al., 1990
B5	Gamborg et al. 1968
FMN6	Mejza *et al.*, 1993
A2	Touraev et al., 1996
MMS3	Hu and Kasha, 1997
NPB-99	Liu et al., 2002

Table 1. The media that are used for androgenic embryogenesis (Kahrizi et al., 2007)

5. Spontaneous chromosome doubling in androgenic embryogenesis

Haploid induction during anther or microspore culture begins with some form of stress applied at a critical stage before or during the culture of the microspores.

Chromosome doubling of microspore-derived from plantlets and embryos is a critical step in haploid breeding programs. In many plants microspores are doubled spontaneously. Spontaneous chromosome doubling rates among microspore-derived from wheat plants are 15-25%. (Kahrizi et al., 2009). It has been revealed that spontaneous chromosome doubling in barley constituted 70-80% of regenerated population and only 15-20% plantlets were haploids (Kahrizi & Mohammadi, 2009; Kahrizi, 2009). (Figures 1 and 2).

Plant	Number of studied genotypes	Responded genotypes[1] (%)	Genotypes with superior response[2] (%)	Regenerated Genotypes (%)	Reference
Barley	11	100	100	100	Logue *et al.*, 1993
	16	100	100	100	Hou *et al.*,1994
Wheat	31	97	77	77	Masojc *et al.*, 1993
	60	98	23	35	Orlav *et al.*,1993
Corn	40	60	3.0	19	Potelino and Jones, 1986
	55	47	4.0	7.0	Hangchang *et al.*, 1991

Table 2. The comparison of androgenic capacity for embryogenesis in barley, wheat and corn (Kahrizi et al., 2007)

The mechanism of chromosome doubling has been one of much speculation and the relationship to the influence of pretreatments is obscure, with endoreduplication and nuclear fusion as the most likely methods. A C-mitosis, such as occurs during colchicine treatment, may result in a simple restitution nucleus with a doubled chromosome number. In *Datura*, it was proposed that both endoreduplication and nuclear fusion were involved in chromosome doubling and that the combination of both methods could explain the ploidy levels obtained that were higher than diploid. Nuclear fusion was described as occurring when two nuclei synchronously entered into division, formed a common metaphase plate and spindle and resulted in two nuclei, each with more than one set of chromosomes. If one or both of the nuclei had undergone endoreduplication prior to nuclear fusion, triploid or higher ploidy level plants could be formed. Sunderland also showed clear evidence of endoreduplication from the generative nucleus and chromosomes from different nuclei on a common metaphase plate.

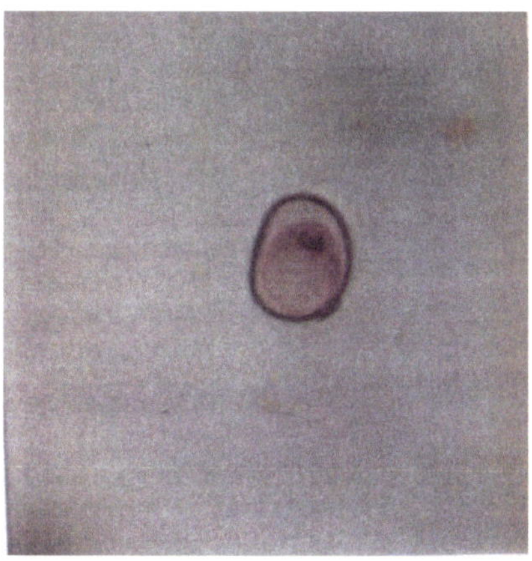

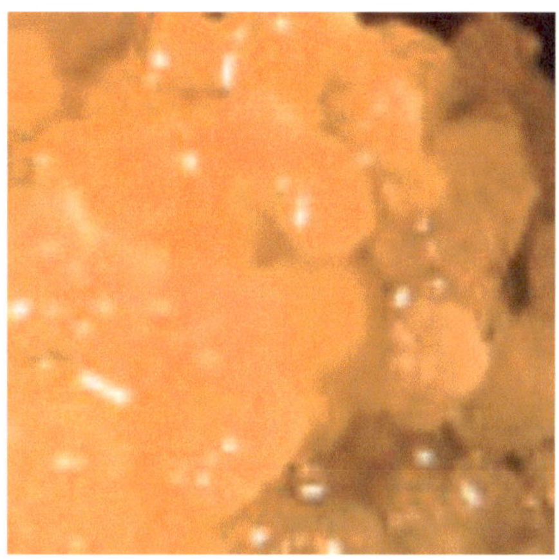

Fig. 1. Isolated microspore culture of barley. Cultured microspore after 4 days (left), Embryoid formation from cultured microspore in liquid medium (right).

[1] Formation at least one embryoid in 100 cultured anthers

[2] Formation at least 10 embryoids in 100 cultured anthers

Both the stage of the microspore when collected for pretreatment and the pathway of nuclear development have also been considered to influence the frequency of doubling. He concluded that microspores collected at uninucleate stages 1-3 (early, mid and late, respectively) resulted in mostly haploid and doubled haploid plants while those collected at later stages (4–6, mitosis and binucleate) resulted in mostly doubled haploids as well as some triploid and tetraploid plants. It has also been demonstrated in wheat that the pretreatment method will influence the pathway along which the nuclei will develop.

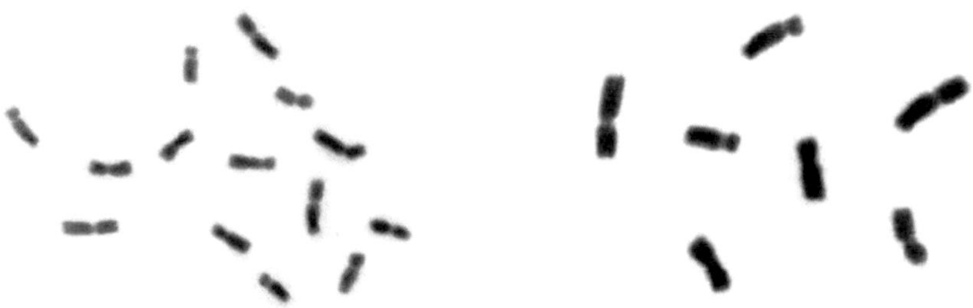

Fig. 2. Cytogenetic test for androgenetic plantlets in barley. The majority of plantlets were spontaneous doubled haploid (A) and Low percents of them were haploid (B) . Kahrizi D (2009).

Development from the normal gametophytic to an embryogenic (sporophytic) switch can be induced by the pretreatment of anthers or spikes. Pretreatments also influence the stage of microspores. Hu and Kasha found that uninucleate microspores of wheat completed the first mitotic division during both the 28 d cold pretreatment and the 6–7 d 0.4 M mannitol pretreatment at 28 °C (Hu and Kasha, 1999). It was also reported that a spike pretreatment combining 0.4 M mannitol solution and cold pretreatment for 4 d in wheat essentially blocked the mitotic division of the nucleus, keeping all microspores at the same stage during pretreatment, and also resulted in the formation of large numbers of true embryo-like structures (ELS) (Hu & Kasha, 1999).

6. Genetic control of microspore embryogenesis

Both environmental and genetic factors contribute significantly to the androgenic responses. The influence of environmental factors has been widely reviewed elsewhere. All three components in androgenesis, embryoid induction, total plant regeneration and green / albino plant ratio have been determined to be independently inherited traits. The inheritable nature of androgenic traits provides the basis for introducing these traits into non-responsive genotypes. In most cases, the genetic component of culturability is attributed to additive gene effects, although epistatic and dominant effects have also been observed. The dominant and additive gene effects provide opportunity to improve androgenic response through cross breeding and recurrent selection. In addition, significant interactions exist between nuclear genes and cytoplasm type for all three components of the androgenic response.

7. References

Bajaj,Y.P.S. (1990). In vitro production of haploids and their use in cell genetics and plant breeding, Biotechnology in Agriculture and Forestry, vol. 12, Haploids in Crop Improvement I. 372–380.

Barnabás, B., Pfahler, P. L. & Kovács, G. (1991): Direct effect of colchicine on the microspore embryogenesis to produce dihaploid plants in wheat (*Triticum aestivum* L.). Theor. Appl. Genet., 81, 675-678.

Burton, G. W. & de Vane, R. W. (1953): Estimating heritability in tall fescue (*Festuca arundinaceia*) from replicated clonal material. Agron. J., 45, 478-481.

Carlson, A. R. (1998): Visual selection of transgenic barley (*Hordeum vulgare*) structures and their regeneration into green plants. Thesis, University of Guelph.

Castillo, A. M., Valles, M. P. & Cistue, L. (2000): Comparison of anther and isolated microspore cultures in barley. Effects of culture density and regeneration medium. Euphytica, 113, 1-8.

Chaleff, R.S. & Stolarz, A. (1981) Factors influencing the frequency of callus formation among cultured rice (*Oryza sativa* L.) anthers. Physiol. Plant. 51 : 201 - 206.

Chu, C. (1978) The N6 medium and its applications to anther culture of cereal crops. In: Proc Symp Plant Tissue Culture. Science Press, Peking, pp 43–50

Chu, C.C., Hill, R.D. & Brûlí-Babel, A.L. (1990) . High frequency of pollen embryoid formation and plant regeneration in *Triticum aestivum* L. on monosaccharide containing media. Plant Science, 66: 255-262.

Chu, C.C., Hill, R.D. & Brûlí-Babel, A.L. (1990) . High frequency of pollen embryoid formation and plant regeneration in *Triticum aestivum* L. on monosaccharide containing media. Plant Science, 66: 255-262.

Dieu P & Beckert M (1986) Further studies of androgenetic embryo production and plant regeneration from *in vitro* cultured anthers in maize (*Zea mays* L.). Maydica 31: 245-259.

Gamborg OL, Miller RA. & Ojima K (1968) Nutrient requirement suspension cultures of soybean root cells. Exp Cell Res 50:151-158.

Genovesi AD & Collins GB (1982) *In vitro* production of haploid plant of corn via anther culture. Crop Sci. 22: 1137 - 1144.

Gustafson VD, Baenziger PS, Wright MS, Stroup W.W. & Yen Y (1995). Isolated wheat microspore culture. Plant Cell Tissue Organ Cult. 42: 207-213.

Hagio, T., Hirabayashi, T., Machii, H. & Tomotsune, H. (1995): Production of fertile transgenic barley (*Hordeum vulgare* L.) plants using the hygomycin-resistance marker. Plant Cell Rep., 14, 329-334.

Hansen, N. J. P. & Anderson, S. B. (1998a): In vitro chromosome doubling with colchicine during microspore culture in wheat (*Triticum aestivum* L.). Euphytica, 102, 101-108.

Hansen, N. J. P. & Anderson, S. B. (1998b): *In vitro* chromosome doubling potential of colchicine, oryzaline, trifuralin and APM in *Brassica napus* microspore culture. Euphytica, 88, 159-164.

Hoekstra, S., van Zijderwold, M. H., Louwerse, J. D., Heidekamp, F. & Vandermark, F. (1992): Anther and microspore culture of *Hordeum vulgare* L. cv. Igri. Plant Sci., 86, 89-96.

Hoekstra, S., Van Zijderwold, M. H.,Heidekamap, F. L. & Roue, C. (1993): Microspore culture of *Hordeum vulgare* L.: the influence of density and osmolality. Plant Cell Rep., 12, 661-665.

Hu T. & Kasha KJ (1997). Improvement of isolated microspore culture of wheat (*Triticum aestivum* L.) through ovary co-culture. Plant Cell Rep. 16: 520-525.

Hu, T. C., Kasha, K. J. (1999): A cytological study of pretreatment effects on isolated microspore culture of wheat *Triticum aestivum* cv. Chris. Genome, 42, 432-441.

Hunter CP (1988). Plant regeneration from microspores of baley (*Hordeum vulgare*). Ashford, Kent: University of London. 1988. PhD Thesis. Wye College , UK, 110 P.

Inagaki, M. (1985): Chromosome doubling of wheat haploids obtained from crosses with *Hordeum bulbosum* L. Jpn. J. Breed., 35, 193-195.

Jähne, A., Lörz, H. (1995): Cereal microspore culture (Review). Plant Sci., 109, 1–12. Johnson, H. W.,

Kahrizi D (2009). Study of Androgenesis and Spontaneous Chromosome Doubling in Barley (*Hordeum vulgare* L.) Advanced Line Using Isolated Microspore Culture. International Journal of Plant Breeding. (3) 2: 111-114.

Kahrizi D & Mohammadi, R (2009). Study of Androgenesis and Spontaneous Chromosome Doubling in Barley (*Hordeum vulgare* L.) genotypes using Isolated Microspore Culture. Acta Agronomica Hungarica, 57(2): 155–164.

Kahrizi, D., Arminian, A., Masumi Asl, A. (2007): *In vitro* Plant Breeding. Razi University Press, Razi, Iran (in Persian).

Kahrizi, D., Moieni, A. and Bozorgipour, R. (2000): Effect of genotype and carbohydrate source on androgenesis of hexaploid wheat (*Triticum aestivum* L.). Seed Plant, 16, 41–51 (in Persian).

Kahrizi, D., Zebarjadi, A. R., Jalali Honarmand, S., Khah, E. M. & Motamedi J. (2009) . Study of Spontaneous Chromosome Doubling in Wheat (*Triticum aestivum* L.) Genotypes Using Androgenesis . World Academy of Science , Engineering and Technology 57: 1162-1166.

Kahrizi, D.,Mahmoodi, S. Bakhshi Khaniki G.R. & Mirzaei, M. (2011). .Effect of genotype on androgenesis in barley (*Hordeum vulgare* L.). Biharean Biologist 5(2): 132-134.

Kahrizi, D., Mahmoodi, S.,Bakhshi Khaniki, B.K. & Mirzaei, M. (2011). Effect of genotype on androgenesis in barley (*Hordeum vulgare* L.). Biharean Biologist. 5(2): 132-134.

Kasha KJ, Ziauddin A & Cho UH (1990) Haploids in Cereal improvement: anther and microspore culture. In: Gustafson JP (ed) Gene Manipulation in Plant Improvement II (pp. 213-235). Plenum Press, New York.

Kasha, K. J., Hu, T. C., Oro, R., Simion, E. & Shim, Y. S. (2001): Nuclear fusion leads to chromosome doubling during mannitol pretreatment of barley (*Hordeum vulgare* L.) microspores. J. Exp. Bot., 52, 1227–1238.

Liu W, Zheng MY, Polle EA. & Konzak C.F. (2002). Highly efficient doubled-haploid production in wheat (*Triticum aestivum* L.) via induced microspore embryogenesis. Crop Sci. 42: 686-692.

Mejza SJ, Morgant V, DiBona DE & Wong JR (1993). Plant regeneration from isolated microspores of *Triticum aestivum* L. Plant Cell Rep. 12: 149-153.

Murashige, T., & Skoog, F. (1962). A revised medium for rapid growth and bioassays with tobacco tissue cultures. Phisiol Plant. 15: 473-497.

Nitsch C, Andersen S, Godrad M, Neutter MG & Sheridan WF (1982) Production of haploid plants of *Zea mays* L. and *Pennisetum* through androgenesis. In: Earle ED & Demarly Y (eds.) Variability in plant regeneration from tissue culture. Praeger, New York. pp. 69 - 91.

Picard EJ & De Buyser (1975) Nouveaux resultants concernant la culture d'antheres in vitro de ble tendure (Triticum aestivum L.). Effects d'un choe thermique at de la position de I'anthere dans I'epis. C.R. Acad. Sci. (Paris), 280D : 127 - 130.

Sunderland N & Roberts M (1977) New approach to pollen culture. Nature 270: 236-238

Touraev A, Indrianto A, Wratschko I, Vicente O. & Heberle-Bors E (1996). Efficient microspore embryogenesis in wheat (*Triticum aestivum* L.) induced by starvation at high temperature. Sex. Plant Reprod. 9: 209-215.

Zheng MY, Liu W, Weng Y, Polle E & Konzak CF (2001). Culture of freshly isolated wheat (*Triticum aestivum* L.) microspores treated with inducer chemicals. Plant Cell Rep. 20: 685-690.

14

Cellular Markers for Somatic Embryogenesis

Ewa U. Kurczynska, Izabela Potocka, Izabela Dobrowolska,
Katarzyna Kulinska-Lukaszek, Katarzyna Sala and Justyna Wrobel
*Laboratory of Cell Biology, Faculty of Biology and Environmental Protection,
University of Silesia, Katowice,
Poland*

1. Introduction

Somatic embryogenesis (SE) is a process in which somatic cells under special conditions develop into embryos and - in the end - into a plant. That is why SE is a good model system for studying the genetic, molecular, physiological, biochemical, histological and cellular mechanisms underlying not only somatic but also zygotic embryogenesis and the totipotency of plant cells. SE begins with a transition of somatic cells to an embryogenic state and it can be induced under certain *in vitro* conditions. The mechanisms which determine SE induction - the transition of cells from the vegetative to the embryogenic state and the conditions underlying such changes - are the main questions of developmental biology (for a review see: de Jong et al., 1993; von Arnold et al., 2002; Fehér et al., 2003; Namasivayam, 2007; Yang & Zhang, 2010).

A description of the events taking place during SE requires the application of different scientific methods such as genetic, molecular or biochemical analysis and also histological studies of explant cells. Moreover, the morphological, histological and cytological analysis of SE is also an object of studies leading to an understanding of the basis of the totipotency, differentiation, dedifferentiation, redifferentiation and changes in cell fate (Quiroz-Figueroa et al., 2006). It could help us to understand the developmental processes taking place during plant growth and development, including pattern formation.

In this review we describe the cellular markers which can be used to identify different groups of cells within the explant during the process of SE. The aim of this review is to summarise information concerning the morphology and histology of explant cells, such as changes in the apoplast and symplast of explants, which can be used as markers to identify a cell/cells which changed their fate from the somatic to the embryogenic state.

2. Definitions

The first information about somatic embryo development in *in vitro* conditions was presented by Steward and co-workers (1958). From that moment on, this kind of plant propagation forced many scientists to study the mechanisms involved in changes from the somatic to the embryogenic state and to improve the efficiency of this process as a method for plant propagation. Since during SE different processes leading to changes in cell fate are taking place, some important definitions concerning this phenomenon are reminded below.

Somatic embryogenesis is divided into direct and indirect embryogenesis (DSE and ISE respectively; Sharp et al., 1980; Evans & Sharp, 1981). In DSE, somatic embryos develop directly from the somatic cells of explants, and in ISE they develop from callus cells. Somatic embryogenesis is also divided depending upon the type of explants. If somatic embryos develop from primary explants it is called primary somatic embryogenesis; if they develop from primary somatic embryos, this is called secondary somatic embryogenesis.

In normal plant development, cells differentiate from an unspecialised to a mature state with the determined function. The term 'cell differentiation' can be interpreted as spatiotemporal and it focuses on the diverging path of differentiation among the constituent cells in a population (Romberger et al., 2004).

During SE, some explant cells change the direction of differentiation. For example, the epidermal cell is the "source" of the somatic embryo, and the parenchyma cell becomes a callus cell and afterwards develops into a somatic embryo. The processes by which cells can change their state of development are dedifferentiation, transdifferentiation and redifferentiation. It is well-documented that most of plant cells retain the possibility to dedifferentiate and as a consequence to change their fate (Grafi, 2004). Such changes are possible because plant cells are totipotent (or at least most of them are), where totipotency is the property of the cell which retains the potential for developing into a complete adult organism (Verdeil et al., 2007). For the most recent analysis of the definitions mentioned above, the article written by Sugimoto and co-workers (2011) is recommended.

According to Nagata (2010) and Grafi (2004), dedifferentiation is the process where differentiated non-dividing cells become meristematic. This concept explains many observations which had shown that cells divisions precede changes in the direction of their differentiation. During dedifferentiation, cells return to the undifferentiated, meristematic state. Transdifferentiation involves processes which lead cells or tissues from one differentiated state of development into a new one, and probably - first of all - such cells dedifferentiate and then redifferentiate along another developmental path (Thomas et al., 2003; Gunawardena et al., 2004). Redifferentiation is the ability of non-differentiated, meristematic cells to differentiate into a new direction, e.g., into new plant organs.

It is worth reminding ourselves of another definition concerning SE. According to Verdeil and co-workers (2007), the embryogenic callus is an undifferentiated, unorganised tissue enriched in embryogenic cells, and the embryogenic cell is a cell that requires no further external stimulus to produce a somatic embryo.

3. General description of SE

During SE, changes in explant tissues cause the development of the somatic embryo. Many studies have shown that somatic embryos are going through the same developmental stages as their zygotic counterparts, which in dicotyledonous plants are called the globular, heart, torpedo and cotyledonary stages (Fig. 1; sometimes such stages were named differently, as with, e.g., Quiroz-Figueroa et al., 2006).

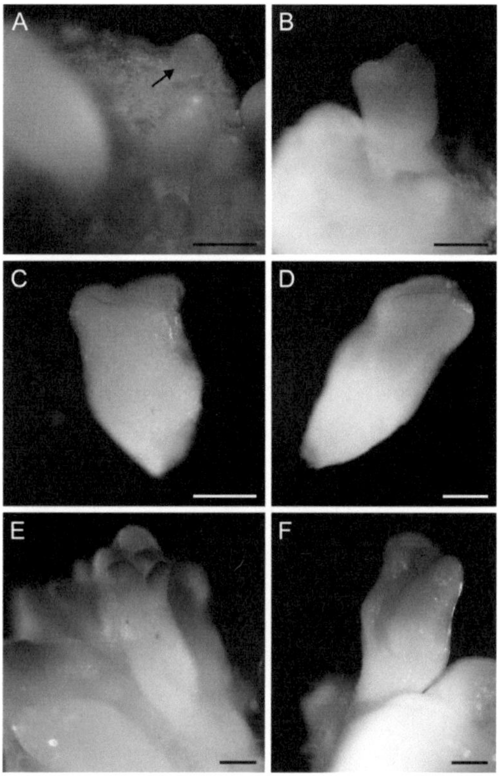

Fig. 1. Different developmental stages of somatic embryos from the example of *Arabidopsis* (A-globular; B-heart; C-torpedo; D-late torpedo; E and F-mature; bar = 200 μm).

Different parts of plant organs or zygotic embryos are used as an explant for the induction of SE. The literature describing this aspect of SE is huge and it is not possible to even mention here most of them. In some species, zygotic embryos are the best source of somatic ones and the explant organs involved in SE are cotyledons or shoot apical meristem (e.g. Canhoto & Cruz, 1996; Gaj, 2001; Kurczyńska et al., 2007; Raghavan, 2004; Rocha et al., 2011). Cultures of leafs, stems and roots parts are also efficient in SE induction (Mathews et al., 1993; Quiroz-Figueroa et al., 2002). In some cases, the production of protoplasts from different plant tissues or suspension cultures is the best for SE (Pennel et al., 1992; Quiroz-Figueroa et al., 2002).

Somatic embryos have a single-cell or multicellular origin. Analyses performed by Canhoto & Cruz (1996) on *Feijoa sellowiana* cotyledons of zygotic embryos, as an explant, showed that somatic embryos developed from a single protodermal cell or from a group of cells including sub-protodermis. Similar results were obtained during the histological analysis of somatic embryogenesis of *Arabidopsis thaliana*, where the single-cell and multicellular origins of somatic embryos were also detected (Kurczyńska et. al., 2007). Cork oak somatic embryos are of a multicellular origin or a single-cell origin depending on the explant cells which participated in the embryo's formation (Puigderrajols et al., 2001). The single- and multicellular origins of somatic embryos was also described (among others) in *Borago officinalis* (Quinn et al., 1989), *Camellia japonica* (Barciela & Vieitez, 1993), *Elaeis guinnesis* (Schwendiman et al., 1990) and

Theobroma cacao (Pence et al., 1980). The unicellular origins of somatic embryos was described (among others) in the leaf explant of *Coffea arabica* (Quiroz-Figueroa et al., 2002), coconut (Verdeil et al., 2001) and *Dactylis glomerata* (Trigiano et al., 1989). In some species, only the multicellular origins of somatic embryos were described, as, for example, in *Carya illinoinensis* (Rodriguez & Wetzstein, 1998) and *Passiflora cincinnata* (Rocha et al., 2011).

It is well-documented that dividing explant cells (e.g., in callus cultures) can follow different developmental pathways, such as organogenesis, SE or unorganised growth (Fehér et al., 2003). Distinguishing between somatic embryo and organ-like structural development within explants can sometimes be difficult. The most distinctive features in the histology of somatic embryos are the anatomically closed radicular end and the lack of a vascular connection with the maternal tissues (Fig. 2 A, B). Moreover, analysis of the distribution of starch in the radicular pole of the embryo showed that starch was present in both zygotic embryos and their somatic counterparts (Fig. 2 C). Using such a criterion it is much easier to distinguish somatic embryo formation from organogenesis, which can take place within the same explant.

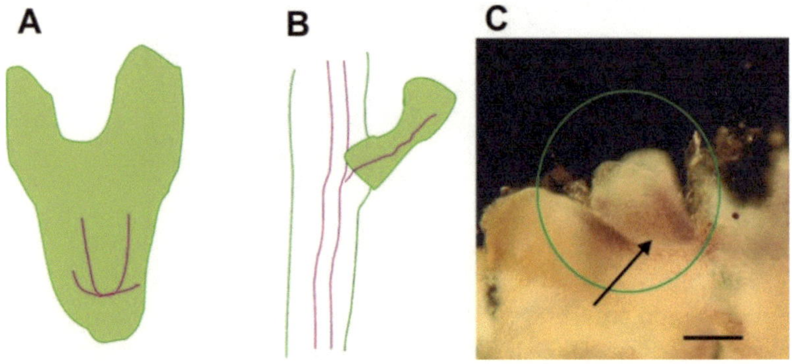

Fig. 2. Schematic differences in the histology of the basal region of the embryo (A) and buds (B; this resembles organogenesis) and starch distribution in the radicular pole of *Arabidopsis* somatic embryo (the red lines on A and B represent the vascular tissue; C – brownish colour after staining with Lugol solution marks starch; bar = 150 μm).

In the case of *Arabidopsis thaliana* (a system described by Gaj, 2001), somatic embryos develop via a DSE from explant cells located on the adaxial side in the cotyledon node (Fig. 3; Kurczyńska et al., 2007).

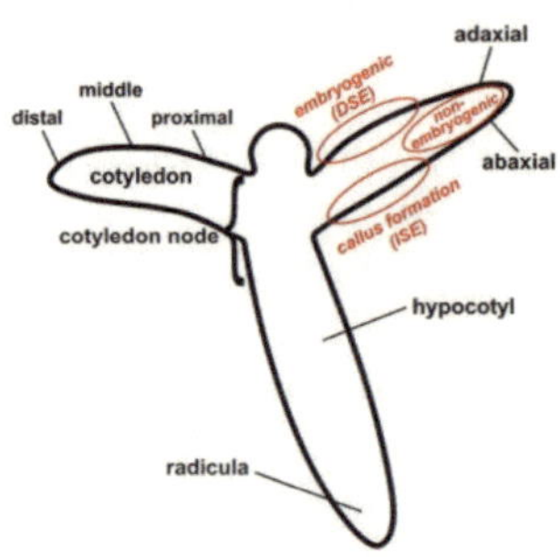

Fig. 3. Schematic representation of a longitudinal section through *Arabidopsis* explants. The location of the embryogenic and non- embryogenic regions is indicated.

From many observations and histological analysis, it appears that in this system only those cells located on the adaxial side of cotyledons undergo transition from a somatic to embryogenic state in the manner of DSE. Sometimes, if zygotic embryos are cultured in a different way, somatic embryos which developed from the callus were also detected (Fig. 4).

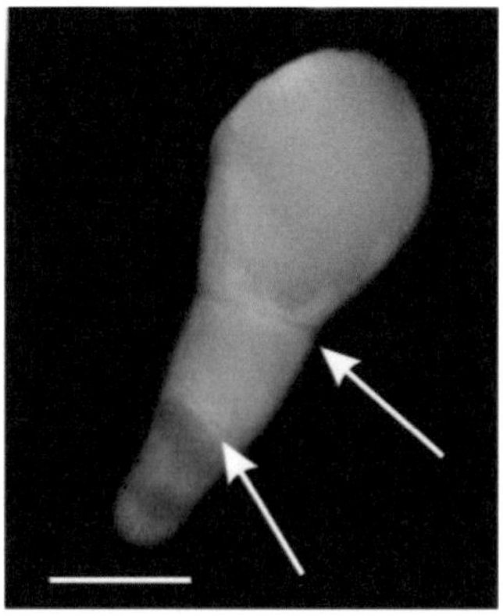

Fig. 4. Structure detected within the callus during SE in an *Arabidopsis* explants, which resembles a very early stage (a few cells) of a somatic embryo developed via an ISE (bar = 10 μm).

4. Changes in cell fate during SE

In the process of somatic embryogenesis, some somatic cells start to divide, becoming totipotent, and then enter the new pathway which is SE (Fehér et al., 2002). The most important question concerns the mechanisms underlying the changes (the transition) of the differentiated state of the plant cell into a totipotent and finally an embryogenic state (Fehér et. al., 2002). It was documented that during DSE somatic cells acquire their embryogenic competence through dedifferentiation (Harada, 1999; Fehér et al., 2003; Steinmacher et al., 2011). Such big changes in cell fate depend on the possibility of acquiring the ability to divide (Nagata, 2010). It is accepted that dedifferentiation is preceded by cell divisions (Fehér et al., 2002; Nagata et al., 1994; Wang et al., 2011) and it is postulated that existing developmental information must be changed so as to allow cells to respond to new signals (Fehér et al., 2002).

The transition from the somatic to the embryogenic state requires the induction of embryogenic competence (Verdeil et al., 2001). How should one recognise this stage of SE? The answer to this question is still far away, as it is very difficult to recognise the very early stages of somatic embryo development, starting from the changes in competence and transition from the somatic to the embryogenic state. Some studies were undertaken to answer this question and the results and the conclusions drawn from them are described below.

4.1 Cell division

From studies on the explants of different species it appears that the direction of cell division can be a marker of cells undergoing changes in cell fate. In *Arabidopsis* explants, during DSE, the protodermal cell is involved in somatic embryo formation and divides periclinally (Kulinska-Lukaszek et al., in press; Kurczyńska et al., 2007). Such a direction of cell division in the protodermal cell is unusual. In normal conditions, epidermal cells divide anticlinally (Considine & Knox, 1981) and periclinal division means that the phenotype of the protodermal cells was changed. This kind of division can be also called asymmetric (asymmetric does not necessarily mean that cells are of a different size after a division) because two daughter cells after periclinal division have a different neighbourhood; one of them still is in contact with the external environment while the other one is not. Other examples where unusual and asymmetric division was detected during SE were described in the case of the development of the secondary somatic embryos of *Trifolium repens* (Meheswaran & Williams, 1985), *Juglans regia* and *Medicago sativa* (Polito et al., 1989; Uzelac et al., 2007) and in the case of *Helianthus annuus* x *H. tuberossus* (Chiappetta et al., 2009).

4.2 Meristematic and embryogenic cells within explants

From many studies, it appears that the development of somatic embryos begins from the explant areas which are described as meristematic. Such a characteristic is typical not only for DSE but also for ISE.

The question now arises whether meristematic cells are histologically, morphologically and ultrastructurally equal to embryogenic ones? Next, how can we recognise meristematic and embryogenic explant cells?

Histological and ultrastructural analysis during the SE of pineapple guava showed that meristematic cells are rich in cytoplasm and containing many ribosomes, some amyloplasts and numerous mitochondria (Canhoto & Cruz, 1996; Canhoto et al., 1996). In this system, meristematic cells were similar on the ultrastructural level to embryogenic (proembryo) cells, with the only exception that the meristematic cells were more vacuolated. In the case of coconut, the meristematic cells were also characterised by dense cytoplasm, many ribosomes, reduced vacuole and a voluminous central nucleus with one or two nucleoli (Fig. 5 A; Verdeil et al., 2001). Cells with the same characteristics were described for *Carya* (Rodriguez & Wetzstein, 1998).

According to many studies, the most widely-described characteristic of the embryogenic cells involved in somatic embryo development are as follows: small cells with an isodiametric shape with dense cytoplasm, a nucleus located in the cell centre with a highly visible nucleolus and with small starch grains and vacuoles (Fig. 5 B; C; Canhoto & Cruz, 1996; Namasivayam et al., 2006; Verdeil et al., 2001). Pasternak and co-workers (2002) have also shown that embryogenic cells can be distinguished from non-embryogenic cells in the case of *Medicago* by the character of these cells. The embryogenic ones are characterised by their small size, with rich cytoplasm and filled with starch. The similar character of embryogenic cells was described in *Passiflora cincinnata* (Rocha et al., 2011) and cork oak (Puigderrajols et al., 2001). Cells with the same characteristics were described for the embryogenic parts of the explants of *Carya* (Rodriguez & Wetzstein, 1998). Nomura and Komamine (1985, 1995) have shown that isolated, small, cytoplasm-rich carrot cells have the ability to develop into somatic embryos. In carrot cultures, several phenotypes of cells capable for SE (embryogenic) were described (Toonen et al., 1994) but the efficiency of SE was highest in cells with a small size, a rich cytoplasm and which are spherical. The comparison of the embryogenic and non-embryogenic parts of explants is much easier as the non-embryogenic parts of explants are highly vacuolated (Fig. 5 D).

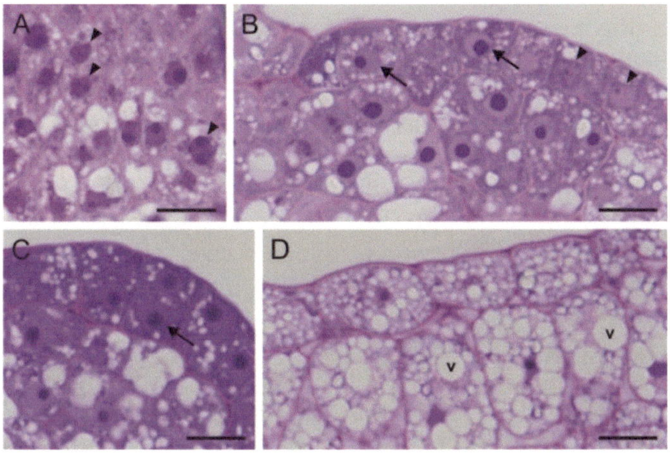

Fig. 5. Semi-thin sections through the *Arabidopsis* explant showing the examples of meristematic (A), meristematic and embryogenic (B), embryogenic (C) and non-embryogenic cells (D; the arrows point to embryogenic cells; arrowheads - to meristematic, note several nucleoli; V - vacuoles; sections stained with toluidine blue; bar = 10 μm; author - Izabela Potocka).

From the features of meristematic and embryogenic cells presented above, it appears that these differences are not distinct. According to Verdeil and co-workers (2007), some other features can be used for better distinguishing between meristematic and embryogenic cells, being the shape and the structure of the nucleus. In meristematic (in that case, the authors described the meristematic cells of shoot meristem) cells, the nucleus is spherical, with several nucleoli and heterochromatin (electron-dense areas under TEM) uniformly distributed within the nucleus. In the case of embryogenic cells, the nucleus is irregular in shape and contains one large nucleolus (Verdeil et al., 2007).

Some observations point to changes in the cell cytoskeleton which in embryogenic cells is organised in a different manner in comparison to non-embryogenic cells (Dijak & Simmonds, 1988; Dudits et al., 1991).

In conclusion: during the analysis of the cell morphology of explants during SE, one must remember that not all meristematic cells become an embryogenic cell, and not all embryogenic cells develop into somatic embryos. The direction of cell division within an explant can be a marker of cells which changed their direction of differentiation. The main features of embryogenic cells are their small size, low elongation rate, their small vacuoles, cells reach with cytoplasm, the high cytoplasm-nucleus ratio, changes in the nucleus and the nuclear envelope and their starch content.

5. Apoplast and symplast during SE

Between the somatic and embryogenic states of development, crucial processes called the transition and induction of embryogenic competence take place. This step is the most important, but at the same time it is less understood (Verdeil et al., 2001). During this step, competent cells are those which are in a transitional state and which still require some stimuli to become embryogenic cells (Namasivayam, 2007). It is not clear how the embryogenic cells originate within the explants and what mechanisms control this process. Changes in cell fate and the direction of differentiation rely on the erasing of the genetic developmental program and switching on of a new one. How this is realised by explant cells is unclear. Some studies indicate that changes in the developmental program rely on physical isolation of a cell or a group of cells from the surroundings. This process may proceed by the isolation of the symplast and/or apoplast. The analysis of these plant compartments has shown that there are some features of the transition from the somatic to the embryogenic state on the cellular and histological level which allows the recognition of this developmental stage.

5.1 Changes in apoplast as a markers for SE

A unique feature of plants is the presence of a system of cell walls which is called 'apoplast'. For many years, apoplast has not been perceived as an important part of plant organisms. At present, it is no longer a dead part of the plant body but a temporally and spatially changing extracellular matrix. It is well-known that many processes depend not only on changes in the chemical and structural composition of the cell wall, but that the cell wall is a place where signal transduction takes place (Fry et al., 1993). If so, also process of SE was investigated from that point of view.

Studies with the secondary embryogenesis of *Brassica napus* have shown some features which should be convenient for the recognition of the transitional stage from the somatic to the embryogenic state (Namasivayam et al., 2006). It was shown that the explant epidermal cells involved in somatic embryogenesis were irregular in shape and size and covered by a layer of additional material deposited on their surface, while such material was not found in the non-embryogenic tissue (Namasivayam et al., 2006). What is interesting is that this material disappeared in the adult somatic embryos, suggesting that such a feature of embryogenic tissue could be a cellular marker for cells which changes their way of development. The staining of this material with AzurII/methylene blue suggested the presence of a mucilage/polysaccharide component (Namasivayam et al., 2006). A similar substance at the surface of the pre-embryogenic tissues was present in *Coffea arabica* (Sondahl et al., 1979), *Cichorium* (Chapman et al., 2000a, 2000b; Dubois et al. 1991, 1992), *Camellia japonica* (Pedroso & Pais, 1992, 1995), *Drosera* (Bobák et al., 2003; Šamaj et al., 1995), *Zea mays* (Šamaj et al., 1995), *Papaver* (Ovečka et al., 1997; Šamaj et al., 1994), *Pinus* (Jasik et al., 1995), *Citrus* (Chapman et al., 2000a) and coconut (Verdeil et al., 2001). The detected material was present only up to the globular stage of embryo development. Because of the time of its appearance and the location, it is postulated that this material is a cellular marker for the acquisition of embryogenic competency (Namasivayam et al., 2006). In some cases, this structure was called a 'supraembryonic network' (Chapman et al., 2000a, 2000b) or an 'extracellular matrix' (Namasivayam et al., 2006).

Another feature of apoplast during SE are the changes in the thickness of the cell wall (Fig. 6). Information about the necessity of the presence of the thick cell wall around developing somatic embryos showed that in some examples such an isolation is necessary (Dubois et al., 1991; Schwendiman et al., 1990; Verdeil et al., 2001). The thickening of the cell walls in the explants' tissues was described for *Gentiana punctata* (Mikuła et al., 2004) and *Feijoa sellowiana*, where thick cell walls were detected around the proembryos (Canhoto & Cruz, 1996).

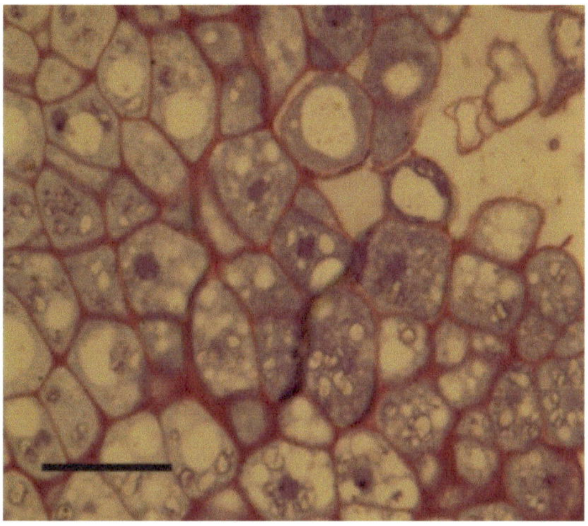

Fig. 6. Differences in wall thickness between cells within the explant through the example of *Arabidopsis* (PAS+toluidine blue staining; bar = 20 µm; author - Czekała).

It seems that the thicker cell walls surrounding the cell with a morphology which is typical for the embryogenic state is the result of the origin of these cells. Namely, if an embryo develops from the one cell and successive cell walls are formed within this mother cell, it is obvious that the cell wall at the surface of the proembryo is thicker, as is the older wall in such a complex. According to Williams and Meheswaran (1986), such isolation is necessary only if the embryogenic cells are surrounded by non-embryogenic ones.

5.1.1 Lipid transfer proteins

The lipid transfer proteins (LTPs) are proteins which can be divided into two classes, depending on the molecular weight. In *in vitro* conditions, it was shown that these proteins are able to transfer phospholipids between cellular membranes (Kader, 1997). The role of LTPs in the process of somatic embryogenesis was shown for the first time in the case of carrot embryos (Sterk et al., 1991). It is postulated that LTPs are involved in cutin biosynthesis and that they can be used as a cellular marker for the development of protodermis in somatic embryos (for a review, see Zimmerman, 1993). LTPs were also found in the extracellular proteins secreted by grapevine somatic embryos (Coutos-Thevenot et al., 1993). In *Arabidopsis* culture, LTPs were also observed outside the meristematic explant cells, which may indicate that LTPs can be used as a cellular marker during the transition from the somatic to the embryogenic state (Fig. 7).

Analysis of the presence of LTPs during somatic embryogenesis has rarely been performed, but studies on gene expression were more abundant and have shown that taking this expression pattern it is possible to distinguish between the embryogenic and non-embryogenic parts of a *Dactylis glomerata* suspension culture (Tchorbadjieva et al., 2005). Similar results indicating the role of LTPs in SE were performed on *Camellia* leaf cultures (Pedroso & Pais, 1995) and cotton (Zeng et al., 2006).

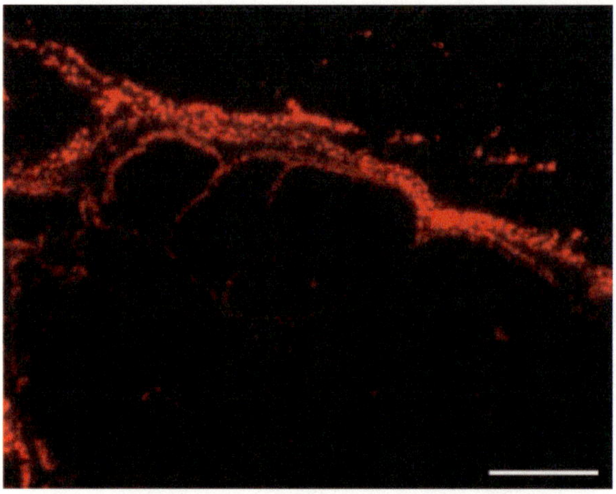

Fig. 7. The distribution of LTP1 epitopes (red dots) in the embryogenic area of *Arabidopsis* explant (LR White resin section-stained with the polyclonal anti-AtLTP1 antibody; bar = 10 μm; author - Potocka).

5.1.2 Arabinogalactan proteins (AGPs)

Arabinogalactan proteins are the group of extracellular and membrane-bound proteins which are very diverse in their composition and which are involved in many morphogenetic processes in plants, such as growth and development, cell expansion, cell proliferation and zygotic and somatic embryogenesis (Kreuger & van Holst, 1993; Qin & Zhao, 2006; for a review, see Seifert & Roberts, 2007). Many antibodies against different AGP epitopes have been introduced in order to study the role of this class of proteins in plant development. The role of AGP is postulated both during the early stages of embryogenesis and in the different developmental stages of the embryo (Stacey et al., 1990). It is also known that AGP secreted into the culture medium can promote the production of somatic embryos (Egertsdotter & von Arnold, 1995; Hengel et al., 2001; Kreuger & van Holst, 1993).

Developmental changes during somatic embryogenesis were described in detail in the case of *Daucus carota* and showed that cells "decorated" by the JIM8 antibody developed into somatic embryos, which suggests that this AGP epitope can serve as a cellular/wall marker for the very early transitional cell stage into an embryogenic pathway (Pennell et al., 1992).

The AGP epitope which was recognised by the JIM8 antibody was able to force the somatic cell of *Daucus carota* to produce somatic embryos, which points to the role of AGP in somatic embryogenesis (McCabe et al., 1997). Within the explant cells of *Arabidopsis*, only some of them during the culture period are characterised by the presence in their wall of AGP epitopes recognised by the JIM8 antibody (Fig. 8).

It was shown that the JIM4 monoclonal antibody can be an early marker for the development of somatic embryos (Stacey et al., 1990). Analysis with the use of the JIM13 antibody showed that in PEM (proembryogenic masses), in the case of *Picea abies* culture, this kind of AGP epitope was present in PEM cell walls and was not found in young somatic embryos, suggesting that this AGP epitope can be a good cellular marker for distinguishing between PEM and somatic embryos (Filonova et al., 2000).

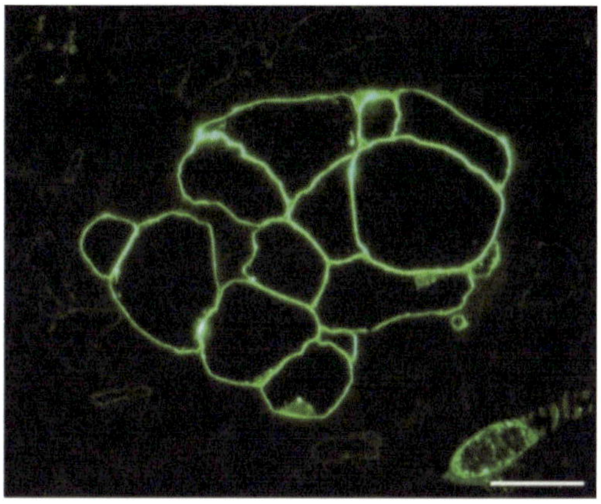

Fig. 8. A group of cells within an *Arabidopsis* explant with the presence of AGP epitope recognized by the JIM8 antibody (bar = 20 μm; author - Potocka).

5.1.3 Pectic epitopes

Pectins are the main component of the middle lamella and the primary cell wall. Pectins are acidic polysaccharides with a heterogeneous nature. The most important function of pectins is the attachment of cells.

During immunohistological studies of *Cichorium* SE with the use of the JIM5 antibody, the pectic epitopes recognised by this antibody were present in the supraembryonic network which covered the embryogenic parts of explant. It was postulated that unesterified pectic epitopes can be used as an early marker of SE (Chapman et al., 2000b).

Detected differences between the embryogenic and non-embryogenic calluses of *Daucus carota* in the amount of neutral sugars of pectin in comparison to the acidic parts of pectin are postulated as a marker for embryogenic cells (Kikuchi et al., 1995).

High levels of esterified pectins were detected during the embryogenesis of *Capsicum annuum* (Bárány et al., 2010), indicating that such a composition of cell walls is not only marker of cell proliferation but also an early marker of microspore reprogramming for embryogenesis.

In the *Arabidopsis* explants, the distribution of pectin epitopes recognised by the JIM5 and JIM7 antibodies was almost the same, but what is interesting in those parts of the explant which do not participate in embryogenesis is that neither pectin epitope was detected in the cells' walls (Fig. 9).

5.1.4 Callose

Callose is a (1→3)-β-D-linked homopolymer of glucose (Gibeaut & Carpita, 1994) present in different plant cells and what is most interesting is synthesized in response to wounding or other stress treatments (Fortes et al., 2002). However, the role of callose is not well-understood and - as was pointed out by Fortes and co-workers (2002) - in some tissues callose can prevent the absorption of water and in others it can enhance this process, which can also be important during SE.

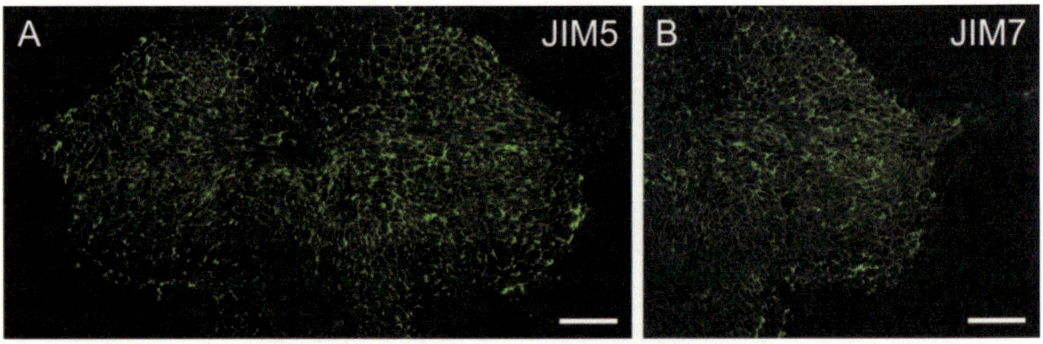

Fig. 9. The distribution of low- (left) and high-esterified (right) pectic epitopes within the *Arabidopsis* explant's cells (bar = 100 µm; author – Potocka).

The deposition of callose in the vicinity of plasmodesmata disturbs symplasmic communication (this will be described in detail below) between cells and - in this manner - influences the exchange of signals through plasmodesmata (Fig. 10 A). When callose is deposited in the cell wall it can interrupt the exchange of signals through the apoplast (Fig. 10 B).

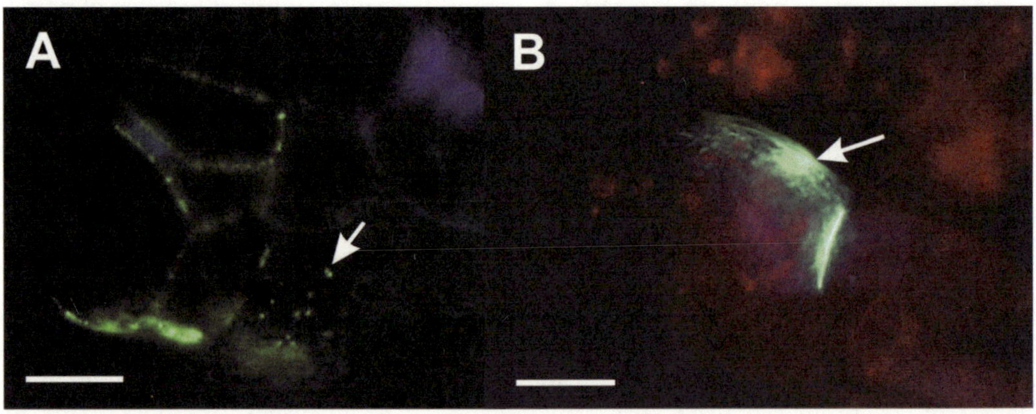

Fig. 10. The deposition of callose in the plasmodesmata regions, suggesting the closure of plasmodesmata only between some of the explants' cells (A), and in the cell wall, suggesting the isolation of neighbouring cells via apoplast (B) (*Arabidopsis* explants during SE; hand-cut sections stained with aniline blue; bar = 15 µm).

Studies with *Cichorium* and *Camellia japonica* showed that the deposition of callose is a prerequisite for somatic embryogenesis (Dubois et al., 1990; Pedroso & Pais, 1992). The same results were described for *Trifolium* (Meheswaran & Williams, 1985) and coconut (Verdeil et al., 2001).

Ultrastructural and histological studies on *Cichorium* during SE have shown that the first sign of SE is the deposition of callose in the cell wall (Verdus et al., 1993). Analysis performed on *Eleutherococcus senticosus* explants showed that after plasmolysis the amount of callose increased in comparison with untreated explants and - moreover - it was shown that callose is deposited between the plasma membrane and the cell wall (You et al., 2006).

5.1.5 Lipid substances

The deposition of lipid substances in the form of lamellae within the cell walls is postulated as being an important factor in the isolation of cells undergoing changes in their fate (Pedroso & Pais, 1992, 1995). It is postulated that apoplast isolation through the deposition of lipid substances is necessary for the abortion of the exchange of molecules through the cell wall. That is why this marker can be used in the detection of cells during the transition from the somatic to the embryogenic state. Unfortunately, there is not much information on the presence of lipid lamellae during the acquisition of embryogenic competence of explant cells.

Histological analysis of the series of a section of the *Arabidopsis* explant showed that within the callus cells some of them are isolated from the others by the lipid lamellae within the cell walls (Fig. 11). If this feature is characteristic of cells in their transition state then it requires further study.

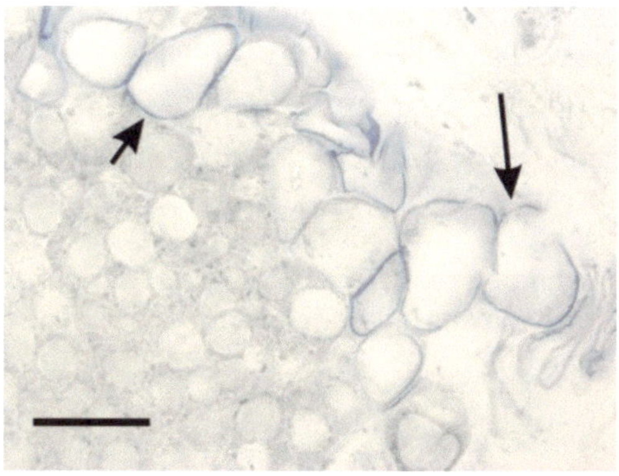

Fig. 11. The presence of lipid substances in some *Arabidopsis* explant cells during the process of SE (Sudan black staining; the arrows point to some of the cells with lipid lamellae in the wall; bar = 10 µm; author - Potocka).

In conclusion

The markers for the early stages of SE during the transition from the somatic to the embryogenic stage of cell development are present within the cell walls. These markers refer to the chemical composition of the extracellular matrix of a cell undergoing the process of transition, which involves changes in AGP and LTP, pectic epitopes, and callose and lipid substances deposited within the cell wall.

5.2 Changes in symplasm during SE

During SE, not only do changes in apoplast take place but changes also take place within the symplasm. Among the different mechanisms which control the process of plant development, including zygotic and non-zygotic embryogenesis (somatic embryogenesis and androgenesis), symplasmic communication/isolation is also postulated (Gisel et al., 1999; Kurczyńska et. al., 2007, Wrobel et al., 2011). This process is an important mechanism for the exchange of information between cells within a plant body. Such exchange of information is also a part of pattern formation within the plant organism, as it is known that the process of cell differentiation relies on the cell's position (for a review, see Scheres, 2001). The exchange of information is important and it allows cells to realise the proper developmental program.

Symplasmic communication relies on a unique feature of plant organisms - the presence of plasmodesmata (PD) which links the cytoplasm of neighbouring cells and which creates the system called 'symplasm' (Romberger et al., 2004). It should be noticed that during plant growth and development, the connection through PD between cells changes and depends on the stage of development. As a result, plant organisms can be divided into symplasmic domains and subdomains (Zambryski & Crawford, 2000). Symplasmic domains present in the plant body can be permanent (for example stomata; Fig. 12 A). Symplasmic subdomains can be also temporal, which means that they changed spatially and temporally and may be composed of several cells or just one cell (Fig. 12). Analysis of the symplasmic tracer distribution within the protodermal cells of *Arabidopsis* explants showed that fluorochrome was present only in some cells (Fig. 12 B, C). What is interesting is that after the division of mother cell, only one of the daughter cells was filled with a fluorochrome, which suggests that communication between these cells is restricted (Fig. 12 B).

The main characteristic of PD is the upper limit of the molecules' size that can freely diffuse through PD, which is called the 'Size Exclusion Limit' (SEL). It was shown that SEL changed during the development because the PD diameter can be changed temporally, spatially and physiologically (Zambryski & Crawford, 2000). PD also can disappear during the development or may be created *de novo*. Thus, the limitation in symplasmic communication is a result of PD disappearance, lowering of their number or else the downregulation of SEL.

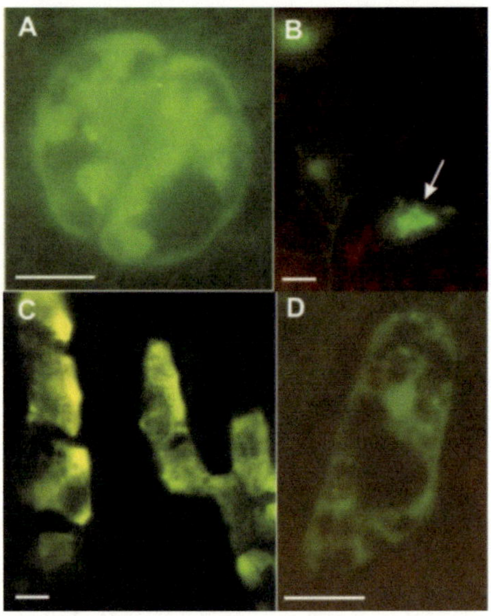

Fig. 12. The distribution of the symplasmic tracer (HPTS -8-hydroxypyrene-1,3,6-trisulfonic acid) within the protodermal cells of *Arabidopsis* explants. A – stomata as an example of the permanent symplasmic domain. B-C examples of the temporal symplasmic domains composed of a few cells (C) or in a single cell (D; as to B, note the unequal distribution of fluorochromes in the daughter cells after a division - arrow; bar = 10 μm).

As is known, molecules which can be exchanged between neighbouring cells through PD are not only ions, hormones, minerals, amino acids and sugars, but also proteins, transcriptional factors and different types of RNA (Kempers & van Bell, 1997; Lucas et al., 1993; Roberts & Oparka, 2003). This indicates that PD can regulate cell-to-cell movement and in this way participates in the regulation and coordination of plant development. It is known that PD plays an important role during the zygotic embryogenesis of *Arabidopsis thaliana* (Kim et al., 2002). Studies of the role of symplasmic communication during zygotic embryogenesis were based on the analysis of the movement of fluorochromes, dextrans conjugated to fluorescein and GFP (Green Fluorescent Protein) between embryo cells in different stages of their development. It appeared that the *Arabidopsis* embryo is one symplasmic domain up to the mid-torpedo stage (Kim et al., 2002). From that moment of development, the embryo is no longer a single symplast and the movement of symplasmic transport tracers of different molecular weights is restricted to different symplasmic domains and subdomains which correlate with the development of primary tissues and organs. This means that the downregulation of PD as the embryo develops is important for proper embryogenesis (Zambryski & Crawford, 2000). The studies mentioned above also indicate that disturbance in the normal permeability of PD leads to disorder in the development of *Arabidopsis*. The changes in PD permeability also took place when embryo changed its development from radial to bilateral symmetry (Kim & Zambryski, 2005). Detailed analysis of the GFP movement between cells also revealed the existence of subdomains which correspond to the establishment of the apical-basal axis of the *Arabidopsis* embryo (Kim et al., 2005b). These results clearly show that the regulation of embryogenesis is based (among others) on changes in symplasmic transport between embryo cells and they reveal the temporal and spatial correlation between the stages of embryo development and the formation of symplasmic domains and subdomains (Kim et al., 2002; Kim et al., 2005a; Kim et al., 2005b; Kim & Zambryski 2005; Stadler et al., 2005).

It is worth noting that there are some similarities between PD in plant organisms and the gap junctions in animal organisms. Namely, gap junctions play a control role during animal development (Warner, 1992).

The role of the disruption of symplasmic connection between cells which undergo different fate of differentiation has been postulated for many years. It is suggested that such a disruption allows those cells which are no longer connected by PD to differentiate in independent ways. Such physiological isolation is needed for reprogramming the cells. The question is: is the closing or decreasing of symplasmic communication a prerequisite for changing in direction of cell differentiation or is it the result of other changes which lead to the downregulation of symplasmic communication? The answer is not obvious. Some reports point to the first possibility while the other may suggest that it is a secondary cell reaction.

Symplasmic communication within explant cells during the initiation and development of somatic embryos was not intensively studied. Analysis of the distribution of CFDA (fluorescent tracer 5-(and-6) Carboxyfluorescein Diacetate) during the DSE in *Arabidopsis* explants showed the presence of the fluorochrome only in the protodermis and sub-protodermis of the explants, indicating that the downregulation of plasmodesmata connection within an explant took place (Kurczyńska et al., 2007).

Studies on the explants of *Panax ginseng* have shown that the disruption of plasmodesmata generated more somatic embryos than in normal conditions, indicating that cell-to-cell communication must be decreased for obtaining more efficient somatic embryogenesis (Choi & Soh, 1997). Similar results were obtained in *Morus alba* (Agarwal et al., 2004).

In the case of coconut, the cells forming the meristematic layer were connected by plasmodesmata, indicating that symplasmic communication between the cells in this layer is present (Verdeil et al., 2001). As somatic embryogenesis proceeds, the decreasing in symplasmic communication between proembryo and meristematic cells occurred, but plasmodesmata within the proembryo and embryo were present (Verdeil et al., 2001). This is an example that cells belonging to the same developmental stage - which is at the beginning of somatic embryo formation - are connected by plasmodesmata but are isolated from their neighbours.

Studies on the zygotic embryos of *Eleutherococcus senticosus* as explants showed that the disruption of plasmodesmata between explants cells promotes the formation of somatic embryos even on the medium without auxin (You et al., 2006). The interpretation of these results is as follows: the interruption of symplasmic communication stimulates the reprogramming of cells into cells competent for the embryogenic pathway (You et al., 2006).

In *Ranunculus*, analysis of the formation of somatic embryos showed that at the early stages of embryoid connection development by plasmodesmata between the embryoid and surrounding tissues were present, but in the latter stage the connection was disturbed (Konar et al., 1972). The isolation of competent cells during the formation of proembryos by disrupting plasmodesmata was also postulated by Yeung (1995). In *Gentiana punctata*, the disappearance of plasmodesmata during somatic embryogenesis was also detected (Mikuła et al., 2004).

Timmers and co-workers (1996), during the analysis of the level of calcium ions in the cells of *Daucus carota* culture, have also shown that an increasing level of these ions can cause the closure of the plasmodesmata between embryogenic cells and the proembryogenic mass.

The analysis of the presence of plasmodesmata in the callus cells of *Cichorium* shows the disappearance of connection by plasmodesmata during somatic embryogenesis, indicating that cells which will undergo new a physiological state are isolated from their neighbouring cells (Sidikou-Seyni et al., 1992). Similar results were described in the case of grasses, where the plasmodesmata connection existed only between cells belonging to the same group of cells creating aggregates (Karlsson & Vasil, 1986).

However, not all of the results described so far are in agreement with those presented above. In the case of *Pineapple guava* symplasmic, isolation was not detected during the formation of somatic embryos (Canhoto et al., 1996). Plasmodesmata were present between the cells of the embryo, but also between the embryo and the surrounding cells. This suggests that symplasmic isolation is not a prerequisite for somatic embryo formation (Canhoto et al., 1996). In other tissue culture systems, the same conclusion was drawn (Jasik et al., 1995; Thorpe, 1980; Williams & Meheswaran, 1986).

Symplasmic communication within somatic embryos is also not well-described. It was shown for barley androgenic embryos that the symplasmic barrier exists between protodermis and the underlying tissues up to the late globular stage, in the isolation of meristematic cells of the embryo in the transitional and coleoptilar stage, and between the embryo proper and the scutellum and the coleorhizae at the mature stage of the embryo (Wrobel et al., 2011). In the case of *Arabidopsis*, symplasmic isolation was correlated with the morphogenesis of somatic embryos (Fig. 13; Wrobel, 2010). In the case of *Cephalotaxus harringtonia*, numerous plasmodesmata connecting the embryo cells were noticed (Rohr et al., 1997). Similar results were described when the secondary somatic embryos of *Eucalyptus globulus* were investigated (Pinto et al., 2008).

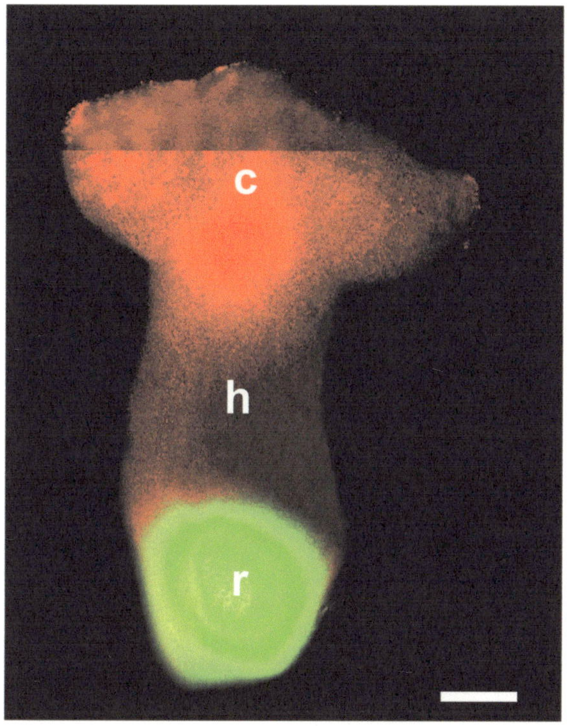

Fig. 13. The distribution of the symplasmic tracer (CMNB - caged fluorescein (fluorescein bis-(5-carboxymethoxy-2-nitrobenzyl ether, dipotassium salt) within the *Arabidopsis* somatic embryo, showing a border in symplasmic communication between the root meristem and other parts of the somatic embryo, which indicates that the symplasmic subdomains correspond with the main morphological parts of the embryo (fluorescence microscope; h - hypocotyl, c - cotyledon, r - root; bar = 150 µm; author - Wrobel, PhD thesis).

6. Conclusions

Knowledge of the cellular markers of somatic embryogenesis from the very early stages of changes in the direction of cell differentiation is important not only from a biotechnological point of view but also in helping in the understanding of the mechanisms underlying the changes in the direction of cell differentiation in general and the transition from the somatic to the embryogenic stage in particular.

It seems that promising cellular markers of cell fate changes exist at the ultrastructural and molecular level (Kiyosue et al., 1992; Pennell et al., 1992; Schmidt et al., 1997; Yeung, 1995).

The analysis of the cell wall's components and symplasmic communication during the changes in the direction of cell differentiation requires further study. Probably, both symplasm and apoplast are involved in the control of the synchronisation of cell division, histodifferentiation and primary organ development.

7. Acknowledgement

This work was supported in part by grant N303092 32/3176 from the Ministry of Science and Higher Education of Poland. We would like to apologise that not every wonderful paper describing somatic embryogenesis has been mentioned in the text, but the only cause of this was a lack of space.

8. References

Agarwal, S., Kanwar, K. & Sharma, D.R. (2004). Factors affecting secondary somatic embryogenesis and embryo maturation in *Morus alba* L. *Scientia Horticulturae*, Vol. 102, No. 3, (November 2004), pp. 359–368, ISSN 0304-4238

Bárány, I., Fadón, B., Risueño, M.C. & Testillano, P.S. (2010). Cell wall components and pectin esterification levels as markers of proliferation and differentiation events during pollen development and pollen embryogenesis in *Capsicum annuum* L. *Journal of Experimental Botany* Vol. 61, No. 4, (January 2010), pp. 1159-1175, ISSN 0022-0957

Barciela, J. & Vieitez, A.M. (1993). Anatomical sequence and morphometric analysis during somatic embryogenesis on cultured cotyledon explants of *Camellia japonica* L. *Annals of Botany*, Vol. 71, No. 5, (May 1993), pp. 395-404, ISSN 0305-7364

Bobák, M., Šamaj, J., Hlinková, E., Hlavačka, A. & Ovečka, M. (2003) Extracellular matrix in early stages of direct somatic embryogenesis in leaves of *Drosera spathulata*. *Biologia Plantarum*, Vol. 47, No. 2, (September 2003), pp. 161-166, ISSN 0006-3134

Canhoto, J.M. & Cruz, G.S. (1996). Histodifferentiation of somatic embryos in cotyledons of pineapple guava (*Feijoa sellowiana* Berg). *Protoplasma*, Vol. 191, Nos. 1-2, (March 1996), pp. 34-45, ISSN 0033-183X

Canhoto, J.M., Mesquita, J.F & Cruz, G.S. (1996). Ultrastructural changes of pineapple guava (Myrtaceae) during somatic embryogenesis. *Annals of Botany*, Vol. 78, No. 4, (October 1996), pp. 513-521, ISSN 0305-7364

Chapman, A., Blervacq, A.-S., Tissier, J.-P., Delbreil, B., Vasseur, J. & Hilbert, J.-L. (2000a). Cell wall differentiation during early somatic embryogenesis in plants. I. Scanning and transmission electron microscopy study on embryos originating from direct, indirect, and adventitious pathways. *Canadian Journal of Botany*, Vol. 78, No. 6, (June 2000), pp. 816-823, ISSN 0008-4026

Chapman, A., Blervacq, A.-S., Hendriks, T., Slomianny, C., Vasseur, J., Hilbert, J.-L. (2000b). Cell wall differentiation during early somatic embryogenesis in plants. II. Ultrastructural study and pectin immunolocalization on chicory embryos. *Canadian Journal of Botany*, Vol. 78, No. 6, (June 2000), pp. 824-831, ISSN 0008-4026

Chiappetta, A., Fambrini, M., Petrarulo, M., Rapparini, F., Michelotti, V., Bruno, L., Greco, M., Baraldi, R., Salvini, M., Pugliesi, C. & Bitonti, M.B. (2009). Ectopic expression of *LEAFY COTYLEDON1-LIKE* gene and localized auxin accumulation mark embryogenic competence in epiphyllous plants of *Helianthus annuus* × *H. tuberosus*. *Annals of Botany, Vol. 103, No. 5, (March 2009), pp. 735-747, ISSN* 0305-7364

Choi, Y.-E. & Soh, W.-Y. (1997). Enhanced somatic single embryo formation by plasmolyzing pretreatment from cultured ginseng cotyledons. *Plant Science*, Vol. 130, No. 2, (December 1997), pp. 197-206, ISSN 0168-9452

Considine, J.A. & Knox, R.B. (1981). Tissue origins, cell lineages and patterns of cell division in the developing dermal system of the fruit of *Vitis vinifera* L. *Planta*, Vol. 151, No. 5, (May 1981), pp. 403-412, ISSN 0032-0935

Coutos-Thevenot, P., Jouenne, T., Maes, O., Guerbette, F., Grosbois, M., Le Caer, J.P., Boulay, M., Deloire, A., Kader, J.C. & Guern, J. (1993). Four 9-kDa proteins excreted by somatic embryos of grapevine are isoforms of lipid-transfer proteins. *European Journal of Biochemistry*, Vol. 217, No. 3, (November 1993), pp. 885-889, ISSN 0014-2956

de Jong, A.J., Schmidt, E.D.L. & de Vries, S.C. (1993). Early events in higher-plant embryogenesis. *Plant Molecular Biology*, Vol. 22, No. 2, (May 1993), pp. 367-377, ISSN 0167-4412

Dijak, M. & Simmonds, D.H. (1988). Microtubule organization during early direct embryogenesis from mesophyll protoplasts of *Medico sativa* L. *Plant Science*, Vol. 58, No. 2, pp. 183-191, ISSN 0168-9452

Dubois, T., Guedira, M., Dubois, J. & Vasseur, J. (1990). Direct somatic embryogenesis in roots of *Cichorium*: is callose an early marker? *Annals of Botany*, Vol. 65, No. 5, (May 1990), pp. 539-545, ISSN 0305-7364

Dubois, T., Guedira, M., Dubois, J. & Vasseur, J. (1991). Direct somatic embryogenesis in leaves of *Cichorium*. A histological and SEM study of early stages. *Protoplasma*, Vol. 162, No. 2-3, (June 1991), pp. 120-127, ISSN 0033-183X

Dubois, T., Dubois, J., Guedira M., Diop, A. & Vasseur, J. (1992). SEM characterization of an extracellular matrix around somatic proembryos in roots of *Cichorium*. *Annals of Botany*, Vol. 70, No. 2, (August 1992), pp. 119-124, ISSN 0305-7364

Dudits, D., Bögre, L. & Györgyey, J. (1991). Molecular and cellular approaches to the analysis of plant embryo development from somatic cells in vitro. *Journal of Cell Science*, Vol. 99, No. 3 (July 1991), pp. 475-484, ISSN 0021-9533

Egertsdotter, U. & von Arnold, S. (1995). Importance of arabinogalactan proteins for the development of somatic embryos of Norway spruce (*Picea abies*). *Physiologia Plantarum*, Vol. 93, No. 2, (February, 1995), pp. 334-345, ISSN: 0031-9317

Evans, D.A. & Sharp, W.R. (1981). Plant regeneration from cell cultures [Methodology, genetic regulation]. *Horticultural reviews*, Vol. 3, (January, 1981), pp. 214-314, ISSN: 0163-7851

Fehér A., Pasternak T., Otvos K., Miskolczi P., Dudits D. (2002). Induction of embryogenic competence in somatic plant cells: a review. *Biologia*, Vol. 57, No.1, pp. 5-12, ISSN 1335-6372

Fehér, A., Pasternak, T. P., Dudits D. (2003). Transition of somatic plant cells to an embryogenic state. *Plant Cell, Tissue and Organ Culture*, Vol. 74, No. 3, (September, 2003), pp.201-228, ISSN: 0167-6857

Filonova, L.H., Bozhkov, P.V. & von Arnold, S. (2000). Developmental pathway of somatic embryogenesis in *Picea abies* as revealed by time-lapse tracking. *Journal of Experimental Botany*, Vol. 51, No. 343, (February, 2000), pp. 249-264, ISSN: 0022-0957

Fortes, A.M., Testillano, P.S., Risueno, M.D. & Pais, M.S. (2002). Studies on callose and cutin during the expression of competence and determination for organogenic nodule formation from internodes of *Humulus lupulus* var. Nugget. *Physiologia Plantarum*, Vol. 116, No. 1, (September, 2002), pp. 113-120, ISSN: 0031-9317

Fry, S.C., Aldington, S., Hetherington, P.R. & Aitken, J. (1993). Oligosaccharides as signals and substrates in the plant cell wall. *Plant Physiology*, Vol. 103, No. 1 (September 1993), pp. 1-5, ISSN 0032-0889

Gaj, M.D. (2001). Direct somatic embryogenesis as a rapid and efficient system for *in vitro* regeneration of *Arabidopsis thaliana*. *Plant cell, tissue and organ culture*, Vol. 64, No. 1, (January, 2001), pp. 39-46, ISSN: 0167- 6857

Gibeaut, D.M. & Carpita, N.C. (1994). Biosynthesis of plant cell wall polysaccharides. *The FASEB Journal*, Vol. 8, No. 12, (September, 1994), pp. 904-915, ISSN: 0892-6638

Gisel, A., Barella, S., Hempel, F.D. & Zambryski, P.C. (1999) Temporal and spatial regulation of symplasmic trafficking during development in *Arabidopsis thaliana* apices. *Development*, Vol. 126, No. 9, (May, 1999), pp. 1879-1889, ISSN: 0950-1991

Grafi, G. (2004). How cell dedifferentiate: a lesson from plants. *Developmental Biology*, Vol. 268, No. 1, (April 2004), pp. 1-6, ISSN: 0012-1606

Gunawardena, A.H.L.A.N., Greenwood, J.S. & Dengler, N.G. (2004). Programmed cell death remodels lace plant leaf shape during development. *Plant Cell*, Vol. 16, No. 1, (January 2004), pp. 60-73, ISSN 1040-4651

Harada, J.J. (1999). Signaling in plant embryogenesis. *Current Opinion in Plant Biology*, Vol. 2, No. 1, (February, 1999), pp. 23-27, ISSN: 1369-5266

Hengel Van, A.J., Tadesse, Z., Immerzeel, P., Schols, H., Kammen Van, A. & de Vries, S.C. (2001). N-acetylglucosamine and glucosamine-containing arabinogalactan proteins control somatic embryogenesis. *Plant Physiology*, Vol. 125, No. 4, (April, 2001), pp. 1880-1890, ISSN: 0032-0889

Jasik, J., Salajova, T. & Salaj, J. (1995). Developmental anatomy and ultrastructure of early somatic embryos in European black pine (*Pinus nigra* Arn.). *Protoplasma*, Vol. 185, Nos. 3-4 (September 1995), pp. 205-211, ISSN 0033-183X

Kader, J.-C. (1997). Lipid-transfer proteins: a puzzling family of plant proteins. *Trends in Plant Science*, Vol. 2, No. 2 (February 1997), pp. 66-70, ISSN 1360-1385

Karlsson, S.B. & Vasil, I.K. (1986). Morphology and ultrastructure of embryogenic cell suspension cultures of *Panicum maximum* (Guinea Grass) and *Pennisetum purpureum* (Napier Grass). *American Journal of Botany*, Vol. 73, No. 6 (June 1986), pp. 894-901, ISSN 00029122

Kempers, R. & van Bell, A.J.E. (1997). Symplasmic connections between sieve element and companion cell in the stem phloem of *Vicia faba* L. have a molecular exclusion limit of at least 10 kDa. *Planta*, Vol. 201, No. 2, (June 1997), pp. 195-201, ISSN 0032-0935

Kim, I., Hempel, F.D., Sha, K., Pfluger, J. & Zambryski, P.C. (2002). Identification of a developmental transition in plasmodesmatal function during embryogenesis in *Arabidopsis thaliana*. *Development*, Vol. 129, No. 5, (March 2002), pp. 1261-1272, ISSN 0950-1991

Kim, I., Cho, E., Crawford, K., Hempel, F.D & Zambryski, P.C. (2005a). Cell-to-cell movement of GFP during embryogenesis and early seedling development in *Arabidopsis*. *Proceedings of the National Academy of Sciences of the United States of America*, Vol. 102, No. 6, (February 2005), pp. 2227-2231, ISSN 0027-8424

Kim, I., Kobayashi, K., Cho, E. & Zambryski, P.C. (2005b). Subdomains for transport via plasmodesmata corresponding to the apical-basal axis established during *Arabidopsis* embryogenesis. *Proceedings of the National Academy of Sciences of the United States of America*, Vol. 102, No. 33, (August 2005), pp. 11945-11950, ISSN 0027-8424

Kim, I. & Zambryski, P.C. (2005). Cell-to-cell communication via plasmodesmata during *Arabidopsis* embryogenesis. *Current Opinion in Plant Biology*, Vol. 8, No. 6, (December 2005), pp. 593-599, ISSN 1369-5266

Kiyosue, T., Yamaguchi-Shinozaki, K., Shinozaki, K., Higashi, K., Satoh, S., Kamada, H., & Harada, H. (1992). Isolation and characterization of a cDNA that encodes ECP31, an embryogenic-cell protein from carrot. *Plant Molecular Biology*, Vol. 19, No. 2 (May 1992), pp. 239-249, ISSN 0167-4412

Konar, R.N., Thomas, E., & Street, H.E. (1972). Origin and structure of embryoids arising from epidermal cells of the stem of *Ranunculus sceleratus* L. *Journal of Cell Science*, Vol. 11 No. 1 (July 1972), pp. 77-93, ISSN 0021-9533

Kreuger, M. & van Holst, G.J. (1993). Arabinogalactan proteins are essential in somatic embryogenesis of *Daucus carota* L. *Planta*, Vol. 189, No. 2 (February 1993), pp. 243–248, ISSN 0032-0935

Kulinska-Lukaszek, K., Tobojka, M., Adamiok, A. & Kurczynska, E.U. (in press). Spatio-temporal expression of the *BBM* gene in explants and embryos during somatic embryogenesis of *Arabidopsis*. *Biologia Plantarum*, in press, ISSN: 0006-3134

Kurczyńska, E.U., Gaj, M.D., Ujczak, A. & Mazur, E. (2007). Histological analysis of direct somatic embryogenesis in *Arabidopsis thaliana* (L.) Heynh. *Planta*, Vol. 226, No. 3 (August 2007), pp. 619-628, ISSN 0032-0935

Lucas, W.J., Ding, B. & van der Shoot, C. (1993). Plasmodesmata and the supracellular nature of plants. *New Phytologist*, Vol. 125, No. 3, (November 1993), pp. 435-476, ISSN 0028-646X

Kikuchi, A., Satoh, S., Nakamura, N. & Fujii, T. (1995). Differences in pectic polysaccharides between carrot embryogenic and nonembryogenic calli. *Plant Cell Reports* Vol. 14, No. 5, (February 1995), pp. 279–284, ISSN 0721-7714

Maheswaran, G. & Williams, E.G. (1985). Origin and development of somatic embryoids formed directly on immature embryos of *Trifoliumrepensin vitro*. *Annals of Botany*, Vol. 56, No. 5, (November 1985), pp. 619-630, ISSN 0305-7364

Mathews, H., Schöpke, C., Carcamo, R., Chavarriago, P., Fauquet, C. & Beachy, R.N. (1993). Improvement of somatic embryogenesis and plant recovery in cassava. *Plant Cell Reports*, Vol. 12, No. 6 (April 1993), pp. 328-333, ISSN 0721-7714

McCabe, P.F., Valentine, T.A., Forsberg, L.S., & Pennell, R.I. (1997). Soluble signals from cells identified at the cell wall establish a developmental pathway in carrot. *The Plant Cell* Vol. 9, No. 12, (December 1997), pp. 2225-2241, ISSN 1040-4651

Mikuła, A., Tykarska, T., Zielińska, M., Kuraś, M. & Rybczyński, J.J. (2004). Ultrastructural changes in zygotic embryos of *Gentiana punctata* L. during callus formation and somatic embryogenesis. *Acta Biologica Cracoviensia, Series Botanica*, Vol. 46, pp. 109-120, ISSN 0001-5296

Nagata, T., Ishida, S., Hasezawa, S. & Takahashi, Y. (1994). Genes involved In the dedifferentiation of plant cells. *International Journal of Developmental Biology*, Vol. 38, No. 2 (June 1994), pp. 321-327, ISSN 0214-6282

Nagata, T. (2010). A journey with plant cell division: reflection at my halfway stop. In: *Progress in Botany*, Lüttge, U., Beyschlag, W., Büdel, B., Francis, D. (Eds.), Vol. 71, pp. 5-21, Springer-Verlag, ISBN 978-3-642-02166-4, Berlin, Heidelberg

Namasivayam, P., Skepper, J. & Hanke, D. (2006). Identification of a potential structural marker for embryogenic competency in the *Brassica napus* ssp. *Oleifera* embryogenic tissue. *Plant Cell Reports*, Vol. 25, No. 9 (September 2006), pp. 887-895, ISSN 0721-7714

Namasivayam, P. (2007). Acquisition of embryogenic competence during somatic embryogenesis. *Plant Cell, Tissue and Organ Culture*, Vol. 90, No. 1 (July 2007), pp. 1-8, ISSN 0167-6857

Nomura, K. & Komamine, A. (1985). Identification and isolation of single cells that produce somatic embryos at a high frequency in a carrot cell suspension culture. *Plant Physiology*, Vol. 79, No. 4 (December 1985), pp. 988-991, ISSN 0032-0889

Nomura, K. & Komamine, A. (1995). Physiological and biological aspects of somatic embryogenesis. In: *In vitro embryogenesis in plants*, Thorpe, T.A. (Ed.), pp. 249-266, Kluwer Academic Publishers, ISBN 0-7923-3149-4, Dordrecht, The Netherlands

Ovečka, M., Bobák, M., Blehová, A. & Krištín, J. (1997). *Papaversomniferum* regeneration by somatic embryogenesis and shoot organogenesis. *Biologia Plantarum*, Vol. 40, No. 3 (November 1997), pp. 321-328, ISSN 0006-3134

Pasternak, T.P., Prinsen, E., Ayaydin, F., Miskolczi, P., Potters, G., Asard, H., Van Onckelen, H.A., Dudits, D. & Fehér, A. (2002). The role of auxin, pH, and stress in the activation of embryogenic cell division in leaf protoplast-derived cells of alfalfa. *Plant Physiology*, Vol. 129, No.4 (August 2002), pp. 1807-1819, ISSN 0032-0889

Pedroso, M.C. & Pais, M.S. (1992). A scanning electron microscope and x-ray microanalysis study during induction of morphogenesis in *Camellia japonica* L. *Plant Science*, Vol. 87, No. 1, pp. 99-108, ISSN 0168-9452

Pedroso, M.C. & Pais, M.S. (1995). Factors controlling somatic embryogenesis. Cell wall changes as an *in vivo* marker of embryogenic competence. *Plant, Cell, Tissue and Organ Culture*, Vol. 43, No. 2 (November 1995), pp. 147-154, ISSN 0167-6857

Pence, V.C., Hasegawa, P.M. & Janick, J. (1980). Initiation and development of asexual embryos of *Theobroma cacao* L. *in vitro*. *ZeitschriftfuerPflanzenphysiologie*, Vol. 98, No. 1 (June 1980), pp. 1-14, ISSN 0044-328X

Pennell, R.I., Janniche, L., Scofield, G.N., Booij, H., de Vries, S.C. & Roberts, K. (1992). Identification of a transitional cell state in the developmental pathway to carrot somatic embryogenesis. *The Journal of Cell Biology*, Vol. 119, No. 5 (December 1992), pp. 1371-1380, ISSN 0021-9525

Pinto, G., Silva, S., Park, I.-S., Neves. L., Araújo C. & Santos, C. (2008). Factors influencing somatic embryogenesis induction in *Eucalyptus globulus* Labill.: basal medium and anti-browning agents. Plant, Cell, Tissue and Organ Culture, Vol. 95, No. 1 (October 2008), pp. 79-88, ISSN 0167-6857

Polito, V.S., McGranahan, G., Pinney, K. & Leslie, C. (1989). Origin of somatic embryos from repetitively embryogenic cultures of walnut (*Juglans regia* L.): implications for *Agrobacterium*-mediated transformation. *Plant Cell Reports*, No. 8 (December 1989), pp. 219-221, ISSN 0721-7714

Puigderrajols, P., Mir, G. & Molinas, M. (2001). Ultrastructure of early secondary embryogenesis by multicellular and unicellular pathways in cork oak (*Quercus suber* L.). *Annals of Botany*, Vol. 87, No. 2 (February 2001), pp. 179-189, ISSN 0305-7364

Qin, Y. & Zhao, J. (2006). Localization of arabinogalactan proteins in egg cells, zygotes, and two-celled proembryos and effects of β-D-glucosyl Yariv reagent on egg cell fertilization and zygote division in *Nicotiana tabacum* L. *Journal of Experimental Botany*, Vol. 57, No. 9, (June 2006), pp. 2061-2074, ISSN 0022-0957

Quinn, J., Simon, J.E. & Janick, J. (1989). Histology of zygotic and somatic embryogenesis in borage. Journal of the American Society for Horticultural Science, Vol. 114, No. 3, (May 1989), pp. 516-520, ISSN 0003-1062

Quiroz-Figueroa, F.R., Fuentes-Cerda, C.F.J., Rojas-Herrera, R. & Loyola-Vargas, V.M. (2002). Histological studies on the developmental stages and differentiation of two different somatic embryogenesis systems of *Coffea arabica*. *Plant Cell Reports*, Vol. 20, No. 12, (June 2002), pp. 1141-1149, ISSN 0721-7714

Quiroz-Figueroa, F.R., Rojas-Herrera, R., Galaz-Avalos, R.M. & Loyola-Vargas, V.M. (2006). Embryo production through somatic embryogenesis can be used to study cell differentiation in plants. *Plant Cell, Tissue and Organ Culture*, Vol. 86, No. 3, (September 2006), pp. 285-301, ISSN 0167-6857

Raghavan, V. (2004). Somatic embryogenesis, In: *Journey of a single cell to plant*, Murch, S.J. & Saxena, P.K., pp. 203-226, Oxford & IBH Publishing, ISBN 1578083524, New Delhi, India

Roberts, A.G. & Oparka, K.J. (2003). Plasmodesmata and the control of symplasmic transport. *Plant, Cell & Environment*, Vol. 26, No. 1, (January 2003), pp. 103-124, ISSN 0140-7791

Rocha, D.I., Vieira, L.M., Tanaka, F.A.O., da Silva, L.C. & Otoni, W.C. (2011). Somatic embryogenesis of a wild passion fruit species *Passiflora Cincinnata* Masters: histocytological and histochemical evidences. *Protoplasma*, (17 September 2011), doi: 10.1007/s00709-011-0318-x, ISSN 1615-6102

Rodriguez, A.P.M. & Wetzstein H.Y. (1998). A morphological and histological comparison of the initiation and development of pecan (*Carya illinoinensis*) somatic embryogenic cultures induced with naphthaleneacetic acid or 2,4-dichlorophenoxyacetic acid. *Protoplasma*, Vol. 204, No. 1-2 (March 1998), pp. 71-83, ISSN 0033-183X

Rohr, R., Piola, F. & Pasquier P. (1997). Somatic embryogenesis in *Cephalotaxus harringtonia* embryo-megagametophyte co-culture. *Journal of Forest Research*, Vol. 2, No. 2 (May 1997), pp. 69-73, ISSN 1341-6979

Romberger, J.A., Hejnowicz, Z. & Hill, J.F. (2004). *Plant structure: function and development. A treatise on anatomy and vegetative development, with special reference to woody plants* (Reprint of First Edition), The Blackburn Press, ISBN 1-930665-95-4, New Jersey, U.S.A.

Šamaj, J., Bobák, M., Ovečka, M., Krištin, J. & Blehová A. (1994). Extracellular matrix in early stages of plant regeneration *in vitro*. *Cell Biology International*, Vol. 18, No. 5 (May 1994), p. 545, ISSN 1065-6995

Šamaj, J., Bobák, M., Krištin, J. & Auxtová- Šamajová, O. (1995). Developmental SEM observations on an extracellular matrix in embryogenic calli of *Drosera rotundifolia* and *Zea mays*. *Protoplasma*, Vol. 186, No. 1-2 (March 1995), pp. 45-49, ISSN 0033-183X

Scheres, B. (2001). Plant cell identity. The role of position and lineage. *Plant Physiology,* Vol. 125, No. 1 (January 2001), pp. 112-114, ISSN 0032-0889

Schmidt, E.D.L., Guzzo, F., Toonen, M.A.J. & de Vries, S. (1997). A leucine-rich repeat containing receptor-like kinase marks somatic plant cells competent to form embryos. *Development,* Vol. 124, No. 10 (May 1997), pp. 2049-2062, ISSN 0950-1991

Schwendiman, J., Pannetier, C. & Michaux-Ferriere, N. (1990). Histology of embryogenic formations during *in vitro* culture of oil palm *Elaeis guineensis* Jacq. *Oléagineux,* Vol. 45, No. 10, pp. 409-418, ISSN 0030-2082

Seifert, G.J. & Roberts, K. (2007). The biology of arabinogalactan proteins. *Annual Review of Plant Biology,* Vol. 58 (January 2007), pp. 137-161, ISSN 1543-5008

Sharp, W.R., Sondahl, M.R., Caldas, L.S. & Maraffa, S.B. (1980). The physiology of *in vitro* asexual embryogenesis. *Horticultural Reviews,* Vol. 2, pp. 268-310, ISSN 0163-7851

Sidikou-Seyni, R., Rambaud, C., Dubois, J. & Vasseur, J. (1992). Somatic embryogenesis and plant regeneration from protoplasts of *Cichorium intybus* L. x *Cichorium endivia* L. *Plant Cell, Tissue and Organ Culture,* Vol. 28, No. 1 (January 1992), pp. 83-91, ISSN 0167-6857

Sondahl, M.R., Salisbury, J.L. & Sharp, W.R. (1979). SEM characterization of embryogenic tissue and globular embryos during high-frequency somatic embryogenesis in coffe callus cells. *Zeitschrift für Pflanzenphysiologie,* Vol. 94, pp. 94, ISSN 0044-328X

Stacey, N.J., Roberts, K. & Knox, J.P. (1990). Patterns of expression of the JIM4 arabinogalactan-protein epitope in cell cultures and during somatic embryogenesis in *Daucus carota* L. *Planta,* Vol. 180, No. 2 (January 1990), pp. 285-292, ISSN 0032-0935

Stadler, R., Lauterbach, C. & Sauer, N. (2005). Cell-to-cell movement of green fluorescent protein reveals post-phloem transport in the outer integument and indentifies symplasmic domains in Arabidopsis seeds and embryos. *Plant Physiology,* Vol. 139, No. 2, (October 2005), pp. 701-712, ISSN 0032-0889

Steinmacher, D.A., Guerra, M.P., Saare-Surminski, K. & Lieberei, R. (2011). A temporary immersion system improves *in vitro* regeneration of peach palm through secondary somatic embryogenesis. *Annals of Botany,* (25 February 2011), doi: 10.1093/aob/mcr033, ISSN 1095-8290

Sterk, P., Booij, H., Schellekens, G.A., van Kammen, A. & de Vries, S.C. (1991). Cell-specific expression of the carrot EP2 lipid transfer protein gene. *The Plant Cell,* Vol. 3, No. 9 (September 1991), pp. 907-921, ISSN 1040-4651

Steward, F.C., Mapes, M.O. & Mears, K. (1958). Growth and organized development of cultured cells. I. Growth and division of freely suspended cells. *American Journal of Botany,* Vol. 45, No. 9 (November 1958), pp. 693-703, ISSN 0002-9122

Sugimoto, K., Gordon, S.P. & Meyerowitz, E.M. (2011). Regeneration in plants and animals: dedifferentiation, transdifferentiation, or just differentiation? Trends in Cell Biology, Vol. 21, No. 4(April 2011), pp. 212-218, ISSN 0962-8924

Tchorbadjieva, M., Kalmukova, R., Pantchev, I. & Kyurchiev, S. (2005). Monoclonal antibody against a cell wall marker protein for embryogenic potential of *Dactylis glomerata* L. suspension cultures. *Planta,* Vol. 222, No. 5 (November 2005), pp. 811-819, ISSN 0032-0935

Thomas, H., Ougham, H.J., Wagstaff, C & Stead, A.D. (2003). Defining senescence and death. *Journal of Experimental Botany*, Vol. 54, No. 385 (April 2003), pp. 1127-1132, ISSN 0022-0957

Thorpe, T.A. (1980). Organogenesis *in vitro:* structural, physiological and biochemical aspects. In: *Perspectives in plant cell and tissue culture. International Review of Cytology - Supplement* 11A, Vasil, I.K. (Ed.), pp. 71-111, ISSN 0074-770X New York Academics Press

Timmers, A.C.J., Reiss, H.-D., Bohsung, J., Traxel, K. & Schel, J.H.N. (1996). Localization of calcium during somatic embryogenesis of carrot (*Daucus carota* L.). *Protoplasma,* Vol. 190, No. 1-2 (March 1996), pp. 107-118, ISSN 0033-183X

Toonen, M.A.J., Hendriks, T., Schmidt, E.D.L., Verhoeven, H.A., van Kammen, A. & de Vries S.C. (1994). Description of somatic-embryo-forming single cells in carrot suspension cultures employing video cell tracking. *Planta*, Vol. 194, No. 4 (December 1994), pp. 565-572, ISSN 0032-0935

Trigiano, R.N., Gray, D.J., Conger, B.V. & McDaniel, J.K. (1989). Origin of direct somatic embryos from cultured leaf segments of *Dactylis glomerata. Botanical Gazette*, Vol. 150, No. 1, (March 1989), pp. 72-77, ISSN 0006-8071

Uzelac, B., Ninković, S., Smigocki, A. & Budimir S. (2007). Origin and development of secondary somatic embryos in transformed embryogenic cultures of *Medicago sativa. Biologia Plantarum,* Vol. 51, No. 1, pp. 1-6, ISSN 0006-3134

Verdeil, J.L., Hocher, V., Huet, C., Grosdemange, F., Escoute, J, Ferriere, N. & Nicole, M. (2001). Ultrastructural Changes in Coconut Calli Associated with the Acquisition of Embryogenic Competence. *Annals of Botany*, Vol. 88, No. 1, (July 2001), pp. 9-18, ISSN 0305-7364

Verdeil, J.L., Alemanno, L., Niemenak, N. & Trambarger, T.J. (2007). Pluripotent versus totipotent plant stem cells: dependence versus autonomy? *TRENDS in Plant Science*, Vol. 12, No. 6 (May 2007), pp. 245-252, ISSN 1360-1385

Verdus, M.C., Dubois, T., Dubois, J. & Vasseur, J. (1993). Ultrastructural Changes in Leaves of *Cicorium* during Somatic Embryogenesis. *Annals of Botany*, Vol. 72, No. 4, (April 1993), pp. 375-383, ISSN 0305-7364

von Arnold, S., Sabala, I., Bozhkov, P., Dyachok, J. & Filonova, L. (2002). Developmental pathways of somatic embryogenesis. *Plant Cell, Tissue and Organ Culture*, Vol. 69, No. 3, (June 2002), pp. 233-249, ISSN 0167-6857

Wang, X.D., Nolan, K.E., Irwanto, R.R., Sheahan, M.B. & Rose, R.J. (2011). Ontogeny of embryogenic callus in *Medicago truncatula*: the fate of the pluripotent and totipotent stem cells. *Annals of Botany*, Vol. 107, No. 4, (April 2011), pp. 599-609

Williams, E.G. & Maheswaran, G. (1986). Somatic embryogenesis: factors influencing coordinated behavior of cells as an embryogenic group. *Annals of Botany*, Vol. 57, No. 4, (October 1985), pp. 443-462, ISSN 0305-7364

Warner, A. (1992). Gap junctions in development-a perspective. *Seminars in Cell Biology*, Vol. 3, No. 1, (February 1992), pp. 81-91, ISSN 1043-4682

Wrobel, J. (2010). Symplasmic communication during somatic embryogenesis of chosen species. PhD thesis, University of Silesia, Katowice, Poland

Wrobel, J., Barlow, P.W., Gorka, K., Nabialkowska, D. & Kurczynska, E.U. (2011). Histology and symplasmic tracer distribution during development of barley androgenic embryos. *Planta*, Vol. 233, No. 5, (May 2011), pp. 873-881, ISSN 0032-0935

Yang, X. & Zhang, X. (2010). Regulation of Somatic Embryogenesis in Higher Plants. *Critical Reviews in Plant Science*, Vol. 29, No. 1-3, (January 2010), pp. 36-57, ISSN 0735-2689

Yeung, E.C. (1995). Structural and developmental patterns in somatic embryogenesis. *In vitro* embryogenesis in plants. In: *Kluwer Academic Publishers*, Thorpe, T.A. (Ed.), pp. 205-247, Netherlands

You, X.L., Yi, J.S. & Choi, Y.E. (2006). Cellular change and callose accumulation in zygotic embryos of *Eleutherococcus senticocus* caused by plasmolyzing pretreatment result in high frequency of single-cell-derived somatic embrygenesis. *Protoplasma*, Vol. 227, No. 5, (May 2006), pp. 105-112, ISSN 0033-183x

Zambryski, P. & Crawford, K. (2000). Plasmodesmata: gatekeepers for cell-to-cell transport of developmental signals in plants. *Annual Review of Cell and Developmental Biology*, Vol. 16, (November 2000), pp. 393-421, ISSN 1081-0706

Zeng, F., Zhang, X., Zhu, L., Tu, L., Guo X., & Nie Y. (2006). Isolation and characterization of genes associated to cotton somatic embryogenesis by suppression subtractive hybridization and macroarray. *Plant Molecuar Biology* Vol. 60, No. 2, (January 2006), pp. 167-183, ISSN 0167-4412

Zimmerman, J.L. (1993). Somatic Embryogenesis: A Model for Early Development in Higher Plants. *The Plant Cell*, Vol. 5, No. 10, (October 1993), pp. 1411-1423, ISSN 1040-4651

15

Genomic Integrity of Mouse Embryonic Stem Cells

Luc Leyns and Laetitia Gonzalez
Vrije Universiteit, Brussel
Belgium

1. Introduction

Embryonic stem (ES) cells are isolated from the inner cell mass (ICM) of a blastocyst stage embryo, which consists of a layer of trophoblast cells lining the ICM and blastocoel or blastocyst cavity. The ICM and trophoblast cells give rise to the embryo proper and extra-embryonic tissue, respectively. Thirthy years ago the *in vitro* culture of mouse ES (mES) cells was first described (Evans and Kaufman, 1981; Martin, 1981) and later in 1998 also human ES (hES) cells were derived (Thomson et al. 1998). ES cells are characterized by the unique properties of unlimited self-renewal without senescence and pluripotency. The latter infers that ES cells give rise to all cell types of the body. These specific properties led to the great scientific interest in ES cell either for their potential medical applications or as models to address more fundamental questions in development.

Maintenance of the genomic integrity of ES cells is of major importance considering that these cells are the precursors of all cells making up the adult body. Any unrepaired DNA damage at the ES cell level could lead to mutations, giving rise to congenital disorders or embryonic lethality. Indeed, a lower spontaneous mutation frequency has been observed in mouse ES (mES) cells compared to somatic cells (Cervantes et al. 2002). Mutation frequencies are generally quantified using mutation reporter genes such as adenine phosphoribosyltransferase (Aprt), located on chromosome 8 or hypoxanthine-guanine phosphoribosyltransferase (Hprt), located on the X chromosome, which encode ubiquitously expressed purine salvage enzymes. Mutations at the heterozygous Aprt or hemizygous Hprt locus, leading to loss of the enzyme activity, can be detected based on the resistance of the cells to toxic purine analogs, such as 2-fluoroadenine or 2,6- diaminopurine for Aprt and 6-thioguanine, 8-azaguanine and 6-mercaptopurine for Hprt. The Aprt system allows detection of point mutations, small deletions/insertions or larger chromosomal events, such as mitotic recombination, chromosome loss and multilocus deletions, all leading to loss of heterozygosity (LOH). Hprt mutations are restricted to intragenic events and cannot be caused by large chromosomal changes such as multilocus deletions or chromosome loss. As it is X-linked and hemizygous Hprt cannot undergo mitotic recombination in XY mES cells.

The spontaneous mutation frequencies at the heterozygous Aprt locus of mES cells were shown to be markedly lower compared to somatic cells (mouse embryonic fibroblasts) i.e.

10^{-6} and 10^{-4}, respectively (Cervantes et al. 2002). Besides the 100-fold lower mutation frequency observed in mES cells, a different origin of the mutations was noted. Both for somatic and mES cells mutations were attributed to 80% of LOH and 20% of point mutations. However, in somatic cells the LOH was the result of mitotic recombination while in mES cells the cause of LOH was more diverse. Mitotic recombination, multilocus deletions and chromosome loss/nondisjunction accounted for 41%, 2% and 57% of the LOH, respectively (Cervantes et al. 2002). Moreover, no spontaneous mutations ($<10^{-8}$) were observed in the hemizygous Hprt locus of mES cells compared to $\sim10^{-5}$ in mouse embryonic fibroblasts (MEF). Although no spontaneous Hprt mutations were recorded in mES cells, these cells are able to undergo Hprt mutations as evidenced by the dose dependent increase upon treatment with alkylating agents such as ethyl methanesulfonate (EMS) and N-ethyl-N-nitrosurea (ENU) (Chen et al. 2000; Cervantes et al. 2002).

A lower mutation frequency could be the result of a lower sensitivity of the cells to a genotoxic insult, caused by better protective mechanisms such as f.e. antioxidant defences, an increased repair capacity compared to somatic cells or additional mechanisms for the prevention of mutation events (induction of apoptosis and /or differentiation). Cairns proposed in 1975 the immortal strand hypothesis as a mechanism to avoid mutations in adult stem cells. This hypothesis postulates that adult stem cells have a specific mechanism for DNA segregation where the template DNA is retained by one daughter cell, the self renewing stem cell, and the newly synthesised DNA potentially containing replication errors segregates to the differentiating daughter cell (Cairns, 2006; Rando et al. 2007; Lew et al. 2008). There is evidence supporting the immortal strand hypothesis in some cell types such as muscle stem cells (Conboy et al. 2007) and intestinal stem cells (Potten et al. 2002). There is, however, no evidence to assume that this immortal strand hypothesis is also at play in embryonic stem cells (Lansdorp, 2007).

This chapter focuses on the mechanisms responsible for the lower mutation frequency in mES cells. mES cells and somatic cells will be compared on basis of the extent of DNA damage, the cell cycle control mechanisms that are involved, the efficiency of the DNA repair and apoptosis induction. Furthermore mES cells have an additional mechanism to avoid passing on mutations to their progeny, i.e. induction of differentiation. A review of these issues in other embryonic stem cell types, more specifically hES cells and induced pluripotent stem cells, will be briefly discussed. Finally, the relation between these mES cell features and the *in vivo* situation will be described.

2. DNA damage, DNA repair mechanisms and cell cycle control

2.1 DNA damage

DNA damaging agents can arise from endogenous (e.g. reactive oxygen/nitrogen species (ROS/RNS)) or exogenous sources (alkylating agents, irradiation,...) leading to different DNA lesions, including base modifications, alkali-labile sites, single and double strand breaks, bulky adducts, intra- and inter-strand crosslinks. In this section the cell survival of mES cells and somatic cells exposed to these endogenous and exogenous genotoxicants has been evaluated.

Endogenous DNA damaging agents are ROS or RNS, which are the result of cellular metabolism. Among the ROS, hydroxyl radicals ($HO\cdot$), peroxynitrite (ONO_2^-) and the diffusible hydrogen peroxide (H_2O_2) are inducing base oxidation (Marnett, 2000). Challenging mES cells with ± 50 µM H_2O_2 showed an approximately 50% reduction of cell viability after 24h as assessed by toluidine blue staining, that stains dead cells (Guo et al. 2010). This concentration falls within the range of EC50-values (concentration at which a 50% effect is observed) in differentiated cell types (Table 1). Fifty percent toxicity was observed at a concentration of 30 µM in mouse leukemic P388 cells (Kanno et al. 2003) and at a concentration above 200 µM in two human gastric adenocarcinoma cell lines, MKN-45 and 23132/87 (Gencer et al. 2011). Based on this data no marked difference in cell survival between mES cells and somatic cell lines can be concluded.

	Cell type	EC50 (µM)	Test method	Reference
mES cells				
	ns	± 50	Toluidine blue staining	Guo et al. 2010
Somatic cells				
	P388 mouse leukemic cells	30	MTT assay	Kanno et al. 2003
	human gastric adenocarcinoma cell line MKN-45	> 200	MTT assay	Gencer et al. 2011
	human gastric adenocarcinoma cell line 23132/87	> 200	MTT assay	Gencer et al. 2011

Table 1. Comparison of the EC50 after 24h treatment of mES cells and somatic cells with H_2O_2. MTT, 3-(4,5-dimethylthiazol-2-yl)-2,5-diphenyl tetrazolium bromide; ns, not specified.

The cell survival of mES cells after an exogenous genotoxic insult compared to somatic cells has been investigated for a number of genotoxicants. Comparison with mouse embryonic fibroblasts (MEF) revealed a lower cell survival of mES cells after γ-ray irradiation, inducing oxidative lesions and DNA breaks, after mitomycin C treatment, inducing interstrand crosslinks, mono adducts and oxidative DNA damage and after UV irradiation, inducing DNA lesions with DNA helix distorting properties such as cyclobutane pyrimidine dimers and (6-4) photoproducts (van Sloun et al. 1999; de Waard 2008). Also treatment with N-methyl-N-nitro-N-nitrosoguanidine, that induces a whole range of DNA lesions including O^6-methylguanine that leads to DNA mispairing, increased cytotoxicity in mES cells compared to Swiss Albino 3T3 mouse fibroblasts (SA 3T3 cells) (Roos et al. 2007).

However, one should not confound cell viability with sensitivity of the cells. The sensitivity of the mES cells should be related to the amount of DNA damage induced. Unfortunately, studies comparing the extent of DNA damage in mES cells with somatic cells under the same experimental conditions are scarce.

Under cell culture conditions (pO_{2gas} of 142mm Hg) Guo et al. demonstrated that 25 µM of H_2O_2 did not induce increases in relative tail length in mES cells as measured by alkaline comet assay. This assay enables the detection of single and double strand breaks as well as alkali-labile sites. The methodology is based on the migration of DNA by electrophoresis, revealing a higher capacity for DNA migration with increased DNA strand breaks and alkali-labile sites (Box1). However, 85 and 150 μM induced a 1.3 and 1.6 fold induction of relative tail length. When combining the Comet assay with formamidopyrimidine DNA glycosylase (FPG) enzymatic treatment, which enables the detection of oxidized purines, a 1.6 and 2.3 fold induction was observed after treatment with 85 and 150 μM H_2O_2 respectively (Powers et al. 2008). In contrast, in P388 cells an increase in DNA migration of approximately 15-fold and 30-fold has been observed after 1h incubation with 30μM and 100μM H_2O_2, respectively (Kanno et al. 2003).

Combining the data on cell survival and amount of DNA damage obtained by the alkaline comet assay, one can conclude that mES cells are indeed more sensitive than differentiated or somatic cells, as fewer lesions lead to similar cell toxicity. In agreement with this, upon UV-C treatment, in mES cells only half of photoproducts (cyclobutane pyrimidine dimers and (6-4) photoproducts) are induced (Van Sloun 1999) and at the same time a higher level of cell death is observed compared to somatic cells (de Waard et al. 2008). Therefore the same amount of DNA lesions, induces a higher level of cell death in mES cells compared to somatic cells. Moreover, by using cell survival to compare the sensitivity of cell types, the sensitivity is underestimated. However, to enable a sound comparison of the sensitivity of mES cells and somatic cells, one should perform the appropriate genotoxicity assays at the appropriate dose (Box1).

Box 1: Commonly-used genotoxicity assays

Alkaline comet assay

The comet or single-cell gel electrophoresis assay was developed during the late 1970s and 1980s. The main principle of the methodology is that when single and/or double strand DNA breaks are induced, this leads to increased relaxation of the supercoiled DNA forming DNA loops. These relaxed negatively-charged DNA loops migrate to a higher extent towards the positive pole compared to supercoiled DNA during electrophoresis, resulting in the characteristic 'comet tails' (Collins et al. 2008).

Several variations on the methodology exist. The methodology that is used most commonly to date was described by Singh et al. in 1988. This comet assay, also referred to as the alkaline comet assay, introduces electrophoresis at alkaline conditions (pH > 13). The alkaline comet assay enables the detection of single (SS) and double strand (DS) DNA breaks as well as alkali-labile sites. Other variations are the neutral comet assay and the neutral comet assay with a lysis step at 50°C. Both variations are able to detect DS breaks, however the lysis at high temperature disrupts the nuclear matrix, thereby eliminating interference of SS breaks (for review Collins, 2004; Møller, 2006). The extent of DNA damage can be expressed in different ways, i.e. tail length (TL), percentage of tail DNA (%TD) or tail moment (TM). Tail moment is the TL multiplied by % TD. Several arguments are in favor of the use of % TD. De Boeck et al. (2000) demonstrated less inter-electrophoresis and inter-experimenter variability when using % TD compared to TL (De Boeck et al. 2000). Collins (2004) argues that TL can be useful at low DNA damage levels, but not at higher levels of DNA damage and that TL is more sensitive to background and threshold settings of the image analysis (Collins, 2004). Furthermore the %TD has a linear dose-response relationship with known DNA break-inducing agents (Collins, 2004; Møller, 2006).

Additional use of enzymes enables the detection of specific lesions. The most commonly used enzymes are endonuclease III (endoIII) for the detection of oxidized pyrimidines, formamidopyrimidine DNA glycosylase (FPG) and human 8-hydroxyguanine DNA glycosylase (hOGG1) for the detection of oxidized purines, T4 endonuclease V for the detection of UV-induced cyclobutane pyrimidine dimers and Alk A for the detection of 3-methyladenines. Each of these enzymes introduces a strand break at the enzyme-sensitive site (for review Collins, 2004). Smith et al. (2006) found that hOGG1 detected oxidized purines with greater specificity and sensitivity compared to endoIII and FPG. Recently, the European Comet Assay Validation Group (ECVAG) performed a study for validation of the comet assay. The inter-laboratory study retrieved dose-response relationships for oxidative DNA damage by assessment of FPG sensitive-sites in coded samples (Johansson et al. 2010; Møller et al. 2010).

It has been shown that mES have a high level of spontaneously induced DNA strand breaks as detected by alkaline comet assay. However, global chromatin decondensation seems involved rather than high levels of DNA strand break formation (Banath et al. 2009).

***In vitro* micronucleus assay**

Micronuclei (MN) are small, extra-nuclear bodies, containing chromosome/chromatid fragments or entire chromosomes/chromatids. MN are formed during cell division, when during anaphase chromosome/chromatid fragments or entire chromosomes/chromatids are not pulled to the spindle poles and lag behind. These acentric fragments or entire chromosomes/chromatids are not incorporated in the two daughter nuclei when the nuclear envelope is reassembled during telophase. MN can occur spontaneously or can be mutagen-induced. Exposure to clastogen can lead to MN containing acentric chromosome or chromatid fragments through different mechanisms. Misrepair of double strand breaks, simultaneous base excision repair in close proximity and on opposite complementary DNA strands and fragmentation of nucleoplasmic bridges may lead to the formation of acentric chromosome/chromatid fragments (for review Fenech et al. 2011; Kirsch-Volders et al. 2011a, 2011b).

Exposure to aneugens leads to MN containing entire chromosomes. Several mechanisms are responsible for aneuploidy. Hypomethylation of cytosine in centromeric and pericentromeric regions lead to chromosome malsegregation/loss probably due to defects in kinetochore assembly. Defects in spindle assembly, mitotic checkpoints and centrosome amplification are also related to increased incidence of aneuploidy. Furthermore dicentric chromosomes, when the centromeres are pulled to opposite poles, can detach from the spindle during anaphase and lead to chromosome-containing MN (for review Fenech et al. 2011; Kirsch-Volders et al. 2011a).

Since cell division is a prerequisite for MN expression, identification of mitosis is crucial. Until 1985, the method was hampered by the difficulty to identify the cells that divided in culture. Fenech and Morley introduced in 1985 the cytokinesis block in the methodology. The CBMN assay is based on the addition of cytochalasin-B, an actin inhibitor and therefore an inhibitor of cytokinesis, allowing the discrimination between cells that did not divide (mononucleated cells or MONO) and cells that divided once (binucleated cells or BN) or more (multinucleated cells) during *in vitro* culture. MN in mononucleated cells can represent the background frequency of MN (the frequency of MN that was present before treatment when considering cell lines or before *in vitro* culture when considering primary cells) or cells that did escape cytokinesis block (Kirsch-Volders and Fenech, 2001). In addition, mononucleated cells with MN can be indicative of mitotic slippage (Elhajouji et al. 1998). In the absence of a functional spindle, cells can exit mitosis without chromatid segregation and immediately proceed to the next interphase, yielding tetraploid cells. This was shown by Elhajouji et al. (1998) in lymphocytes after treatment with nocodazole (Elhajouji et al. 1998).

The number of mono-, bi- and multinucleated cells allows the calculation of the cytokinesis-block proliferation index or CBPI, a measure for cell proliferation, which is a requirement for the expression of MN. Besides MN, other biomarkers of cytogenetic damage (NPB and NBUD) as well as apoptosis and necrosis can be evaluated simultaneously. Discrimination between MN containing acentric fragments and whole chromosomes/chromatids provides useful information on the mode of action of the mutagen and hence, its classification as a clastogen or aneugen, respectively. Information on the MN content can be obtained in different ways. The use of antibodies against the kinetochore has the disadvantage that with this technique whole chromosomes with defective centromeres, and hence, absent centromeres are not detected. Furthermore, test chemicals interfering with mRNA responsible for kinetochore protein production could lead to false negatives when using antibodies against the kinetochore. The size of the MN can be indicative of its content, but is not definitive. The most commonly used method fluorescence *in situ* hybridisation (FISH) with pancentromeric or chromosome specific probes. Pancentromeric probes allow discrimination between centromere-negative MN, indicating clastogenicity, and centromere-positive MN, indicating aneugenicity. Chromosome-specific probes can additionally detect non-disjunction or unequal distribution of chromosomes in the two daughter nuclei (Elhajouji et al. 1995, 1997).

No data is available on micronucleus frequencies in mES cells, either spontaneously induced frequencies (or background levels) or frequencies induced by genotoxicants. This assay has the great advantage to discriminate chromosome breakage and chromosome loss events and could therfore greatly contribute to our understanding of DNA damage responses.

Detection of γ-H2AX

Histone protein H2AX is phosphorylated on serine 139 (γ-H2AX) at sites flanking double strand breaks. Detection of these γ-H2AX foci, using antibodies against the phosphorylated form of the protein, can be used as a measure of double strand breaks in cells. These foci can be quantified by microscopical methods or FACS analysis. It has been shown that mES cells show a high number of spontaneous γ-H2AX foci, which appears to be related to global chromatin decondensation rather than spontaneous or pre-existing DNA damage (Banath et al. 2009).

2.2 Repair mechanisms

Repair of DNA lesions is achieved through different repair mechanisms, i.e. base excision repair (BER), nucleotide excision repair (NER), mismatch repair (MMR) and double strand break repair (DSBR) or the combinations of different repair mechanisms dependent on the type of damage. Lesions where only one of the two DNA strands are affected are repaired by base excision repair (BER) or nucleotide excision repair (NER). BER is involved in the repair of lesions as a result of oxidative damage, alkylation, deamination and depurination/depyrimidination and single strand breaks (SSB). NER repairs lesions that impair transcription and replication by interfering with the DNA helical conformation, such as bulky adducts, intra- and interstrand crosslinks, UV induced pyrimidine dimers and photoproducts. Some oxidative lesions, such as cyclopurines are repaired by NER, either by global genome repair (GGR) recognising strand distortions or transcription coupled repair (TCR) removing lesions that block RNA polymerases. DSBR repairs double strand breaks (DSB) as well as SSB converted into DSB after replication. Double strand breaks are repaired by two main mechanisms, i.e. non-homologous end-joining (NHEJ) and homologous recombination (HR). Damage that disturbs replication can be repaired or bypassed by homologous recombination (template switching and strand displacement) or by translesional synthesis (TLS). MMR removes mispaired nucleotides as a consequence of base deamination, oxidation or methylation or replication errors (for review Hoeijmakers, 2001; Garinis et al. 2008, Decordier et al. 2010).

Base excision repair. BER consists of different steps. The first step involves recognition, base removal and incision. Damaged or incorrect bases are recognised by DNA glycosylases that remove bases through hydrolyzing the N-glycosidc bond leaving an apurinic/apyrimidinic (AP) site. Some DNA glycosylases (f.e. OGG1) have endogenous 3'-endonuclease activity leading to formation of a single strand break. In a next step polymerase β inserts the nucleotide. Depending on the state of the 5' deoxyribose phosphate (5'dRP) terminus, either short-patch BER or long-patch BER will be induced. Oxidised or reduced AP sites will undergo long-patch BER whereas unaltered AP sites will be repaired through short-patch BER. Finally ligation is performed either by ligase I, interacting with PCNA and polymerase β in long-patch repair, or ligase III, interacting with XRCC1, polymerase β and poly(ADP-ribose)polymerase-1 (PARP) for short-patch BER (Figure 1) (Christmann et al. 2003; Hegde et al. 2008).

The BER capacity in mES cells is greater compared to MEF. It has been shown that proteins involved in BER, f.e. Ape1, DNA ligase III, Parp1, Pcna, Ung2, Xrcc1, are expressed to a higher extent in mES cells. Furthermore a BER incorporation assay and a DNA incision assay have shown a higher BER activity. The latter assay revealed a six-fold greater level of incision production in mES cells compared to MEF cells (Tichy et al. 2011).

Nucleotide excision repair. The NER mechanism consists of the removal of a short stretch of DNA containing the lesion and the subsequent restoration of this lesion using the non-damaged DNA strand as a template. NER is divided into two distinct pathways, the global genome NER (GG-NER) and the transcription-coupled NER (TC-NER). GG-NER is largely transcription-independent and removes lesions in non-transcribed domains of the genome or non-transcribed strands in the transcribed domains. In contrast TC-NER removes lesions from the transcribed strand of active genes. In GG-NER, DNA damage recognition is performed by the XPC-HR23B and UV-DDB complex. TC-NER is triggered by the blockage of the RNA polymerase. In both NER pathways, the transcription factor TFIIH as well as XPA and RPA are recruited to the lesion for verification of the lesion. After dual incision around the lesion, mediated by XPF-ERCC1 and XPG, the single strand gap is filled by DNA polymerase δ, PCNA and RFC. Ligation occurs through DNA ligase III-XRCC1 activity. In dividing cells, additionally ligase I and DNA polymerase ε play a role (Figure 2) (Fousteri and Mullenders, 2008).

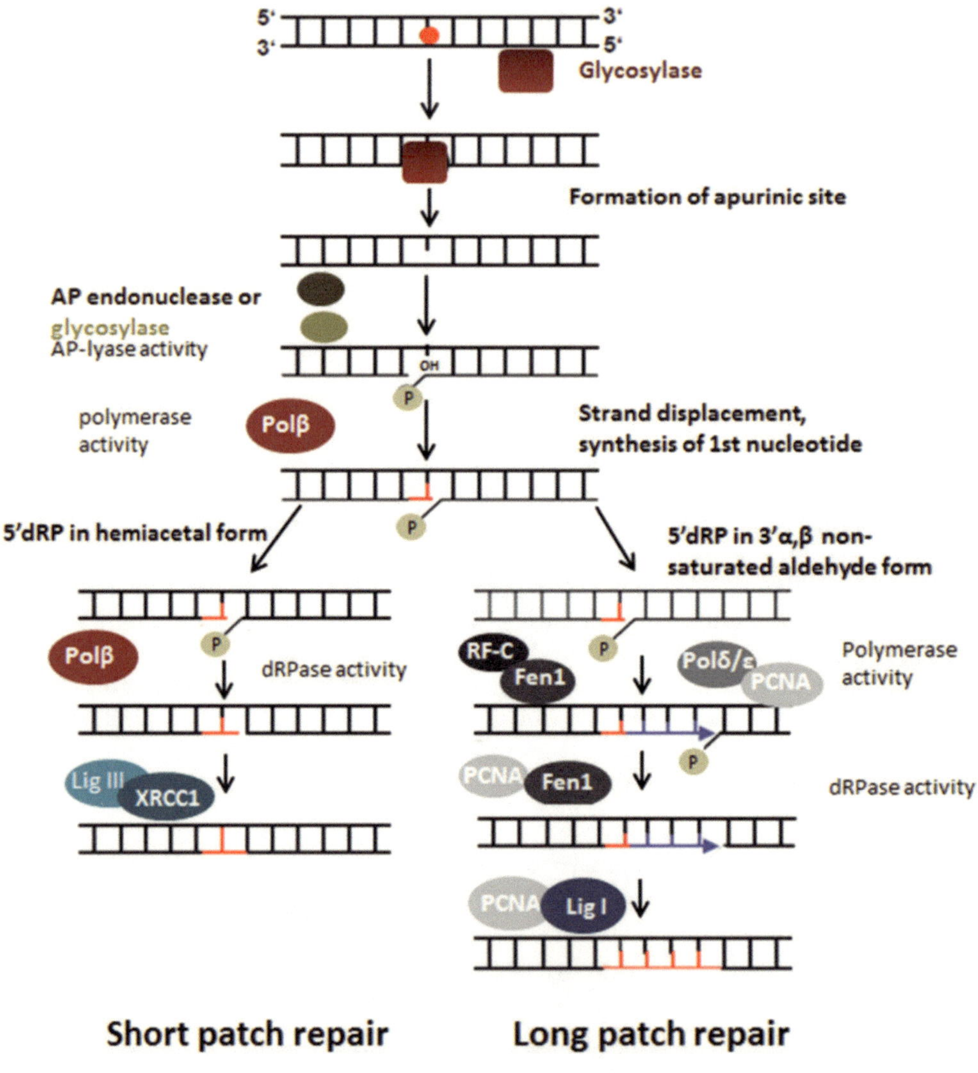

Fig. 1. Schematic representation of base excision repair (BER) mechanism. BER consists of two main pathways, short patch repair(left) and long patch repair (right). The first step of BER involves recognition, base removal and incision. The choice between short-patch BER or long-patch BER depends on the state of the 5′ deoxyribose phosphate (5′dRP) terminus. In the final step ligation is performed (modified from Christmann et al. 2003).

Analysis of gene-specific removal of UV-C induced photolesions showed a lower NER activity in mES cells compared to MEF. In mES cells, UV-C induced cyclobutane pyrimidine dimers were not removed and (6-4) photoproducts were removed up to 30% compared to MEF that are able to remove 40-70% of (6-4) photoproducts and 80% of cyclobutane pyrimidine dimers (Van Sloun 1999). Furthermore a saturation of the NER activity was observed already at effective dose 5J/m² of UV-C corresponding to three-fold lower dose than in MEF (Van Sloun 1999, van der Wees, 2007). The contribution of both types of NER, GGR and TCR, was investigated using ES cell lines deficient in repair specific genes (Xpa for total NER, Csb for TCR and Xpc for GGR). This study showed that GGR played a greater role in the survival of mES cells after UV radiation, although TCR is functional in mES cells (de Waard, 2008). In addition, the observation that $Xpc^{-/-}$ cells are hypersensitive but do not undergo apoptosis, leads to the conclusion that Xpc might play a role in both DNA damage sensing and the induction of apoptosis (de Waard et al.2008).

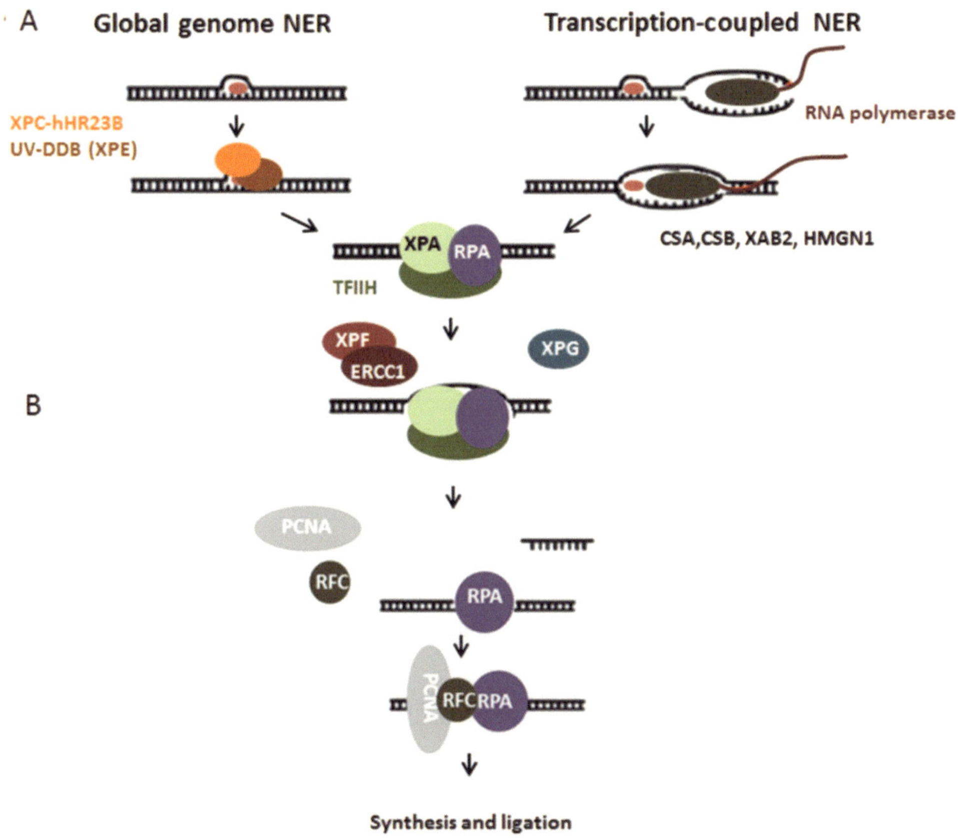

Fig. 2. The two main pathways of nucleotide excision repair (NER), global genome repair (GG-NER) and transcription-coupled repair (TC-NER) (A) and the common NER pathway. The NER mechanism consists of the removal of a short stretch of DNA containing the lesion and the subsequent restoration of this lesion using the non-damaged DNA strand as a template. GG-NER removes lesions in non-transcribed domains of the genome or non-transcribed strands in the transcribed domains; TC-NER removes lesions from the transcribed strand of active genes (modified from Fousteri and Mullenders, 2008).

Mismatch repair. Recognition of the mismatches or chemically modified bases is mediated by MSH2 and MSH6 proteins that form the MutSα complex. This complex requires phosphorylation for efficient binding to base-base and insertion/deletion mismatches.

Alternatively MSH2 can form together with MSH3 the MutSβ complex, which is able to bind to insertion/deletion mismatches. In the next step the daughter strand is identified by non-ligated single strand breaks. Two proposed models exist, i.e. the molecular switch model and the hydrolysis-driven translocation model. The former implies that MutSα-ADP binding leads to ADP-ATP transition and the formation of a hydrolysis-independent sliding clamp, followed by the binding of the MutLα complex (MLH1-MLH2). The latter model proposes that ATP hydrolysis induces translocation of MutSα along the DNA. In both cases after the association of MutSα with MutLα, excision is performed by exonuclease I and ligation by DNA polymerase δ (Figure 3) (Christmann et al. 2003).

Mismatch recognition proteins, Msh2 and Msh6, and accessory proteins, Pms2 and Mlh1, are expressed at higher level in mES cells compared to MEFs. Also mRNA levels were elevated but not to the same extent, indicating that a mechanism beyond mere higher transcription was underlying the elevated levels of MMR proteins. MMR capacity, as assessed using a MMR reporter plasmid, was shown to be 30-fold and 2-fold higher compared controls in mES cells and MEF transfected with a control vector, respectively, indicating a significantly more active repair in mES cells (Tichy et al. 2011).

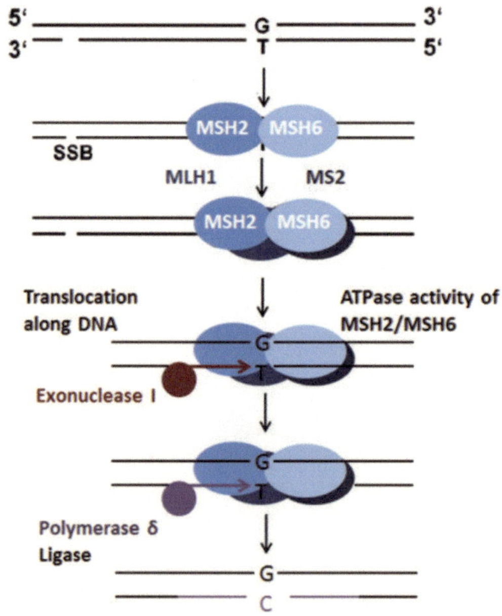

Fig. 3. Schematic representation of mismatch repair. Recognition of the mismatches or chemically modified bases is mediated by MSH2 and MSH6 proteins that form the MutSα complex. In the next step the daughter strand is identified by non-ligated single strand breaks. MutLα complex (MLH1-MLH2) associates with MutSα, excision is performed by exonuclease I and ligation by DNA polymerase δ (adapted from Christmann et al. 2003).

Double strand break repair. There are two main pathways for DSBR, error-prone non-homologous end-joining (NHEJ) and error-free homologous recombination (HR). NHEJ seems to be the predominant pathway in mammalian cells, however cell cycle phase also plays a role in the choice of pathway. NHEJ occurs in G0/G1, whereas HR occurs in late S and G2 phase. NHEJ initiates through binding of the Ku70-Ku80 complex to damaged DNA and subsequent binding of DNA-PK leading to the formation of the DNA-PK holoenzyme. Processing of the DSB is performed by the MRE11-Rad50-NBS1 complex that has exonuclease, endonuclease and helicase activity and Artemis that acts in complex with DNA-PK. After processing, XRCC4-Ligase IV binds to the DNA end and performs ligation (Figure 4A) (Christmann et al. 2003).

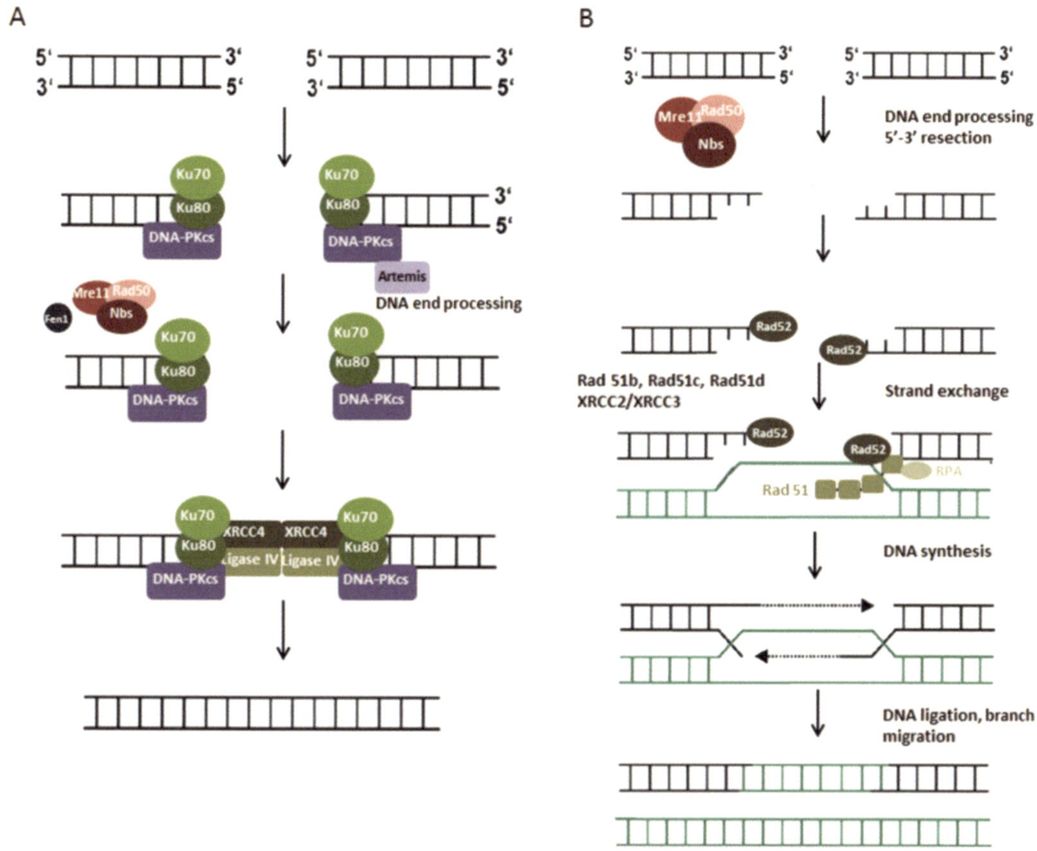

Fig. 4. Two pathways of double strand break repair: (A) non homologous end joining and (B) homologous recombination. NHEJ initiates through binding of the Ku70-Ku80 complex to damaged DNA and subsequent binding of DNA-PK leading to the formation of the DNA-PK holoenzyme. Processing of the DSB is performed by the MRE11-Rad50-NBS1 complex that has exonuclease, endonuclease and helicase activity and Artemis that acts in complex with DNA-PK. After processing, XRCC4-Ligase IV binds to the DNA end and performs ligation. HR starts with the resection of the DNA ends at the double strand breaks. This is mediated by the MRN complex (MRE11-Rad50 and NBS). The resulting single strand DNA tails are coated with RPA protein and the resulting nucleoprotein invades the complementary sequence of the sister chromatid forming heteroduplex DNA. Both Rad51 and BRCA2, involved in controlling the recombinase activity of Rad 51, are required for this process. Other proteins are also involved BRCA1, Rad52, Rad54 and Rad51 paralogues (adapted from Christmann et al. 2003).

HR starts with the resection of the DNA ends at the double strand breaks. This is mediated by the MRN complex (MRE11-Rad50 and NBS). Recruitment of this complex is promoted through binding of NBS to phosphorylated histone H2AX. The resulting single strand DNA tails are coated with RPA protein and the resulting nucleoprotein invades the complementary sequence of the sister chromatid forming heteroduplex DNA. Both Rad51 and BRCA2, involved in controlling the recombinase activity of Rad 51, are required for this process. Other proteins are also involved BRCA1, Rad52, Rad54 and Rad51 paralogues (Figure 4B) (Altieri et al. 2008).

No direct comparison of the DSBR in mES cells and somatic cells could be found in the published literature. Nonetheless, DSBR seems active in mES cells. Chuykin et al. reported induction of γ-H2AX foci after γ-irradiation (1 Gy) with a maximal number of foci obtained after 2h. Subsequently the number of foci decreased, suggesting DSBR is activated in mES (Chuykin et al. 2008).

2.3 Cell cycle control

The cell cycle of somatic cells and mES cells differs markedly both in length and cell cycle phase distribution. The mES cells are characterised by a short cell cycle of 11 to 16 hours (Orford and Scadden, 2008). Cell cycle distribution analysis showed that 10%, 75% and 15% of mES cells are respectively in G1, S and G2/M phase, indicating a very brief G1 phase (~1.5h) compared to somatic cells (~10h) (Savatier et al. 1996; Chuykin et al. 2008). In contrast, embryonic fibroblasts show a cell cycle distribution of 70%, 25%, and 5% of cells in G1, S and G2/M phase, respectively. In this section an overview and comparison of the cell cycle control pathways that are at play in mES cells and somatic cells is given.

In somatic cells, G1/S transition is mediated through the activation of Cdk4/6 and Cdk2 kinases. Upon binding to cyclin-D Cdk4/6 is activated, leading to the phosphorylation of proteins of the retinoblastoma family (pRB). This, in turn, leads to a partial inhibition of RB and the release of E2F transcription factors. The latter induces the transcription of E2F targets such as E-type cyclins. Type E-cyclins activate Cdk2 upon binding, leading to additional phosphorylation of pRB and phosphorylation of other targets important in S-phase progression. Furthermore as a consequence of the full release of E2F genes required for S-phase progression are transcribed (Figure 5A) (Wang and Blelloch, 2009). In mES cells, the G1/S transition is regulated in a different way. The Cdk4/6-Cyclin D complex is absent and the Cdk2-Cyclin E is constitutively active (Figure 5B) (Savatier et al. 1996; Wang and Blelloch, 2009).

Upon DNA damage, G1 arrest can be achieved through two main pathways in somatic cells. Double strand breaks are sensed by MRE11, a member of the MRN complex (MRE11, Nijmegen breakage syndrome and Rad50), which activates ATM. ATM autophosphorylates and phosphorylates p53 and Chk2. p53 phosphorylated by ATM and Chk2 activates the transcription of p21, that is a Cdk inhibitor, leading to G1 arrest. Active Chk2 also leads to the degradation of Cdc25 that is responsible for Cdk2 dephosphorylation necessary for G1/S phase transition (Figure 6A) (Hong and Stambrook, 2004; Stambrook, 2007). In contrast, in mES cells the G1/S checkpoint is lacking (Aladjem et al. 1998). It has been shown that in mES cells DNA damage induced by ionising irradiation does not lead to the degradation of Cdc25, as is the case in MEF. Therefore upstream events were examined, revealing that Chk2 is localised at the centrosomes and not intranuclear like in MEF, thereby unable to phosphorylate Cdc25 (Figure 6B) (Hong and Stambrook, 2004).

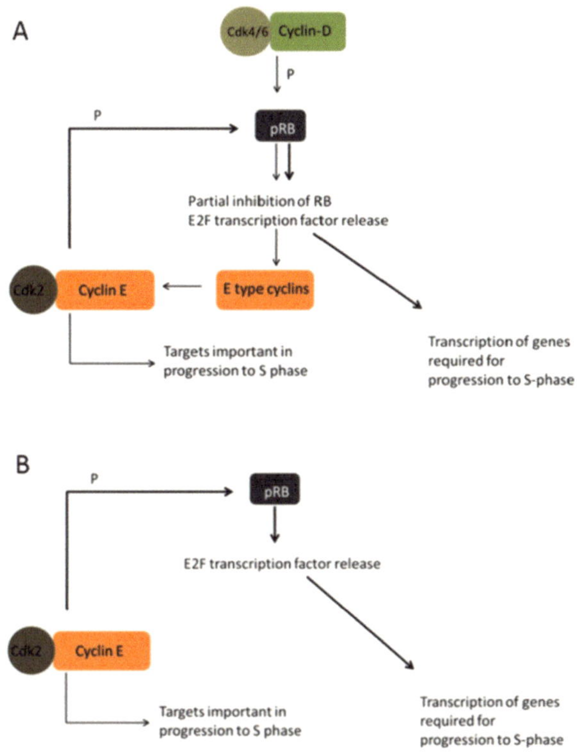

Fig. 5. Regulation of G1/S phase transition in somatic cells (A) and mES cells (B). In mES cells the Cdk4/6-Cyclin D complex is absent and the Cdk2-Cyclin E is constitutively active.

The pathway involving phosphorylation of p53 and subsequent transcription of p21 in mES cells remains unclear as data is contradictory. The amount of p53 protein is much higher in mES cells than in MEF (27-fold higher) (Sabapathy et al. 1997) or NIH3T3 cells (Solozobova et al. 2010). The higher amount of p53 proteins in mES cells was not due to a higher stability in the protein, however, both RNA content and RNA stability were increased compared to MEF cells. The cause of the higher p53 protein content was due to an enhanced translation of p53 in mES cells as well as a lower expression of miRNA 125a and miRNA125b in mES cells compared to differentiated cells (Solozobova et al. 2010).

p53 is located in the cytoplasm in undifferentiated mES cells (Solozobova et al. 2009) and is translocated to the nucleus upon challenge with IR or UV. Depending on the type of genotoxic insult the temporal pattern of p53 presence in the nucleus differs. For instance, IR induces the nuclear translocation of p53 after 1h while after 8h all p53 had disappeared from the nucleus, to reappear again in the nucleus after 24h. In contrast, upon UV light exposure p53 remained in the nucleus up till 24h (Solozobova et al. 2009). Treatment of mES cells with the antimetabolite n-phosphonacetyl-L-aspartate (PALA) leading to rNTP depletion did not induce efficient translocation of p53 to the nucleus resulting in a significant heterogeneity in PALA-treated cells (Aladjem et al. 1998).

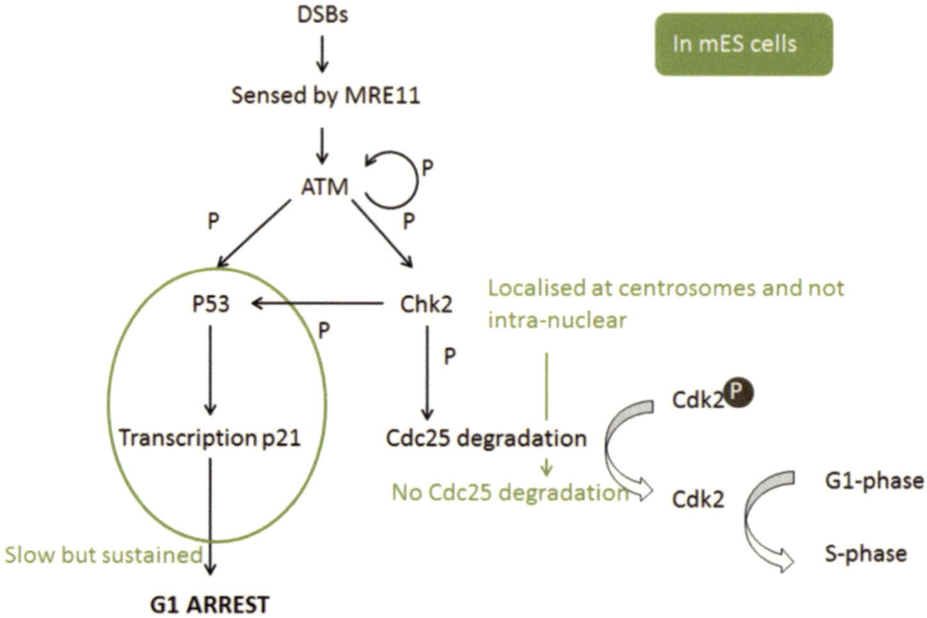

Fig. 6. Schematic representation of G1/S checkpoint in somatic cells. Differences in mES cells are depicted in green.

The transcriptional activity of p53 in mES cells is another subject of debate. On the one hand there is data supporting the transcriptional activation of p21 by p53 in mES cells. p53 activity was demonstrated using a p53-specific reporter plasmid in untreated and UV-C treated ES cells, indicating that there is a p53 baseline activity (Prost et al. 1998). Roos et al. found that upon treatment with the methylating agent N-methyl-N-nitro-N-nitrosoguanine p53 was stabilized in mES cells, which was not observed in SA 3T3 cells. Furthermore an upregulation of p21 protein was observed (Roos et al. 2007). Solozobova et al. demonstrated that p21 RNA was present and this in a comparable amount to 3T3. Furthermore p21 RNA levels further increased after ionizing radiation. However, at protein level p21 was not detectable before or after treatment with ionizing radiation, suggesting that post-transcriptional regulation plays an important role (Solozobova et al. 2009). Indeed it has been shown that micro RNAs regulate p21 expression. Members of the miR-290 cluster directly target and suppress p21, thereby modulating cell cycle progression (Wang and Blelloch, 2009).

In contrast, there is data supporting that p53 is not a transcriptional activator of p21 in mES cells. Aladjem et al. did not detect p21 expression by immunoblots, immunofluorescence or northern hybridization analysis (Aladjem et al. 1998). This is in agreement with earlier findings of Savatier et al. that did not detect p21 RNA or proteins (Savatier et al. 1996).

The G2/M checkpoint and spindle assembly checkpoint (SAC) are far less studied in mES cells. Both checkpoints are functional in mES cells (Hirao et al. 2000). It has been shown that 12h after a 10 Gy dose of γ-irradiation cells were arrested in G2-phase (Hirao et al. 2000). Furthermore at lower dose of γ-irradiation (1Gy) mES cells underwent a G2/M delay (Chuykin et al. 2008). Chk-1 is required for the initiation of the G2 arrest (Liu et al. 2000), whereas Chk-2 has been shown to play a role in the maintenance of this arrest (Hirao et al. 2000). Treatment with nocodazole, a microtubule assembly inhibitor, induced mitotic arrest in 35% of the cells after 12h, indicating that the spindle assembly checkpoint was functional (Hirao et al. 2000).

2.4 Induction of apoptosis in mES cells

In somatic cells, p53 is stabilised and activated upon genotoxic stress which can lead to cell cycle arrest, senescence or apoptosis. Upon stress p53 activates the transcription of many genes such as p21, Mdm2, Noxa and Puma that mediate the cell cycle arrest, senescence and apoptotic processes. Apoptosis can also be induced in a p53-dependent but transcription-independent manner by targeting the mitochondria thereby inducing cytochrome-C release (Zhao and Xu, 2010).

Roos et al. demonstrated the induction of p53-dependent apoptosis through p53 transcriptional activation in mES cells. Upon induction of O^6-methylguanine by treatment with N-methyl-N-nitro-N-nitrosoguanidine, apoptosis seemed activated via the Fas death pathway as the Fas receptor, which is transcriptionally regulated by p53, was upregulated and caspase-3 and -7 were activated. The lack of cytochrome-C release and the increase of the Bcl-2/Bax fraction, indicative of protection against mitochondrial-mediated apoptosis, demonstrate the inactivity of this latter apoptotic pathway (Roos et al. 2007).

mES cells have been shown to undergo apoptosis in a p53-dependent as well as in a p53-independent way. Corbet *et al.* demonstrated that upon UV treatment the majority of the cells underwent apoptosis within 36h whereas treatment with γ-irradiation induced less than 25% apoptosis within 72h corresponding to control values. This corresponded with the induction of p53 expression that was induced 4h after UV treatment and returned to basal levels after 48h. Upon γ-irradiation no overall increase in p53 protein expression was observed. Exposing $p53^{-/-}$ mES cells to UV treatment reduced apoptosis to the background level confirming the p53 dependency. However, these p53 $^{-/-}$ cells still showed a low but significant level of apoptosis, indicative of a p53-independent pathway (Corbet et al. 1999).

Aladjem *et al.* demonstrated, using p53 $^{+/+}$ and p53 $^{-/-}$ mES cells, similar kinetics in the apoptotic response upon treatment with Adriamycin, a DNA intercalating agent and inhibitor of macromolecular biosynthesis. Together with the observation that p53 was not functioning as an efficient transcriptional activator, this indicates that mES cells undergo p53-independent apoptosis (Aladjem et al. 1998).

3. DNA damage and its role in differentiation/pluripotency

One way to deal with DNA damage for ES cells is to induce the process of differentiation in order to avoid pass mutations to their progeny. A key player in this process is p53.

It has been shown that p53 induces differentiation of mES cells through suppression of Nanog, a gene required for mES cell renewal. Four hours after DNA damage, induced by UV light or doxorubicin, an increase in the level of p53 is induced. Suppression of Nanog is mediated by binding of p53 to its promotor region, leading to the differentiation of mES cells. However, this decrease in Nanog expression was not due to the expression of Oct3/4, another marker for undifferentiated mES cells. Differentiation of mES cells into other cell types upon DNA damage can therefore be a mechanism by which damaged mES cells are removed from the proliferative pool and are more efficiently subjected to p53-dependent apoptosis or cell cycle arrest (Lin et al. 2005).

Surprisingly, another target of p53 in mES cells, but not in mES cell-derived neural progenitor cells or in MEF, has been shown to be the Wnt pathway. Five Wnt ligands (Wnt3, Wnt3a, Wnt8a, Wnt8b and Wnt9a), five Wnt receptors (Fz1, Fz2, Fz6, Fz8 and Fz10), one component of the Lef1/Tcf complex (Lef1) and nine putative regulators or downstream targets of the Wnt signalling pathway (Ppp3cb, Nfatc1, Ccnd2, Ppard, Smad3, FosL1 and PPP2r2c) were identified as targets of p53. Lee et al. demonstrated that this induction of Wnt genes is not restricted to a genotoxic response (doxorubicin and UV treatment), but rather a general p53-mediated stress response as the Wnt gene expression was also induced after the use of a non-genotoxic p53 inducer, nutilin, and decreased after the reduction of p53 expression through siRNA treatment. Furthermore the induction of Wnt genes was not dependent of the induction of apoptosis or of the repression of Nanog. Wnt pathway activation leads to the inhibition of mES cell differentiation and promotion of cell proliferation. Conditioned medium of mES cells treated with UV light (CM with UV) was used to grow mES cells and lead to an increase in Nanog-positive (~29%) and Oct3/4-positive (~41%) cells, two markers of undifferentiated mES cells. Furthermore they demonstrated that cell proliferation was induced as the number of mES cells, grown in CM with UV, was two times higher after 7 days of culture in absence of leukemia inhibitory factor (LIF) as the number of mES cells, grown in CM without UV (Lee et al. 2010).

To explain these both seemingly contradictory observations, i.e. the induction of differentiation through the repression of Nanog and the antidifferentiation signals through Wnt pathway activation, the following model has been proposed. Upon DNA damage, p53 is activated to induce differentiation and apoptosis in order to prevent the DNA damage to be passed on to the progeny. To avoid differentiation and/or cell death of the entire mES cell population, as mES cells are hypersensitive to DNA damage, Wnt secretion by stressed mES cells inhibit differentiation and promote proliferation presumably of the other undamaged mES cells in order to maintain cell population numbers (Lee et al. 2010).

Box 2: Human embryonic stem cells and induced pluripotent stem cells

Human embryonic stem cells

hES cells have a higher repair capacity for different types of DNA damage compared to human primary fibroblasts. This has been shown for hES cells exposed to H_2O_2, UV-C, ionizing radiation and psoralen. In all cases, except one, the repair capacity in hES cells was higher. Only after UV-C treatment Hela cells, but not WI-38 and hs27 cells, demonstrated enhanced repair capacity compared to hES cells (Maynard et al. 2008). Furthermore, Maynard et al. demonstrated that although the level of 8-oxoG, a common oxidative lesion in DNA, was significantly lower in hES cells compared to WI-38 cells, this was not due to a higher activity of OGG1, a key component of BER. Other genes were shown to be upregulated in the different repair pathways: BER (Fen1, Lig3, Mpg, Nthl1 and Ung), NER (Rpa3), DSBR (Brca1 and Xrcc5) and interstrand crosslink repair (Blm, Fancg, Fancl and Wrn) (Maynard et al. 2008).

The G1/S checkpoint is lacking in mES cells. Whether the G1/S checkpoint exists in hES cells is a matter of debate. Data supporting the existence of the G1/S checkpoint arises from experiments using synchronized hES cells. These synchronized cells were subjected to 15 J/m^2 UVC light and were shown to accumulate in G1-phase (47% of hES cells compared to 19% in controls). Cdk2 was reduced in G1-arrested hES cells. Both potential pathways in which G1 arrest is induced, i.e. p53 transcriptional activation of p21 and the pathway involving Cdc25 degradation, were investigated. Barta et al. demonstrated that upon UVC treatment Cdc25 is downregulated in a dose-dependent manner. Furthermore inhibition of Chk1 and Chk2 demonstrated that both play a redundant role in the regulation of cell cycle progression of hES cells after UV treatment (Barta et al. 2010). Others state that the G1/S checkpoint is not functional in hES cells. Filion et al. came to this conclusion as they did not observe increases in G1-phase cells after treatment of hES cells with γ-irradiation. They did, however, observe G2-arrest, indicating that G2/M checkpoint is functional (Filion et al. 2009). In agreement with this, Sokolov et al. observed a G2-arrest, but no G1-arrest after treatment of hES cells with 1Gy dose of X-rays (Sokolov et al. 2011).

It has been shown that in hES cells apoptosis is not induced through p53 transcriptional activation. p53 protein levels are enhanced after UV irradiation and γ-irradiation, however the expression level of p53 target genes, mdm2, p21, bax and puma are down-regulated. p21 seems to be post-transcriptionally regulated as p21 protein levels were increased 2-fold after UV treatment. Apoptosis in hES cells is induced through the mitochondrial pathway. p53 was shown to accumulate in the mitochondrial fraction and caspase-9activity increased 3-fold upon UV treatment. Furthermore p53 knockdown rescued 40 % of hES cells from apoptosis and inhibited caspase-9 increase by 50%, indicating a p53 dependent apoptosis. The use of pifithrin-μ, a molecule specifically inhibiting binding of p53 to the mitochondria, resulted in an increased survival of hES cells, confirming the mitochondrial pathway apoptosis (Qin et al. 2007).

Induced pluripotent stem cells (iPS cells)

Induced pluripotent stem cells are somatic cells that have been reprogrammed with a set of transcription factors. Combinations of Oct4, Sox2, Klf4 and c-Myc or Oct-4, Nanog, Sox2 and Lin28 have been successful to transform somatic cells into cells with the same key features as ES cells, i.e. pluripotency, self-renewal and the expression of the pluripotency markers, Oct4, Nanog, Sox2 and SSEA-4. Some of these inducing transcription factors (e.g. c-Myc, Klf4, Oct4 and Lin28), however, have known oncogenic activity. Some studies have demonstrated a higher incidence of aneuploidy such as chromosome 12 duplications which might increase tumorigenicity (Mayshar et al. 2010; Pasi et al. 2011). Moreover, inactivation of p53 has been shown to increase reprogramming efficiency (Krizhanovsky and Lowe, 2009). Therefore assessing the genomic integrity in these iPS cells is of great importance for further development of applications (Sarig and Rotter, 2011). However, to date data on DNA damage responses in iPS cells is scarce.

After 1Gy of γ-irradiation, the induction of γ-H2AX foci, indicating the presence of double strand breaks, was observed in iPS cells. These foci returned to basal level within 6h after treatment. Repair of these double strand breaks appeared to be mediated by homologous recombination (HR), evidenced by the formation of Rad51 foci, a recombinase that is essential for HR. Moreover, the capacity of HR in iPS cells was similar to hES cells (Momcilovic et al. 2010). Upon γ-irradiation the activation of the checkpoint signalling cascade was induced as evidenced by phosphorylation of ATM and target proteins, such as p53. However, no G1-arrest was induced after treatment of iPS cells with 1Gy of γ-irradiation. Nine hours after treatment 77% of iPS cells were arrested in G2-phase and after 24h the cell cycle distribution resembled non-irradiated cells. iPS cells detached from the substrate which is indicative of apoptosis. In support of this, an increase in cleaved caspase-3 (more pronounced in detached cells) 4h after γ-irradiation was observed (Momcilovic et al. 2010).

4. DNA damage in embryonic development

In this section, some similarities between genotoxic effects seen in mES cells and mouse embryos are highlighted, for an extensive review of all effects caused by genotoxicants in mouse embryos I refer to some excellent reviews on the effects of ionizing radiation (De Santis et al. 2007) and oxidative stress (Wells et al. 2010).

4.1 DNA damage and repair in mouse embryos

It has been well established that exposing pregnant mice to genotoxicants leads to adverse effects in their offspring. As for mES cells, assessment of the actual extent of DNA damage in mouse embryos upon genotoxic stress is, however, scarce. A summary of the findings available in literature is given in table 2. Mainly the amount or induction of γ-H2AX foci, indicating the formation and repair of double strand breaks has been investigated in these studies (Adiga et al. 2007; Yukawa et al. 2007; Luo et al. 2006). The formation and/or repair of double strand breaks is not detected in one- and two cell stage embryos after *in* or *ex utero* exposure of the embryos to ionizing radiation, and seems therefore developmental stage-dependent. One study investigated the extent of DNA migration by alkaline comet assay after exposure of pregnant mice to pyrimethamine, a dihydrofolate reductase inhibitor used for prophylaxis and treatment of malaria and toxoplasmosis. This study showed an induction of DNA strand breakage and alkali-labile sites in the embryo at day 13 of embryonic development (E13) (Tsuda et al. 1998). The presence of DNA repair pathways is essential for correct response of mouse embryos to genotoxicants, as shown by exposure of mice bearing null mutations in genes involved in DNA repair pathways to different toxicants. These experiments demonstrated a greater susceptibility of mice bearing null mutations in DNA repair-related genes. Both knockouts of OGG1, involved in base excision repair, and CSB, involved in transcription-coupled nucleotide excision repair, showed greater susceptibility to *in utero* exposure of mice to metamphetamine (Pachowski et al. 2011).

4.2 The role of p53 in the mouse embryo stress response

The role of p53 during mouse embryo development has been investigated by generation of a p53 null mutant mice and analysis of their development. Donehower et al. demonstrated that p53 null mice develop normally, but they spontaneously develop tumours, most frequently malignant lymphomas, by 6 months of age (Donehower et al. 1992). Other studies have shown developmental defects in p53 null mice at high incidence, such as exencephaly (Armstrong et al. 1995; Sah et al. 1995).

These p53 null embryos are great tools for elucidating the role of p53 in the response of embryos to DNA damage. Heyer et al. demonstrated that p53 and the upstream activator

Genotoxicant	Exposure	Analysis of embryo	Extent of DNA damage	Remarks	Reference
Ionizing radiation	In utero exposure 3, 5, 10, 15 Gy of γ-rays	γ-H2AX foci in one-cell stage embryos 30 min after exposure	No detection of γ-H2AX foci after 3-10 Gy treatment, detection of γ-H2AX foci after 15 Gy treatment	13.3 % of blastomeres were γ-H2AX positive 72h after fertilization	Adiga et al. 2007
	In utero exposure 3 Gy of γ-rays	γ-H2AX foci in two-cell stage embryos 30 min after exposure	No detection of γ-H2AX foci after 3 Gy treatment	79% γ-H2AX positive 48h after fertilization	Adiga et al. 2007
	In utero exposure 3 Gy of γ-rays	γ-H2AX foci in six- eight -cell stage embryos 30 min after exposure	Detection of γ-H2AX foci after 3 Gy treatment		Adiga et al. 2007
	In utero exposure 3 Gy of γ-rays	γ-H2AX foci in blastocyst stage embryos 30 min after exposure	Detection of γ-H2AX foci after 3 Gy treatment		Adiga et al. 2007
Ionizing radiation	Ex utero exposure with 10 Gy γ-rays	γ-H2AX foci detection in embryos of different stages	No detection of γ-H2AX foci in one- or two-cell embryos 4-cell stage, morula stage and blastocyst stage embryos have a marked increased number of γ-H2AX foci compared to untreated controls		Yukawa et al. 2007
Electromagnetic field	Ex utero exposure with 0.5mT 50Hz electromagnetic field for 24h	γ-H2AX foci in two-cell embryos γ-H2AX foci in eight-cell embryos	6.25-fold increase in γ-H2AX foci 11.9- fold increase in γ-H2AX foci	Similar results after 48h of exposure	Luo et al. 2006
Pyrimethamine (PYR)	Oral treatment of pregnant mice with 50mg PYR/kg	E13, alkaline comet assay 6h after treatment E13, alkaline comet assay 16h after treatment	~18 and ~28 times higher DNA migration in head and body, respectively ~3 and ~19 times higher DNA migration in head and body, respectively		Tsuda et al 1998

Table 2. Summary of studies investigating the extent of DNA damage in embryos exposed to genotoxicants.

ATM are required for the embryonic response upon relatively low dose irradiation (0.5 Gy X-rays) as apoptosis was induced in wild-type embryos but not in p53 null or Atm null embryos. Heterozygous embryos showed an intermediate apoptotic response. It should also be noted that apoptosis occurred in the embryonic region and not in the extra-embryonic region. Another study by Norimura et al. demonstrated that upon 2 Gy of X-radiation, E3.5 and E9 embryos had a differential outcome depending on their p53-status. p53 null embryos had a lower incidence of death compared to their wildtype counterparts. 44% of p53 null embryos irradiated at E3.5 died before day 9 of gestation, whereas the incidence of death was 73% in wild type embryos. E9.5 p53 null embryos exposed to 2 Gy of X-rays died during gestation with a frequency of 7% compared to 60 % for their wildtype counterparts. but the incidence of malformations was higher. However, the incidence of malformations in p53 null embryos was higher with frequencies of 22% in E3.5 and 70% in E9.5 p53 null embryos and 0% in E3.5 and 20 % in E9.5 wild type embryos. Therefore they concluded that p53 suppresses teratogenesis by removing injured cells by apoptosis (Norimura et al. 1996). Others have shown that mice lacking p53 are more sensitive to alkylating agents such as cyclophosphamide, as they demonstrated grosser limb malformations (Moallem and Hales, 1998). The presence of p53 and p53-dependent apoptosis during organogenesis is therefore required for teratogenesis suppression. Also exposure to benzo[a]pyrene leads to a 3.6-fold increase in embryo resorption or *in utero* death in $p53^{-/-}$ mice compared to their wildtype counterparts (Nicol et al. 1995).

In contrast, Pekar et al. demonstrated that the teratogenic effects of cyclophosphamide are mediated by the induction of a p53-dependent apoptotic response (Pekar et al. 2007). Therefore p53 could also act an inducer of teratogenesis. Torchinsky and Toder (2010) proposed a model to explain this duality. This model describes two pathways, one pathway where p53 acts as a teratogenesis suppressor through activation of DNA repair, cell cycle arrest and suppression of ROS formation. A second pathway where p53 acts as a teratogenesis activator through induction of apoptosis is described. However, this model does not take into account the dosage and type of stress, as well as the timing of exposure. Therefore, as for mES cells, the exact role of p53 in embryo stress responses is not elucidated yet.

5. Conclusion

Genomic integrity of the mouse embryo is crucial for correct development. The genome maintenance of embryonic stem cells was discussed here, as they are models for early development and are used for medical applications. It has been demonstrated that mES cells are more sensitive than somatic cells. However, to define the difference in sensitivity, accurate assessment of the extent of DNA damage is imperative in mES cells as well as in the mouse embryo. The *in vitro* micronucleus assay could be an excellent tool to achieve this, as it enables the detection of chromosome breakage (clastogenicity) and chromosome loss (aneuploidy). Besides difference in sensitivity to genotoxic agents, mES cells have a generally higher DNA repair capacity, contributing to the maintenance of their genomic integrity, compared to somatic cells. Furthermore the cell cycle and cell cycle control in mES cells are regulated in a distinct way with the major feature being the lack of a G1/S checkpoint. Other cell cycle checkpoints (G2/M and the spindle assembly checkpoint), however, have been far less studied. The role of p53 in cell cycle control, apoptosis and differentiation vs. pluripotency is subject of some controversy. Because of contradictory results the exact role of p53, both in mES cells as well as in the embryo, remains unclear and deserves further attention.

6. Acknowledgment

This work was funded by European Union small or medium-scale focused research project ENPRA (grant number NMP-2008-1.3-2). LG received a postdoctoral fellowship from the Fund for Scientific Research–Flanders (FWO-Vlaanderen). Corresponding author: Laetitia Gonzalez, Laboratory of Cell Genetics, Department of Biology, Vrije Universiteit Brussel, Pleinlaan 2, 1050 Brussels, Belgium. Email: lgonzale@vub.ac.be

7. References

Adiga, S.K., Toyoshima, M., Shimura, T., Takeda, J., Uematsu, N. and Niwa, O. (2007). Delayed and stage specific phosphorylation of H2AX during preimplantation development of gamma-irradiated mouse embryos. *Reproduction*. Vol. 133 No. 2 pp. ISSN 415-422 1470-1626

Aladjem, M.I., Spike, B.T., Rodewald, L.W., Hope, T.J., Klemm, M., Jaenisch, R. and Wahl, G.M. (1998). ES cells do not activate p53-dependent stress responses and undergo p53-independent apoptosis in response to DNA damage. *Curr Biol*. Vol. 8 No. 3 pp. 145-155 ISSN 0960-9822

Altieri, F., Grillo, C., Maceroni, M. and Chichiarelli, S. (2008). DNA damage and repair: from molecular mechanisms to health implications. *Antioxid Redox Signal*. Vol. 10 No. 5 pp. 891-937 ISSN 1523-0864

Armstrong, J.F., Kaufman, M.H., Harrison, D.J. and Clarke, A.R. (1995). High-frequency developmental abnormalities in p53-deficient mice. *Curr Biol*. Vol. 5 No. 8 pp. 931-936 ISSN 0960-9822

Banath, J.P., Banuelos, C.A., Klokov, D., MacPhail, S.M., Lansdorp, P.M. and Olive, P.L. (2009). Explanation for excessive DNA single-strand breaks and endogenous repair foci in pluripotent mouse embryonic stem cells. *Exp Cell Res*. Vol. 315 No. 8 pp. 1505-1520 ISSN 1090-2422

Barta, T., Vinarsky, V., Holubcova, Z., Dolezalova, D., Verner, J., Pospisilova, S., Dvorak, P. and Hampl, A. (2010). Human embryonic stem cells are capable of executing G1/S checkpoint activation. *Stem Cells*. Vol. 28 No. 7 pp. 1143-1152 ISSN 1549-4918

Cairns, J. (2006). Cancer and the immortal strand hypothesis. *Genetics*. Vol. 174 No. 3 pp. 1069-1072 ISSN 0016-6731

Cervantes, R.B., Stringer, J.R., Shao, C., Tischfield, J.A. and Stambrook, P.J. (2002). Embryonic stem cells and somatic cells differ in mutation frequency and type. *Proc Natl Acad Sci U S A*. Vol. 99 No. 6 pp. 3586-3590 ISSN 0027-8424

Chen, Y., Yee, D., Dains, K., Chatterjee, A., Cavalcoli, J., Schneider, E., Om, J., Woychik, R.P. and Magnuson, T. (2000). Genotype-based screen for ENU-induced mutations in mouse embryonic stem cells. *Nat Genet*. Vol. 24 No. 3 pp. 314-317 ISSN 1061-4036

Christmann, M., Tomicic, M.T., Roos, W.P. and Kaina, B. (2003). Mechanisms of human DNA repair: an update. *Toxicology*. Vol. 193 No. 1-2 pp. 3-34 ISSN 0300-483X

Chuykin, I.A., Lianguzova, M.S., Pospelova, T.V. and Pospelov, V.A. (2008). Activation of DNA damage response signaling in mouse embryonic stem cells. *Cell Cycle*. Vol. 7 No. 18 pp. 2922-2928 ISSN 1551-4005

Collins, A.R., Oscoz, A.A., Brunborg, G., Gaivao, I., Giovannelli, L., Kruszewski, M., Smith, C.C. and Stetina, R. (2008). The comet assay: topical issues. *Mutagenesis*. Vol. 23 No. 3 pp. 143-151 ISSN 1464-3804

Conboy, M.J., Karasov, A.O. and Rando, T.A. (2007). High incidence of non-random template strand segregation and asymmetric fate determination in dividing stem cells and their progeny. *PLoS Biol*. Vol. 5 No. 5 pp. e102 ISSN 1545-7885

Corbet, S.W., Clarke, A.R., Gledhill, S. and Wyllie, A.H. (1999). P53-dependent and -independent links between DNA-damage, apoptosis and mutation frequency in ES cells. *Oncogene*. Vol. 18 No. 8 pp. 1537-1544 ISSN 0950-9232

De Boeck, M., Touil, N., De Visscher, G., Vande, P.A. and Kirsch-Volders, M. (2000). Validation and implementation of an internal standard in comet assay analysis. *Mutat Res*. Vol. 469 No. 2 pp. 181-197 ISSN 0027-5107

De Santis, M., Cesari, E., Nobili, E., Straface, G., Cavaliere, A.F. and Caruso, A. (2007). Radiation effects on development. *Birth Defects Res C Embryo Today*. Vol. 81 No. 3 pp. 177-182 ISSN 1542-975X

de Waard, H., Sonneveld, E., de Wit, J., Esveldt-van Lange, R., Hoeijmakers, J.H., Vrieling, H. and van der Horst, G.T. (2008). Cell-type-specific consequences of nucleotide excision repair deficiencies: Embryonic stem cells versus fibroblasts. *DNA Repair (Amst)*. Vol. 7 No. 10 pp. 1659-1669 ISSN 1568-7864

Decordier, I., Loock, K.V. and Kirsch-Volders, M. (2010). Phenotyping for DNA repair capacity. *Mutat Res*. Vol. 705 No. 2 pp. 107-129 ISSN 0027-5107

Donehower, L.A., Harvey, M., Slagle, B.L., McArthur, M.J., Montgomery, C.A., Jr., Butel, J.S. and Bradley, A. (1992). Mice deficient for p53 are developmentally normal but susceptible to spontaneous tumours. *Nature*. Vol. 356 No. 6366 pp. 215-221 ISSN 0028-0836

Elhajouji, A., Cunha, M. and Kirsch-Volders, M. (1998). Spindle poisons can induce polyploidy by mitotic slippage and micronucleate mononucleates in the cytokinesis-block assay. *Mutagenesis*. Vol. 13 No. 2 pp. 193-198 ISSN 0267-8357

Elhajouji, A., Tibaldi, F. and Kirsch-Volders, M. (1997). Indication for thresholds of chromosome non-disjunction versus chromosome lagging induced by spindle inhibitors in vitro in human lymphocytes. *Mutagenesis*. Vol. 12 No. 3 pp. 133-140 ISSN 0267-8357

Elhajouji, A., Van Hummelen, P. and Kirsch-Volders, M. (1995). Indications for a threshold of chemically-induced aneuploidy in vitro in human lymphocytes. *Environ Mol Mutagen*. Vol. 26 No. 4 pp. 292-304 ISSN 0893-6692

Evans, M.J. and Kaufman, M.H. (1981). Establishment in culture of pluripotential cells from mouse embryos. *Nature*. Vol. 292 No. 5819 pp. 154-156 ISSN 0028-0836

Fenech, M., Kirsch-Volders, M., Natarajan, A.T., Surralles, J., Crott, J.W., Parry, J., Norppa, H., Eastmond, D.A., Tucker, J.D. and Thomas, P. (2011). Molecular mechanisms of micronucleus, nucleoplasmic bridge and nuclear bud formation in mammalian and human cells. *Mutagenesis*. Vol. 26 No. 1 pp. 125-132 ISSN 1464-3804

Filion, T.M., Qiao, M., Ghule, P.N., Mandeville, M., van Wijnen, A.J., Stein, J.L., Lian, J.B., Altieri, D.C. and Stein, G.S. (2009). Survival responses of human embryonic stem cells to DNA damage. *J Cell Physiol*. Vol. 220 No. 3 pp. 586-592 ISSN 1097-4652

Fousteri, M. and Mullenders, L.H. (2008). Transcription-coupled nucleotide excision repair in mammalian cells: molecular mechanisms and biological effects. *Cell Res*. Vol. 18 No. 1 pp. 73-84 ISSN 1748-7838

Garinis, G.A., van der Horst, G.T., Vijg, J. and Hoeijmakers, J.H. (2008). DNA damage and ageing: new-age ideas for an age-old problem. *Nat Cell Biol*. Vol. 10 No. 11 pp. 1241-1247 ISSN 1476-4679

Gencer, S. and Irmak Yazicioglu, M.B. (2011). Differential response of gastric carcinoma MKN-45 and 23132/87 cells to H2O2 exposure. *Turk J Gastroenterol*. Vol. 22 No. 2 pp. 145-151 ISSN 1300-4948

Guo, Y.L., Chakraborty, S., Rajan, S.S., Wang, R. and Huang, F. (2010). Effects of oxidative stress on mouse embryonic stem cell proliferation, apoptosis, senescence, and self-renewal. *Stem Cells Dev*. Vol. 19 No. 9 pp. 1321-1331 ISSN 1557-8534

Hegde, M.L., Hazra, T.K. and Mitra, S. (2008). Early steps in the DNA base excision/single-strand interruption repair pathway in mammalian cells. *Cell Res*. Vol. 18 No. 1 pp. 27-47 ISSN 1748-7838

Hirao, A., Kong, Y.Y., Matsuoka, S., Wakeham, A., Ruland, J., Yoshida, H., Liu, D., Elledge, S.J. and Mak, T.W. (2000). DNA damage-induced activation of p53 by the checkpoint kinase Chk2. *Science*. Vol. 287 No. 5459 pp. 1824-1827 ISSN 0036-8075

Hoeijmakers, J. H.(2001). Genome maintenance mechanisms for preventing cancer. *Nature* Vol. 411 No.6835 pp. 366-74 ISSN 0028-0836

Hong, Y. and Stambrook, P.J. (2004). Restoration of an absent G1 arrest and protection from apoptosis in embryonic stem cells after ionizing radiation. *Proc Natl Acad Sci U S A*. Vol. 101 No. 40 pp. 14443-14448 ISSN 0027-8424

Johansson, C., Moller, P., Forchhammer, L., Loft, S., Godschalk, R.W., Langie, S.A., Lumeij, S., Jones, G.D., Kwok, R.W., Azqueta, A., Phillips, D.H., Sozeri, O., Routledge, M.N., Charlton, A.J., Riso, P., Porrini, M., Allione, A., Matullo, G., Palus, J., Stepnik, M., Collins, A.R. and Moller, L. (2010). An ECVAG trial on assessment of oxidative damage to DNA measured by the comet assay. *Mutagenesis*. Vol. 25 No. 2 pp. 125-132 ISSN 1464-3804

Kanno, S., Shouji, A., Asou, K. and Ishikawa, M. (2003). Effects of naringin on hydrogen peroxide-induced cytotoxicity and apoptosis in P388 cells. *J Pharmacol Sci*. Vol. 92 No. 2 pp. 166-170 ISSN 1347-8613

Kirsch-Volders, M., Decordier, I., Elhajouji, A., Plas, G., Aardema, M.J. and Fenech, M. (2011). In vitro genotoxicity testing using the micronucleus assay in cell lines, human lymphocytes and 3D human skin models. *Mutagenesis*. Vol. 26 No. 1 pp. 177-184 ISSN 1464-3804

Kirsch-Volders, M. and Fenech, M. (2001). Inclusion of micronuclei in non-divided mononuclear lymphocytes and necrosis/apoptosis may provide a more comprehensive cytokinesis block micronucleus assay for biomonitoring purposes. *Mutagenesis*. Vol. 16 No. 1 pp. 51-58 ISSN 0267-8357

Kirsch-Volders, M., Plas, G., Elhajouji, A., Lukamowicz, M., Gonzalez, L., Vande Loock, K. and Decordier, I. (2011). The in vitro MN assay in 2011: origin and fate, biological significance, protocols, high throughput methodologies and toxicological relevance. *Arch Toxicol*. Vol. 85 No. 8 pp. 873-899 ISSN 1432-0738

Krizhanovsky, V. and Lowe, S.W. (2009). Stem cells: The promises and perils of p53. *Nature*. Vol. 460 No. 7259 pp. 1085-1086 ISSN 1476-4687

Lansdorp, P.M. (2007). Immortal strands? Give me a break. *Cell*. Vol. 129 No. 7 pp. 1244-1247 ISSN 0092-8674

Lee, K.H., Li, M., Michalowski, A.M., Zhang, X., Liao, H., Chen, L., Xu, Y., Wu, X. and Huang, J. (2010). A genomewide study identifies the Wnt signaling pathway as a major target of p53 in murine embryonic stem cells. *Proc Natl Acad Sci U S A*. Vol. 107 No. 1 pp. 69-74 ISSN 1091-6490

Lew, D.J., Burke, D.J. and Dutta, A. (2008). The immortal strand hypothesis: how could it work? *Cell*. Vol. 133 No. 1 pp. 21-23 ISSN 1097-4172

Lin, T., Chao, C., Saito, S., Mazur, S.J., Murphy, M.E., Appella, E. and Xu, Y. (2005). p53 induces differentiation of mouse embryonic stem cells by suppressing Nanog expression. *Nat Cell Biol*. Vol. 7 No. 2 pp. 165-171 ISSN 1465-7392

Liu, Q., Guntuku, S., Cui, X.S., Matsuoka, S., Cortez, D., Tamai, K., Luo, G., Carattini-Rivera, S., DeMayo, F., Bradley, A., Donehower, L.A. and Elledge, S.J. (2000). Chk1 is an essential kinase that is regulated by Atr and required for the G(2)/M DNA damage checkpoint. *Genes Dev*. Vol. 14 No. 12 pp. 1448-1459 ISSN 0890-9369

Luo, Q., Yang, J., Zeng, Q. L., Zhu, X. M., Qian, Y. L. &Huang, H. F.(2006). 50-Hertz electromagnetic fields induce gammaH2AX foci formation in mouse preimplantation embryos in vitro. *Biol Reprod* Vol. 75 No.5 pp. 673-80 ISSN 0006-3363

Marnett, L.J. (2000). Oxyradicals and DNA damage. *Carcinogenesis*. Vol. 21 No. 3 pp. 361-370 0143-3334

Martin, G.R. (1981). Isolation of a pluripotent cell line from early mouse embryos cultured in medium conditioned by teratocarcinoma stem cells. *Proc Natl Acad Sci U S A*. Vol. 78 No. 12 pp. 7634-7638 ISSN 0027-8424

Maynard, S., Swistowska, A.M., Lee, J.W., Liu, Y., Liu, S.T., Da Cruz, A.B., Rao, M., de Souza-Pinto, N.C., Zeng, X. and Bohr, V.A. (2008). Human embryonic stem cells have enhanced repair of multiple forms of DNA damage. *Stem Cells*. Vol. 26 No. 9 pp. 2266-2274 ISSN 1549-4918

Mayshar, Y., Ben-David, U., Lavon, N., Biancotti, J.C., Yakir, B., Clark, A.T., Plath, K., Lowry, W.E. and Benvenisty, N. (2010). Identification and classification of chromosomal aberrations in human induced pluripotent stem cells. *Cell Stem Cell*. Vol. 7 No. 4 pp. 521-531 ISSN 1875-9777

Moallem, S.A. and Hales, B.F. (1998). The role of p53 and cell death by apoptosis and necrosis in 4-hydroperoxycyclophosphamide-induced limb malformations. *Development*. Vol. 125 No. 16 pp. 3225-3234 ISSN 0950-1991

Moller, P. (2006). The alkaline comet assay: towards validation in biomonitoring of DNA damaging exposures. *Basic Clin Pharmacol Toxicol*. Vol. 98 No. 4 pp. 336-345 ISSN 1742-7835

Moller, P., Moller, L., Godschalk, R.W. and Jones, G.D. (2010). Assessment and reduction of comet assay variation in relation to DNA damage: studies from the European Comet Assay Validation Group. *Mutagenesis*. Vol. 25 No. 2 pp. 109-111 ISSN 1464-3804

Momcilovic, O., Knobloch, L., Fornsaglio, J., Varum, S., Easley, C. and Schatten, G. (2010). DNA damage responses in human induced pluripotent stem cells and embryonic stem cells. *PLoS One*. Vol. 5 No. 10 pp. e13410 ISSN 1932-6203

Nicol, C.J., Harrison, M.L., Laposa, R.R., Gimelshtein, I.L. and Wells, P.G. (1995). A teratologic suppressor role for p53 in benzo[a]pyrene-treated transgenic p53-deficient mice. *Nat Genet*. Vol. 10 No. 2 pp. 181-187 ISSN 1061-4036

Norimura, T., Nomoto, S., Katsuki, M., Gondo, Y. and Kondo, S. (1996). p53-dependent apoptosis suppresses radiation-induced teratogenesis. *Nat Med*. Vol. 2 No. 5 pp. 577-580 ISSN 1078-8956

Orford, K.W. and Scadden, D.T. (2008). Deconstructing stem cell self-renewal: genetic insights into cell-cycle regulation. *Nat Rev Genet.* Vol. 9 No. 2 pp. 115-128 ISSN 1471-0064

Pachkowski, B. F., Guyton, K. Z. &Sonawane, B.(DNA repair during in utero development: a review of the current state of knowledge, research needs, and potential application in risk assessment. *Mutat Res* Vol. 728 No.1-2 pp. 35-46 ISSN 0027-5107

Pasi, C.E., Dereli-Oz, A., Negrini, S., Friedli, M., Fragola, G., Lombardo, A., Van Houwe, G., Naldini, L., Casola, S., Testa, G., Trono, D., Pelicci, P.G. and Halazonetis, T.D. (2011). Genomic instability in induced stem cells. *Cell Death Differ.* Vol. 18 No. 5 pp. 745-753 ISSN 1476-5403

Pekar, O., Molotski, N., Savion, S., Fein, A., Toder, V. and Torchinsky, A. (2007). p53 regulates cyclophosphamide teratogenesis by controlling caspases 3, 8, 9 activation and NF-kappaB DNA binding. *Reproduction.* Vol. 134 No. 2 pp. 379-388 ISSN 1470-1626

Potten, C.S., Owen, G. and Booth, D. (2002). Intestinal stem cells protect their genome by selective segregation of template DNA strands. *J Cell Sci.* Vol. 115 No. Pt 11 pp. 2381-2388 ISSN 0021-9533

Powers, D.E., Millman, J.R., Huang, R.B. and Colton, C.K. (2008). Effects of oxygen on mouse embryonic stem cell growth, phenotype retention, and cellular energetics. *Biotechnol Bioeng.* Vol. 101 No. 2 pp. 241-254 1097-0290

Prost, S., Bellamy, C.O., Clarke, A.R., Wyllie, A.H. and Harrison, D.J. (1998). p53-independent DNA repair and cell cycle arrest in embryonic stem cells. *FEBS Lett.* Vol. 425 No. 3 pp. 499-504 ISSN 0014-5793

Qin, H., Yu, T., Qing, T., Liu, Y., Zhao, Y., Cai, J., Li, J., Song, Z., Qu, X., Zhou, P., Wu, J., Ding, M. and Deng, H. (2007). Regulation of apoptosis and differentiation by p53 in human embryonic stem cells. *J Biol Chem.* Vol. 282 No. 8 pp. 5842-5852 ISSN 0021-9258

Rando, T.A. (2007). The immortal strand hypothesis: segregation and reconstruction. *Cell.* Vol. 129 No. 7 pp. 1239-1243 ISSN 0092-8674

Roos, W.P., Christmann, M., Fraser, S.T. and Kaina, B. (2007). Mouse embryonic stem cells are hypersensitive to apoptosis triggered by the DNA damage O(6)-methylguanine due to high E2F1 regulated mismatch repair. *Cell Death Differ.* Vol. 14 No. 8 pp. 1422-1432 ISSN 1350-9047

Sabapathy, K., Klemm, M., Jaenisch, R. and Wagner, E.F. (1997). Regulation of ES cell differentiation by functional and conformational modulation of p53. *EMBO J.* Vol. 16 No. 20 pp. 6217-6229 ISSN 0261-4189

Sah, V.P., Attardi, L.D., Mulligan, G.J., Williams, B.O., Bronson, R.T. and Jacks, T. (1995). A subset of p53-deficient embryos exhibit exencephaly. *Nat Genet.* Vol. 10 No. 2 pp. 175-180 ISSN 1061-4036

Sarig, R. and Rotter, V. (2011). Can an iPS cell secure its genomic fidelity? *Cell Death Differ.* Vol. 18 No. 5 pp. 743-744 ISSN 1476-5403

Savatier, P., Lapillonne, H., van Grunsven, L.A., Rudkin, B.B. and Samarut, J. (1996). Withdrawal of differentiation inhibitory activity/leukemia inhibitory factor up-regulates D-type cyclins and cyclin-dependent kinase inhibitors in mouse embryonic stem cells. *Oncogene.* Vol. 12 No. 2 pp. 309-322 ISSN 0950-9232

Singh, N.P., McCoy, M.T., Tice, R.R. and Schneider, E.L. (1988). A simple technique for quantitation of low levels of DNA damage in individual cells. *Exp Cell Res.* Vol. 175 No. 1 pp. 184-191 ISSN 0014-4827

Smith, C.C., O'Donovan, M.R. and Martin, E.A. (2006). hOGG1 recognizes oxidative damage using the comet assay with greater specificity than FPG or ENDOIII. *Mutagenesis*. Vol. 21 No. 3 pp. 185-190 ISSN 0267-8357

Sokolov, M.V., Panyutin, I.V., Panyutin, I.G. and Neumann, R.D. (2011). Dynamics of the transcriptome response of cultured human embryonic stem cells to ionizing radiation exposure. *Mutat Res*. Vol. 709-710 No. pp. 40-48 ISSN 0027-5107

Solozobova, V. and Blattner, C. (2010). Regulation of p53 in embryonic stem cells. *Exp Cell Res*. Vol. 316 No. 15 pp. 2434-2446 ISSN 1090-2422

Solozobova, V., Rolletschek, A. and Blattner, C. (2009). Nuclear accumulation and activation of p53 in embryonic stem cells after DNA damage. *BMC Cell Biol*. Vol. 10 No. pp. 46 ISSN 1471-2121

Stambrook, P.J. (2007). An ageing question: do embryonic stem cells protect their genomes? *Mech Ageing Dev*. Vol. 128 No. 1 pp. 31-35 ISSN 0047-6374

Thomson, J.A., Itskovitz-Eldor, J., Shapiro, S.S., Waknitz, M.A., Swiergiel, J.J., Marshall, V.S. and Jones, J.M. (1998). Embryonic stem cell lines derived from human blastocysts. *Science*. Vol. 282 No. 5391 pp. 1145-1147 ISSN 0036-8075

Tichy, E.D., Liang, L., Deng, L., Tischfield, J., Schwemberger, S., Babcock, G. and Stambrook, P.J. (2011). Mismatch and base excision repair proficiency in murine embryonic stem cells. *DNA Repair (Amst)*. Vol. 10 No. 4 pp. 445-451 ISSN 1568-7856

Torchinsky, A. and Toder, V. (2010). Mechanisms of the embryo's response to embryopathic stressors: a focus on p53. *J Reprod Immunol*. Vol. 85 No. 1 pp. 76-80 ISSN 1872-7603

Tsuda, S., Kosaka, Y., Matsusaka, N. and Sasaki, Y.F. (1998). Detection of pyrimethamine-induced DNA damage in mouse embryo and maternal organs by the modified alkaline single cell gel electrophoresis assay. *Mutat Res*. Vol. 415 No. 1-2 pp. 69-77 ISSN 0027-5107

van der Wees, C., Jansen, J., Vrieling, H., van der Laarse, A., Van Zeeland, A. and Mullenders, L. (2007). Nucleotide excision repair in differentiated cells. *Mutat Res*. Vol. 614 No. 1-2 pp. 16-23 ISSN 0027-5107

Van Sloun, P.P., Jansen, J.G., Weeda, G., Mullenders, L.H., van Zeeland, A.A., Lohman, P.H. and Vrieling, H. (1999). The role of nucleotide excision repair in protecting embryonic stem cells from genotoxic effects of UV-induced DNA damage. *Nucleic Acids Res*. Vol. 27 No. 16 pp. 3276-3282 ISSN 1362-4962

Wang, Y. and Blelloch, R. (2009). Cell cycle regulation by MicroRNAs in embryonic stem cells. *Cancer Res*. Vol. 69 No. 10 pp. 4093-4096 ISSN 1538-7445

Wells, P.G., McCallum, G.P., Lam, K.C., Henderson, J.T. and Ondovcik, S.L. (2010). Oxidative DNA damage and repair in teratogenesis and neurodevelopmental deficits. *Birth Defects Res C Embryo Today*. Vol. 90 No. 2 pp. 103-109 ISSN 1542-9768

Yukawa, M., Oda, S., Mitani, H., Nagata, M. and Aoki, F. (2007). Deficiency in the response to DNA double-strand breaks in mouse early preimplantation embryos. *Biochem Biophys Res Commun*. Vol. 358 No. 2 pp. 578-584 ISSN 0006-291X

Zhao, T. and Xu, Y. (2010). p53 and stem cells: new developments and new concerns. *Trends Cell Biol*. Vol. 20 No. 3 pp. 170-175 ISSN 1879-3088

16

Bamboo Regeneration via Embryogenesis and Organogenesis

Xinchun Lin[1], Lichun Huang[2] and Wei Fang[1]
[1]*The Nurturing Station for the State Key Laboratory of Subtropical Silviculture, Zhejiang Agriculture and Forestry University, Zhejiang,*
[2]*Institute of Plant and Microbial Biology, Academia Sinica, Taibei, Taiwan, China*

1. Introduction

Bamboo is a member of grass family (Poaceae: Bambusoideae) (Wu & Raven, 2006). With the characteristics of short rotation, marketability of culms every year and immediate returns, bamboos are the fast growing multipurpose plants of high economic and environmental value that converts solar radiation into useful goods and services better than most tree species (Franklin, 2006; Kassahun, 2000). Besides producing fresh edible shoots and culms for timber, furniture and handicraft or as a raw material for pulping, bamboo serves as an efficient agent for conservation of water and soil (Christanty et al., 1996, 1997; Kassahun, 2003; Kleinhenz & Midmore, 2001; Mailly et al., 1997). Additionally, new products such as bamboo charcoal, bamboo vinegar, bamboo juice, bamboo healthy food, bamboo fiber product have been developed. World-wide interest in bamboo as a source of biofuel or bioenergy has also increased rapidly in recent years (Fu, 2001; Scurlock, 2000).

There are about 88 genera and 1400 recorded species of bamboo in the world, 34 genera and 534 species of which are in China (Wu & Raven, 2006). Bamboo is found in an area of more than 14 million ha throughout the tropics, subtropics and temperate zones of the world. Eighty percent of the species and area are confined to South and Southeast Asia, and largely in China, India, and Myanmar. China, with the richest resources and largest bamboo industry worldwide, possesses 5 million ha of bamboo forests (Bystriakova et al., 2003; McNeely, 1999).

Because bamboos flowering is unpredictable and has a long interval, the manipulation of bamboo crossbreeding is difficult (Lin et al, 2010a, 2010b; Lu et al., 2009). Gene transformation is another efficient approach to increase productivity and quality in plants. However, there have been no successful reports on bamboo gene transformation till now, because a stable and efficient regeneration system, the prerequisite to bamboo gene transformation, is still not completely established yet (Huang et al., 1989; Zhang et al., 2010; Zuo & Liu, 2004).

2. Process of bamboo regeneration and influencing factor

2.1 Regeneration process

Shoot, seeds, mature zygotic embryo, immature embryo, anther and inflorescence (Figure 1) can be used as explants of bamboo regeneration (Huang & Murashige, 1983; Pei et al.,

2011; Saxena & Dhawan, 1999; Zhang et al., 2010). After inoculation, calli are induced in the medium with a high concentration of 2,4-dichlorophenoxyacetic acid (2,4-D) usually. The quantity and quality of calli differ significantly between different concentration of 2,4-D in the medium. Three kinds of calli are often observed after treated by 2,4-D: (1) Yellowish, granular, and compact calli, with good potential regeneration ability (Fig.2a); (2) Pale-yellow, translucent, watery, and sticky calli, unable to regenerate generally (Fig.2b); (3) Creamy-yellow, compact, and non-embryogenic calli (Fig.2c), unable to regenerate. The yellowish, granular, and compact calli will proliferate after treatment in the callus growth maintenance medium with no or lower levels of 2,4-D compared with callus initiation medium. Then the calli will develop into adventitious shoots, embryo or adventitious roots, after subjected to the differentiated medium, and the callus with adventitious roots (Fig.2d) will not usually continue to differentiate. The destiny of calli is determined by different kinds of plant growth regulators (PGRs) such as 2-isopentenyladenine (2iP), thidiazuron (TDZ), zeatin (ZT), 6-benzyladenine (BA), kinetin (KT), naphthaleneacetic acid (NAA), and indole-3-butyricacid (IBA), etc., and high cytokinin/low auxin will result in adventitious shoot formation. Embryoids have radicles (Fig.2e-g), while adventitious shoot need to root before transplantation. Some shoots will produce roots naturally without any treatment, but others need to be treated with high auxin and minimal or no cytokinin during root development (Fig.2h-i). After rooting, the plantlet can be transferred to potting soil in the greenhouse (Fig.2j). (Huang et al., 1989; Yeh & Chang, 1986a, 1986b, 1987; Zhang et al., 2010).

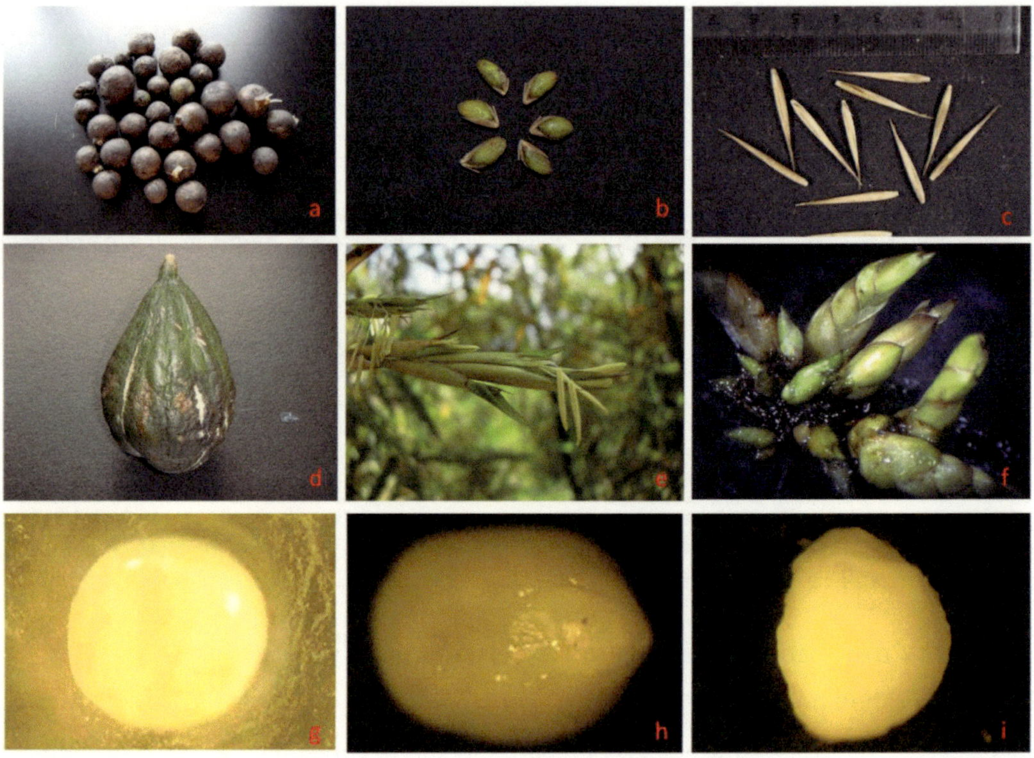

Fig. 1. Explants of bamboos.

a) Seeds of *Melocalamus compactiflorus*; b) Seeds of *Qiongzhurea tumidinoda*; c) Seeds of *Phyllostachys edulis*; d) The seed of *Melocanna baccifera*; e) The inflorescence of *Phyllostachys violascens*; f) Flower buds proliferation of *Bambusa oldhamii*; g) The globular embryo of *Phyllostachys violascens*; h) The cotyledon embryo of *Phyllostachys violascens*; i) The mature embryo of *Dendrocalamus hamiltonii*.

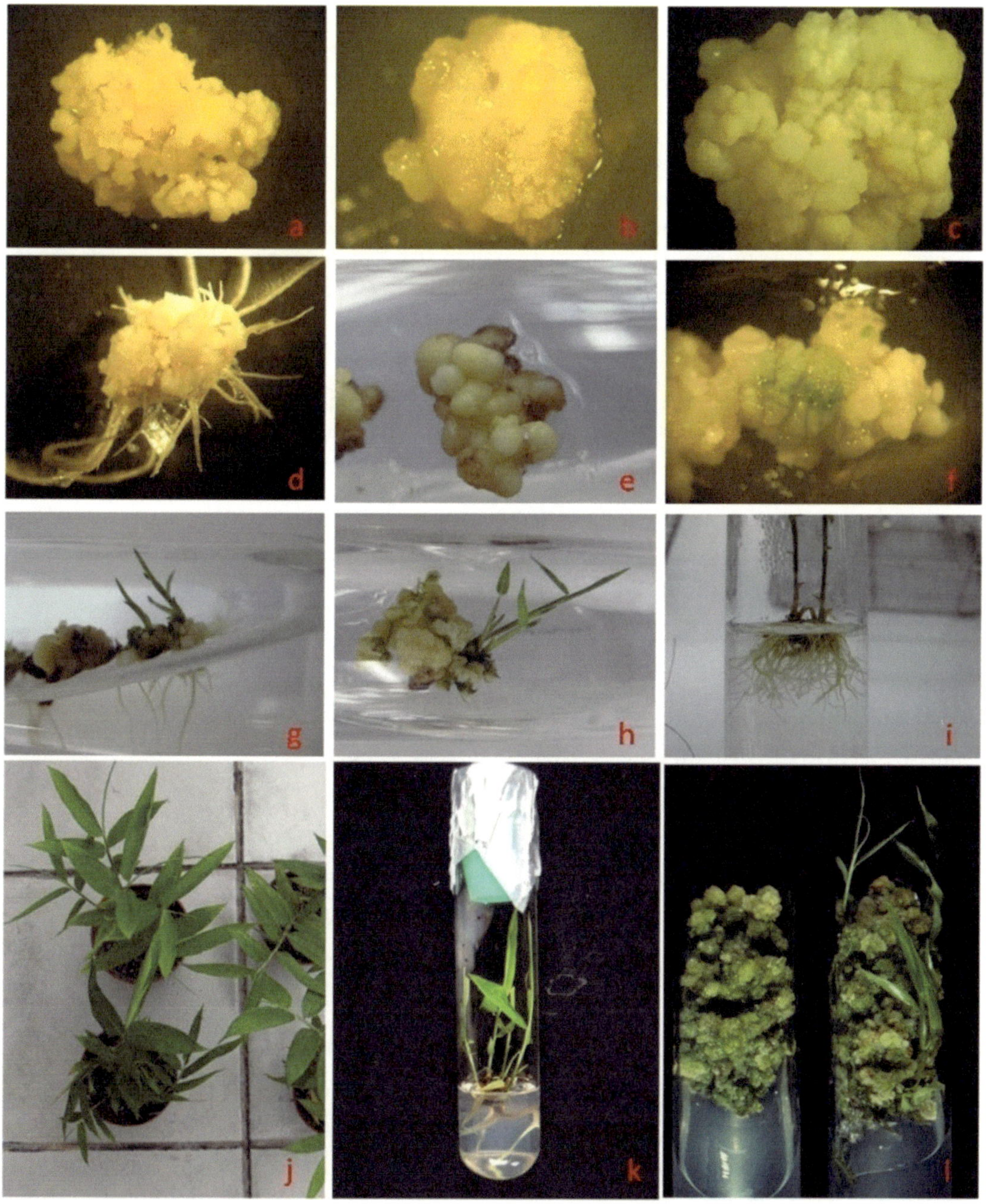

Fig. 2. The somatic embryogenesis and organogenesis of Bamboos.

a-c) Three kinds of calli of *Dendrocalamus hamiltonii;* d) Adventitious roots differentiation of *Dendrocalamus hamiltonii;* e-g) Embryogenesis of *Dendrocalamus hamiltonii;* h-i) Organogenesis of *Dendrocalamus hamiltonii;* j) Transplanted plantlets of *Dendrocalamus hamiltonii;* k) Organogenesis of *Bambusa oldhamii;* l) Organogenesis of *Phyllostachys aurea.*

2.2 Regeneration type

Bamboo can regenerate via embryogenesis and organogenesis (Fig.2e-k), and the frequency of embryogenesis is lower than that of organogenesis (Ramanayake & Wanniarachchi, 2003; Woods et al., 1992; Zhang et al., 2010).

During the bamboo embryogenesis, the embryoids initiate and develop from somatic cells. Compared with organogenesis, somatic embryogenesis is characterized by the formation of a bipolar structure, which will develop into plumule and radicle (Fig.2e-g). Histological analysis reveals that embryogenic cells are small in size, isodiametric with dense cytoplasm, generally locate along the periphery of calli, distribute in clusters, and intersperse with large parenchymal cells. Somatic embryos gradually developed from the granular onsite to heart-shaped, torpedo-shaped, and final cotyledons (Zhang et al., 2010).

In contrasted to the embryogenesis, organogenesis occurs via apparent shoot meristem or leaf primordial (Fig.2h-i). Histological analysis shows that non-embryogenic cells are large, and vacuolated parenchymal cells contain few plastids (Zhang et al., 2010). Callus will differentiate into adventitious shoots, and develop with subsequent formation of adventitious roots.

2.3 Factors affecting regeneration

The bamboo embryogenesis and organogenesis will be affected by many factors such as bamboo species (including cultivars, genotypes and ecotypes), type and age of explants, type of basal media, type and concentration of plant growth regulators, etc. (Godbole et al., 2002; Hassan & Debergh, 1987). Serious browning and difficult differentiation are popular in bamboo regeneration experiments (Huang & Murashige, 1983).

3. Innovative approaches about bamboo regeneration

To establish a stable and efficient regeneration system of bamboo, some efficient measures are proposed as follows:

3.1 Screening of bamboo species

About 20 bamboo species are used for regeneration system establishment in our lab, and we find that the bamboo regeneration ability differs significantly in different kinds of bamboo species, and the sympodial bamboo is easier to regenerate than monopodial bamboo. There are about 1400 kinds of bamboo species in the world, the successful reports about bamboo regeneration mainly focus on the species of *Bambusa* and *Dendrocalamus* (*Sinocalamus* is the anonymus of *Dendrocalamus*), so we can select the bamboo species which are easy to regenerate for overcoming the obstacle of bamboo gene transformation at first.

In addition to the difference among different kinds of species, genotype has distinct influence on the efficiency of plant regeneration via organogenesis or embryogenesis of various plant species such as soybean (*Glycine max*), rapeseed (*Brassica napus*), rice (*Oryza sativa*), etc. (Akasaka-Kennedy et al., 2005; Bailey et al., 1993; Hoque & Mansfield, 2004). Screening of bamboo genotypes or cultivars with strong regeneration ability may be a good choose for setting up an efficient system for bamboo gene transformation.

3.2 Selection of explants

Mature embryos, immature embryos, shoot tips, leaves, young inflorescences, hypocotyls, flower stalks, cotyledons, anthers and nodal segments are the common explants in plant regeneration. Most of those explants (Fig.1) are also efficient during the bamboo regeneration experiments (Lin et al, 2003, 2004; Rout & Das, 1994; Yuan et al., 2009). Within a species, the age of explants is important, loss of competence is correlated with maturation extent of explants, i.e. extent of differentiation, developmentally immature organs (or less differentiated cells) are most likely to contain morphogenetically competent cells. The regeneration ability of mature embryos, immature embryos, shoot tips and flower buds as explants of bamboo regeneration are tested in our lab. We find that the induction and differentiation of shoot tips of young bamboo seedling are easier than those of adult bamboo plants, and embryos, especially for immature embryos, are more efficient than other kinds of explants. Using the immature embryos (Fig.1g-h) as the explants, we have succeeded in setting up a regeneration system of *Phyllostachys violascens*, a species of monopodial bamboo (Pei et al., 2011). However, the materials related to bamboo flowers and seeds such as embryos, inflorescences and anthers are difficult to get for bamboo seldom flowering, shoots which are easier to obtain would be a better choice as the explants.

3.3 Selection of media

The components of media are also important during bamboo callus induction, callus growth maintenance, shoot differentiation, and root development. MS, NB(including N6's macrosalts, B5's microsalts and organic compounds), N6, HB and B5 basal media have been used in bamboo regeneration, and MS basal medium is the most common (Rao et al., 1985; Sun et al., 1999; Tsay et al., 1990; Wu & Chen, 1987; Zhang et al., 2010).

Different kinds of plant growth regulators are needed in different stage of bamboo regeneration, and auxin and cytokinin are the critical components for the morphogenesis in vitro. Besides, ethylene, abscisic acid (ABA) and brassinosteroid (BR) will also have different effects on embryogenesis and organogenesis (Aydin et al., 2006; Torrizo & Zapata, 1986; Vain et al., 1989).

3.4 Complementary approaches for advancing regeneration ability

3.4.1 *NiR* gene

Nitrate assimilation is an important process in rice regeneration. A quantitative trait loci gene encoding the ferrodoxin-nitrite reductase (*NiR*), an enzyme that catalyzes the reduction of nitrite to ammonium leading to the accumulation of toxic nitrite in culture media, was isolated from the high-regeneration rice strain Kasalath. The level of *NiR* expression in the

Koshihikari, a notorious poor rice line for genetic transformation, may result in lower enzymatic activity, and the enzymatic activity is correlated with the regeneration ability. With the introduction of Kasalath *NiR* gene encoding high enzymatic activity, the regeneration ability of low-regeneration rice strain Koshihikari had been improved (Nishimura et al., 2005). The *NiR* gene cloned from the high-regeneration rice strain Konansou has the similar function with that of Kasalath (Ozawa & Kawahigashi, 2006). However, *NiR* gene based improvement method will be suitable for the major Japonica rice varieties but not Indica rice varieties for having high *NiR* activity (Nishimura et al., 2006). In addition, the *NiR* gene can be used as a selection marker for rice gene transformation (Nishimura et al., 2005; Ozawa & Kawahigashi, 2006). The *NiR* gene isolated from the high–regeneration rice line may be useful in promoting the regeneration capacity during bamboo regeneration and gene transformation.

3.4.2 *ipt* gene

Cytokinins play a vital role in the differentiation process of plants. The isopentenyl transferase (*ipt*) gene, isolated from *Agrobacterium tumefaciens*, encodes for isopentenyltransferase which catalyzes the condensation of adenosine - 5′ - monophosphate and isopentenylpyrophosphate to isopentenyladenosine - 5′ - monophosphate (Akiyoshi et al. 1984). Integrating with the *ipt* gene, a cytokinin biosynthetic gene, the transformed cells present higher concentrations of endogenous cytokinins, and lead to higher frequencies of differentiation and transformation than untransformed control cells (Endo et al., 2002; Lopez-Noguera et al., 2009; Smigocki & Owens, 1988). Overexpression of *ipt* gene driven by a strong constitutive promoter favors plant regeneration, and the transformed plants exhibit abnormal morphogenetic variations such as an increased rate of branching, shorter stem internodes and little or no root formation. These morphogenetic changes can be used as selective markers during gene transformation, but these changes, especially for rooting difficultly, also disturb the normal development of transformed plants (Endo et al., 2001; Molinier et al., 2002; Smigocki & Owens, 1988). These defects derived from overexpression of *ipt* gene can be amended by gene deletor technology to delete the exogenous *ipt* gene. (Luo et al., 2007, 2008). It may be a good choose integrating those genes advancing regeneration frequency such as the *ipt* gene with objective genes during bamboo gene transformation.

In addition to *ipt* gene, a number of genes involved in hormone signal transduction have been indentified to influence the regenerative competence of plant cells for somatic embryogenesis and/or adventitious shoot formation (Sakamoto et al., 2006; Srinivasan et al., 2007, 2011).

*KNOX1*genes regulate the shoot apical meristem differentiation, and upregulate cytokinin biosynthesis and decrease gibberellin accumulation in plants, ectopic expression of *KNOX1* genes induces adventitious shoot regeneration in vitro-cultured explants (Sakamoto et al., 2006; Srinivasan et al., 2011).

Heterologous expression of the *BABY BOOM* (*BBM*) AP2/ERF transcription factor enhances the competence of tissues to undergo organogenesis and somatic embryogenesis (Srinivasan et al., 2007).

Identification and application of those genes regulating plant development and regeneration may lead to new approaches for plant regeneration in vitro.

3.4.3 Chemical additives

Many chemical additives including osmoticums, antioxidants, ethylene inhibitors, etc. have the good effects on plant regeneration, and may be used for increasing the efficiency of bamboo regeneration.

Osmotic pressure is correlated with plant development and differentiation, appropriate treatment by the common osmoticums such as sucrose, mannitol and polyethylene glycol (PEG) enhances the embryogenesis and organogenesis in *Solanum melongena* (Mukherjee et al.,1991), *Brassica napus* (Ferrie & Keller, 2007) and white spruce (*Picea glauca*) (Misra et al., 1993).

Tissue browning is the major problem of bamboo regeneration. Oxidized phenolic compounds produced from the damaged explants will suppress enzyme activity, darken the culture medium, and lead to the death of the explants. Treated with antioxidants and absorbents such as cysteine and ascorbic acid, polyvinylpyrrolidone (PVP) and activated carbon, will alleviate the phenolic oxidation and favor the plant regeneration (Abdelwahd et al., 2008; Sanyal et al., 2005; Toth et al., 1994).

Ethylene plays an important role in plant morphogenesis, and has a negative effect on plant regeneration, ethylene inhibitors such as AgNO3 and AVG promote the callus initiation and plant regeneration in cabbage, tobacco, maize and wheat accordingly. The silver ion is reported to be an inhibitor of ethylene action by competitively binding to ethylene receptors which are located predominantly at the intracellular membrane, while AVG inhibits ethylene biosynthesis directly (Vain et al., 1989; Zhang et al., 1998). In addition to silver ion, other heavy metals including Cu and other ethylene inhibitors (Co and Ni), also significantly facilitate the regeneration and somatic embryogenesis (Purnhauser & Gyulai, 1993; Roustan et al. 1989).

3.4.4 Partial desiccation

Partial desiccation has been reported to accelerate plant organogenesis or embryogenesis and results in high regeneration ability significantly in grape (Gray, 1989), wheat (Cheng et al., 2003), *Brassica napus* (Kott & Beversdorf, 1990), rice (Rance et al., 1994; Saharan et al., 2004; Tsukahara & Hirosawa, 1992) and cassava (Mathews et al., 1993). The possible mechanism about its promotion on plant regeneration capacity may be that partial desiccation terminates the developmental mode and "switches" the embryo into a germination mode (Attree et al., 1991). Partial desiccation not only enhances the plant regeneration efficiency, but also benefits the plant organogenesis or embryogenesis and subsequent differentiated stage, and thus reduces the whole time in plant tissue culture (Rance et al., 1994). In addition to the positive effect on wheat organogenesis or embryogenesis, partial desiccation during co-culture greatly enhances the transformation efficiency through inhibiting the growth of Agrobacterium which will suppress the recovery of wheat tissue, and favoring the transfer DNA (T-DNA) delivery (Cheng et al., 2003). Partial desiccation may be also beneficial in bamboo differentiation.

4. Somaclonal variation

Somaclonal variation is the common phenomenon during plant tissue culture. Being high efficient, time-saving and low cost, somaclonal variation has become a useful tool to creating new germplasms with beneficial economic traits of the breeding process in rice, potato, maize, barley and sugar cane, etc. (Karp et al., 1995; Larkin & Scowcroft, 1981). Somaclonal variation, such as mosaic leaf, albino, etiolated shoots, polyploidization and early flowering in vitro etc., also occurs during bamboo embryogenesis and organogenesis (Fig.3), and the frequency of variation will increase after continuous subculture. Most of those bamboo variants can grow normally, but is generally difficult in root formation (Zhang et al., 2010). Compared with poplar and other economic tree species, the process of bamboo breeding is slower for its peculiar flowering characteristics, screening of somaclonal variants with stable and valuable traits may be an alternative choose for bamboo improvement.

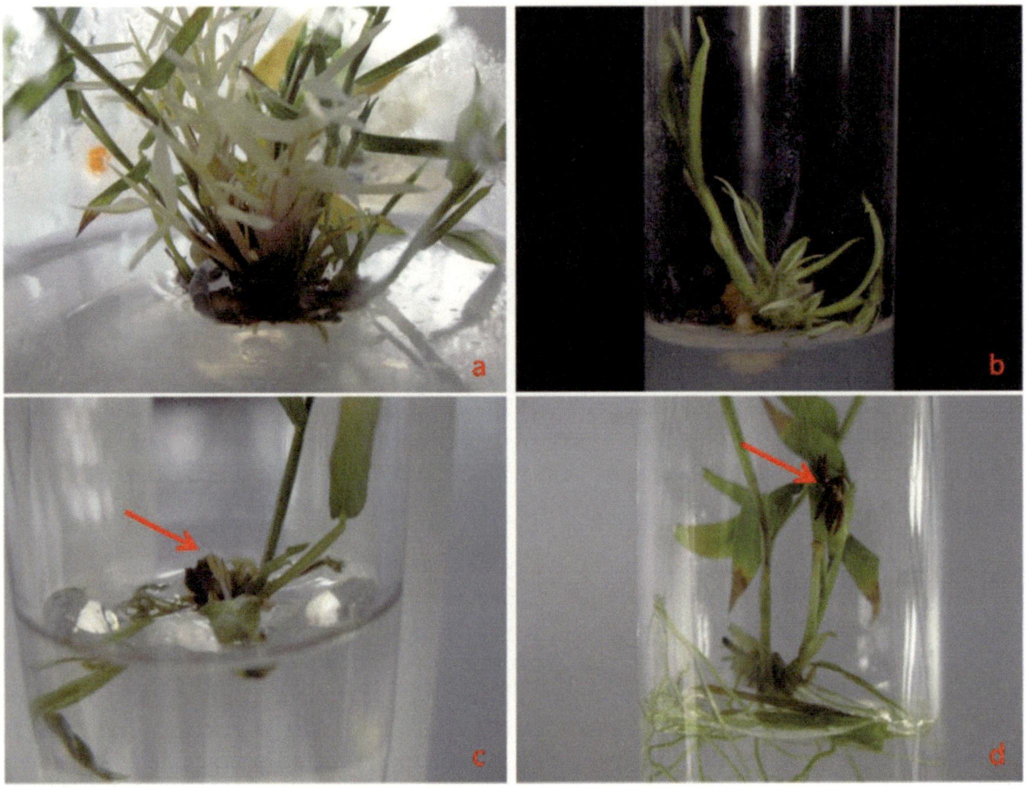

Fig. 3. Somaclonal variation during regeneration of *Dendrocalamus hamiltonii.*

a) Albino plantlets; b) The plantlet with mosaic leaf; c-d) Plantlets flowering in vitro, as indicated with red arrows.

5. Genetic transformation

Using the regeneration system of *Dendrocalamus hamiltonii* of our lab, we tried to establish a bamboo genetic transformation system. After pre-culture for 4 days, good calli were infected by Agrobacterium strains *EHA105* habouring the *pCAMBIA 1301* vector. After co-culture, for 3 days, the calli were transferred to the recovery medium for 8 days, then the calli were transferred to the selection medium with hygromycin selection. The resistant calli produced and then differentiate shoots and plantlets. To determine the genetic transformation frequency, 10 resistant plantlets were examined by PCR, and all of them are positive, which shows that *Hygromycin B phosphotransferase* (*HPT*) gene of *pCAMBIA 1301* was successfully integrated into the genome of *Dendrocalamus hamiltonii* via agrobacterium, the result was further verified through sequencing the PCR products.

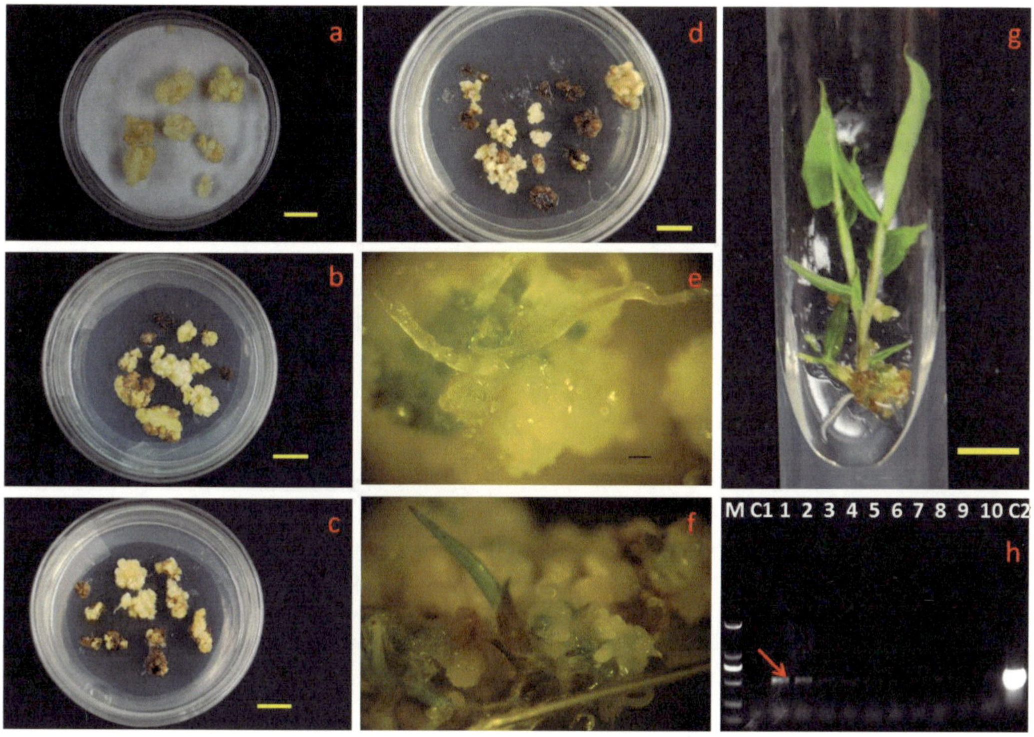

Fig. 4. The genetic transformation and PCR detection of *Dendrocalamus hamiltonii*.

a) Co-culture; b) First selection culture; c) Second selection culture; d) Third selection culture; e-f) Resistant calli differentiate shoots; g) Resistant plantlet; h) PCR detection of plantlets. M: marker; C1: Untransferred plantlet; 1-10: Resistant plantlets; C2: Positive control. Obiective bands were indicated with red arrows.6. Conclusions and prospects

6. Conclusions and prospects

Gene transformation has been proved to be efficient in plant breeding (Nishimura et al., 2006; Varshney et al., 2007). Being one of the most challenging aspects of the gene transformation protocol, a stable and efficient regeneration system must be developed. Lack of a well established regeneration system is the main obstacle for bamboo gene transformation. Understanding bamboo regeneration process and adopting innovative approaches about it will help to enhance the regeneration ability of bamboos and make breakthrough in bamboo gene transformation. The application of gene transformation will open up a new field for bamboo breeding.

Although we have succeeded in establishing a genetic transformation for *Dendrocalamus hamiltonii* at the first time, there are still many problems during the bamboo genetic transformation process such as serious browning, low differentiate frequency, etc (Zuo & Liu, 2004). More effort is needed to establish a stable and efficient genetic transformation system about bamboos.

7. Acknowledgements

This study is supported by research grants from the Natural Science Foundation of Zhejiang Province [Grant No. Z3100366] and the Ministry of Science and Technology of China (Grant No. 2012CB723008).

8. References

Akasaka-Kennedy, Y., Yoshida, H. & Takahata, Y. (2005). Efficient plant regeneration from leaves of rapeseed (*Brassica napus* L.): the influence of AgNO3 and genotype. Plant Cell Reports, 24: 649-654

Akiyoshi, D.E., Klee, H., Amasino, R.M., Nester, E.W. & Gordon, M.P. (1984). T-DNA of *Agrobacterium tumefaciens* encodes an enzyme of cytokinin biosynthesis. Proceedings of the National Academy of Science USA, 81:5994–5998

Attree, S.M., Moore, D., Sawhney, V.K. & Fowke, L.C. (1991). Enhanced maturation and desiccation tolerance of white spruce [*Picea glauca* (Moench.) Voss] somatic embryos: Effects of a non-plasmolysing water stress and abscisic acid. Annals of Botany, 68: 519-525

Aydin, Y., Talas-Ogras, T., Ipekçi-Altas, Z. & Gözükirmizi, N. (2006). Effects of brassinosteroid on cotton regeneration via somatic embryogenesis. Biologia, 61(3): 289-293

Bailey, M.A., Boerma H.R. & Parrot D.W.A. (1993). Genotype effects on proliferative embryogenesis and plant regeneration of soybean. In Vitro Cellular & Developmental Biology - Plant, 29(3): 102-108

Bystriakova, N., Kapos, V., Lysenko, I. & Stapleton, C.M.A. (2003). Distribution and conservation status of forest bamboo biodiversity in the Asia-Pacific Region. Biodiversity and Conservation, 12: 1833–1841

Cheng, M., Hu, T., Layton, J., Liu, C.N. & Fry, J. E. (2003). Desiccation of plant tissues post-Agrobacterium infection enhances T-DNA delivery and increases stable transformation efficiency in wheat. In Vitro Cellular & Developmental Biology-Plant, 39: 595–604

Christanty, L., Mailly, D. & Kimmins, J. P. (1996). "Without bamboo, the land dies": Biomass, litterfall, and soil organic matter dynamics of a Javanese bamboo talun-kebun system. Forest Ecology and Management, 87: 75-88.

Christanty, L., Kimmins, J. P. & Mailly, D. (1997). "Without bamboo, the land dies": A conceptual model of the biogeochemical role of bamboo in an Indonesian agroforestry system. Forest Ecology and Management, 91: 83-91.

Endo, S., Kasahara, T., Sugita, K., Matsunaga, E. & Ebinuma, H. (2001). The isopentenl-transferase gene is effective as a selectable marker gene for plant transformation in tobacco (*Nicotiana tabacum* cv. Petite Havana SRI). Plant Cell Reports, 20(1): 60-66

Endo, S., Kasahara, T., Sugita, K. & Ebinuma, H. (2002). A new GST-MAT vector containing both *ipt* and *iaaM/H* genes can produce marker-free transgenic tobacco plants with high frequency. Plant Cell Reports, 20(10): 923-928

Ferrie, A. M. R. & Keller, W. A. (2007). Optimization of methods for using polyethylene glycol as a non-permeating osmoticum for the induction of microspore embryogenesis in the Brassicaceae. In Vitro Cellular & Developmental Biology-Plant, 43: 348–355

Franklin, D.C. (2006). Wild bamboo stands fail to compensate for a heavy 1-year harvest of culm shoots. Forest Ecology and Management, 237:115-118

Fu, J. (2001). Bamboo Juice, Beer and Medicine. The Magazine of The American Bamboo Society, 22(5): 16

Godbole, S., Sood, A., Thakur, R., Sharma, M. & Ahuja, P.S. (2002). Somatic embryogenesis and its conversion into plantlets in a multipurpose bamboo, *Dendrocalamus hamiltonii* Nees et Arn. Ex Munro. Current Science, 83: 885-889

Gray, D.J. (1989). Effects of dehydration and exogenous growth regulators on dormancy, quiescence and germination of grape somatic embryos. In Vitro Cellular & Developmental Biology-Plant, 25: 1173-1178

Hassan, A.E. & Debergh, P. (1987). Embryogenesis and plantlet development in the bamboo *Phyllostachys viridis* (Young) McClure. Plant cell Tissue and Organ Culture, 10: 73-77

Hoque, M.E. & Mansfield, J.W. (2004). Effect of genotype and explant age on callus induction and subsequent plant regeneration from root-derived callus of Indica rice genotypes. Plant Cell, Tissue and Organ Culture, 78: 217–223

Huang, L.C. & Murashige, T. (1983). Tissue culture investigation of bamboo I: Callus culture of *Bambusa, Phyllostachys* and *Sasa*. Academia Sinica Institute of Botany Bulletin, 24:31-52

Huang, L.C., Huang, B.L. & Chen, W.L. (1989). Tissue culture investigations of bamboo IV: Organogenesis leading to adventitious shoots and plants in excised shoot apices. Environmental and Experimental Botany, 29: 307-315.

Karp, A. (1995). Somaclonal variation as a tool for crop improvement. Euphytica, 85: 295-302

Kassahun, E. (2000). The indigenous bamboo forests of Ethiopia: an overview. Ambio, 29: 518-521.

Kassahun, E. (2003). Ecological aspects and resource management of bamboo forests in Ethiopia. PhD Dissertation. Swedish University of Agricultural Sciences, Uppsala

Kleinhenz, V. & Midmore, D.J. (2001). Aspects of bamboo agronomy. Advances in Agronomy, 74: 99-145.

Kott, L.S. & Beversdorf, W.D. (1990). Enhanced plant regeneration from microspore-derived embryos of *Brassica napus* by chilling, partial desiccation and age selection. Plant Cell, Tissue and Organ Culture, 23: 187-192

Larkin, P.J. & Scowcroft, W.P. (1981). Somaclonal variation-novel source of variability from cell culture for plant improvement. Theoretical and Applied Genetics, 60: 197-214

Lin, C.S., Lin, C.C. & Chang, W.C. (2003). In vitro flowering of *Bambusa edulis* and subsequent plantlet survival. Plant Cell, Tissue and Organ Culture, 72: 71-78

Lin, C.S., Lin, C.C. & Chang, W.C. (2004). Effect of thidiazuron on vegetative tissue-derived somatic embryogenesis and flowering of bamboo *Bambusa edulis*. Plant Cell, Tissue and Organ Culture, 76: 75-82

Lin, X.C., Chow, T.Y., Chen H.H., Liu, C.C., Chou, S.J., Huang, B.L., Kuo, C.I., Wen, C.K., Huang, L.C. & Fang, W. (2010a). Understanding bamboo flowering based on large-scale analysis of expressed sequence tags. Genetics and Molecular Research, 9(2): 1085-1093

Lin, X.C., Lou, Y.F., Liu, J., Peng, J.S., Liao, G.L. & Fang, W. (2010b). Crossbreeding of *Phyllostachys* species (Poaceae) and identification of their hybrids using ISSR markers. Genetics and Molecular Research, 9(3): 1398-1404

Lopez-Noguera, S., Petri, C. & Burgos, L. (2009). Combining a regeneration-promoting *ipt* gene and site-specific recombination allows a more efficient apricot transformation and the elimination of marker genes. Plant Cell Reports, 28:1781–1790

Luo, K., Duan, H., Zhao, D., Zheng, X., Deng, W., Chen, Y., Jr, C.N.S., McAvoy, R., Jiang, X., Wu, Y., He, A., Pei, Y. & Li, Y. (2007). 'GM-gene-deletor' for transgenic plants: fused *loxP-FRT* recognition sequences dramatically improve the efficiency of *FLP* or *CRE* recombinase on transgene excision from pollen and seed of tobacco plants. Plant Biotechnology Journal, 5: 263-274

Luo, K., Sun, M., Deng, W. & Xu, S. (2008). Excision of selectable marker gene from transgenic tobacco using the GM-gene-deletor system regulated by a heat-inducible promoter. Biotechnology Letters, 30(7): 1295-1302

Lu, J.J., Yoshinaga, K., Fang, W. & Tang, D.Q. (2009). Identification of the hybrid bamboo F1 by SSR markers, Scientia Silvae Sinicae, 45(3): 29-34.

Mailly, D., Christanty, L. & Kimmins, J. P. (1997). "Without bamboo, the land dies": nutrient cycling and biogeochemistry of a Javanese bamboo talun-kebun system. Forest Ecology and Management, 91: 155-173.

Mathews, H., Schopke, C., Carcamo, R., Chavarriaga, P., Fauquet, C. & Beachy R.N. (1993). Improvement of somatic embryogenesis and plant recovery in cassava. Plant Cell Reports, 12: 328-333

McNeely, J.A. (1999). Biodiversity and bamboo genetic resources in Asia: in situ, community-based and *ex situ* approaches to conservation. Chinese biodiversity, 7(1): 38-51

Misra, S., Attree, S. M., Leal, I. & Fowke, L.C. (1993). Effect of abscisic acid, osmoticum, and desiccation on synthesis of storage proteins during the development of white spruce somatic embryos. Annals of Botany, 71:11-22

Molinier, J., Thomas, C., Brignou, M. & Hahne, G. (2002). Transient expression of *ipt* gene enhances regeneration and transformation rates of sunflower shoot apices (*Helianthus annuus* L.). Plant Cell Reports, 21:251–256

Mukherjee, S. K., Rathinasabapathi, & Gupta, N. (1991). Low sugar and osmotic requirements for shoot regeneration from leaf pieces of *Solanum melongena* L.. Plant Cell, Tissue and Organ Culture, 25: 13-16

Nishimura, A., Aichi, I. & Matsuoka, M. (2006). A protocol for Agrobacterium-mediated transformation in rice. Nature Protocols, 1(6): 2796-2802

Nishimura, A., Ashikari, M., Lin, S.Y., Takashi, T., Angeles, E.R., Yamamoto, T. & Matsuoka, M. (2005). Isolation of a rice regeneration quantitative trait loci gene and its application to transformation systems. Proceedings of the National Academy of Science USA, 102(33): 11940-11944

Ozawa, K. & Kawahigashi, H. (2006). Positional cloning of the nitrite reductase gene associated with good growth and regeneration ability of calli and establishment of a new selection system for Agrobacterium-mediated transformation in rice (*Oryza sativa* L.). Plant Science, 170: 384-393

Pei, H.Y., Lin, X.C., Fang, W. & Huang, L.C. (2011). A preliminary study of somatic embryogenesis of *Phyllostachys violascens* in vitro. Chinese Bulletin of Botany, 46 (2): 170-178

Purnhauser, L. & Gyulai, G. (1993). Effect of copper on shoot and root regeneration in wheat, triticale, rape and tobacco tissue cultures. Plant Cell, Tissue and Organ Culture, 35: 131-139

Ramanayake, S.M.S.D. & Wanniarachchi, W.A.V.R. (2003). Organogenesis in callus derived from an adult giant bamboo (*Dendrocalamus giganteus* Wall. ex Munro). Scientia Horticulturae, 98:195-200

Rance, I.M., Tian, W., Mathews, H., Kochko, A. d., Beachy, R.N. & Fauquet, C. (1994). Partial desiccation of mature embryo-derived caili, a simple treatment that dramatically enhances the regeneration ability of indica rice. Plant Cell Reports, 13: 647-651

Rao, I.U., Rao, I.V.R. & Narang, V. (1985). Somatic embryogenesis and regeneration of plants in the bamboo *Dendrocalamus strictus*. Plant Cell Reports, 4:191-194

Roustan, J.P., Latche, A. & Fallot, J. (1989). Stimulation of *Daucus carota* somatic embryogenesis by inhibitors of ethylene synthesis: cobalt and nickel. Plant Cell Reports, 8:182-185

Rout, G.R. & Das, P. (1994). Somatic embryogenesis and *in vitro* flowering of 3 species of bamboo. Plant Cell Reports, 13:683-686

Saharan, V., Yadav, R.C., Yadav, N.R. & Chapagain, B.P. (2004). High frequency plant regeneration from desiccated calli of indica rice (*Oryza sativa* L.). African Journal of Biotechnology, 3(5): 256-259

Sakamoto, T., Sakakibara, H., Kojima, M., Yamamoto, Y., Nagasaki, H., Inukai, Y., Sato, Y. & Matsuoka, M. (2006). Ectopic expression of *KNOTTED1*-like homeobox protein induces expression of cytokinin biosynthesis genes in rice. Plant Physiology, 142: 54–62

Sanyal, I., Singh, A.K., Kaushik, M. & Amla, D.V. (2005). Agrobacterium mediated transformation of chickpea (*Cicer arietinum* L.) with Bacillus thuringiensis *cry1Ac* gene for resistance against pod borer insect *Helicoverpa armigera*. Plant Science, 168: 1135-1146.

Saxena, S. & Dhawan, V. (1999). Regeneration and large-scale propagation of bamboo (*Dendrocalamus strictus* Nees) through somatic embryogenesis. Plant Cell Reports, 18:438-443

Scurlock, J.M.O., Dayton, D.C. & Hames B. (2000). Bamboo: an overlooked biomass resource? Biomass and Bioenergy, 19: 229-244

Smigocki, A. & Owens, L. (1988). Cytokinin gene fuses with a strong promoter enhances shoot organogenesis and zeatin level in transformed plant cells. Proceedings of the National Academy of Science USA, 85: 5131-5135

Srinivasan, C., Liu, Z., Heidmann, I., Supena, E.D.J., Fukuoka H., Joosen, R., Lambalk, J., Angenent, G., Scorza, R., Custers, J.B.M. & Boutilier, K. (2007) Heterologous expression of the *BABY BOOM* AP2/ERF transcription factor enhances the regeneration capacity of tobacco (Nicotiana tabacum L.). Planta, 225: 341-351

Srinivasan, C., Liu, Z., & Scorza, R. (2011) Ectopic expression of class 1 *KNOX* genes induce adventitious shoot regeneration and alter growth and development of tobacco

(*Nicotiana tabacum* L) and European plum (*Prunus domestica* L). Plant Cell Reports, 30: 655–664

Sun, G.Z., Ma, M.Q., Zhang, Y.Q., Xie, X.L., Cai, J.F., Li, X.P., Yin, Z.M., Qin, J., Zhang, R., Xu, D., Yang, J.Y. & Wang, H.B. (1999). A suitable medium for callus induction and maintenance for wheat. Journal of Hebei Agriculture Science, 3: 224-226

Toth, K., Haapala, T. & Hohtola, A. (1994). Alleviation of browning in oak explants by chemical pretreatments. Biologia Plantarum, 36: 511-517

Torrizo, L. B. & Zapata, F. J. (1986). Anther culture in rice: IV. The effect of abscisic acid on plant regeneration. Plant Cell Reports, 5(2): 136-139

Tsay, H.S., Yeh, C.C. & Hsu, J.Y. (1990). Embryogenesis and plant regeneration from anther culture of bamboo (*Sinocalamus latiflora* (Munro) McClure). Plant Cell Reports, 9:349-351

Tsukahara, M. & Hirosawa, T. (1992). Simple dehydration treatment promotes plantlet regeneration of rice (*Oryza sativa* L.) callus. Plant Cell Reports, 11: 550-553

Vain, P., Yean, H. & Flament, P. (1989). Enhancement of production and regeneration of embryogenic type II callus in *Zea mays* L. by AgNO3. Plant Cell, Tissue and Organ Culture, 18:143-151

Varshney, R. K., Langridge, P. & Graner, A. (2007). Application of genomics to molecular breeding of wheat and barley. Advances in Genetics, 58: 121-155

Woods, S.H., Phillips, G.C., Woods, J.E. & Collins, G.B. (1992). Somatic embryogenesis and plant regeneration from zygotic embryo explants in Mexican weeping bamboo, *Otatea acuminate aztecorum*. Plant Cell Reports, 11:257-261

Wu, C.Y. & Chen, Y. (1987). A study on the genotypical differences in anther culture of Keng rice (*Oryza sativa* subsp. *keng*). Acta Genetica Sinica, 14: 168-174

Wu, Z.Y. & Raven, P.H., eds. (2006). Flora of China: Poaceae. Vol. 22. Beijing: Science Press, St. Louis: MBG Press.

Yeh, M. & Chang, W.C. (1986a). Plant regeneration through somatic embryogenesis in callus culture of green bamboo (*Bambusa oldhamii* Munro). Theoretical and Applied Genetics, 73:161-163

Yeh, M. & Chang, W.C. (1986b). Somatic embryogenesis and subsequent plant regeneration from inflorescence callus of *Bambusa beecheyana* Munro var. *beecheyana*. Plant Cell Reports, 5:409-411

Yeh, M. & Chang, W.C. (1987). Plant regeneration via somatic embryogenesis in mature embryo-derived callus culture of *Sinocalamus latiflora* (Munro) McClure. Plant Science,51: 93-96

Yuan, J.L., Gu, X.P., Li, L.B., Yue, J.J., Yao, N. & Guo, G.P. (2009). Induction and plantlet regeneration of *Bambusa multiplex*. Scientia Silvae Sinicae, 3:35- 40

Zhang, F.L., Takahata, Y. & Xu, J.B. (1998). Medium and genotype factors influencing shoot regeneration from cotyledonary explants of Chinese cabbage (*Brassica campestris* L. ssp. *pekinensis*). Plant Cell Reports, 17: 780–786

Zhang, N., Fang, W., Shi, Y., Liu, Q.Q., Yang, H.Y., Gui, R.Y. & Lin, X.C. (2010). Somatic embryogenesis and organogenesis in *Dendrocalamus hamiltonii*. Plant Cell, Tissue and Organ Culture, 103: 325–332.

Zhuo, R.Y. & Liu, X.G. (2004). Factors effecting transgenic breeding of *Dendrocalamus latiflorus*. Acta Agriculturae Universitatis Jiangxiensis, 26: 551-554.

17

Role of Polyamines in Efficiency of Norway Spruce (Hurst Ecotype) Somatic Embryogenesis

J. Malá[1], M. Cvikrová[2], P. Máchová[1] and L. Gemperlová[2]
[1]*Forestry and Game Management Research Institute, Jíloviště*
[2]*Institute of Experimental Botany, Academy of Sciences of the Czech Republic, Praha*
Czech Republic

1. Introduction

Somatic embryogenesis is considered as to be an advantageous methodology for plant micropropagation *in vitro*, particularly for conifers. It offers, moreover, a row of possibilities to study developmental processes during the embryo differentiation, and it enables also more detailed analyses of the mechanisms of embryo conversion.

Somatic embryogenesis can be divided into several stages, which are comparable to the stages in zygotic embryogenesis (Atree & Fowke, 1993). However, since somatic embryos develop without the protective environment of the surrounding maternal tissue, there is a need to supply developing embryos both the nutrients and the regulatory compounds exogenously. Induction and continuous proliferation requires the auxins and the cytokinins, whereas the further growth and maturation of embryos depends on the abscisic acid (Attree et al., 1991). By the end of the maturation stage, all structures of the embryo are morphologically fully developed (Find, 1997) but the embryo becomes biochemically mature after a desiccation processing (Flinn et al., 1993).

Somatic embryogenesis in some coniferous species provides sufficient numbers of fully developed embryos usable for propagation. On the other hand, the yield of converted somatic embryos in other species is often too low for practical applications (Igasaki et al., 2003). In some instances, the successful somatic embryogenesis is a question of the selection of responsible clones within the range of a coniferous species. Research of somatic embryogenesis in conifers has increased rapidly since the eighties of the last century. Promising results were achieved especially with Norway spruce (*Picea abies* (L.) Karst.), in which the successful regeneration of complete plants was obtained (Attree & Fowke, 1993; Bornman, 1985; Chalupa, 1985; Chalupa et al., 1990; Hakman et al., 1985; Malá et al., 1995). The process of somatic embryogenesis in Norway spruce can be divided into four stages characterized by the different degree of embryonic tissue differentiation: the induction of embryogenic tissue, the proliferation of somatic embryos, maturation, and finally, the conversion of mature embryos into complete plants.

The induction of embryogenic tissues can be achieved by applying phytohormones on mature or immature zygotic embryos. The initiation rate is higher when immature zygotic embryos are used; however, it is difficult to determine an optimal cone harvest time (Chalupa, 1985). The transfer of embryogenic tissue from proliferation onto maturation medium leads to the induction of embryo development. Despite of the successful protocol for establishment of Norway spruce somatic embryogenesis technique, there is a lack of data concerning the endogenous composition of biologically active compounds both in somatic and zygotic embryos. Generally, the development of embryos as well as their conversion into complete plantlets is closely associated with changes in endogenous phytohormone levels. Changes in endogenous hormone levels (IAA, ABA, and ethylene) during Norway spruce somatic embryo development and maturation have been recently reported (Vágner et al., 2005).

Beside the key roles of auxins and cytokinins, very important function during growth and differentiation of plant tissues belongs to polyamines (PAs) (Mattoo et al., 2010; Vera-Sirera et al., 2010). PAs have a wide spectrum of action with some similarities with plant phytohormones. In cooperation with auxins and cytokinins, PAs modulate morphogenetic processes (Altamura et al., 1993). From this point of view PAs could be considered as new category of plant hormones acting particularly as regulators of such processes as gene expression, cell proliferation, cell wall formation, etc. (Cohen, 1998). PAs are involved also in the transmission of cellular signals. They regulate the synthesis of nitric oxide, which is known as a plant signaling molecule (Besson-Bard et al., 2008).

PAs are small polycationic molecules with several amino groups, which are ubiquitous in both prokaryotes and eukaryotes (Cohen, 1998; Tiburcio et al., 1997). Also the mechanisms of PAs synthesis, transport, and catabolism are conserved from bacteria to animals and plants (Kusano et al., 2008; Tabor & Tabor, 1984). Most of the biological functions of PAs can be explained by their polycationic nature, which allows interactions with anionic macromolecules such as DNA, RNA, and with negative groups of cellular membrane components. The synthesis of PAs within various plant tissues depends on a great variety of physiological growth regulatory stimuli as well as on various external influences as periodicity or stressing conditions (humidity, droughts), and environmental damaging factors, too.

PAs are essential compounds for life. Decrease or arrest of internal PA production inhibits a row of cellular functions, e. g. cell growth. Therefore, in the case of PAs deficiency, plant cells are equipped with a high efficient system for transfer and functional utilization of PA molecules from external sources (Cohen, 1998, Hanfrey et al., 2001, Kusano et al., 2008).

Three commonly occurring PAs in plants are diamine putrescine (Put), triamine spermidine (Spd) and tetramine spermine (Spm). All these compounds are present in the free form or as conjugates with other low molecular substances (e. g. phenolic acids) or macromolecules (proteins, nucleoproteins). They are found in cell walls, vacuoles, mitochondria, chloroplasts and cytoplasm (Kaur-Sawhney et al., 2003). PAs are detected in increased amounts within actively differentiating and growing plant tissues. Also their activity increases mainly in growing plant tissues, during embryogenesis, root formation and stem elongation, fruit development and ripening, and during response to abiotic and biotic stress factors, too (Kumar et al., 1997).

Polyamines play a fundamental role in the regulation of somatic and zygotic embryogenesis (Kong et al., 1998; Silveira et al., 2004). The role of PAs during *in vivo* and *in vitro* development, including somatic embryogenesis, were recently reviewed (Baron & Stasolla, 2008). The accumulation of high levels of PAs in somatic embryos contributes to their reserve consisting predominately of proteins and triglycerides, which are utilized during embryo germination. PAs changes were studied in embryogenic cultures of *Picea abies* (R. Minocha et al., 1993; Serapiglia et al., 2008; Vondráková et al., 2010), *Picea rubens* (R. Minocha et al., 1993), *Pinus taeda* (Silveira et al., 2004), and *P. radiata* (R. Minocha et al., 1999). Polyamine profiles in germinating somatic embryos derived from long term cultivated embryogenic mass and germinating zygotic embryos of Norway spruce were studied by Gemperlová et al. (2009). There are also several reports indicating the participation of PAs in somatic embryo development of some coniferous species (R. Minocha et al., 1999; Santanen & Simola, 1992; Silveira et al., 2004) but the mechanism of how polyamines regulate cell differentiation processes is not fully elucidated up to the present.

Norway spruce is the most important forest tree species in the Czech Republic, both economically and due to its representation. However, only few populations can be regarded autochthonous. These populations are irreplaceable in the future, not only for maintenance and natural regeneration of the biotope, but also as an important source of genetic material needed for the breeding programs which are aimed to preserve the valuable forest sources for the future generations. The Hurst ecotype of Norway spruce is considered to be autochthonous and it is rarely preserved at the altitudes over 700 m. Reproduction of these populations is really difficult due to the high age of the trees and longer and lengthening flushing intervals. For conifers and mainly for Norway spruce, micropropagation technologies, mainly somatic embryogenesis, represent very suitable methods of reproduction and preservation of valuable genotypes.

The aim of this study was to compare PA levels during development of somatic embryos of high responsible AFO 541 cell line with less responsible cell lines derived from the Hurst ecotype of *Picea abies*. The results obtained could help to a better understanding of PAs function in regulation of plant tissue differentiation processes and contribute to improving the micropropagation of less responsible Hurst Norway spruce by somatic embryogenesis.

2. Experimental part

2.1 Materials and methods

2.1.1 Cell lines

Picea abies (L.) Karst. embryogenic cultures of high responsible cell line AFO 541 (AFOCEL, Nangis, France) and five less responsible cell lines (L10, L13, L16, L17, L28) derived from a *P. abies* Hurst ecotype were used.

2.1.2 Hurst cell lines initiation

Immature cones of 140 years old elite open pollinated Hurst Norway Spruce growing in the conservation area Labské Pískovce (Northern Bohemia, CR) were collected in late July 2006 and stored at 4 °C. To induce embryogenic tissue differentiation, the immature embryos extirpated from sterilized seeds (1% NaClO, Savo, Biochemie, CR) were cultivated in darkness at 24 °C on the modification of solid E medium (Gupta & Durzan,

1986) with 0.2 mg.l^{-1} gelerit (Sigma-Aldrich, Germany) and phytohormones (0.5 mg.l^{-1} of BAP, 1.0 mg.l^{-1}of 2,4-D, and 0.5 mg.l^{-1} of Kin), pH adjusted to 5.8 prior to the medium autoclaving (Malá, 1991).

In a preliminary experiment the embryogenic capacity (i.e. the ability of the ESM to produce mature somatic embryos) were determined in 45 cell lines of Hurst Norway Spruce ESM. Five of them, with diverse characteristics, were further selected for the subsequent experiments.

2.1.3 Induction of proliferation

The cultures of embryogenic mass were after 4 wks of induction transferred onto fresh E medium of the same composition and cultured in the same conditions as previously. The embryogenic cultures were maintained by subculturing weekly.

2.1.4 Maturation of somatic embryos

After 12 wks of cultivation on proliferation medium were the cultures transferred onto maturation medium (solid E medium without phytohormones, supplemented with 8 mg.l^{-1} of ABA (Sigma, Chemical Co., USA) and 20 mg.l^{-1} of PEG (m. w. 3350, Sigma, Chemical Co., USA). Cultures were kept in same conditions as described above and subcultured every week. After 2 wks, the somatic embryo cultures were transferred onto solid E medium containing 0.1mg.l^{-1} of IBA (Sigma Chemical Co., USA) and 20 mg.l^{-1} of PEG and cultured under white fluorescent light (30 µmol.m^{-2}.s^{-1}) and 16 h photoperiod. After 3-4 wks the somatic embryos were harvested for desiccation.

2.1.5 Desiccation

Only the fully developed embryos were desiccated. The embryos were carefully transferred on the dry paper in small Petri dishes (3cm in diameter). Open dishes were placed into large Petri dishes (18cm in diameter) with several paper layers wetted by sterile water Large Petri dishes were covered by lids and sealed by parafilm. They were kept under the light regime of 12 hours of light and 12 hours of darkness, at 20±1^{0}C for 2 wks.

2.1.6 Material for biochemical analyses

The contents of PAs were determined in the course of somatic embryo development. The samples were immediately frozen in liquid nitrogen and stored at –80 °C until determination.

2.1.7 Polyamine analysis

The cells were ground in liquid nitrogen and extracted overnight at 4 °C with 1 ml of 5% perchloric acid (PCA) per 100 mg fresh weight tissue. 1,7-Diaminoheptane was added as an internal standard, and the extracts were centrifuged at 21 000 x *g* for 15 min. PCA-soluble free PAs were determined in one-half volume of the supernatant. The remaining supernatant and pellet were acid hydrolysed in 6 M HCl for 18 h at 110 °C to obtain PCA-soluble and PCA-insoluble conjugates of PAs as described by Slocum et al. (1989). Standards (Sigma-Aldrich, Prague, Czech Republic) and PCA-soluble free PAs, and acid hydrolysed PA conjugates were benzoylated according to the method of Slocum et al. (1989), and the resulting benzoyl-amines were analyzed by HPLC using a Beckman chromatographic system equipped with a 125S Gradient Solvent Delivery Module, 507 Variable Mode Injection Autosampler, and 168 Diode Array Detector (Beckman Instruments, Inc., Fullerton, CA, USA). A Gold Nouveau software data system was used to collect, integrate and analyse the chromatographic data. A C18 column (Phenomenex Aqua, 5 μm, 125A, 250x4.6 mm, Phenomenex, Utrecht, NL) was used for the separation of polyamines. Elution was carried out at a flow rate of 0.4 mL min^{-1} at 45 °C. Standard sample (5 μl and 10 μl) was injected for a single run. The mobile phase consisted of solvent A (10% v/v methanol) and solvent B (80% v/v methanol). The gradient program (expressed as percentages of solvent A) was as follows: 0–10 min, 45% to 0%; 10-30 min, isocratic 0%; 30-40 min, 0% to 45%. Column was washed with 45% solvent A for 30 min between samples. Eluted polyamines were detected by UV detector at 254 nm by comparing of their R_t values with those of standards (Sigma-Aldrich, Prague, the Czech Republic).

2.1.8 Statistical analyses

Two independent experiments were carried out. Analogous results were obtained in both experiments. Means ± S.E. of one experiment (with 3 replicates) are shown in the figures. Data were analyzed using the Student's *t* distribution criteria.

2.2 Results and discussion

Tissue culture approaches, in particular somatic embryogenesis, is considered as the advantageous technique for *in vitro* propagation and gene conservation of conifers. Generally, the development of embryos and their conversion into plantlets is closely associated with changes in endogenous phytohormone levels, including polyamines. Positive correlation between embryogenic capacity and total content of free PAs confirmed to a crucial role of PAs (with Spd predominating, Figs 1, 2, 3) during somatic embryo development in *Picea* as previously described (Gemperlová et al., 2009; S.C. Minocha & Long, 2004). On transfer from proliferation to maturation medium the levels of Put and Spd in the culture of highly responsible cell line AFO 541 were almost equal while in less responsible cultures of Hurst ecotype significantly higher levels of Put than Spd were determined as is apparent from the Put/Spd ratios in the embryogenic suspensor masses (ESM) of six cell lines of Norway spruce (AFO 541 and five of Hurst ecotype) grown on solid proliferation medium (Figs 1, 2). The contents of Put, Spd and Spm in highly responsible cell line AFO 541 steadily increased during maturation from ESM until early cotyledonary stage (Fig. 3). This stage of embryo development was characterized by very high Spd contents. On the contrary to Put and Spd, the level of Spm significantly increased during the desiccation phase (Fig. 3). The increase in Spm level in this phase might result from „certain" abiotic stress in the course of desiccation. The decline in PA contents in mature embryos was probably due to the increased catabolism of Put and Spd during the later stages of embryo development, as previously described in *Picea abies* (Santanen & Simola, 1992).

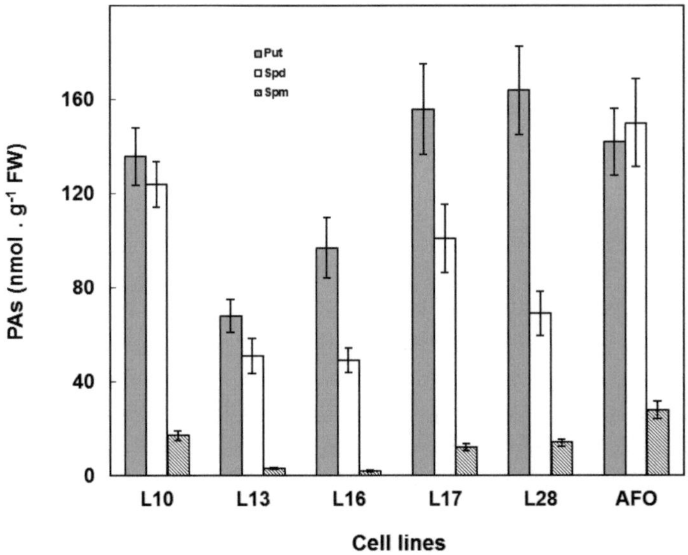

Fig. 1. Comparison of the contents of free putrescine (Put), spermidine (Spd) and spermine (Spm) in the ESMs of six cell lines of Norway spruce (AFO 541 and five of Hurst ecotype) grown on solid proliferation medium (before transfer to maturation medium). Bars represent SE of three replicates. ESM, embryogenic suspensor mass.

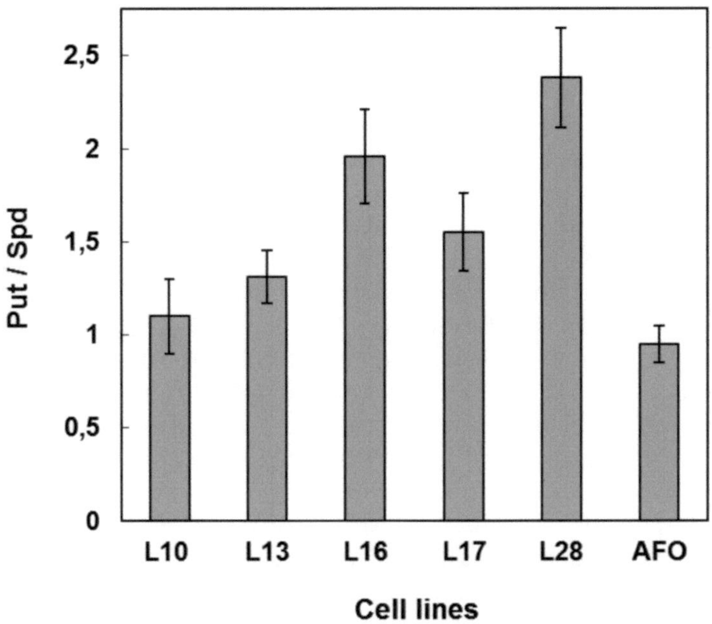

Fig. 2. Comparison of putrescine/spermidine (Put/Spd) ratios in the ESMs of six cell lines of Norway spruce (AFO 541 and five of Hurst ecotype) grown on solid proliferation medium (before transfer to maturation medium). Bars represent SE of three replicates. ESM, embryogenic suspensor mass.

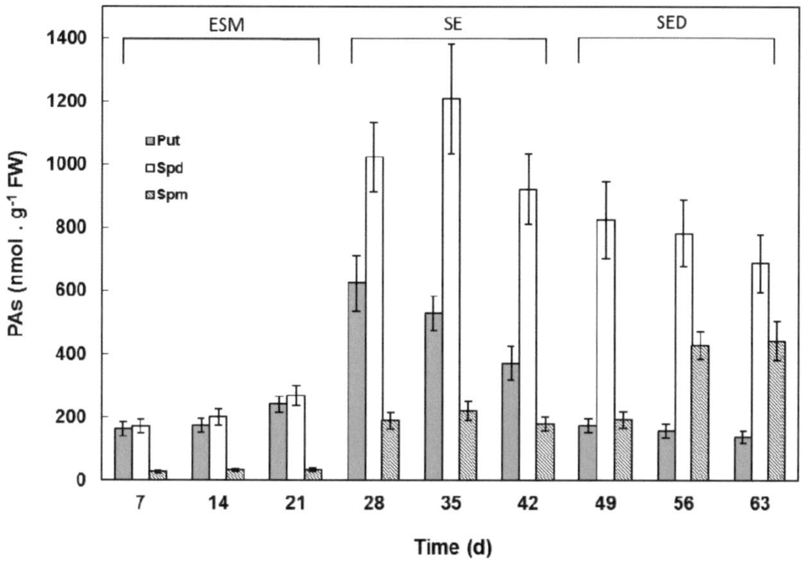

Fig. 3. Changes in cellular levels of free putrescine (Put), spermidine (Spd) and spermine (Spm) during Norway spruce (AFO 541) somatic embryo development from proliferation to desiccation. Bars represent SE of three replicates. ESM, embryogenic suspensor mass; SE, somatic embryo; SED, somatic embryo during desiccation; d, days.

Parallel rises in the content of Spd occurred during the 6 weeks of embryo development of Hurst ecotype cell lines. At this stage of somatic embryo development the predominant PA was Spd followed by Put (Fig. 4), although the mature embryos of highly responsible cell line AFO 541 contained still significantly higher level of Spd. Cell line AFO 514 and Hurst ecotype cell line L10 were characterized by high content of Spd and represented plant material with stable rapid growth during proliferation and a huge yield of somatic embryos was obtained at the end of maturation of cell line L10 (Fig. 5). On the contrary, rather low yield of less matured embryos was found in the remaining studied cell lines of less responsible ecotypes (L16 and L28) which contained lower level of Spd (Fig. 6). However, a high level of free PAs is not the only important PA-related factor in somatic embryogenesis, and (for instance) it has been proposed that an inadequate Spd/Put ratio may be causally linked to abnormal growth and disorganized cell proliferation of grape somatic embryos with high free PA contents (Faure et al., 1991). Less matured somatic embryos and lower yield of embryos in the remaining studied cell lines L13 and L17 (in comparison with the yield of embryos in the cell line L10) might coincide with the inadequate Put/Spd ratio determined in the embryos.

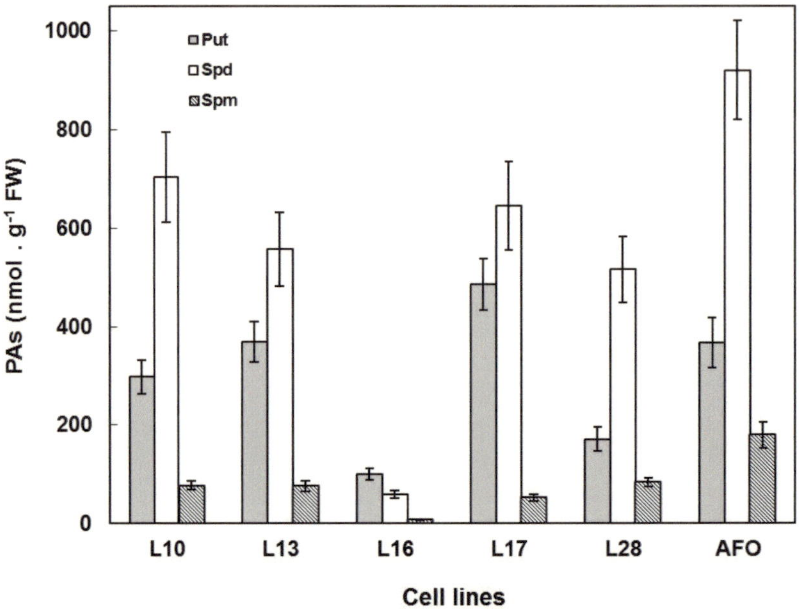

Fig. 4. Comparison of the contents of free putrescine (Put), spermidine (Spd) and spermine (Spm) in 6 week-old somatic embryos of six cell lines of Norway spruce (AFO 541 and five of Hurst ecotype) grown on solid maturation medium.

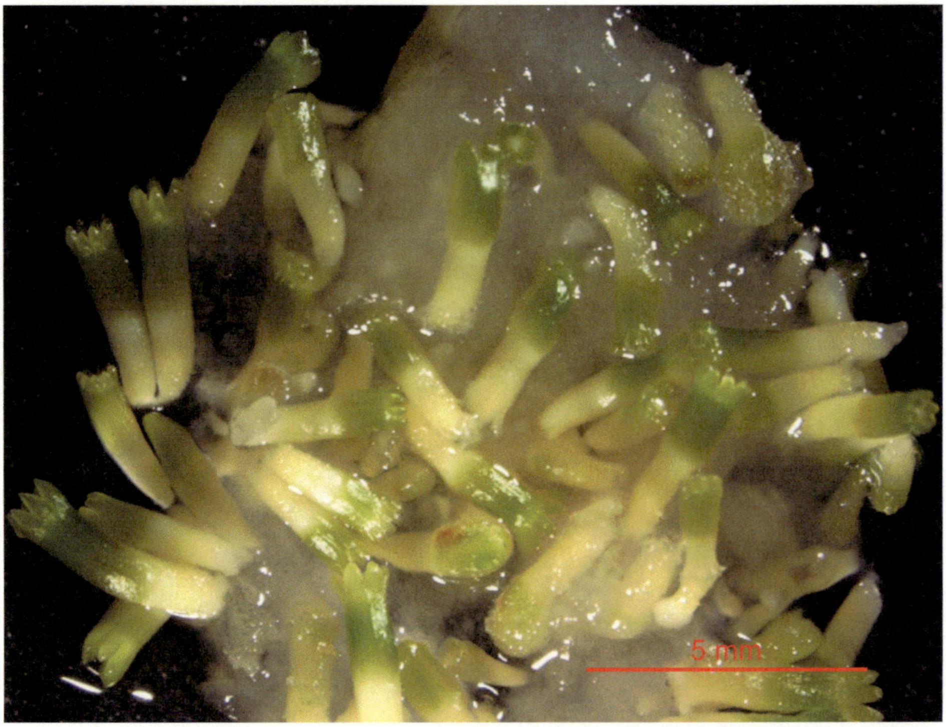

Fig. 5. Mature somatic embryos (6 week-old) of Hurst ecotype of Norway spruce L10.

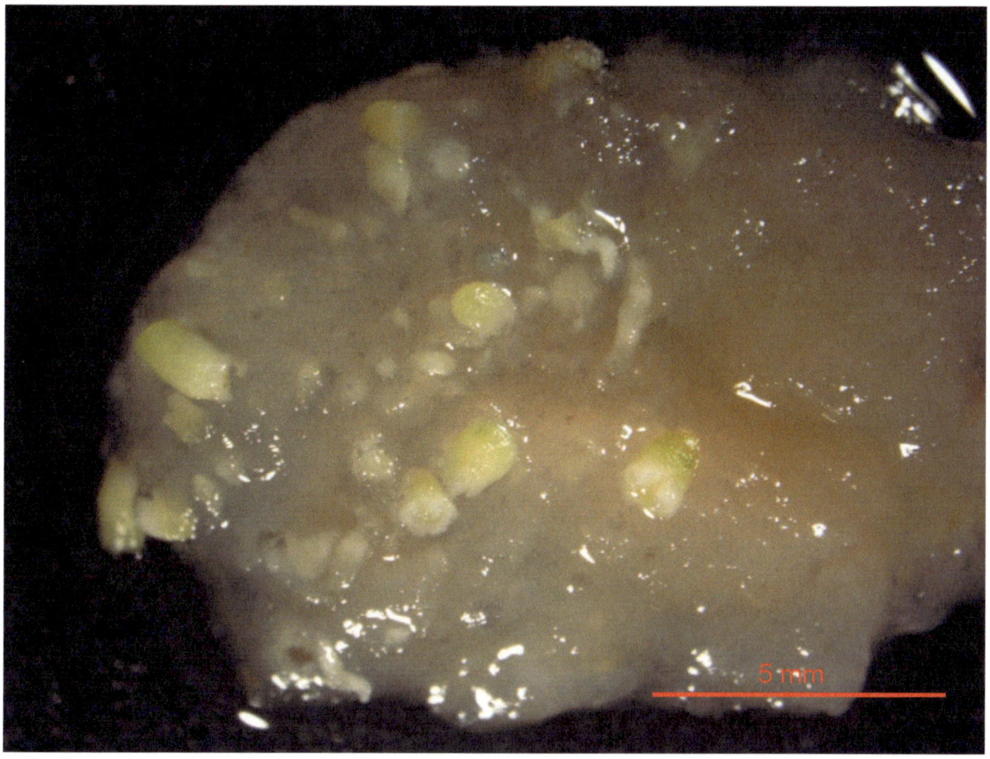

Fig. 6. Mature somatic embryos (6 week-old) of Hurst ecotype of Norway spruce L28.

Similarly, contents of PAs (higher Spd than Put levels) could be used as criteria for the physiological characterization of somatic embryogenesis in *Pinus nigra* Arn. (Noceda et al., 2009). Furthermore, the important role of cellular levels of metabolically active free PAs, especially contents of Spd, was shown to be essential for preservation of embryogenic potential of Norway spruce cultures after cryopreservation (Vondráková et al., 2010). The formation of somatic embryos in tissue cultures of wild carrot seemed to be also associated with high Spd level and much more Spd than Put was found in torpedo stage of these embryos (Mengoli et al., 1989). Especially Spd was implicated in somatic embryogenesis in tissue cultures of *Vigna aconitifolia* (Kaur-Sawhney et al., 1985), *Hevea brasiliensis* (El Hadrami & D'Auzac, 1992) and in the development of globular pro-embryos in alfalfa (Cvikrová et al., 1999). However, it is not always Spd, which is the dominant polyamine in somatic embryos of conifers. Putrescine was the most abundant PA in the embryogenic suspension culture of *Pinus taeda* (Silveira et al., 2004), whereas the development of both somatic and zygotic embryos of *Pinus radiata* was characterized by high level of Spd and its concentration positively correlated with the embryo development (R. Minocha et al., 1999). High level of Put was determined in pro-embryogenic tissue of *Picea rubens*, while Spd was predominant during embryo development in this culture (S.C. Minocha & Long, 2004).

As we have already mentioned in the Introduction, embryo maturation and low germination frequencies are main limitations for a broader use of somatic embryogenesis in practice. Requirement of exogenous phytohormones for efficient somatic embryogenesis is well established. Exogenously supplied polyamines might therefore affect and improve the induction and somatic embryo development in less responsible plant genotypes. It has been found that the exogenous application of Spd in the initiation phase significantly increased the production of embryos in *Panax ginseng* cultures (Kevers et al., 2000). This knowledge led as to try to improve the efficiency of somatic embryogenesis of less responsible genotypes by application of PAs into the growth medium. The studies of the possibility of improving the method of somatic embryogenesis in less responsible Hurst ecotype of Norway spruce are now in progress in our laboratory. Preliminary experiments (results not shown) reveal that low exogenous application of Put (0.1 and 0.01 mM) increased the number of early forms of embryos. However, on the bases of these results the effect of PA application into the growth medium in order to improve the efficiency of somatic embryogenesis of Norway spruce can not be generalized and further experiments are necessary.

The results presented here indicate a direct role for Spd and adequate Put/Spd ratio in somatic embryogenesis. Cell lines AFO 514 and L10, characterized by high content of Spd, represented plant material with stable rapid growth during proliferation and a huge yield of somatic embryos was obtained at the end of maturation. Less matured somatic embryos and rather low yield of embryos in the remaining studied cell lines (L13, L16, L17 and L28) might coincide with the lower level of Spd and/or inadequate Put/Spd ratio determined in these embryos.

3. Conclusion

Micropropagation technologies represent a powerful tool for improvement and acceleration of tree breeding programs in forestry. Tissue culture approaches, in particular somatic embryogenesis, hold considerable promise for breeding programs of coniferous trees. Utilization of somatic embryogenesis could facilitate reproduction of rare or selected coniferous genotypes. Despite the availability of a successful protocol for generating Norway spruce plants using a somatic embryogenesis technique, there is a lack of data concerning the endogenous composition of biologically active compounds in somatic embryos. Beside the key roles of auxins and cytokinins, very important function in differentiation processes belongs to polyamines although the mechanism of their action is still not fully cleared. Positive correlation between embryogenic capacity and total content of free PAs confirmed crucial role of PAs during somatic embryo development.

It was shown that the predominant PAs in somatic embryos of highly responsible Hurst ecotype of Norway spruce (L10) was spermidine, while embryos of less responsible ecotype (L13, L16, L17 and L28) contained lower level of Spd and/or inadequate Put/Spd ratio. Exogenously supplied PAs might therefore affect and improve the induction and somatic embryo development in less responsible plant genotypes. The studies related to the improving of somatic embryogenesis method in less responsible Hurst ecotype of Norway spruce are now in progress in our laboratory.

4. Acknowledgments

The authors acknowledge the funding of the Ministry for Agriculture (Project number QH 82303) and Institutional Grant AV0Z 50380511.

5. Abbreviations

ABA - abscisic acid, BAP - 6-benzylaminopurine, 2,4-D - 2,4 dichlorfenoxy acid, ESM - embryogenic suspensor mass, IBA - indolylbutyric acid, Kin - kinetin, PAs - polyamines, Put - putrescine, Spd - spermidine, Spm - spermine

6. References

Altamura, M.M.; Torrigiani, P.; Falasca, G.; Rossini, P. & Bagni, N. (1993). Morpho-functional gradients in superficial and deep tissues along tobacco stem: polyamine levels, biosynthesis and oxidation, and organogenesis in vitro. *Journal of Plant Physiology*, Vol. 142, pp. 543–551, ISSN 0176-1617.

Attree, S.M. & Fowke, L.C. (1993). Embryogeny of gymnosperms:advances in synthetic seed technology of conifers. *Plant Cell, Tissue and Organ Culture*, Vol. 35, No. 1, pp 1–35, ISSN: 0167-6857.

Attree, S.M.; Moore, D.; Sawhney, V.K. & Fowke, L.C. (1991). Enhanced maturation and desiccation tolerance of white spruce (*Picea glauca* [Moench.] Voss.) somatic embryos: effects of a nonplasmolysing water stress and abscisic acid. *Annals of Botany*, Vol. 68, No. 6, pp 519–525, ISSN 0305-7364.

Baron, K. & Stasolla, C. (2008). The role of polyamines during *in vivo* and *in vitro* development. *In Vitro Cellular & Developmental Biology – Plant*, Vol. 44, No. 5, pp 384-395, ISSN 1054-5476.

Besson-Bard, A.; Courtois C.; Gauthier, A.; Dahan, J.; Dobrowolska, G.; Jeandroz, S.; Pugin, A. & Wendehenne D. (2008). Nitric oxide in plants: production and cross-talk with Ca^{2+} signaling. *Molecular Plant*, Vol. 1, No. 2, pp 218-228, ISSN 1674-2052.

Bornman, C.H. (1985). Hormonal control of growth and differentiation in conifer tissues in vitro. *Biologia Plantarum*, Vol. 27, No. 4-5, pp 249–256, ISSN 006-3134.

Chalupa, V. (1985). Somatic embryogenesis and plantlet regeneration from cultured immature and mature embryos of *Picea abies*/L./Karst. *Communicationes Instituti Forestalis Cechoslovaca*, Vol. 14, pp 65–90, ISSN: 1211-2992.

Chalupa, V.; Malá, J. & Dujíčková, M. (1990). Somatic embryogenesis and regeneration of spruce *(Picea abies* /L./Karst.) and oak *(Quercus robur* L.). In: „Manipulation *in vitro* in higher plants", Proc. Conf. Inst. Exp. Botany, Prague, CSAS, Olomouc, CR: p. 98.

Cohen, S.S. (1998). A guide to the polyamines. pp. 1-595, Oxford university Press, New York, NY.

Cvikrová, M.; Binarová, P.; Eder, J.; Vágner, M.; Hrubcová, M.; Zon, J. & Macháčková, I. (1999). Effect of inhibition of phenylalanine ammonia-lyase activity on growth of alfalfa cell suspension culture: alterations in mitotic index, ethylene production, and contents of phenolics, cytokinins, and polyamines. *Physiologia Plantarum*, Vol 107, No. 3, pp 329–337, ISSN 1399-3054.

El Hadrami, M.I. & D'Auzac, J. (1992). Effects of polyamine biosynthetic inhibitors on somatic embryogenesis and cellular polyamines in *Hevea brasiliensis*. *Journal of Plant Physiology*. Vol. 140, pp 33–36, ISSN 0176-1617.

Find, J.I. (1997). Changes in endogenous ABA levels in developing somatic embryos of Norway spruce (*Picea abies* (L.) Karst.) in relation to maturation medium, dessication and germination. *Plant Science*, Vol. 128, No. 1, pp 75-83, , ISSN 0168-9452.

Flinn, B.S.; Roberts D.R.; Newton C.H.; Cyr D.R.; Webster F.B. & Taylor I.E.P. (1993). Storage protein gene expression in zygotic and somatic embryos of interior spruce. *Physiologia Plantarum*. Vol. 89, No. 4, pp 719-730, ISSN 1399-3054.

Faure, O.; Mengoli, M.; Nougarede A. & Bagni. N.(1991). Polyamine pattern and biosynthesis in zygotic and somatic embryo stages of *Vitis vinifera*. *Journal of Plant Physiology*, Vol. 138, pp 545-549, ISSN 0176-1617.

Gemperlová, L.; Fisherová, L.; Cvikrová, M.; Malá, J.; Vondráková, Z.; Martincová, O. & Vágner, M. (2009). Polyamine profiles and biosynthesis in somatic embryo development and comparison of germinating somatic and zygotic ambryos of Norway spruce. *Tree Physiology*, Vol. 29, No. 10, pp 1287-1298, ISSN 0829-318X.

Gupta, P. K. & Durzan, D. J. (1986). Somatic polyembryogenesis from callus of mature sugar pine embryos. *Bio/technology*, Vol. 4, pp 643-645.

Hakman, I.; Fowke, L.C.; Von Arnold, S. & Eriksson, T. (1985). The development of somatic embryos of *Picea abies* (Norway spruce). *Plant Science*, Vol. 38, No. 1, pp 53-59, ISSN 0168-9452.

Hanfrey, C.; Sommer, S.; Mayer, M.J.; Burtin, D. & Michael, A.J. (2001). Arabidopsis polyamine biosynthesis: absence of ornithine decarboxylase and the mechanism of arginine decarboxylase activity. The Plant Journal, Vol. 27, No. 6, pp 551-560, ISSN 1365-313X.

Igasaki, T.; Sato, T.; Akashi, N.; Mohri, T.; Maruyama, E.; Kinoshita, I.; Walter C. & Shinohara, K. 2003. Somatic embryogenesis and plant regeneration from immature zygotic embryos of *Cryptomeria japonica* D. Don. *Plant Cell Reports*, Vol. 22, No. 4, pp 239-243, ISSN 0721-7714.

Kaur-Sawhney, R.; Shekhawat, N.S. & Galston, A.W. (1985). Polyamine levels as related to growth, differentiation and senescence in protoplast-derivated cultures of *Vigna-aconitifolia* and *Avena-sativa*. *Plant Growth Regulation*, Vol. 3, No. 3-4, pp 329-337, ISSN 0167-6903.

Kaur-Sawhney, R.; Tiburcio, A.F.; Altabella, T. & Galston, A.W. (2003). Polyamines in plants: An overwiew. *Journal of Cell and Molecular Biology*, Vol. 2, No. 1, pp 1-12, ISSN 1303-3646.

Kevers, C.; Le Gal, N.; Monteiro, M.; Dommes, J. & Gaspar, T. (2000). Somatic embryogenesis of *Panax ginseng* in liquid cultures: a role polyamines and their metabolic pathways. *Plant Growth Regulation*, Vol. 31, No. 3, pp 209-214, ISSN 0167-6903.

Kong, L.; Attree, S.M. & Fowke, L.C. (1998). Effects of polyethylene glycol and methylglyoxal bis(guanylhydrazone) on endogenous polyamine levels and somatic embryo maturation in white spruce (*Picea glauca*). *Plant Science*, Vol. 133, No. 2, pp 211-220, ISSN 0168-9452.

Kusano, T.; Berberich, T.; Tateda, C. & Takahashi, Y. (2008). Polyamines: essential factors for growth and survival. *Planta*, Vol. 228, No. 3, pp 367-381, ISSN 0032-0935.

Kumar, A.; Altabella, T.; Taylor, M. & Tiburcio, A.F. (1997). Recent advances in polyamine research. *Trends in Plant Science*, Vol. 2, No. 4, pp. 124-130, ISSN 1360-1385.

Malá, J. (1991). Organogenesis and somatic embryogenesis in Norway spruce. *Communicationes Instituti Forestalis Cechoslovaca*, Vol. 17, pp 59–72, ISSN: 1211-2992.

Malá, J.; Dujíčková, M. & Kálal, J. (1995). The development of encapsulated somatic embryos of Norway Spruce (*Picea abies* /L./Karst.). *Communicationes Instituti Forestalis Bohemicae*, Vol. 18, pp 59-73, ISSN: 1211-2992.

Mattoo, A.K.; Minocha, S.C.; Minocha, R. & Handa, A.K. (2010). Polyamines and cellular metabolism in plants: transgenic approaches reveal different responses to diamine putrescine versus higher polyamines spermidine and spermine. *Amino Acids*, Vol. 38, No. 2, pp 405-413, ISSN 0939-4451.

Mengoli, M.; Pistocchi, R. & Bagni, N. (1989). Effect of long-term treatment of carrot cell-cultures with millimolar concentrations of putrescin. *Plant Physiology and Biochemistry*, Vol. 27, No. 1, pp 1-8, ISSN 0981-9428.

Minocha, R.; Kvaalen, H.; Minocha, S.C. & Long, S. (1993). Polyamines in embryogenic cultures of Norway spruce (*Picea abies*) and red spruce (*Picea rubens*). *Tree Physiology*, Vol. 13, No. 4, pp. 365-377, ISSN 0829-318X.

Minocha, R.; Smith, D.R.; Reeves, C.; Steele, K.D. & Minocha, S.C. (1999). Polyamine levels during the development of zygotic and somatic embryos of *Pinus radiata*. *Physiologia Plantarum*, Vol. 105, No. 1, pp 155-164, ISSN 1399-3054.

Minocha, S.C & Long, S. (2004). Polyamines and their biosynthetic enzymes during somatic embryo development in red spruce (*Picea rubens* Sarg.) *In Vitro Cellular & Developmental Biology-Plant*, Vol. 40, No. 6, pp 572-580, ISSN 1054-5476.

Noceda, C.; Salaj, T.; Pérez, M.; Viejo, M.; Cańal, M.J.; Salaj, J. & Rodriguez R. (2009). DNA demethylation and decrease on free polyamines is associated with embryogenic capacity of *Pinus nigra* Arn. cell culture. *Trees – Structure and Function*, Vol. 23, No. 6, pp 1285-1293, ISSN 0931-1890.

Santanen, A. & Simola, L.K. (1992). Changes in polyamine metabolism during somatic embryogenesis in *Picea abies*. *Journal of Plant Physiology*. Vol.140, pp 475-480, ISSN 0176-1617.

Serapiglia, M.J.; Minocha, R. & Minocha, S.C. (2008). Changes in polyamines, inorganic ions and glutamine synthetase activity in response to nitrogen avaibility and form in red spruce (*Picea rubens*). *Tree Physiology*, Vol. 28, No. 12, pp 1793-1803, ISSN 0829-318X.

Silveira, V.; Floh, E.I.S.; Handro, W. & Guerra, M.P. (2004). Effect of plant growth regulators on the cellular growth and levels of intracellular proteins, starch and polyamines in embryogenic suspension cultures of *Pinus taeda*. *Plant Cell, Tissue and Organ Culture*, Vol. 76, No. 1, pp 53-60, ISSN 0167-6857.

Slocum, R.D.; Flores, H.E.; Galston, A.W. & Weinstein, L.H. (1989). Improved method for HPLC analysis of polyamines, agmatine and aromatic monoamines in plant tissue. *Plant Physiology*, Vol. 89, No. 2, pp 512–517, ISSN 0032-0889.

Tabor, C.W. & Tabor, H. (1984). Polyamines. *Annual Review of Biochemistry*, Vol. 53, pp 749-790, ISSN 0066-4154.

Tiburcio, A.F.; Altabella, T.; Borrell, A. & Masgrau, C. (1997). Polyamine metabolism and its regulation. *Physiologia. Plantarum*, Vol. 100, No. 3, pp 664-674, ISSN 1399-3054

Vágner, M.; Vondráková, Z.; Fischerová, L.; Vičánková, A. & Malbeck, J. (2005). Endogenous phytohormones during Norway spruce somatic embryogenesis. Procceding COST 843 and 851 Action, Stará Lesná (28.6.-3.7.), pp. 162-164.

Vera-Sirera, F.; Minquet, E.G., Singh, S.K.; Ljung, K., Tuominen, H., Blazquez, M.A. & Carbonell, J. (2010). Role of polyamines in plant vascular development. *Plant Physiology and Biochemistry,* Vol. 48, No. 7, pp 534-539, ISSN 0981-9428.

Vondráková, Z.; Cvikrová, M.; Eliášová, K., Martincová, O. & Vágner, M. (2010). Cryotolerance in Norway spruce and its association with growth rates, anatomical features and polyamines of embryogenic cultures. *Tree Physiology.* Vol. 30, No 10, pp 1335-1348, ISSN 0829-318X.

18

Somatic Embryogenesis and Efficient Plant Regeneration in Japanese Cypresses

Tsuyoshi E. Maruyama and Yoshihisa Hosoi
Forestry and Forest Products Research Institute, Department of Molecular and Cell Biology, Tsukuba, Japan

1. Introduction

There are six species in the genus *Chamaecyparis* worldwide, of which two, namely the Hinoki cypress (*Chamaecyparis obtusa* Sieb. *et* Zucc.) and Sawara cypress (*Chamaecyparis pisifera* Sieb. *et* Zucc.) are distributed in Japan (Maruyama *et al.*, 2002). The Hinoki cypress is one of the most important commercial timber trees in Japan, representing about 25% of the plantation area in the country. However, the plantation areas are subject to various pests and diseases. In addition, Hinoki cypress pollinosis is reportedly one of the most serious allergic diseases in Japan (Maruyama *et al.*, 2005). The wood quality of Sawara cypress is considered inferior to Hinoki cypress, but grows faster (Fukuhara, 1978), is highly adaptable to humid and poor soils, and is considered more resistant to termite injury (Maeta, 1982) and far more tolerant to cold than the Hinoki cypress (Fukuhara, 1978). Fukuhara (1989) and Yamamoto and Fukuhara (1980) reported the possibility of obtaining natural hybrids between *C. obtusa* and *C. pisifera*.

We are interested in the development of a transgenic Japanese cypress with disease resistance and allergen-free pollen grains. Genetic engineering offers a significant tool to improve forest trees within a relatively short period. However, unfortunately, the major limitation to transformation is the difficulty in regenerating whole plants from target cells, making it vital to develop an efficient and stable plant regeneration system for genetic engineering and somatic hybridization breeding in order to develop disease-resistant hybrids. Somatic embryogenesis is an ideal procedure for effective propagation; not only of plus trees but also target tissue for genetic transformation. Since somatic embryogenesis and the plantlet regeneration of gymnosperm woody species was first reported in Norway spruce (*Picea abies* L. Karst.) (Hakman *et al.*, 1985; Chalupa, 1985; Hakman and von Arnold, 1985), studies in many other conifers have been reported (Tautorus *et al.*, 1991; Attree and Fowke, 1993; Gupta and Grob, 1995; Jain *et al.*, 1995; Hay and Charest, 1999). However, except for the *Larix* or *Picea* species and *Pinus radiata* (Lelu *et al.*, 1994a; Lelu *et al.*, 1994b; Klimaszewska *et al.*, 1997; Kong and Yeung, 1992; Kong and Yeung, 1995; Walter *et al.*, 1998), the regeneration of plants for most species is sometimes difficult or poor and effective utilization remains problematic.

In this chapter we describe a stable and efficient plant regeneration system for the Hinoki and Sawara cypress via somatic embryogenesis. The initiation of embryogenic cultures (EC), their maintenance and proliferation, maturation of somatic embryos, germination and plant conversion, and *ex vitro* acclimatization and field transfer will be discussed in subsequent sections.

2. Embryogenic culture initiation (ECI)

Immature open-pollinated cones of the Hinoki and Sawara cypress (Fig. 1A and Fig. 2A) were collected in June and July from plus mother trees. The collected cones were subsequently disinfected by 1 min immersion in 99.5% ethanol and dried in the laminar flow cabinet before dissection. The excised seeds were disinfected with 1% (w/v available chlorine) sodium hypochlorite solution for 15 min and then rinsed five times with sterile distilled water. After the seed coats had been removed, the megagametophytes containing immature zygotic embryos were used as explants for ECI initiation.

The explants were cultured in 24-well tissue culture plates (one per well) containing 1/2 MS medium (Murashige and Skoog medium)(Murashige and Skoog, 1962)(MS medium with basal salts reduced to half the standard concentration but replacing all NH_4NO_3 with 1000 mgL^{-1} glutamine) or 1/2 EM medium (Embryo Maturation medium) (Maruyama *et al.*, 2000) (EM medium with basal salts, vitamins, and myo-inositol reduced to half the standard concentration and with KCl concentration reduced to 40 mgL^{-1}), supplemented with 0.5 gL^{-1} casein hydrolysate, 1.0 gL^{-1} glutamine, 10 µM 2,4-dichlorophenoxyacetic acid (2,4-D), 5 µM 6-benzylaminopurine (BAP), 10 gL^{-1} sucrose, and 3 gL^{-1} gelrite. The pH of the media was adjusted to 5.8 prior to autoclaving for 15 min at 121°C. The cultures were kept in darkness at 25±1°C. The presence or absence of the distinct early stages of embryos characterized by an embryonal head with a suspensor system (Fig. 1C and Fig. 2C) from the explants was observed under an inverted microscope weekly for up to 3 months.

Embryogenic tissues (ET) extruding from the micropylar ends of explants appeared mostly after 2-4 weeks of culture, while the mean initiation frequency of ET from immature seeds of the Sawara cypress (Fig. 1B) varied from 12.5 to 33.3%. Initiation of ET was also possible in the absence of exogenous plant growth regulators (PGR) as reported for pine species (Smith, 1996; Lelu *et al.* 1999). In the Hinoki cypress, a medium without PGR containing 2 gL^{-1} activated charcoal (AC) was also effective for the induction of EC. The mean initiation frequencies of ET on a medium with and without PGR were 14.5 and 17.2%, respectively, which indicated that when explants are cultured at the appropriate developmental stage, the absence of exogenous PGR did not impede ECI.

The results of experiments for somatic embryogenesis initiation in both cypresses, where relatively small variations were achieved, suggested that the medium was not the most critical factor for ECI when explants were collected from late June to early July. The induction response and the beginning of germination were observed in some explants collected in mid-July. Since the physiological maturation of a seed is determined by its ability to germinate, this result indicates that the zygotic embryos from immature seeds collected in mid-July was the critical limit for ECI on a medium with no PGR. At this time, no germination was observed on PGR-supplemented medium. Among the factors influencing the somatic embryogenesis initiation, the appropriate developmental stage of zygotic embryos seemed the most critical. The optimal developmental stage for many conifer species has been reported in terms of seed collection date or time after fertilization (Becwar *et al.*, 1990; Tautorus *et al.*, 1991; Lelu *et al.*, 1994b; Jain *et al.*, 1995; Zoglauer *et al.*, 1995; Klimaszewska *et al.*, 1997; Lelu *et al.*, 1999; Kim *et al.*, 1999). However, due to the

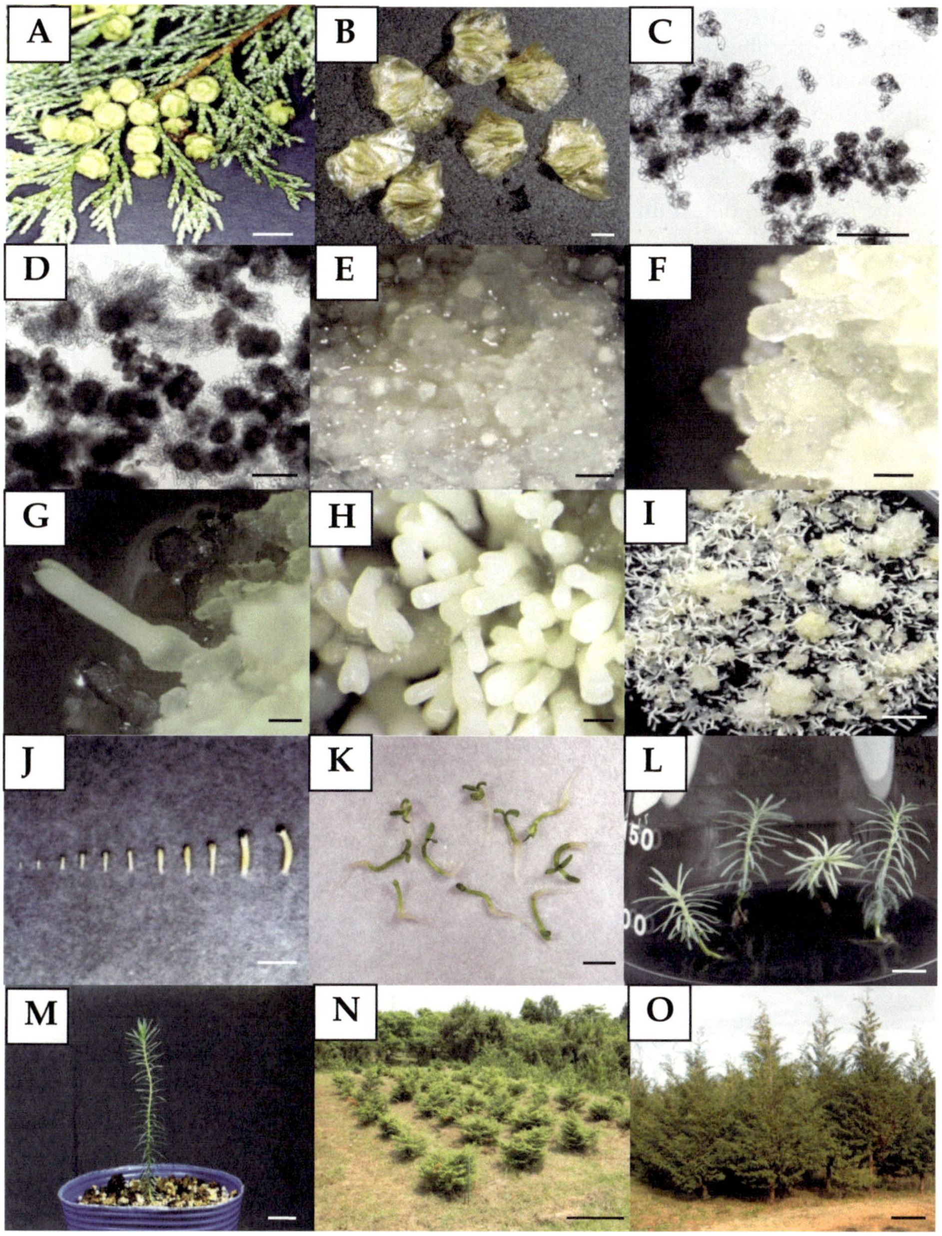

Fig. 1. Somatic embryogenesis in Sawara cypress.
A: Open-pollinated cones. B: Excised immature seeds. C: Embryogenic cells. D-F: Development of embryogenic cells. G-I: Embryo maturation. J: Different maturated embryo sizes in function to PEG concentration in maturation media. K: Germination. L: Plant conversion. M: Acclimatized plant derived from a somatic embryo. N-O: Somatic plants growing out in the field. *Bars* 1mm (B-H), 1cm (A, I-M), 1m (N-O)

difficulty in determining the precise time of fertilization in open-pollinated cones and the fact that the variation in the zygotic embryo development depends on weather and location, the criteria for explant collection for ECI cannot be easily generalized. In addition, variation in the developmental stage of embryos may be observed among trees and even the same tree when individual cones are compared. In the case of the Hinoki and Sawara cypress, most of the immature embryos collected from late June to early July seemed at the late embryogeny stage. Observation of the developmental stage of individual embryos is thus likely to be the most appropriate method to determine the optimal time for embryo selection.

In the present study, relatively high initiation frequencies were achieved for both species and almost all the initiated lines continued to proliferate, even after several years of culture, resulting in stable embryogenic lines. Sometimes however, the initiation of somatic embryogenesis may not result in the establishment of an embryogenic line because the ensuing ET ceases to proliferate, making it important to distinguish between the initial extrusion from an explants and continuous growth, when assessing the success rate (Klimaszewka *et al.*, 2007). Kim *et al.* (1999) reported that from 294 lines initiated in *Larix leptolepis*, only one embryogenic cell line could be proliferated. These results suggest that the capture of stable cell lines should be the optimal criterion by which to compare the ability of somatic embryogenesis initiation among species and families.

3. Maintenance and proliferation of embryogenic cultures

The maintenance and proliferation of EC was possible in several media containing a combination of 2,4-D plus BAP. The principal characteristics of these media were the reduction in the concentration of inorganic components from the standard and the addition of glutamine as an organic nitrogen source. The growth and proliferation of EC on media with a high concentration of inorganic components as a nitrogen source was suboptimal. These media supported growth only for short culturing whereupon the cell condition deteriorated over time. A similar response was also observed for the Japanese cedar EC (Maruyama *et al.*, 2000).

The positive effect of organic nitrogen sources in the medium on the maintenance and proliferation of EC have been reported for many species (Boulay *et al.*, 1988; Finer *et al.*, 1989; Becwar *et al.*, 1990; Gupta and Pullman, 1991; Tremblay and Tremblay, 1991; Smith, 1996; Klimaszewska and Smith, 1997). In our study, filter-sterilized glutamine in a medium combined with a reduction of the nitrate content increased the proliferation rate and the number of mature cotyledonary embryos of the Sawara cypress. In contrast, Zoglauer *et al.* (1995) reported that the continuous subculture of embryogenic suspensions of *Larix decidua* on organic nitrogen-supplemented medium resulted in a dramatic decline in the number of mature embryos obtained. Jalonen and von Arnold (1991) demonstrated the dependence of embryo maturation on the type of embryo morphology during proliferation.

In our culture routines, EC were maintained and proliferated by 2 to 3-week interval subcultures on 90-mm diameter Petri dishes containing 1/2 EM medium or 1/2 LP medium (Aitken-Christie and Thorpe, 1984) supplemented with 30 gL^{-1} sucrose, 3 μM 2,4-D, 1 μM BAP, and 1.5 gL^{-1} glutamine. These media supported the growth of the embryogenic cell lines captured. ET proliferated readily and retained their original translucent and mucilaginous appearance. The fresh weight of ET on the maintenance-proliferation medium increased about 5- to 12-fold after a 2- to 3-wk culture period. In general, solid media were used for the maintenance routine and liquid media for rapid proliferation of the cultures. The low-density subculture helped maintain suitable conditions for EC (densely embryonal head with a distinct suspensor system) in the suspension culture. Before the maturation step, about 10-20 mg FW of ET from the solid medium were transferred to a 100 mL flask containing 30-40 mL of medium (of a composition equivalent to that used for the maintenance and proliferation but without gelrite) and cultured for about 2 weeks on a rotary shaker at 50-70 rpm, in darkness at 25±1°C.

Although the initiation of ET was also possible without any additional auxin and cytokinin supplements required, exogenous PGR were found to be essential for the continuous maintenance and proliferation of ET (Fig. 2B). Conversely, the maintenance and proliferation of EC on media with no PGR was reported for *Pinus radiata* (Smith, 1996). He indicated that the use of PGR is not necessary, and that some cell lines maintained on a medium with 2,4-D and BAP lose their plant-forming potential much sooner than others, which have been maintained on a medium without PGR. However, in our experiments, the EC of Japanese cypresses maintained in the absence of PGR showed a tendency to embryo development and a decline in proliferation over time. This result was consistent with the results reported for other Japanese conifers (Maruyama *et al.*, 2000; Maruyama *et al.*, 2005; Maruyama *et al.*, 2007).

4. Maturation of somatic embryos

About 100-200 mg FW of ET suspended in 2-3 mL of medium were plated on 70-mm diameter filter paper disks over 90-mm diameter Petri dishes containing 30-40 mL of maturation medium that contained sugar, abscisic acid (ABA), AC, polyethylene glycol 4,000 (PEG), and EMM amino acids (Smith, 1996) (gL^{-1}: glutamine 7.3, asparagine 2.1, arginine 0.7, citrulline 0.079, ornithine 0.076, lysine 0.055, alanine 0.04, and proline 0.053). The petri dishes were sealed with Novix-II film (Iwaki Glass Co., Ltd., Chiba, Japan) and kept in darkness at 25±1°C for 6-12 weeks.

4.1 Effect of kind and concentration of sugar

Table 1 shows the effect of different kinds of sugar on the maturation of Sawara cypress somatic embryos. At the tested sugar concentrations, optimal results were achieved by using maltose as a carbohydrate source. Although 30 and 50 gL^{-1} did not result in any statistical difference in terms of cotyledonary embryos per Petri dish, the peak embryo maturation frequency resulted from the medium containing 50 gL^{-1} maltose with an average of 372 mature embryos. In contrast, when sucrose was used, 50 gL^{-1} resulted in a decrease of maturation frequency. Maltose has been considered a better carbohydrate and/or osmoticant source than sucrose or glucose for embryo maturation (Uddin *et al.*, 1990; Uddin, 1993). Similarly, Nørgaard and Krogstrup (1995) reported the beneficial effect of maltose for embryo maturation of *Abies* spp. A medium containing maltose as a carbohydrate source and PEG as osmoticum was reported as an effective combination to enhance somatic embryo maturation in the Loblolly pine (Li *et al.*, 1998). These authors inferred that about a 10-fold enhancement was achieved by using maltose to replace sucrose, and that the morphology of cotyledonary embryos was improved. In our results, the morphologies of cotyledonary embryos induced on the medium with sucrose or maltose were relatively similar. The main difference came in terms of the embryo maturation efficiency.

Kind of sugar	Concentration of sugar	
	30 gL^{-1}	50 gL^{-1}
Sucrose	108 B	158 B
Maltose	316 A	387 A

[1] Cotyledonary embryos per Petri dish. Means followed by same letter are not significantly different at $p < 0.05$. Three dishes for each treatment were used.

Table 1. Effect of kind and concentration of sugar on maturation of Sawara cypress somatic embryos[1]

4.2 Effects of ABA and AC

Table 2 showed the beneficial effect of increased ABA content in media supplemented with AC on the maturation of Sawara cypress somatic embryos. The best result was achieved with 100 μM ABA in the presence of AC, obtaining an average of 348 cotyledonary embryos per petri dish. The higher the ABA concentration, the greater the number of mature embryos. A similar result was reported in *Pinus strobus* (Klimaszewska and Smith, 1997), *Picea glauca-engelmannii* complex (Roberts *et al.*, 1990a), and *P. glauca* (Dunstan *et al.*, 1991). The addition of AC into the media notably enhanced the maturation efficiency, with around a 4-fold enhancement achieved by using 33.3 to 100 μM in combination with 2 gL^{-1} AC. Pullman and Gupta (1991) reported further improved Loblolly pine embryo development using a combination of ABA and AC, while Gupta *et al.* (1995) reported further improved quality of cotyledonary embryos of Douglas-fir (*Pseudotsuga menziesii*) by a combination of ABA, AC, and PEG. Similarly, Lelu-Walter el al. (2006) indicated that coating the cells with AC reduced ET proliferation and significantly enhanced the maturation of maritime pine somatic embryos. AC is widely used in tissue culture media, where it is believed to function as an adsorbent for toxic metabolic products and residual hormones (von Aderkas *et al.*, 2002; Pullman and Gupta, 1991).

ABA-free media or those supplemented with a low concentration (10 μM) failed to stimulate appropriate embryo maturation, producing only a few mature cotyledonary embryos (Table 2). Embryogenic cells on media without ABA did not develop beyond the embryo stage 1, as described elsewhere (von Arnold and Hakman, 1988). Most of the proembryos arrested development, with the proliferation of EC evident. Lelu *et al.* (1999) reported that mature embryos of *Pinus sylvestris* and *P. pinaster* were produced in far higher numbers and that the development of cotyledonary somatic embryos versus abnormal, shooty ones was enhanced with the addition of 60 μM ABA in comparison with media without ABA. Somatic embryos of the hybrid larch (*Larix x leptoeuropaea*) developed normally on a medium supplemented with 60 μM ABA, but abnormally on a medium with no ABA (Gutmann *et al.*, 1996). Most of the studies on somatic embryogenesis in conifers have reported ABA as a key hormone in embryo development and that the number and quality of embryo produced was vastly reduced in its absence (Durzan and Gupta, 1987; von Arnold and Hakman, 1988; Hakman and von Arnold, 1988; Attree and Fowke, 1993; Dunstan *et al.*, 1998).

ABA (μM)	AC (0 gL^{-1})	AC (2 gL^{-1})
0	1 D	3 D
10	7 D	16 D
33.3	48 CD	178 B
100	84 C	348 A

[1] Cotyledonary embryos per Petri dish. Means followed by same letter are not significantly different at $p < 0.05$. Three dishes for each treatment were used.

Table 2. Effect of ABA and AC on maturation of Sawara cypress somatic embryos [1]

Several authors have suggested that the role of ABA in somatic embryogenesis is to inhibit cleavage polyembryony with the consequent development of individual somatic embryos (Durzan and Gupta, 1987; Boulay *et al.*, 1988; Krogstrup *et al.*, 1988; Gupta *et al.*, 1991), to stimulate the accumulation of nutrients, lipids, proteins, and carbohydrates (Hakman and von Arnold, 1988), and suppress precocious germination (Roberts *et al.*, 1990a). In addition, Gupta *et al.* (1993) reported improved desiccation tolerance to less than 10% water content with 80 to 90% germination rates in Norway spruce embryos produced with a combination of ABA and AC. The use of ABA for somatic embryo maturation in gymnosperms is extensively reported in the compilation of Jain *et al.* (1995).

4.3 Effect of PEG

As shown in Table 3, the addition of PEG stimulated the mature embryo production of Sawara cypress (Fig.1D-I), with a higher concentration of PEG in the medium resulting in a higher maturation frequency. The best result was obtained at a concentration of 150 gL^{-1} with an average number of 1,043 cotyledonary embryos collected per Petri dish, in comparison with 382, 215, and 13 embryos per dish at concentrations of 75, 50, and 0 gL^{-1}, respectively. In the absence of PEG, most of the proembryos did not develop into cotyledonary embryos. Embryogenic cell proliferation was evident and most of them developed into structures consisting of small embryonal heads from which elongated suspensors extended (stage 1 somatic embryos).

Although in recent years, several studies have reported promotion of the maturation of somatic embryos by the addition of ABA into media solidified with a high concentration of gellan gum (gelrite) in the absence of PEG (Klimaszewska and Smith, 1997; Lelu *et al.*, 1999), the use of PEG in combination with ABA has become routine for stimulating somatic embryo maturation in many gymnosperms. In our study, a high concentration of gellan gum in the absence of PEG was not effective in promoting the somatic embryo maturation of Hinoki and Sawara cypress as described above (data not shown). In contrast, some authors have reported that PEG promotes maturation but inhibits the further development of *Picea glauca* (Kong and Yeung, 1995) and *P. abies* somatic embryos (Bozhkov and von Arnold, 1998). The results of our experiments indicated that the positive effect of PEG on maturation did not inhibit the further development of somatic embryos in Japanese cypresses. Almost all mature cotyledonary embryos germinated (Fig. 1K) and developed normal plants (Fig. 1L). The beneficial effect of PEG on embryo maturation may be related to a water stress induction similar to that generated by desiccation (Attree and Fowke, 1993), to an increase in the accumulation of storage reserves, such as storage proteins, lipids, and polypeptides (Roberts *et al.*, 1990a; Attree *et al.*, 1992; Misra *et al.*, 1993), and to a tolerance to water loss (Attree *et al.*, 1991).

Morphological differences among somatic embryos of Sawara cypress obtained on media supplemented with different concentrations of PEG was restricted to size (Fig. 1J). The higher the PEG concentration, the smaller the resulting embryos (Table 3). However, the embryo size was not found to be influential in germination and subsequently plant conversion. Cotyledonary embryos germinated and converted in plants at high frequencies independent of their size (Table 3). More compact PEG-treated embryos were also reported for *Larix laricina* (Klimaszewska *et al.*, 1997) and *Picea abies* (Find, 1997). Iraki *et al.* (1989) reported that small cell size was a typical symptom of PEG-induced osmotic stress. Low external osmotic potential may have led to alterations in the cell wall composition, decreasing the ratio of cellulose to hemicellulose. This results in decreased cell wall tensile strength and the reduced ability of cells to expand (Iraki *et al.*, 1989). Therefore, the presence of PEG in the maturation medium may have influenced the subsequent growth of somatic embryos. Bozhkov and von Arnold (1998) determined that the morphology of mature somatic embryos of *Picea abies* had changed after PEG-treatment (smaller, irregularly shaped embryos, smaller cell size, larger root caps with intercellular spaces in pericolumn, degraded quiescent center), which could further restrict the embryo growth. However, in our study the subsequent development of PEG-treated embryos was no different to untreated ones. Germination frequencies and plant conversion rates of Sawara cypress were similar in somatic embryos derived from different PEG-treated media (Table 3).

PEG (gL^{-1})	Somatic embryos	Size range (mm)	Germination (%)	Conversion (%)
0	13 C	3-10	97 A	92 A
50	215 BC	2- 8	98 A	93 A
75	382 B	2- 6	97 A	93
150	1,043 A	1- 3	97 A	92 A

[1] Cotyledonary embryos per Petri dish. Means followed by same letter are not significantly different at $p < 0.05$. Three dishes for each PEG concentration were used.

Table 3. Effect of PEG concentration in maturation media on production, size, germination and plant conversion of Sawara cypress somatic embryos [1]

The development of a proembryo mass of Hinoki cypress was encouraged by the transfer of EC onto a PGR free-medium. Cells developed gradually to form an individual and compact mass showing the early stages of somatic embryos going to a mature stage (Fig. 2D-E). Embryo maturation was induced by the transfer of cultures onto a medium containing maltose, PEG, AC, ABA and a higher concentration of amino acids. The embryos continue to develop and after 3-4 weeks of culture the initial formation of the cotyledonary embryo was observed (Fig. 2F). For most cell lines, the development of somatic embryos to the cotyledonary stage was observed after about 6-8 weeks of culture (Fig. 2G).

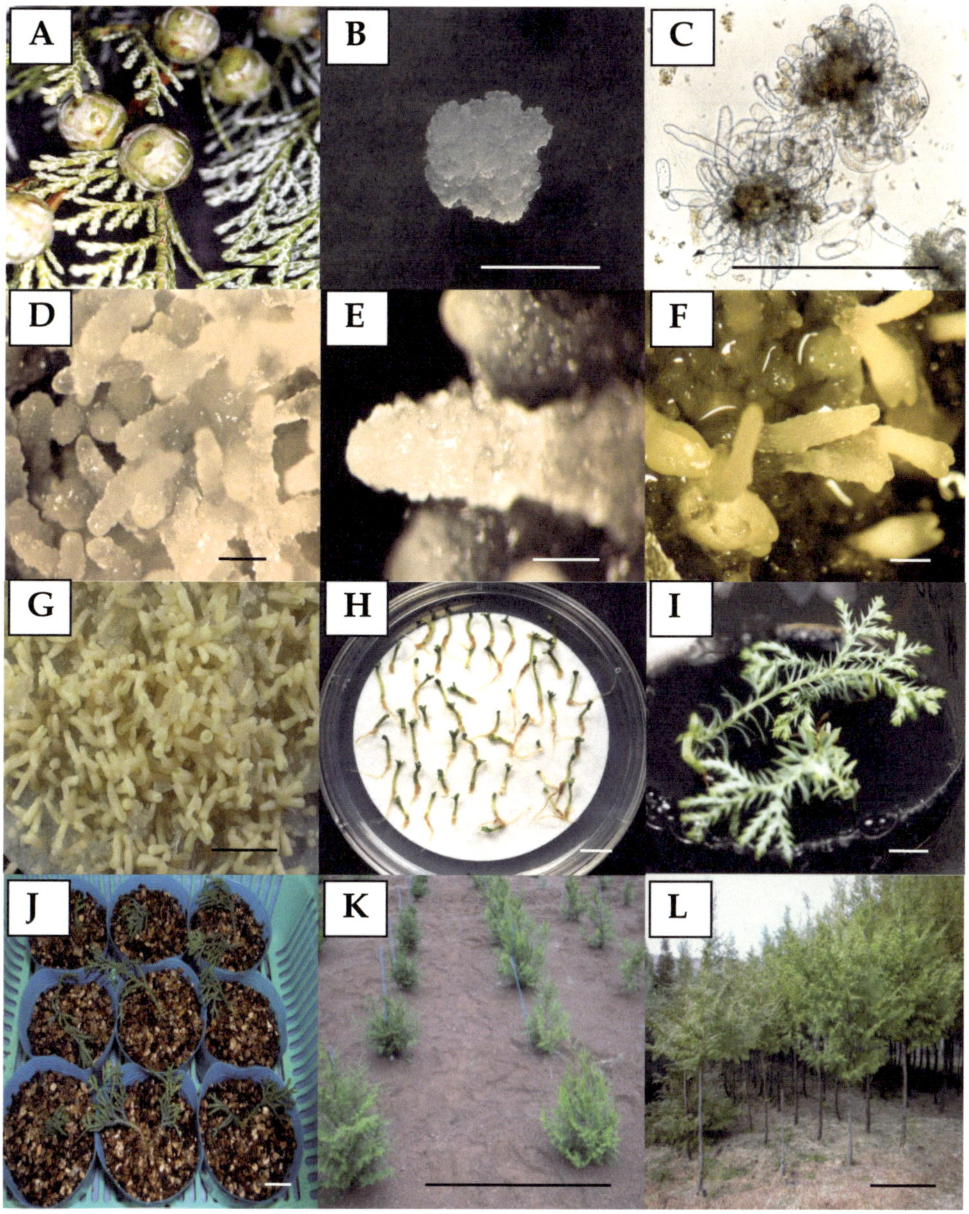

Fig. 2. Somatic embryogenesis in Hinoki cypress. A: Collected open-pollinated cones. B: Proliferation of induced embryogenic tissue on medium containing auxin and cytokinin. C: Embryogenic cells. D-F: Different developmental maturation stages of somatic embryos. G: Production of somatic embryos. H: Germination of somatic embryos. I: Plantlets growing *in vitro*. J: Acclimatized plants derived from somatic embryos. K-L: Somatic plants growing out in the field. *Bars* 1mm (C-F), 1cm (A-B, G-J), 1m (K-L)

Cell line	Total number of somatic embryos	Number of somatic embryos per Petri dish (Mean ± SE [1])	Germination frequency (%) (germinants/total tested)	Conversion frequency (%) (plants/total tested)
HNO7-1	1403	467.7 ± 21.3	94 (659/700)	91 (637/700)
HNO7-2	32	10.7 ± 1.2	50 (5/10)	40 (4/10)
HNO7-3	450	150.0 ± 15.0	82 (41/50)	78 (39/50)
HNO7-4	312	104.0 ± 18.6	83 (33/40)	80 (32/40)
HH2-1	47	15.7 ± 4.3	80 (8/10)	80 (8/10)
HH2-2	30	10.0 ± 1.7	70 (7/10)	70 (7/10)
HN1-1	54	18.0 ± 5.7	50 (5/10)	40 (4/10)
HN1-2	57	19.0 ± 3.8	76 (38/50)	72 (36/50)
HHA2-1	1536	512.0 ± 34.8	93 (219/236)	91 (215/236)
HHA2-2	188	62.7 ± 22.6	86 (43/50)	80 (40/50)
HHA2-5	14	4.7 ± 1.2	70 (7/10)	60 (6/10)
HHA2-6	1724	574.7 ± 78.3	94 (317/336)	92 (308/336)
HF4-1	565	188.3 ± 34.6	95 (123/130)	94 (122/130)
HF4-11	12	4.0 ± 2.1	NT[2]	NT
HF4-15	170	56.7 ± 9.0	98 (47/48)	96 (46/48)
HF4-19	181	60.3 ± 11.8	90 (18/20)	90 (18/20)
HF4-21	7	2.3 ± 1.9	NT	NT
HK7-17	4	1.3 ± 0.9	NT	NT
HK7-25	209	69.7 ± 11.0	93 (28/30)	93 (28/30)
HK7-29	8	2.7 ± 1.5	NT	NT
HK7-30	1511	503.7 ± 86.0	100 (130/130)	100 (130/130)
HK7-33	1052	350.7 ± 47.7	99 (286/290)	97 (280/290)
HK7-39	33	11.0 ± 1.0	70 (7/10)	60 (6/10)
HK7-45	19	6.2 ± 1.9	50 (5/10)	50 (5/10)
HK7-46	3	1.0 ± 0.6	NT	NT
HK7-57	280	93.3 ± 19.3	98 (41/42)	95 (40/42)
HK7-58	10	3.3 ± 0.3	NT	NT
HK7-60	18	6.0 ± 2.6	NT	NT
HK7-72	10	3.3 ± 1.9	NT	NT
HK7-75	1428	476.0 ± 56.0	100 (50/50)	100 (50/50)
HK7-83	7	2.3 ± 1.5	NT	NT
HK7-88	30	10.0 ± 5.1	NT	NT
HK7-105	66	22.0 ± 6.2	NT	NT
HK7-107	66	22.0 ± 1.5	60 (6/10)	60 (6/10)
Total	11536	113.1±18.1	93 (2123/2282)	91 (2067/2282)

[1]SE: standard errors of means of 3 replicates for each cell line
[2]NT: non-tested

Table 4. Somatic embryo production, germination and plant conversion for 34 cell lines of Hinoki cypress

Mature cotyledonary embryos were produced in 34 of 50 embryogenic cells lines tested (68%), and the mean number of somatic embryos per Petri dish produced varied from 1 to 575 (Table 4). This result indicates that the potential to develop cotyledonary somatic embryos varied among the cell lines. Similar results were reported for the Japanese cedar (Igasaki *et al.*, 2003), maritime pine (Ramarosandratana *et al.*, 2001; Miguel *et al.*, 2004; Lelu-Walter *et al.*, 2006), and Japanese pines (Maruyama *et al.*, 2005; Maruyama *et al.*, 2007).

5. Germination and plant conversion

Mature cotyledonary somatic embryos were collected from the maturation medium and transferred to the germination medium (1/2 LP or a 1/2 EM PGR free-medium with 2 gL^{-1} AC and 10 gL^{-1} agar). Cultures were kept at 25±1°C under a photon flux density of about 65 $\mu mol\ m^{-2}s^{-1}$ with cooling and fluorescent lamps for 16 h daily.

The start of germination (Fig. 2H) was observed as early as 3-5 days after transfer to the germination medium, and after 2-4 weeks of culture, most of the somatic embryos germinated and were converted into plantlets. The mature cotyledonary somatic embryos from 23 embryogenic cell lines of the Hinoki cypress were tested, with mean germination and plantlet conversion frequencies of 93 and 91%, respectively (Table 4). This result was similar to that achieved for the Sawara cypress (Table 3). No morphological difference among the germinants and plantlets was observed among the genotypes.

Regenerated emblings of Hinoki (Fig. 2I) and Sawara cypress (Fig. 1L) were transferred to 300 ml flasks containing 100 mL of fresh medium (same composition used for the germination and conversion but with 30 gL^{-1} sucrose and 5 gL^{-1} AC) and kept under the same conditions described above for 8-12 weeks before *ex vitro* acclimatization.

6. *Ex vitro* acclimatization and field transfer

The developed emblings of the Hinoki (Fig.2J) and Sawara cypress (Fig.1M) were transplanted into plastic pots filled with vermiculite and acclimatized in plastic boxes inside a growth cabinet. During the first 2 weeks, emblings were kept under high relative humidity by covering the plastic boxes with transparent plastic covers and irrigating with tap water. Subsequently, the cover was gradually opened and the pots were fertilized with a nutrient solution modified from Nagao (1983) containing in mgL^{-1}: NH_4NO_3 143, $NaH_2PO_4 \cdot 2H_2O$ 55.1, KCl 47.1, $CaCl_2 \cdot 2H_2O$ 52.5, $MgSO_4 \cdot 7H_2O$ 61, Fe-III EDTA 25, Cu EDTA 0.1, Mn EDTA 0.1, Zinc EDTA 0.1, H_3BO_3 1.5, KI 0.01, $CoCl_2 \cdot 6H_2O$ 0.005, and MoO_3 0.005. The covers were completely removed about 4 weeks after transplanting. Survival rates ranging from 90 to 100% were achieved after acclimatization. Subsequently, the acclimatized plants were transferred to a greenhouse and grown under controlled conditions for 6-8 months before transplanting to the field. No indication of any morphological abnormality was reported, and the growth of established plants is currently being monitored in the field (Fig. 1N-O and Fig. 2K-L).

7. Concluding remarks

An effective plant regeneration system has been achieved for Japanese cypresses via the specified procedure. In addition to high somatic embryo maturation efficiency, the subsequent high germination and plant conversion frequencies attained demonstrated the high quality of the somatic embryos produced. These somatic embryos have a zygotic embryo-like morphology, are generally longer than they are wide, with radial symmetry, and have the ability to produce normal plants like the zygotic one. The maturation frequency and the quality of embryo produced are the key criteria for the optimization of an efficient plant regeneration system via somatic embryogenesis. The cotyledonary somatic embryos of the Hinoki and Sawara cypress readily germinated after transfer to a PGR-free medium without any kind of post-maturation treatment, as was previously reported as necessary to promote the germination of somatic embryos of some other species (Roberts *et al.*, 1990b; Roberts *et al.*, 1991; Kong and Yeung, 1992; Kong and Yeung, 1995; Jones and van Staden, 2001). Thus, most of the germinants developed epycotyl and grew into normal plants. The present system should permit, in the near future, the large-scale clonal propagation of selected trees and the genetic engineering of Japanese cypresses.

8. References

Aitken-Christie, J. and Thorpe, T, A. (1984) Clonal Propagation: Gymnosperms. *In* Cell Culture and Somatic Cell Genetics of Plants, Vol. 1., Vasil, I.K. (Ed.), 480pp, Academic Press Inc., San Diego, 82-95.

Attree, S.M. and Fowke, L.C. (1993) Somatic embryogenesis and synthetic seeds of conifers. Plant Cell Tiss. Org. Cult., 35: 1-35.

Attree, S.M., Moore, D., Sawhney, V.K., and Fowke, L.C. (1991) Enhanced maturation and desiccation tolerance of white spruce [*Picea glauca* (Moench) Voss] somatic embryos: effects of a non-plasmolysing water stress and abscisic acid. Ann. Bot., 68: 519-525.

Attree, S.M., Pomeroy, M.K., and Fowke, L.C. (1992) Manipulation of conditions for the culture of somatic embryos of white spruce for improved triacylglycerol biosynthesis and desiccation tolerance. Planta, 187: 395-404.

Becwar, M.R., Nagmani, R., and Wann, S.R. (1990) Initiation of embryogenic cultures and somatic embryo development in loblolly pine (*Pinus taeda*). Can. J. For. Res., 20: 810-817.

Boulay, M.P., Gupta, P.K., Krogstrup, P., and Durzan, D.J. (1988) Development of somatic embryos from cell suspension cultures of Norway spruce (*Picea abies* Karst.). Plant Cell Rep., 7: 134-137.

Bozhkov, P.V. and von Arnold, S. (1998) Polyethylene glycol promotes maturation but inhibits further development of *Picea abies* somatic embryos. Physiol. Plant., 104: 211-224.

Chalupa, V. (1985) Somatic embryogenesis and plantlet regeneration from cultured immature and mature embryos of *Picea abies* (L.). Karst. Communi. Inst. For. Cech., 14: 57-63.

Dunstan, D.I., Bekkaoui, F., Pilon, M., Fowke, L.C., and Abrams, S.R. (1998) Effects of abscisic acid and analogues on the maturation of white spruce (*Picea glauca*) somatic embryos. Plant Sci., 58: 77-84.

Dunstan, D.I., Bethune, T.D., and Abrams, S.R. (1991) Racemic abscisic acid and abscisyl alcohol promote maturation of white spruce (*Picea glauca*) somatic embryos. Plant Sci., 76: 219-228.

Durzan, D.J. and Gupta, P.K. (1987) Somatic embryogenesis and polyembryogenesis in Douglas-fir cell suspension cultures. Plant Sci., 52: 229-235.

Find, J.I. (1997) Changes in endogenous ABA levels in developing somatic embryos of Norway spruce (*Picea abies* [L.] Karts.) in relation to maturation medium, desiccation and germination. Plant Sci., 128: 75-83.

Finer, J.J., Kriebel, H.B., and Becwar, M.R. (1989) Initiation of embryogenic callus and suspension cultures of easter white pine (*Pinus strobus* L.). Plant Cell Rep., 8: 203-206.

Fukuhara, N. (1978) Meiotic observation in the pollen mother cell of interspecific hybrid between *Chamaecyparis obtusa* and *C. pisifera*. J. Jpn. For. Soc., 60: 437-441.

Fukuhara, N. (1989) Fertility in interspecific-crossing between hinoki (*Chamaecyparis obtusa* Endl.) and Sawara (*C. pisifera* Endl.) and identification of the hybrids. Bulletin of the Forestry and Forest Products Research Institute, 354: 1-38.

Gupta, P.K. and Grob, J.A. (1995) Somatic embryogenesis in conifers. *In* Somatic embryogenesis in woody plants, Vol. 1., Jain, S.M. *et al.* (Eds.), 460pp, Kluwer Academic Publishers, Netherlands, 81-89.

Gupta, P.K. and Pullman, G.S. (1991) Method for reproducing coniferous plants by somatic embryogenesis using abscisic acid and osmotic potential variation. United States Patent # 5,036,007.

Gupta, P.K., Pullman, G., Timmis, R., Kreitinger, M., Carlson, W., Grob, J., and Welty, E. (1993) Forestry in the 21st century: The biotechnology of somatic embryogenesis. Bio/Technology, 11: 454-459.

Gupta, P.K., Timmis, R., Timmis, K.A., Carlson, W.C., and Welty, E.D.E. (1995) Somatic embryogenesis in Douglas-fir (*Pseudotsuga menziessi*). *In* Somatic Embryogenesis in Woody Plants, Vol. 3, Gymnosperms. Jain, S.M., Gupta, P.K., and Newton, R. (Eds.), 388pp, Kluwer Academic Publishers, Netherlands, 303-313.

Gutmann, M., von Aderkas, P., Label, P., and Lelu, M.-A. (1996) Effects of abscisic acid on somatic embryo maturation of hybrid larch. J. Exp. Bot., 35: 1905-1917.

Hakman, I., Fowke, L.C., von Arnold, S., and Eriksson, T. (1985) The development of somatic embryos in tissue cultures initiated from immature embryos of *Picea abies* (Norway spruce). Plant Sci., 38: 53-59.

Hakman, I. and von Arnold, S. (1985) Plantlet regeneration through somatic embryos in *Picea abies* (Norway spruce). J. Plant Physiol., 121: 149-158.

Hakman, I. and von Arnold, S. (1988) Somatic embryogenesis and plant regeneration from suspension cultures of *Picea glauca* (white spruce). Physiol. Plant., 72: 579-587.

Hay, E.I. and Charest, P.J. (1999) Somatic embryo germination and desiccation tolerance in conifers. *In* Somatic Embryogenesis in Woody Plants, Vol. 4. Jain, S.M. *et al.* (ed), 547 pp, Kluwer Academic Publishers, Dordrecht, 61-96.

Igasaki, T., Sato, T., Akashi, N., Mohri, T., Maruyama, E., Kinoshita, I., Walter, C., Shinohara, K. (2003) Somatic embryogenesis and plant regeneration from immature zygotic embryos of *Cryptomeria japonica* D. Don. Plant Cell Rep., 22: 239-243.

Iraki, N.M., Bressan, R.A., Hasegawa, P.M., and Carpita, N.C. (1989) Alteration of the physical and chemical structure of the primary cell wall of growth-limited plant cells adapted to osmotic stress. Plant Physiol., 91: 39-47.

Jain, S.M., Gupta, P.K., and Newton, R. (1995) Somatic embryogenesis in woody plants, Vol. 3, Gymnosperms, 388 pp. Kluwer Academic Publishers, Netherlands.

Jalonen, P. and von Arnold, S. (1991) Characterization of embryogenic cell lines of *Picea abies* in relation to their competence for maturation. Plan Cell Rep., 10: 384-387.

Jones, N.B. and van Staden, J. (2001) Improved somatic embryo production from embryogenic tissue of *Pinus patula*. In Vitro Cell. Dev. Biol.-Plant, 37:543-549

Kim, Y.W., Youn, Y., Noh, E.R., and Kim, J.C. (1999) Somatic embryogenesis and plant regeneration from immature zygotic embryos of Japanese larch (*Larix leptolepis*). Plant Cell Tiss. Org. Cult., 55: 95-101.

Klimaszewska, K., Devantier, Y., Lachance, D., Lelu, M.-A., and Charest, P.J. (1997) *Larix laricina* (tamarack): somatic embryogenesis and genetic transformation. Can. J. For. Res., 27: 538-550.

Klimaszewska, K. and Smith, D.R. (1997) Maturation of somatic embryos of *Pinus strobus* is promoted by a high concentration of gellam gum. Physiol. Plant., 100: 949-957.

Klimaszewska, K., Trontin, J-F., Becwar M.R., Devillard, C., Park, Y-S., Lelu-Walter, M-A. (2007) Recent progress in somatic embryogenesis of four *Pinus* spp. Tree and Forestry Science and Biotechnology, 1:11-25.

Kong, L. and Yeung, E. (1992) Development of white spruce somatic embryos: II. Continual shoot meristem development during germination. *In vitro* Cell. Dev. Biol., 28P: 125-131.

Kong, L. and Yeung, E. (1995) Effects of silver nitrate and polyethylene glycol on white spruce (*Picea glauca*) somatic embryo development: enhancing cotyledonary embryo formation and endogenous ABA content. Physiol. Plant., 93: 298-304.

Krogstrup, P., Eriksen, E.N., Moller, J.D., and Roulund, H. (1988) Somatic embryogenesis in Sitka spruce (*Picea sitchensis* (Bong.) Carr.). Plant Cell Rep., 7: 594-597.

Lelu, M.-A., Bastien, C., Drugeault, A., Gouez, M.-L., and Klimaszewska, K. (1999) Somatic embryogenesis and plantlet development in *Pinus sylvestris* and *Pinus pinaster* on medium with and without growth regulators. Physiol. Plant., 105: 719-728.

Lelu, M.-A., Bastien, C., Klimaszewska, K., and Charest, P.J. (1994a) An improved method for somatic plantlet production in hybrid larch (*Larix* x *leptoeuropaea*). Part 2. Control of germination and plantlet development. Plant Cell Tiss. Org. Cult., 36:117-127.

Lelu, M.-A., Bastien, C., Klimaszewska, K., Ward, C., and Charest, P.J. (1994b) An improved method for somatic plantlet production in hybrid larch (*Larix* x *leptoeuropaea*). Part 1. Somatic embryo maturation. Plant Cell Tiss. Org. Cult., 36:107-115.

Lelu-Walter, M.A., Bernier-Cardou, M., and Klimaszewska, K. (2006) Simplified and improved somatic embryogenesis for clonal propagation of *Pinus pinaster*. Plant Cell Rep., 25:767-776.

Li, X.Y., Huang, F.H., Murphy, J.B., and Gbur, E.E.JR. (1998) Polyethylene glycol and maltose enhance somatic embryo maturation in loblolly pine (*Pinus taeda* L.). *In vitro* Cell. Dev. Bio.-Plant, 34: 22-26.

Maeta, T. (1982) Effects of gamma-rays irradiation on interspecific hybridization between *Chamaecyparis obtusa* S. et Z. and *C. pisifera* S. et Z. Hoshasen Ikusyujo Kenkyu Hokoku 5: 1-87 (in Japanese).

Maruyama, E., Hosoi, Y., and Ishii, K. (2002) Somatic embryogenesis in Sawara cypress (*Chamaecyparis pisifera* Sieb. et Zucc.) for stable and efficient plant regeneration, propagation and protoplast culture. J. For. Res., 7: 23-34.

Maruyama, E., Hosoi, Y., and Ishii, K. (2003) Somatic embryo culture for propagation, artificial seed production, and conservation of Sawara cypress (*Chamaecyparis pisifera* Sieb. et Zucc.). J. For. Res., 8: 1-8.

Maruyama, E., Hosoi, Y., and Ishii, K. (2005) Somatic embryo production and plant regeneration of Japanese black pine (*Pinus thunbergii*). J. For. Res., 10: 403-407.

Maruyama, E., Hosoi, Y., and Ishii, K. (2007) Somatic embryogenesis and plant regeration in yakutanegoyou, *Pinus armandii* Franch. var. *amamiana* (Koidz.) Hatusima, an endemic and endangered species in Japan. In Vitro Cell. Dev. Biol.-Plant, 43:28-34.

Maruyama, E., Ishii, K., and Hosoi, Y. (2005) Efficient plant regeneration of Hinoki cypress (*Chamaecyparis obtusa*) via somatic embryogenesis. J. For. Res., 10:73-77.

Maruyama, E., Tanaka, T., Hosoi, Y., Ishii, K., and Morohoshi, N. (2000) Embryogenic cell culture, protoplast regeneration, cryopreservation, biolistic gene transfer and plant regeneration in Japanese cedar (*Cryptomeria japonica* D. Don). Plant Biotechnology, 17: 281-296.

Miguel, C., Gonçalves, S., Tereso, S., Marum, L., Maroco, J., and Olivera, M.M. (2004) Somatic embryogenesis from 20 open-pollinated families of Portuguese plus trees of maritime pine. Plant Cell Tiss. Orga.Cult., 76:121-130.

Misra, S., Attree, S.M., Leal, I., and Fowke, L.C. (1993) Effects of abscisic acid, osmoticum and desiccation on synthesis of proteins during the development of white spruce somatic embryos. Ann. Bot., 71: 11-22.

Murashige, T. and Skoog, F. (1962) A revised medium for rapid growth and bioassays with tobacco cultures. Physiol. Plant., 15: 473-497.

Nagao, A. (1983) Differences of flower initiation of *Cryptomeria japonica* under various alternating temperatures. J. Jap. For. Soc., 65: 335-338 (in Japanese).

Nørgaard, J.V. and Krogstrup, P. (1995) Somatic embryogenesis in *Abies* spp. *In* Somatic Embryogenesis in Woody Plants, Vol. 3, Gymnosperms. Jain, S.M., Gupta, P.K., and Newton, R. (Eds.), 388pp, Kluwer Academic Publishers, Netherlands, 341-355.

Pullman, G.S. and Gupta, P.K. (1991) Method for reproducing coniferous plants by somatic embryogenesis using absorbent materials in the development stage media. U.S. Patent No. 5,034,326.

Ramarosandratana, A., Harvengt, L., Bouvet, A., Calvayrac, R., and Pâques, M. (2001) Effect of carbohydrate source, polyethylene glycol and gellum gum concentration on embryonal-suspensor mass (ESM) proliferation and maturation of maritime pine somatic embryos. In Vitro Cell. Dev. Biol.-Plant., 37:29-34.

Roberts, D.R., Flinn, B.S., Webb, D.T., Webster, F.B., and Sutton, B.C.S. (1990a) Abscisic acid and indole-3-butyric acid regulation of maturation and accumulation of storage proteins in somatic embryos of interior spruce. Physiol. Plant., 78: 355-360.

Roberts, D.R., Lazaroff, W.R., and Webster, F.B. (1991) Interaction between maturation and high relative humidity treatments and their effects on germination of Sitka spruce somatic embryos. J. Plant Physiol., 138: 1-6.

Roberts, D.R., Sutton, B.C.S., and Flinn, B.S. (1990b) Synchronous and high frequency germination of interior spruce somatic embryos following partial drying at high relative humidity. Can. J. Bot., 68: 1086-1090.

Smith, D.R. (1996) Growth medium. U. S. Patent No. 5,565,455.

Tautorus, T.E., Fowke, L.C., and Dunstan, D.I. (1991) Somatic embryogenesis in conifers. Can. J. Bot., 69: 1873-1899.

Tremblay, l. and Tremblay, F.M. (1991) Carbohydrate requirements for the development of black spruce (*Picea mariana*) and red spruce (*P. rubens*) somatic embryos, Plant Cell Tiss. Org. Cult., 27: 95-103.

Uddin, M. (1993) Somatic embryogenesis in Gymnosperms. U.S. Patent No. 5,187,092.

Uddin, M.R., Dinus, R.J., and Webb, D.T. (1990) Effects of different carbohydrates on maturation of *Pinus taeda* somatic embryos. Abstracts VII International Congress on Plant Tissue and Cell Culture, Amsterdam, Netherlands, p. 272.

von Aderkas, P., Label P., and Lelu, M.A. (2002) Charcoal effects on early developmental and hormonal levels of somatic embryos of hybrid larch. Tree Physiology, 22:431-434.

von Arnold, S., and Hakman, I. (1988) Regulation of somatic developments in *Picea abies* by abscisic acid (ABA). J. Plant Physiol., 132:164-169.

Walter, C., Grace, L.J., Wagner, A., White, D.W.R., Walden, A.R., Donaldson, S.S., Hinton, H., Gardner, R.C., Smith, D.R. (1998) Stable transformation and regeneration of transgenic plants of *Pinus radiata* D. Don. Plant Cell Rep., 17: 460-468.

Yamamoto, Ch. and Fukuhara, N. (1980) Cone and seed yields after open-, self-, intraspecific-, and interspecific-pollinations in *Chamaecyparis obtusa* (Sieb. et Zucc.) Endl. and *C. pisifera* (Sieb. et Zucc.) Endl. Bulletin of the Forestry and Forest Products Research Institute, 311: 65-92.

Zoglauer, K., Dembny, H., Behrendt, U., and Korlach, J. (1995) Developmental patterns and regulating factors in direct somatic embryogenesis of European larch (*Larix decidua* Mill.). Med. Fac. Landbouww. Univ. Gent, 60: 1627-1636.

19

Mechanisms of Lumen Development in *Drosophila* Tubular Organs

Na Xu[1,2,*], Carolyn Pirraglia[1,*], Unisha Patel[1] and Monn Monn Myat[1]
[1]*Department of Cell and Developmental Biology, Weill Medical College of Cornell University, New York*
[2]*Department of Cell Biology, Albert Einstein College of Medicine, New York*
USA

1. Introduction

Tubular organs of both invertebrate and vertebrate animals serve many important physiological functions, such as the delivery of gases, nutrients and hormones and removal of waste. All tubular organs contain a central lumen that is formed through a variety of mechanisms and whose size and shape is essential for organ function. While some lumens form from pre-polarized cells, others form *de novo* from single cells or solid cords of cells (Andrew and Ewald, 2010). Studies of lumen formation in tubular organs in the *Drosophila* embryo have benefited from the genetic analysis available in *Drosophila* and the advent of sophisticated microscopic techniques that allow lumen formation to be visualized *in vivo* in real time in a developing embryo. In this chapter we will review recent advances on the cellular and molecular mechanisms by which lumens form and their size is controlled in the salivary gland, trachea and dorsal vessel of the *Drosophila melanogaster* embryo.

2. Dorsal vessel

The *Drosophila* cardiac tube, or dorsal vessel, is a hemolymph pumping organ that constitutes the entire cardiovascular system of the *Drosophila* open circulatory system. The dorsal vessel is established during embryogenesis and is composed of two rows of 52 contractile myoendothelial cells (cardioblasts [CBs]) enclosing a central lumen surrounded by loosely attached non-muscular pericardial cells (Figure 1A and B) (Tao and Schulz, 2007). The dorsal vessel is derived from mesodermal cells that acquire certain epithelial characteristics to form two bilateral rows of CBs that migrate dorsally and meet at the dorsal midline to create a lumen exclusively formed by the membrane walls of the CBs (Figure 1B). At the end of cardiac morphogenesis, the posterior portion of the dorsal vessel becomes enlarged and constitutes the definitive heart, whereas the anterior portion has a narrow diameter and is equivalent to the aorta (Figure 1A). The heart is the only region of the dorsal vessel that exhibits automatic and synchronized beating to act as a myogenic pump and promote circulation of the hemolymph throughout the cardiovascular system.

---

[*] These authors contributed equally

In this section, we discuss the genetic networks that control lumen formation of the *Drosophila* dorsal vessel. In particular, we discuss the necessary changes in cell shape and cell-cell adhesion that occur during lumen formation, and the requirement of G-protein signaling for maintenance of the cardiac tube.

2.1 Dorsal vessel lumen formation

The cardiac myoendothelium originates from mesodermal cells that form two bilateral rows of CBs. During dorsal closure, when the dorsal epidermis from opposing sides of the embryo migrates as a sheet to seal the opening at the dorsal surface, the two rows of aligned CBs, together with adjacent pericardial cells, migrate as a sheet of cells, in association and in coordination, with the overlying ectoderm towards the dorsal midline. Lateral alignment and dorsal migration of CBs are critical for the proper formation of the mature dorsal vessel, as mutations in genes that regulate these processes result in structural and lumenal defects (Reim and Frasch, 2010; Tao and Schulz, 2007). As the lateral rows of CBs approach the dorsal midline, the CBs adopt a pear-like shape through constriction of their cellular surfaces facing the dorsal midline (Figure 1C) (Medioni et al., 2008; Santiago-Martinez et al., 2008). Actin-rich protrusions extend from this membrane domain, which constitutes the leading edge of the dorsally migrating CBs (Medioni et al., 2008). CBs from each of the two lateral rows initiates contact with its contralateral counterpart at their dorsal-most leading edge and join at the dorsal midline. Subsequently, the CBs adopt a crescent-like shape, thereby allowing contralateral CBs to join ventrally to close the tube and form a central lumen (Figure 1C) (Medioni et al., 2008; Santiago-Martinez et al., 2008).

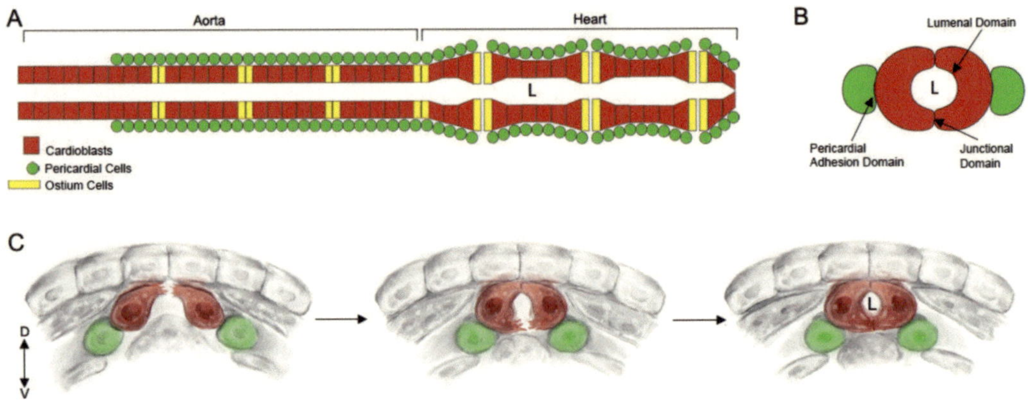

Fig. 1. Lumen formation in the dorsal vessel.

(A) The *Drosophila* embryonic dorsal vessel consists of the aorta and the heart proper where the lumen is lined by cardioblasts (red) and ostium cells (yellow) which in turn are surrounded by the pericardial cells (green). (B) Cross section of the dorsal vessel with a central lumen (L) showing the lumenal and junctional domains of the cardioblasts (red) and the pericardial adhesion domain between the cardioblasts and pericardial cells (green). (C) Lumen formation in the dorsal vessel is preceded by the dorsal migration of a row of cardioblasts (red) in contact with pericardial cells (green) on each side of the embryo, followed by cell-cell contact at the dorsal and then the ventral sides of the cardioblasts to form a central lumen. D: dorsal; V: ventral. Panel C was kindly provided by F. Macabenta and S. Kramer.

Concomitant with these cell shape changes, the membrane domains of CBs undergo significant remodeling to alter their cellular polarity. As CBs approach the dorsal midline, proteins required for cell adhesion, junctional domain formation and attractive/repulsive signals become sub-localized within distinct CB membrane domains. The lumenal domain, which encloses the lumen itself, is characterized by the presence of basal membrane matrix proteins, including Dystroglycan and Perlecan, and the attractant/repellant proteins, Slit and Roundabout (Robo) (Figure 1B). The junctional domain, located at the ventral and dorsal membrane regions, is characterized by the accumulation of adherens junction (AJ) proteins, such as E-Cadherin, Discs-Large and β-catenin. The pericardial adhesion domain, which exists at the contact points between the CBs and the pericardial cells (PCs), is distinguished by the presence of extracellular matrix (ECM) proteins, such as pericardin (Chartier et al., 2002).

The specification and maintenance of these distinct membrane domains and the dynamic changes in cell shape require specific genetic regulators, the loss of which disrupts lumen formation. *Shotgun* (*shg*), which encodes the *Drosophila* homolog of E-cadherin, is specifically required for adhesion of opposing rows of CBs to form the junctional domain (Haag et al., 1999; Santiago-Martinez et al., 2008). The loss of *shg* function results in a loss of adhesion between contralateral CBs, whereas the overexpression of E-cadherin in CBs results in an expansion of the junctional domain and the inability to form a lumen (Haag et al., 1999; Santiago-Martinez et al., 2008). One key regulator of E-cadherin-mediated adhesion between contralateral CBs is the Slit/Robo signaling pathway. Slit is an EGF- and LRR-containing secreted extracellular matrix protein that functions as the ligand for the Robo family of transmembrane receptors and has been shown previously to regulate repulsive axonal guidance in the *Drosophila* nervous system (Kidd et al., 1999; Qian et al., 2005; Rothberg et al., 1990). During migration of the bilateral rows of CBs, Slit and Robo accumulate at the presumptive lumenal domain as the CBs align at the dorsal midline. This polarization of Slit/Robo signaling is critical for its function in regulating lumen formation. In *robo* and *slit* mutants, E-cadherin mediated adhesion between the two opposing CBs is expanded preventing critical cell shape changes and blocking lumen formation (Medioni et al., 2008; Santiago-Martinez et al., 2008). In contrast, when Slit is ectopically expressed on all CB surfaces, a loss of cell adhesion was observed, resulting in the formation of multiple lumens (Santiago-Martinez et al., 2008). These studies indicate that polarized Slit/Robo repulsion is required for inhibition of E-cadherin mediated adhesion at the presumptive lumenal domain to form a central lumen.

Restriction of Slit localization to the lumenal domain is regulated by the transmembrane heparin sulfate proteoglycan, Syndecan (Knox et al., 2011). Syndecans are known to interact with a diversity of extracellular ligands, often in conjunction with other cell surface receptors, and are thought to play a dual role in adhesion and as regulators of signaling from the extracellular matrix (ECM). In *Drosophila*, the single Syndecan homolog, Sdc, regulates axon guidance by acting as a co-receptor with Robo to mediate Slit signaling (Chanana et al., 2009). Embryos that lack Sdc function fail to localize Slit and Robo to the luminal domain and fail to properly form a lumen, indicating that Sdc may also act as a co-receptor for Slit to regulate lumen formation in the dorsal vessel (Knox et al., 2011).

Formation of the dorsal vessel lumen also depends on the transmembrane receptor, Uncoordinated 5 (Unc5). Unc5 represents the single *Drosophila* homolog of a conserved receptor family that binds to the secreted ligand, Netrin (Net) (Keleman and Dickson, 2001). Unc5/Net signaling, like Slit/Robo signaling, plays a role in repulsive axonal guidance and has a localization pattern in the dorsal vessel similar to that of Slit and Robo, where Unc5, and its ligand, NetB, accumulate at the lumenal domain of CBs (Albrecht et al., 2011; Keleman and Dickson, 2001; von Hilchen et al., 2010). In embryos mutant for *unc5* or *netB*, CBs migrate and initiate contact with their contralateral counterparts normally but fail to form a central lumen (Albrecht et al., 2011). Thus, Unc5/Netrin acts as a repulsive force to inhibit contralateral CBs from attaching to one another at their presumptive lumenal domains.

2.2 Maintenance of the dorsal vessel

Genetic analysis has identified the mechanisms by which the lumen of the dorsal vessel is maintained. In particular, at the end of dorsal vessel development, the pericardial cells and CBs must adhere tightly to maintain the structure and integrity of the dorsal vessel. The loss of pericardial and CB adhesion results in the disruption of the dorsal vessel lumen and loss of cardiac function (Yi et al., 2006). The mevalonate pathway, which is important for the synthesis of isoprene derivatives that modify the C termini of proteins containing a CAAX motif (C, cysteine; A, aliphatic amino acids; X, any amino acid), is required for proper pericardial and CB adhesion and dorsal vessel maintenance. In mutants for HMGCR (hydroxymethylglutaryl (HMG)-coenyme A (CoA) reductase), an important regulator of the mevalonate pathway, CBs and pericardial cells properly align at the dorsal midline to form a central lumen; however, at the end of embryogenesis, pericardial cells dissociate from the CBs resulting in CB misalignment and loss of lumen integrity (Yi et al., 2006).

Dorsal vessel defects of *HMGCR* mutant embryos result from the failure of G protein γ subunit 1 (Gγ1) to be post-translationally modified with a geranylgeranyl moiety (Yi et al., 2006; Yi et al., 2008). G proteins form heterotrimers with subunits designated α, β and γ and act as intracellular effectors of G protein coupled receptors (GPCRs) (Malbon, 2005). Gγ1 functions with the β and α subunits, Gβ13F and G-oα47A, respectively, to regulate dorsal vessel maintenance, where loss of Gβ13F or G-oα47A results in pericardial cell-CB dissociation (Yi et al., 2008). Genetic analysis indicates that regulation between the Gα and Gβγ subunits, in coordination with Loco, a member of the regulators of G-protein signaling (RGS) protein family, ensure proper maintenance of the dorsal vessel (Yi et al., 2008). One mechanism by which heterotrimeric G proteins regulate CB-pericardial cell adhesion is by regulating septate junction (SJ) components (Yi et al., 2008). In *Drosophila*, SJs are spoke and ladder septa that connect adjacent plasma membranes and are functionally similar to tight junctions in mammalian systems (Banerjee et al., 2006). Although SJs are absent in the embryonic dorsal vessel, SJ proteins are present, suggesting that SJ proteins perform non-canonical functions during dorsal vessel morphogenesis. Gγ1 regulates the cellular localization of the SJ proteins, Coracle (Cora), Sinuous (Sinu), Neurexin-IV (Nrx-IV) and Nervana2 (Nrv2), and mutants for these SJ proteins have defects in pericardial cell-CB adhesion (Yi et al., 2008). In embryos mutant for SJ proteins, CBs properly align and adhere their ventral and lateral membrane domains at the dorsal midline to form a central lumen; however, the lumen is not maintained and becomes twisted and flattened (Yi et al., 2008). This is in contrast to embryos mutant for AJ proteins, where CBs fail to initialize adhesion with contralateral CBs at the dorsal midline.

These studies suggest a novel pathway in which heterotrimeric G-protein signaling controls proper localization and function of SJ proteins at the pericardial adhesion domain of CBs, which leads to the establishment of stable "SJ-like" adhesive contacts with pericardial cells to maintain the mature dorsal vessel lumen.

3. Salivary gland

The *Drosophila* salivary gland is a secretory organ and consists of a pair of elongated secretory tubes (hereafter referred to the salivary gland) that are connected to the larval mouth through the finer set of duct tubes. The glands are formed during embryogenesis and become functional in the larval stage when they synthesize and secrete proteins necessary for lubrication, digestion and taste. The salivary gland consists of a layer of polarized epithelial cells surrounding a central lumen that is formed from two placodes of epithelial cells, approximately 100 cells each. Salivary glands invaginate through constriction of apical domains and basal migration of nuclei to form a tube that is initially oriented dorsally. After all salivary gland cells have invaginated, the gland turns and migrates posteriorly until it reaches its final position in the embryo (Pirraglia and Myat, 2010). In this section, we will focus on our current understanding of how the salivary gland lumen achieves and maintains its size and shape.

3.1 Growth and remodeling of the apical membrane

The salivary gland lumen forms concomitantly with invagination of gland cells from the embryo surface. During the early migratory step of salivary gland development when the internalized gland turns and migrates posteriorly, gland lumen length doubles and lumen width in the proximal region (the region closest to the ventral surface) is reduced by half (Figure 2A-C) (Pirraglia et al., 2010). Salivary gland lumen size is controlled, at least in part, by the dynamic growth and remodeling of the apical membrane. Transmission electron micrographs (TEMs) revealed that after all salivary gland cells have invaginated from the embryo surface, the gland lumen is characterized by abundant apical protrusions into the luminal space (Myat and Andrew, 2002). Measurements of the length of the apical surface membrane per individual salivary gland cell showed an increase in apical surface membrane, suggesting dramatic growth of the apical membrane (Myat and Andrew, 2002). This rapid phase of membrane growth is followed by elongation of the apical domain of individual gland cells in the proximal-distal (Pr-Di) direction, the direction in which the salivary gland lumen elongates concomitant with posterior migration of the gland (Figure 2D) (Myat and Andrew, 2002; Pirraglia et al., 2010). The Sp1/egr-like transcription factor, Huckebein (Hkb), regulates the size and shape of the salivary gland lumen through control of apical membrane growth (Myat and Andrew, 2000a; Myat and Andrew, 2002). In *hkb* mutant salivary gland cells, the apical surface membrane fails to grow and the apical domain fails to elongate resulting in spherical lumens (Myat and Andrew, 2002).

In the salivary gland placode, the pattern of *hkb* RNA precedes the order in which salivary gland cells invaginate (Myat and Andrew, 2000a). This pattern of *hkb* RNA expression is controlled by Hairy, a basic helix-loop-helix (bHLH) transcription factor (Carroll et al., 1988; Hooper et al., 1989). In *hairy* mutant embryos, *hkb* RNA is expressed in all gland cells and

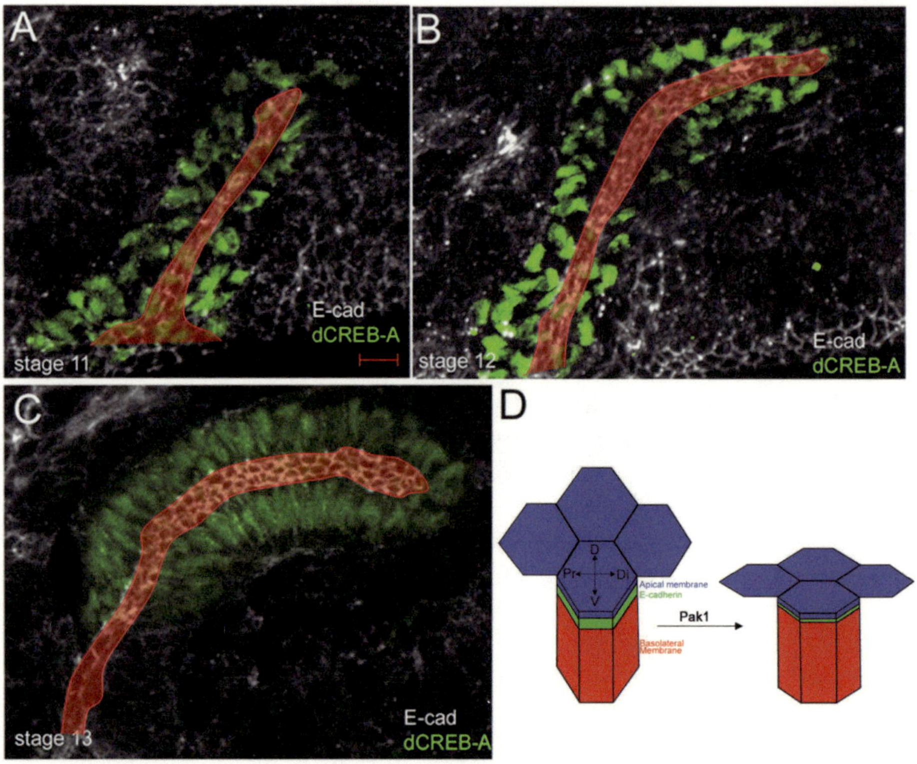

Fig. 2. Lumen elongation in the *Drosophila* embryonic salivary gland.

(A) The salivary gland lumen is formed as salivary gland cells invaginate from the embryo surface at stage 11. (B and C) As the gland migrates posteriorly, lumen length increases. (D) Apical domain elongation is controlled by differential localization of E-cadherin in a Pak1-dependent manner. Panels in A-C are projected confocal images of wild-type embryos stained for dCREB-A (green) to mark the gland nuclei and E-cadherin (E-cad; white) to mark the gland lumen that is outlined in red. Scale bar in A represents 5 μm.

the lumens that form are expanded or branched (Myat and Andrew, 2002). Similar to loss of *hairy* function, overexpression of *hkb* in salivary gland cells leads to expanded and rounded lumens, instead of elongated lumens, but not branched lumens (Myat and Andrew, 2002). Hkb controls salivary gland lumen size through two downstream target genes, *klarsicht* (*klar*), which encodes a *Drosophila* KASH (Klar, Anc-1, Syne-1 homology) domain protein (Mosley-Bishop et al., 1999), and *crumbs* (*crb*), which encodes an apical transmembrane protein that confers apical identity (Myat and Andrew, 2002; Wodarz et al., 1995). In *Drosophila* ovaries and eye, Klar is present on the nuclear envelope and is required for nuclear migration whereas in the early embryo, Klar localizes to lipid droplets and is required for lipid droplet transport (Guo et al., 2005; Kracklauer et al., 2007; Welte et al., 1998). Similar to Klar, the mammalian KASH domain proteins, such as Nesprins, localize to nuclear membranes (Zhang et al., 2001) and regulate nuclear positioning (Zhang et al., 2010). Crumbs (Crb) is important for the establishment and maintenance of apical polarity in both *Drosophila* and mammalian epithelia and photoreceptor cells (Bulgakova and Knust, 2009; Izaddoost et al., 2002; Pellikka et al., 2002; Tepass et al., 1996; Tepass and Knust, 1990;

Wodarz et al., 1995). Hkb regulates not only the levels of *crb* RNA in salivary gland cells but also Crb protein level and/or localization together with Klar (Myat and Andrew, 2002). Considering Klar likely mediates dynein-dependent cargo transport along microtubules (Mosley-Bishop et al., 1999; Welte et al., 1998), it is thought that Hkb mediates the apical delivery of vesicles, such as those containing Crb, through Klar, to promote apical membrane growth and polarized elongation of apical domains during salivary gland lumen elongation.

3.2 Ribbon function in salivary gland lumen elongation

crb RNA expression in salivary gland cells is also controlled by Ribbon (Rib), a BTB (bric-a-brac, tramtrack, broad-complex)/POZ (poxvirus and zinc finger) domain transcription factor required for the proper morphology of multiple tubular organs in *Drosophila*, such as the salivary gland, trachea, Malpighian tubules and the hindgut (Blake et al., 1998; Bradley and Andrew, 2001; Jack and Myette, 1997; Kerman et al., 2008; Shim et al., 2001). In salivary gland cells, Rib controls lumen elongation by simultaneously promoting *crb* RNA expression and limiting apical localization of active phosphorylated Moesin (Moe), a *Drosophila* Ezrin-Radixin-Moesin (ERM) family protein that links the actin cytoskeleton to the plasma membrane (Kerman et al., 2008). The salivary gland phenotype of *rib* mutants is phenocopied by gland specific expression of Moe^{T559D}, a phosphomimetic mutation in Moe where threonine (T) 559 is replaced by aspartic acid (D) and functions as a constitutively-active form of Moe in *Drosophila* developing eyes (Karagiosis and Ready, 2004; Kerman et al., 2008). Since Moe normally links the actin cytoskeleton to the plasma membrane, it is thought that inhibition of Moe activity by Rib decreases the linkage of the apical membrane to the actin cytoskeleton, which in turn, reduces apical membrane stiffness to allow lumen elongation. Furthermore, Rib may control lumen elongation by promoting Rab11-dependent delivery of apically targeted vesicles since *rib* mutant gland cells have a reduced number of apical Rab-11 positive vesicles (Kerman et al., 2008). Rab11 is a small GTPase that mediates apical trafficking of cargo proteins through recycling endosomes or directly from the Golgi (Satoh et al., 2005). Based on these observations, a model for Rib regulation of salivary gland lumen elongation is proposed where Rib promotes *crb* RNA expression and Rab11-dependent apical vesicle delivery to facilitate apical membrane growth, and limits apical Moe activity to reduce apical membrane stiffness which allows the salivary gland lumen to elongate (Kerman et al., 2008). This model is supported by computational models based on live imaging, which suggest that *rib* mutant salivary glands have increased apical stiffness and apical viscosity compared to wild-type salivary glands (Cheshire et al., 2008).

3.3 Pak1 is required for correct salivary gland lumen width

Recent studies from our laboratory demonstrate an essential role for the p21 activated kinase (Pak) 1 in control of salivary gland lumen size through the cell-cell adhesion protein, E-cadherin. Pak proteins are serine-threonine kinases that control vascular integrity in zebrafish blood vessels (Buchner et al., 2007; Liu et al., 2007) and lumen formation by human endothelial cells cultured in three-dimensional collagen matrices (Koh et al., 2008; Koh et al., 2009). In the *Drosophila* embryonic salivary gland, Pak1 functions downstream of the small

GTPase, Cdc42, to regulate gland lumen size (Pirraglia et al., 2010). Loss of *pak1* results in expansion of lumen diameter in the medial and distal regions of the gland without affecting lumen length. The widened lumen of *pak1* mutant salivary glands is not due to increased cell proliferation, and instead, is due to failure to limit apical domain size and to elongate the apical domain in the direction of lumen elongation. These changes in apical domain size and elongation in *pak1* mutant gland cells is accompanied by increased localization of E-cadherin, at the adherens junctions (AJs) and reduced localization at the basolateral membrane (Figure 2D). Pak1 controls this differential localization of E-cadherin in salivary gland cells through Rab5- and Dynamin-dependent endocytosis; not only does inhibition of either *Rab5* or Dynamin in salivary gland cells phenocopy the *pak1* mutant lumen defects, but expression of constitutively-active *Rab5* in *pak1* mutant gland cells restores normal distribution of E-cadherin and restores normal apical domain size and elongation (Pirraglia et al., 2010). Pak1 may regulate E-cadherin endocytosis indirectly through its downstream effector Merlin, the *Drosophila* homologue of the human neurofibromatosis 2 gene (McClatchey and Fehon, 2009), since expression of dominant-negative Merlin phenocopies the salivary gland lumen defects of *pak1* and *Rab5* mutant embryos. Thus, Pak1-dependent localization of E-cadherin at the AJs and at the basolateral membrane is important for apical domain elongation and control of salivary gland lumen size (Figure 2D). A role for Pak1 in lumen size control through membrane transport of E-cadherin is further supported by the demonstration that expression of an activated membrane-bound form of Pak1 in the salivary gland forms multiple intercellular lumens instead of a single central lumen. Induction of multiple intercellular lumens by activated Pak1 is due to the internalization of E-cadherin and apical membrane proteins into early endosomes (Pirraglia et al., 2010).

3.4 Control of salivary gland lumen size through secretory activity

While dynamic changes at the apical membrane and differential localization of E-cadherin control salivary gland lumen size early in gland development, directed secretion into the lumenal space expands lumen width and allows formation of a patent lumen in the mature gland. Secretory products are detected as electron dense material by TEM within apical vesicular structures and in the luminal space. As embryogenesis proceeds, the salivary gland lumen continues to fill with electron-dense secreted products and lumen width increases uniformly throughout the length of the lumen (Myat and Andrew, 2002; Seshaiah et al., 2001). Secretory function of salivary gland cells is controlled by *pasilla* (*ps*) which encodes a *Drosophila* homologue of the human Nova family RNA-binding proteins that function in RNA splicing (Jensen et al., 2000; Seshaiah et al., 2001), and by *PH4αSG1* and *PH4αSG2*, which encode homologues of the α-subunit of resident endoplasmic reticulum enzymes that hydroxylate proline in select secreted proteins (Abrams et al., 2006; Kivirikko and Pihlajaniemi, 1998). In *ps* mutant salivary glands, secretory contents within the lumen and apical vesicles is reduced, and the lumen fails to expand uniformly (Seshaiah et al., 2001). Similar to *ps* mutant embryos, *PH4αSG1* and *PH4αSG2* mutant embryos have reduced secretory products in the salivary gland lumens and are characterized by abnormally shaped lumens with regions of expansion, constriction and closure (Abrams et al., 2006). Together these studies show that *ps*, *PH4αSG*1 and *PH4αSG2* control salivary gland lumen size at later stages of embryogenesis by affecting secretion into the gland lumen.

The expression of *PH4αSG1* and *PH4αSG2* is regulated by the single *Drosophila* FoxA family transcription factor Fork head (Fkh), that affects 59% of gene expression in the salivary gland (Maruyama et al., 2011) and is required for cell survival and cell shape change during salivary gland invagination (Myat and Andrew, 2000b). Fkh regulates the expression of *sage,* encoding a salivary gland specific basic helix-loop-helix (bHLH) protein, and functions with Sage to directly regulate the expression of *PH4αSG2* and to indirectly regulate the expression of *PH4αSG1* (Abrams et al., 2006). In addition to Fkh, secretory activity in the *Drosophila* salivary glands is controlled by CrebA which belongs to the CrebA/Creb3-like family of bZip transcription factors (Abrams and Andrew, 2005; Andrew et al., 1997; Fox et al., 2010). CrebA can bind directly to the enhancers of genes encoding components in secretory pathways and upregulate the expression of genes encoding both the general protein machinery required for secretion and of cell type-specific secreted proteins (Fox et al., 2010). Consistent with the role of CrebA in salivary gland secretion, lumens of CrebA mutant embryos are smaller and have reduced secretory material (Fox et al., 2010).

In summary, salivary gland lumen size in early stages of gland development is controlled by apical membrane growth and apical domain elongation in individual gland cells through processes regulated by transcription factors, Hairy, Hkb and Rib, and their downstream targets, Klar, Crb and Moe as well as by Cdc42 and its effector Pak1 through differential localization of E-cadherin. During late embryogenesis, uniform expansion of the gland lumen is controlled by directed secretion into the lumen through the activities of *ps*, *PH4αSG1*, *PH4αSG2* and *CrebA*.

4. Trachea

The *Drosophila* trachea serves as the respiratory organ of the animal, and like the vertebrate lung, salivary gland and vasculature it is a branched network of tubes. The pattern of the larval trachea is established during embryogenesis when cells from ten tracheal placodes or plates of approximately 90 ectodermal epithelial cells on each side of the embryo, invaginate into the underlying mesoderm to form elongated sacs (Figure 3A). In response to Fibroblast Growth Factor (FGF) or Branchless (Bnl), which is expressed in surrounding ectodermal and mesodermal cells (Ohshiro et al., 2002; Sutherland et al., 1996; Zhan et al., 2010), the invaginated tracheal cells which express the FGF receptor, Breathless (Btl), migrate towards the Bnl source to form the six primary branches (Figure 3B and C). Some of the primary branches, such as the visceral branch (VB) and the anterior and posterior dorsal trunk (DT), grow along the anterior-posterior axis, whereas other branches, such as the dorsal branch (DB), lateral trunk (LT) and ganglionic branch (GB), grow along the dorsal-ventral axis (Figure 3D). Tracheal cell migration is followed by fusion between the contralateral DBs, DT and LT branches of adjacent segmentally arranged metameres on each side of the embryo to form an interconnected tracheal network with a single central lumen (Figure 3F).

Similar to the *Drosophila* embryonic salivary gland, the lumen of the trachea is formed during the invagination step when cells of the placode become internalized and form elongated sacs (Casanova, 2007). As the internalized tracheal cells migrate out to form the six primary branches, the lumen extends simultaneously with the elongating branches. In this section, we focus on how lumen size is controlled in the trachea and how lumens form *de novo* at two distinct stages of tracheal development, first, during anastomosis of the tracheal DT, and second, during intracellular lumen formation in the specialized terminal cells.

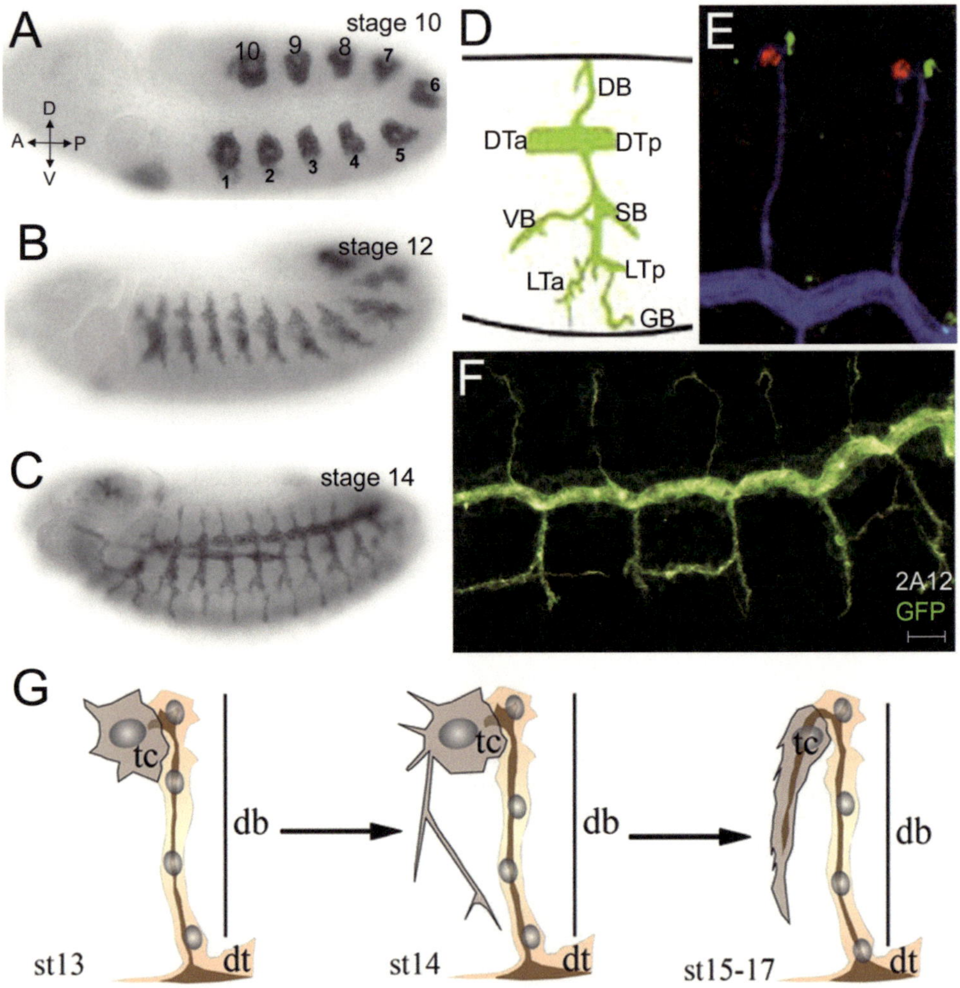

Fig. 3. Lumen formation in the tracheal branches.

(A) The embryonic trachea is formed from 10 placodes of ectodermal cells that invaginate into the interior of the embryo. D: dorsal; V: ventral; A: anterior and P: posterior. (B) Internalized tracheal cells migrate out to form the six primary branches, some of which fuse with branches from adjacent metameres to form an interconnected network (C). (D) Schematic diagram of one tracheal metamere showing the dorsal trunk (anterior and posterior; Dta and Dtp), lateral trunk (anterior and posterior; Lta and Ltp), dorsal branch (DB), visceral branch (VB), spiracular branch (SB) and ganglionic branch (GB). (E) Two DBs, each with a terminal cell (TC, red) and a fusion cell (FC, green). (F) The interconnected tracheal network of a stage 15 embryo has a single central lumen. (G) Terminal cell (TC) forms a lumen *de novo* as the cell elongates; db: dorsal branch, dt: dorsal trunk. Embryos in A-C were processed for RNA *in situ* hybridization to *trachealess* to label tracheal cells. Embryo in E was stained for DSRF (red) to label TC, Dysfusion to label FC (green) and 2A12 (blue) to label the lumen of the DB. Embryo in F was stained for 2A12 (white) to label the lumen and GFP to detect actin-GFP expressed specifically in the trachea with *breathless*-GAL4. Diagram in D is not drawn to scale. Panel G was kindly provided by J. Casanova with permission from the Nature Publishing Group.

4.1 Regulation of tracheal tube/lumen size and shape

Morphometric and genetic analyses in the *Drosophila* embryonic trachea were among the first to show that tube and lumen size are under genetic control. Tracheal tube length increases gradually, whereas tube diameter increases abruptly at distinct times during development. By the larval stage, tracheal tube diameter can be 40x times its original size (Beitel and Krasnow, 2000). These morphometric studies by Beitel and Krasnow (2000) were the first to show that tracheal tube size is not controlled by the number, size or shape of the cells that comprise the tube, and instead, is controlled at the apical surface of the tracheal cells and by the overall identity of each branch. The role of the apical surface membrane in control of tracheal tube size is supported by studies of the *grainy head* (*grh*) mutant (Hemphala et al., 2002). In *grh* mutant embryos, tracheal DT length is increased by 40% and is characterized by the dramatic growth of the apical surface membrane. Grh encodes a transcription factor that is expressed in a number of epithelial tissues (Bray and Kafatos, 1991; Ostrowski et al., 2002), including the epidermis, where Grh controls re-epithelialization during wound healing through the tyrosine kinase Stitcher (Wang et al., 2009). In the trachea, Grh acts downstream of Bnl/FGF signaling to limit lumen elongation and thus, ensure that branches with lumens of the correct size are formed (Hemphala et al., 2002).

A second mechanism by which tracheal lumen size is controlled is through the luminal secretion and modification of chitin, a fibrous substance composed of polysaccharides. Secretion of chitin occurs prior to expansion of the DT lumen and continues throughout growth of the DT lumen. Transient accumulation of chitin is thought to coordinate and stabilize expansion of the lumen (Araujo et al., 2005; Devine et al., 2005; Tonning et al., 2005). While genes encoding proteins that synthesize and secrete chitin control the uniform expansion of tracheal lumen diameter and elongation of lumen length, genes encoding proteins that modify chitin, specifically control lumen length. In mutants where chitin fibers do not form, the DT lumen at points of anastomosis between branches of neighboring hemisegments fail to expand, whereas the lumen throughout the rest of the DT is excessively dilated (Moussian et al., 2006; Tonning et al., 2005). By contrast, in mutants for Vermiform (Verm) and Serpentine (Serp), which encode chitin deacetylating proteins, the DT lumen is excessively elongated (Luschnig et al., 2006; Wang et al., 2006). Restriction of tracheal tube length also depends on genes encoding components of the SJs, a structure located basal to the adherens junctions, which like the vertebrate tight junctions functions as a paracellular diffusion barrier and is comprised in part by the claudin family proteins (Behr et al., 2003; Nelson et al., 2010; Tepass et al., 2001; Wu et al., 2004). Mutations in several SJ proteins affect both tracheal tube length and diameter but not early aspects of tracheal development (Behr et al., 2003; Beitel and Kransnow, 2000; Llimargas et al., 2004; Paul et al., 2003; Wu et al., 2004). One mechanism by which SJ proteins control tracheal tube size is through apical secretion of Verm and Serp (Luschnig et al., 2006; Wang et al., 2006). SJ-associated polarity proteins, such as Discs Large (Dlg) and Scribble (Scrib), also control tracheal tube length independent of chitin and without affecting the paracellular diffusion barrier function (Laprise et al., 2010). The FERM domain protein, Yurt, which belongs to the Yurt/Coracle group of basolateral polarity proteins controls tracheal lumen length by antagonizing the apical determinant protein, Crumbs. However, unlike Yurt, Scrib controls lumen size independent of Crb. The SJ-associated protein, Coracle (Cora), regulates tracheal lumen length by limiting Crb activity independent of Yrt as well as by promoting Verm secretion (Laprise et al., 2010). Thus, independent of Verm/Serp-dependent chitin modification, tracheal lumen length is controlled by a Yurt/Cora pathway dependent on Crb activity, and by a Scrib pathway independent of Crb. SJs likely control tracheal tube size by other mechanisms, such as cell shape since mutations in the SJ proteins, encoded by *megatrachea* and *lachesin*, cause tracheal cells to adopt an irregularly stretched morphology (Behr et al., 2003; Llimargas et al., 2004).

Apical secretion of luminal contents precedes expansion of tube diameter and occurs in a sudden burst through COPI-, COPII- and Sec24-dependent membrane transport (Forster et al., 2010; Grieder et al., 2008; Jayaram et al., 2008; Tsarouhas et al., 2007) and is dependent on Rho-Diaphanous-Myosin V transport (Massarwa et al., 2009). In addition to secretion of chitin, apical secretion may also play a role in tube length by contributing to apical membrane growth and/or targeting other as of yet unidentified, regulators of tube size to the luminal surface. At the end of embryogenesis, the chitin scaffold that has served to control lumen size in the trachea is removed in time for larval hatching when the trachea gets filled with oxygen and other gases. This is achieved through an endocytic pulse that allows the tracheal cells to internalize and clear away the luminal contents (Tsarouhas et al., 2007). The small GTPases, Rab5 and Dynamin are required for the endocytic pulse and luminal protein clearance (Tsarouhas et al., 2007). These studies highlight the important role that chitin plays in tracheal lumen size control; however, it is not known how chitin fibers allow uniform diametric growth of the tracheal tube and restrict tube length. Independent of chitin and SJs, tracheal lumen size is likely to be controlled by additional mechanisms, such as that demonstrated by Convoluted/dALS (Swanson et al., 2009) and by *serrano* mutants which implicate the planar cell polarity pathway in control of tracheal tube length (Chung et al., 2009).

Lumen shape in the tracheal tubes is controlled by receptor tyrosine phosphatases. In embryos double mutant for two receptor-linked protein-tyrosine phosphatases (RPTPs), *Ptp4E* and *Ptp10D*, tracheal branches, such as the ganglionic branches and terminal branches, form large bubble-like cysts with dilated lumens that stain positive for apical marker proteins (Jeon and Zinn, 2009). Cyst size and number are increased upon expression of activated Egfr (epidermal growth factor receptor) and decreased with reduction of Egfr. Thus, proper lumen shape in the trachea is achieved through downregulation of Egfr signaling by the Ptp4E and Ptp10D RPTPs.

4.2 Dorsal trunk anastomosis

During primary branch outgrowth, the tracheal lumen is initially closed at the branch tips. Later in development, a continuous tubular network is formed during anastomosis, when specialized cells, known as fusion cells, which are found at the tips of migrating branches such as the DT and DB, recognize each other's partner in the adjacent metamere and connect to form a continuous lumen (Figure 3E) (Baer et al., 2009). Although these specialized cells are called fusion cells, they, in fact, do not fuse themselves and instead mediate the fusion of two separate tubular structures. The tracheal fusion process occurs in four distinct steps. In the first step, tracheal cells at the tip of adjacent branches contact each other through filopodial extensions. In the second step, fusion cells form a cytoskeletal track at the site of contact consisting of F-actin, microtubules, the plakin Short Stop (Shot) and E-cadherin-based adhesion complexes that are assembled *de novo* at the contact site (Lee and Kolodziej, 2002). Structure function studies showed that distinct sites within the cytoplasmic domain of E-cadherin control the initial assembly of the F-actin track, recruitment of Shot and subsequent maturation of the track in a microtubule-dependent manner (Lee et al., 2003). In the third step, the cytoskeletal track expands to span the fusion cells and bridge the apical surfaces of the DT lumens with apical membrane formed *de novo* at the contact site. In the fourth and final step, the cytoskeletal track disassembles, the apical surfaces become continuous and the narrow lumen that is initially formed expands to its final size (Baer et al., 2009). Connection of the pre-existing DT lumens to the new lumen is dependent on targeted exocytosis and remodeling of the plasma membrane by the Arf-like 3 small GTPase (Arl3) which is known to associate with microtubules and vesicles (Jiang et al., 2007; Kakihara et al., 2008), and the COPI coatomer complex that mediates membrane transport of small vesicles (Grieder et al., 2008). Therefore, tracheal branch fusion is a complex and highly regulated process involving precise coordination of cytoskeletal proteins, adhesion proteins and components of the vesicular trafficking machinery.

4.3 Terminal cell lumen formation

Terminal cells (TCs) at the tips of some tracheal branches form intracellular lumens *de novo* (Figure 3E and G). Although *de novo* lumen formation in TCs was initially thought to occur by the "cell hollowing" mechanism (Lubarsky and Krasnow, 2003), recent studies by Gervais and Casanova (2010) show that the intracellular lumen forms by the inward growth of new apical membrane from the surface that is in contact with the adjacent tracheal cell and not through a cell-hollowing mechanism, shedding significant insight into this process. The TC elongates as its lumen is formed intracellularly and both these processes are accompanied by the asymmetric accumulation of the actin and microtubule cytoskeletal systems (Figure 3G). Genetic perturbation of the microtubule network results in defects in TC lumen elongation suggesting a critical role for microtubules in TC lumen formation. The Bnl/FGF signaling pathway, known to regulate multiple aspects of tracheal morphogenesis as described above, also regulates TC lumen elongation; in embryos with reduced gene dosage of *bnl*, TC lumen length is shortened (Zhan et al., 2010). Bnl/FGF signaling controls TC elongation and intracellular lumen formation by regulating actin and microtubules through Drosophila Serum Response Factor (DSRF) and Enabled, a VASP protein (Gervais and Casanova, 2010); however, DSRF is not required for Bnl-dependent initiation of TC elongation and lumen formation, and instead allows these processes to progress under normal conditions (Gervais and Casanova, 2011).

In addition to the requirement of Bnl signaling for intiation and progression of TC elongation and lumen formation, integrin-mediated adhesion between the terminal branches and the surrounding extracellular matrix is necessary for maintaining these tubes and for proper organization of the intracellular lumen (Levi et al., 2006). The amenability of *Drosophila* to large-scale genetic screens has allowed the generation of many new mutants affecting TC lumen formation (Ghabrial et al., 2011). Analysis of these new mutants is bound to bring novel insights to lumen formation in the tracheal TCs in the years to come.

5. Conclusion

In this chapter, we have reviewed our current understanding of how lumens form and are maintained in the dorsal vessel, salivary gland and trachea of the *Drosophila* embryo. Lumen formation in the *Drosophila* embryonic salivary gland and primary branches of the trachea occurs concomitantly with invagination of the salivary gland and tracheal cells from the embryo surface. Thus, it is not entirely surprising that lumen size control in these two epithelial-based organs share similar cellular and molecular mechanisms, such as the roles of apical membrane growth and luminal secretion in defining tube and lumen size. Although a role for chitin fibers in uniform diametric growth and restriction of tube length has not been documented for the salivary gland as in the trachea, evidence does exist for luminal secretion in forming a patent lumen in the salivary gland.

The dorsal vessel forms by entirely distinct mechanisms from that of the salivary gland and trachea; however, in terms of lumen formation and size control, there are conserved mechanisms between the dorsal vessel and salivary gland and trachea. For example, E-cadherin-mediated cell-cell adhesion is important for correct lumen size in the salivary gland and for forming a luminal space between CBs in the dorsal vessel. Although endocytic trafficking of E-cadherin is important for lumen size control in the salivary gland, it is not known whether Slit/Robo inhibition of E-cadherin occurs by a similar or distinct mechanism. In addition to E-cadherin, SJ proteins, such as Coracle, are required for correct lumen size in the trachea and the dorsal vessel. In the trachea, it is well established that synthesis, secretion and modification of chitin affects tube and lumen size. Although dorsal vessel shape is affected in SJ mutants, it is not known whether vessel diameter and/or length are affected as well. It was recently reported that the lumen of the mouse dorsal aorta forms by a "cord-hollowing" mechanism where lumen formation between two cells is initiated extracellularly through repositioning of cadherin-based adherens junctions and through repulsion of apposed lateral membranes (Lubarsky and Krasnow, 2003; Strillic et al., 2009). Due to the similarities between lumen formation in the *Drosophila* dorsal vessel and the mouse aorta, studies of lumen formation in the *Drosophila* dorsal vessel will continue to yield insight into lumen formation in the vertebrate vasculature.

Studies in the *Drosophila* embryonic salivary gland showed that growth of the apical membrane and modulation of E-cadherin localization at the adherens junctions and the basolateral membrane can influence lumen size and number. In the *Drosophila* embryonic salivary gland, the regulated process of invagination ensures that only a single central lumen is formed; however, the single central lumen can be replaced by multiple intercellular lumens, such as by expression of activated Pak1, as described above. By contrast, the formation of multiple lumens is a normal intermediate step in the formation of a single central lumen during zebrafish gut tube morphogenesis (Bagnat et al., 2007) and in pathological conditions, such as pre-invasive breast cancer, where multiple lumens characterize cribriform ductal carcinoma *in situ* (DCIS) (Jaffar and Bleiweiss, 2002). Thus, understanding the mechanisms by which tubular organs can transition between single and multiple lumens will increase our understanding of more complex processes, such as DCIS.

In the *Drosophila* embryonic trachea, *de novo* lumen formation occurs during anastomosis of specific branches, such as the DT, between adjacent hemisegments. A similar process of *de novo* lumen formation occurs during anastomosis of vascular sprouts during angiogenesis. Like the tracheal tip cells of the *Drosophila* trachea, vascular tip cells extend filopodia to explore the surrounding enrivonment. Moreover, the presence of vascular E-cadherin (VE-cadherin) at the tips of filopodia in cultured human endothelial cells (Almagro et al., 2010) and at tip-tip contact sites between neighboring sprouts during formation of the zebrafish intersegmental vessel (Blum et al., 2008) suggest a role for VE-cadherin in vascular anastomosis that parallels the role played by E-cadherin in *Drosophila* tracheal anastomosis.

Although the structure and function of the *Drosophila* embryonic dorsal vessel, salivary gland and trachea may differ from more complex organs of other organisms, it is clear that there are conserved mechanisms for lumen formation. Thus, the study of tube and lumen formation in *Drosophila* tubular organs will continue to yield novel mechanisms and shed significant insight into how lumens form in more complex organisms.

6. Acknowledgements

We are grateful to F. Macabenta and S. Kramer for providing Figure 1C and for critical reading of the manuscript. We also thank J. Casanova for providing Figure 3G.

7. References

Abrams, E. & Andrew, D. (2005). CrebA regulates secretory activity in the *Drosophila* salivary gland and epidermis. *Development* 132, 2743-2758.

Abrams, E., Milhoulides, W. & Andrew, D. (2006). Fork head and Sage maintain a uniform and patent salivary galnd lumen through regulation of two downstream target genes, PH4alphaSG1 and PH4alphaSG2. *Development* 133, 3517-3527.

Albrecht, S., Altenhein, B. & Paululat, A. (2011). The transmembrane receptor Uncoordinated5 (Unc5) is essential for heart lumen formation in *Drosophila melanogaster*. *Developmental Biology* 350 89-100.

Almagro, S., Durmort, C., Chervin-Petinot, A., Heyraud, S., Dubois, M., Lambert, O., Maillefaud, C., Hewat, E., Schaal, J., Huber, P. et al. (2010). The motor protein myosin-X transports VE-cadherin along filopodia to allow the formation of early endothelial cell-cell contacts. *Mol Cell Biol* 30, 1703-1717.

Andrew, D., Baig, A., Bhanot, P., Smolik, S. & Henderson, K. (1997). The Drosophila dCreb-A gene is required for dorsal/ventral patterning of the larval cuticle. *Development*, 181-193.

Andrew, D. & Ewald, A. (2010). Morphogenesis of epithelial tubes: Insights into tube formation, elongation and elaboration. *Dev Biol* 341, 34-55.

Araujo, S., Aslam, H., Tear, G. & Casanova, J. (2005). mummy/cystic encodes an enzyme required for chitin and glycan synthesis, involved in trachea, embryonic cuticle and CNS development - Analysis of its role in Drosophila tracheal morphogenesis. *Developmental Biology* 288, 179-193.

Baer, M. M., Chanut-Delalande, H. & Affolter, M. (2009). Cellular and Molecular Mechanisms Underlying the Formation of Biological Tubes. *Current Topics in Developmental Biology* 89, 137-162.

Bagnat, M., Cheung, I., Mostov, K. & Stainier, D. (2007). Genetic control of single lumen formation in the zebrafish gut. *Nat Cell Biol* 954-960.

Banerjee, S., Sousa, A. & Bhat, M. (2006). Organization and function of septate junctions: an evolutionary perspective. *Cell Biochem Biophys* 46, 65-77.

Behr, M., Riedel, D. & Schuh, R. (2003). The Claudin-like Megatrachea is essential in septate junctions for the epithelial barrier function in *Drosophila*. *Developmental Cell* 5, 611-620.

Beitel, G. & Krasnow, M. A. (2000). Genetic control of epithelial tube size in the *Drosophila* tracheal system. *Development* 127, 3271-3282.

Blake, K., Myette, G. & Jack, J. (1998). The products of ribbon and raw are necessary for proper cell shape and cellular localization of nonmuscle myosin in *Drosophila*. *Dev Biol* 147, 177-88.

Blum, Y., Belting, H., Ellertsdottir, E., Herwig, L., Luders, F. & Affolter, M. (2008). Complex cell rearrangements during intersegmental vessel sprouting and vessel fusion in the zebrafish embryo. *Dev Biol* 316, 312-322.

Bradley, P. B. & Andrew, D. J. (2001). Ribbon encodes a novel BTB/POZ protein required for directed cell migration in *Drosophila melanogaster*. *Development* 128, 3001-3015.

Bray, S. & Kafatos, F. (1991). Developmental function of Elf-1: an essential transcription factor during embryogenesis in Drosophila. *Genes Dev* 5, 1672-1683.

Buchner, D., Su, F., Yamaoka, J., Kamei, M., Shavit, J., Barthel, L., McGee, B., Amigo, J., Kim, S., Hanosh, A. et al. (2007). pak2a mutations cause cerebral hemorrhage in *redhead* zebrafish. *PNAS* 104, 13996-14001.

Bulgakova, N. & Knust, E. (2009). The Crumbs complex: from epithelial cell-polarity to retinal degeneration. *J Cell Sci* 122, 2587-2596.

Carroll, S., Laughon, A. & Thalley, B. (1988). Expression, function and regulation of the hairy segmentation protein in the *Drosophila* embryo. *Genes and Development* 2, 883-890.

Casanova, J. (2007). The emergence of shape: notions from the study of the Drosophila tracheal system. *EMBO Rep.* 8, 335-339.

Chanana, B., Steigemann, P., Jackle, H. & Vorbruggen, G. (2009). Reception of Slit requires only the chondroitin-sulphate-modified extracellular domain of Syndecan at the target cell surface. *PNAS* 106, 11984-11988.

Chartier, A., Zaffran, S., Astier, M., Semeriva, M. & Gratecos, D. (2002). Pericardin, a *Drosophila* type IV collagen-like protein is involved in the morphogenesis and maintenance of the heart epithelium during dorsal ectoderm closure. *Development* 129, 3241-3253.

Cheshire, A., Kerman, B., Zipfel, W., Spector, A. & Andrew, D. (2008). Kinetic and mechanical analysis of live tube morphogenesis. *Developmental Dynamics*, 2874-2888.

Chung, S., Vining, M., Bradley, P., Chan, C., Wharton, K. J. & Andrew, D. (2009). Serrano (sano) functions with the planar cell polarity genes to control tracheal tube length. *PLoS Genet* 5, e1000746.

Devine, P., Lubarsky, B., Shaw, K., Luschnig, S., Messina, L. & Krasnow, M. A. (2005). Requirement for chitin biosynthesis in epithelial tube morphogenesis. *PNAS* 102, 17014-17019.

Forster, D., Armbruster, K. & Luschnig, S. (2010). Sec24-dependent secretion drives cell-autonomous expansion of tracheal tubes in Drosophila. *Current Biology* 20, 62-68.

Fox, R., Hanlon, C. & Andrew, D. (2010). The CrebA/Creb-like transcription factors are major and direct regulators of secretory capacity. *J Cell Biol* 191, 479-92.

Gervais, L. & Casanova, J. (2010). In vivo coupling of cell elongation and lumen formation in a single cell. *Current Biology* 20, 359-366.

Gervais, L. & Casanova, J. (2011). The Drosophila homologue of SRF acts as a boosting mechanism to sustain FGF-induced terminal branching in the tracheal system. *Development* 138, 1269-1274.

Ghabrial, A., Levi, B. & Krasnow, M. (2011). A systematic screen for tube morphogenesis and branching genes in the Drosophila tracheal system. *PLoS Genet* 7, e1002087.

Grieder, N. C., Caussinus, E., Parker, D. S., Cadigan, K. & Affolter, M. (2008). γCOP is required for apical secretion and epithelial morphogenesis in *Drosophila melanogaster*. *PLoS One* 3, e3241.

Guo, Y., Jangi, S. & Welte, M. (2005). Organelle-specific control of intracellular transport: distinctly targeted isoforms of the regulator Klar. *Mol Biol Cell.* 16, 1406-1416.

Haag, T., Haag, N., Lekven, A. & Hartenstein, V. (1999). The Role of Cell Adhesion Molecules in *Drosophila* Heart Morphogenesis: *Faint Sausage*, *Shotgun*/DE-Cadherin, and *Laminin A* Are Required for Discrete Stages in Heart Development. *Developmental Biology* 208, 56-69.

Hemphala, J., Uv, A., Cantera, R., Bray, S. & Samakovlis, C. (2002). Grainy head controls apical membrane growth and tube elongation in response to Branchless/FGF signaling. *Development* 130, 249-258.

Hooper, K. L., Parkhurst, S. M. & Ish-Horowicz, D. (1989). Spatial control of *hairy* protein expression during embryogenesis. *Development* 107, 489-504.

Izaddoost, S., Nam, S. C., Bhat, M. A., Bellen, H. J. & Choi, K. W. (2002). *Drosophila* crumbs is a positional cue in photoreceptor adherens junctions and rhabdomeres. *Nature* 416, 178-183.

Jack, J. & Myette, G. (1997). The genes raw and ribbon are required for proper shape of tubular epithelial tissues in *Drosophila. Genetics* 147, 243-253.

Jaffar, S. & Bleiweiss, I. (2002). Histologic classification of ductal carcinoma in situ. *Microscopy research and technique* 59, 92-101.

Jayaram, S., Senti, K., Tiklova, K., Tsahouras, V., Hemphala, J. & Samakovlis, C. (2008). COPI vesicle transport is a common requirement for tube expansion in Drosophila. *PLoS One* 3, e1964.

Jensen, K., Dredge, B., Stefani, G., Zhong, R., Buckanovich, R., Okano, H., Yang, Y. & Darnell, R. (2000). Nova-1 regulates neuron-specific alternative splicing and is essential for neuronal specificity. *Neuron* 25, 359-371.

Jeon, M. & Zinn, K. (2009). Receptor tyrosine phosphatases control tracheal tube geometries through negative regulation of Egfr signaling. *Development* 136, 3121-3129.

Jiang, L., Rogers, S. L. & Crews, S. T. (2007). The *Drosophila* dead end Arf-like 3 GTPase controls vesicle trafficking during tracheal fusion cell morphogenesis. *Dev. Biol* 311, 487-499.

Kakihara, K., Shinmyozu, K., Kato, K., Wada, H. & Hayashi, S. (2008). Conversion of plasma membrane topology during epithelial tube connection requires Arf-like 3 GTPase in *Drosophila. Mechanisms of Development* 125, 325-336.

Karagiosis, S. & Ready, D. (2004). Moesin contributes an essential structural role in *Drosophila* photoreceptor morphogenesis. *Development* 131, 725-32.

Keleman, K. & Dickson, B. (2001). Short- and Long-Range Repulsion by the *Drosophila* Unc5 Nectrin Receptor. *Neuron* 32, 605-617.

Kerman, B., Chesire, A., Myat, M. & Andrew, D. (2008). Ribbon modulates apical membrane during tube elongation through Crumbs and Moesin. *Developmental Biology* 320, 278-288.

Kidd, T., Bland, K. & Goodman, C. (1999). Slit is the midline repellent for the robo receptor in *Drosophila. Cell* 96, 785-94.

Kivirikko, K. & Pihlajaniemi, T. (1998). Collagen hydroxylases and the protein disulfide isomerase subunit of prolyl 4-hydroxylases. *Adv Enzymol Relat Areas Mol Biol* 72, 325-98.

Knox, J., Moyer, K., Yacoub, N., Soldaat, C., Komosa, M., Vassilieva, K., Wilk, R., Hu, J., de Lourdes Vasquez Pas, L., Syed, Q. et al. (2011). Syndecan contributes to heart cell specification and lumen formation during *Drosophila* cardiogenesis. *Developmental Biology* 356, 279-290.

Koh, W., Mahan, R. & Davis, G. (2008). Cdc42- and Rac1-mediated endothelial lumen formation requires Pak2, Pak4 and Par3, and PKC-dependent signaling. *J Cell Sci* 121, 989-1001.

Koh, W., Sachidanandam, K., Stratman, A., Sacharidou, A., Mayo, A., Murphy, E., Cheresh, D. &Davis, G. (2009). Formation of endothelial lumens requires a coordinated PKC_{E-}, Src-, Pak- and Raf- kinase-dependent signaling cascade downstream of Cdc42 activation. *J Cell Sci* 122, 1812-1822.

Kracklauer, M., Banks, S., Xie, X., Wu, Y. & Fischer, J. (2007). Drosophila klaroid encodes a SUN domain protein required for Klarsicht localization to the nuclear envelope and nuclear migration in the eye. *Fly (Austin)* 1, 75-85.

Laprise, P., Paul, S., Boulanger, J., Robbins, R., Beitel, G. J. & Tepass, U. (2010). Epithelial polarity proteins regulate *Drosophila* tracheal tube size in parallel to the luminal matrix pathway. *Current Biology* 20, 55-61.

Lee, M., Lee, S., Zadesh, A. D. & Kolodziej, P. A. (2003). Distinct sites in E-cadherin regulate different steps in *Drosophila* tracheal tube fusion. *Development* 130, 5989-5999.

Lee, S. & Kolodziej, P. A. (2002). The plakin Short Stop and the RhoA GTPase are requiered for E- cadherin-dependent apical surface remodeling during tracheal tube fusion. *Development* 129, 1509-1520.

Levi, B., Ghabrial, A. & Krasnow, M. A. (2006). Drosophila talin and integrin genes are required for maintenance of tracheal terminal branches and luminal organization. *Development* 133, 2383-93.

Liu, J., Fraser, S., Faloon, P., Rollins, E., Vom Berg, J., Starovic-Subota, O., Laliberte, A., Chen, J., Serluca, F. & Childs, S. (2007). A betaPix pak2a signaling pathway regulates cerebral vascular stability in zebrafish. *Proc Natl Acad Sci USA* 104, 13990-13995.

Llimargas, M., Strigini, M., Katidou, M., Karagogeos, D. & Casanova, J. (2004). Lachesin is a component of a septate junction-based mechanism that controls tube size and epithelial integrity in the *Drosophila* tracheal system. *Development* 131, 181-190.

Lubarsky, B. & Krasnow, M. A. (2003). Tube morphogenesis: making and shaping biological tubes. *Cell* 112, 19-28.

Luschnig, S., Batz, T., Armbruster, K. & Krasnow, M. A. (2006). Serpentine and Vermiform encode matrix proteins with chitin binding and deacetylation domains that limit tracheal tube length in *Drosophila. Current Biology* 16, 186-194.

Malbon, C. (2005). G proteins in development *Nat Rev Mol Cell Biol* 6, 689-701.

Maruyama, R., Grevengoed, E., Stempniewicz, P. & Andrew, D. (2011). Genome-wide analysis reveals a major role in cell fate maintenance and an unexpected role in endoreduplication for the Drosophila FoxA gene Fork head. *PLoS One* 6, e20901.

Massarwa, R., Schejter, E. & Shilo, B. (2009). Apical secretion in epithelial tubes of the Drosophila embryo is directed by the Formin-family protein Diaphanous. *Dev Cell.* 16, 877-888.

McClatchey, A. & Fehon, R. (2009). Merlin and the ERM proteins--regulators of receptor distribution and signaling at the cell cortex. *Trends Cell Biol* 19, 198-206.

Medioni, C., Astier, M., Zmojdzian, M., Jagla, K. & Semeriva, M. (2008). Genetic control of cell morphogenesis during *Drosophila melanogaster* cardiac tube formation. *J Cell Biol* 182, 249-261.

Mosley-Bishop, K. L., Li, Q., Patterson, L. & Fischer, J. A. (1999). Molecular analysis of the *klarsicht* gene and its role in nuclear migration within differentiating cells of the *Drosophila* eye. *Current Biology* 9, 1211-1220.

Moussian, B., Tang, E., Tonning, A., Helms, S., Schwarz, H., Nusslein-Volhard, C. & Uv, A. (2006). Drosophila Knickkopf and Retroactive are needed for epithelial tube growth and cuticle differentiation through their specific requirement for chitin filament organization. *Development* 133, 163-171.

Myat, M. M. & Andrew, D. J. (2000a). Organ shape in the *Drosophila* salivary gland is controlled by regulated, sequential internalization of the primordia. *Development* 127, 679-691.

Myat, M. M. & Andrew, D. J. (2000b). Fork head prevents apoptosis and promotes cell shape change during formation of the *Drosophila* salivary glands. *Development* 127, 4217-4226.

Myat, M. M. & Andrew, D. J. (2002). Epithelial tube morphology is determined by the polarized growth and delivery of apical membrane. *Cell* 111, 879-891.

Nelson, K., Furuse, M. & Beitel, G. (2010). The Drosophila Claudin Kune-kune is required for septate junction organization and tracheal tube size control. *Genetics* 185, 831-839.

Ohshiro, T., Emori, Y. & Saigo, K. (2002). Ligand-dependent activation of breathless FGF receptor gene in *Drosophila* developing trachea. . *Mechanisms of Development* 114, 3-11.

Ostrowski, S., Dierick, H. & Bejsovec, A. (2002). Genetic control of cuticle formation during embryonic development of Drosophila melanogaster. *Genetics* 161, 171-182.

Paul, S. M., Ternet, M., Salvaterra, P. M. & Beitel, G. J. (2003). The Na+/K+ ATPase is required for septate junction function and epithelial tube-size control in the *Drosophila. Development* 130, 4963-4974.

Pellikka, M., Tanentzapf, G., Pinto, M., Smith, C., McGlade, C. J., Ready, D. F. & Tepass, U. (2002). Crumbs, the *Drosophila* homologue of human CRB1/RP12, is essential for photoreceptor morphogenesis. *Nature* 416, 143-149.

Pirraglia, C. & Myat, M. M. (2010). Genetic Regulation of Salivary Gland Development in *Drosophila melanogaster*. In *Salivary Glands: Development, Adaptations and Disease.*, vol. 14 (ed. A. Tucker and I. Miletich), pp. 32-47: S. Karger.

Pirraglia, C., Walters, J. & Myat, M. M. (2010). Pak1 control of E-cadherin endocytosis regulates salivary gland lumen size and shape. *Development* 137, 4177-4189.

Qian, L., Liu, J. & Bodmer, R. (2005). Slit and Robo Control Cardiac Cell Polarity and Morphogenesis. *Current Biology* 15, 2271-2278.

Reim, I. & Frasch, M. (2010). Genetic and genomic dissection of cardiogenesis in the Drosophila model. *Pediatr Cardiol* 31, 325-334.

Rothberg, J., Jacobs, J., Goodman, C. & Artavanis-Tsakonas, S. (1990). Slit: an extracellular protein necessary for development of the midline glia and commissural axon pathway contains both EGF and LRR domains. *Genes and Development* 4, 2169-2187.

Santiago-Martinez, E., Soplop, N., Patel, R. & Kramer, S. (2008). Repulsion by Slit and Roundabout prevents Shotgun/E-cadherin-mediated cell adhesion during *Drosophila* heart tube lumen formation. *J Cell Biol* 182, 241-248.

Satoh, A., O'Tousa, J., Ozaki, K. & Ready, D. (2005). Rab11 mediates post-Golgi trafficking of rhodopsin to the photosensitive apical membrane of Drosophila photoreceptors. *Development* 132, 1487-97.

Seshaiah, P., Miller, B., Myat, M. M. & Andrew, D. J. (2001). Pasilla, the *Drosophila* homologue of the human Nova-1 and Nova-2 proteins, is required for normal secretion in the salivary gland. *Developmental Biology* 239, 309-22.

Shim, K., Blake, K. J., Jack, J. & Krasnow, M. A. (2001). The *Drosophila* ribbon gene encodes a nuclear BTB domain protein that promotes epithelial migration and morphogenesis. *Development* 128, 4923-4933.

Strillic, B., Kucera, T., Eglinger, J., Huges, M., McNagny, K., Tsukita, S., Dejana, E., Ferrara, N. & Lamert, E. (2009). The molecular basis of vascular lumen formation in the developing mouse aorta. *Developmental Cell* 17, 505-515.

Sutherland, D., Samakovlis, C. & Kransnow, M. A. (1996). Branchless encodes a *Drosophila* FGF homolog that controls tracheal cell migration and the pattern of branching. *Cell* 87, 1091-1101.

Swanson, L., Yu, M., Nelson, K., Laprise, P., Tepass, U. & Beitel, G. (2009). Drosophila convoluted/dALS is an essential gene required for tracheal tube morphogenesis and apical matrix organization. *Genetics* 181, 1281-1290.

Tao, Y. & Schulz, R. (2007). Heart development in *Drosophila. Seminars in Cell & Developmental Biology* 18, 3-15.

Tepass, U., Gruszynski-DeFeo, E., Haag, T. A., Omatyar, L., Torok, T. & Hartenstein, V. (1996). Shotgun encodes *Drosophila* E-cadherin and is preferentially required during cell rearrangement in the neurectoderm and other morphogenetically active epithelia. *Genes & Development* 10, 672-685.

Tepass, U. & Knust, E. (1990). Phenotypic and developmental analysis of mutations at the crumbs locus, a gene required for the development of epithelia in *Drosophila* melanogaster. *Roux's Arch Dev Biol* 199, 189-206.

Tepass, U., Tanentzapf, G., Ward, R. & Fehon, R. (2001). Epithelial cell polarity and cell junctions in *Drosophila. Annu Rev Genet* 35, 747-784.

Tonning, A., Hemphala, J., Tang, E., Nannmark, U., Samakovlis, C. & Uv, A. (2005). A transcient luminal chitinous matrix is required to model epithelial tube diameter in the *Drosophila* Trachea. *Developmental Cell* 9, 423-430.

Tsarouhas, V., Senti, K., Jayaram, S., Tiklova, K., Hemphala, J., Adler, J. & Samakovlis, C. (2007). Sequential pulses of apical epithelial secretion and endocytosis drive airway maturation in drosophila. *Dev Cell* 13.,214-225.

von Hilchen, C., Hein, I., Technau, G. & Altenhein, B. (2010). Netrins guide migration of distinct glial cells in the *Drosophila* embryo. *Development* 137, 1251-1262.

Wang, S., Jayaram, S., Hemphala, J., Senti, K., Tsarouhas, V., Jin, H. & Samakovlis, C. (2006). Septate- junction-dependent luminal deposition of chitin deacetylases restricts tube elongation in the *Drosophila* trachea. *Current Biology* 16, 180-185.

Wang, S., Tsahouras, V., Xylourgidis, N., Sabri, N., Tiklova, K., Nautiyal, N., Gallio, M. & Samakovlis, C. (2009). The tyrosine kinase Stitcher activates Grainy head and epidermal wound healing in Drosophila. *Nat Cell Biol* 11, 890-895.

Welte, M. A., Gross, S. P., Postner, M., Block, S. M. & Wieschaus, E. F. (1998). Developmental Regulation of Vesicle Transport in *Drosophila* Embryos: Forces and Kinetics. *Cell* 92, 547-557.

Wodarz, A., Hinz, U., Engelbert, M. & Knust, E. (1995). Expression of Crumbs confers apical character on plasma membrane domains of ectodermal epithelia of *Drosophila. Cell* 82, 67-76.

Wu, V. M., Schulte, J., Hirschi, A., Tepass, U. & Beitel, G. J. (2004). Sinuous is a *Drosophila* claudin required for septate junction organization and epithelial tube size control. *The Journal of Cell Biology* 164, 313-323.

Yi, P., Han, Z., Li, X. & Olson, E. (2006). The Mevalonate Pathway Controls Heart Formation in Drosophila by Isoprenylation of Gγ1. *Science* 313, 1301-1303.

Yi, P., Johnson, A., Han, Z., Wu, J. & Olson, E. (2008). Heterotrimeric G Proteins Regulate a Noncanonical Function of Septate Junction Proteins to Maintain Cardiac Integrity in *Drosophila. Developmental Cell* 15, 704-713.

Zhan, Y., Maung, S. W., Shao, B. & Myat, M. M. (2010). The bHLH transcription factor, hairy, refines the terminal cell fate in the *Drosophila* embryonic trachea. *PLoS One* 5, e14134.

Zhang, J., Felder, A., Liu, Y., Guo, L., Lange, S., Dalton, N., Gu, Y., Peterson, K., Mizisin, A., Shelton, G. et al. (2010). Nesprin 1 is critical for nuclear positioning and anchorage. *Hum Mol Genet* 19, 329-41.

Zhang, Q., Skepper, J., Yang, F., Davies, J., Hegyi, L., Roberts, R., Weissberg, P., Ellis, J. & Shanahan, C. (2001). Nesprins: a novel family of spectrin-repeat-containing proteins that localize to the nuclear membrane in multiple tissues. *J Cell Sci* 114, 4485-98.

20

Somatic Embryogenesis in Forest Plants

Katarzyna Nawrot-Chorabik
Department of Forest Pathology, Faculty of Forestry,
University of Agriculture in Kraków, Kraków
Poland

1. Introduction

Somatic embryogenesis has become an increasingly applied *in vitro* method in plant breeding in many laboratories across the world. It provides potentially high micropropagation efficiency and other possibilities, such as: cryopreservation of plant material (Hargreaves & Menzies 2007, Misson *et al*. 2006), obtaining secondary metabolites (Mulabagal & Tsay 2004), obtaining valuable and selected planting stock in short time (Rodriguez *et al*. 2007), obtaining transformed plants (Walters *et al*. 2005) and conducting studies on pathogenicity on embryonic level (Hendry *et al*. 1993; Nawrot-Chorabik *et al*. 2011). Hence, there is considerable interest in application of this vegetative micropropagation method in many tree species.

When defining the method of somatic embryogenesis, it needs to be stressed, that this is an *in vitro* morphogenesis, in which adventive embryos, which are not the product of gametic fusion, are formed from plant somatic cells. This method is based on a theory of plant cell totipotency, according to which there is unlimited ability of living cells to divide and to reproduce the whole organism.

The first research on somatic embryogenesis was carried out in the 50s of the 20th century, when the first somatic embryos were obtained in carrot (*Daucus carota*) (Steward 1958). Seven years later embryos of a deciduous species – sandalwood (*Santalum album*) were obtained (Rao 1965). Pioneering studies on somatic embryogenesis in conifers were conducted in Canada in the period of 1968–1980 (Durzan & Steward 1968, Chalupa & Durzan 1973, Durzan & Chalupa 1976). In 1985 Hakman *et al*. (1985) and Chalupa (1995) initiated somatic embryogenesis in European spruce. In recent years *in vitro* studies of woody plants have become more important, since they created new perspectives for development of many industries, such as: pharmacy (e.g. obtaining Taxol from European yew) (Cusidó *et al*. 1999), cosmetology (e.g. obtaining Juglone from walnut and saponins from Conker tree) (Wilkinson and Brown 1999) or production of Christmas trees and decorations (establishment of plantation areas of Nordmann fir) (Misson *et al*. 2006).

Intensive research on improving and on the potential of somatic embryogenesis of economically important tree species are carried out on the following genera: *Abies* (Nawrot-Chorabik 2008; 2009; Salaj & Salaj 2003/4), *Picea* (Klimaszewska *et al*. 2010; Mihaljević & Jelaska 2005), *Pinus* (Lelu-Walter *et al*. 2008; Klimaszewska *et al*. 2001), *Taxus* (Nhut *et al*.

2007), *Acer* (Ďurkovič & Mišalová 2008), *Castanea* (Corredoira *et al.* 2003), *Quercus* (Toribo *et al.* 2005), *Salix* (Naujoks 2007) and *Ulmus* (Ďurkovič & Mišalová 2008; Mala *et al.* 2007).

Before entering the material from *in vitro* cultures into a commercial scale, it is required to conduct long-term observation of growth and development of large amount of somatic seedlings, that represent significant number of genotypes. This allows valuable species of trees to be produced *in vitro* in commercial tissue culture laboratories around the world, i.e. in United States of America (Plant Tissue Cultures Lab - West Lafayette) and in Canada, where Park et al. (2001) included somatic seedlings of white spruce (*Picea glauca*) – the most widespread species in this country - into the program of forest tree breeding and selection. Moreover, somatic seedlings are produced in Great Britain (Date Palm Developments), Israel (Ginosa Tissue Culture Nurseries Ltd.), France – planting stock of *Pinus pinaster* for establishment of forest cultivation (Cyr & Klimaszewska 2002) and in Poland (Tissue culture laboratory Vitroflora in Łochowo), in Italy (Department of Plant Production Di.Pro.Ve.) and in many other countries.

The purpose of this chapter is to present information on somatic embryogenesis of trees in a concise manner, which should introduce the reader into the most important aspects related to this topic. Various stages of the method will be explained indicating the difficulties encountered during *in vitro* culture of trees. Additionally, external factors affecting the breeding success will be discussed. Finally, a short history of research on somatic embryogenesis will be presented.

Concisely presented information on somatic embryogenesis of trees will introduce the reader to key concepts of this topic, briefly present the history of the research on this method, it will also explain each stage of the process indicating the difficulties encountered during *in vitro* cultures of trees with somatic embryogenesis and discuss external factors affecting the success of cultures.

All these aspects will help to identify the most appropriate future research directions in *in vitro* cultures of trees and to introduce the importance of somatic embryogenesis as an alternative method for vegetative reproduction and its contribution to the plant biotechnology development.

2. Material and experimental procedures

2.1 Primary explants used for initiation of *in vitro* cultures with somatic embryogenesis

The term "primary explant" refers to the initial plant material inoculated on a medium, i.e. a fragment of a plant from which the *in vitro* culture was initiated (other plant fragments are called secondary explants). The following types of primary explants may be used in the somatic embryogenesis method: mature zygotic embryos isolated from mature seeds of trees, megagametophytes - immature seeds collected from immature cones with embryo and endosperm, buds, needles or leaves of trees and progenitor cells. Next, the following aspects need to be considered when choosing the primary explant: age of tissues and organs of the parent plants. Most preferably, young organs should be collected, because they have grater potential for development. The minimum storage time, particularly for megagametophytes and seeds of coniferous trees, needs to be reduced. The highest frequency of embryogenesis is obtained from "fresh" seeds and megagametophytes. The location within the plant is also important - in the case of buds - initial, developed leaf buds should be collected. Moreover, the location of primary explant on the medium is significant too - zygotic embryos should be placed on solidified media in a horizontal position, since there is variation in the explants' development on media, which results from natural polarity of plant fragments (Tab. 2). The Author's own research showed, that mature zygotic embryos of silver fir, which did not adhere strictly to the medium, did not produce callus or the initiated callus tissue quickly decays. Another significant factor is the date of explant collection. Generally: in a temperate climate buds need to be collected in the early spring, megagametophytes should be collected from closed cones in June, while mature zygotic embryos should be isolated from non-stored seeds, acquired immediately after physiological maturity. This phenomenon is associated with the natural biological rhythm of parent plants, which affects the effect of embryogenesis. From a physiological point of view this is associated with the period of intensity of most metabolic and enzymatic activity of cells, which is the most intensive in spring. For example, the ability of the explants of white poplar (*Populus alba*) to form callus is maintained at high levels from spring to autumn, while it decreases in winter.

2.2 Disinfection of plant material

In the case of forest trees it is difficult to optimize the method of explants' disinfection due to large contamination of most plant organs with bacteria and endophytic fungi (Kowalski & Kehr 1992). The disinfection procedure should be optimized for a specific tree species, and even for the type of primary explant, for which the chemical agent will be effective against microorganisms. Disinfection of forest trees' explants needs to be conducted in several stages. Disinfection time is sometimes quite long (up to 2-day). Based on many experiments, the Author recommends that during disinfection the seeds of coniferous trees should be kept at 4°C for 24 hours in sterile water with the addition of ascorbic acid or PVP (Polyvinylpyrrolidone), which act as antioxidants. This promotes easier isolation of zygotic embryos, but also embryos inoculated onto media produce smaller amount of phenolic glycosides, which disrupt the process of callogenesis (Pict. 1d). Disinfecting solutions should be supplied with substances that reduce surface tension and facilitate the penetration of the surface of plant material, e.g. Tween 80. In specific cases, plant material is additionally disinfected with solutions of fungicides or antibiotics, which may sometimes have negative impact on reducing the frequency of callus initiation.

Explants' disinfection stages of forest trees can be presented in the following way:

- initial disinfection: explants should be rinsed with running water in temperature about 18°C for 30 minutes (by the end with the addition of Tween 80) to get rid of the resin which in varying degrees covers the ligneous plant material. In some cases it is recommended to use brushes and sometimes even 2-second flaming is recommended to remove the epidermal products.
- proper disinfection: it is performed under sterile conditions in a laminar air flow chamber Biohazard, in 70% solution of ethyl alcohol, followed by the selected disinfectant, e.g. sodium hypochlorite - NaOCl, calcium hypochlorite - $Ca(OCl)_2$, hydrogen peroxide – H_2O_2 or mercuric chloride (sublimate) – $HgCl_2$ (Tab. 2). Finally, the explants should be 3-5 times rinsed with sterile deionized water. Seeds should be tightly closed in a beaker with sterile deionized water with the addition of ascorbic acid

or PVP and placed at 4°C. After 24 hours in sterile conditions the primary explants are inoculated on the medium for initiation.

2.3 Chemical composition of media

Choosing the right type of culture medium, that contains the optimum concentrations of growth regulators for the species, is a key factor to achieve the desired effects in *in vitro* cultures of trees. In almost every step of somatic embryogenesis the composition of basic media needs to be modernized and plant hormone concentrations need to be adjusted. Culture media applied for woody species are rich in macro- and microelements, vitamins, carbon source and growth and development regulators, and sometimes a source of amino acids (enzymatic digest of casein) (Tab. 1).. Activated charcoal– AC is used in some stages of somatic embryogeniesis, usually during the change in the medium composition between the successive stages of embryogenesis. The consistency of media is usually solid and in bioreactors media are liquid. The pH of media is within the range of 5.6 – 5.8. Macro-and micronutrients and vitamins are prepared in a concentrated form of so-called stock solutions, that can be portioned in 10 or 100 dm^3 and stored at minus 20°C in plastic bags.

Macronutrients (N, K, P, Ca, Mg, S) are added in concentrations up to $3000 mg \times dm^{-3}$ in the form of inorganic salts. For induction of somatic embryogenesis it is necessary to maintain balance between cations – NH_4^+ and anions – NO_3^-. Macronutrients are necessary for synthesis of proteins, nucleic acids and for proper functioning of the water balance of plant cells. They ensure appropriate cytoplasmic membrane permeability and are involved in the synthesis of chlorophyll.

Micronutrients (Fe, Cu, Zn, Mn, B, Mo, I, Al) are added to media in concentrations from 0.03 to 100 $mg \times dm^{-3}$, in the form of inorganic salts. However, too low concentration of micronutrients in a medium may inhibit proliferation of embryogenic callus or its dieback. The Author's own research indicates that frequency and quality of embryogenic callus of trees may be increased by adding higher concentrations of zinc (Zn) in hydrated form into the media: $ZnSO_4 \times 7H_2O$. Micronutrients are essential for the synthesis of chlorophyll, they are involved in the functioning of chloroplasts, and assimilation of atmospheric nitrogen.

Vitamins such as thiamine (vitamin B_1), nicotinic acid (vitamin B_3), pyridoxine (vitamin B_6), folic acid (vitamin B_9) and myo-inositol (isomeric form of vitamin B_8, precursor of vitamins) and biotin (vitamin H) aim to improve the physiological condition of cells, they are also necessary for the proliferation of fir (*Abies*) and pine (*Pinus*) callus.

Disaccharides, mainly sucrose and sometimes maltose, are the carbon source in the media, necessary for synthesis of organic compounds. Carbohydrates act also as osmotic balance stabilizers of the media, which affect the absorbance of substances influencing the embryogenic cells' development (Tab. 1).

Substances that solidify media for forest trees are most frequently Phytagel and less frequently agar – natural extract from red algae. The concentration of these substances in the medium is important for the correct development of callus. Too high concentration hinders diffusion, and hence reduces the availability of nutrients for cells, while too low concentration favors the occurrence of "vitreous" explants i.e. callus is too hydrated, it is characterized by anatomical and physiological anomalies. Genus *Pinus* is an exception among coniferous trees, for which the medium should be less solidified. Based on the own research, the Author recommends application of Phytogel (Sigma-Aldrich) for the genus *Pinus* in the concentration of 3.8 g x dm^{-3}.

Growth regulators, so called phytohormones - auxins, cytokines, gibberellins and inhibitors affect callus growth and development through regulation of gene expression. An auxin to cytokine ratio is of particular importance in the early stages of embryogenesis. The presence of auxins: 2,4–D (2,4-dichlorophenoxy acetic acid), IBA (indolyl-3-butyric acid), picloram (4-amino-3,5,6-trichloro-2-pyridinecarboxylic acid) is essential for the induction of somatic embryogenesis and rooting of somatic embryos in the cotyledonary stage. The role of auxins is to stimulate the differentiation of primary explants, which leads to unleashing the embryogenic potential of cells. Such cells rapidly divide and form clusters of embryonic cells. Cytokines such as BA (benzylaminopurine), KIN (kinetin), TDZ (thidiazuron) promote the proliferation of callus and somatic embryo formation in the globular stage. Cytokines stimulate the biosynthesis of nucleic acids, structural proteins and enzymes, inhibit the activity of ribonuclease and protease, and accelerate cell division.

On the other hand, inhibitors such as ABA (abscisic acid) are used in the further stages of somatic embryogenesis. They cause the maturation of somatic embryos through globular, heart-shaped, torpedo and cotyledonary stages (Fig. 1), and in the final stage - their development into the seedling. Moreover, ABA increases the resistance of cells to stress conditions.

3. Stages of somatic embryogenesis of trees

The method of somatic embryogenesis is a multi-stage process. It consists of 5 basic phases (Fig. 1). For a planned outcome of the subsequent stages of embryogenesis, the media need to be selected and optimized for each phase separately. The selected medium, whose composition depends on the species of a tree, must be enriched with optimized concentration of growth regulators to enforce specific organogenetic changes in the plant material. Furthermore, one needs to determine what environmental conditions should be adjusted for the success of *in vitro* culture for each morphogenetic level.

3.1 Embryogenic callus initiation

Initiation, also called indution, is a process of unleashing the embryogenic potential of a single cell or a group of cells. Embryogenic callus, in trees having the form of floculent, usually transparent or white, often viscous, well-hydrated mass, originates on the initial explant (Pict. 1a). The first formed embryogenic cells are called proembryogenic masses (PEM). For about 2-3 weeks the initiated embryogenic callus grows on the initiation medium and then embryogenic cell mass is formed, otherwise known as embryogenic suspensor mass (ESM) (Pict. 1b). It creates a shapeless mass of rapidly dividing cells differentiated in size and shape (from izometric cells to loosely bound, large cells). Callus initiated on a single explant is called a line, which is a single genotype with single set of chromosomes. In this phase, it must be determined whether the callus is embryogenic, by staining with acetocarmine and microscopic observations of proembryos (Gupta & Durzan 1987), (Pict. 1c). In the callus of gymnosperm trees, zones of embryogenic masses may be distinguished – small cells whose nuclei stain red and long, colorless cells with small nuclei and large vacuoles. In some cases, one can find polyploid cells in the callus, originating from selective effect of cytokines, which favors the development of micro-seedlings with unfavorable characteristics.

Components:	Gupta & Durzan (1985) **DCR**	Litvay et al. (1985) **LV**	Bornman & Jansson (1981) **MCM**	Murashige & Skoog (1962) **MS**	Schenken & Hildebrandt (1972) **SH**
Macronutrients [mg/dm³]					
NH_4NO_3	400	1601	-	1650	-
KNO_3	340	2022	2000	1900	2500
$CaCl_2 \times 2H_2O$	85	22		440	200
$Ca(NO_3)_2 \times 4H_2O$	556	-	500	-	-
$MgSO_4 \times 7H_2O$	370	1849	125	370	400
KH_2PO_4	170	408	135	170	-
$(NH_4)_2SO_4$	-	-	400	-	-
$NH_4H_2\ PO_4$	-	-	-	-	300
$Na\ H_2\ PO_4 \times H_2O$	-	-	-	-	-
$FeCL_3 \times 6H_2O$	-	-	-	-	-
$K_2\ SO_4$	-	-	-	-	-
KCl	-	-	75	-	-
Micronutrietns [mg/dm³]					
KI	0.83	4.1	0.25	0.83	1.0
H_3BO_3	6.20	30.9	1.5	6.2	5.0
$MnSO_4 \times 4H_2O$	-	27.9	0.17	22.3	13.2
$MnSO_4 \times H_2O$	22.30	-	-	-	-
$ZnSO_4 \times 7H_2O$	86.5*	86.5*	3.0	8.6	86.5*
$Na_2MoO_4 \times 2H_2O$	0.25	1.21	0.25	0.25	0.1
$CuSO_4 \times 5H_2O$	0.25	0.5	0.025	0.025	0.2
$CoCl_2 \times 6H_2O$	0.03	0.12	0.025	0.025	0.1
$Na_2 \times EDTA$	37.30	37.3	37.25	37.3	20.0
$FeSO_4 \times 7H_2O$	27.80	27.8	27.85	27.8	15.0
Vitamins and other organic compounds [mg/dm³]					
Meso-inositol	-	99.1	90	100	1000
Nicotinic acid	0.5	0.49	0.6	0.5	5.0
Pyridoxine	0.5	0.1	1.2	0.5	0.5
HCl	1.0	0.1	1.7	0.1	5.0
Thiamine HCl	2.0	-	2.0	2.0	-
Glycine Panthoten	-	-	0.5	-	-
Biotine	-	-	0.125	-	-
Folic acid	-	-	1.1	-	-
Glutamine	50.0		500	-	-
Enzymatic digest of casein	1000*	1500*	-	-	1500*
Sucrose	10 g ×l-1	20 g×l-1	20 g×l-1	30 g×l-1	20 g×l-1
pH	5.8	5.7	5.6	5.8	5.6

Table 1. Examples of media used for embryogenic callus *in vitro* initiation (Author's own modification *)

Tree (Genus)	**Primary explant**	**Disinfectant/ time of disinfection**	**Initiation medium**
Coniferous trees:			
Abies	embryos isolated from mature seeds; megagametophytes	sodium hypochlorite - NaOCl 5 - 10% (5 - 30 min.)	SH[1], MCM[2],
Picea	embryos isolated from mature seeds; leaf buds; protoplasts	sodium hypochlorite 10% (15 min.) calcium hypochlorite 7% (20 min.)	MS[3], BM-3[4]
Pinus	embryos isolated from mature seeds;	hydrogen peroxide – H_2O_2 7 - 12% (5 - 15 min.)	DCR[5], LV[6]
Taxus	embryos isolated from mature seeds	sodium hypochlorite - NaOCl 5 - 10% (5 - 30 min.); calcium hypochlorite - $Ca(OCl)_2$ 5 - 10% (5 - 30 min.)	MS, WPM[7]
Deciduous trees:			
Betula	leaves, seeds	sodium hypochlorite 3 – 10%; calcium hypochlorite 7%	WPM, MS, N7[8]
Castanea	leaves	sodium hypochlorite 3 – 10%	GD[9], MS
Fagus	immature zygotic embryos isolated from seeds	commercial bleach (40 g x dm^{-3})	WMP (1/2 concentration)
Quercus	mature embryos regenerating into shoot	mercuric chloride 0,1%	WPM

[1] - Schenken & Hildebrandt (1972); [2] – Bornman & Jansson (1981);
[3] - Murashige & Skoog (1972); [4]- Gupta & Durzan (1986); [5]- Gupta & Durzan (1985);
[6] - Litvay et al. (1985); [7] - Lyoyd & McCown's (1981); [8] – Simola (1985);
[9] - Gresshoff & Doy (1972)

Table 2. Most commonly used types of primary explants, disinfectants and media for the initiation of *in vitro* culture by somatic embryogenesis, depending on the generic name of a tree

3.2 Callus proliferation

Callus proliferation is necessary to obtain suitable quantities of embryogenic tissue. Cell proliferation is a result of callus passages (each 2–3 weeks) onto fresh media of identical or amended composition in relation to the composition of initial medium. Increasing the concentration of cytokines in the medium for propagation has a beneficial effect on callogenesis because these regulators stimulate cell division processes. Enzymatic digest of casein added to the medium in quantities of 1000 – 1500 mg x dm^3, particularly in the case of gymnosperm trees, often has a beneficial effect on proliferation of callus (Nawrot-Chorabik 2008), (Fig. 1).

Not all callus lines are embryogenic and are capable of intensive proliferation. Only certain genotypes are characterized by high frequency of embryogenesis (Pict. 1e). The origin of plant material, particularly seeds, has a significant impact on embryogenic capacity of callus. First somatic embryos are formed in a globular stage. This is the induction of somatic embryos (Pict. 1f). Also the explant itself, e.g. a leaf, has a particular meaning in the process of embryo induction on a proliferated callus. Younger – the innermost leaf tissues (constituting the primary explant) produce callus with large quantities of somatic embryos, while further - more external - parts of leaves may produce smaller callus or the embryos are induced directly on this leaf fragment (Trigiano & Gray 2011).

3.3 Conversion of somatic embryos, gene expresion

Globally speaking, the phenomenon of conversion is understood in two ways – as the development of somatic embryos into plants of identical genotype as initial explant capable of *ex vitro* growth and development, morphologically developed - with a root, apical bud and first assimilation organs (Becwar et al. 1989) - and more rarely as survivability of seedlings regenerated after inoculation and adaptation to *ex vitro* conditions. For somatic embryogenesis of forest trees conversion also refers to the successive stages of somatic embryos' development. The following stages may be distinguished: globular, heart-shaped, torpedo, early-cotyledonary and cotyledonary (Fig. 1, Pict. 1 g, h). Subsequent stage of somatic embryos development (maturation) has gained importance due to its aftermath. With proper embryonic morphogenesis in the process of micropropagation one can obtain valuable plants with large capacities for uniform and rapid germination, with normal growth in the broadly understood range of environmental factors. Properly developed seedlings in terms of physiology are formed not only from embryos, that have the appropriate morphology, but also that gathered the necessary amount of reserve material. Otherwise, often only a rootless shoot is developed. In woody plants the embryo development starts from small clusters of embryogenic cells called proembryogenic masses (PEM I), composed of cells with dense cytoplasm, adjacent to a single vacuolated cell showing tendency to elongation. After about three days further elongated cells develop from a group of cells with dense cytoplasm and form PEM II. Then, after about two weeks large aggregates of cells are formed, classified as PEM III (von Arnold & Clapham 2008). Reducing the amount of auxins and cytokines sometimes stimulates the differentiation of somatic embryos, but the rule is that the addition of abscisic acid (ABA) to the medium is necessary to obtain a cotyledonary embryo. The first visible response of somatic embryos to abscisic acid is their change to colorless. From this point the embryo begins to elongate and form cotyledons.

During the conversion of somatic embryos **gene expression** occurs – which, if started at the right time, ensures proper construction and development of the embryo. So far the following types of genes have been identified: genes responsible for cell cycle and cell wall synthesis, genes responsive to hormones and transcription process associated with somatic embryogenesis. Cell division and growth requires a strict control in time and space.

Expression of genes responsible for cell-cycle process is therefore important for the further development of the embryo. Genes responsible for cell wall synthesis are also important, as somatic embryogenesis depends on proper formation of cell wall components. Among others, the following genes are included in the group responsible for cell-cycle and cell wall synthesis: cdc2M, CEM6, SERP, AGP. The expression of these genes at the right time ensures proper construction of the embryo (Yiang & Zhang 2011). Induction and growth of somatic cells can be stimulated by appropriate hormones that affect hormone-sensitive genes, among which one can distinguish genes responsive to abscisic acid (ABA) e.g. LEA, but also genes responsive to auxins (indolyl-3-acetic acid - IAA and picloram - PIC). These genes include GH3, PIN, ARF, SAUR. The proper course of somatic embryogenesis requires genes that regulate the individual stages and the entire process. These include transcription factors associated with somatic embryogenesis, such as LEC, BBM, WUC, AGL15. All these factors ensure the proper development of somatic embryo (Yiang & Zhang 2011).

3.4 *In vitro* seedling rhizogenesis

Only somatic embryos in cotyledonary stage with clearly developed cotyledons, hypocotyl and primordial root, with morphology similar or identical to zygotic embryo, will germinate and develop into somatic seedlings. Such embryos are transferred onto germination medium. The majority of these are media poor in macro- and micronutrients and sugar, often without growth regulators. These media should be supplemented with auxin, which acts as root inducer - *indole-3-butyric acid* (IBA). Some species, particularly gymnosperm trees, require additional treatments during the rhizogenesis stage, such as drying of embryos (so called desiccation) under conditions of high humidity (ca. 95%) or higher concentrations of solidifiers in the culture media. These treatments cause that the developed embryos in the cotyledonary stage have proper turgidity, which enhances their ability to germinate. According to the literature, the germination ability of somatic embryos obtained by somatic embryogenesis is relatively low and the average is around 15% (Cornu & Geoffrion 1990; Salajova et al. 1995).

3.5 Acclimation to environmental conditions

Adaptation of developed forest tree seedlings to *ex vitro* conditions is difficult due to physiological determinants of young tree seedlings. Their slenderness due to lack of woody tissue and the covering tissue - cuticle, poorly developed root system and assimilation apparatus and significant hydration of the tissues causes instability of seedlings in a new medium - cellulose-peat pots. The cultivated seedlings are transferred from media to pots with a volume of 0.065 liters distributed under different names, e.g. Fetlipots, Finnpots, Jiffypots. The substrate in pots should be watered with basic medium diluted in a 1:1 ratio. Due to the above-mentioned physiological determinants of seedlings, the following treatments should be used to facilitate acclimation: undercooling (important for conifer species) that prevent growth interruption, increasing the light intensity and the use of fogging and variable conditions of light (photoperiod) and temperature in computer-controlled greenhouses. One can also introduce LED (Light Emitting Diode) illumination. For better growth and development of seedlings of gymnosperm species, the Author recommends white LED light with color temperature of 5000 - 6500 K.

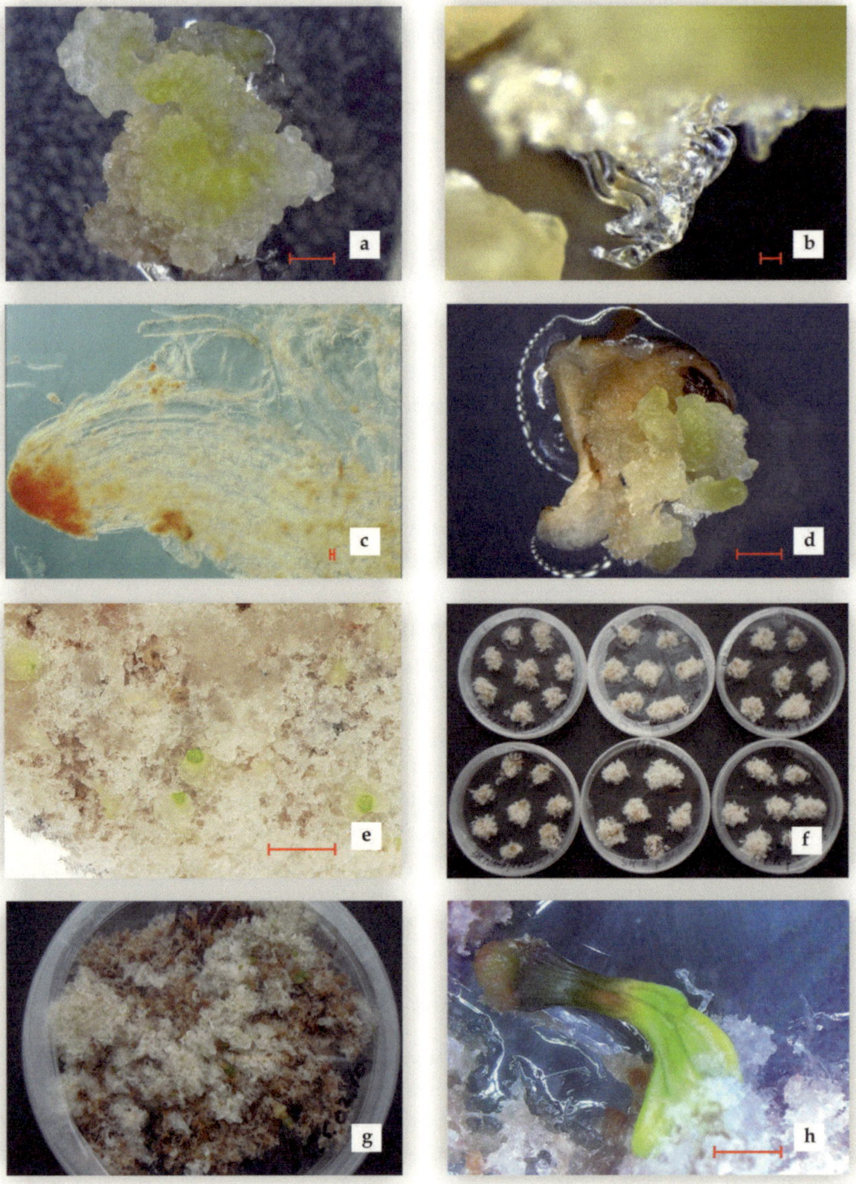

Picture 1. Initiated embryogenic callus on a zygotic embryo of *P. sylvestris* **(a)**; characteristic, hydrated embryogenic callus of gymnosperm trees, the example of *P. sylvestris* **(b)**; elongated embryogenic cells of *Abies alba* **(c)**; callus of *Pinus sylvestris* with evident brown fragments resulting from the produced polyphenols **(d)**; proliferated clones of *Abies nordmaniana* - genotype No. 19 **(e)**; embryogenic callus of *Abies nordmaniana* with induced somatic embryos in globular stage **(f)**; embryogenic callus of *Abies nordmaniana* with embryo in torpedo stage **(g);** embryogenic callus of *Abies nordmaniana* with embryos in cotyledonary stage **(h);** Bars a, d = 10 mm; Bar b = 5000 μm; Bar c = 1000 μm; Bar e, h = 15 mm; (Pictures: **a – d, h** T. Kowalski; **e – g** B. Chorabik)

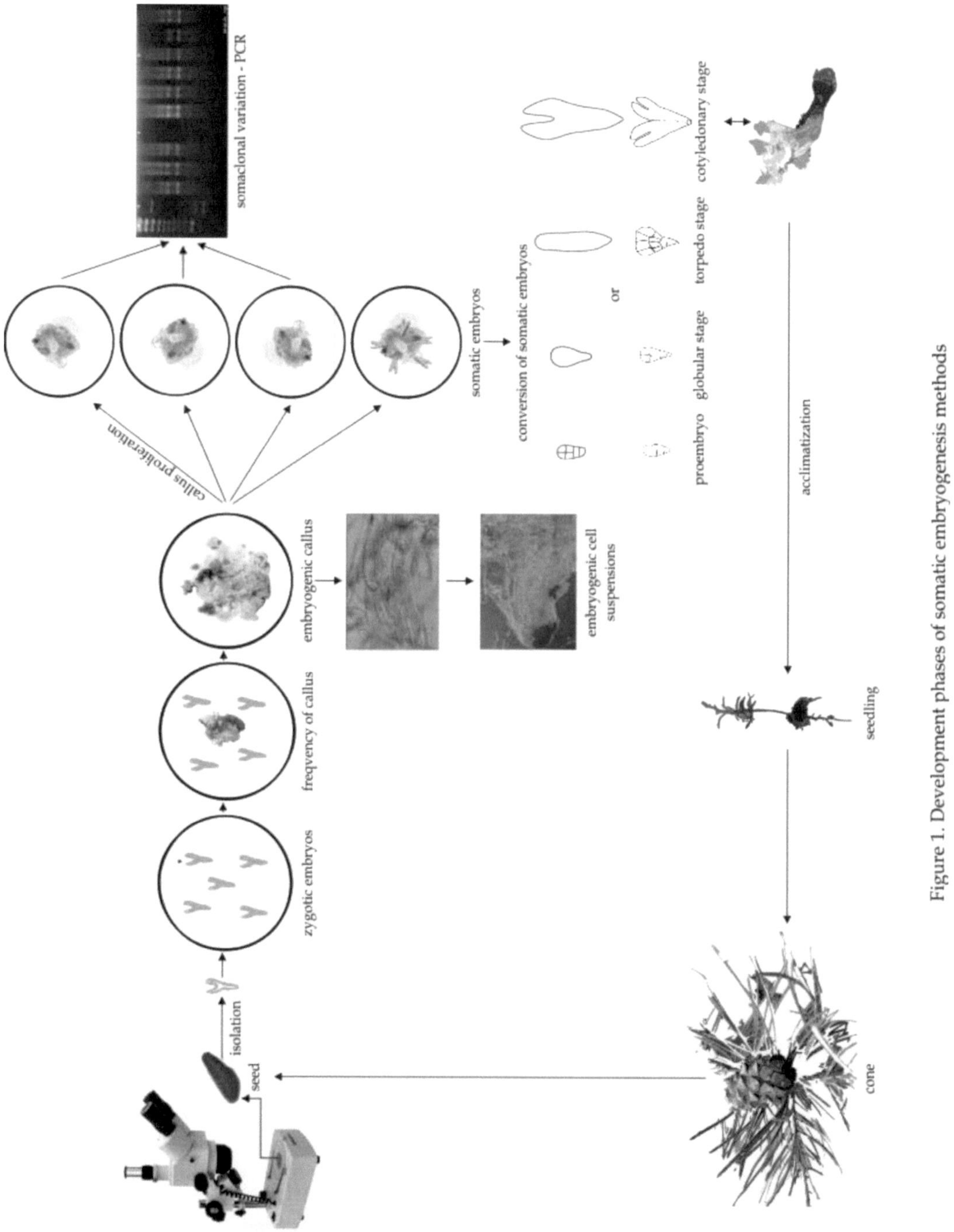

Fig. 1. Development phases of somatic embryogenesis methods

4. Physical conditions of *in vitro* cultures

The physical conditions affecting the state of *in vitro* culture during plant tissue morphogenesis are the abiotic factors such as temperature, light, relative humidity, pH, oxygen and carbon dioxide concentration. These factors must be closely coordinated, but also they must be coordinated with other chemical factors such as e.g. composition of media. For the somatic embryogenesis culture to be successful, usually a constant **temperature** is maintained *in vitro* both during the day and night. Only in rare cases it is necessary to apply proper temperature variation. Most frequently the temperature in a phytotron chamber varies from 23 to 25°C. The optimum temperature, however, should be determined experimentally, depending on the tested species and primary explant. Each stage of the culture may require different temperature. Furthermore, it should be noted that the temperature inside the room with cultures is a few degrees lower than inside the vessel with explants. Therefore, tree explants respond better to the temperature slightly decreased in relation to its optimum temperature than to increased temperature. The **light** impacts the morphogenetic changes, that often are induced by this important factor. The first two stages of somatic embryogenesis in most species of trees progress without light, due to the fact that development process of embryogenic callus does not require intensive photosynthesis. Biotechnological Laboratory of *in vitro* Cultures in the Department of Forest Pathology, University of Agriculture in Cracow, carries out research on the impact of light wavelength and light intensity on the morphogenetic changes in embryogenic callus with somatic embryos of basic, forest-forming gymnosperm tree species of Poland (fir, spruce, pine). It was found that white, diffused, low intensity LED light, which is a mixture of various wavelengths (380–780 nm), in 12-hours' photoperiod is needed only during the conversion of embryos. White light is the most favorable due to the similarity to the prevailing natural conditions. It matches the range of photosynthetically active light (Photosynthetically Active Radiation - PAR) with a wavelength of 400 - 700 nm. It affects the induction of chlorophyll synthesis, chloroplast development and formation of adventitious organs from callus cells. In the beginning of later stages, namely during rhizogenesis, darkness is required (similarly to initiation and proliferation of callus). Only after 10-14 days, the seedlings need to be transferred to white LED light (about 10 times lower intensity than in natural conditions). During the acclimation of somatic seedlings the plants should be placed in a higher intensity white LED light - of intensity similar to natural conditions, optimal for each species. Moreover, it was experimentally demonstrated that blue LED light in the wavelength of 440-490 nm, used for the 12-hour photoperiod has beneficial effect on callus with forming embryos. Embryogenic callus passaged onto activated charcoal medium without plant hormones for the period of 10 - 14 days, kept in blue light, is easier to purify from growth regulators obtained from proliferation medium. Thanks to blue light in the later stage, i.e. conversion, morphogenetic processes are launched more rapidly and the matured somatic embryos are correctly transformed into somatic seedlings in cotyledonary stage (Nawrot-Chorabik, unpublished data). The mechanism of biochemical processes occurring in embryogenic callus with developing embryos exposed to light of different wavelengths is not fully understood, therefore this issue should be carefully investigated. Other light wavelengths, i.e. green light (490-560 nm) and yellow light (560-590 nm) sometimes stimulates formation of adventitious buds from hypocotyl fragments. Conducting *in vitro* culture with different wavelengths argues for the introduction of light parameters (wavelength, light intensity and exposure time) control in phytotrons for better plant growth. **Relative humidity** - RH determines the content of water vapor in the gas phase of the vessel in which the culture is conducted (above the medium surface). RH depends among others on the temperature, chemical composition of a medium, size of explants and vessels. Once the medium and the interior of e.g. a Petri dish have the same temperature, and the vessel is sealed, then the relative humidity should theoretically be 98-99%. However, glass and plastic materials used *in vitro* are not sufficiently leakproof and water vapor gradually escapes on the outside. Therefore, phytotrons with humidity settings should be used, which in the case of micropropagation of trees should oscillate between 50 and 70%. A **pH** of media has significant impact on *in vitro* cultures of trees. Callus and somatic embryos of woody species are formed in acidic pH, i.e. within the range of pH 5.6 - 5.8. pH of a medium may change during the culture. Such changes may be observed particularly in liquid media, and in solid media they may result from too rarely conducted passages. **Oxygen** (product of photosynthesis) and **carbon dioxide** (product of respiration) are two gasses, components of air occurring at a concentration of 21% and 0.036%. However, in Petri dishes or in Erlenmeyer's flasks, in which the culture is carried out, the concentration of these gasses depends among others on: the size of explant, and thus the intensity of photosynthesis, respiration or transpiration and the composition of media (mainly carbohydrate content), light, temperature and the size and shape of the vessel. It is most preferred to maintain oxygen concentration in the vessel at a level higher than its concentration in the air. It was demonstrated that under such conditions, i.e. at the concentration of oxygen within the range of 60-70%, intensive cell divisions occur and the amount of callus, adventitious shoots and somatic embryos increases. Lower than in the air oxygen concentration generally inhibits the plant development. Even roots, which naturally grow in conditions of oxygen deprivation, develop more intensively on the medium in sufficient oxygen supply. Characteristic and frequently observed growth of roots over the level of the medium suggests a lack of oxygen. Sometimes, however, low level of oxygen (7.8%) induces formation of lower amounts of callus, but with the majority of embryogenesis-competent cells. Proper CO_2 concentration primarily determines the proper course of photosynthesis. It has been shown that concentration of this gas higher than in the air (approximately 1-5%) stimulates the explants. It accelerates the intensity of photosynthesis, the cell proliferation intensity in suspension and callus proliferation (Woźny & Przybył 2004).

5. Application of bioreactors

In large production *in vitro* laboratories somatic embryogenesis method is used for reproduction of selected tree species by using bioreactors. In the early stages of micropropagation, embryogenesis is induced on solid media, and after a certain time embryogenic tissue is transferred to liquid media, where it is propagated in the cell suspension in bioreactors. Bioreactors are constructed to enable conducting cell cultures under conditions appropriate to minimize or completely eliminate the possibility of infection. They allow not only the commercial tissue culture, but also the production of somatic embryos. They also allow to obtain embryogenic cells from non-embryogenic ones and to carry out microbiological and enzymatic processes. Bioreactors contain a number of control and measurement sensors, that measure and continuously maintain the following parameters: speed of mixing and aeration, concentration of dissolved oxygen, concentration of dissolved carbon dioxide, the amount of foam, overpressure in the tank, but also oxygen and carbon dioxide concentration in exhaust gasses. This is ensured by appropriate technological parameters and modern design solutions of bioreactors by applying specialized computer software. Bioreactors allow to precisely control the metabolism of plants and processes of proliferation and development of callus. The basic requirements for bioreactors designed for *in vitro* culture are: high efficiency of oxygen exchange and discharge of secreted heat. Air lift bioreactors are now the largest group, since they are very versatile. On the other hand, balloon-type bubble bioreactors are practical because of their shape which prevents media foaming. Bioreactors without forced mixing seem to be particularly useful in cell, tissue and plant organ cultures, as they do not generate the stress of mechanical or pneumatic agitation. The current review of bioreactors used in research and practice was presented in the papers by: Paek & Chakrabarty (2003), and Ziv (2005).

6. Cryopreservation as a method for long-term storage of material obtained by *in vitro* cultures

Cryopreservation is considered the best method for the long-term storage of plant tissues cultured *in vitro* at the temperature of liquid nitrogen (-196°C). When plant material is kept at such low temperature, cell divisions and metabolic processes are stopped for an indefinite time. Additional advantages of this method is low storage space and relatively low costs. Cryopreservation is a method of storage of callus, somatic embryos, pollen, buds and tree seeds in Dewar flasks. As a result of biotechnology development, genetic resources in gene banks have been supplemented with new, valuable genotypes of endangered, economically and ecologically important tree species. The success of cryopreservation depends on increasing tissue tolerance to dehydration stress and the stress caused by rehydration after thawing. Physical state that ensures cell survival in the process of dehydration and freezing is non-crystalline state i.e. vitrification. Under the stress of dehydration, the protein-lipid cytoplasmic membranes are the most vulnerable to damage, since polynusaturated fatty acids of membrane phospholipids are easily peroxidized during desiccation. Moreover, during freezing and thawing of plant material, spontaneous mutations as well as biochemical and structural changes at the cellular level may occur. Therefore, before and after freezing, the plant material should be analyzed using molecular biology techniques, e.g. by checking the somaclonal variation of embryogenic callus (Nawrot-Chorabik 2009).

Cryopreservation process may be carried out in different ways from placing the cryo-tubes in a Mr. Frosty vessel (NALGENE™ W USA), which ensure a slow temperature decrease by 1°C to the use of computerized cryobath equipment (CryolLogic) with freeze control system.

7. Short review of economically important coniferous and deciduous trees micropropagated with somatic embryogenesis including difficulties encountered during *in vitro* cultures

Pioneering studies on somatic embryogenesis of coniferous trees were carried out in 1968-1980, when the development and metabolism of callus and suspended cells was studied (Durzan & Steward 1968, Chalupa & Durzan 1973, Durzan & Chalupa 1976). Thorpe & Biondi (1984), Dunstan (1988) and Becwar et al. (1988) paid attention to the potential of a method, which could be used for vegetative proliferation of gymnosperm species. They conducted the *in vitro* culture of selected species of conifers. However, the first studies on deciduous trees originate from the forties, when reports on the *in vitro* regeneration of adventitious buds from the callus tissue of field elm (*Ulmus campestris*) were published (Gautheret 1940). Experiments on *in vitro* organogenesis of field elm were also conducted in 1949 by Jacquiot (1949). Results of his study were similar to the results obtained nine years earlier by Gautheret (1940) (Szczygieł 2005 after Gautheret 1940). It should be noted that field elm was cultivated in the forties as park and avenue tree. Currently this species is endangered due to its susceptibility to Dutch elm disease. Jacquiot (1949) simultaneously conducted research on organogenesis of silver birch (*Betula verrucosa*). Apart from adventitious buds Jacquiot (1949) obtained the beginnings of roots, however, he did not manage to grow fully developed plants (Szczygieł 2005). The first complete plant, which was obtained during this intensive research, was common aspen (*Populus tremula*) regenerated from a leaf in 1970 by Winton (1970). This achievement initiated greater interest in the method of vegetative *in vitro* propagation of trees.

Currently over 300 plant species, including 120 species of deciduous trees, are propagated by somatic embryogenesis (Bajaj 1995). Some of them are forest trees, such as: European beech (*Fagus sylvatica)*, English oak (*Quercus robur)*, ash (*Fraxinus* spp.), small-leaved lime (*Tilia cordata*), walnut tree (*Juglans* spp.), poplar (*Populus* spp.) and locust tree (*Robinia*). Among all *in vitro* propagated plants there are 50 coniferous trees, e.g.: European silver fir (*Abies alba*), European larch (*Larix decidua*), larch hybrids, Norway spruce (*Picea abies*), white spruce (*Picea glauca*), black spruce (*Picea mariana*), sugar cone pine (*Pinus lambertiana*), Caribbean pine (*Pinus caribea*), Loblolly pine (*Pinus taeda*) and others.

As indicated in Chapter 2.1, in order to initiate embryogenic tissue of coniferous trees, mature and immature zygotic embryos are mainly used as primary explants. The cotyledons of 7-day germinated embryos were used for initiation of embryogenic callus of *Picea abies* (Krogstrup 1986, Lelu et al. 1990), and 12-day cotyledons were used for initiation of *Picea glauca* and *Picea mariana* (Lelu & Bornman 1990). Other researchers applied also cotyledons of 12-30-day seedlings of *Picea glauca* and *Picea mariana* (Attree et al. 1990). Ruaud et al. (1992) used hypocotyls and cotyledons of 1-month somatic and zygotic seedlings and needles of 14-months somatic seedlings cultured in a greenhouse, as well as needles of 7-56 - day somatic and zygotic seedlings for initiation of embryogenic callus of *Picea abies* (Ruaud 1993). Harvengt et al. (2001) obtained embryogenic tissue on 3-year needles of somatic seedlings of *Picea abies*. These needles are the oldest spruce explant, from which embryogenic tissue was obtained (Szczygieł 2005). Nagmani & Bonga (1985) in *Larix decidua* and von Aderkas et al. (1990) in *L. decidua* and *L. leptolepis* used megagametophytes with removed immature embryos for initiation of haploid embryogenic tissue and megagametophytes with immature embryos to initiate diploid embryogenic callus. For initiation of somatic embryogenesis also protoplasts were used (Attree et al. 1987, Klimaszewska 1989, von Aderkas et al. 1990). Attree et al. (1987) regenerated somatic embryos from protoplasts isolated from embryogenic tissue of *Picea glauca* and Klimaszewska (1989) cultured seedlings of *Larix decidua* x *L. leptolepis* hybrid also using protoplasts from embryogenic tissue as explants in somatic embryogenesis. Similarly, von Aderkas et al. (1990) regenerated seedlings from protoplasts isolated from haploid callus of *Larix decidua*. Higher frequency of embryogenic callus initiation was obtained using immature emryos as explants. However, more practical is the use of mature zygotic embryos, isolated from seeds stored in cold rooms. Embryogenic tissue on mature zygotic embryos of European silver fir (*Abies alba*) was initiated by Hristoforoglu et al. (1995) in 40%, Szczygieł (2005) after Braumüller et al. (2001) in 52% and Nawrot - Chorabik (2008) in 6%. Currently, other sources of explants (needles, cotyledons, hypocotyls) and new, synthetic growth regulators that stimulate the process of somatic embryogenesis initiation are searched for (Szczygieł 2005). The first reports on somatic embryogenesis of Scots pine were focused predominantly on initiation from immature seeds and on studying the reactions of cut zygotic embryos at several developmental stages on various culture media (Lelu et al. 1999). The efforts during the regeneration of a small amount of somatic seedlings and young trees were not aimed at the development of mature somatic embryos, but the creation of a protocol for the efficient production of large amounts of plant clones. In another case, crossbreeding was conducted among selected parent trees in order to assess the impact of genotype of parents on somatic embryogenesis (Niskanen et al. 2004). During initiation, maternal effect was clearly visible, while paternal effect was predominantly invisible. A similar conclusion was reached during somatic embryogenesis studies in *Pinus taeda* (MacKay et al. 2006). In other conducted experiments the impact of several factors on the maturation of somatic embryos was investigated. These factors are: age of the culture, abscisic acid and sucrose concentration in the medium (Lelu-Walter et al. 2008). The most current research on somatic embryogenesis in genus *Pinus* has concentrated on examining the impact of parental genotypes and initiation that origin from controlled crossing between maternal trees, that had previously been tested for their response to initiation (Lelu et al. 1999).

The research on somatic embryogenesis in deciduous trees has shown that during *in vitro* culture many difficulties may be encountered. Based on the vine, it was found that although somatic and zygotic embryos are nearly identical in structural and functional characteristics, the ontogeny of somatic embryos tends to be more variable. Somatic embryos of most species, including grapevine (*Vitis* spp.), tend to exhibit several typical morphological abnormalities such as variation in shape, size, and number of cotyledons. In most species, somatic embryos are larger than zygotic embryos, and their regeneration rates are lower. For instance, in *Vitis rupestris* Scheele, only 3% of somatic embryos were capable of developing into complete plants (Jayasankar et al. 2003). This kind of abnormalities may also be found in forest tree species.

Penduculate oak (*Quercus robur*) is an endangered species due to the periodic dieback of oak stands in ecosystems of Troncais forest in France, but also in Austria, Hungary, Romania, Northern Germany, Russia and Ukraine. Oaks die also in Poland in The Krotoszyn Plateau and within the area of Mediterranean Basin. Oaks reproduce in nature by acorns, which are very sensitive to drying during storage, therefore their ability to germinate drops significantly. For this reason, this species should definitely be rescued by micropropagation in *in vitro* laboratories, although the oak is less susceptible to tissue cultures. Such attempt was undertaken in Slovakia, where the method of somatic embryogenesis was used for micropropagation of oak (*Querkus* spp.). Callus was initiated on mature oak seeds. Disinfection of seeds was slightly different than in the case of conifers, i.e.: the seeds were washed in 70% ethanol, extending the duration of the alcohol to 10 minutes and then they were treated for 15–20 with 0.1% solution of mercuric chloride. Embryogenic axes were aseptically isolated from the surrounding cotyledons with preservation of cotyledonary nodes and plumule. Isolated explants were treated with 100 mg x dm^{-3} solution of ascorbic acid to prevent oxidation for 30 min. For the cultivation of embryogenic axes in *Quercus* spp. WPM medium (Lyoyd & McCown 1980) with 20 g x dm^{-3} sucrose and 6 g x dm^{-3} Difco-Bacto Agar, supplemented with 1 mg x dm^{-3} BA and 0.01 mg x dm^{-3} NAA was used. In all experiments the medium pH was adjusted to 5.5 - 5.7. The culture required less frequent passages than in the case of conifers, i.e. in 4-5 week intervals. The number of shoots per explant formed during the subculture was recorded (Ostrolucká et al. 2007).

Silver birch (*Betula pendula*) is one of the most important birch species. It naturally occurs throughout Europe and in central parts of Asia. Silver birch is economically significant because of its medicinal properties. Birch leaves, that contain saponins, flavonoids and terpene compounds are used as medicinal substances. Chaga mushroom was used in folk medicine as an anticancer agent. Its therapeutic properties have been confirmed by research conducted in Poland and Russia. Forest yield can be enhanced significantly by large-scale multiplication of selected genotypes with improved growth rates, valuable quality of wood and high stress and disease tolerance. Vegetative propagation is an important tool of preserving unique characteristics of some of the selected trees of Silver birch (Chalupa 1995). In 1990 Kurtén et al. (1990) induced somatic embryogenesis of *B. pendula* using eight different families, obtained by crossing parent plants with different herbivore resistance. Embryogenic culture was initiated from seeds, seedlings and leaves from 1-year-old plants. Sodium hypochlorite was used for explant disinfection (leaves for 10 min., seeds for 30 min.), and N7 basal medium was used as the medium for initiation (Simola 1985). Nuutila et al. (1991) studied effect of different sugar and inorganic nitrogen concentrations in *in vitro* cultures of birch. Embryogenic callus was initiated on N7 medium, on which somatic embryos were obtained in a later stage (Simola 1985). The first stage of *in vitro* culture (callus initiation) and maturation of somatic embryos was carried out on solidified medium, while the second stage (proliferation) was carried out in liquid medium. Embryogenic tissue of birch in Chalupa's cultures (1987) was characterized by regions of meristematic cells, which were small, thin-walled and highly cytoplasmic. Globular somatic embryos developed at the periphery of the meristematic regions and consisted of densely cytoplasmic cells. At later stages, embryos were surrounded by epidermic cells. Late heart-shaped embryos developed only in small part of callus initiated from explants. Somatic embryos matured after 4 - 6 weeks (Chalupa 1987).

Sweet chestnut (*Castanea sativa*) is the tree valued mostly because of its fruit (chestnuts). This species of *Fagaceae* family occurs naturally in the Mediterranean Basin, Asia Minor and the Caucasus. A major limitation of the embryogenic systems used in chestnut is the maitenance of embryogenic competance and the low conversion rate of somatic embryos into plants. Experiments were performed to determine the influence of proliferation medium on the maintenance of embryogenic competence and on repetitive embryogenesis in *C. sativa* somatic embryos derived from leaf explants. Somatic embryo proliferation was carried out by both direct secondary embryogenesis and by the culture of nodular callus tissue originated from cotyledons of somatic embryos. Both systems led to the production of cotyledonary somatic embryos on MS proliferation medium supplemented with 0.1 mg x dm^{-3} BA and 0.1 mg x dm^{-3} NAA. A total of 39% of embryos eventually produced plants either through conversion to plantlets or indirectly through rooting of shoots. Shoots formed by somatic embryos could be excised, multiplied and rooted following the micropropagation procedures (Corredoira et al. 2003).

European beech (*Fagus sylvatica*) occurs almost in the whole Europe. Its wood is hard, compact, with no heartwood, which causes the beech to be the most commonly used in the art and practice of utility (high calorific value). Therefore, the trees selected for desirable genotypes can be cloned by *in vitro* cultures developing an efficient method of micropropagation. Until now, very few researchers dealt with this economically significant species. Among them were Vieitez et al. (1992) and Naujoks (2001). Vieitez et al. (1992) isolated immature embryos from seeds disinfected in commercial bleach (40 g x dm^{-3}). The culture was established on WPM medium with addition of 2,4-D (0.45; 2.36; 4.52 µM x dm^{-3}) and BA (2.2 µM x dm^{-3}). Embryogenic cell suspensions of 5 genotypes were successfully established in LM medium containing 2,4-D, on which the secondary explants were passaged. The earliest stage, identified as embryogenic, consisted of single cells, undergoing a first asymmetric division leading to the formation of two daughter cells of unequal size, a small cell with dense cytoplasm and strong affinity for acetocarmine and a larger cell with only slight affinity for acetocarmine. Subsequently, either the smaller cells underwent further polarized divisions to form pro-embryos or both daughter cells underwent a series of anarchical divisions leading to the formation of cell aggregates or proembryogenic masses, from which multiple embryos developed by cleavage polyembryony. Finally, 10% of embryos (63 plantlets from 638 embryos) obtained by somatic embryogenesis had developed roots, shoots and well-formed leaves (Vieitez et al. 1992). On the other hand, the research by Naujoks (2001) showed, that on WPM medium, the somatic embryos regenerated on 4 callus lines among 33 lines analyzed (7.9%). Somatic embryos of beech matured on a medium 50% WPM (with 2,4-D and BA) followed by rooting and acclimation in the ground. However, based on the experience and results gained, it was concluded that the long-term storage of embryogenic lines and somatic embryos should be carried out (Naujoks 2001).

The above examples show that the method of somatic embryogenesis is intensively tested in *in vitro* cultures. However, despite conducting numerous experiments on obtaining micro-seedlings of tree species, some of the issues related to this method remain still unresolved. More attention should be paid to the optimization methods, so that the plant material obtained *in vitro* (somatic embryos, callus tissue and properly developed seedlings) was useful for selection, breeding and molecular biology of forest trees and to be useful in other business sectors.

8. Acknowledgements

The author would like to express their special thanks to Prof. dr hab. Tadeusz Kowalski for the given valuable suggestions and doing microscopic photos.

9. References

Attree, S.M.; Bekkaoui, F.; Dunstan, D.L. & Fowke, L.C. (1987). Regeneration of somatic embryos from protoplasts isolated from an embryogenic suspension culture of white spruce (*Picea glauca*). *Plant Cell Reports,* Vol. 6, pp. 480-483.

Attree, S.M.; Budimir S. & Fowke, L.C. (1990). Somatic embryogenesis and plantlet regeneration from cultured shoots and cotyledons of seedlings from stored seeds of black and white spruce (*Picea mariana* and. *P. glauca*). *Canadian Journal of Botany,* Vol. 68, pp. 30-34.

Bajaj, Y.P.S. (1995). Somatic embryogenesis and its applications for crop improvement. In: Bajaj Y.P.S. (Ed.). Biotechnology in Agriculture and Forestry. Vol. 30, Somatic embryogenesis and synthetic seeds I, pp. 221-233. Springer-Verlag,

Becwar, M.R.; Noland T.J. & Wyckoff, J.L. (1989). Maturation, germination and conversion of Norway spruce (*Picea abies* L.) somatic embryos to plants. *In Vitro Cellular and Developmental Biology – Plant,* Vol. 25, pp. 575-580.

Becwar, M.R.; Wann, S.R.; Johnson, M.A.; Verhagen, S.A.; Feirer R. & Nagmani, R. (1988). Development and characterization of *in vitro* embryogenic systems in conifers. In: Ahuja M.R. (Ed.). Somatic cell genetics and woody plants. Kluwer Academic Publishers, Dordrecht. pp. 1-18.

Bornman, C.H. & Jansson, E. (1981). Regeneration of plants from conifer leaf, with special reference to *Picea abies* and *Pinus sylvestris. Colloque International sur la Culture In Vitro des Essances Forestieres. Fontaineblau,* AFOCEL. Nangis. pp. 41-53.

Braumüller, S.; Ross, H.; Rahmad, A. & Zoglauer, K. (2001). Somatic embryogenesis in silver fir *(Abies alba* Mill.). *International Conference on Wood, Breeding, Biotechnology and Industrial Expectations.* Abstract, Bordeaux, France, pp. 62.

Chalupa, V. & Durzan, D.J. (1973). Growth and development of resting buds of conifers *in vitro. Canadian Journal of Forest Research,* Vol. 3, pp. 196-208.

Chalupa, V. (1985). Somatic embryogenesis and plantlet regeneration from cultured immature and mature embryos of *Picea abies* (L.) Karst. *Communication Institute of Forest Czech Republik,* Vol. 14, pp. 57-63.

Chalupa, V. (1987). Somatic embryogenesis and plant regeneration in *Picea, Quercus, Betula, Tilia, Robinia, Fagus* and *Aesculus. Communication Institute of Forest Czech Republik,* Vol. 15, pp. 133-148.

Chalupa, V. (1995). Somatic embryogenesis in birch (*Betula pendula* Roth.). In: Jain, S.M., Gupta, P.K. & Newton, R.J. (Ed(s).). (1995). Vol. 2: 207-220. Somatic Embryogenesis in Woody Plants. Kluwer Academic Publishers, Dordrecht.

Chen, Z.; Yao, Y. & Zhang, L. (1988). Studies on embryogenesis of woody plants in China. In: Ahuja M.R. (Ed(s).). (1988). Somatic Cell Genetics of Woody Plants. Kluwer Academic Publishers, Dordrecht. pp. 19-25.

Cornu, D. & Geoffrion, C. (1990). Aspects de l'embryogenese somatique chez le meleze. *Bulletin de la Société Botanique de France,* Paris. Vol. 137, pp. 25-34.

Corredoira, E.; Balleste, A. & Vieitez, A.M. (2003). Proliferation, Maturation and Germination of *Castanea sativa* Mill. Somatic Embryos Orginated from Leaf Explants. *Annals of Botany,* Vol. 92, pp. 129-136.

Cusidó, R.M.; Palazón, J.; Navia-Osorio, A.; Mallol, A.; Bonfill, M.; Morales, C. & Piñol, M.T. (1999). Production of Taxol and baccatin III by a selected *Taxus baccata* callus line and its derived cell suspension culture. *Plant Science,* Vol. 146, pp. 101-107.

Cyr, D.R. & Klimaszewska K. (2002). Conifer somatic embryogenesis: II Applications. *Dendrobiology,* Vol. 48, pp. 41-49.

Dunstan, D.I. (1988). Prospects and progress in conifer biotechnology. *Canadian Journal of Forest Research,* Vol. 18, No. 12, pp. 1497-1506.

Ďurkovič, J. & Mišalová, A. (2008). Micropropagation of Temperate Noble Hardwoods: An Overview. *Functional Plant Science and Biotechnology,* Vol. 2, No. 1, pp. 1-9.

Durzan, D.J. & Chalupa, V. (1976). Growth and metabolism of cells and tissue of jack pine (*Pinus banksiana*). 3. Growth of cells in liquid suspension cultures in light and darkness. *Canadian Journal of Botany,* Vol. 54, pp. 456-467.

Durzan, D.J. & Steward, F.C. (1968). Cell and tissue culture of white spruce and jack pine. *Bi-monthly research notes / Canadian Forestry Service,* Vol. 24, pp. 30.

Gautheret, R.J. (1940). Nouvelles recherches sur le bourgeonnernent du tissu cambial d'*Ulmus campestris* cultive *in vitro. C. R. Academy of Science Paris,* 210: 744-746.

Gresshoff, P.M. & Doy, C.H. (1972). Development and differentiation of haploid *Lycopersicon esculentum. Planta,* Vol. 107, pp. 161-170.

Gupta, P.K. & Durzan, D.J. (1985). Shoot multiplication from mature trees of Douglas - fir (*Pseudotsuga menziesii*) and sugar pine (*Pinus lambertiana*). *Plant Cell Reports,* Vol. 4, pp. 177-179.

Gupta, P.K. & Durzan, D.J. (1987). Biotechnology of somatic polyembryogenesis and plantlet regeneration in loblolly pine. *Bio/Technology,* Vol. 5, pp. 147-151.

Gupta, P.K., Durzan, D.J. (1986). Plantlet regeneration via somatic embryogenesis from subcultured callus of mature embryos of *Picea abies* (Norway spruce). *In Vitro Cellular and Developmental Biology Plant,* Vol. 22, pp. 685-688.

Hakman, I.; Fowke, L.C; von Arnold, S. & Eriksson, T. (1985). The development of somatic embryos in tissue cultures initiated from immature embryos of *Picea abies* (Norway spruce). *Plant Science,* Vol. 38, pp. 53-59.

Hargreaves, C. & Menzies, M. (2007). Organogenesis and cryopreservation of juvenile radiata pine. Vol. 6, pp. 51-66. In: Jain, S.M. & Häggman H. (Ed(s).). (2007). *Protocols for Micropropagation of Woody Trees and Fruits,* Springer-Verlag.

Harvengt, L.; Trontin, J.F.; Reymond, L.; Canlet, F. & Paques, M. (2001). Molecular evidence of true-to-type propagation of 3-year old Norway spruce through somatic embryogenesis. *Planta,* Vol. 213, No. 5, pp. 828-832.

Hendry, S.J.; Boddy, L. & Lonsdale, D. (1993). Interactions between callus cultures of European beech, indigenous ascomycetes and derived fungal extracts. *New Phytologist,* Vol. 123, pp. 421-428.

Hristoforoglu, K.; Schmidt, J. & Bolhar-Nordenkampf, H. (1995). Development and germination *of Abies alba* somatic embryos. *Plant Cell Tissue and Organ Culture,* Vol. 40, pp. 277-284.

Jacquiot, C. (1949). Observations sur la neoformation de burgeons chez le tissu cambial d'*Ulmus campestris* cultive *in vitro. C. R. Academy of Science Paris,* Vol. 229, pp. 529-530.

Jayasankar, S.; Bondada, B.R., Li Z. & Gray, D. J. (2003). Comparative anatomy and morphology of *Vitis vinifera* (*Vitaceae*) somatic embryos from solid- and liquid-culture-derived proembryogenic masses. *American Journal of Botany,* Vol. 90, pp. 973-979.

Klimaszewska, K. (1989). Recovery of somatic embryos and plantlets from protoplast cultures of *Larix* x *eurolepsis. Plant Cell Reports,* Vol. 8, pp. 440-444.

Klimaszewska, K.; Overton C.; Stewart D. & Rutledge R.G. (2010). Initiation of somatic embryos and regeneration of plants from primordial shoots of 10-year-old somatic white spruce and expression profiles of 11 genes followed during the tissue culture process. *Planta,* Vol. 233, No. 3, pp. 635-647.

Klimaszewska, K.; Park, Y.-S.; Overton, C.; Maceacheron, I. & Bonga, J.M. (2001). Optimized somatic embryogenesis in *Pinus strobus* L. *In Vitro Cellular and Developmental Biology Plantarum,* Vol. 37, pp. 392-399.

Kowalski, T. & Kehr, R.D. (1992). Endophytic fungal colonization of branch bases in several forest tree species. *Sydowia,* Vol. 44, pp. 137-168.

Krogstrup, P. (1986). Embryo-like structures from cotyledons and ripe embryos of Norway spruce *(Picea abies). Canadian Journal of Forest Research,* 16: 664-668.

Kúrten, U.; Nuutila, A.-M.; Kauppinen, V. & Rousi, M. (1990). Somatic embryogenesis in cell cultures of birch (*Betula pendula* Roth). *Plant Cell Tissue and Organ Cultures,* Vol. 23, pp. 101-105.

Lelu, M.A. & Bornman, C.H. (1990). Induction of somatic embryogenesis in excised cotyledons of *Picea glauca* and *Picea mariana. Plant Physiology and Biochemistry,* Vol. 28, No. 6, pp. 785-791.

Lelu, M.A.; Bastein, K.; Drugeault, A. & Klimaszewska, K. (1999). Somatic embryogenesis and plantles development in *Pinus sylvestris* and *Pinus pinaster* on medium with and without growth regulators. *Physiologia Plantarum,* Vol. 105, pp. 719-728.

Lelu, M.A.; Boulay, M.P. & Bornman, C.H. (1990). Somatic embryogenesis in cotyledons of *Picea abies* is enhanced by an adventitious bud-inducing treatment. *New Forests,* Vol. 4, pp. 125-135.

Lelu-Walter, M.A.; Bernier-Cardou, M. & Klimaszewska, K. (2008). Clonal plant production from self- and cross-pollinated seed families of *Pinus sylvestris* (L.) through somatic embryogenesis. *Plant Cell Tissue and Organ Cultures,* Vol. 92, pp. 31-45.

Litvay, J.D.; Verma, D.C. & Johnson, M.A. (1985). Influence of loblolly pine (*Pinus taeda* L.) culture medium and its components on growth and somatic embryogenesis of wild carrot (*Daucus carota* L.). *Plant Cell Reports,* Vol. 4, pp. 325-328.

Lloyd, G. & McCown, B. (1981). Commercially-feasible micropropagation of Mountain laurel, *Kalmia latifolia* , by use of shoot tip culture. *International Plant Propagators Society,* Vol. 30, pp. 421-427.

MacKay, J.J.; Becwar, M.R. & Park, Y.S. (2006). Genetic control of somatic embryogenesis initiation in loblolly pine and implications for breeding. *Tree Genetics and Genomes,* Vol. 2, pp. 1-9.

Malá, J.; Cvikrová, M. & Chalupa, V. (2007). Micropropagation of mature trees of *Ulmus glabra, Ulmus minor* and *Ulmus laevis.* In: Jain S.M. & Häggman H. (Ed(s).). *Protocols for Micropropagation of Woody Trees and Fruits,* Vol. 22, pp. 237-248. Springer-Verlag.

Mihaljevic, S. & Jelaska, S. (2005). Omorica spruce (*Picea omorica*). In: Jain, S.M. & Gupta P. (Ed(s).). *Protocol for somatic embryogenesis in woody plants. Forestry Sciences,* 77. Vol. 4, pp. 35-46. Springer-Verlag.

Misson, J.-P.; Druart, P.; Panis, B. & Watillon, B. (2006). Contribution to the study of the maintenance of somatic embryos of *Abies nardmaniana* Lk: culture media and cryopreservation method. *Propagation of Ornamental Plants,* Vol. 6, No. 1, pp. 17-23.

Mulabagal, V. & Tsay, H.-S. (2004). Plant Cell Cultures - An Alternative and efficient source for the production of biologically important secondary metabolites. *International Journal of Engineering Science,* Vol. 2, No. 1, pp. 29-48.

Murashige, T. & Skoog, F. (1962). A revised medium for rapid growth and bioassays with tobacco tissue cultures. *Physiologia Plantarum,* Vol. 15, pp. 473-494.

Nagmani, R. & Bonga, J.M. (1985). Embryogenesis in subcultured callus of *Larix decidua. Canadian Forest Research,* Vol. 15, pp. 108-1091.

Naujoks, G. (2001). Investigations on somatic embryogenesis of beech (*Fagus sylvatica* L.). *Poster at the Xth International Conference on Plant Embryology -"From Gametes to Embryos"*, 5. - 8. September 2001, Nitra, Slovak Republik.

Naujoks, G. (2007). Micropropagation of *Salix caprea* L. In: Jain S.M. & Häggman, H. (Ed(s).). *Protocols for Micropropagation of Woody Trees and Fruits,* Vol. 20, pp. 213-220. Springer-Verlag.

Nawrot - Chorabik, K. (2008). Embryogenic callus induction and differentiation in silver fir (*Abies alba* Mill.) tissue culture. *Dendrobiology,* Vol. 59, pp. 31-40.

Nawrot - Chorabik, K. (2009). Somaclonal variation in embryogenic cultures of silver fir (*Abies alba* Mill.). *Plant Biosystems,* Vol. 143, pp. 377-385.

Nawrot - Chorabik, K.; Jankowiak, R. & Grad, B. (2011). Growth of two blue-stain fungi associated with *Tetropium* beetles in the presence of callus cultures of *Picea abies. Dendrobiology,* Vol. 66, pp. 41-47.

Nhut, D.T.; Hien, N.T.T.; Don, N.T. & Khiem, D.V. (2007). *In vitro* shoot development of *Taxus wallichiana* Zucc., a valuable medicinal plant. In: Jain, S.M. & Häggman, H. (Ed(s).). *Protocols for Micropropagation of Woody Trees and Fruits,* Vol. 10, pp. 107-116. Springer-Verlag.

Niskanen, A.M.; Lu, J.; Seitz, S.; Keinonen, K.; Weissenberg, K. & Pappinen, A. (2004). Effect of parent genotype on somatic embryogenesis in Scots pine (*Pinus sylvestris*). *Tree Physiology,* 24, pp. 1259-1265.

Nuutila, A.M.; Kúrten, U. & Kauppinen, V. (1991). Optimization of sucrose and inorganic nitrogen concentration for somatic embryogenesis of birch (*Betula pandula* Roth.) callus cultures: A statistical approach. *Plant Cell, Tissue and Organ Culture,* Vol. 24, pp. 73-77.

Ostrolucká, M.G.; Gajdošová, A. & Libiaková, G. (2007). Protocol for micropropagation of *Quercus* spp. In: Jain S.M. & Häggman H. (Ed(s).). *Protocols for Micropropagation of Woody Trees and Fruits,* Vol. 8, pp. 85–92. Springer-Verlag.

Paek, K.Y. & Chakrabarty, D. (2003). Micropropagation of woody plants using bioreactor. In: Jain, S.M. & Ishii, K. (Ed(s).). (2003) Micropropagation of woody trees and fruits. Dordrecht, The Netherlands: Kluwer Academic Publishers, pp. 735-756.

Park, Y.S. (2001). Implementation of somatic embryogenesis in clonal forestry: technical requirements and deployment strategies. *International Conference on: Wood, Breeding, Biotechnology and Industrial expectations,* Abstract, Bordeaux, France, pp. 106.

Rao, P.S. (1965). *In vitro* induction of embryonal proliferation in *Santalum album* L. *Phytomorphology,* Vol. 15, pp. 175-179.

Rodríguez, R.; Valledor, L.; Sánchez, P.; Fraga, M.F.; Berdasco, M.; Hasbún, R.; Rodríguez, J.L.; Pacheco, J.C.; García, I.; Uribe, M.M.; Ríos, D.; Sánchez-, M.; Materán, M.E.; Walter, C. & Cañal, M.J. (2007). Propagation of selected *Pinus* genotypes regardless of age. In: Jain, S.M. & Häggman, H. (Ed(s).). *Protocols for Micropropagation of Woody Trees and Fruits,* Vol. 13, pp. 137-146. Springer-Verlag.

Ruaud, J.N. (1993). Maturation and conversion into plantlets of somatic embryos derived from needles and cotyledons of 7-56-day old *Picea abies. Plant Sciences,* Vol. 92, pp. 213-220.

Ruaud, J.N.; Bercetche, J. & Paques, M. (1992). First evidence of somatic embryogenesis from needles of 1-yearold *Picea abies* plants. *Plant Cell Reports,* Vol. 11, pp. 563-566.

Salaj, T. & Salaj, J. (2003/4). Somatic embryo formation on mature *Abies alba* × *Abies cephalonica* zygotic embryo explants. *Biologia Plantarum,* Vol. 47, pp. 7- 11.

Salajova, T.; Salaj, J., Jasik, J. & Kormutak, A. (1995). Somatic embryogenesis in *Pinus nigra* Arn. In: Jain, S.M.; Gupta, P.K. & Newton, R.J. (Ed(s).). Somatic Embryogenesis in Woody Plants. Kluwer Academic Publishers, Dordrecht. pp. 207-220.

Schenck, R.U. & Hildebrandt, A.C. (1972). Medium and techniques for induction and growth of monocotyledonous and dicotyledonous plant cell cultures. *Canadian Journal of Botany,* Vol. 50, pp. 199-204.

Simola, L.K. (1985). Propagation of plantlets from leaf callus *Betula pendula* f. *purpurea. Scientia Horticulare,* Vol. 26, pp. 77-85.

Steward, F.C. (1958). Growth and development of cultivated cells. III. Interpretations of the growth from free cell of carrot. *American Journal of Botany,* Vol. 45, pp. 709-713.

Szczygieł, K. (2005). Somatyczna embriogeneza - alternatywny sposób uzyskiwania wyslekcjonowanego materiału sadzeniowego gatunków drzew iglastych. *Leśne Prace Badawcze,* 3: 71-92. [Somatic embryogenesis - alternative way of obtaining selected planting stock of coniferous tree species]. *Forest Research Papers,* Vol. 3, pp. 71-92.

Thorpe, T.A. & Biondi, S. (1984). Conifers. Handbook of plant cell culture. In: Sharp, W.R.; Evans, A.; Ammirato, P.V. & Yamada, Y. (Ed(s).). MacMillian Publishing Company of New York, pp. 435-470.

Toribo, M.; Celestino, C. & Molinas, M. (2005). Cork oak, *Quercus suber* L. In: Jain, SM. & Gupta, P. (Ed(s).). *Protocol for somatic embryogenesis in woody plants. Forestry Sciences 77,* Vol. 35: 445-458. Springer-Verlag.

Trigiano, R.N. & Gray, D.J. (Ed(s).). (2011). Plant Development and Biotechnology. Section IV Propagation and development concepts. CRC PRESS.

Troch, V.; Werbrouck, S.; Geelen D. & Van Labeke, M-Ch. (2009). Optimization of horse chestnut (*Aesculus hippocastanum* L.) somatic embryo conversion. *Plant Cell, Tissue and Organ Culture,* Vol. 98, No. 1, pp. 115-123.

Vieitez, J.F.; Ballester, A. & Vieitez, A.M. (1992). Somatic embryogenesis and plantlet regeneration from cell suspension cultures of *Fagus sylvatica* L. *Plant Cell Reports,* Vol. 11, pp. 609-613.

von Aderkas, P.; Klimaszewska, K. & Bonga, J. (1990). Diploid and haploid embryogenesis in *Larix letlolepis, L. decidua,* and their reciprocal hybrids. *Canadian Forest Research,* Vol. 20, pp. 9-14.

von Arnold, S. & Clapham, D. (2008). Spruce embryogenesis. In: Suárez M.F., & Bozhkov P.V.) (Ed(s).). Methods in molecular biology, *Plant embryogenesis.* Vol. 427, pp. 31-45. *Humana Press,* Inc. in *Totowa, NJ,* US (United States).

Walters, C.; Find, J.I. & Grace, L.J. (2005). Somatic embryogenesis and genetic transformation in *Pinus radiata.* In: Jain S.M. & Gupta P. (Ed(s).). *Protocol for somatic embryogenesis in woody plants. Forestry Sciences* 77, Vol. 2, pp. 11-24. Springer-Verlag.

Wilkinson, J.A. & Brown, A.M.G. (1999). Horse Chestnut - *Aesculus hippocastanum*: Potential applications in cosmetic Skin-care products. *International Journal of Cosmetic Science,* Vol. 21, No. 6, pp. 437-447.

Winton, L.L. (1970). Shoot and tree production from aspen tissue cultures. *American Journal of Botany,* Vol. 57, pp. 904-909.

Woźny, A. & Przybył, K. (Ed(s).). (2004). Komórki roślinne w warunkach stresu. Tom II Komórki *in vitro.* [Plant cells under stress conditions]. Vol. 2. *In vitro* cells. Adam Mickiewicz University. pp. 72-91.

Yang, X. & Zhang, X. (2011). Developmental and molecular aspects of nonzygotic (somatic) embryogenesis In: Trigiano R.N. & Gray D.J. (Ed(s).). (2011). *Plant tissue culture, development, and biotechnology,* CRC Press. pp. 307-326.

Ziv, M. (2005). Simple bioreactors for mass propagation of plants. *Plant Cell, Tissue and Organ Culture,* Vol. 81, pp. 277-285.

21

Phospho-Signaling at Oocyte Maturation and Fertilization: Set Up for Embryogenesis and Beyond Part I. Protein Kinases

A.K.M. Mahbub Hasan[1], Takashi Matsumoto[2], Shigeru Kihira[2], Junpei Yoshida[2] and Ken-ichi Sato[2,*]

[1]*Laboratory of Gene Biology, Department of Biochemistry and Molecular Biology, University of Dhaka, Dhaka,*
[2]*Laboratory of Cell Signaling and Development, Department of Molecular Biosciences, Faculty of Life Sciences, Kyoto Sangyo University, Kamigamo-Motoyama, Kita-ku, Kyoto*
[1]*Bangladesh*
[2]*Japan*

1. Introduction

In the field of developmental biology, day by day data are accumulated to describe the molecular mechanisms involved in gamete cell production (oogenesis and spermatogenesis) and the sperm-egg interaction/fusion (fertilization) leading the formation of zygote to embryo (embryogenesis) that ultimately develop into a complete body. Here, we will review how *oocyte maturation*, sperm mediated *egg activation/fertilization* and early steps of *embryogenesis* are accomplished and regulated through protein phosphorylation(s) highlighting the participating molecules (e.g. protein kinases) (**this chapter**) and their regulators and substrates (**another chapter entitled "Part II. Kinase Regulators and Substrates"**). Meiosis is the process by which diploid germ-line cell reduces their number of chromosomes in half to generate haploid gamete and combine with opposite sex haploid gamete to create a genetically new, diploid individual. Oocyte maturation, which undergoes two meiotic cell cycles that arrest at several stages, has been studied extensively in many species of vertebrates and invertebrates. A lot of review articles on oocyte meiotic maturation of different species have been written (Kang and Han 2011; Liang et al. 2007; Machaca 2007; Madgwick and Jones 2007; Schmitt and Nebreda 2002a; Tripathi et al. 2010). In almost all vertebrates, oocyte meiotic cell cycle starts during fetal life (at 4-5 weeks) but arrest at first in diplotene stage of first meiotic prophase (before the metaphase I or MI) that may last for several months or years in follicular microenvironment depending on the species (Mehlmann and Jaffe 2005; Sirard 2001; Trounson et al. 2001; Wassmann et al. 2003). The progression of meiotic cell cycle is also arrested, in many but not all species, at stages of second meiotic metaphase II (MII) and/or metaphase-like arrest (MIII). During oocyte

* Corresponding Author

maturation different kinds of molecules e.g. second messengers, protein kinases, protein phosphatases and their regulator and/or substrate proteins are involved. Here, the molecular mechanisms involved in the arrest and resumption of these stages will be discussed briefly.

MPF (maturation or M-phase promoting factor), a serine/threonine kinase, is composed of a catalytic subunit cyclin-dependent kinase 1 (Cdc2/CDK1), and a regulatory subunit, cyclin B; are the key components in the maintenance of diplotene arrest. In activated MPF, dephosphorylated CDK1 is associated with cyclin B and both cyclin B synthesis and degradation is required for MPF activity (Clarke and Karsenti 1991; Ledan et al. 2001). Cyclin B is accumulated in diplotene-arrested oocytes due to the presence of early mitotic inhibitor1 (Emi1) that inhibits anaphase promoting complex/cyclosome (APC/C), an ubiquitin ligase complex responsible for the destruction of cyclin B (Marangos et al. 2007). In oocyte, the level of cGMP and cAMP are very high and they are secreted from cumulus and granulosa cells surrounding the oocyte and are essential for the maintenance of meiotic arrest at diplotene stage (Norris et al. 2009; Sirard and Bilodeau 1990b; Sun et al. 2009; Vaccari et al. 2008). The increased level of cGMP inactivates phosphodiesterase 3A (PDE3A) and prevents hydrolysis of cAMP thus further increase its level (Mayes and Sirard 2002; Tsafriri et al. 1996; Vaccari et al. 2008). In diplotene-arrested oocytes, high concentrations of cAMP activate protein kinase A (PKA), and activated PKA phosphorylates two CDK1 regulators such as cell division cycle 25 homologue B (Cdc25B) phosphatase (Pirino et al. 2009) and Wee1/Myt1 (myelin transcription factor 1) kinase (Han and Conti 2006; Stanford and Ruderman 2005). The inactivation of Cdc25B and activation of Wee1/Myt1 kinase ultimately inactivate MPF activity for the maintenance of meiotic arrest at diplotene stage (Han and Conti 2006; Potapova et al. 2009; Solc et al. 2010). Luteinizing hormone (LH) released from surrounding granulosa cells act indirectly on oocytes to resume diplotene arrest at the onset of puberty (Mehlmann 2005; Zhang et al. 2009). LH mediated MAPK activation in granulosa cells interrupts the cells-oocytes communications and the result is the decrease of cAMP and cGMP level in oocytes (Liang et al. 2007; Mehlmann 2005; Norris et al. 2009). Reduced level of intraoocyte cGMP causes the activation of PDE3A activity that further reduces the intra oocyte cAMP level (Tornell et al. 1991; Wang et al. 2008). Net reduction of cAMP in oocytes inhibits PKA actions and dephospho-form of Cdc25B phosphatase remains active (Han and Conti 2006). On the other hand, dephospho-form of Wee1/Myt1 kinase remains inactive (Han and Conti 2006; Liang et al. 2007; Mehlmann et al. 2002; Solc et al. 2010) and finally resumes the diplotene arrest that is morphologically characterized by germinal vesicle breakdown (GVBD).

Getting release from diplotene arrest, activated MAPK through proper organization of metaphase spindle makes the progression of MI when homologous chromosomes are segregated (Sirard and Bilodeau 1990a). Oocytes are arrested at MI until the entire sister chromatids properly attached to the bipolar spindle and aligned at the metaphase plate where spindle assembly checkpoint (SAC) proteins e.g. Mad2 (metaphase arrest deficient 2), Bub1, and Bub3 (budding uninhibited by benzimidazole 1 and 3) act for all the required activities (Hupalowska et al. 2008; Li et al. 2009; Niault et al. 2007; Wassmann et al. 2003). The SAC proteins for accurate homologous chromosome segregation and to delay anaphase onset target APC/C (Brunet and Maro 2005; Homer 2011; Wassmann et al. 2003). Formation of functional spindle, spindle migration correlates with the progressive increase and continuous MPF activity (Brunet and Maro 2005; Madgwick et al. 2004). Mos/MAPK activity is also important in microtubule reorganization and positioning of metaphase spindle to the oocyte cortex (Choi et al. 1996; Verlhac et al. 1996; Zhou et al. 1991). At the end of MI, MPF activity is declined and is characterized by first polar body extrusion. After completion of MI, oocytes undergo some cytoplasmic changes and progress to the arrest at MII with further high MPF activity until fertilization. Stabilization of MPF activity is maintained by CSF (cytostatic factor) activity, not a single molecule but a total activity (Madgwick and Jones 2007; Wu and Kornbluth 2008) and by Mos-mediated MAPK pathway (Perry and Verlhac 2008; Shoji et al. 2006). Emi1 and Emi2 are two members of Emi/Erp family of proteins that has also the CSF activity (Schmidt et al. 2006) and functions in MII arrest (Madgwick and Jones 2007; Schmidt et al. 2006; Shoji et al. 2006; Tang et al. 2008). Complex of dephosphorylated active Emi2 with Cdc20, inhibit APC/C for the maintenance of MII arrest (Shoji et al. 2006). Sperm mediated Ca^{2+} oscillation activates calcium/calmodulin-dependent protein kinase II (CaMKII) and Emi2 can be phosphorylated by activated CaMKII followed by further phosphorylation by polo-like kinase (Hansen et al. 2006; Madgwick and Jones 2007; Masui and Markert 1971; Shoji et al. 2006). Cdc20 is released from Emi2 and subsequently bind with APC/C that results an active APC/C complex (Liu et al. 2006). Activated APC/C induces the degradation of cyclin B and MPF activity is decreased with an exit of egg from MII arrest by a process of sperm-egg interaction and fusion called fertilization. Another mechanism of MII arrest is by Mos (pp39, serine/threonine kinase), a proto-oncogene product act in the upstream of MEK/MAPK pathway that ultimately activates ribosomal protein S6 kinase ($p90^{Rsk}$). $p90^{Rsk}$ induces SAC protein activation and thereby inhibition of APC/C (Madgwick and Jones 2007; Maller et al. 2001) to maintain MII arrest. At fertilization Mos is degraded while the MEK/MAPK/$p90^{Rsk}$ is shortly inactivated and release from MII arrest. To the end of this process the sister chromatids are segregated, second polar body is extruded and the first cleavage starts. Postovulatory oocytes mimic the action of egg activation due to aging, increases cytoplasmic Ca^{2+}, and induces exit from MII arrest but they do not progress further and get arrest again in a new metaphase-like stage called MIII in few vertebrate species though the mechanisms for MIII arrest is not well understood (Chaube et al. 2007; Galat et al. 2007; Vincent et al. 1992; Zernicka-Goetz 1991). In aged eggs insufficient Ca^{2+} release and sufficient CSF activity is still present to stabilize the residual or newly formed MPF activity results in MIII arrest (Kubiak et al. 1992; Vincent et al. 1992).

Sperm-induced release of MII of an egg is also termed as "egg activation" that is characterized by so many biochemical changes e.g. Ca^{2+} oscillations, cortical granules exocytosis to block polyspermy, the formation of polar body and male and female pronuclei, recruitment of maternal mRNAs, initiation of DNA synthesis for mitotic divisions to unveil the complete developmental program (Ducibella 1996; Ducibella and Fissore 2008; Schultz and Kopf 1995). The wave of Ca^{2+} initiates at the site of sperm binding/fusion and soon after a wave of intracellular Ca^{2+} traverses the entire volume of the egg (Gilkey et al. 1978; Miyazaki and Ito 2006; Runft et al. 2002; Steinhardt and Epel 1974; Stricker 1999; Whitaker 2006). It is interesting to note that the increase in Ca^{2+} was reported in lysates of sea urchin eggs more than quarter century ago (Mazia 1937). Several excellent review articles have been published describing how egg becomes active in fertilization dependent manner and unite with sperm nuclei to form a zygote (Ajduk et al. 2008; Ducibella and Fissore 2008; Horner and Wolfner 2008; Miyazaki and Ito 2006; Swann et al. 2006; Townley et al. 2006).

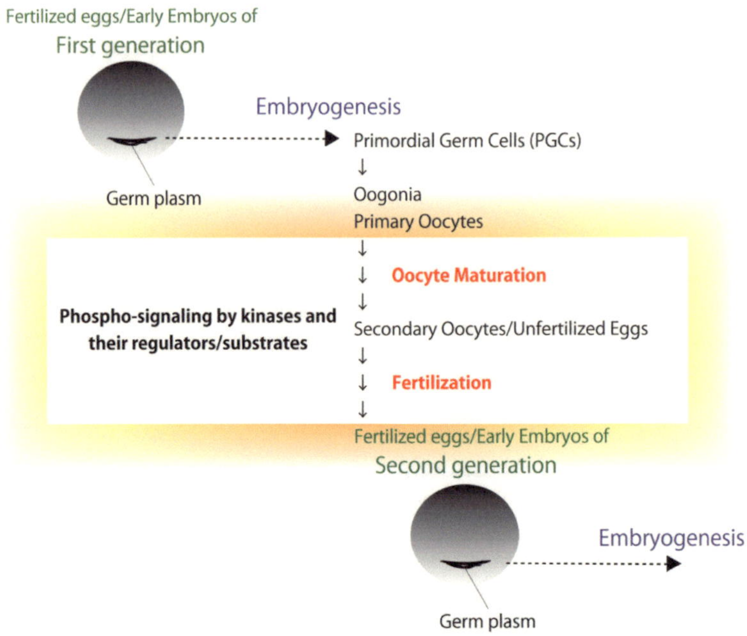

Fig. 1. Germline transmission from one generation to the next generation in sexual reproduction system. In most vertebrate species, the primary oocytes (or immature oocytes) in ovarian tissue pauses their cell cycle at prophase of the first meiosis, resumes the meiosis in response to hormonal signals, re-pauses at metaphase of the second meiotic cell cycle as the secondary oocytes (or mature oocytes), and are subject to ovulation and fertilization. Upon fertilization, eggs undergo a series of extracellular and intracellular reactions/changes, collectively called egg activation that triggers the initiation of development or early embryogenesis. A similar mechanism, although not identical in several species, has been shown to be involved in sexual reproduction system in a diverse array of animal species and maybe in some algae and plants.

Oocyte plasma membrane is surrounded by glycoprotein-rich extracellular matrix called the vitelline envelope (VE) or vitelline membrane (VM) in invertebrates and amphibians, and zona pellucida (ZP) in mammals. Upon fertilization this layer must be modified to prevent additional sperm to bind and fuse to block the polyspermy. Prevention of polyspermy is accomplished in part through Ca^{2+}-dependent cortical granule exocytosis (CGE) (Wessel et al. 2001; Wessel and Wong 2009). Upon egg activation, CGE fuse with the oocyte plasma membrane and release their contents into the perivitelline space that results the biochemical modification of the outer membrane. Ca^{2+}-mediated active CaMKII phosphorylate Emi2 that is further phosphorylated by polo-like kinase and this phosphorylated Emi2 is targeted by APC/C resulting in an active APC/C (Liu and Maller 2005; Rauh et al. 2005). Activated APC/C leads to the degradation of cyclin B that results the inactivation of Cdc2 and might also inactivate the function of Mos (Castro et al. 2001; Madgwick et al. 2006; Madgwick and Jones 2007). Thus, due to the absence of Cdc2/CDK1 activity, meiosis-specific host protein phosphorylations are reduced allowing eggs to exit M-phase. Src family tyrosine kinases (SFKs) are playing important roles in sperm-induced Ca^{2+} oscillation in several species e.g. in starfish (Abassi et al. 2000; Carroll et al. 1999; Giusti et al. 1999a, 1999b), Fyn kinase in sea urchin eggs (Kinsey and Shen 2000) and in rat eggs (Talmor et al. 1998), and Src in frog eggs (Sato et al. 1996; Sato et al. 2006a). In mouse eggs though Src related tyrosine kinase (e.g. Lck, Src) has been reported (Mori et al. 1991) but it is not sufficient or required for fertilization-induced Ca^{2+} oscillation (Kurokawa et al. 2004). In mammals, PLC activity is high enough in sperm that's why even a single sperm equivalent PLC can generate sufficient IP_3 when introduced into the egg cytoplasm (Rice et al. 2000). ζ isoform of PLC present in sperm has been characterized as a soluble sperm factor that evokes Ca^{2+} oscillations in eggs of several mammals e.g. mouse, bovine and human (Malcuit et al. 2005; Rogers et al. 2004; Saunders et al. 2002). Thus upon successful fertilization, the newly formed zygote initiates the developmental program through early stages of embryogenesis until a full different born.

2. Kinases in oocyte maturation, fertilization and activation of development

2.1 Abelson tyrosine kinase (Abl)

Abl has been originally identified as the oncogene product (termed v-Abl) of Abelson murine leukemia virus (Wang et al. 1983). In human, the cellular homolog of v-Abl, c-Abl, is translocated to the Philadelphia chromosome in chronic myelocytic leukemia (so-called Philadelphia syndrome) (de Klein et al. 1982). Gleevec (STI-571), a well-known drug for chronic myeloid leukemia (CML) and some other cancers, has been designed to target the protein product of the CML transforming gene, Bcr (breakpoint cluster region)-Abl (Schindler et al. 2000). In the sea urchin, a 220-kDa Abl-related tyrosine kinase has been identified in the egg cortex. Immunoprecipitation studies demonstrated that it is activated within minutes of fertilization, suggesting a possible role for sperm-induced egg activation, and immunofluorescent studies showed its association with cortical cytoskeleton (Moore and Kinsey 1994; Walker et al. 1996; Wang et al. 1983). However, its mode of activation and physiological substrate has not yet been demonstrated.

2.2 Akt protein kinase (Akt)

The serine/threonine-specific protein kinase **Akt** has been identified first as the oncogene product of murine transforming retrovirus. Because of its structural homology in the catalytic domain to protein kinase A (PKA) and C (PKC), an alternative term "protein kinase B or PKB" is sometimes used. Akt is shown to be involved in several aspects of cellular functions, and most frequently, it is regarded as a kinase that promotes anti-apoptotic growth of cells (Hemmings 1997). Upstream kinases, such as phosphoinositide-dependent protein kinase 1 (PDK1) and mammalian target of rapamycin (mTOR), are responsible for phosphorylation and activation of Akt. Thus, Akt is regulated by metabolism of membrane-bound phosphoinositides as well as extracellular nutrient environments. Akt is shown to be involved in oocyte maturation in some species (e.g. starfish, mouse, and maybe *Xenopus*) (Deng et al. 2011; Feng et al. 2007; Han et al. 2006; Hoshino and Sato 2008; Hoshino et al. 2004; Kalous et al. 2009; Kalous et al. 2006; Mammadova et al. 2009; Okumura et al. 2002; Reddy et al. 2005; Tomek and Smiljakovic 2005; Zhang et al. 2010b). For example, Akt phosphorylation and down-regulation of Myt1, an MPF-inhibitory kinase, and PDE3, a cAMP-antagonizing enzyme, in maturing starfish and mouse oocytes have been demonstrated (Han et al. 2006a). On the other hand, fertilization promotes an activating phosphorylation (on Thr-308) of Akt in *Xenopus* (Mammadova et al. 2009), suggesting its possible role in initiation of development and/or suppression of cell death.

2.3 Adenosine 5'-monophosphate-dependent protein kinase (AMPK)

AMPK is a serine/threonine kinase that is activated in response to high AMP and/or low ATP levels in the cell. AMPK is composed of three subunits; one catalytic subunit and two regulatory subunits, all of which are evolutionary conserved in budding yeast as the SNF1 protein kinase complex (Hardie and Carling 1997). AMPK is phosphorylated and activated by an upstream AMPK kinase. Inhibitory effect of AMP and/or AMPK on oocyte maturation and/or meiotic resumption has been demonstrated in marine worm, starfish, and some mammalian species (Bilodeau-Goeseels et al. 2007; Chen and Downs 2008; Chen et al. 2006; LaRosa and Downs 2006; Stricker 2011; Stricker and Smythe 2006; Stricker et al. 2010b; Tosca et al. 2007). In marine worm, liver kinase B1 (LKB1)-like kinase is likely involved in up-regulation of AMPK (via phosphorylation of Thr-172), and thus suppresses the occurrence of oocyte maturation. On the other hand, MAPK and MPF are shown to simultaneously phosphorylate AMPK on two sites (Ser-485/491), and thereby inactivate the activity of AMPK. Physiological target of AMPK in this species is under investigation.

2.4 Aurora protein kinase (Aurora A/B/C/AIR-2/Eg2/IAK2/Ipl1p)

Aurora is a serine/threonine kinase that has been initially characterized as a protein that regulates proper chromosomal segregation and cytokinesis (Bischoff and Plowman 1999). In *C. elegans*, AIR-2 (homolog of aurora kinase) is involved in the release of chromosomal cohesion. In *Xenopus*, Eg2 (an alternative name of this kinase) has been shown as a component of progesterone-induced maturation of oocytes. H3 histone, a linker histone that regulates the integrity of nucleosome core, has been identified a substrate of aurora in mouse and porcine oocytes. Another substrate known to date includes cytoplasmic polyadenylation element-binding protein (CPEB) that regulates translation of mRNA for Mos, and maskin that regulates the assembly of microtubules. Analyses of cell-free extracts demonstrated that protein phosphatase 2A (PP2A) is responsible for suppression of MPF, which is an upstream activator for aurora kinase. In the meiotic and mitotic exit, aurora undergoes degradation under the control of APC/C interaction with the APC/C recognition domain of aurora kinase. Thus aurora kinase behaves like a component of cytostatic factor (e.g. cyclin, Mos) (Andresson and Ruderman 1998; Detivaud et al. 2003; Ding et al. 2011; Eckerdt et al. 2009; Frank-Vaillant et al. 2000; Hodgman et al. 2001; Jelinkova and Kubelka 2006; Kinoshita et al. 2005; Littlepage and Ruderman 2002; Littlepage et al. 2002; Ma et al. 2003; Maton et al. 2005; Maton et al. 2003; Mendez et al. 2000; Pascreau et al. 2005; Pascreau et al. 2008; Pascreau et al. 2009; Rogers et al. 2002; Roghi et al. 1998; Sardon et al. 2008; Yang et al. 2010b).

2.5 Calmodulin-dependent protein kinase II (CaMKII)

CaMKII is a serine/threonine-specific kinase that is regulated by the intracellular concentration of Ca^{2+} ions. Biochemical analyses demonstrated that the binding of Ca^{2+}/calmodulin to the catalytic core of the kinase as well as the release of an autoinhibitory region from the kinase domain coordinately activates the enzyme (Ishida and Fujisawa 1995). Gene targeting analyses have demonstrated that this kinase is involved in synaptic plasticity such as the long-term potentiation in hippocampus (Silva et al. 1992a; Silva et al. 1992b). In mammalian oocytes and cell-free extracts prepared from *Xenopus* unfertilized eggs, the kinase activity of CaMKII oscillates in response to sperm-induced Ca^{2+} oscillations, well-known phenomenon that is required for the meiotic exit and initiation of embryonic development. The activated CaMKII is believed to be involved in the initiation of signaling cascade involving cyclin/Mos degradation and calcineurin/Rsk activation, both of which leads to the inactivation of Emi2, a suppressor of meiotic exit (Ducibella and Fissore 2008; Hansen et al. 2006; Hudmon et al. 2005; Liu and Maller 2005; Madgwick et al. 2005; Nishiyama et al. 2007b; Nutt et al. 2005).

2.6 Casein kinase II (CKII/CK2)

CKII is a family of serine/threonine-specific kinases that are ubiquitously expressed in eukaryotic organisms including budding yeast (Glover 1998). In the oocyte of *Xenopus*, CKII is shown to localize to the nucleus and transcription factor IIIA has been identified as a substrate of CKII (Leiva et al. 1987; Sanghera et al. 1992; Westmark et al. 2002). CKII can be regulated by PKC and other serine/threonine kinases, and therefore it may be involved in sperm-induced egg activation as well. In this respect, the fact that CKII phosphorylates a serine/threonine residue in the cytoplasmic sequence of uroplakin IIIa (UPIIIa) in uropathological bacteria-infected human urinary bladder cells is interesting. As UPIIIa in *Xenopus* eggs has been suggested to be important for sperm-egg interaction and subsequent phospho-signaling for egg activation (see below) (Mahbub Hasan et al. 2011), CKII may also be an important player in the same system through the phosphorylation of UPIIIa.

2.7 Cyclic AMP-dependent protein kinase (cAPK/PKA)

Inactive **PKA** is a tetrameric protein that is composed of two catalytic subunits and two regulatory (or inhibitory) subunits, latter of which, when cAMP binds, is released from the catalytic subunits. The discovery of AMP as well as PKA as intracellular mediators of several extracellular signal-dependent cellular functions has opened firstly a window of the research field of "phospho-signal transduction" (Robison et al. 1968), followed by discoveries of other important factors such as PKC, receptor/kinase and Src. In vertebrate oocytes, activity of PKA is shown to decrease by phosphodiesterase (PDE)-mediated decrease of intracellular cAMP and then re-increase upon meiotic maturation, and its active state is maintained until fertilization. Upon fertilization, PKA undergoes a rapid decline in its activity. Transition from mitotic phase to interphase in fertilized egg requires MPF-dependent PKA activity. In mammals, maturing oocytes involves PKA phosphorylation of Cdc25B tyrosine phosphatase that leads to up-regulation of MPF activity. In marine worm, AMPK activity has been implicated in oocyte maturation, suggesting that intracellular balance of cAMP and AMP concentrations, as regulated by PDE and adenylate cyclase, is important for oocyte functions (Bornslaeger et al. 1986; Browne et al. 1990; Daar et al. 1993; Faure et al. 1998; Faure et al. 1999; Grieco et al. 1994; Grieco et al. 1996; Matten et al. 1994; Meijer et al. 1989b; Newhall et al. 2006; Pirino et al. 2009; Schmitt and Nebreda 2002a, 2002b; Stricker and Smythe 2006; Stricker et al. 2010b; Wang and Liu 2004; Webb et al. 2008; Yu et al. 2005; Zhang et al. 2008).

2.8 Cyclin-dependent protein kinase (Cdc2/CDK/MPF)

The term "cdc" refers *cell division cycle* and has originally been coined in the study of yeast genetics. While the genetic background as well as biochemical and molecular biological identifications of key regulators for cell division cycle (i.e. several **cdc/CDK** kinases and cyclins) have firstly been demonstrated in the studies of such model organisms as yeast, sea urchin, and clam (Hartwell 1991; Minshull et al. 1989; Nurse 1990), early studies with use of frog oocytes has also contributed to arise a concept of **MPF** (maturation/mitosis-promoting factor) (Masui 1992). It is well known that cdc/CDK kinases are mainly responsible for meiotic cell cycle progression in maturing oocytes, and thereafter acts as an essential component of mitotic cell cycles. Regulatory mechanism of cdc/CDK kinases involves a complex combination of phosphorylation/dephosphorylation on a threonine and tyrosine residues in the ATP-binding pocket (e.g. Wee1, Myt1, Cdc25, PP2A) and a threonine residue in the catalytic domain of cdc/CDK kinase (i.e. CAK kinase), and protein level of activator proteins (e.g. cyclin and RINGO/speedy) and inhibitor proteins (e.g. p16 and p21). Kinase activity of cdc/CDK/MPF has been sometimes regarded as "histone H1 kinase (H1K or HH1K)" because of its in vitro evaluation. Cellular targets of cdc/CDK kinases include aurora kinase and Emi2, which are implicated in chromosomal integrity and meiotic arrest, respectively (Anger et al. 2004; Castilho et al. 2009; Culp and Musci 1999; Eckberg 1997; Edgecombe et al. 1991; Ferrell 1999; Ferrell et al. 1991; Gavin et al. 1999; Grieco et al. 1996; Gutierrez et al. 2006; Karaiskou et al. 1998; Karaiskou et al. 2004; Katsu et al. 1999; Kume et al. 2007; Kuo et al. 2011; Lohka et al. 1988; Masui 2000; Maton et al. 2005; Maton et al. 2003; Meijer et al. 1989a; Meijer et al. 1991; Meijer et al. 1989b; Palmer et al. 1998; Qian et al. 2001; Rime et al. 1994; Ruiz et al. 2008; Sakamoto et al. 1998; Tang et al. 2008; Tokmakov et al. 2005; Wu et al. 2007b; Yu et al. 2005; Yu et al. 2004).

2.9 Dual-specificity tyrosine-regulated kinase 1A/2 (DYRK)/Minibrain-related kinase (Mirk)/MBK-2/Nuclear kinase

DYRK is a dual-specificity protein kinase, whose expression in a wide variety of animal species (e.g. Yak1 in yeast, Mnb in fly, Dyrk1~4 in mammals) has been reported. Tyrosine autophosphorylation in the activation loop is important for enzyme activation of DYRK as a serine/threonine kinase. A similar scheme of kinase regulation has been shown in some other kinases including MAPK, so DYRK is regarded as a member of the MAPK superfamily (Miyata and Nishida 1999). DYRK has been implicated in neurobiological disease such as Down syndrome, cell proliferation and anti-apoptosis in cancer cells, and cell cycle control (Becker 2011; Becker and Sippl 2011). In nematode oocytes, DYRK2/MBK2, a member of DYRK, in cooperation with CDK1 (this kinase catalyses activating phosphorylation of MBK-2 on Ser-68) (Cheng et al. 2009), GSK3, and Kin-19, phosphorylates and promotes degradation of OMA-1 that regulates oocyte-to-embryo transition (Nishi and Lin 2005; Qu et al. 2006; Qu et al. 2007; Stitzel et al. 2007; Stitzel et al. 2006). In *Xenopus* oocytes, Ras-dependent oocyte maturation involves the function of DYRK1A (Qu et al. 2006; Qu et al. 2007).

2.10 Epidermal growth factor receptor (EGFR/HER1)

EGFR is a prototype of the cell surface receptor/kinase that consists of an extracellular ligand -binding domain, a transmembrane hydrophobic sequence, and a cytoplasmic kinase domain that is followed by a non-catalytic sequence, which contains some tyrosine residues to be autophosphorylated in activated molecules. Normally, EGFR is activated by EGF-dependent dimerization (activation as tyrosine kinase) and autophosphorylation (activation as phosphotyrosine-dependent docking protein). Its oncogenic counterpart has been found in avian sarcoma virus that encodes v-erbB, whose protein product lacks entirely the extracellular domain so that the kinase activity is constitutively elevated irrespective of the presence of EGF. While a variety of cellular functions (e.g. normal and malignant growth in several kinds of cells and tissues) have been shown to involve EGF and EGFR, its contribution to oocyte maturation and fertilization remains unclear. In *Xenopus* eggs, ectopically expressed EGFR is capable of inducing egg activation in an EGF-dependent manner (Yim et al. 1994). This could be explained as that active tyrosine kinase can mediate the process of egg activation in this system. In fact, it has been shown that *Xenopus* eggs employ an endogenous tyrosine kinase-dependent egg activation system involving Src and PLCγ.

2.11 ErbB4/HER4

ErbB4 is a member of the EGFR (ErbB1/HER1)/HER family of receptor/tyrosine kinases. Although its involvement in oocyte maturation and fertilization has not yet been shown, implantation of mammalian early embryos involves the actions of ErbB4 and its cognate ligand heparin-binding EGF-like growth factor (HB-EGF) (Chobotova et al. 2002). In this system, metalloproteinase-dependent extracellular shedding of HB-EGF is required for survival of trophoblasts at low oxygen conditions (Armant et al. 2006; Jessmon et al. 2009), one of pro-apoptotic pressures in the embryogenic microenvironment at early stages of pregnancy.

2.12 Focal adhesion kinase (FAK)

FAK is a cytoplasmic tyrosine kinase, whose activity is stimulated by integrin-dependent cell-extracellular matrix (ECM) interactions. Namely, in response to heterodimeric interaction with the ECM-activated integrin α and β subunits, FAK undergoes autophosphorylation and then phosphorylated by Src on tyrosine residues. The activated FAK undergoes a number of molecular interactions with cytoskeletal and signaling proteins, including Src, phosphatidylinositol 3-kinase (PI3K), Grb2, $p130^{Cas}$ and paxillin (Cary and Guan 1999). Recent studies also highlight the interaction of FAK with cell cycle control system (e.g. CDK5), pro-apoptotic system (e.g. p53), and cadherin-dependent cell-cell communications (Golubovskaya and Cance 2010; Quadri 2011; Xie et al. 2003). On the other hand, roles of FAK in gamete interaction and gametogenesis have not yet been fully documented. Developmental expression of FAK in porcine oocytes (Okamura et al. 2001) and in *Xenopus* oocytes and early embryos (Hens and DeSimone 1995; Zhang et al. 1995) have only been reported.

2.13 Fer tyrosine kinase (Fer)

DNA microarray analysis demonstrates that Feline encephalitis virus (FES)-related tyrosine kinase protein, named **FER**, is highly expressed in oocytes of the mouse (McGinnis et al. 2011a). It shows a uniform distribution in the ooplasm of small oocytes, but becomes concentrated in the germinal vesicle (GV) during oocyte growth. Association of FER with spindle bodies is seen after GV breakdown (GVBD), suggesting that it is involved in the control of cell cycle and/or chromosomal dynamics (McGinnis et al. 2011b). In support with this, siRNA-mediated knockdown of FER causes the failure of the oocytes to undergo GVBD or during MI (McGinnis et al. 2011b). While upstream and downstream mediators of FER regulation and functions have not yet been shown, other cell systems so far analyzed demonstrate that phospholipase D (PLD)-phosphatidic acid (PA) pathway is capable of stimulating FER activity (Itoh et al. 2009), and that TATA-element modulatory protein is a substrate of nuclear-localized FER (Schwartz et al. 1998). The former fact is of interest because, in amphibian (*Rana pipiens*) oocytes, progesterone-induced oocyte maturation involves a rapid activation of PLD (Kostellow et al. 1996).

2.14 Fibroblast growth factor receptor-1/-2 (FGFR1/2)

To date, 22 members of FGF family of growth factors and 4 members of **FGFR** family of receptor/tyrosine kinase have been identified in human. The FGF-FGFR system is activated in concert with heparin and heparan sulfate proteoglycan on the cell surface, and phosphorylates a number of intracellular substrate to promote a variety of cellular functions (Eswarakumar et al. 2005). In *Xenopus* maturing oocytes, translational activation of FGFR1 has been demonstrated. In the same system, overexpressed FGFR by itself can promote oocyte maturation in response to FGF stimulation, through interaction and/or phosphorylation of the SNT1/FRS2 adaptor protein. In bovine oocytes, FGF10 is shown to enhance the maturation and developmental competence (Zhang et al. 2010a), suggesting that oocytes contain the endogenous and functional FGFR. Developmental expression of FGFR has also been demonstrated in *Xenopus* and zebrafish. However, its involvement in fertilization has not yet been shown (Cailliau et al. 2003; Culp and Musci 1998; Culp and Musci 1999; Mood et al. 2002; Rappolee et al. 1998; Robbie et al. 1995; Tonou-Fujimori et al. 2002).

2.15 Fyn tyrosine kinase (Fyn)

Fyn, 59-kDa protein, is a member of Src family of non-receptor tyrosine kinases (SFKs). Like Src and Yes, another kind of SFK, Fyn is ubiquitously expressed in human tissues and its pleiotropic contribution to cellular functions (e.g. T-lymphocyte activation, spatial learning, and alcohol sensitivity) has been well documented (Palacios and Weiss 2004; Resh 1998; Trepanier et al. 2011). Oocyte-expressing Fyn and Fyn-related protein have been characterized extensively not only in vertebrates (e.g. mammals and fish) but also in sea invertebrates (sea urchin). In sea urchin, sperm-induced tyrosine phosphorylation of oocyte/egg proteins is mainly due to the activated Fyn and Src (and maybe Abl). In this species, tyrosine phosphorylation of phospholipase Cγ (PLCγ) plays an important role in inositol trisphosphate (IP_3)-induced Ca^{2+} release. A similar tyrosine kinase-PLCγ pathway also operates in starfish, ascidian, fish, and frog. In mice and rats, Fyn is shown to interact with tubulin and involve in cleavage furrow ingression during meiosis and mitosis. Another report demonstrates that Fyn contributes to establish and maintain polarity of the egg cortex. Further, knockdown of FYN kinase by siRNA resulted in an approximately 50% reduction in progression to metaphase II similar to what was observed in oocytes isolated from Fyn-knockout mice matured in vitro. These results clearly demonstrate that involvement of Fyn in oocyte and egg functions vary among species (Eliyahu et al. 2002; Kierszenbaum et al. 2009; Kinsey 1995; Kinsey 1996; Kinsey and Shen 2000; Kinsey et al. 2003; Levi et al. 2010; Luo et al. 2009; McGinnis et al. 2009;

Rongish and Kinsey 2000; Sette et al. 2002; Sharma and Kinsey 2006; Sharma and Kinsey 2008; Steele et al. 1990; Talmor et al. 1998; Talmor-Cohen et al. 2004b; Wu and Kinsey 2000; Wu and Kinsey 2002; Wu and Kinsey 2004).

2.16 Flagellar protein-tyrosine kinase (Flagellar PTK)

Fertilization in the biflagellated green algae, *Chlamydomonas*, is initiated by flagellar adhesion between gametes of opposite mating types: plus (mt+) and minus (mt-). Flagellar adhesion is followed by an increase in cytoplasmic cAMP concentration that is required for gamete fusion. Pharmacological and biochemical studies have demonstrated that a tyrosine kinase activity, named **flagellar PTK**, which acts upstream of the cAMP elevation, is present in adhering bisexual gametes but not in non-adhering, unisexual gametes. A 105-kDa protein has been identified as a substrate of the flagellar PTK. Analyses of temperature-sensitive mutants have shown that kinesin II is an essential component that connects flagellar adhesion and activation of the tyrosine kinase activity (Kurvari and Snell 1996; Kurvari et al. 1996; Wang and Snell 2003).

2.17 Flagellar p48 protein kinase (SksC)

On the contrary to flagellar PTK, another protein kinase activity is shown to decrease rapidly after gamete adhesion in *Chlamydomonas*. The kinase, named **SksC**, is a 48-kDa protein that is capable of autophosphorylating on serine and tyrosine residues, indicating that it is a dual-specificity kinase. Although it's physiological substrate other than SksC by itself has not yet been identified, adhesion-induced SksC down-regulation and flagellar PTK up-regulation may play important roles simultaneously in gamete fusion and activation of embryogenesis (Pan and Snell 2000; Zhang et al. 1996). In this species, a rapid degradation of two gamete-specific proteins, FUS1 and HAP1, occur upon gamete fusion (Liu et al. 2010). This event is required for polyspermy block. However, its relationship to the aforementioned phospho-signaling is not known.

2.18 Fms-like tyrosine kinase/vascular endothelial growth factor receptor (FLT/Colony-stimulating factor receptor-like/VEGFR)

FLT/VEGFR is a receptor/tyrosine kinase, whose extracellular ligand is VEGF (de Vries et al. 1992). The term FLT is coined because it is structurally related to c-fms/macrophage colony-stimulating factor-1 receptor/kinase. The viral counterpart of c-fms in a feline sarcoma virus (McDonough and HZ-5 strain) arises as a result of alterations in receptor coding sequences that affect its activity as a tyrosine kinase (Sherr et al. 1988). Pleiotropic functions of FLT/VEGFR have been well documented and, most of all, its involvement in angiogenesis in normal as well as cancerous cell conditions has been of clinical interest (Shibuya 1995). In bovine cumulus-oocyte complexes and porcine ovary, expression and physiological impact of VEGF and/or FLT/VEGFR have been investigated. The results so far obtained suggest that VEGF-FLA/VEGFR pathway is involved in viability of oocytes (Einspanier et al. 2002; Okamura et al. 2001).

2.19 Glycogen synthase kinase 3 (GSK3/shaggy/GSK3-B)

GSK3, a serine/threonine protein kinase, have the two isoforms GSK3 (p51) and GSK3 (p47) is known to play roles in many biological processes. Mouse eggs contain centrosomal spindle poles when arrested at meiotic metaphase II. Phosphorylated PKC (p-PKC) and GSK3 are enriched at both centrosomal spindle poles and the kinetochore region (Baluch and Capco 2008). p-PKC phosphorylates GSK3 on the Ser-9 position to inactivate GSK3 and consequently maintaining spindle stability during meiotic metaphase arrest (Baluch and Capco 2008). Similarly, in mouse oocytes, p-GSK3 was increased and phospho-MAPK3/MAPK1 was decreased before GVBD and oocytes were mainly arrested at MI (Uzbekova et al. 2009). GSK3 might be also involved in the local activation of Aurora A kinase that controls MI/MII transition (Uzbekova et al. 2009). GSK3/shaggy along with other downstream components of the Wnt pathway mediate patterning along the primary animal-vegetal axis of the sea urchin embryo (Emily-Fenouil et al. 1998) and along the dorsal-ventral axis in *Xenopus*, suggesting a conserved basis for axial patterning between invertebrate and vertebrate. Double phosphorylation (Thr-239 by DYRK kinase MBK-2 and Thr-339 by GSK-3) on OMA-1 is essential for correctly timed degradation of OMA-1 and ensures a normal oocyte-to-embryo transition in *C. elegans* (Nishi and Lin 2005). Even the conserved function of GSK3 is observed in hydra embryogenesis (Rentzsch et al. 2005), and in zebrafish cardiogenesis (Emily-Fenouil et al. 1998; Lee et al. 2007; Liu et al. 2007; Nishi and Lin 2005; Uzbekova et al. 2009).

2.20 Greatwall kinase (Gwl/GWK)

The balance between Cdc2 kinase/cyclin B also known as M-phase-promoting factor (Arceci et al. 1992), and protein phosphatase 2A (PP2A) is crucial to enable in time mitotic entry and exit. Greatwall (Gwl) kinase (**GWK**) has been identified as a key element in M phase initiation and maintenance in *Drosophila, Xenopus* oocytes/eggs, and mammalian cells. GWK is activated by cdk1/cyclin B (Arceci et al. 1992), and promotes the inhibition of protein phosphatase 2A (PP2A) that works on the phosphorylated substrate mediated by CDKs. Activated GWK negatively regulates a crucial phosphatase and thus induce inhibiting phosphorylations of Cdc25 to inhibits M phase induction (Zhao et al. 2008). Thus, mitotic entry and maintenance is not only mediated by the activation of Cdc2 kinase/cyclin B but also by the regulation of PP2A by GWK in *Xenopus* oocytes/eggs (Castilho et al. 2009; Mochida et al. 2010; Vigneron et al. 2009; Yamamoto et al. 2011).

2.21 Histone H1 kinase (HH1K/H1K)

Maturation promoting factor (Arceci et al. 1992) is universally recognized as the biological entity responsible for driving the cell cycle from G2- to M-phase. Histone H1 kinase (**HH1K**) activity is widely accepted as a biochemical indicator of p34Cdc2 protein kinase complex activity and therefore MPF activity. In spontaneously maturing oocytes, HH1K activity increases before GVBD in mouse (Gavin et al. 1994). HH1K activity being higher in the first than in the second cell cycle in mouse embryogenesis that reaches to the basal level (Ciemerych et al. 1998; Fulka et al. 1992). Inhibition of protein phosphatases are correlated with HH1K activity and is sufficient to induce the entry into M-phase during the first cell cycle of the mouse parthenogenetic activated oocyte (Rime and Ozon 1990). In fertilized sea urchin eggs the activity of HH1K oscillates during the cell division cycle and there is a striking temporal correlation between HH1K activation and the accumulation of a phosphorylated form of cyclin (Meijer et al. 1989a; Meijer and Pondaven 1988; Tosuji et al. 2003). HH1K activity correlation with the oocyte maturation and after fertilization were carried out in other species e.g. bovine (Collas et al. 1993), cat fish (Balamurugan and Haider 1998), fish (Yamashita et al. 1992), goldfish (Pati et al. 2000), pig (Kikuchi et al. 1995), rabbit (Jelinkova et al. 1994) and sea star (Arion et al. 1988; Pelech et al. 1987).

2.22 Insulin-like growth factor 1 receptor/kinase (IGF-1R/IGFR)

In somatic cell insulin-like growth factor (IGF) receptor (**IGFR**) has the ability to phosphorylate the overall cellular substrates, in particular PLCγ, annexin II and to activate phosphatidylinositol 3-kinase via insulin receptor substrate 1 (Jiang et al. 1996). *Xenopus* oocytes bear both the IGFR-1 and IGFR-2, where IGFR-1, a tyrosine kinase, has the capability of autophosphorylation (Janicot et al. 1991; Nissley et al. 1985). IGF-1-induced oocyte maturation required IGFR-1-mediated endocytosis in *Xenopus* (Taghon and Sadler 1994). IGFR-1 in *Xenopus* ovarian follicle cells somehow supports the IGF-1-stimulated oocyte maturation (Sadler et al. 2010). Expression of IGFR has been shown in the oocytes of rat (Zhao et al. 2001), in bovine (Nuttinck et al. 2004) and in rainbow trout positively correlated with embryonic survival (Aegerter et al. 2004).

2.23 Insulin receptor/kinase (IR)

Insulin/insulin-like growth factor (IGF)-1 receptor (**IR/IGF1R**), a tyrosine kinase, exerts its cellular functions by the phosphorylation of insulin receptor substrate-1 (IRS-1). Tyrosine phosphorylated form of IRS-1 binds to specific Src homology-2 (SH2) domain-containing proteins including the p85 subunit of phosphatidylinositol (PI) 3-kinase and GRB2, a molecule believed to link IRS-1 to the Ras pathway in *Xenopus* oocyte maturation (Chuang et al. 1994; Chuang et al. 1993; El-Etr et al. 1979; Grigorescu et al. 1994). Insulin through IR has influences on oocyte maturation and embryonic development in mouse (Acevedo et al. 2007). Recently, it has been shown that IR and IGF1R are not required for oocyte growth, differentiation, and maturation in mice using genetically ablated mouse (Pitetti et al. 2009). It was shown that IR is the components of sea urchin eggs plasma membrane (Jeanmart et al. 1976) and insulin like peptide 3 acts through mosquito IR in mosquito egg production (Brown et al. 2008).

2.24 c-Jun N-terminal kinase (JNK)

The c-Jun N-terminal kinase (**JNK**) is member of the mitogen-activated protein kinase family that plays critical roles in stress responses and apoptosis. JNK is activated just prior to germinal vesicle breakdown during *Xenopus* oocyte maturation and remains active until the early gastrula stage of embryogenesis (Bagowski et al. 2001). JNK was activated after the microinjection of Mos (Bagowski et al. 2001). Progesterone mediated *Xenopus* oocyte maturation might involve JNK activation both through the raf/MEK (MAPKK)/p42 MAPK-dependent pathway (Bagowski et al. 2001; Chie et al. 2000) and through MEK/p42 MAPK-independent pathways (Bagowski et al. 2001). JNK2 plays an important role in spindle assembly and first polar body extrusion during mouse oocyte meiotic maturation (Huang et al. 2011). JNK mRNA was detected in mouse eggs and pre-implantation embryos (Zhong et al. 2004).

2.25 c-Kit tyrosine kinase (c-Kit)

The proto-oncogene product **c-Kit**, a transmembrane tyrosine kinase, acts as a receptor in mouse oocytes to communicate with the surrounding granulose cells and for its maturation.

Stem cell factor (SCF), a ligand for c-Kit is required for the production of the mature gametes e.g. the growth and maturation of the oocytes in response to gonadotropic hormones (Sette et al. 2000). The level of c-Kit increases during the maturation of mouse oocytes and following fertilization, it decreases rapidly until the early 2-cell stage but it is not detected in the embryos of 4-cell, 8-cell, and morula stages (Arceci et al. 1992; Horie et al. 1991). It is suggested that Kit-PI3K-Akt-GSK-3 pathway might work in the regulation of mouse oocytes growth (Liu et al. 2007).

2.26 Lck tyrosine kinase (Lck)

Lck, a 56-kDa protein, has originally been characterized as a Src-related tyrosine kinase that is specifically expressed in lymphocytes (Lck is named after lymphocyte kinase). In T-cells, Lck associates with CD4/CD8 cell surface receptor for major histocompatibility complex and, upon interaction with antigen-presenting cells, it will be activated by dephosphorylation in the carboxyl-terminal tyrosine residue, as catalyzed by CD45 phosphatase. In murine eggs, it has been reported that CD4-like structures on the vitelline membranes are involved in gamete interaction, and that Lck-like protein could have been detected in association with those CD4-like structures (Mori et al. 2000; Mori et al. 1991). While these studies have been done with the use of specific monoclonal antibodies (e.g. immunofluorescent and immunochemical approaches), biochemical and molecular biological identifications have not yet been demonstrated.

2.27 p38 MAPK/Mipk/Stress-activated protein kinase (SAPK)/Xp38γ

p38/SAPK, which has initially been identified as a stress-activated protein kinase, belongs to the MAPK superfamily (Miyata and Nishida 1999). In the sea star, a p38-related kinase Mipk (meiosis-inhibited protein kinase) has been identified and characterized. Before oocyte maturation, Mipk is highly phosphorylated on tyrosine residues, and during oocyte maturation and some hours after fertilization, it becomes tyrosine-dephosphorylated and enzymatically inactive, suggesting that inhibition of Mipk is related to cell cycle progression during meiosis (Morrison et al. 2000). However, knockdown of Mipk by antisense oligonucleotide is not effective in inducing oocyte maturation. On the other hand, *Xenopus* p38γ/SAPK3 is a major player in G2/M transition of immature oocytes induced by MKK6, a p38 activator. The activated p38γ/SAPK3 is also shown to phosphorylate Ser-205 of and activate Cdc25C phosphatase (Perdiguero et al. 2003). One another interesting feature of p38 in oocyte/egg system is that it may contribute to apoptotic process in starfish eggs left unfertilized for a long time. In this system, inactivation of MAPK is pre-requisite for inducing activation of caspase, a pro-apoptotic protease. p38 has been shown to activate after the MAPK inactivation and seems to be responsible for apoptotic body formation (Morrison et al. 2000; Perdiguero et al. 2003; Sasaki and Chiba 2004).

2.28 Mitogen-activated protein kinase (p42/p44MAPK/ERK)

MAPK is a serine/threonine kinase that has been originally identified as a microtubule-associated protein 2 (MAP2) kinase (this is also termed "MAPK" or "MAP2 kinase") and then well recognized as a mitogen-activated protein kinase (Maller 1990). MAPK is a component of the MAPK kinase, which consists of at least three steps of phospho-dependent activation of kinases that include MAPK (e.g. Erk, p38, JNK), MAPK kinase (MAPKK: e.g. MEK), and MAPKK kinase (MAPKKK: e.g. Mos, Raf). The MAPK cascade is evolutionarily conserved in a variety of unicellular and multicellular organisms and serves as a trigger of multiple cellular functions such as differentiation, nutrition signals, proliferation, and stress responses. In maturing oocytes of several organisms, stoichiometric activation of MAPK will occur (all-or-none signaling of MAPK activation) (Ferrell and Machleder 1998). This MAPK activation seems to be required for maintaining the maturing oocytes to arrest at the metaphase of second meiosis (in mammals and frog), rather than oocyte maturation itself. This is a so-called cytostatic factor's function. MAPK activation can be evaluated by the phosphorylation of a threonine and tyrosine residues in the MAPK molecule, both of which are catalyzed by an upstream dual-specificity kinase, MAPKK. Fertilization promotes Ca^{2+}-dependent degradation and/or inactivation of upstream kinases Mos and MAPKK, and triggers a rapid dephosphorylation/inactivation of all MAPK (inactivation of cytostatic factor). In the actively dividing embryos, a fraction of MAPK will be transiently activated at mitotic phase, and thereafter serves as a component of checkpoint (Chesnel et al. 1997; Chung et al. 1991; Eckberg 1997; Fabian et al. 1993; Ferrell 1999; Ferrell et al. 1991; Gavin et al. 1999; Git et al. 2009; Gross et al. 2000; Huo et al. 2004; Ito et al. 2010; Iwasaki et al. 2008; Katsu et al. 1999; Keady et al. 2007; Kosako et al. 1992; Lee et al. 2006; Lu et al. 2002; Palmer et al. 1998; Philipova and Whitaker 1998; Sackton et al. 2007; Sadler et al. 2004; Sasaki and Chiba 2004; Sato et al. 2001; Sato et al. 2003; Sato et al. 2000; Shibuya et al. 1992; Shibuya et al. 1996; Stricker 2009; Sun et al. 1999; Tokmakov et al. 2005; Verlhac et al. 1996; Zhang et al. 2006).

2.29 MAPK kinase (MAPKK/MEK)

MAPKK is a serine/threonine kinase that will be activated by MAPKKK phosphorylation of its serine residues in the catalytic domain. The activated MAPKK is capable of phosphorylating threonine and tyrosine residues in the catalytic domain of a downstream kinase MAPK, thus MAPKK is a dual-specificity kinase. MAPKK is well known as a mediator of Mos-dependent activation of MAPK cascade in maturing oocytes (Kosako et al. 1992; Xiong et al. 2008).

2.30 Meiosis inhibited protein kinase (MIPK)

p38 type of MAPK is a member of the mitogen-activated protein kinase (MAPK) is usually activated in response to cytokines and various stresses and plays a role in the inhibition of cell proliferation and tumor progression, but its role in oocyte maturation is described recently. In *Xenopus* oocytes, p38MAPK phosphorylated Cdc25C for the meiotic G_2/M progression and this required neither protein synthesis nor activation of p42MAPK-$p90^{Rsk}$ pathway (Perdiguero et al. 2003). The function of p38MAPK in accurate chromosome segregation during mouse oocyte meiotic maturation has also been described (Ou et al. 2010). In porcine oocytes, active phosphorylated p38MAPK accumulated in the nucleus before GVBD and remained active through MI to MII (Villa-Diaz and Miyano 2004). A p38MAPK homolog **Mipk** (meiosis-inhibited protein kinase) was highly tyrosine phosphorylated in immature sea star oocytes and subsequently dephosphorylated during the arrest at the G_2/M transition of meiosis I (Morrison et al. 2000). Dephosphorylated Mipk was maintained until the maturation of oocytes and the early mitotic cell divisions but was re-phosphorylated at the time of differentiation and acquisition of G phases in the developing embryos (Morrison et al. 2000).

2.31 Mos protein kinase (Mos)

Mos, a mitogen-activated protein (MAP) kinase kinase kinase that activates the MAPK pathway, is normally expressed only in vertebrate oocytes and take part in their maturation. Cytoplasmic polyadenylation element binding (CPEB) factor is essential for the polyadenylation of c-Mos mRNA and its subsequent translation (Mendez et al. 2000). Early phosphorylation of CPEB is catalyzed by Eg2, a member of the Aurora family of serine/threonine protein kinases (Mendez et al. 2000). Mos in coordination with Cdc2 regulate the translational activation of a maternal FGF receptor-1 (FGFR) mRNA during *Xenopus* oocyte maturation (Culp and Musci 1999). Mos contribute in the first cycle of *Xenopus* embryogenesis (Murakami and Vande Woude 1998) and act like Mos/Raf-1/MAPK pathway (Muslin et al. 1993) or without Raf like Mos/MAPK pathway both in *Xenopus* (Shibuya et al. 1996) and mouse (Verlhac et al. 1996). Mos is also involved in MAPK cascade in the control of microtubule and chromatin organization during meiosis in mouse oocytes (Chesnel et al. 1997; Culp and Musci 1999; Daar et al. 1993; Faure et al. 1998; Mendez et al. 2000; Murakami and Vande Woude 1998; Muslin et al. 1993; Shibuya et al. 1992; Shibuya et al. 1996; Tang et al. 2008; Verlhac et al. 1996; Wu et al. 2007a).

2.32 Myelin basic protein kinase (MBPK)

MBPK is present during maturation and early embryogenesis of the sea star. A meiosis-activated MBP kinase (MBPK) was purified from maturing oocytes of the sea star that rapidly undergo autophosphorylation on serine/threonine residues (Sanghera et al. 1990). MBPK remained highly active until 12 h post-fertilization (Arceci et al. 1992), after which it declined (Lefebvre et al. 1999). During maturation of sea star oocytes, MBPK-II (p110) was fully activated at the time of GVBD, whereas peak activation of MBPK-I (p45) occurred after this event (Pelech et al. 1988). Inhibiting an upstream phosphorylation event in the MBPK activation pathway the sea urchin embryo mitotic cycle at metaphase can be blocked (Pesando et al. 1999). The MBPK activity was at approximately the same high level in all categories (medium, small and tiny) of bovine oocytes after 24 h of culture and remained stable until 40 h (Pavlok et al. 1997; Pelech et al. 1988; Sanghera et al. 1990).

2.33 Myt1 protein kinase (Myt1)

Activation of MPF (composed of cyclin B and Cdc2 kinase) is required to entry into M-phase in all animals. The inhibitory kinase **Myt1**, a member of Wee1 family phosphorylates Cdc2 kinase to keep MPF in an inactive state. During *Xenopus* oocyte maturation MAPK phosphorylates and activates $p90^{Rsk}$ and that $p90^{Rsk}$ in turn down-regulates Myt1 by phosphorylation, leading to the activation of Cdc2 kinase/cyclin B (Palmer et al. 1998; Ruiz et al. 2010). Alternatively, Mos triggers Myt1 phosphorylation, even in the absence of MAPK activation in a mechanism that directly activates MPF in *Xenopus* oocytes (Peter et al. 2002). Recent model is that up-regulation of cyclin B synthesis causes rapid inactivating phosphorylation of Myt1, mediated by Cdc2 and without any significant contribution of Mos/MAPK or Plx1 (Gaffre et al. 2011). Non-cyclin proteins RINGO/Speedy can phosphorylate Ser residue in the regulatory domain of Myt1 and lead the activation of CDK during G2/M transition in *Xenopus* oocytes (Burrows et al. 2006; Inoue and Sagata 2005; Oh et al. 2010; Palmer et al. 1998; Ruiz et al. 2008).

2.34 Nemo-like kinase 1 (NLK1)

NLK Nemo-like kinase (NLK) is an evolutionary conserved MAPK-like kinase, an atypical MAPK that phosphorylates several transcription factors and is known to function in multiple developmental processes in vertebrates and invertebrates (Ota et al. 2011a; Ota et al. 2011b). Activated NLK directly phosphorylates microtubule-associated protein-1B (MAP1B) and the focal adhesion adaptor protein, paxillin (Ishitani et al. 2009). Inactive NLK1 in immature *Xenopus* oocytes becomes active during maturation depending on Mos protein synthesis but not on p42 MAPK activation (Ota et al. 2011b). NLK1 acts as a kinase downstream of Mos and catalyzes the phosphorylation of Pumilio 1 (Pum1), Pum2, and cytoplasmic polyadenylation element-binding protein (CPEB) to regulate the translation of mRNAs, including cyclin B1 mRNA, stored in oocytes (Ota et al. 2011b). NLK may play a role in neural development together with Sox11 during early *Xenopus* embryogenesis (Hyodo-Miura et al. 2002). NLK appears to function as a positive regulator of Wnt signaling during early zebrafish development (Thorpe and Moon 2004).

2.35 Nerve growth factor receptor (NGFR/TrkA/TrkB)

NGFR, the nerve growth factor (NGF) receptor (NGFR), an integral single membrane protein that is phosphorylated and heavily glycosylated in *Xenopus* oocytes and potentiates the ability of progesterone to induce maturation (Sehgal et al. 1988). NGF treatment on *Xenopus* oocytes results the tyrosine phosphorylation of ectopically expressed human Trk, a proto-oncogene product ($p140^{proto\text{-}Trk}$), and meiotic maturation, as determined by germinal vesicle breakdown and the activation of MPF (Nebreda et al. 1991). Thus, the Trk proto-oncogene product can act as a receptor for NGF (Nebreda et al. 1991). In human ovaries, NGF and TrkA (NGF's high-affinity receptor) were detected in granulose cells of preantral and antral follicles and in thecal cells of antral follicles (Salas et al. 2006). NGF/TrkA is present in bovine sperm and might have roles in regulation of sperm physiology relevant to male fertility and infertility (Li et al. 2010).

2.36 Neu tyrosine kinase

$p185^{Neu}$, the protein product of the neu gene, is a tyrosine kinase receptor that has the structural similarity to EGFR. The transformed/activated form of $p185^{Neu}$ tyrosine kinase (Val664Glu) facilitates the oocyte maturation events reducing the half-life from approximately 9 h to 5 h that are elicited by some steroids (e.g. progesterone) (Narasimhan et al. 1992). However, the activated $p185^{Neu}$ tyrosine kinases are not able to mimic the EGF-stimulated EGF receptor tyrosine kinase in triggering oocyte maturation, which suggests that the EGF receptor and the $p185^{Neu}$ tyrosine kinase do not work in the same pathways in *Xenopus* oocytes (Narasimhan et al. 1992). But in mouse embryo culture cells, it was shown that mutationally activated Neu protein can substitute the ligand-activated EGF receptor activity to reflect the structural similarity and EGF induced phosphorylation and regulation of $p185^{Neu}$ (Kokai et al. 1988; Shirahata et al. 1990).

2.37 p21-activated protein kinase (PAK)

PAK is a serine/threonine kinase that will be activated by its interaction with a small GTP-binding protein (e.g. Rac, Cdc42) and has been implicated in cytoskeletal dynamics and cell motility, transcription through MAPK cascades, death and survival signaling, and cell-cycle progression (Bokoch 2003). In *Xenopus* oocytes, microinjection of catalytically inactive mutant of PAK-related kinase (X-PAK) accelerates cell cycle progression from GV through MII stages. On the other hand, catalytically active mutant of X-PAK is shown to suppress progesterone-induced Mos accumulation and MAPK activation. These data suggest that the endogenous PAK activity is involved in the cell cycle arrest before maturation (Faure et al. 1997; Faure et al. 1999). An inhibitory effect of X-PAK on oocyte maturation seems to be due to a PKA-like mechanism of suppression of the PLK-induced activation of Cdc25 phosphatase, which is a trigger of the activation of Cdc2/cyclin complex (i.e. MPF) (Faure et al. 1999).

2.38 Phosphoinositide-dependent protein kinase 1 (PDK1)

PDK is a serine/threonine kinase that is regulated by a lipid activator phosphatidylinositol 3,4,5-trisphosphate (PIP_3), a product of PI3K phosphorylation of phosphatidylinositol 4,5-bisphosphate (PIP_2) (Toker and Newton 2000). In general, PDK consists of two distinct gene products, PDK1 and PDK2. In 1-methyladenine (1-MA)-dependent maturing starfish oocytes, Akt kinase is responsible for activation of MPF. Akt kinase is, as described above, regulated by upstream kinases such as PDK and mTOR. In fact, starfish PDK1, but not PDK2, is required for 1-MA-induced Akt activation and cell cycle progression (Hiraoka et al. 2004). PI3K-PDK-Akt axis has also been shown in other organisms such as nematode *C. elegans* (Hertweck et al. 2004), however, their involvement in oocyte and egg functions is not yet known.

2.39 Polo-like protein kinase-1 (Plk/1PLK-1/Plx1)

PLK, polo-like kinase, a serine/threonine kinase, is implicated in the regulation of cell cycle progression in all eukaryotes (Sumara et al. 2002). Polo-like kinase type 1 (plk1) is present during meiotic maturation, fertilization, and early embryo cleavage in mouse (Pahlavan et al. 2000; Tong et al. 2002; Xiong et al. 2008), rat (Fan et al. 2003), porcine (Anger et al. 2004; Yao et al. 2003) and parasite trematode oocytes (Long et al. 2010). Though all three *Xenopus* type Plk (Plx); Plx1, Plx2 and Plx3 are observed in oocytes and unfertilized eggs but Plx2 and Plx3 in embryos strongly suggests that individual Plk family members perform distinct functions at later stages of development (Duncan et al. 2001). Plx1 is required for activation of the phosphatase Cdc25C and cyclin B-Cdc2 in *Xenopus* oocytes (Liu and Maller 2005; Qian et al. 2001). The APC/C inhibitor Emi2 or XErp1, a pivotal CSF component, required to maintain metaphase II arrest and rapidly destroyed in response to Ca^{2+} signaling through phosphorylation by Plx1 (Hansen et al. 2006). Interestingly, Plx1 kinase that is required for Cdc25 activation and MPF auto-amplification in fully-grown oocytes is not expressed at the protein level in small stage IV oocytes (Karaiskou et al. 2004). Plx1 acts as a direct inhibitory kinase of Myt1 in the mitotic cell cycles in *Xenopus* (Anger et al. 2004; Eckerdt et al. 2009; Fan et al. 2003; Hansen et al. 2006; Inoue and Sagata 2005; Ito et al. 2008; Karaiskou et al. 2004; Liu and Maller 2005; Pahlavan et al. 2000; Qian et al. 2001; Sumara et al. 2002; Tong et al. 2002; Wianny et al. 1998; Xiong et al. 2008; Yao et al. 2003).

2.40 Protein kinase C (PKC)

PKC is a family of serine/threonine kinase that is primarily regulated by diacylglycerol (DG), a phospholipase C-hydrolyzed product of PIP_2, and intracellular Ca^{2+} (Nishizuka 1984; Nishizuka 1986; Nishizuka 1988). Classical or typical PKCs (α, βI/βII, γ) are also known as an intracellular receptor for phorbol ester, a tumor promoter. Other subfamily members of PKC (atypical or novel types: e.g. δ, ε, ζ) have other mechanisms of enzyme regulation such as tyrosine phosphorylation. Live cell imaging studies demonstrated that spatial distribution of PKCs, which differ in both PKC subfamily members and cellular environments, is crucial for PKC activation and its access to substrates. In eggs/oocytes of several organisms (e.g. mammals, marine worms, frog, and sea urchin), activation and PKC(s) and its contribution to oocyte maturation, fertilization, and initiation of development have been well documented. Cellular functions regulated by PKC(s) include the onset of anaphase I, sperm-induced activation of respiratory burst oxidase, MAPK inactivation, reorganization of cytoskeleton, exocytosis of cortical granules, and pronucleus formation (Akabane et al. 2007; Baluch et al. 2004; Capco 2001; Capco et al. 1992; de Barry et al. 1997; Diaz-Meco et al. 1994; Ducibella and LeFevre 1997; Eliyahu et al. 2001; Eliyahu and Shalgi 2002; Eliyahu et al. 2002; Eliyahu et al. 2005; Fan et al. 2002; Gallicano et al. 1995; Gallicano et al. 1997; Haberman et al. 2011; Halet 2004; Heinecke et al. 1990; Kalive et al. 2010; Lu et al. 2002; Luria et al. 2000; Madgwick et al. 2005; Nakaya et al. 2000; Olds et al. 1995; Pauken and Capco 2000; Quan et al. 2003; Sakuma et al. 1997; Sanghera et al. 1992; Shen and Buck 1990; Stricker 2009; Swann et al. 1989; Tatone et al. 2003; Viveiros et al. 2004; Viveiros et al. 2003; Yang et al. 2004; Yu et al. 2004; Yu et al. 2008). In rat eggs, PKC interaction and phosphorylation of RACK (receptor for C-kinase) has been suggested (Haberman et al. 2011). In *Xenopus* oocytes, hormone-induced maturation is accompanied by polarized localization and interaction of atypical PKC(s) and ASIP/PAR-3, a cell polarity regulator, suggesting their involvement in establishing animal-vegetal asymmetry before fertilization (Nakaya et al. 2000).

2.41 Protein kinase M (PKM)

PKM is a catalytic fragment of PKC, produced by a limited proteolysis (probably by calpain, a Ca^{2+}-dependent protease) of the molecule. It has been shown that PKM contributes to the remodeling of cytoskeleton during egg activation in the mouse (Gallicano et al. 1995). Its physiological target (i.e. substrate) is not yet known.

2.42 Proline-rich tyrosine kinase2 (Pyk2)

Pyk2 is a non-receptor tyrosine kinase related to the focal adhesion kinase (FAK; p125) that is rapidly phosphorylated on tyrosine residues in response to various stimuli that elevate the intracellular calcium ion concentration (Lev et al. 1995). Pyk2 is up-regulated in various types of tumors like hepatocellular carcinoma (HCC) (Sun et al. 2011; Sun et al. 2007) and small cell lung cancer (SCLC) (Roelle et al. 2008). Activation of Pyk2 leads to the activation of the MAPK signaling pathways. PYK2 is present in mouse spermatocytes and spermatids (Chieffi et al. 2003). Pyk2 plays a dynamic role during rat oocyte meiotic maturation by regulating the organization of actin filaments (microfilaments) from GV stage to telophase (Meng et al. 2006). Pyk2 has ligand sequences for Src homology 2 and 3 (SH2 and SH3), and has binding sites for paxillin (Li and Earp 1997) and $p130^{Cas}$ (Astier et al. 1997).

2.43 Raf protein kinase (A-Raf/B-Raf/Raf-1)

Raf is a serine/threonine kinase that has been originally identified as an oncogene that acts in concert with Myc transcription factor. Raf can be activated by PKC phosphorylation, and the activated Raf acts as a MAPKKK that activates MAPKK-MAPK pathway. Therefore, Raf is a mediator of transmembrane signaling involving hydrolysis of phospholipids and subsequent cytoplasmic kinase cascade. In *Xenopus* oocytes, Raf-1 is shown to act downstream of Mos, another kind of MAPKKK specific to oocyte maturation system, to promote MAPK activation and rearrangement of intracellular pH (from 7.2 to 7.7) in response to progesterone or insulin. The latter phenomenon involves phospho-dependent regulation of Na^+/H^+ exchanger. Whether Raf is responsible for this phosphorylation is unknown (Chesnel et al. 1997; Fabian et al. 1993; Kang et al. 1998; MacNicol et al. 1995; Muslin et al. 1993; Shibuya et al. 1996). Developmental expression of Raf has also been demonstrated in *Xenopus*; however, its role in fertilization has not yet been shown (MacNicol et al. 1995).

2.44 RET tyrosine kinase (Ret)

Receptor tyrosine kinase are rearranged during transfection (**RET**) for activation and about 15 RET gene rearrangement was identified in papillary thyroid carcinoma (PTC) among which RET/PTC1 and RET/PTC3 are the most common type (Marotta et al. 2011). RET was detected in mammalian (human) oocytes (Farhi et al. 2010) and are expressed in embryos throughout the early development with an increase after the early blastocyst stage (Kawamura et al. 2008). Glial cell line-derived neurotrophic factor (GDNF) and both its co-receptors, GDNF family receptor alpha-1 (GFR alpha-1) and RET receptor affect porcine oocyte maturation and pre-implantation embryo developmental competence in a follicular stage-dependent manner (Linher et al. 2007). Receptor tyrosine kinase (RTK1) that is highly similar to RET kinase was not detected in sea urchin unfertilized eggs and was activated after blastula stage (Sakuma et al. 1997).

2.45 S6 kinase (S6K)/ Rsk protein kinase I/II (Rsk)

Several 40S ribosomal protein kinases in vertebrate/frog oocyte stage 6 (**S6K**) are directly phosphorylated and activated by MAPK in order to activate MPF (Barrett et al. 1992; Erikson and Maller 1988). Some S6Ks have been identified and characterized for example in progesterone- and insulin-treated *Xenopus* eggs termed S6K II (S6K II, p92) different from S6K I (Erikson et al. 1987), differential role in *Xenopus* embryogenesis (S6K; p70) (Schwab et al. 1999), in *Rana* oocytes (S6K; p83) (Byun et al. 2002), in porcine oocytes (Sugiura et al. 2002), and G1 phase after completion of meiosis II in starfish unfertilized eggs (Mori et al. 2006) but not in mouse oocytes (Dumont et al. 2005). S6K ($p90^{Rsk}$) inhibits the degradation of cyclin B by anaphase-promoting complex/cyclosome (APC/C) and results the second meiotic metaphase arrest (Maller et al. 2001). S6K phosphorylates and activates the Bub1 protein kinase, which may cause metaphase arrest due to the inhibition of APC (Maller et al. 2001). Mos-dependent phosphorylation of Erp1 by $p90^{Rsk}$ at Thr-336, Ser-342 and Ser-344 is crucial for both stabilizing Erp1 that inhibits cyclin B degradation by binding the APC/C and establishing CSF arrest in meiosis II of *Xenopus* oocytes (Nishiyama et al. 2007a).

2.46 Src tyrosine kinase (Src)

Src has been firstly identified as an oncogene of Rous sarcoma virus and thereafter discovered as a normal cellular gene that encodes a 60-kDa protein-tyrosine kinase (Brown and Cooper 1996; Jove and Hanafusa 1987; Thomas and Brugge 1997) that is distributed in a wide range of animal species from a unicellular organism (i.e. *Monosiga ovata*) through multicellular organisms including human (Segawa et al. 2006). In human, Src is ubiquitously expressed in several tissues and seems to be involved in several cellular functions as well (e.g. lymphocyte activation, neuronal signal transduction). In some sea invertebrates (sea urchin, starfish, ascidian, and others) (Abassi et al. 2000; Belton et al. 2001; Dasgupta and Garbers 1983; Giusti et al. 1999a; Giusti et al. 1999b; Giusti et al. 2000a; Giusti et al. 2003; Giusti et al. 2000b; Kamel et al. 1986; O'Neill et al. 2004; Runft et al. 2004; Runft and Jaffe 2000; Runft et al. 2002; Sakuma et al. 1997; Shen et al. 1999; Shilling et al. 1994; Stricker et al. 2010a; Townley et al. 2006; Townley et al. 2009), fish (zebrafish) (in this case, Fyn tyrosine kinase) and frog (African clawed frog) (Glahn et al. 1999; Iwasaki et al. 2008; Iwasaki et al. 2006; Kushima et al. 2011; Mahbub Hasan et al. 2011; Mahbub Hasan et al. 2007; Mahbub Hasan et al. 2005; Mammadova et al. 2009; Sakakibara et al. 2005; Sato et al. 1996; Sato et al. 2006a; Sato et al. 1999; Sato et al. 2004; Sato et al. 2002; Sato et al. 2001; Sato et al. 2003; Sato et al. 2000; Sato et al. 2006b; Steele 1985; Steele et al. 1989b; Tokmakov et al. 2002), the oocyte-expressing Src is suggested to be involved in the initiation of sperm-induced egg activation through the phosphorylation and activation of oocyte proteins such as phospholipase Cγ (thereby promoting IP_3-dependent Ca^{2+} release). Progesterone-induced oocyte maturation in *Xenopus* also seems to involve the activity of Src (Tokmakov et al. 2005). In mammalian species (i.e. mouse and rat), chromosomal dynamics, rather than sperm-induced Ca^{2+} release (Kurokawa et al. 2004b; McGinnis et al. 2007; Mehlmann and Jaffe 2005; Reut et al. 2007; Tomashov-Matar et al. 2008), seems to be regulated by Src and/or other Src-related kinases (e.g. Fyn) in fertilized oocytes.

2.47 Src64/DSrc

Src64 is a *Drosophila* homolog of the tyrosine kinase Src and is required for ovarian ring canal morphogenesis during oogenesis. Tec29 tyrosine kinase interacts with Src64 and contributes to ring canal development. The Src64-Tec29 axis is also involved in microfilament contraction during cellularization, a *Drosophila*-specific phenomenon. Although the cellular target of Src64 phosphorylation is not yet clearly shown, its upstream regulators such as csk homolog-mediated phosphorylation and phosphoinositide-dependent activation mechanism have been demonstrated (Dodson et al. 1998; Lu et al. 2004; O'Reilly et al. 2006).

2.48 Stigmatic S receptor kinase (SRK)

SRK is a transmembrane receptor/kinase that works as a female determinant for self-incompatibility/self-sterility to prevent inbreeding in *Brassica*, a flowering plant. Upon self-pollination, the pollen-borne ligand S locus protein 11/SCR interacts with SRK expressed in stigma, which in turn autophosphorylates and promotes Ca^{2+}-dependent signal transduction that culminates in self-pollen rejection (Murase et al. 2004). Another protein kinase, named M locus protein kinase, has also been identified as a cytoplasmic mediator of self-incompatibility in this species (Kakita et al. 2007). This is the first example that explains how self-incompatibility, in other words, allogenic authentication, is made possible in sexual reproduction of hermaphrodite organism. More recent studies have demonstrated that a similar system of the allogenic authentication (that utilizes gamete coat/membrane-associated proteins) is also present in animal hermaphrodite organisms (e.g. ascidian) (Harada et al. 2008). Whether such animal system involves protein kinase signaling is unknown.

2.49 T-Cell Origin Protein Kinase/ T-LAK cell-originated protein kinase (TOPK)

TOPK (T-LAK cell-originated protein kinase) is distributed in lymphokine-activated killer T (T-LAK) cell, testis, activated lymphoid cells, and lymphoid tumors, and is related to the dual specific mitogen-activated protein kinase kinase (MAPKK) (Abe et al. 2000). TOPK protein is expressed mainly in the cytosol of spermatocytes and spermatids to support the testicular functions (Fujibuchi et al. 2005). During mitosis, TOPK-Thr-9 was phosphorylated by cdk1/cyclin B and TOPK significantly associates with mitotic spindles (Matsumoto et al. 2004). Insulin-matured *Xenopus* oocytes showed much higher expression of TOPK and nuclear kinase (DYRK1A) but neither of these kinases activates or is activated by MAPK and is therefore unique to insulin-activated wild-type $p21^{Ras}$-induced oocyte maturation via the activation of Raf (Qu et al. 2006; Qu et al. 2007). The functions of insulin-activated wild-type $p21^{Ras}$ do not depend on the two classic Raf targets, MEK and MAPK (MAPK or ERK) (Qu et al. 2006; Qu et al. 2007).

2.50 $p65^{tpr\text{-}met}$, a fused tyrosine kinase (Tpr-Met)

Tpr-met ($p65^{tpr\text{-}met}$, a fused tyrosine kinase) efficiently induced meiotic maturation in *Xenopus* oocytes and activate MPF through a Mos-dependent pathway (Daar et al. 1991; Park et al. 1986). During *Xenopus* oocyte maturation, receptor tyrosine kinase (RTK) pathway including tpr-met takes part in the activation of MPF that requires activation of Raf and MAPK (Fabian et al. 1993). Aberrant or activated expression of Met receptor (Tpr-Met) in *Xenopus* embryonic system induces ectopic morphogenetic structures during *Xenopus* embryogenesis where recruitment of either the Grb2 or the Shc adaptor protein is sufficient to induce ectopic structures and anterior reduction but the role of PI 3-kinase and PLC recruitment are unclear (Ishimura et al. 2006). Grb2-associated binder 1 (Gab1) when overexpressed in *Xenopus* oocyte is crucial for Tpr-Met-mediated morphological transformation (Mood et al. 2006). Thus, to induce such structure Ras/Raf/MAPK pathway is important.

2.51 Vaccinia-related kinase 1 (VRK1)/*Drosophila* NHK-1

VRK1, a member of the casein kinase I (Minshull et al. 1989) family is a serine/threonine kinase related to vaccinia virus B1R serine/threonine kinase (Klerkx et al. 2009), has been identified as an early response gene required for cyclin D1 expression. VRK1 controls cell survival by phosphorylation of p53, chromatin condensation by phosphorylation of histone, and nuclear envelope assembly by phosphorylation of BANF1 (Valbuena et al. 2011). It is also involved in fragmentation of Golgi apparatus in the G2 phase-cell cycle. In *Drosophila* oocytes, nucleosomal histone kinase-1 (*Drosophila* homolog of VRK1) regulates chromosome-nuclear envelope association via phosphorylation of BAF protein (barrier to auto-integration factor), thereby supports the meiotic progression (karyosome formation) (Lancaster et al. 2007). In the mouse, target disruption of VRK1 causes a delay in meiotic progression and results in the appearance of lagging chromosomes during formation of the metaphase plate (Schober et al. 2011), suggesting that function of VRK1 is evolutionarily conserved, although its substrate has not yet been demonstrated.

2.52 Wee1 protein kinase (Wee1)

Weel, a protein tyrosine kinase, is the key regulator of cell cycle progression by phosphorylating and inhibiting Cdc2. Weel, an inhibitor of Cdc2/cyclin B kinase, is decreased for mammalian oocytes meiotic competence (Mitra and Schultz 1996). Weel activity is necessary for the control of the first embryonic cell cycle following the fertilization of meiotically mature *Xenopus* oocytes where the protein accumulation is regulated at the level of mRNA translation (Charlesworth et al. 2000). p42 MAPK was found to phosphorylate and activate Weel activity towards Cdc2, thus Weel might work in the downstream of Mos/MEK/p42 MAPK (Walter et al. 2000). Basically in *Xenopus*, eukaryotic Weel homologue, termed WeelA functions in pre-gastrula embryos with rapid cell cycle and zygotic isoform WeelB functions post-gastrula embryos where WeelB inhibits Cdc2 activity and oocyte maturation much more strongly than WeelA (Okamoto et al. 2002). PKA also involved in the inactive state of Cdc2/cyclin B kinase by regulating Weel kinase (Han and Conti 2006).

2.53 Yes tyrosine kinase (Yes/c-Yes)

The egg cortex is known to be rich in cortical structures such as actin cytoskeleton forming microfilaments and cortical vesicles and they are important in many dynamic events in mammalian egg maturation and fertilization, such as sperm incorporation, cortical granule exocytosis, polar body emission, etc. SFKs have been shown to be associated with a wide range of cytoskeletal components and/or to phosphorylate them (Thomas and Brugge 1997). It has demonstrated that Fyn, **c-Yes** and c-Src are distributed throughout the rat egg cytoplasm, but Fyn and c-Yes are tend to concentrate at the egg cortex whereas only Fyn is localized to the spindle (Talmor-Cohen et al. 2004a). Localization of c-Src, c-Yes and Fyn to different compartments within the egg indicates that these proteins may have different functions within the egg. No change in the subcellular distribution of the three kinases has been observed throughout the stages of the fertilization process, or after parthenogenetic activation (Talmor-Cohen et al. 2004a). Though Yes kinase activity was decreased at fertilization in Zebra fish but it was concentrated in blastoderm cells and maintained the high activity throughout the gastrulation (Tsai et al. 2005). It is possible that the intracellular distribution of c-Src, c-Yes and Fyn imply their association with the cytoskeleton. The involvement of SFKs in reorganization of the cytoskeleton might be involved in egg fertilization. (Steele et al. 1989a; Tsai et al. 2005)

3. Conclusion

For conclusion, please refer to the section 3 of the chapter entitled "Phospho-signaling at Oocyte Maturation and Fertilization: Set Up for Embryogenesis and Beyond Part II. Kinase Regulators and Substrates" by Mahbub Hasan et al.

4. Acknowledgements

We apologize to those whose work was not cited or insufficiently cited. This work is supported by a Grant-in-Aid on Innovative Areas (22112522), and a grant for Private University Strategic Research Foundation Support Program (S0801060) from the Ministry of Education, Culture, Sports, Science and Technology, Japan to K.S.

5. References

Abassi YA, Carroll DJ, Giusti AF, Belton RJ, Jr., Foltz KR. 2000. Evidence that Src-type tyrosine kinase activity is necessary for initiation of calcium release at fertilization in sea urchin eggs. Dev Biol 218(2):206-219.

Abe Y, Matsumoto S, Kito K, Ueda N. 2000. Cloning and expression of a novel MAPKK-like protein kinase, lymphokine-activated killer T-cell-originated protein kinase, specifically expressed in the testis and activated lymphoid cells. J Biol Chem 275(28):21525-21531.

Acevedo N, Ding J, Smith GD. 2007. Insulin signaling in mouse oocytes. Biol Reprod 77(5):872-879.

Aegerter S, Jalabert B, Bobe J. 2004. Messenger RNA stockpile of cyclin B, insulin-like growth factor I, insulin-like growth factor II, insulin-like growth factor receptor Ib, and p53 in the rainbow trout oocyte in relation with developmental competence. Mol Reprod Dev 67(2):127-135.

Ajduk A, Malagocki A, Maleszewski M. 2008. Cytoplasmic maturation of mammalian oocytes: development of a mechanism responsible for sperm-induced Ca2+ oscillations. Reprod Biol 8(1):3-22.

Akabane H, Fan J, Zheng X, Zhu GZ. 2007. Protein kinase C activity in mouse eggs regulates gamete membrane interaction. Mol Reprod Dev 74(11):1465-1472.

Anderson RG. 1998. The caveolae membrane system. Annu Rev Biochem 67:199-225.

Andresson T, Ruderman JV. 1998. The kinase Eg2 is a component of the Xenopus oocyte progesterone-activated signaling pathway. EMBO J 17(19):5627-5637.

Anger M, Klima J, Kubelka M, Prochazka R, Motlik J, Schultz RM. 2004. Timing of Plk1 and MPF activation during porcine oocyte maturation. Mol Reprod Dev 69(1):11-16.

Arceci RJ, Pampfer S, Pollard JW. 1992. Expression of CSF-1/c-fms and SF/c-kit mRNA during preimplantation mouse development. Dev Biol 151(1):1-8.

Arion D, Meijer L, Brizuela L, Beach D. 1988. cdc2 is a component of the M phase-specific histone H1 kinase: evidence for identity with MPF. Cell 55(2):371-378.

Armant DR, Kilburn BA, Petkova A, Edwin SS, Duniec-Dmuchowski ZM, Edwards HJ, Romero R, Leach RE. 2006. Human trophoblast survival at low oxygen concentrations requires metalloproteinase-mediated shedding of heparin-binding EGF-like growth factor. Development 133(4):751-759.

Astier A, Manie SN, Avraham H, Hirai H, Law SF, Zhang Y, Golemis EA, Fu Y, Druker BJ, Haghayeghi N, Freedman AS, Avraham S. 1997. The related adhesion focal tyrosine kinase differentially phosphorylates p130Cas and the Cas-like protein, p105HEF1. J Biol Chem 272(32):19719-19724.

Bagowski CP, Xiong W, Ferrell JE, Jr. 2001. c-Jun N-terminal kinase activation in Xenopus laevis eggs and embryos. A possible non-genomic role for the JNK signaling pathway. J Biol Chem 276(2):1459-1465.

Balamurugan K, Haider S. 1998. Partial purification of maturation-promoting factor from catfish, Clarias batrachus: identification as the histone H1 kinase and its periodic activation. Comp Biochem Physiol C Pharmacol Toxicol Endocrinol 120(3):329-342.

Baluch DP, Capco DG. 2008. GSK3 beta mediates acentromeric spindle stabilization by activated PKC zeta. Dev Biol 317(1):46-58.

Baluch DP, Koeneman BA, Hatch KR, McGaughey RW, Capco DG. 2004. PKC isotypes in post-activated and fertilized mouse eggs: association with the meiotic spindle. Dev Biol 274(1):45-55.

Barrett CB, Erikson E, Maller JL. 1992. A purified S6 kinase kinase from Xenopus eggs activates S6 kinase II and autophosphorylates on serine, threonine, and tyrosine residues. J Biol Chem 267(7):4408-4415.

Becker W. 2011. Recent insights into the function of DYRK1A. FEBS J 278(2):222.

Becker W, Sippl W. 2011. Activation, regulation, and inhibition of DYRK1A. FEBS J 278(2):246-256.

Belton RJ, Jr., Adams NL, Foltz KR. 2001. Isolation and characterization of sea urchin egg lipid rafts and their possible function during fertilization. Mol Reprod Dev 59(3):294-305.

Bilodeau-Goeseels S, Sasseville M, Guillemette C, Richard FJ. 2007. Effects of adenosine monophosphate-activated kinase activators on bovine oocyte nuclear maturation in vitro. Mol Reprod Dev 74(8):1021-1034.

Bischoff JR, Plowman GD. 1999. The Aurora/Ipl1p kinase family: regulators of chromosome segregation and cytokinesis. Trends Cell Biol 9(11):454-459.

Bokoch GM. 2003. Biology of the p21-activated kinases. Annu Rev Biochem 72:743-781.

Bornslaeger EA, Mattei P, Schultz RM. 1986. Involvement of cAMP-dependent protein kinase and protein phosphorylation in regulation of mouse oocyte maturation. Dev Biol 114(2):453-462.

Brown MR, Clark KD, Gulia M, Zhao Z, Garczynski SF, Crim JW, Suderman RJ, Strand MR. 2008. An insulin-like peptide regulates egg maturation and metabolism in the mosquito Aedes aegypti. Proc Natl Acad Sci U S A 105(15):5716-5721.

Brown MT, Cooper JA. 1996. Regulation, substrates and functions of src. Biochim Biophys Acta 1287(2-3):121-149.

Browne CL, Bower WA, Palazzo RE, Rebhun LI. 1990. Inhibition of mitosis in fertilized sea urchin eggs by inhibition of the cyclic AMP-dependent protein kinase. Exp Cell Res 188(1):122-128.

Brunet S, Maro B. 2005. Cytoskeleton and cell cycle control during meiotic maturation of the mouse oocyte: integrating time and space. Reproduction 130(6):801-811.

Burrows AE, Sceurman BK, Kosinski ME, Richie CT, Sadler PL, Schumacher JM, Golden A. 2006. The C. elegans Myt1 ortholog is required for the proper timing of oocyte maturation. Development 133(4):697-709.

Byun HM, Kang SG, Kang HM. 2002. Cloning of ribosomal protein S6 kinase cDNA and its involvement in meiotic maturation in Rana dybowskii oocytes. Mol Cells 14(1):16-23.

Cailliau K, Le Marcis V, Bereziat V, Perdereau D, Cariou B, Vilain JP, Burnol AF, Browaeys-Poly E. 2003. Inhibition of FGF receptor signalling in Xenopus oocytes: differential effect of Grb7, Grb10 and Grb14. FEBS Lett 548(1-3):43-48.

Capco DG. 2001. Molecular and biochemical regulation of early mammalian development. Int Rev Cytol 207:195-235.

Capco DG, Tutnick JM, Bement WM. 1992. The role of protein kinase C in reorganization of the cortical cytoskeleton during the transition from oocyte to fertilization-competent egg. J Exp Zool 264(4):395-405.

Carroll DJ, Albay DT, Terasaki M, Jaffe LA, Foltz KR. 1999. Identification of PLCgamma-dependent and -independent events during fertilization of sea urchin eggs. Dev Biol 206(2):232-247.

Cary LA, Guan JL. 1999. Focal adhesion kinase in integrin-mediated signaling. Front Biosci 4:D102-113.

Castilho PV, Williams BC, Mochida S, Zhao Y, Goldberg ML. 2009. The M phase kinase Greatwall (Gwl) promotes inactivation of PP2A/B55delta, a phosphatase directed against CDK phosphosites. Mol Biol Cell 20(22):4777-4789.

Castro A, Peter M, Magnaghi-Jaulin L, Vigneron S, Galas S, Lorca T, Labbe JC. 2001. Cyclin B/cdc2 induces c-Mos stability by direct phosphorylation in Xenopus oocytes. Mol Biol Cell 12(9):2660-2671.

Charlesworth A, Welk J, MacNicol AM. 2000. The temporal control of Wee1 mRNA translation during Xenopus oocyte maturation is regulated by cytoplasmic polyadenylation elements within the 3'-untranslated region. Dev Biol 227(2):706-719.

Chaube SK, Dubey PK, Mishra SK, Shrivastav TG. 2007. Verapamil reversibly inhibits spontaneous parthenogenetic activation in aged rat eggs cultured in vitro. Cloning Stem Cells 9(4):608-617.

Chen J, Downs SM. 2008. AMP-activated protein kinase is involved in hormone-induced mouse oocyte meiotic maturation in vitro. Dev Biol 313(1):47-57.

Chen J, Hudson E, Chi MM, Chang AS, Moley KH, Hardie DG, Downs SM. 2006. AMPK regulation of mouse oocyte meiotic resumption in vitro. Dev Biol 291(2):227-238.

Cheng KC, Klancer R, Singson A, Seydoux G. 2009. Regulation of MBK-2/DYRK by CDK-1 and the pseudophosphatases EGG-4 and EGG-5 during the oocyte-to-embryo transition. Cell 139(3):560-572.

Chesnel F, Bonnec G, Tardivel A, Boujard D. 1997. Comparative effects of insulin on the activation of the Raf/Mos-dependent MAP kinase cascade in vitellogenic versus postvitellogenic Xenopus oocytes. Dev Biol 188(1):122-133.

Chie L, Amar S, Kung HF, Lin MC, Chen H, Chung DL, Adler V, Ronai Z, Friedman FK, Robinson RC, Kovac C, Brandt-Rauf PW, Yamaizumi Z, Michl J, Pincus MR. 2000. Induction of oocyte maturation by jun-N-terminal kinase (JNK) on the oncogenic ras-p21 pathway is dependent on the raf-MEK signal transduction pathway. Cancer Chemother Pharmacol 45(6):441-449.

Chieffi P, Barchi M, Di Agostino S, Rossi P, Tramontano D, Geremia R. 2003. Prolin-rich tyrosine kinase 2 (PYK2) expression and localization in mouse testis. Mol Reprod Dev 65(3):330-335.

Chobotova K, Spyropoulou I, Carver J, Manek S, Heath JK, Gullick WJ, Barlow DH, Sargent IL, Mardon HJ. 2002. Heparin-binding epidermal growth factor and its receptor ErbB4 mediate implantation of the human blastocyst. Mech Dev 119(2):137-144.

Choi T, Rulong S, Resau J, Fukasawa K, Matten W, Kuriyama R, Mansour S, Ahn N, Vande Woude GF. 1996. Mos/mitogen-activated protein kinase can induce early meiotic phenotypes in the absence of maturation-promoting factor: a novel system for analyzing spindle formation during meiosis I. Proc Natl Acad Sci U S A 93(10):4730-4735.

Chuang LM, Hausdorff SF, Myers MG, Jr., White MF, Birnbaum MJ, Kahn CR. 1994. Interactive roles of Ras, insulin receptor substrate-1, and proteins with Src homology-2 domains in insulin signaling in Xenopus oocytes. J Biol Chem 269(44):27645-27649.

Chuang LM, Myers MG, Jr., Backer JM, Shoelson SE, White MF, Birnbaum MJ, Kahn CR. 1993. Insulin-stimulated oocyte maturation requires insulin receptor substrate 1 and interaction with the SH2 domains of phosphatidylinositol 3-kinase. Mol Cell Biol 13(11):6653-6660.

Chung J, Pelech SL, Blenis J. 1991. Mitogen-activated Swiss mouse 3T3 RSK kinases I and II are related to pp44mpk from sea star oocytes and participate in the regulation of pp90rsk activity. Proc Natl Acad Sci U S A 88(11):4981-4985.

Ciemerych MA, Tarkowski AK, Kubiak JZ. 1998. Autonomous activation of histone H1 kinase, cortical activity and microtubule organization in one- and two-cell mouse embryos. Biol Cell 90(8):557-564.

Clarke PR, Karsenti E. 1991. Regulation of p34cdc2 protein kinase: new insights into protein phosphorylation and the cell cycle. J Cell Sci 100 (Pt 3):409-414.

Collas P, Sullivan EJ, Barnes FL. 1993. Histone H1 kinase activity in bovine oocytes following calcium stimulation. Mol Reprod Dev 34(2):224-231.

Culp PA, Musci TJ. 1998. Translational activation and cytoplasmic polyadenylation of FGF receptor-1 are independently regulated during Xenopus oocyte maturation. Dev Biol 193(1):63-76.

Culp PA, Musci TJ. 1999. c-mos and cdc2 cooperate in the translational activation of fibroblast growth factor receptor-1 during Xenopus oocyte maturation. Mol Biol Cell 10(11):3567-3581.

Daar I, Yew N, Vande Woude GF. 1993. Inhibition of mos-induced oocyte maturation by protein kinase A. J Cell Biol 120(5):1197-1202.

Daar IO, White GA, Schuh SM, Ferris DK, Vande Woude GF. 1991. tpr-met oncogene product induces maturation-producing factor activation in Xenopus oocytes. Mol Cell Biol 11(12):5985-5991.

Dasgupta JD, Garbers DL. 1983. Tyrosine protein kinase activity during embryogenesis. J Biol Chem 258(10):6174-6178.

de Barry J, Kawahara S, Takamura K, Janoshazi A, Kirino Y, Olds JL, Lester DS, Alkon DL, Yoshioka T. 1997. Time-resolved imaging of protein kinase C activation during sea urchin egg fertilization. Exp Cell Res 234(1):115-124.

de Klein A, van Kessel AG, Grosveld G, Bartram CR, Hagemeijer A, Bootsma D, Spurr NK, Heisterkamp N, Groffen J, Stephenson JR. 1982. A cellular oncogene is translocated to the Philadelphia chromosome in chronic myelocytic leukaemia. Nature 300(5894):765-767.

de Vries C, Escobedo JA, Ueno H, Houck K, Ferrara N, Williams LT. 1992. The fms-like tyrosine kinase, a receptor for vascular endothelial growth factor. Science 255(5047):989-991.

Deng X, Feng C, Wang EH, Zhu YQ, Cui C, Zong ZH, Li GS, Liu C, Meng J, Yu BZ. 2011. Influence of proline-rich inositol polyphosphate 5-phosphatase, on early development of fertilized mouse eggs, via inhibition of phosphorylation of Akt. Cell Prolif 44(2):156-165.

Detivaud L, Pascreau G, Karaiskou A, Osborne HB, Kubiak JZ. 2003. Regulation of EDEN-dependent deadenylation of Aurora A/Eg2-derived mRNA via phosphorylation and dephosphorylation in Xenopus laevis egg extracts. J Cell Sci 116(Pt 13):2697-2705.

Diaz-Meco MT, Lozano J, Municio MM, Berra E, Frutos S, Sanz L, Moscat J. 1994. Evidence for the in vitro and in vivo interaction of Ras with protein kinase C zeta. J Biol Chem 269(50):31706-31710.

Ding J, Swain JE, Smith GD. 2011. Aurora kinase-A regulates microtubule organizing center (MTOC) localization, chromosome dynamics, and histone-H3 phosphorylation in mouse oocytes. Mol Reprod Dev 78(2):80-90.

Dodson GS, Guarnieri DJ, Simon MA. 1998. Src64 is required for ovarian ring canal morphogenesis during Drosophila oogenesis. Development 125(15):2883-2892.

Ducibella T. 1996. The cortical reaction and development of activation competence in mammalian oocytes. Hum Reprod Update 2(1):29-42.

Ducibella T, Fissore R. 2008. The roles of Ca2+, downstream protein kinases, and oscillatory signaling in regulating fertilization and the activation of development. Dev Biol 315(2):257-279.

Ducibella T, LeFevre L. 1997. Study of protein kinase C antagonists on cortical granule exocytosis and cell-cycle resumption in fertilized mouse eggs. Mol Reprod Dev 46(2):216-226.

Dumont J, Umbhauer M, Rassinier P, Hanauer A, Verlhac MH. 2005. p90Rsk is not involved in cytostatic factor arrest in mouse oocytes. J Cell Biol 169(2):227-231.

Duncan MJ, Li G, Shin JS, Carson JL, Abraham SN. 2004. Bacterial penetration of bladder epithelium through lipid rafts. J Biol Chem 279(18):18944-18951.

Duncan PI, Pollet N, Niehrs C, Nigg EA. 2001. Cloning and characterization of Plx2 and Plx3, two additional Polo-like kinases from Xenopus laevis. Exp Cell Res 270(1):78-87.

Eckberg WR. 1997. MAP and cdc2 kinase activities at germinal vesicle breakdown in Chaetopterus. Dev Biol 191(2):182-190.

Eckerdt F, Pascreau G, Phistry M, Lewellyn AL, DePaoli-Roach AA, Maller JL. 2009. Phosphorylation of TPX2 by Plx1 enhances activation of Aurora A. Cell Cycle 8(15):2413-2419.

Edgecombe M, Patel R, Whitaker M. 1991. A cyclin-abundance cycle-independent p34cdc2 tyrosine phosphorylation cycle in early sea urchin embryos. EMBO J 10(12):3769-3775.

Einspanier R, Schonfelder M, Muller K, Stojkovic M, Kosmann M, Wolf E, Schams D. 2002. Expression of the vascular endothelial growth factor and its receptors and effects of VEGF during in vitro maturation of bovine cumulus-oocyte complexes (COC). Mol Reprod Dev 62(1):29-36.

El-Etr M, Schorderet-Slatkine S, Baulieu EE. 1979. Meiotic maturation in Xenopus laevis oocytes initiated by insulin. Science 205(4413):1397-1399.

Eliyahu E, Kaplan-Kraicer R, Shalgi R. 2001. PKC in eggs and embryos. Front Biosci 6:D785-791.

Eliyahu E, Shalgi R. 2002. A role for protein kinase C during rat egg activation. Biol Reprod 67(1):189-195.

Eliyahu E, Talmor-Cohen A, Shalgi R. 2002. Signaling through protein kinases during egg activation. J Reprod Immunol 53(1-2):161-169.

Eliyahu E, Tsaadon A, Shtraizent N, Shalgi R. 2005. The involvement of protein kinase C and actin filaments in cortical granule exocytosis in the rat. Reproduction 129(2):161-170.

Emily-Fenouil F, Ghiglione C, Lhomond G, Lepage T, Gache C. 1998. GSK3beta/shaggy mediates patterning along the animal-vegetal axis of the sea urchin embryo. Development 125(13):2489-2498.

Erikson E, Maller JL. 1988. Substrate specificity of ribosomal protein S6 kinase II from Xenopus eggs. Second Messengers Phosphoproteins 12(2-3):135-143.

Erikson E, Stefanovic D, Blenis J, Erikson RL, Maller JL. 1987. Antibodies to Xenopus egg S6 kinase II recognize S6 kinase from progesterone- and insulin-stimulated Xenopus oocytes and from proliferating chicken embryo fibroblasts. Mol Cell Biol 7(9):3147-3155.

Eswarakumar VP, Lax I, Schlessinger J. 2005. Cellular signaling by fibroblast growth factor receptors. Cytokine Growth Factor Rev 16(2):139-149.

Fabian JR, Morrison DK, Daar IO. 1993. Requirement for Raf and MAP kinase function during the meiotic maturation of Xenopus oocytes. J Cell Biol 122(3):645-652.

Fan HY, Tong C, Li MY, Lian L, Chen DY, Schatten H, Sun QY. 2002. Translocation of the classic protein kinase C isoforms in porcine oocytes: implications of protein kinase C involvement in the regulation of nuclear activity and cortical granule exocytosis. Exp Cell Res 277(2):183-191.

Fan HY, Tong C, Teng CB, Lian L, Li SW, Yang ZM, Chen DY, Schatten H, Sun QY. 2003. Characterization of Polo-like kinase-1 in rat oocytes and early embryos implies its functional roles in the regulation of meiotic maturation, fertilization, and cleavage. Mol Reprod Dev 65(3):318-329.

Farhi J, Ao A, Fisch B, Zhang XY, Garor R, Abir R. 2010. Glial cell line-derived neurotrophic factor (GDNF) and its receptors in human ovaries from fetuses, girls, and women. Fertil Steril 93(8):2565-2571.

Faure S, Morin N, Doree M. 1998. Inactivation of protein kinase A is not required for c-mos translation during meiotic maturation of Xenopus oocytes. Oncogene 17(10):1215-1221.

Faure S, Vigneron S, Doree M, Morin N. 1997. A member of the Ste20/PAK family of protein kinases is involved in both arrest of Xenopus oocytes at G2/prophase of the first meiotic cell cycle and in prevention of apoptosis. EMBO J 16(18):5550-5561.

Faure S, Vigneron S, Galas S, Brassac T, Delsert C, Morin N. 1999. Control of G2/M transition in Xenopus by a member of the p21-activated kinase (PAK) family: a link between protein kinase A and PAK signaling pathways? J Biol Chem 274(6):3573-3579.

Feng C, Yu A, Liu Y, Zhang J, Zong Z, Su W, Zhang Z, Yu D, Sun QY, Yu B. 2007. Involvement of protein kinase B/AKT in early development of mouse fertilized eggs. Biol Reprod 77(3):560-568.

Ferrell JE, Jr. 1999. Xenopus oocyte maturation: new lessons from a good egg. Bioessays 21(10):833-842.

Ferrell JE, Jr., Machleder EM. 1998. The biochemical basis of an all-or-none cell fate switch in Xenopus oocytes. Science 280(5365):895-898.

Ferrell JE, Jr., Wu M, Gerhart JC, Martin GS. 1991. Cell cycle tyrosine phosphorylation of p34cdc2 and a microtubule-associated protein kinase homolog in Xenopus oocytes and eggs. Mol Cell Biol 11(4):1965-1971.

Frank-Vaillant M, Haccard O, Thibier C, Ozon R, Arlot-Bonnemains Y, Prigent C, Jessus C. 2000. Progesterone regulates the accumulation and the activation of Eg2 kinase in Xenopus oocytes. J Cell Sci 113 (Pt 7):1127-1138.

Fujibuchi T, Abe Y, Takeuchi T, Ueda N, Shigemoto K, Yamamoto H, Kito K. 2005. Expression and phosphorylation of TOPK during spermatogenesis. Dev Growth Differ 47(9):637-644.

Fulka J, Jr., Jung T, Moor RM. 1992. The fall of biological maturation promoting factor (MPF) and histone H1 kinase activity during anaphase and telophase in mouse oocytes. Mol Reprod Dev 32(4):378-382.

Gaffre M, Martoriati A, Belhachemi N, Chambon JP, Houliston E, Jessus C, Karaiskou A. 2011. A critical balance between Cyclin B synthesis and Myt1 activity controls meiosis entry in Xenopus oocytes. Development 138(17):3735-3744.

Galat V, Zhou Y, Taborn G, Garton R, Iannaccone P. 2007. Overcoming MIII arrest from spontaneous activation in cultured rat oocytes. Cloning Stem Cells 9(3):303-314.

Gallicano GI, McGaughey RW, Capco DG. 1995. Protein kinase M, the cytosolic counterpart of protein kinase C, remodels the internal cytoskeleton of the mammalian egg during activation. Dev Biol 167(2):482-501.

Gallicano GI, McGaughey RW, Capco DG. 1997. Activation of protein kinase C after fertilization is required for remodeling the mouse egg into the zygote. Mol Reprod Dev 46(4):587-601.

Gavin AC, Cavadore JC, Schorderet-Slatkine S. 1994. Histone H1 kinase activity, germinal vesicle breakdown and M phase entry in mouse oocytes. J Cell Sci 107 (Pt 1):275-283.

Gavin AC, Ni Ainle A, Chierici E, Jones M, Nebreda AR. 1999. A p90(rsk) mutant constitutively interacting with MAP kinase uncouples MAP kinase from p34(cdc2)/cyclin B activation in Xenopus oocytes. Mol Biol Cell 10(9):2971-2986.

Gilkey JC, Jaffe LF, Ridgway EB, Reynolds GT. 1978. A free calcium wave traverses the activating egg of the medaka, Oryzias latipes. J Cell Biol 76(2):448-466.

Git A, Allison R, Perdiguero E, Nebreda AR, Houliston E, Standart N. 2009. Vg1RBP phosphorylation by Erk2 MAP kinase correlates with the cortical release of Vg1 mRNA during meiotic maturation of Xenopus oocytes. RNA 15(6):1121-1133.

Giusti AF, Carroll DJ, Abassi YA, Foltz KR. 1999a. Evidence that a starfish egg Src family tyrosine kinase associates with PLC-gamma1 SH2 domains at fertilization. Dev Biol 208(1):189-199.

Giusti AF, Carroll DJ, Abassi YA, Terasaki M, Foltz KR, Jaffe LA. 1999b. Requirement of a Src family kinase for initiating calcium release at fertilization in starfish eggs. J Biol Chem 274(41):29318-29322.

Giusti AF, Foltz KR, Jaffe LA. 2000a. The role of Src family kinases in starfish egg fertilisation. Zygote 8 Suppl 1:S16-17.

Giusti AF, O'Neill FJ, Yamasu K, Foltz KR, Jaffe LA. 2003. Function of a sea urchin egg Src family kinase in initiating Ca2+ release at fertilization. Dev Biol 256(2):367-378.

Giusti AF, Xu W, Hinkle B, Terasaki M, Jaffe LA. 2000b. Evidence that fertilization activates starfish eggs by sequential activation of a Src-like kinase and phospholipase cgamma. J Biol Chem 275(22):16788-16794.

Glahn D, Mark SD, Behr RK, Nuccitelli R. 1999. Tyrosine kinase inhibitors block sperm-induced egg activation in Xenopus laevis. Dev Biol 205(1):171-180.

Glover CV, 3rd. 1998. On the physiological role of casein kinase II in Saccharomyces cerevisiae. Prog Nucleic Acid Res Mol Biol 59:95-133.

Golubovskaya VM, Cance W. 2010. Focal adhesion kinase and p53 signal transduction pathways in cancer. Front Biosci 15:901-912.

Grieco D, Avvedimento EV, Gottesman ME. 1994. A role for cAMP-dependent protein kinase in early embryonic divisions. Proc Natl Acad Sci U S A 91(21):9896-9900.

Grieco D, Porcellini A, Avvedimento EV, Gottesman ME. 1996. Requirement for cAMP-PKA pathway activation by M phase-promoting factor in the transition from mitosis to interphase. Science 271(5256):1718-1723.

Grigorescu F, Baccara MT, Rouard M, Renard E. 1994. Insulin and IGF-1 signaling in oocyte maturation. Horm Res 42(1-2):55-61.

Gross SD, Schwab MS, Taieb FE, Lewellyn AL, Qian YW, Maller JL. 2000. The critical role of the MAP kinase pathway in meiosis II in Xenopus oocytes is mediated by p90(Rsk). Curr Biol 10(8):430-438.

Gutierrez GJ, Vogtlin A, Castro A, Ferby I, Salvagiotto G, Ronai Z, Lorca T, Nebreda AR. 2006. Meiotic regulation of the CDK activator RINGO/Speedy by ubiquitin-proteasome-mediated processing and degradation. Nat Cell Biol 8(10):1084-1094.

Haberman Y, Alon LT, Eliyahu E, Shalgi R. 2011. Receptor for activated C kinase (RACK) and protein kinase C (PKC) in egg activation. Theriogenology 75(1):80-89.

Halet G. 2004. PKC signaling at fertilization in mammalian eggs. Biochim Biophys Acta 1742(1-3):185-189.

Han SJ, Conti M. 2006. New pathways from PKA to the Cdc2/cyclin B complex in oocytes: Wee1B as a potential PKA substrate. Cell Cycle 5(3):227-231.

Han SJ, Vaccari S, Nedachi T, Andersen CB, Kovacina KS, Roth RA, Conti M. 2006a. Protein kinase B/Akt phosphorylation of PDE3A and its role in mammalian oocyte maturation. EMBO J 25(24):5716-5725.

Hansen DV, Tung JJ, Jackson PK. 2006. CaMKII and polo-like kinase 1 sequentially phosphorylate the cytostatic factor Emi2/XErp1 to trigger its destruction and meiotic exit. Proc Natl Acad Sci U S A 103(3):608-613.

Harada Y, Takagaki Y, Sunagawa M, Saito T, Yamada L, Taniguchi H, Shoguchi E, Sawada H. 2008. Mechanism of self-sterility in a hermaphroditic chordate. Science 320(5875):548-550.

Hardie DG, Carling D. 1997. The AMP-activated protein kinase--fuel gauge of the mammalian cell? Eur J Biochem 246(2):259-273.

Hartwell LH. 1991. Twenty-five years of cell cycle genetics. Genetics 129(4):975-980.

Heinecke JW, Meier KE, Lorenzen JA, Shapiro BM. 1990. A specific requirement for protein kinase C in activation of the respiratory burst oxidase of fertilization. J Biol Chem 265(14):7717-7720.

Hemmings BA. 1997. Akt signaling: linking membrane events to life and death decisions. Science 275(5300):628-630.

Hens MD, DeSimone DW. 1995. Molecular analysis and developmental expression of the focal adhesion kinase pp125FAK in Xenopus laevis. Dev Biol 170(2):274-288.

Hertweck M, Gobel C, Baumeister R. 2004. C. elegans SGK-1 is the critical component in the Akt/PKB kinase complex to control stress response and life span. Dev Cell 6(4):577-588.

Hiraoka D, Hori-Oshima S, Fukuhara T, Tachibana K, Okumura E, Kishimoto T. 2004. PDK1 is required for the hormonal signaling pathway leading to meiotic resumption in starfish oocytes. Dev Biol 276(2):330-336.

Hodgman R, Tay J, Mendez R, Richter JD. 2001. CPEB phosphorylation and cytoplasmic polyadenylation are catalyzed by the kinase IAK1/Eg2 in maturing mouse oocytes. Development 128(14):2815-2822.

Homer H. 2011. New insights into the genetic regulation of homologue disjunction in mammalian oocytes. Cytogenet Genome Res 133(2-4):209-222.

Horie K, Takakura K, Taii S, Narimoto K, Noda Y, Nishikawa S, Nakayama H, Fujita J, Mori T. 1991. The expression of c-kit protein during oogenesis and early embryonic development. Biol Reprod 45(4):547-552.

Horner VL, Wolfner MF. 2008. Transitioning from egg to embryo: triggers and mechanisms of egg activation. Dev Dyn 237(3):527-544.

Hoshino Y, Sato E. 2008. Protein kinase B (PKB/Akt) is required for the completion of meiosis in mouse oocytes. Dev Biol 314(1):215-223.

Hoshino Y, Yokoo M, Yoshida N, Sasada H, Matsumoto H, Sato E. 2004. Phosphatidylinositol 3-kinase and Akt participate in the FSH-induced meiotic maturation of mouse oocytes. Mol Reprod Dev 69(1):77-86.

Huang X, Tong JS, Wang ZB, Yang CR, Qi ST, Guo L, Ouyang YC, Quan S, Sun QY, Qi ZQ, Huang RX, Wang HL. 2011. JNK2 participates in spindle assembly during mouse oocyte meiotic maturation. Microsc Microanal 17(2):197-205.

Hudmon A, Schulman H, Kim J, Maltez JM, Tsien RW, Pitt GS. 2005. CaMKII tethers to L-type Ca2+ channels, establishing a local and dedicated integrator of Ca2+ signals for facilitation. J Cell Biol 171(3):537-547.

Huo LJ, Fan HY, Zhong ZS, Chen DY, Schatten H, Sun QY. 2004. Ubiquitin-proteasome pathway modulates mouse oocyte meiotic maturation and fertilization via regulation of MAPK cascade and cyclin B1 degradation. Mech Dev 121(10):1275-1287.

Hupalowska A, Kalaszczynska I, Hoffmann S, Tsurumi C, Kubiak JZ, Polanski Z, Ciemerych MA. 2008. Metaphase I arrest in LT/Sv mouse oocytes involves the spindle assembly checkpoint. Biol Reprod 79(6):1102-1110.

Hyodo-Miura J, Urushiyama S, Nagai S, Nishita M, Ueno N, Shibuya H. 2002. Involvement of NLK and Sox11 in neural induction in Xenopus development. Genes Cells 7(5):487-496.

Inoue D, Sagata N. 2005. The Polo-like kinase Plx1 interacts with and inhibits Myt1 after fertilization of Xenopus eggs. EMBO J 24(5):1057-1067.

Ishida A, Fujisawa H. 1995. Stabilization of calmodulin-dependent protein kinase II through the autoinhibitory domain. J Biol Chem 270(5):2163-2170.

Ishimura A, Lee HS, Bong YS, Saucier C, Mood K, Park EK, Daar IO. 2006. Oncogenic Met receptor induces ectopic structures in Xenopus embryos. Oncogene 25(31):4286-4299.

Ishitani T, Ishitani S, Matsumoto K, Itoh M. 2009. Nemo-like kinase is involved in NGF-induced neurite outgrowth via phosphorylating MAP1B and paxillin. J Neurochem 111(5):1104-1118.

Ito J, Yoon SY, Lee B, Vanderheyden V, Vermassen E, Wojcikiewicz R, Alfandari D, De Smedt H, Parys JB, Fissore RA. 2008. Inositol 1,4,5-trisphosphate receptor 1, a widespread Ca2+ channel, is a novel substrate of polo-like kinase 1 in eggs. Dev Biol 320(2):402-413.

Ito J, Yoshida T, Kasai Y, Wakai T, Parys JB, Fissore RA, Kashiwazaki N. 2010. Phosphorylation of inositol 1,4,5-triphosphate receptor 1 during in vitro maturation of porcine oocytes. Anim Sci J 81(1):34-41.

Itoh T, Hasegawa J, Tsujita K, Kanaho Y, Takenawa T. 2009. The tyrosine kinase Fer is a downstream target of the PLD-PA pathway that regulates cell migration. Sci Signal 2(87):ra52.

Iwasaki T, Koretomo Y, Fukuda T, Paronetto MP, Sette C, Fukami Y, Sato K. 2008. Expression, phosphorylation, and mRNA-binding of heterogeneous nuclear ribonucleoprotein K in Xenopus oocytes, eggs, and early embryos. Dev Growth Differ 50(1):23-40.

Iwasaki T, Sato K, Yoshino K, Itakura S, Kosuge K, Tokmakov AA, Owada K, Yonezawa K, Fukami Y. 2006. Phylogeny of vertebrate Src tyrosine kinases revealed by the epitope region of mAb327. J Biochem 139(3):347-354.

Janicot M, Flores-Riveros JR, Lane MD. 1991. The insulin-like growth factor 1 (IGF-1) receptor is responsible for mediating the effects of insulin, IGF-1, and IGF-2 in Xenopus laevis oocytes. J Biol Chem 266(15):9382-9391.

Jeanmart J, Uytdenhoef P, De Sutter G, Legros F. 1976. Insulin receptor sites as membrane markers during embryonic development. I. Data obtained with unfertilized and fertilized sea urchin eggs. Differentiation 7(1):23-30.

Jelinkova L, Kubelka M. 2006. Neither Aurora B activity nor histone H3 phosphorylation is essential for chromosome condensation during meiotic maturation of porcine oocytes. Biol Reprod 74(5):905-912.

Jelinkova L, Kubelka M, Motlik J, Guerrier P. 1994. Chromatin condensation and histone H1 kinase activity during growth and maturation of rabbit oocytes. Mol Reprod Dev 37(2):210-215.

Jessmon P, Leach RE, Armant DR. 2009. Diverse functions of HBEGF during pregnancy. Mol Reprod Dev 76(12):1116-1127.

Jiang Y, Chan JL, Zong CS, Wang LH. 1996. Effect of tyrosine mutations on the kinase activity and transforming potential of an oncogenic human insulin-like growth factor I receptor. J Biol Chem 271(1):160-167.

Jove R, Hanafusa H. 1987. Cell transformation by the viral src oncogene. Annu Rev Cell Biol 3:31-56.

Kakita M, Murase K, Iwano M, Matsumoto T, Watanabe M, Shiba H, Isogai A, Takayama S. 2007. Two distinct forms of M-locus protein kinase localize to the plasma membrane and interact directly with S-locus receptor kinase to transduce self-incompatibility signaling in Brassica rapa. Plant Cell 19(12):3961-3973.

Kalive M, Faust JJ, Koeneman BA, Capco DG. 2010. Involvement of the PKC family in regulation of early development. Mol Reprod Dev 77(2):95-104.

Kalous J, Kubelka M, Solc P, Susor A, Motlik J. 2009. AKT (protein kinase B) is implicated in meiotic maturation of porcine oocytes. Reproduction 138(4):645-654.

Kalous J, Solc P, Baran V, Kubelka M, Schultz RM, Motlik J. 2006. PKB/AKT is involved in resumption of meiosis in mouse oocytes. Biol Cell 98(2):111-123.

Kamel C, Veno PA, Kinsey WH. 1986. Quantitation of a src-like tyrosine protein kinase during fertilization of the sea urchin egg. Biochem Biophys Res Commun 138(1):349-355.

Kang MK, Han SJ. 2011. Post-transcriptional and post-translational regulation during mouse oocyte maturation. BMB Rep 44(3):147-157.

Kang MG, Kulisz A, Wasserman WJ. 1998. Raf-1 kinase, a potential regulator of intracellular pH in Xenopus oocytes. Biol Cell 90(6-7):477-485.

Karaiskou A, Cayla X, Haccard O, Jessus C, Ozon R. 1998. MPF amplification in Xenopus oocyte extracts depends on a two-step activation of cdc25 phosphatase. Exp Cell Res 244(2):491-500.

Karaiskou A, Lepretre AC, Pahlavan G, Du Pasquier D, Ozon R, Jessus C. 2004. Polo-like kinase confers MPF autoamplification competence to growing Xenopus oocytes. Development 131(7):1543-1552.

Katsu Y, Minshall N, Nagahama Y, Standart N. 1999. Ca2+ is required for phosphorylation of clam p82/CPEB in vitro: implications for dual and independent roles of MAP and Cdc2 kinases. Dev Biol 209(1):186-199.

Kawamura K, Ye Y, Kawamura N, Jing L, Groenen P, Gelpke MS, Rauch R, Hsueh AJ, Tanaka T. 2008. Completion of Meiosis I of preovulatory oocytes and facilitation of preimplantation embryo development by glial cell line-derived neurotrophic factor. Dev Biol 315(1):189-202.

Keady BT, Kuo P, Martinez SE, Yuan L, Hake LE. 2007. MAPK interacts with XGef and is required for CPEB activation during meiosis in Xenopus oocytes. J Cell Sci 120(Pt 6):1093-1103.

Kierszenbaum AL, Rivkin E, Talmor-Cohen A, Shalgi R, Tres LL. 2009. Expression of full-length and truncated Fyn tyrosine kinase transcripts and encoded proteins during spermatogenesis and localization during acrosome biogenesis and fertilization. Mol Reprod Dev 76(9):832-843.

Kikuchi K, Naito K, Daen FP, Izaike Y, Toyoda Y. 1995. Histone H1 kinase activity during in vitro fertilization of pig follicular oocytes matured in vitro. Theriogenology 43(2):523-532.

Kinoshita K, Noetzel TL, Pelletier L, Mechtler K, Drechsel DN, Schwager A, Lee M, Raff JW, Hyman AA. 2005. Aurora A phosphorylation of TACC3/maskin is required for centrosome-dependent microtubule assembly in mitosis. J Cell Biol 170(7):1047-1055.

Kinsey WH. 1995. Differential phosphorylation of a 57-KDa protein tyrosine kinase during egg activation. Biochem Biophys Res Commun 208(1):204-209.

Kinsey WH. 1996. Biphasic activation of Fyn kinase upon fertilization of the sea urchin egg. Dev Biol 174(2):281-287.

Kinsey WH, Shen SS. 2000. Role of the Fyn kinase in calcium release during fertilization of the sea urchin egg. Dev Biol 225(1):253-264.

Kinsey WH, Wu W, Macgregor E. 2003. Activation of Src-family PTK activity at fertilization: role of the SH2 domain. Dev Biol 264(1):255-262.

Klerkx EP, Lazo PA, Askjaer P. 2009. Emerging biological functions of the vaccinia-related kinase (VRK) family. Histol Histopathol 24(6):749-759.

Kokai Y, Wada T, Myers JN, Brown VI, Dobashi K, Cohen J, Hamuro J, Weiner DB, Greene MI. 1988. The role of the neu oncogene product in cell transformation and normal development. Princess Takamatsu Symp 19:45-57.

Kosako H, Gotoh Y, Matsuda S, Ishikawa M, Nishida E. 1992. Xenopus MAP kinase activator is a serine/threonine/tyrosine kinase activated by threonine phosphorylation. EMBO J 11(8):2903-2908.

Kostellow AB, Ma GY, Morrill GA. 1996. Progesterone triggers the rapid activation of phospholipase D in the amphibian oocyte plasma membrane when initiating the G2/M transition. Biochim Biophys Acta 1304(3):263-271.

Kubiak JZ, Weber M, Geraud G, Maro B. 1992. Cell cycle modification during the transitions between meiotic M-phases in mouse oocytes. J Cell Sci 102 (Pt 3):457-467.

Kume S, Endo T, Nishimura Y, Kano K, Naito K. 2007. Porcine SPDYA2 (RINGO A2) stimulates CDC2 activity and accelerates meiotic maturation of porcine oocytes. Biol Reprod 76(3):440-447.

Kuo P, Runge E, Lu X, Hake LE. 2011. XGef influences XRINGO/CDK1 signaling and CPEB activation during Xenopus oocyte maturation. Differentiation 81(2):133-140.

Kurokawa M, Sato K, Smyth J, Wu H, Fukami K, Takenawa T, Fissore RA. 2004. Evidence that activation of Src family kinase is not required for fertilization-associated [Ca2+]i oscillations in mouse eggs. Reproduction 127(4):441-454.

Kurvari V, Snell WJ. 1996. SksC, a fertilization-related protein kinase in Chlamydomonas, is expressed throughout the cell cycle and gametogenesis, and a phosphorylated form is present in both flagella and cell bodies. Biochem Biophys Res Commun 228(1):45-54.

Kurvari V, Zhang Y, Luo Y, Snell WJ. 1996. Molecular cloning of a protein kinase whose phosphorylation is regulated by genetic adhesion during Chlamydomonas fertilization. Proc Natl Acad Sci U S A 93(1):39-43.

Kushima S, Mammadova G, Mahbub Hasan AK, Fukami Y, Sato K. 2011. Characterization of Lipovitellin 2 as a tyrosine-phosphorylated protein in oocytes, eggs and early embryos of Xenopus laevis. Zoolog Sci 28(8):550-559.

Lancaster OM, Cullen CF, Ohkura H. 2007. NHK-1 phosphorylates BAF to allow karyosome formation in the Drosophila oocyte nucleus. J Cell Biol 179(5):817-824.

LaRosa C, Downs SM. 2006. Stress stimulates AMP-activated protein kinase and meiotic resumption in mouse oocytes. Biol Reprod 74(3):585-592.

Ledan E, Polanski Z, Terret ME, Maro B. 2001. Meiotic maturation of the mouse oocyte requires an equilibrium between cyclin B synthesis and degradation. Dev Biol 232(2):400-413.

Lee B, Vermassen E, Yoon SY, Vanderheyden V, Ito J, Alfandari D, De Smedt H, Parys JB, Fissore RA. 2006. Phosphorylation of IP3R1 and the regulation of [Ca2+]i responses at fertilization: a role for the MAP kinase pathway. Development 133(21):4355-4365.

Lee HC, Tsai JN, Liao PY, Tsai WY, Lin KY, Chuang CC, Sun CK, Chang WC, Tsai HJ. 2007. Glycogen synthase kinase 3 alpha and 3 beta have distinct functions during cardiogenesis of zebrafish embryo. BMC Dev Biol 7:93.

Lefebvre DL, Charest DL, Yee A, Crawford BJ, Pelech SL. 1999. Characterization of fertilization-modulated myelin basic protein kinases from sea star: regulation of Mapk. J Cell Biochem 75(2):272-287.

Leiva L, Carrasco D, Taylor A, Veliz M, Gonzalez C, Allende CC, Allende JE. 1987. Casein kinase II is a major protein phosphorylating activity in the nuclei of Xenopus laevis oocytes. Biochem Int 14(4):707-717.

Lev S, Moreno H, Martinez R, Canoll P, Peles E, Musacchio JM, Plowman GD, Rudy B, Schlessinger J. 1995. Protein tyrosine kinase PYK2 involved in Ca(2+)-induced regulation of ion channel and MAP kinase functions. Nature 376(6543):737-745.

Levi M, Maro B, Shalgi R. 2010. Fyn kinase is involved in cleavage furrow ingression during meiosis and mitosis. Reproduction 140(6):827-834.

Li M, Li S, Yuan J, Wang ZB, Sun SC, Schatten H, Sun QY. 2009. Bub3 is a spindle assembly checkpoint protein regulating chromosome segregation during mouse oocyte meiosis. PLoS One 4(11):e7701.

Li C, Sun Y, Yi K, Ma Y, Zhang W, Zhou X. 2010. Detection of nerve growth factor (NGF) and its specific receptor (TrkA) in ejaculated bovine sperm, and the effects of NGF on sperm function. Theriogenology 74(9):1615-1622.

Li X, Earp HS. 1997. Paxillin is tyrosine-phosphorylated by and preferentially associates with the calcium-dependent tyrosine kinase in rat liver epithelial cells. J Biol Chem 272(22):14341-14348.

Liang CG, Su YQ, Fan HY, Schatten H, Sun QY. 2007. Mechanisms regulating oocyte meiotic resumption: roles of mitogen-activated protein kinase. Mol Endocrinol 21(9):2037-2055.

Linher K, Wu D, Li J. 2007. Glial cell line-derived neurotrophic factor: an intraovarian factor that enhances oocyte developmental competence in vitro. Endocrinology 148(9):4292-4301.

Littlepage LE, Ruderman JV. 2002. Identification of a new APC/C recognition domain, the A box, which is required for the Cdh1-dependent destruction of the kinase Aurora-A during mitotic exit. Genes Dev 16(17):2274-2285.

Littlepage LE, Wu H, Andresson T, Deanehan JK, Amundadottir LT, Ruderman JV. 2002. Identification of phosphorylated residues that affect the activity of the mitotic kinase Aurora-A. Proc Natl Acad Sci U S A 99(24):15440-15445.

Liu J, Grimison B, Lewellyn AL, Maller JL. 2006. The anaphase-promoting complex/cyclosome inhibitor Emi2 is essential for meiotic but not mitotic cell cycles. J Biol Chem 281(46):34736-34741.

Liu J, Maller JL. 2005. Calcium elevation at fertilization coordinates phosphorylation of XErp1/Emi2 by Plx1 and CaMK II to release metaphase arrest by cytostatic factor. Curr Biol 15(16):1458-1468.

Liu L, Rajareddy S, Reddy P, Jagarlamudi K, Du C, Shen Y, Guo Y, Boman K, Lundin E, Ottander U, Selstam G, Liu K. 2007. Phosphorylation and inactivation of glycogen synthase kinase-3 by soluble kit ligand in mouse oocytes during early follicular development. J Mol Endocrinol 38(1-2):137-146.

Liu Y, Misamore MJ, Snell WJ. 2010. Membrane fusion triggers rapid degradation of two gamete-specific, fusion-essential proteins in a membrane block to polygamy in Chlamydomonas. Development 137(9):1473-1481.

Lohka MJ, Hayes MK, Maller JL. 1988. Purification of maturation-promoting factor, an intracellular regulator of early mitotic events. Proc Natl Acad Sci U S A 85(9):3009-3013.

Long T, Cailliau K, Beckmann S, Browaeys E, Trolet J, Grevelding CG, Dissous C. 2010. Schistosoma mansoni Polo-like kinase 1: A mitotic kinase with key functions in parasite reproduction. Int J Parasitol 40(9):1075-1086.

Lu N, Guarnieri DJ, Simon MA. 2004. Localization of Tec29 to ring canals is mediated by Src64 and PtdIns(3,4,5)P3-dependent mechanisms. EMBO J 23(5):1089-1100.

Lu Q, Smith GD, Chen DY, Han ZM, Sun QY. 2002. Activation of protein kinase C induces mitogen-activated protein kinase dephosphorylation and pronucleus formation in rat oocytes. Biol Reprod 67(1):64-69.

Luo J, McGinnis LK, Kinsey WH. 2009. Fyn kinase activity is required for normal organization and functional polarity of the mouse oocyte cortex. Mol Reprod Dev 76(9):819-831.

Luria A, Tennenbaum T, Sun QY, Rubinstein S, Breitbart H. 2000. Differential localization of conventional protein kinase C isoforms during mouse oocyte development. Biol Reprod 62(6):1564-1570.

Ma C, Cummings C, Liu XJ. 2003. Biphasic activation of Aurora-A kinase during the meiosis I- meiosis II transition in Xenopus oocytes. Mol Cell Biol 23(5):1703-1716.

Machaca K. 2007. Ca2+ signaling differentiation during oocyte maturation. J Cell Physiol 213(2):331-340.

MacNicol AM, Muslin AJ, Howard EL, Kikuchi A, MacNicol MC, Williams LT. 1995. Regulation of Raf-1-dependent signaling during early Xenopus development. Mol Cell Biol 15(12):6686-6693.

Madgwick S, Hansen DV, Levasseur M, Jackson PK, Jones KT. 2006. Mouse Emi2 is required to enter meiosis II by reestablishing cyclin B1 during interkinesis. J Cell Biol 174(6):791-801.

Madgwick S, Jones KT. 2007. How eggs arrest at metaphase II: MPF stabilisation plus APC/C inhibition equals Cytostatic Factor. Cell Div 2:4.

Madgwick S, Nixon VL, Chang HY, Herbert M, Levasseur M, Jones KT. 2004. Maintenance of sister chromatid attachment in mouse eggs through maturation-promoting factor activity. Dev Biol 275(1):68-81.

Madgwick S, Levasseur M, Jones KT. 2005. Calmodulin-dependent protein kinase II, and not protein kinase C, is sufficient for triggering cell-cycle resumption in mammalian eggs. J Cell Sci 118(Pt 17):3849-3859.

Mahbub Hasan AK, Fukami Y, Sato KI. 2011. Gamete membrane microdomains and their associated molecules in fertilization signaling. Mol Reprod Dev. 78(10-11):814-830.

Mahbub Hasan AK, Ou Z, Sakakibara K, Hirahara S, Iwasaki T, Sato K, Fukami Y. 2007. Characterization of Xenopus egg membrane microdomains containing uroplakin Ib/III complex: roles of their molecular interactions for subcellular localization and signal transduction. Genes Cells 12(2):251-267.

Mahbub Hasan AK, Sato K, Sakakibara K, Ou Z, Iwasaki T, Ueda Y, Fukami Y. 2005. Uroplakin III, a novel Src substrate in Xenopus egg rafts, is a target for sperm protease essential for fertilization. Dev Biol 286(2):483-492.

Malcuit C, Knott JG, He C, Wainwright T, Parys JB, Robl JM, Fissore RA. 2005. Fertilization and inositol 1,4,5-trisphosphate (IP3)-induced calcium release in type-1 inositol 1,4,5-trisphosphate receptor down-regulated bovine eggs. Biol Reprod 73(1):2-13.

Maller JL. 1990. Xenopus oocytes and the biochemistry of cell division. Biochemistry 29(13):3157-3166.

Maller JL, Schwab MS, Roberts BT, Gross SD, Taieb FE, Tunquist BJ. 2001. The pathway of MAP kinase mediation of CSF arrest in Xenopus oocytes. Biol Cell 93(1-2):27-33.

Mammadova G, Iwasaki T, Tokmakov AA, Fukami Y, Sato K. 2009. Evidence that phosphatidylinositol 3-kinase is involved in sperm-induced tyrosine kinase signaling in Xenopus egg fertilization. BMC Dev Biol 9:68.

Marangos P, Verschuren EW, Chen R, Jackson PK, Carroll J. 2007. Prophase I arrest and progression to metaphase I in mouse oocytes are controlled by Emi1-dependent regulation of APC(Cdh1). J Cell Biol 176(1):65-75.

Marotta V, Guerra A, Sapio MR, Vitale M. 2011. RET/PTC rearrangement in benign and malignant thyroid diseases: a clinical standpoint. Eur J Endocrinol 165(4):499-507.

Masui Y, Markert CL. 1971. Cytoplasmic control of nuclear behavior during meiotic maturation of frog oocytes. J Exp Zool 177(2):129-145.

Masui Y. 1992. Towards understanding the control of the division cycle in animal cells. Biochem Cell Biol 70(10-11):920-945.

Masui Y. 2000. The elusive cytostatic factor in the animal egg. Nat Rev Mol Cell Biol 1(3):228-232.

Maton G, Lorca T, Girault JA, Ozon R, Jessus C. 2005. Differential regulation of Cdc2 and Aurora-A in Xenopus oocytes: a crucial role of phosphatase 2A. J Cell Sci 118(Pt 11):2485-2494.

Maton G, Thibier C, Castro A, Lorca T, Prigent C, Jessus C. 2003. Cdc2-cyclin B triggers H3 kinase activation of Aurora-A in Xenopus oocytes. J Biol Chem 278(24):21439-21449.

Matsumoto S, Abe Y, Fujibuchi T, Takeuchi T, Kito K, Ueda N, Shigemoto K, Gyo K. 2004. Characterization of a MAPKK-like protein kinase TOPK. Biochem Biophys Res Commun 325(3):997-1004.

Matten W, Daar I, Vande Woude GF. 1994. Protein kinase A acts at multiple points to inhibit Xenopus oocyte maturation. Mol Cell Biol 14(7):4419-4426.

Mayes MA, Sirard MA. 2002. Effect of type 3 and type 4 phosphodiesterase inhibitors on the maintenance of bovine oocytes in meiotic arrest. Biol Reprod 66(1):180-184.

Mazia D. 1937. The release of calcium in *Arbacia* eggs upon fertilization. J Cell and Comp Phys 10(3):291-304.

McGinnis LK, Albertini DF, Kinsey WH. 2007. Localized activation of Src-family protein kinases in the mouse egg. Dev Biol 306(1):241-254.

McGinnis LK, Carroll DJ, Kinsey WH. 2011a. Protein tyrosine kinase signaling during oocyte maturation and fertilization. Mol Reprod Dev. 78(10-11):831-845.

McGinnis LK, Hong X, Christenson LK, Kinsey WH. 2011b. Fer tyrosine kinase is required for germinal vesicle breakdown and meiosis-I in mouse oocytes. Mol Reprod Dev 78(1):33-47.

McGinnis LK, Kinsey WH, Albertini DF. 2009. Functions of Fyn kinase in the completion of meiosis in mouse oocytes. Dev Biol 327(2):280-287.

Mehlmann LM. 2005. Stops and starts in mammalian oocytes: recent advances in understanding the regulation of meiotic arrest and oocyte maturation. Reproduction 130(6):791-799.

Mehlmann LM, Jaffe LA. 2005. SH2 domain-mediated activation of an SRC family kinase is not required to initiate Ca2+ release at fertilization in mouse eggs. Reproduction 129(5):557-564.

Mehlmann LM, Jones TL, Jaffe LA. 2002. Meiotic arrest in the mouse follicle maintained by a Gs protein in the oocyte. Science 297(5585):1343-1345.

Meijer L, Arion D, Golsteyn R, Pines J, Brizuela L, Hunt T, Beach D. 1989a. Cyclin is a component of the sea urchin egg M-phase specific histone H1 kinase. EMBO J 8(8):2275-2282.

Meijer L, Azzi L, Wang JY. 1991. Cyclin B targets p34cdc2 for tyrosine phosphorylation. EMBO J 10(6):1545-1554.

Meijer L, Dostmann W, Genieser HG, Butt E, Jastorff B. 1989b. Starfish oocyte maturation: evidence for a cyclic AMP-dependent inhibitory pathway. Dev Biol 133(1):58-66.

Meijer L, Pondaven P. 1988. Cyclic activation of histone H1 kinase during sea urchin egg mitotic divisions. Exp Cell Res 174(1):116-129.

Mendez R, Hake LE, Andresson T, Littlepage LE, Ruderman JV, Richter JD. 2000. Phosphorylation of CPE binding factor by Eg2 regulates translation of c-mos mRNA. Nature 404(6775):302-307.

Meng XQ, Zheng KG, Yang Y, Jiang MX, Zhang YL, Sun QY, Li YL. 2006. Proline-rich tyrosine kinase2 is involved in F-actin organization during in vitro maturation of rat oocyte. Reproduction 132(6):859-867.

Minshull J, Pines J, Golsteyn R, Standart N, Mackie S, Colman A, Blow J, Ruderman JV, Wu M, Hunt T. 1989. The role of cyclin synthesis, modification and destruction in the control of cell division. J Cell Sci Suppl 12:77-97.

Mitra J, Schultz RM. 1996. Regulation of the acquisition of meiotic competence in the mouse: changes in the subcellular localization of cdc2, cyclin B1, cdc25C and wee1, and in the concentration of these proteins and their transcripts. J Cell Sci 109 (Pt 9):2407-2415.

Miyata Y, Nishida E. 1999. Distantly related cousins of MAP kinase: biochemical properties and possible physiological functions. Biochem Biophys Res Commun 266(2):291-295.

Miyazaki S, Ito M. 2006. Calcium signals for egg activation in mammals. J Pharmacol Sci 100(5):545-552.

Mochida S, Maslen SL, Skehel M, Hunt T. 2010. Greatwall phosphorylates an inhibitor of protein phosphatase 2A that is essential for mitosis. Science 330(6011):1670-1673.

Mood K, Friesel R, Daar IO. 2002. SNT1/FRS2 mediates germinal vesicle breakdown induced by an activated FGF receptor1 in Xenopus oocytes. J Biol Chem 277(36):33196-33204.

Mood K, Saucier C, Bong YS, Lee HS, Park M, Daar IO. 2006. Gab1 is required for cell cycle transition, cell proliferation, and transformation induced by an oncogenic met receptor. Mol Biol Cell 17(9):3717-3728.

Moore KL, Kinsey WH. 1994. Identification of an abl-related protein tyrosine kinase in the cortex of the sea urchin egg: possible role at fertilization. Dev Biol 164(2):444-455.

Mori M, Hara M, Tachibana K, Kishimoto T. 2006. p90Rsk is required for G1 phase arrest in unfertilized starfish eggs. Development 133(9):1823-1830.

Mori T, Guo MW, Sato E, Baba T, Takasaki S, Mori E. 2000. Molecular and immunological approaches to mammalian fertilization. J Reprod Immunol 47(2):139-158.

Mori T, Wu GM, Mori E. 1991. Expression of CD4-like structure on murine egg vitelline membrane and its signal transductive roles through p56lck in fertilization. Am J Reprod Immunol 26(3):97-103.

Morrison DL, Yee A, Paddon HB, Vilimek D, Aebersold R, Pelech SL. 2000. Regulation of the meiosis-inhibited protein kinase, a p38(MAPK) isoform, during meiosis and following fertilization of seastar oocytes. J Biol Chem 275(44):34236-34244.

Murakami MS, Vande Woude GF. 1998. Analysis of the early embryonic cell cycles of Xenopus; regulation of cell cycle length by Xe-wee1 and Mos. Development 125(2):237-248.

Murase K, Shiba H, Iwano M, Che FS, Watanabe M, Isogai A, Takayama S. 2004. A membrane-anchored protein kinase involved in Brassica self-incompatibility signaling. Science 303(5663):1516-1519.

Muslin AJ, MacNicol AM, Williams LT. 1993. Raf-1 protein kinase is important for progesterone-induced Xenopus oocyte maturation and acts downstream of mos. Mol Cell Biol 13(7):4197-4202.

Nakaya M, Fukui A, Izumi Y, Akimoto K, Asashima M, Ohno S. 2000. Meiotic maturation induces animal-vegetal asymmetric distribution of aPKC and ASIP/PAR-3 in Xenopus oocytes. Development 127(23):5021-5031.

Narasimhan V, Hamill O, Cerione RA. 1992. The effects of the normal and oncogenic forms of the neu tyrosine kinase, and the corresponding forms of an immunoglobulin E receptor/neu tyrosine kinase fusion protein, on Xenopus oocyte maturation. FEBS Lett 303(2-3):164-168.

Nebreda AR, Martin-Zanca D, Kaplan DR, Parada LF, Santos E. 1991. Induction by NGF of meiotic maturation of Xenopus oocytes expressing the trk proto-oncogene product. Science 252(5005):558-561.

Newhall KJ, Criniti AR, Cheah CS, Smith KC, Kafer KE, Burkart AD, McKnight GS. 2006. Dynamic anchoring of PKA is essential during oocyte maturation. Curr Biol 16(3):321-327.

Niault T, Hached K, Sotillo R, Sorger PK, Maro B, Benezra R, Wassmann K. 2007. Changing Mad2 levels affects chromosome segregation and spindle assembly checkpoint control in female mouse meiosis I. PLoS One 2(11):e1165.

Nishi Y, Lin R. 2005. DYRK2 and GSK-3 phosphorylate and promote the timely degradation of OMA-1, a key regulator of the oocyte-to-embryo transition in C. elegans. Dev Biol 288(1):139-149.

Nishiyama T, Ohsumi K, Kishimoto T. 2007a. Phosphorylation of Erp1 by p90rsk is required for cytostatic factor arrest in Xenopus laevis eggs. Nature 446(7139):1096-1099.

Nishiyama T, Yoshizaki N, Kishimoto T, Ohsumi K. 2007b. Transient activation of calcineurin is essential to initiate embryonic development in Xenopus laevis. Nature 449(7160):341-345.

Nishizuka Y. 1984. The role of protein kinase C in cell surface signal transduction and tumour promotion. Nature 308(5961):693-698.

Nishizuka Y. 1986. Studies and perspectives of protein kinase C. Science 233(4761):305-312.

Nishizuka Y. 1988. The molecular heterogeneity of protein kinase C and its implications for cellular regulation. Nature 334(6184):661-665.

Nissley SP, Haskell JF, Sasaki N, De Vroede MA, Rechler MM. 1985. Insulin-like growth factor receptors. J Cell Sci Suppl 3:39-51.

Norris RP, Ratzan WJ, Freudzon M, Mehlmann LM, Krall J, Movsesian MA, Wang H, Ke H, Nikolaev VO, Jaffe LA. 2009. Cyclic GMP from the surrounding somatic cells regulates cyclic AMP and meiosis in the mouse oocyte. Development 136(11):1869-1878.

Nurse P. 1990. Universal control mechanism regulating onset of M-phase. Nature 344(6266):503-508.

Nutt LK, Margolis SS, Jensen M, Herman CE, Dunphy WG, Rathmell JC, Kornbluth S. 2005. Metabolic regulation of oocyte cell death through the CaMKII-mediated phosphorylation of caspase-2. Cell 123(1):89-103.

Nuttinck F, Charpigny G, Mermillod P, Loosfelt H, Meduri G, Freret S, Grimard B, Heyman Y. 2004. Expression of components of the insulin-like growth factor system and gonadotropin receptors in bovine cumulus-oocyte complexes during oocyte maturation. Domest Anim Endocrinol 27(2):179-195.

O'Neill FJ, Gillett J, Foltz KR. 2004. Distinct roles for multiple Src family kinases at fertilization. J Cell Sci 117(Pt 25):6227-6238.

O'Reilly AM, Ballew AC, Miyazawa B, Stocker H, Hafen E, Simon MA. 2006. Csk differentially regulates Src64 during distinct morphological events in Drosophila germ cells. Development 133(14):2627-2638.

Oh JS, Han SJ, Conti M. 2010. Wee1B, Myt1, and Cdc25 function in distinct compartments of the mouse oocyte to control meiotic resumption. J Cell Biol 188(2):199-207.

Okamoto K, Nakajo N, Sagata N. 2002. The existence of two distinct Wee1 isoforms in Xenopus: implications for the developmental regulation of the cell cycle. EMBO J 21(10):2472-2484.

Okamura Y, Myoumoto A, Manabe N, Tanaka N, Okamura H, Fukumoto M. 2001. Protein tyrosine kinase expression in the porcine ovary. Mol Hum Reprod 7(8):723-729.

Okumura E, Fukuhara T, Yoshida H, Hanada Si S, Kozutsumi R, Mori M, Tachibana K, Kishimoto T. 2002. Akt inhibits Myt1 in the signalling pathway that leads to meiotic G2/M-phase transition. Nat Cell Biol 4(2):111-116.

Olds JL, Favit A, Nelson T, Ascoli G, Gerstein A, Cameron M, Cameron L, Lester DS, Rakow T, De Barry J, et al. 1995. Imaging protein kinase C activation in living sea urchin eggs after fertilization. Dev Biol 172(2):675-682.

Ota R, Kotani T, Yamashita M. 2011a. Biochemical characterization of Pumilio1 and Pumilio2 in Xenopus oocytes. J Biol Chem 286(4):2853-2863.

Ota R, Kotani T, Yamashita M. 2011b. Possible involvement of Nemo-like kinase 1 in Xenopus oocyte maturation as a kinase responsible for Pumilio1, Pumilio2, and CPEB phosphorylation. Biochemistry 50(25):5648-5659.

Ou XH, Li S, Xu BZ, Wang ZB, Quan S, Li M, Zhang QH, Ouyang YC, Schatten H, Xing FQ, Sun QY. 2010. p38alpha MAPK is a MTOC-associated protein regulating spindle assembly, spindle length and accurate chromosome segregation during mouse oocyte meiotic maturation. Cell Cycle 9(20):4130-4143.

Pahlavan G, Polanski Z, Kalab P, Golsteyn R, Nigg EA, Maro B. 2000. Characterization of polo-like kinase 1 during meiotic maturation of the mouse oocyte. Dev Biol 220(2):392-400.

Palacios EH, Weiss A. 2004. Function of the Src-family kinases, Lck and Fyn, in T-cell development and activation. Oncogene 23(48):7990-8000.

Palmer A, Gavin AC, Nebreda AR. 1998. A link between MAP kinase and p34(cdc2)/cyclin B during oocyte maturation: p90(rsk) phosphorylates and inactivates the p34(cdc2) inhibitory kinase Myt1. EMBO J 17(17):5037-5047.

Pan J, Snell WJ. 2000. Signal transduction during fertilization in the unicellular green alga, Chlamydomonas. Curr Opin Microbiol 3(6):596-602.

Park M, Dean M, Cooper CS, Schmidt M, O'Brien SJ, Blair DG, Vande Woude GF. 1986. Mechanism of met oncogene activation. Cell 45(6):895-904.

Pascreau G, Delcros JG, Cremet JY, Prigent C, Arlot-Bonnemains Y. 2005. Phosphorylation of maskin by Aurora-A participates in the control of sequential protein synthesis during Xenopus laevis oocyte maturation. J Biol Chem 280(14):13415-13423.

Pascreau G, Delcros JG, Morin N, Prigent C, Arlot-Bonnemains Y. 2008. Aurora-A kinase Ser349 phosphorylation is required during Xenopus laevis oocyte maturation. Dev Biol 317(2):523-530.

Pascreau G, Eckerdt F, Lewellyn AL, Prigent C, Maller JL. 2009. Phosphorylation of p53 is regulated by TPX2-Aurora A in xenopus oocytes. J Biol Chem 284(9):5497-5505.

Pati D, Lohka MJ, Habibi HR. 2000. Time-related effect of GnRH on histone H1 kinase activity in the goldfish follicle-enclosed oocyte. Can J Physiol Pharmacol 78(12):1067-1071.

Pauken CM, Capco DG. 2000. The expression and stage-specific localization of protein kinase C isotypes during mouse preimplantation development. Dev Biol 223(2):411-421.

Pavlok A, Kalab P, Bobak P. 1997. Fertilisation competence of bovine normally matured or aged oocytes derived from different antral follicles: morphology, protein synthesis, H1 and MBP kinase activity. Zygote 5(3):235-246.

Pelech SL, Meijer L, Krebs EG. 1987. Characterization of maturation-activated histone H1 and ribosomal S6 kinases in sea star oocytes. Biochemistry 26(24):7960-7968.

Pelech SL, Tombes RM, Meijer L, Krebs EG. 1988. Activation of myelin basic protein kinases during echinoderm oocyte maturation and egg fertilization. Dev Biol 130(1):28-36.

Perdiguero E, Pillaire MJ, Bodart JF, Hennersdorf F, Frodin M, Duesbery NS, Alonso G, Nebreda AR. 2003. Xp38gamma/SAPK3 promotes meiotic G(2)/M transition in Xenopus oocytes and activates Cdc25C. EMBO J 22(21):5746-5756.

Perry AC, Verlhac MH. 2008. Second meiotic arrest and exit in frogs and mice. EMBO Rep 9(3):246-251.

Pesando D, Pesci-Bardon C, Huitorel P, Girard JP. 1999. Caulerpenyne blocks MBP kinase activation controlling mitosis in sea urchin eggs. Eur J Cell Biol 78(12):903-910.

Peter M, Labbe JC, Doree M, Mandart E. 2002. A new role for Mos in Xenopus oocyte maturation: targeting Myt1 independently of MAPK. Development 129(9):2129-2139.

Philipova R, Whitaker M. 1998. MAP kinase activity increases during mitosis in early sea urchin embryos. J Cell Sci 111 (Pt 17):2497-2505.

Pirino G, Wescott MP, Donovan PJ. 2009. Protein kinase A regulates resumption of meiosis by phosphorylation of Cdc25B in mammalian oocytes. Cell Cycle 8(4):665-670.

Pitetti JL, Torre D, Conne B, Papaioannou MD, Cederroth CR, Xuan S, Kahn R, Parada LF, Vassalli JD, Efstratiadis A, Nef S. 2009. Insulin receptor and IGF1R are not required for oocyte growth, differentiation, and maturation in mice. Sex Dev 3(5):264-272.

Potapova TA, Daum JR, Byrd KS, Gorbsky GJ. 2009. Fine tuning the cell cycle: activation of the Cdk1 inhibitory phosphorylation pathway during mitotic exit. Mol Biol Cell 20(6):1737-1748.

Qian YW, Erikson E, Taieb FE, Maller JL. 2001. The polo-like kinase Plx1 is required for activation of the phosphatase Cdc25C and cyclin B-Cdc2 in Xenopus oocytes. Mol Biol Cell 12(6):1791-1799.

Qu Y, Adler V, Chu T, Platica O, Michl J, Pestka S, Izotova L, Boutjdir M, Pincus MR. 2006. Two dual specificity kinases are preferentially induced by wild-type rather than by oncogenic RAS-P21 in Xenopus oocytes. Front Biosci 11:2420-2427.

Qu Y, Adler V, Izotova L, Pestka S, Bowne W, Michl J, Boutjdir M, Friedman FK, Pincus MR. 2007. The dual-specificity kinases, TOPK and DYRK1A, are critical for oocyte maturation induced by wild-type--but not by oncogenic--ras-p21 protein. Front Biosci 12:5089-5097.

Quadri SK. 2011. Cross talk between focal adhesion kinase and cadherins: Role in regulating endothelial barrier function. Microvasc Res.

Quan HM, Fan HY, Meng XQ, Huo LJ, Chen DY, Schatten H, Yang PM, Sun QY. 2003. Effects of PKC activation on the meiotic maturation, fertilization and early embryonic development of mouse oocytes. Zygote 11(4):329-337.

Rappolee DA, Patel Y, Jacobson K. 1998. Expression of fibroblast growth factor receptors in peri-implantation mouse embryos. Mol Reprod Dev 51(3):254-264.

Rauh NR, Schmidt A, Bormann J, Nigg EA, Mayer TU. 2005. Calcium triggers exit from meiosis II by targeting the APC/C inhibitor XErp1 for degradation. Nature 437(7061):1048-1052.

Reddy P, Shen L, Ren C, Boman K, Lundin E, Ottander U, Lindgren P, Liu YX, Sun QY, Liu K. 2005. Activation of Akt (PKB) and suppression of FKHRL1 in mouse and rat oocytes by stem cell factor during follicular activation and development. Dev Biol 281(2):160-170.

Rentzsch F, Hobmayer B, Holstein TW. 2005. Glycogen synthase kinase 3 has a proapoptotic function in Hydra gametogenesis. Dev Biol 278(1):1-12.

Resh MD. 1998. Fyn, a Src family tyrosine kinase. Int J Biochem Cell Biol 30(11):1159-1162.

Reut TM, Mattan L, Dafna T, Ruth KK, Ruth S. 2007. The role of Src family kinases in egg activation. Dev Biol 312(1):77-89.

Rice A, Parrington J, Jones KT, Swann K. 2000. Mammalian sperm contain a Ca(2+)-sensitive phospholipase C activity that can generate InsP(3) from PIP(2) associated with intracellular organelles. Dev Biol 228(1):125-135.

Rime H, Huchon D, De Smedt V, Thibier C, Galaktionov K, Jessus C, Ozon R. 1994. Microinjection of Cdc25 protein phosphatase into Xenopus prophase oocyte activates MPF and arrests meiosis at metaphase I. Biol Cell 82(1):11-22.

Rime H, Ozon R. 1990. Protein phosphatases are involved in the in vivo activation of histone H1 kinase in mouse oocyte. Dev Biol 141(1):115-122.

Robbie EP, Peterson M, Amaya E, Musci TJ. 1995. Temporal regulation of the Xenopus FGF receptor in development: a translation inhibitory element in the 3' untranslated region. Development 121(6):1775-1785.

Robison GA, Butcher RW, Sutherland EW. 1968. Cyclic AMP. Annu Rev Biochem 37:149-174.

Roelle S, Grosse R, Buech T, Chubanov V, Gudermann T. 2008. Essential role of Pyk2 and Src kinase activation in neuropeptide-induced proliferation of small cell lung cancer cells. Oncogene 27(12):1737-1748.

Rogers E, Bishop JD, Waddle JA, Schumacher JM, Lin R. 2002. The aurora kinase AIR-2 functions in the release of chromosome cohesion in Caenorhabditis elegans meiosis. J Cell Biol 157(2):219-229.

Rogers NT, Hobson E, Pickering S, Lai FA, Braude P, Swann K. 2004. Phospholipase Czeta causes Ca2+ oscillations and parthenogenetic activation of human oocytes. Reproduction 128(6):697-702.

Roghi C, Giet R, Uzbekov R, Morin N, Chartrain I, Le Guellec R, Couturier A, Doree M, Philippe M, Prigent C. 1998. The Xenopus protein kinase pEg2 associates with the centrosome in a cell cycle-dependent manner, binds to the spindle microtubules and is involved in bipolar mitotic spindle assembly. J Cell Sci 111 (Pt 5):557-572.

Rongish BJ, Kinsey WH. 2000. Transient nuclear localization of Fyn kinase during development in zebrafish. Anat Rec 260(2):115-123.

Ruiz EJ, Hunt T, Nebreda AR. 2008. Meiotic inactivation of Xenopus Myt1 by CDK/XRINGO, but not CDK/cyclin, via site-specific phosphorylation. Mol Cell 32(2):210-220.

Ruiz EJ, Vilar M, Nebreda AR. 2010. A two-step inactivation mechanism of Myt1 ensures CDK1/cyclin B activation and meiosis I entry. Curr Biol 20(8):717-723.

Runft LL, Carroll DJ, Gillett J, Giusti AF, O'Neill FJ, Foltz KR. 2004. Identification of a starfish egg PLC-gamma that regulates Ca2+ release at fertilization. Dev Biol 269(1):220-236.

Runft LL, Jaffe LA. 2000. Sperm extract injection into ascidian eggs signals Ca(2+) release by the same pathway as fertilization. Development 127(15):3227-3236.

Runft LL, Jaffe LA, Mehlmann LM. 2002. Egg activation at fertilization: where it all begins. Dev Biol 245(2):237-254.

Sackton KL, Buehner NA, Wolfner MF. 2007. Modulation of MAPK activities during egg activation in Drosophila. Fly (Austin) 1(4):222-227.

Sadler KC, Yuce O, Hamaratoglu F, Verge V, Peaucellier G, Picard A. 2004. MAP kinases regulate unfertilized egg apoptosis and fertilization suppresses death via Ca2+ signaling. Mol Reprod Dev 67(3):366-383.

Sadler SE, Angleson JK, Dsouza M. 2010. IGF-1 receptors in Xenopus laevis ovarian follicle cells support the oocyte maturation response. Biol Reprod 82(3):591-598.

Sakakibara K, Sato K, Yoshino K, Oshiro N, Hirahara S, Mahbub Hasan AK, Iwasaki T, Ueda Y, Iwao Y, Yonezawa K, Fukami Y. 2005. Molecular identification and characterization of Xenopus egg uroplakin III, an egg raft-associated transmembrane protein that is tyrosine-phosphorylated upon fertilization. J Biol Chem 280(15):15029-15037.

Sakamoto I, Takahara K, Yamashita M, Iwao Y. 1998. Changes in cyclin B during oocyte maturation and early embryonic cell cycle in the newt, Cynops pyrrhogaster: requirement of germinal vesicle for MPF activation. Dev Biol 195(1):60-69.

Sakuma M, Onodera H, Suyemitsu T, Yamasu K. 1997. The protein tyrosine kinases of the sea urchin Anthocidaris crassispina. Zoolog Sci 14(6):941-946.

Salas C, Julio-Pieper M, Valladares M, Pommer R, Vega M, Mastronardi C, Kerr B, Ojeda SR, Lara HE, Romero C. 2006. Nerve growth factor-dependent activation of trkA receptors in the human ovary results in synthesis of follicle-stimulating hormone receptors and estrogen secretion. J Clin Endocrinol Metab 91(6):2396-2403.

Sam MR, Elliott BE, Mueller CR. 2007. A novel activating role of SRC and STAT3 on HGF transcription in human breast cancer cells. Mol Cancer 6:69.

Sanghera JS, Charlton LA, Paddon HB, Pelech SL. 1992. Purification and characterization of echinoderm casein kinase II. Regulation by protein kinase C. Biochem J 283 (Pt 3):829-837.

Sanghera JS, Paddon HB, Bader SA, Pelech SL. 1990. Purification and characterization of a maturation-activated myelin basic protein kinase from sea star oocytes. J Biol Chem 265(1):52-57.

Sardon T, Peset I, Petrova B, Vernos I. 2008. Dissecting the role of Aurora A during spindle assembly. EMBO J 27(19):2567-2579.

Sasaki K, Chiba K. 2004. Induction of apoptosis in starfish eggs requires spontaneous inactivation of MAPK (extracellular signal-regulated kinase) followed by activation of p38MAPK. Mol Biol Cell 15(3):1387-1396.

Sato K, Aoto M, Mori K, Akasofu S, Tokmakov AA, Sahara S, Fukami Y. 1996. Purification and characterization of a Src-related p57 protein-tyrosine kinase from Xenopus oocytes. Isolation of an inactive form of the enzyme and its activation and translocation upon fertilization. J Biol Chem 271(22):13250-13257.

Sato K, Fukami Y, Stith BJ. 2006a. Signal transduction pathways leading to Ca2+ release in a vertebrate model system: lessons from Xenopus eggs. Semin Cell Dev Biol 17(2):285-292.

Sato K, Iwao Y, Fujimura T, Tamaki I, Ogawa K, Iwasaki T, Tokmakov AA, Hatano O, Fukami Y. 1999. Evidence for the involvement of a Src-related tyrosine kinase in Xenopus egg activation. Dev Biol 209(2):308-320.

Sato K, Iwasaki T, Hirahara S, Nishihira Y, Fukami Y. 2004. Molecular dissection of egg fertilization signaling with the aid of tyrosine kinase-specific inhibitor and activator strategies. Biochim Biophys Acta 1697(1-2):103-121.

Sato K, Iwasaki T, Ogawa K, Konishi M, Tokmakov AA, Fukami Y. 2002. Low density detergent-insoluble membrane of Xenopus eggs: subcellular microdomain for tyrosine kinase signaling in fertilization. Development 129(4):885-896.

Sato K, Ogawa K, Tokmakov AA, Iwasaki T, Fukami Y. 2001. Hydrogen peroxide induces Src family tyrosine kinase-dependent activation of Xenopus eggs. Dev Growth Differ 43(1):55-72.

Sato K, Tokmakov AA, He CL, Kurokawa M, Iwasaki T, Shirouzu M, Fissore RA, Yokoyama S, Fukami Y. 2003. Reconstitution of Src-dependent phospholipase Cgamma phosphorylation and transient calcium release by using membrane rafts and cell-free extracts from Xenopus eggs. J Biol Chem 278(40):38413-38420.

Sato K, Tokmakov AA, Iwasaki T, Fukami Y. 2000. Tyrosine kinase-dependent activation of phospholipase Cgamma is required for calcium transient in Xenopus egg fertilization. Dev Biol 224(2):453-469.

Sato K, Yoshino K, Tokmakov AA, Iwasaki T, Yonezawa K, Fukami Y. 2006b. Studying fertilization in cell-free extracts: focusing on membrane/lipid raft functions and proteomics. Methods Mol Biol 322:395-411.

Saunders CM, Larman MG, Parrington J, Cox LJ, Royse J, Blayney LM, Swann K, Lai FA. 2002. PLC zeta: a sperm-specific trigger of Ca(2+) oscillations in eggs and embryo development. Development 129(15):3533-3544.

Schindler T, Bornmann W, Pellicena P, Miller WT, Clarkson B, Kuriyan J. 2000. Structural mechanism for STI-571 inhibition of abelson tyrosine kinase. Science 289(5486):1938-1942.

Schmitt A, Nebreda AR. 2002b. Inhibition of Xenopus oocyte meiotic maturation by catalytically inactive protein kinase A. Proc Natl Acad Sci U S A 99(7):4361-4366.

Schmidt A, Rauh NR, Nigg EA, Mayer TU. 2006. Cytostatic factor: an activity that puts the cell cycle on hold. J Cell Sci 119(Pt 7):1213-1218.

Schmitt A, Nebreda AR. 2002a. Signalling pathways in oocyte meiotic maturation. J Cell Sci 115(Pt 12):2457-2459.

Schober CS, Aydiner F, Booth CJ, Seli E, Reinke V. 2011. The kinase VRK1 is required for normal meiotic progression in mammalian oogenesis. Mech Dev 128(3-4):178-190.

Schultz RM, Kopf GS. 1995. Molecular basis of mammalian egg activation. Curr Top Dev Biol 30:21-62.

Schwab MS, Kim SH, Terada N, Edfjall C, Kozma SC, Thomas G, Maller JL. 1999. p70(S6K) controls selective mRNA translation during oocyte maturation and early embryogenesis in Xenopus laevis. Mol Cell Biol 19(4):2485-2494.

Schwartz Y, Ben-Dor I, Navon A, Motro B, Nir U. 1998. Tyrosine phosphorylation of the TATA element modulatory factor by the FER nuclear tyrosine kinases. FEBS Lett 434(3):339-345.

Segawa Y, Suga H, Iwabe N, Oneyama C, Akagi T, Miyata T, Okada M. 2006. Functional development of Src tyrosine kinases during evolution from a unicellular ancestor to multicellular animals. Proc Natl Acad Sci U S A 103(32):12021-12026.

Sehgal A, Wall DA, Chao MV. 1988. Efficient processing and expression of human nerve growth factor receptors in Xenopus laevis oocytes: effects on maturation. Mol Cell Biol 8(5):2242-2246.

Sette C, Dolci S, Geremia R, Rossi P. 2000. The role of stem cell factor and of alternative c-kit gene products in the establishment, maintenance and function of germ cells. Int J Dev Biol 44(6):599-608.

Sette C, Paronetto MP, Barchi M, Bevilacqua A, Geremia R, Rossi P. 2002. Tr-kit-induced resumption of the cell cycle in mouse eggs requires activation of a Src-like kinase. EMBO J 21(20):5386-5395.

Sharma D, Kinsey WH. 2006. Fertilization triggers localized activation of Src-family protein kinases in the zebrafish egg. Dev Biol 295(2):604-614.

Sharma D, Kinsey WH. 2008. Regionalized calcium signaling in zebrafish fertilization. Int J Dev Biol 52(5-6):561-570.

Shen SS, Buck WR. 1990. A synthetic peptide of the pseudosubstrate domain of protein kinase C blocks cytoplasmic alkalinization during activation of the sea urchin egg. Dev Biol 140(2):272-280.

Shen SS, Kinsey WH, Lee SJ. 1999. Protein tyrosine kinase-dependent release of intracellular calcium in the sea urchin egg. Dev Growth Differ 41(3):345-355.

Sherr CJ, Roussel MF, Rettenmier CW. 1988. Colony-stimulating factor-1 receptor (c-fms). J Cell Biochem 38(3):179-187.

Shibuya EK, Boulton TG, Cobb MH, Ruderman JV. 1992. Activation of p42 MAP kinase and the release of oocytes from cell cycle arrest. EMBO J 11(11):3963-3975.

Shibuya EK, Morris J, Rapp UR, Ruderman JV. 1996. Activation of the Xenopus oocyte mitogen-activated protein kinase pathway by Mos is independent of Raf. Cell Growth Differ 7(2):235-241.

Shibuya M. 1995. Role of VEGF-flt receptor system in normal and tumor angiogenesis. Adv Cancer Res 67:281-316.

Shilling FM, Carroll DJ, Muslin AJ, Escobedo JA, Williams LT, Jaffe LA. 1994. Evidence for both tyrosine kinase and G-protein-coupled pathways leading to starfish egg activation. Dev Biol 162(2):590-599.

Shirahata S, Rawson C, Loo D, Chang YJ, Barnes D. 1990. ras and neu oncogenes reverse serum inhibition and epidermal growth factor dependence of serum-free mouse embryo cells. J Cell Physiol 144(1):69-76.

Shoji S, Yoshida N, Amanai M, Ohgishi M, Fukui T, Fujimoto S, Nakano Y, Kajikawa E, Perry AC. 2006. Mammalian Emi2 mediates cytostatic arrest and transduces the signal for meiotic exit via Cdc20. EMBO J 25(4):834-845.

Silva AJ, Paylor R, Wehner JM, Tonegawa S. 1992a. Impaired spatial learning in alpha-calcium-calmodulin kinase II mutant mice. Science 257(5067):206-211.

Silva AJ, Stevens CF, Tonegawa S, Wang Y. 1992b. Deficient hippocampal long-term potentiation in alpha-calcium-calmodulin kinase II mutant mice. Science 257(5067):201-206.

Sirard MA. 2001. Resumption of meiosis: mechanism involved in meiotic progression and its relation with developmental competence. Theriogenology 55(6):1241-1254.

Sirard MA, Bilodeau S. 1990a. Effects of granulosa cell co-culture on in-vitro meiotic resumption of bovine oocytes. J Reprod Fertil 89(2):459-465.

Sirard MA, Bilodeau S. 1990b. Granulosa cells inhibit the resumption of meiosis in bovine oocytes in vitro. Biol Reprod 43(5):777-783.

Solc P, Schultz RM, Motlik J. 2010. Prophase I arrest and progression to metaphase I in mouse oocytes: comparison of resumption of meiosis and recovery from G2-arrest in somatic cells. Mol Hum Reprod 16(9):654-664.

Stanford JS, Ruderman JV. 2005. Changes in regulatory phosphorylation of Cdc25C Ser287 and Wee1 Ser549 during normal cell cycle progression and checkpoint arrests. Mol Biol Cell 16(12):5749-5760.

Steele RE. 1985. Two divergent cellular src genes are expressed in Xenopus laevis. Nucleic Acids Res 13(5):1747-1761.

Steele RE, Deng JC, Ghosn CR, Fero JB. 1990. Structure and expression of fyn genes in Xenopus laevis. Oncogene 5(3):369-376.

Steele RE, Irwin MY, Knudsen CL, Collett JW, Fero JB. 1989a. The yes proto-oncogene is present in amphibians and contributes to the maternal RNA pool in the oocyte. Oncogene Res 4(3):223-233.

Steele RE, Unger TF, Mardis MJ, Fero JB. 1989b. The two Xenopus laevis SRC genes are co-expressed and each produces functional pp60src. J Biol Chem 264(18):10649-10653.

Steinhardt RA, Epel D. 1974. Activation of sea-urchin eggs by a calcium ionophore. Proc Natl Acad Sci U S A 71(5):1915-1919.

Stitzel ML, Cheng KC, Seydoux G. 2007. Regulation of MBK-2/Dyrk kinase by dynamic cortical anchoring during the oocyte-to-zygote transition. Curr Biol 17(18):1545-1554.

Stitzel ML, Pellettieri J, Seydoux G. 2006. The C. elegans DYRK Kinase MBK-2 Marks Oocyte Proteins for Degradation in Response to Meiotic Maturation. Curr Biol 16(1):56-62.

Stricker SA. 1999. Comparative biology of calcium signaling during fertilization and egg activation in animals. Dev Biol 211(2):157-176.

Stricker SA. 2009. Interactions between mitogen-activated protein kinase and protein kinase C signaling during oocyte maturation and fertilization in a marine worm. Mol Reprod Dev 76(8):708-721.

Stricker SA. 2011. Potential upstream regulators and downstream targets of AMP-activated kinase signaling during oocyte maturation in a marine worm. Reproduction 142(1):29-39.

Stricker SA, Carroll DJ, Tsui WL. 2010a. Roles of Src family kinase signaling during fertilization and the first cell cycle in the marine protostome worm Cerebratulus. Int J Dev Biol 54(5):787-793.

Stricker SA, Smythe TL. 2006. Differing mechanisms of cAMP- versus seawater-induced oocyte maturation in marine nemertean worms I. The roles of serine/threonine kinases and phosphatases. Mol Reprod Dev 73(12):1578-1590.

Stricker SA, Swiderek L, Nguyen T. 2010b. Stimulators of AMP-activated kinase (AMPK) inhibit seawater- but not cAMP-induced oocyte maturation in a marine worm: Implications for interactions between cAMP and AMPK signaling. Mol Reprod Dev 77(6):497-510.

Sugiura K, Naito K, Iwamori N, Kagii H, Goto S, Ohashi S, Naruoka H, Yada E, Yamanouchi K, Tojo H. 2002. Activation of ribosomal S6 kinase (RSK) during porcine oocyte maturation. Zygote 10(1):31-36.

Sumara I, Vorlaufer E, Stukenberg PT, Kelm O, Redemann N, Nigg EA, Peters JM. 2002. The dissociation of cohesin from chromosomes in prophase is regulated by Polo-like kinase. Mol Cell 9(3):515-525.

Sun CK, Ng KT, Lim ZX, Cheng Q, Lo CM, Poon RT, Man K, Wong N, Fan ST. 2011. Proline-rich tyrosine kinase 2 (Pyk2) promotes cell motility of hepatocellular carcinoma through induction of epithelial to mesenchymal transition. PLoS One 6(4):e18878.

Sun CK, Ng KT, Sun BS, Ho JW, Lee TK, Ng I, Poon RT, Lo CM, Liu CL, Man K, Fan ST. 2007. The significance of proline-rich tyrosine kinase2 (Pyk2) on hepatocellular carcinoma progression and recurrence. Br J Cancer 97(1):50-57.

Sun QY, Rubinstein S, Breitbart H. 1999. MAP kinase activity is downregulated by phorbol ester during mouse oocyte maturation and egg activation in vitro. Mol Reprod Dev 52(3):310-318.

Sun QY, Miao YL, Schatten H. 2009. Towards a new understanding on the regulation of mammalian oocyte meiosis resumption. Cell Cycle 8(17):2741-2747.

Swann K, Igusa Y, Miyazaki S. 1989. Evidence for an inhibitory effect of protein kinase C on G-protein-mediated repetitive calcium transients in hamster eggs. EMBO J 8(12):3711-3718.

Swann K, Saunders CM, Rogers NT, Lai FA. 2006. PLCzeta(zeta): a sperm protein that triggers Ca2+ oscillations and egg activation in mammals. Semin Cell Dev Biol 17(2):264-273.

Taghon MS, Sadler SE. 1994. Insulin-like growth factor 1 receptor-mediated endocytosis in Xenopus laevis oocytes. A role for receptor tyrosine kinase activity. Dev Biol 163(1):66-74.

Talmor A, Kinsey WH, Shalgi R. 1998. Expression and immunolocalization of p59c-fyn tyrosine kinase in rat eggs. Dev Biol 194(1):38-46.

Talmor-Cohen A, Tomashov-Matar R, Eliyahu E, Shapiro R, Shalgi R. 2004a. Are Src family kinases involved in cell cycle resumption in rat eggs? Reproduction 127(4):455-463.

Talmor-Cohen A, Tomashov-Matar R, Tsai WB, Kinsey WH, Shalgi R. 2004b. Fyn kinase-tubulin interaction during meiosis of rat eggs. Reproduction 128(4):387-393.

Tang W, Wu JQ, Guo Y, Hansen DV, Perry JA, Freel CD, Nutt L, Jackson PK, Kornbluth S. 2008. Cdc2 and Mos regulate Emi2 stability to promote the meiosis I-meiosis II transition. Mol Biol Cell 19(8):3536-3543.

Tatone C, Delle Monache S, Francione A, Gioia L, Barboni B, Colonna R. 2003. Ca2+-independent protein kinase C signalling in mouse eggs during the early phases of fertilization. Int J Dev Biol 47(5):327-333.

Thomas SM, Brugge JS. 1997. Cellular functions regulated by Src family kinases. Annu Rev Cell Dev Biol 13:513-609.

Thorpe CJ, Moon RT. 2004. nemo-like kinase is an essential co-activator of Wnt signaling during early zebrafish development. Development 131(12):2899-2909.

Toker A, Newton AC. 2000. Cellular signaling: pivoting around PDK-1. Cell 103(2):185-188.

Tokmakov A, Iwasaki T, Itakura S, Sato K, Shirouzu M, Fukami Y, Yokoyama S. 2005. Regulation of Src kinase activity during Xenopus oocyte maturation. Dev Biol 278(2):289-300.

Tokmakov AA, Sato KI, Iwasaki T, Fukami Y. 2002. Src kinase induces calcium release in Xenopus egg extracts via PLCgamma and IP3-dependent mechanism. Cell Calcium 32(1):11-20.

Tomashov-Matar R, Levi M, Shalgi R. 2008. The involvement of Src family kinases (SFKs) in the events leading to resumption of meiosis. Mol Cell Endocrinol 282(1-2):56-62.

Tomek W, Smiljakovic T. 2005. Activation of Akt (protein kinase B) stimulates metaphase I to metaphase II transition in bovine oocytes. Reproduction 130(4):423-430.

Tong C, Fan HY, Lian L, Li SW, Chen DY, Schatten H, Sun QY. 2002. Polo-like kinase-1 is a pivotal regulator of microtubule assembly during mouse oocyte meiotic maturation, fertilization, and early embryonic mitosis. Biol Reprod 67(2):546-554.

Tonou-Fujimori N, Takahashi M, Onodera H, Kikuta H, Koshida S, Takeda H, Yamasu K. 2002. Expression of the FGF receptor 2 gene (fgfr2) during embryogenesis in the zebrafish Danio rerio. Mech Dev 119 Suppl 1:S173-178.

Tornell J, Billig H, Hillensjo T. 1991. Regulation of oocyte maturation by changes in ovarian levels of cyclic nucleotides. Hum Reprod 6(3):411-422.

Tosca L, Uzbekova S, Chabrolle C, Dupont J. 2007. Possible role of 5'AMP-activated protein kinase in the metformin-mediated arrest of bovine oocytes at the germinal vesicle stage during in vitro maturation. Biol Reprod 77(3):452-465.

Tosuji H, Fusetani N, Seki Y. 2003. Calyculin A causes the activation of histone H1 kinase and condensation of chromosomes in unfertilized sea urchin eggs independently of the maturation-promoting factor. Comp Biochem Physiol C Toxicol Pharmacol 135(4):415-424.

Townley IK, Roux MM, Foltz KR. 2006. Signal transduction at fertilization: the Ca2+ release pathway in echinoderms and other invertebrate deuterostomes. Semin Cell Dev Biol 17(2):293-302.

Townley IK, Schuyler E, Parker-Gur M, Foltz KR. 2009. Expression of multiple Src family kinases in sea urchin eggs and their function in Ca2+ release at fertilization. Dev Biol 327(2):465-477.

Trepanier CH, Jackson MF, Macdonald JF. 2011. Regulation of NMDA receptors by the tyrosine kinase Fyn. FEBS J.

Tripathi A, Kumar KV, Chaube SK. 2010. Meiotic cell cycle arrest in mammalian oocytes. J Cell Physiol 223(3):592-600.

Trounson A, Anderiesz C, Jones G. 2001. Maturation of human oocytes in vitro and their developmental competence. Reproduction 121(1):51-75.

Truong LD, Shen SS. 2011. Immunohistochemical diagnosis of renal neoplasms. Arch Pathol Lab Med 135(1):92-109.

Tsafriri A, Chun SY, Zhang R, Hsueh AJ, Conti M. 1996. Oocyte maturation involves compartmentalization and opposing changes of cAMP levels in follicular somatic and germ cells: studies using selective phosphodiesterase inhibitors. Dev Biol 178(2):393-402.

Tsai WB, Zhang X, Sharma D, Wu W, Kinsey WH. 2005. Role of Yes kinase during early zebrafish development. Dev Biol 277(1):129-141.

Uzbekova S, Salhab M, Perreau C, Mermillod P, Dupont J. 2009. Glycogen synthase kinase 3B in bovine oocytes and granulosa cells: possible involvement in meiosis during in vitro maturation. Reproduction 138(2):235-246.

Vaccari S, Horner K, Mehlmann LM, Conti M. 2008. Generation of mouse oocytes defective in cAMP synthesis and degradation: endogenous cyclic AMP is essential for meiotic arrest. Dev Biol 316(1):124-134.

Valbuena A, Sanz-Garcia M, Lopez-Sanchez I, Vega FM, Lazo PA. 2011. Roles of VRK1 as a new player in the control of biological processes required for cell division. Cell Signal 23(8):1267-1272.

Vigneron S, Brioudes E, Burgess A, Labbe JC, Lorca T, Castro A. 2009. Greatwall maintains mitosis through regulation of PP2A. EMBO J 28(18):2786-2793.

Villa-Diaz LG, Miyano T. 2004. Activation of p38 MAPK during porcine oocyte maturation. Biol Reprod 71(2):691-696.

Vincent C, Cheek TR, Johnson MH. 1992. Cell cycle progression of parthenogenetically activated mouse oocytes to interphase is dependent on the level of internal calcium. J Cell Sci 103 (Pt 2):389-396.

Viveiros MM, O'Brien M, Eppig JJ. 2004. Protein kinase C activity regulates the onset of anaphase I in mouse oocytes. Biol Reprod 71(5):1525-1532.

Viveiros MM, O'Brien M, Wigglesworth K, Eppig JJ. 2003. Characterization of protein kinase C-delta in mouse oocytes throughout meiotic maturation and following egg activation. Biol Reprod 69(5):1494-1499.

Walker G, Burgess D, Kinsey WH. 1996. Fertilization promotes selective association of the Abl [correction of AbI] kinase with the egg cytoskeleton. Eur J Cell Biol 70(2):165-171.

Walter SA, Guadagno SN, Ferrell JE, Jr. 2000. Activation of Wee1 by p42 MAPK in vitro and in cycling xenopus egg extracts. Mol Biol Cell 11(3):887-896.

Wang JY, Prywes R, Baltimore D. 1983. Structure and function of the Abelson murine leukemia virus transforming gene. Prog Clin Biol Res 119:57-63.

Wang Q, Snell WJ. 2003. Flagellar adhesion between mating type plus and mating type minus gametes activates a flagellar protein-tyrosine kinase during fertilization in Chlamydomonas. J Biol Chem 278(35):32936-32942.

Wassmann K, Niault T, Maro B. 2003. Metaphase I arrest upon activation of the Mad2-dependent spindle checkpoint in mouse oocytes. Curr Biol 13(18):1596-1608.

Westmark CJ, Ghose R, Huber PW. 2002. Phosphorylation of Xenopus transcription factor IIIA by an oocyte protein kinase CK2. Biochem J 362(Pt 2):375-382.

Wessel GM, Brooks JM, Green E, Haley S, Voronina E, Wong J, Zaydfudim V, Conner S. 2001. The biology of cortical granules. Int Rev Cytol 209:117-206.

Wessel GM, Wong JL. 2009. Cell surface changes in the egg at fertilization. Mol Reprod Dev 76(10):942-953.

Whitaker M. 2006. Calcium at fertilization and in early development. Physiol Rev 86(1):25-88.

Wianny F, Tavares A, Evans MJ, Glover DM, Zernicka-Goetz M. 1998. Mouse polo-like kinase 1 associates with the acentriolar spindle poles, meiotic chromosomes and spindle midzone during oocyte maturation. Chromosoma 107(6-7):430-439.

Wojcik EJ, Sharifpoor S, Miller NA, Wright TG, Watering R, Tremblay EA, Swan K, Mueller CR, Elliott BE. 2006. A novel activating function of c-Src and Stat3 on HGF transcription in mammary carcinoma cells. Oncogene 25(19):2773-2784.

Wu JQ, Hansen DV, Guo Y, Wang MZ, Tang W, Freel CD, Tung JJ, Jackson PK, Kornbluth S. 2007a. Control of Emi2 activity and stability through Mos-mediated recruitment of PP2A. Proc Natl Acad Sci U S A 104(42):16564-16569.

Wu JQ, Kornbluth S. 2008. Across the meiotic divide - CSF activity in the post-Emi2/XErp1 era. J Cell Sci 121(Pt 21):3509-3514.

Wu Q, Guo Y, Yamada A, Perry JA, Wang MZ, Araki M, Freel CD, Tung JJ, Tang W, Margolis SS, Jackson PK, Yamano H, Asano M, Kornbluth S. 2007b. A role for Cdc2- and PP2A-mediated regulation of Emi2 in the maintenance of CSF arrest. Curr Biol 17(3):213-224.

Wu W, Kinsey WH. 2000. Fertilization triggers activation of Fyn kinase in the zebrafish egg. Int J Dev Biol 44(8):837-841.

Wu W, Kinsey WH. 2002. Role of PTPase(s) in regulating Fyn kinase at fertilization of the zebrafish egg. Dev Biol 247(2):286-294.

Wu W, Kinsey WH. 2004. Detection and measurement of membrane-bound protein tyrosine kinases in the zebrafish egg. Methods Mol Biol 253:273-283.

Wu XR, Kong XP, Pellicer A, Kreibich G, Sun TT. 2009. Uroplakins in urothelial biology, function, and disease. Kidney Int 75(11):1153-1165.

Wu XR, Lin JH, Walz T, Haner M, Yu J, Aebi U, Sun TT. 1994. Mammalian uroplakins. A group of highly conserved urothelial differentiation-related membrane proteins. J Biol Chem 269(18):13716-13724.

Wu XR, Manabe M, Yu J, Sun TT. 1990. Large scale purification and immunolocalization of bovine uroplakins I, II, and III. Molecular markers of urothelial differentiation. J Biol Chem 265(31):19170-19179.

Xie Z, Sanada K, Samuels BA, Shih H, Tsai LH. 2003. Serine 732 phosphorylation of FAK by Cdk5 is important for microtubule organization, nuclear movement, and neuronal migration. Cell 114(4):469-482.

Xiong B, Sun SC, Lin SL, Li M, Xu BZ, OuYang YC, Hou Y, Chen DY, Sun QY. 2008. Involvement of Polo-like kinase 1 in MEK1/2-regulated spindle formation during mouse oocyte meiosis. Cell Cycle 7(12):1804-1809.

Xu X, Sun TT, Gupta PK, Zhang P, Nasuti JF. 2001. Uroplakin as a marker for typing metastatic transitional cell carcinoma on fine-needle aspiration specimens. Cancer 93(3):216-221.

Yamamoto TM, Blake-Hodek K, Williams BC, Lewellyn AL, Goldberg ML, Maller JL. 2011. Regulation of Greatwall kinase during Xenopus oocyte maturation. Mol Biol Cell 22(13):2157-2164.

Yamashita M, Fukada S, Yoshikuni M, Bulet P, Hirai T, Yamaguchi A, Yasuda H, Ohba Y, Nagahama Y. 1992. M-phase-specific histone H1 kinase in fish oocytes. Purification, components and biochemical properties. Eur J Biochem 205(2):537-543.

Yang D, Hinton SD, Eckberg WR. 2004. Regulation of cleavage by protein kinase C in Chaetopterus. Mol Reprod Dev 69(3):308-315.

Yang KT, Li SK, Chang CC, Tang CJ, Lin YN, Lee SC, Tang TK. 2010b. Aurora-C kinase deficiency causes cytokinesis failure in meiosis I and production of large polyploid oocytes in mice. Mol Biol Cell 21(14):2371-2383.

Yao LJ, Fan HY, Tong C, Chen DY, Schatten H, Sun QY. 2003. Polo-like kinase-1 in porcine oocyte meiotic maturation, fertilization and early embryonic mitosis. Cell Mol Biol (Noisy-le-grand) 49(3):399-405.

Yim DL, Opresko LK, Wiley HS, Nuccitelli R. 1994. Highly polarized EGF receptor tyrosine kinase activity initiates egg activation in Xenopus. Dev Biol 162(1):41-55.

Yu B, Wang Y, Liu Y, Li X, Wu D, Zong Z, Zhang J, Yu D. 2005. Protein kinase A regulates cell cycle progression of mouse fertilized eggs by means of MPF. Dev Dyn 232(1):98-105.

Yu BZ, Zheng J, Yu AM, Shi XY, Liu Y, Wu DD, Fu W, Yang J. 2004. Effects of protein kinase C on M-phase promoting factor in early development of fertilized mouse eggs. Cell Biochem Funct 22(5):291-298.

Yu Y, Halet G, Lai FA, Swann K. 2008. Regulation of diacylglycerol production and protein kinase C stimulation during sperm- and PLCzeta-mediated mouse egg activation. Biol Cell 100(11):633-643.

Zernicka-Goetz M. 1991. Spontaneous and induced activation of rat oocytes. Mol Reprod Dev 28(2):169-176.

Zhang K, Hansen PJ, Ealy AD. 2010a. Fibroblast growth factor 10 enhances bovine oocyte maturation and developmental competence in vitro. Reproduction 140(6):815-826.

Zhang L, Liang Y, Liu Y, Xiong CL. 2010b. The role of brain-derived neurotrophic factor in mouse oocyte maturation in vitro involves activation of protein kinase B. Theriogenology 73(8):1096-1103.

Zhang WL, Huitorel P, Geneviere AM, Chiri S, Ciapa B. 2006. Inactivation of MAPK in mature oocytes triggers progression into mitosis via a Ca2+ -dependent pathway but without completion of S phase. J Cell Sci 119(Pt 17):3491-3501.

Zhang M, Ouyang H, Xia G. 2009. The signal pathway of gonadotrophins-induced mammalian oocyte meiotic resumption. Mol Hum Reprod 15(7):399-409.

Zhang X, Wright CV, Hanks SK. 1995. Cloning of a Xenopus laevis cDNA encoding focal adhesion kinase (FAK) and expression during early development. Gene 160(2):219-222.

Zhang Y, Luo Y, Emmett K, Snell WJ. 1996. Cell adhesion-dependent inactivation of a soluble protein kinase during fertilization in Chlamydomonas. Mol Biol Cell 7(4):515-527.

Zhang Y, Zhang Z, Xu XY, Li XS, Yu M, Yu AM, Zong ZH, Yu BZ. 2008. Protein kinase A modulates Cdc25B activity during meiotic resumption of mouse oocytes. Dev Dyn 237(12):3777-3786.

Zhao J, Taverne MA, Van Der Weijden GC, Bevers MM, Van Den Hurk R. 2001. Insulin-like growth factor-I (IGF-I) stimulates the development of cultured rat pre-antral follicles. Mol Reprod Dev 58(3):287-296.

Zhao Y, Haccard O, Wang R, Yu J, Kuang J, Jessus C, Goldberg ML. 2008. Roles of Greatwall kinase in the regulation of cdc25 phosphatase. Mol Biol Cell 19(4):1317-1327.

Zhong W, Sun T, Wang QT, Wang Y, Xie Y, Johnson A, Leach R, Puscheck EE, Rappolee DA. 2004. SAPKgamma/JNK1 and SAPKalpha/JNK2 mRNA transcripts are expressed in early gestation human placenta and mouse eggs, preimplantation embryos, and trophoblast stem cells. Fertil Steril 82 Suppl 3:1140-1148.

Zhou RP, Oskarsson M, Paules RS, Schulz N, Cleveland D, Vande Woude GF. 1991. Ability of the c-mos product to associate with and phosphorylate tubulin. Science 251(4994):671-675.

22

Phospho-Signaling at Oocyte Maturation and Fertilization: Set Up for Embryogenesis and Beyond Part II. Kinase Regulators and Substrates

A.K.M. Mahbub Hasan[1], Takashi Matsumoto[2],
Shigeru Kihira[2], Junpei Yoshida[2] and Ken-ichi Sato[2,*]
[1]Laboratory of Gene Biology, Department of Biochemistry and Molecular Biology, University of Dhaka, Dhaka,
[2]Laboratory of Cell Signaling and Development, Department of Molecular Biosciences, Faculty of Life Sciences, Kyoto Sangyo University, Kamigamo-Motoyama, Kita-ku, Kyoto
[1]Bangladesh
[2]Japan

1. Introduction

This chapter is the sequel to the chapter entitled "Phospho-signaling at Oocyte Maturation and Fertilization: Set Up for Embryogenesis and Beyond Part I. Protein Kinases" by Mahbub Hasan et al.

2. Kinase regulators and substrates in oocyte maturation, fertilization and activation of development

2.1 Actin

Filamentous actin or **F-actin** is a major component of stress fibers and involved in cellular architecture. Its dynamic rearrangement supports not only cellular morphology but also intracellular signal transduction that regulate cell-cell or cell-extracellular matrix interactions, cell motility, and proliferation. Several lines of evidence demonstrate that, in several organisms, oocyte cortical cytoskeleton involving F-actin network undergoes a dynamic rearrangement during meiosis/oocyte maturation and that this is often involving phosphorylation of actin and/or actin-interacting proteins (e.g. ADF/coffilin, see below) catalyzed by PKC (in Tubifex, *Xenopus*) (Capco et al. 1992; Shimizu 1997). In *Drosophila*, PKC phosphorylation of a tumor suppressor protein-homolog named Lgl (lethal (2) giant larvae) is responsible for actin-dependent oocyte polarity formation (Tian and Deng 2008). In mammalian oocytes (rat), F-actin has been implicated in tyrosine kinase-dependent

* Corresponding Author

rearrangement of cortical structures (Meng et al. 2006). In unfertilized rat eggs, F-action is in association with PKC and RACKS and thought to suppress the cortical granule to exocytose, and after fertilization, PKC-dependent phosphorylation releases the actin suppression and cortical granule exocytosis occurs (Eliyahu et al. 2005).

2.2 ADF/coffilin

Actin-depolymerizing factor (**ADF**)/**coffilin** are an evolutionarily conserved F-actin-binding protein, whose function is essential for cortical actin cytoskeleton. It is well known that the actin-binding ability of ADF/coffilin can be regulated by its phosphorylation and dephosphorylation (Bamburg et al. 1999). This type of regulation of ADF/coffilin has been reported in maturing oocytes of starfish, where active transport of MPF from nucleus to cytoplasm is required for oocyte maturation (Santella et al. 2003), and dividing embryos of *Xenopus*, where cytokinesis involves the function of ADF/coffilin (Abe et al. 1996; Chiu et al. 2010; Tanaka et al. 2005). In the former case, MPF has been identified as a kinase for ADF/coffilin. In the latter case, protein phosphatase Slingshot is involved in Rho-dependent inactivation of ADF/coffilin, thereby promotes the rearrangement of actin cytoskeleton essential for cytokinesis.

2.3 ASIP/PAR-3

ASIP/PAR-3 (atypical PKC isotype-specific interacting protein/partitioning defective 3) is a PDZ-domain-containing adaptor protein that has been initially identified as a downstream element of PAR-6 in early embryos of the nematode *C. elegans* (Watts et al. 1996). Further studies have demonstrate the importance of PAR3 as an atypical PKC (aPKC)-interacting protein functioning in establishing asymmetric cell division and polarized cell structures in *C. elegans* and *Drosophila* embryos, and mammalian epithelial cells (Joberty et al. 2000). In *Xenopus* immature oocytes, ASIP/PAR-3 is shown to localize to animal hemisphere in association with aPKC, and upon hormone-induced oocyte maturation, aPKC undergoes kinase activity-dependent re-localization. These results suggest a potential role of ASIP/PAR-3 as a regulator and/or substrate of aPKC (Nakaya et al. 2000). Although phosphorylation of Ser-827 in ASIP/PAR-3 by aPKC has been shown in mammalian somatic cell systems (Hirose et al. 2002), its occurrence in oocyte/egg system is not yet demonstrated.

2.4 Astrin

Astrin is a spindle-associated non-motor protein that regulates mitotic cell cycle progression. In the meiosis of mouse oocytes, where centrioles are missing but multiple microtubule-organizing centers (MTOCs) are present, proper lining and segregation of homologous chromosomes and sister chromatids require the precise regulation of MTOCs by centrosomal protein kinases such as Aurora kinase and PLK1. It has been shown that inhibition of Astrin function by RNAi-mediated knockdown or overexpression of a coiled-coil domain of Astrin results in a defect in spindle disorganization, chromosome misalignment and meiosis progression arrest (Yuan et al. 2009). As Astrin localizes to the spindle apparatus, it is suggested that Astrin is a substrate of Aurora/PLK1. In support with this idea, site-directed mutation of Thr-24, Ser-66 or Ser-447, potential PLK1 phosphorylation sites in Astrin, causes oocyte meiotic arrest at metaphase I with highly disordered spindles and disorganized chromosomes (Yuan et al. 2009).

2.5 Bad

Bad is a member of BH3 (Bcl-2 homology 3) family proteins, the other members of which include Bax, Bak, Bik, Bid and Hrk. While Bcl-2, a firstly identified BH3 and other BH domain (BH1 and BH2)-containing protein, and its relative proteins (e.g. Bcl-xL) act as anti-apoptosis components, Bad and other BH3-only proteins participate in pro-apoptotic cellular functions (e.g. activation of caspases) (Danial 2008; Lutz 2000). Most of these anti-apoptotic or pro-apoptotic proteins localize to mitochondrial outer membranes and function as a sensor of intracellular damage as well as a trigger of mitochondrial death/survival pathway. Several species ranging from nematode, *Drosophila* and sea invertebrates to vertebrates including mammals undergo germline or ovarian/postovulatory oocyte apoptosis in an age-dependent or -independent manner (Buszczak and Cooley 2000; Chiba 2004; Morita and Tilly 1999). In particular, Bad has recently been identified as a factor for phospho-dependent mechanism of egg apoptosis in *Xenopus* (Du Pasquier et al. 2011). Bad in ovarian oocytes at the first meiotic propahse is negatively regulated by inhibitory phosphorylation on Ser-112 and Ser-136 by unknown mechanism (maybe PKA phosphorylation). Upon oocyte maturation, Bad becomes further phosphorylated on Ser-128 in a CDK- and JNK-dependent manner. The Ser-128 phosphorylation, if it exceeds the extent of those of Ser-112/Ser-136 phosphorylations during a long period of oocyte maturation in the absence of fertilizing sperm, will allow Bad to trigger a mitochondrial apoptotic pathway involving cytochrome c release and caspase activation. Whether normal process of oocyte maturation and fertilization involves anti-apoptotic mechanism is not known.

2.6 Brain-derived neurotrophic factor (BDNF)

BDNF is a member of neurotropic family of growth factors that include nerve growth factor (NGF). Its cellular functions are exerted by cell surface receptors such as TrkB, a tyrosine kinase/receptor, and p75 low-affinity NGF receptor (Chao and Hempstead 1995). In mammals including human, ovarian BDNF has been implicated in oogenesis, oocyte maturation, and pre-implantation embryogenesis (Kawamura et al. 2005; Zhang et al. 2010). In vitro maturation of mouse oocytes in the presence of cumulus cells is accompanied by BDNF-dependent activation of Akt/PKB and MAPK and its maintenance has been demonstrated (Zhang et al. 2010). Pharmacological experiments suggest that the Akt/PKB activation involves TrkB function (TrkB-PI3K-PIP_3 pathway), while the MAPK does not.

2.7 Bub1/BubR1

Bub1 and **BubR1** (Mad3 in yeast, worms and plants) are multidomain-containing protein-serine/threonine kinases that have been characterized as components of the mitotic checkpoint of spindle assembly (Bolanos-Garcia and Blundell 2011). In mouse oocytes, BubR1 is shown to act as a spindle assembly checkpoint protein in the first meiotic arrest (Homer et al. 2009; Jones and Holt 2010; Schwab et al. 2001; Wei et al. 2010). In maturing *Xenopus* oocytes, Bub1 is activated by MAPK-dependent $p90^{Rsk}$ phosphorylation, and is suggested to be involved in spindle assembly checkpoint and, in collaboration with cdk2/cyclin E complex, cytostatic arrest of the meiosis II (Schwab et al. 2001; Tunquist et al. 2002). Precise mechanism of the cytostatic arrest, i.e. inhibition of anaphase-promoting complex, is not known, because a substrate of Bub1 has not yet been identified. In mammals, first meiotic anaphase also seems to be regulated by Bub1-dependent mechanism (McGuinness et al. 2009).

2.8 Calcineurin

Calcineurin is a protein serine/threonine-specific phosphatase that can be up-regulated by the binding of Ca^{2+}/calmodulin (Pallen and Wang 1985), another target of which is CaMKII. In *Xenopus* eggs and cell-free egg extracts, Ca^{2+}-dependent exit of meiosis II involves transient activation of calcineurin. When the activation of calcineurin is blocked, inactivation of MPF by means of cyclin degradation does not occur and sperm nuclei remains condensed. In addition, cortical contraction of the pigmented granules in the animal hemisphere is also blocked. On the other hand, if the activity of calcineurin is artificially kept up-regulated for a prolonged period, growth of sperm aster is inhibited and fusion of the female and male pronuclei is also inhibited. It has been shown that calcineurin dephosphorylates Cdc20, a key regulator of the anaphase-promoting factor that is a substrate of MAPK (Mochida and Hunt 2007; Nishiyama et al. 2007). These results highlight a requirement of calcineurin for Ca^{2+}-dependent inactivation of cytostatic factor and for the onset of the mitotic cell cycle in the early embryos.

2.9 Caspase 2

Caspase 2 is a member of caspase family, which regulates and/or triggers the apoptotic cell death in response to a wide variety of extracellular and intracellular signals. It has been shown that in caspase 2-deficient mice, excess number of ovarian oocytes is a major cause, suggesting that caspase 2 is involved in ovarian oocyte apoptosis. Oocytes deficient in caspase 2 expression also exhibit a marked resistance to cell death induced by chemicals (Bergeron et al. 1998; Morita and Tilly 1999). Further insight into the roles of caspase 2 in the control of oocyte survival has been demonstrated by the studies with use of cell-free extracts prepared form *Xenopus* eggs. In this system, glucose-6-phosphate has been identified as an important component to drive continual operation of the pentose phosphate pathway that prolongs cell survival. In addition, NADPH generation by this pathway is critical for promoting CaMKII-dependent inhibitory phosphorylation of caspase 2 (Nutt et al. 2005). As CaMKII is known as a crucial component that inactivates CSF activity in frog and mammals, it is intriguing whether the CaMKII-caspase 2 axis also functions at fertilization.

2.10 Cdc20/Fizzy

Cdc20 is an activator of anaphase-promoting complex (APC) that directs the onset and progression of the meiotic and mitotic cell cycle (Chung and Chen 2003; Rudner and Murray 2000; Shteinberg et al. 1999; Tang et al. 2004; Weinstein 1997). In *Drosophila,* Cdc20-related gene Fizzy serves a similar function (Dawson et al. 1993; Pesin and Orr-Weaver 2008). The activity of Cdc20 is negatively regulated by phosphorylation on its serine and threonine residues: in case of *Xenopus* Cdc20, Ser-50, Thr-64, Thr-68 and Thr-79. In *Xenopus* maturing oocytes, phosphorylation of Cdc20 is catalyzed by MAPK, a component of cytostatic factor, and/or Bub1/BubR1 kinases, key regulators of spindle checkpoint, and it is involved in the maintenance of cytostatic factor activity that involves the inactivation of APC. Analyses using cell-free extracts prepared from unfertilized *Xenopus* eggs demonstrate that the phosphorylated form of Cdc20 is a target of calcineurin, whose phosphatase activity is transiently activated in response to Ca^{2+} signals (Mochida and Hunt 2007).

2.11 Cdc25 phosphatase (Cdc25A/B/C)

Cdc25 is a protein-tyrosine phosphatase that has been originally identified and characterized as a yeast cell cycle regulator (Fleig and Gould 1991). A major target of this phosphatase is the Cdc2 protein-serine/threonine kinase, its cyclin-associated form of which functions as MPF. Before oocyte maturation in vertebrates, the activity of Cdc2 protein is down-regulated by the absence of cyclin and by phosphorylation by Myt1/Wee1 dual-specificity kinases on Thr-14 and Tyr-15 residues. During oocyte maturation, however, both accumulation of newly synthesized cyclin as well as removal of the phosphates from Cdc2 ensures the Cdc2 activation (Karaiskou et al. 1998; Kim et al. 1999b; Oh et al. 2010; Perdiguero and Nebreda 2004; Perdiguero et al. 2003; Pirino et al. 2009; Qian et al. 2001; Rime et al. 1994; Zhang et al. 2008; Zhao et al. 2008). There are several types of Cdc25: e.g. Cdc25A, Cdc25B, and Cdc25C. PKA phosphorylation and activation of Cdc25B has been reported in mammals (Pirino et al. 2009). In *Xenopus*, Cdc25C is up-regulated by Plx1-mediated phosphorylation on Ser-287 (Qian et al. 2001). Other reports have shown that Xp38γ/SAPK (Perdiguero et al. 2003) and Greatwall kinase (Zhao et al. 2008) can be responsible for the stimulatory phosphorylation of Cdc25C. Cdc25A has been implicated in embryonic cell cycle regulation (Kim et al. 1999b).

2.12 Cdh1/Cort/Fzy

Cdh1 is an activator of anaphase promoting complex/cyclosome (APC/C), an E3 ubiquitin ligase that regulates the onset of anaphase during meiotic and mitotic cell cycle (Visintin et al. 1997). Several cell cycle regulators are subjected to Cdh1- and proteasome-dependent degradation, by which APC/C-dependent cell cycle progression through anaphase is triggered. In *Xenopus* egg cell-free extracts, Cdh1-dependent degradation of Aurora A kinase plays an important role in mitotic exit (Littlepage and Ruderman 2002). The Aurora A-Cdh1 interaction requires the phosphorylation of Aurora A on Ser-53 residue, which is a substrate of M-phase-activated kinase(s). On the other hand, APC-independent cellular function involving Cdh1 has also been suggested in *Xenopus* oocyte maturation (Papin et al. 2004). In immature mouse oocytes, where the meiotic cell cycle is paused at the prophase I, Emi1-dependent mechanism of cdh1 inhibition (thereby inhibition of APC/C) functions for the MI arrest (Marangos et al. 2007). In *Drosophila* and *C. elegans*, Cdc20/Cdh1-related protein, Cort and Fzy, respectively, controls the meiotic cell cycle progression in a Cdh1-like manner (Kitagawa et al. 2002; Marangos et al. 2007; Swan and Schupbach 2007).

2.13 Cohesin/SCC1/Rec-8

Cohesin is a chromosome-binding protein that is involved in meiotic and mitotic assembly and segregation of sister chromatids (Heck 1997). In many vertebrate species, cell cycle progression through anaphase involves a proteolytic cleavage of cohesin, as catalyzed by separase and subsequent release of cohesin from the sister chromatids, so that the chromosomal segregation occurs. In *Xenopus*, however, proteolysis-independent release of cohesin from sister chromatids is working and it involves polo-like kinase phosphorylation of cohesin (Sumara et al. 2002). A similar phospho-dependent release of chromosome cohesion has been demonstrated in *C. elegans*, where the AIR-2 kinase (Aurora B kinase in this species) phosphorylation of the nematode cohesion Rec-8 (Rogers et al. 2002).

2.14 Crk adaptor protein (Crk/CRKL)

Crk is an SH2/SH3-containing adaptor protein that has been originally identified as an oncogene product (viral Crk or v-Crk) of avian sarcoma virus CT10 (Feller et al. 1994; Mayer et al. 1988; Mayer and Hanafusa 1990). Its SH2 domain-dependent phosphotyrosine-binding property and SH3 domain-dependent binding to proline-rich sequences in other molecules are required for malignant cell transformation. Three cellular homologues of v-Crk have been found in mammals: c-Crk I, c-Crk II, and c-Crk-like (CRKL). These cellular Crk family proteins have been identified as a major substrate of Bcr-Abl tyrosine kinase that causes chronic myeloid leukemia (CML) (Feller et al. 1998). Another aspect of Crk function has been demonstrated in the studies of *Xenopus* egg cell-free extract: apoptosis in aged egg extracts is shown to involve interaction between the SH2 domain of Crk and the tyrosine-phosphorylated form of Wee1 dual-specificity kinase (Evans et al. 1997; Smith et al. 2000). Further study has demonstrated that the SH3 domain of Crk is important for interacting with the nuclear export factor Crm1, an antagonistic factor for apoptosis in cell-free extract, and that mutually exclusive interaction between Crk and Crm1 or Wee1 in the nucleus regulates the onset of apoptosis.

2.15 Cyclin B

Cyclin is a family of CDK activator proteins, whose first example has been discovered in fertilized sea urchin eggs (Evans et al. 1983) and starfish maturing oocytes (Evans et al. 1983; Standart et al. 1987). Cyclin family consists of several proteins: cyclin A, B, D, E and others, and cyclin B are a component of MPF, another subunit of which is Cdc2/CDK1 serine/threonine-specific protein kinase (Hunt 1989; Maller 1990). In many species, hormone-induced MPF activity in maturing oocytes is generally dependent on *de novo* synthesis and accumulation of cyclin B (and subsequent phospho-dependent regulation of Cdc2/CDK1 by the actions of Wee1/Myt1 kinases and Cdc25 phosphatase is also important) (Gaffre et al. 2011). Fertilization triggers an ubiquitin/proteasome-dependent degradation of cyclin B that causes a rapid decrease of MPF activity (Edgecombe et al. 1991; Huo et al. 2004b; Lapasset et al. 2005; Lapasset et al. 2008; Meijer et al. 1989a; Meijer et al. 1991; Meijer et al. 1989b; Sakamoto et al. 1998). Other cyclins (e.g. cyclin A, D) serve a similar CDK-activating property, but have distinct physiological functions (e.g. G_1/S transition, spindle checkpoint) by interacting with a specific CDK member(s) (e.g. CDK2, CDK5).

2.16 *sn*-1,2-diacylglycerol (DG)

DG is one of two hydrolyzed products by phospholipase C of phosphatidylinositol 4,5-bisphosphate, another product of which is inositol 1,4,5-trisphosphate (IP_3). DG serve as a second messenger in a variety of extracellular signals such as hormones and neurotransmitters, and is well characterized as a direct activator for PKC, a family of serine/threonine kinase (Nishizuka 1984; Nishizuka 1986). DG also acts as a substrate of DG kinase that produces phosphatidic acid or PA, which has pleiotropic cellular functions. In *Xenopus* eggs, fertilization promotes a rapid increase in intracellular DG concentration, a large part of which seems to be due to phospholipase D (PLD)-mediated cleavage of phosphatidylcholine (PC) (but not PIP_2). In support of this, choline, another product of PC hydrolysis by PLD, is also accumulating in a similar time course of fertilization. Whether DG is involved in the activation of egg PKC remains to be clarified (Stith et al. 1997). Production of DG has also been examined in mouse eggs (Stith et al. 1997; Yu et al. 2008). In this species, sperm-derived PLCζ seems to be mainly responsible for DG production and subsequent PKC activation.

2.17 Initiation factor 4E-binding protein (4E-BP)

4E-BP is a binding protein for eukaryotic initiation factor 4E (eIF4E), an mRNA cap-binding protein that facilitates the initiation of protein synthesis in association with eIF4F. The interaction between 4E-BP and eIF4E depends on the phosphorylation state of 4E-BP: hypo-phosphorylated form of 4E-BP has an ability to bind to and inhibit eIF4E, whereas the phosphorylated form of 4E-BP releases eIF4E so that eIF4E-eIF4F complex is formed and promotes active translation of mRNA (Lasko 2003). In sea urchin eggs, fertilization is accompanied by a rapid burst of protein synthesis. It has been shown that fertilization also promotes a rapid decrease in 4E-BP as well as an increase in phosphorylated form of 4E-BP (Cormier et al. 2001). Two-dimensional electrophoresis demonstrated that 4E-BP is phosphorylated on multiple sites after fertilization. In mitotic sea urchin embryos, further decrease in 4E-BP expression has been demonstrated and it is mediated by a rapamycin-sensitive mechanism of proteolysis of 4E-BP (Salaun et al. 2003), suggesting that mTOR (mammalian target of rapamycin)-like kinase is involved in the phosphorylation of 4E-BP. A rapamycin-sensitive mechanism of global protein synthesis involving 4E-BP regulation (but not translation of some proteins such as cyclin B and Mos, whose translational control involves the phosphorylation of CPEB phosphorylation) has also been demonstrated in maturing oocytes of starfish (Lapasset et al. 2008).

2.18 EGG-3/4/5

C. elegans **EGG-3** is a member of protein-tyrosine phosphatase-like (PTPL) family, whose mutant egg undergoes fertilization normally but has a defect in polarized dispersal of F-actin, formation of chitin eggshell, and production of polar bodies (Maruyama et al. 2007). Although enzymatic substrate for EGG-3 has not yet been demonstrated (PTPL proteins are supposed to be pseudo-phosphatase), its functional interaction with CHS-1, which is required for deposition of egg shell, plays a role for proper distribution of MBK-2 kinase that regulates degradation of maternal proteins and egg-to-embryo transition (Nishi and Lin 2005; Qu et al. 2006; Qu et al. 2007; Stitzel et al. 2007; Stitzel et al. 2006). Other members of PTPL family such as EGG-4 and EGG-5 have also been characterized as components of meiotic cell cycle progression and egg-to-embryo transition. These two EGG proteins have no phosphatase activity, however, interact with YTY motif of MBK-2 kinase, which is autophosphorylated in the active kinase, and inhibit the kinase activity (Cheng et al. 2009; Parry et al. 2009).

2.19 Emi1 and Emi2/xErp1

In vertebrate unfertilized eggs, cytostatic factor (CSF) is responsible for maintaining the meiotic cell cycle at MII (metaphase of second meiosis) (Masui 2000; Tunquist and Maller 2003). As a candidate of molecule involved in CSF activity, several kinase proteins have been suggested and evaluated (e.g. Mos, MAPK, Rsk). On the other hand, APC/C (anaphase promoting complex/cyclosome) has been identified an initiator of meiotic resumption (thus, as a disruptor of CSF-mediated arrest or a main target of CSF activity). **Emi1** has been identified first as a negative regulator of APC/C in *Xenopus* eggs and cell-free extracts (Reimann et al. 2001a; Reimann et al. 2001b; Reimann and Jackson 2002). Thereafter, an Emi1-related protein named **Emi2/xErp1** has been identified and characterized as an essential component of CSF inhibition of APC/C (Hansen et al. 2006; Liu and Maller 2005; Rauh et al. 2005; Tang et al. 2008; Tung et al. 2005; Wu et al. 2007a; Wu et al. 2007b). In the current scenario, CSF arrest by Emi2/xErp1 of APC/C involves recruitment of PP2A to the Rsk-phosphorylated Emi2/xErp1 (this phosphorylation has stabilizing effect on Emi2/xErp1) and its phosphatase action on other phosphates in Emi2/xErp1 catalyzed by Cdc2/cyclin B complex (this phosphorylation weakens Emi2/xErp1). After fertilization, CaMKII and Plx1 phosphorylation promotes ubiquitin-dependent proteolysis of Emi2/xErp1, thereby APC/C is released from the inhibitory interaction with Emi2/xErp1 (Wu and Kornbluth 2008).

2.20 FKHRL1/FOXO3a

FKHRL (forkhead in rhabdomyosarcoma) is a transcription factor, whose activation has been implicated in the onset of apoptosis and Akt phosphorylation (on Thr-24, Ser-256, and Ser-319) leads to suppression of its function (Brunet et al. 1999; Tang et al. 1999). Its genetic loss or ablation can be a trigger of carcinogenesis, thus FKHRL is a tumor suppressor (Gallego Melcon and Sanchez de Toledo Codina 2007). Akt-dependent phosphorylation of FKHRL1 has been demonstrated in follicular oocytes that receive stem cell factor (SCF) for mammalian oocyte development (Reddy et al. 2005). SCF is a ligand for c-Kit receptor/tyrosine kinase that, upon its ligand-induced activation, promotes sequential activation of PI3K, PDK, and Akt. Thus, follicular development of oocytes involves the suppression of pro-apoptotic signal transduction by FKHRL1. In support of this, FKHRL1 gene-deficient mice exhibited excessive activation from primordial to primary follicles as well as enlarged oocyte sizes (Reddy et al. 2005). A similar pathway involving FOXO3a, a rat homologue of FKHRL transcription factor, has been shown in rat oocytes (Liu et al. 2009).

2.21 XGef

XGef is a *Xenopus* homologue of mammalian guanine nucleotide exchanging factor, RhoGEF that activates Rho-family small GTP-binding protein such as Cdc42. XGef has been initially identified as a CPEB-binding protein and in fact, it has been shown that XGef is involved in polyadenylation and translation of Mos mRNA during oocyte maturation (Reverte et al. 2003). GEF activity of XGef is required for Mos synthesis. In addition, interaction between XGef is responsible for an increase in CPEB phosphorylation during oocyte maturation, which is important for CPEB activation (Martinez et al. 2005). Further studies have shown that MAPK interacts with XGef and acts as a kinase of CPEB on Thr-22,

Thr-164, Ser-184, and Ser-248 (Keady et al. 2007). These phosphorylation sites seem to be required for another and most important phosphorylation event on CPEB: Ser-174 phosphorylation (maybe catalyzed by XRINGO/CDK1 kinase complex) (Kuo et al. 2011).

2.22 Grb2/7/10/14

Grb is a growth factor receptor-bound protein family that has one or more phosphotyrosine-binding and proline-rich interacting domains (i.e. SH2 and SH3 domains) and plays crucial roles in tyrosine kinase receptor-dependent signal transduction (Rozakis-Adcock et al. 1993). There are several Grb family members (e.g. Grb2), most well known of which is Grb2, whose *Drosophila* homologue is *drk* (Olivier et al. 1993). Grb2/*drk* directly interacts to receptor/tyrosine kinase with phosphotyrosine residue(s) (e.g. EGFR in mammals, *sevenless* in *Drosophila*). Because Grb2 interacts constitutively with Sos (*son of sevenless* in *Drosophila*), a guanine nucleotide-exchanging factor (GEF) for Ras, its recruitment to the plasma membranes leads to Ras activation and subsequent MAPK cascade propagation. In *Xenopus* oocytes expressing fibroblast growth factor receptor/kinase (FGFR), some Grb family members (Grb7, Grb10, and Grb14) have been implicated in tyrosine kinase-dependent signal transduction (Cailliau et al. 2003). Microinjection of Grb2 into immature *Xenopus* oocytes has been shown to cause oocyte maturation in a Ras-dependent manner (Browaeys-Poly et al. 2007; Cailliau et al. 2001). In this unusual, but interesting oocyte maturation system, SH2 domains and SH3 domain of Grb2 interact with tyrosine-phosphorylated lipovitellin 1 and PLCγ, respectively. Whether hormone-induced oocyte maturation involves Grb protein is not yet clear.

2.23 Heparin-binding and EGF-like growth factor (HB-EGF)

HB-EGF is a member of EGFR/Erb/HER ligand family, other members of which include EGF, transforming growth factor α, and heregulin. HB-EGF is initially expressed as a membrane-associated precursor and its mature form is secreted outside the cells is done by extracellular shedding as mediated by matrix metalloproteinases (MMPs). HB-EGF participates in several biological processes, including heart development and maintenance, skin wound healing, eyelid formation, progression of atherosclerosis and tumor formation (Miyamoto et al. 2006). In mammals, implantation of early embryos have been shown to involve the action of HB-EGF secreted from the surrounding epithelium as well as those autocrined (Lim and Dey 2009). In this system, HB-EGF exerts its biological functions through activation of intracellular Ca^{2+}-dependent pathways and MAPK cascade. Human trophoblast survival, where anti-apoptosis in low oxygen environment is a key event, has been shown to involve HB-EGF function (Armant et al. 2006). In other species such chicken and fish, expression of HB-EGF in oocytes is supposed to be required for ovarian follicle cell proliferation (Tse and Ge 2009; Wang et al. 2007).

2.24 Heterogenous nuclear ribonucleoprotein K (hnRNP K)

hnRNP K is a K homology (KH) domain-containing RNA-binding protein of the HnRNP family, other KH-containing RNA-binding proteins of which include hnRNP E1/E2 and Sam68 (Bomsztyk et al. 2004; Dreyfuss et al. 2002; Mattick 2004). hnRNP K binds to RNA through its three KH domains and serves multiple functions related to transcription and posttranscriptional regulation of mRNAs (e.g. splicing, translation). In *Xenopus* unfertilized eggs, hnRNP K is phosphorylated on serine and/or threonine residue(s). This phosphorylation seems to be done by MAPK, because a MAPKK inhibitor U0126, but not other inhibitors for MPF (Cdc2/cyclin B) and PKA, diminishes the signals. Consistently, fertilization results in a rapid decrease of the MAPK phosphorylation of hnRNP K. At the same time, hnRNP K becomes tyrosine-phosphorylated, most likely because of sperm-induced Src activation (Iwasaki et al. 2008). These MAPK and Src phosphorylation of hnRNP K has also been demonstrated in mammalian cell systems, in which RNA-binding property (i.e. inhibition of translation) of hnRNP K is up-regulated by MAPK and down-regulated by Src (Habelhah et al. 2001; Ostareck-Lederer et al. 2002). In *Xenopus* eggs and embryos (before mid-blastula transition, where zygotic transcription is activated), maternal mRNAs will be subjected to active protein synthesis to support embryonic development. Data obtained so far suggest that hnRNP K is involved in the suppression and release of specific subset of maternal mRNAs for its active translation (Iwasaki et al. 2008).

2.25 Heterotrimeric and monomeric GTP-binding proteins

G-proteins constitute a large family of proteins that includes small G-proteins and trimeric G-proteins, each of which act as a transducer for extracellular and/or intracellular signals (Gilman 1987; Kaziro et al. 1991). In the case of small G-proteins, a monomeric G-protein (e.g. Ras) is regulated by cell surface receptor-mediated modulation of GAP (GTPase-activating protein) and GEF (guanine nucleotide exchanging factor) activities, and the GTP-bound, active form interacts with effector molecules (e.g. Raf kinase) and regulates cellular functions. Trimeric G-proteins (e.g. Gi, Gs) consist of three subunits: α, β, and γ. Before activation, these three subunits containing GDP-bound form of a subunit are present in a tight complex. Upon activation of cognate cell surface receptors, they become dissociated and each of the subunit (GTP-bound form of α subunit and β/γ complex) exerts its cellular function. In some species, introduction of non-hydrolysable GTPγS or expression of G-protein-coupled cell surface receptor and its ligand activation, which promotes a constitutive activation of (mainly heterotrimeric) G-proteins, is shown to cause egg activation-like phenomena such as repetitive increase in intracellular Ca^{2+} concentration (in mammals) (Swann et al. 1989), cortical reactions (in *Xenopus*) (Kline et al. 1991), and DNA synthesis (in starfish) (Shilling et al. 1994). While involvement of some specific G-proteins (e.g. Gq) in the process of sperm-induced egg activation have been negatively evaluated (Runft et al. 1999; Williams et al. 1998), the fact that the *Xenopus* egg membrane-associated Src activity can be directly stimulated by GTPγS suggests that one or more unknown G-protein(s) serve as a signal transducer of gamete interaction (Sato et al. 2003; Shilling et al. 1994; Swann et al. 1989). Involvement of trimeric G-proteins in oocyte maturation is much more convincing in some species (Mehlmann 2005). Starfish and mouse oocyte meiotic arrest and/or maturation is shown to involve G-protein that directs PI3K-dependent or independent mechanism of Akt/MAPK/MPF/PKA activities (Han et al. 2006; Kalinowski et al. 2004; Kishimoto 2011; Mehlmann et al. 2004; Okumura et al. 2002). *Xenopus* oocyte maturation also seems to involve progesterone-induced membrane receptor activation that leads to modulation of G-protein (maybe Gs, not Gi)/adenylate cyclase pathway (Gallo et al. 1995; Kalinowski et al. 2003).

2.26 Histone H3

Histone is a family of basic polypeptides with ~130 amino acids and has been well characterized as DNA-binding proteins. Nucleosome, a complex of DNA-histones, is organized by an octamer of histone H2A, H2B, H3, and H4. Posttranslational modifications such as acetylation, methylation, and phosphorylation regulate the DNA-binding property of histones including H3. In some mammalian species, phosphorylation of H3 by aurora kinase and an adjacent dimethylated lysine residue are coordinately involved in chromosomal condensation during oocyte maturation (Bui et al. 2007; Ding et al. 2011; Eberlin et al. 2008; Gu et al. 2008; Jelinkova and Kubelka 2006; Maton et al. 2003; Swain et al. 2007; Wang et al. 2006).

2.27 Inositol trisphosphate receptor (IP3R)

Fertilization induces oscillation of inositol 1,4,5-trisphosphate receptor (**IP3R**)-dependent intracellular Ca^{2+} that is responsible for initiating oocyte maturation, egg activation and early embryogenesis. Three isoforms of IP3R have been detected. IP3R is dynamically regulated during meiotic maturation and is required for fertilization induced Ca^{2+} release in *Xenopus* (Kume et al. 1997; Runft et al. 1999). Developmentally regulated type 1 IP3R is up-regulated in oocytes at fertilization and down-regulated after fertilization and this down-regulation is mediated by degradation in proteasome pathway in mouse (Fissore et al. 1999; Jellerette et al. 2000; Parrington et al. 1998; Wakai et al. 2011) and bovine (Malcuit et al. 2005). IP3R1 is phosphorylated during both maturation and the first cell cycle mediated by M-phase kinases e.g. MAPK/ERK2 or polo-like kinase 1 and this is vital for IP3R function in optimum Ca^{2+} release at fertilization in *Xenopus*, mouse and pig (Ito et al. 2008; Ito et al. 2010; Lee et al. 2006; Sun et al. 2009; Vanderheyden et al. 2009). Type 1 IP3R is differentially distributed during human oocyte maturation through GV to MII stage and after fertilization in both peripheral and central in the zygotes and early 2-4-cell embryos and in perinuclear in the 6-8-cell embryos (Goud et al. 1999).

2.28 Insulin

Insulin is a peptide hormone and is crucial for follicular cell growth and development. The addition of insulin to the serum- and hormone-free maturation medium though does not improve the maturation but improves the fertilization rate of bovine oocytes in vitro (Matsui et al. 1995). Artificially induced impaired insulin secretion had a lower percentage of zygotes and a higher percentage of unfertilized and degenerated oocytes in mouse (Vesela et al. 1995). Mouse oocyte has the insulin receptor-beta and highly elevated insulin influences oocyte meiosis, chromatin remodeling, and embryonic developmental competence (Acevedo et al. 2007). Insulin did not activate MPF might be primarily due to the inability of the peptide to activate Ras and to stimulate Mos synthesis in *Xenopus* stage IV but successfully induced maturation of stage VI oocyte (Chesnel et al. 1997). Binding of insulin was revealed in oocytes, granulosa and theca internal cells of healthy pre-antral and antral follicles implying its function in these cells of swine (Quesnel 1999). Insulin increased the developmental potential of porcine oocytes and embryo (Lee et al. 2005). In insulin induced carp oocyte maturation, PI3K is an initial component of the signal transduction pathway, which proceeds, MAPK, and MPF activation (Paul et al. 2009).

2.29 Insulin-like growth factor -1 (IGF-1)

Insulin-like growth factor-1 (**IGF-1**) is primarily synthesized in liver and secreted in circulation that mediate endocrine signal important for the early embryonic development. In *in vitro* reconstructed horse oocytes, IGF-1 induced a bigger accumulation of MAPK (especially ERK2) in the cytoplasm that undergoes nuclear remodeling like a normal embryo following somatic cell nuclear transfer (Li et al. 2004). IGF-1 acts differentially to induce oocyte maturation competence but not meiotic resumption by IGF-1 in white bass (Weber and Sullivan 2005) and white perch (Weber et al. 2007). IGF-1 as like insulin also mediates its action through the activity of IRS-1 in *Xenopus* oocyte maturation (Chuang et al. 1993b). IGF-1 induced mammalian oocyte maturation and subsequently the embryo development e.g. in bovine (Bonilla et al. 2011; Stefanello et al. 2006; Wasielak and Bogacki 2007), mouse (Inzunza et al. 2010) and even human (Coppola et al. 2009).

2.30 Insulin receptor substrate-1 (IRS-1)

Insulin and insulin-like growth factor-1 (IGF-1) receptors (IR and IGFR-1) possess tyrosine-kinase enzymatic activity that is essential for signal transduction to mediate the putative effects of these hormones on oocyte maturation, fetal growth and development. This causes rapid tyrosine phosphorylation of a high-molecular-weight substrate termed insulin receptor substrate-1 (**IRS-1**), a docking protein that can bind with Src homology 2 domain containing molecules e.g. PI 3-kinase, Grb2. Insulin-induced maturation of *Xenopus* oocytes involve the activation of IRS-1 and PI 3-kinase where activation of PI 3-kinase might act upstream of mitogen-activated protein kinase activation and p70 S6K activation (Chuang et al. 1994; Chuang et al. 1993a; Chuang et al. 1993b; Liu et al. 1995; Yamamoto-Honda et al. 1996). IRS-1 is expressed maternally and constantly during *Xenopus* embryogenesis and is important for eye development (Bugner et al. 2011).

2.31 Integrin β1

Integrins are a family of cell surface receptors that mediate cell-cell and cell-matrix interactions in different cellular systems. Variety of integrins is differentially expressed during development, consistent with diverse roles for integrins in embryogenesis. **Integrin β1** (this subunit can interact with α6) is present on the mouse egg surface that increases the rate of sperm attachment but does not alter the total number of sperm that can attach or fuse to the egg (Baessler et al. 2009; Tarone et al. 1993). Integrin α6β1 in association with tetraspanin CD151 and CD9 complex do function in human and mouse gamete fusion (Ziyyat et al. 2006). In *Xenopus*, integrin β1 is present on the oocyte membrane throughout oogenesis and during maturation it is localized in several membrane vesicles in the cytoplasm might be to provide the material source for the rapid membrane formation during cleavage (Muller et al. 1993). Even integrin α6β1 might serve as potential clinical marker for evaluating sperm quality in men (Reddy et al. 2003).

2.32 Interleukin-7 (IL-7)

Interleukin-7 (**IL-7**, pre-B-cell growth factor) is playing its role not only as immunomodulator but also in the beginning of development. IL-7 in together with IL-8 inhibited the gamete interaction of hamster egg and sperm (Lambert et al. 1992). The role of

IL-7 was tested in differentiation during embryonic development e.g. in mouse: development of thymus (Wiles et al. 1992) and lymph node (Coles et al. 2006). IL-7 could be also a good marker of the embryo quality for implantation (Achour-Frydman et al. 2010). In rat granulosa cell culture of early antral and preovulatory follicles, IL-7 stimulated the phosphorylation of AKT, glycogen synthase kinase (GSK3B), and STAT5 proteins in a time- and dose-dependent manner (Cheng et al. 2011). It is concluded that oocyte-derived IL-7 act on neighboring granulosa cells as a survival factor and promote the nuclear maturation of pre-ovulatory oocytes through activation of the PIK3/AKT pathway (Cheng et al. 2011).

2.33 Lipovitellin (LV)

LV1 and **LV2** are components of crystallized yolk platelet in vertebrate oocytes, eggs, and embryos. Precursor protein of LVs, vitellogenin, is synthesized in a highly phosphorylated form in liver of adult and transferred to ovarian tissue, where growing oocytes actively incorporate vitellogenin through the action of specific oocyte membrane receptors (Bergink and Wallace 1974). The incorporated vitellogenin is subjected to partial proteolysis so that LV2 and other fragments such as lipovitellin 1, phosvitin, and pp25 are formed (Finn 2007). A similar set of yolk-associated proteins is also found in invertebrates including insect (e.g. vitelline). It is well known that phosvitin and pp25 are highly serine/threonine-phosphorylated proteins that serve as an energy source of oogenesis and early embryogenesis. On the other hand, tyrosine phosphorylation of LV1 (Browaeys-Poly et al. 2007) and LV2 (Kushima et al. 2011) has recently been demonstrated in *Xenopus*. In particular, tyrosine phosphorylation of LV2 is unusually stable during oogenesis, oocyte maturation, and early embryogenesis until the removal of yolk-associated materials from swimming tadpole (Kushima et al. 2011). Possible function of tyrosine-phosphorylated form of *Xenopus* LV1 and LV2 so far suggested is oocyte maturation (Browaeys-Poly et al. 2007; Kushima et al. 2011), although it's upstream (liver or oocyte) kinase and downstream cellular function is uncertain.

2.34 Maskin/Cytoplasmic polyadenylation element (CPE)-binding protein (CPEB)/TACC3/p82

Maskin is a cytoplasmic polyadenylation element-binding protein-associated factor. Dormant state of maternal mRNAs in immature oocytes is maintained by an abortive interaction of this protein with the eukaryotic initiation factors 4E and 4G. Phosphorylation of maskin promotes the dissociation of this interaction, thereby allows the dormant mRNAs to be translated actively. Aurora phosphorylation of maskin is reported to be involved in protein synthesis in maturing clam and *Xenopus* oocytes and in centrosome-dependent microtubule assembly at mitosis (Kinoshita et al. 2005; Pascreau et al. 2005).

2.35 Myosin regulatory light chain (MRLC)

Myosin regulatory light chain (**MRLC**) or, in short, myosin light chain (MLC) is a component of myosin that regulates the function of actin and actin filaments (see above) through the binding to the actin molecule. Unfertilized eggs of sea urchin undergo cortical contraction in response to calyculin A, an inhibitor for protein phosphates. The results suggest that an egg protein(s), in its phosphorylated form(s), is capable of inducing cortical contraction in this system. As a candidate phosphoprotein for this phenomenon, MRLC has been identified (Asano and Mabuchi 2001). Further biochemical experiments have demonstrated that CK2 (casein kinase 2) is a responsible kinase for the phosphorylation of MRLC (Komaba et al. 2001). Phosphorylation of MRLC in sea urchin eggs occurs on Ser-19 and Thr-18 residues, both of which are stimulatory phosphorylation sites (Asano and Mabuchi 2001). On the other hand, MRLC has also been identified as a phosphoprotein in cell-free extracts prepared form sea urchin eggs. In this system, phosphorylation of MRLC occurs at mitotic phase of cell cycle on Ser-1/2 and Thr-9, all of which are canonical PKC sites, and it is suggested that MPF is the responsible kinase (Totsukawa et al. 1996). In *Drosophila,* phosphorylation of Ser-21 of MRLC-homologue (*sqh,* spaghetti squash gene product) has been implicated as an important event for oogenesis (Jordan and Karess 1997).

2.36 Na^+/H^+ antiporter/exchanger

On fertilization there are marked changes in the cytoplasmic ionic concentration e.g. Ca^{2+}, H^+, are necessary and sufficient to constitute the egg activation and beyond. A second messenger type substance that stimulates protein kinase C linked the activation of the Na^+/H^+ exchange to the calcium transient and ultimately the protein synthesis is increased and the cytoplasmic alkalinization occur in sea urchin eggs (Swann and Whitaker 1985). In sea urchin eggs, though the **Na^+/H^+ exchanger** is regulated by PKC or Ca^{2+}/CaMK activities but fertilization mediated activation of this exchanger is Ca^{2+}, CaM-dependent (Shen 1989). G proteins activated Na^+/H^+ antiporter mediated by PKA and/or PKC in *Xenopus* oocytes (Busch 1997; Busch et al. 1995). A typical Na^+/H^+ exchanger mediated increased intracellular pH though activate the surf clam oocytes but is neither sufficient nor required for GVBD (Dube and Eckberg 1997). The function of Na^+/H^+ exchanger has also been described even for later stage of development e.g. blastocyst of mouse (Barr et al. 1998), bovine embryos (Lane and Bavister 1999) and human pre-implantation embryos (Phillips et al. 2000).

2.37 OMA-1

In *C. elegans,* two CCCH-type zinc finger proteins **OMA-1** and OMA-2 are expressed specifically in maturing oocytes and are functionally redundant during maturation. Both Oma-1 and Oma-2 mutant oocytes arrest at a defined point in prophase I and the removal of Myt1-like kinase Wee-1.3 results the release of prophase I arrest (Detwiler et al. 2001). As WEE-1.3 functions as a negative regulator, OMA-1 and OMA-2 either function upstream of WEE-1.3 or in parallel with WEE-1.3 as positive regulators of prophase progression (Detwiler et al. 2001). OMA-1 protein is largely reduced because of rapid degradation after the first mitotic division and this is necessary for the early embryonic development by regulating the temporal degradation of maternal proteins in early *C. elegans* embryos (Lin 2003; Shimada et al. 2006; Shirayama et al. 2006). OMA-1 is directly phosphorylated (Thr-239) by DYRK kinase MBK-2 that facilitates subsequent phosphorylation (Thr-339) by another kinase GSK-3 and these precisely timed phosphorylation events are important for its function in 1-cell embryo and degradation after first mitosis (Nishi and Lin 2005).

2.38 p53

The **p53** protein family includes three transcription factors-p53, p63 and p73 that play roles in both cancer and normal development (Levine et al. 2011). Mostly stable p53 protein is synthesized during late oogenesis and stage VI oocyte and even after fertilization at least until the tadpole stage during *Xenopus* development (Tchang et al. 1993). After fertilization, part of the largely stored p53 is imported into the nucleus and associates both with decondensed DNA and the nuclear lamina envelope but not with any replication complexes during *Xenopus* early development (Tchang and Mechali 1999). In the absence of TPX2 (targeting protein for Xklp2), p53 can inhibit Aurora A, a serine/threonine kinase, activity (Eyers and Maller 2004). TPX2 is required for Aurora A activation and for p53 synthesis and phosphorylation during *Xenopus* oocyte maturation (Pascreau et al. 2009). The tumor suppressor protein p53 regulates the efficiency of human reproduction. The p53 allele encoding proline at 72 (Pro72) was found to be significantly higher (P=0.003) over the allele encoding arginine (Arg72) among women experiencing recurrent implantation failure (Kang et al. 2009; Kay et al. 2006; Levine et al. 2011)

2.39 p95

Several studies showed that in mammals, egg-specific extracellular matrix zona pellucida component ZP3 regulates an essential event in sperm function. Mouse zona pellucida glycoprotein ZP3 regulates acrosomal exocytosis by aggregating its corresponding receptors located in the mouse sperm plasma membrane e.g. a protein **p95** that might serve as a substrate for a tyrosine kinase in response to zona pellucida binding or itself act as tyrosine kinase (Saling 1991). A phosphotyrosine containing receptor tyrosine kinase was identified in human sperm that is similar to mouse sperm protein, p95, having tyrosine kinase activity and human ZP3 stimulate the tyrosine kinase activity of this protein (Burks et al. 1995; Naz and Ahmad 1994). Acrosome reaction was induced with increased tyrosine phosphorylation of p95 epitope only in capacitated human spermatozoa (Brewis et al. 1998).

2.40 Paxillin

Paxillin is a prominent focal adhesion docking protein that regulates somatic and germ cell signaling. Paxillin was shown as one of the major tyrosine kinase substrates during rat chick embryogenesis (Turner 1991) and regulator of Rho and Rac signaling during *Drosophila* development (Chen et al. 2005). It was described that paxillin is required for synthesis and activation of Mos (the germ cell Raf homolog), that promotes MEK and subsequently Erk signaling and then possibly Erk mediate the phosphorylation of paxillin required for steroid (testosterone)-induced *Xenopus* oocyte maturation (Rasar et al. 2006). In prostate cancer cell, EGFR-induced Erk activation requires Src-mediated phosphorylation of paxillin but paxillin was not involved in PKC-induced Erk signal (Sen et al. 2010). Erk-mediated phosphorylation of paxillin was necessary for both EGFR- and PKC-mediated cellular proliferation indicate that paxillin serves as a specific upstream regulator of Erk in response to receptor-tyrosine kinase activity but as a general regulator of downstream Erk actions regardless of agonist (Sen et al. 2010).

2.41 Peptidylarginine deiminase (PAD)

Peptidylarginine deiminase (PAD) catalyzes the post-translational modification of protein converting the arginine to citrulline in the presence of calcium ions. PAD is present in the cortical granules of mouse oocytes, is released extracellularly during the cortical reaction, and remains associated as a peripheral membrane protein until the blastocyst stage (Liu et al. 2005). In mouse peptidylarginine deiminase-like protein termed ePAD (p75) was expressed in immature oocyte, mature egg, and until the blastocyst stage of embryonic development (Wright et al. 2003). Peptidylarginine deiminase 6 (PAD6) is uniquely expressed in male and female germ cells but the inactivation of PAD6 gene leads to female infertility whereas male fertility is not affected (Esposito et al. 2007) and its transcript is detectable at embryonic day 16.5 in mouse (Choi et al. 2010). Mouse oocyte cytoplasmic sheet-associated PADI6 undergoes developmental change in phosphorylation that might be linked to interaction between PAD16-YWHA during oocyte maturation (Snow et al. 2008). PADI6-deficient mice are also infertile might be due to disruption of development beyond the two-cell stage (Snow et al. 2008).

2.42 Phosphodiesterase 3A (PDE3A)

Intracellular concentration of the second messenger cAMP is the key signaling molecules in the control of oocyte meiotic resumption mediated by the activity of phosphodiesterases (**PDEs**). cAMP blocks meiotic maturation of oocytes of a broad spectrum of species and cyclic nucleotide phosphodiesterase 3A (PDE3A) is primarily responsible for oocyte cAMP hydrolysis. The PDE3A activity in the regulation of oocyte maturation of several species has been studied extensively e.g. in rodent (Wiersma et al. 1998), rat (Richard et al. 2001), mouse (Masciarelli et al. 2004; Nogueira et al. 2003b; Nogueira et al. 2005), monkey (Jensen et al. 2005), porcine (Sasseville et al. 2006; Sasseville et al. 2007), bovine (Mayes and Sirard 2002; Thomas et al. 2002), and human (Nogueira et al. 2003a). Various PDE3 inhibitors were used like org9935, cilostamide, or milrinone. PDE3 activity is required for insulin/insulin-like growth factor-1 stimulation of *Xenopus* oocyte meiotic resumption. It should be note that the activation of PDE3A by PKB/Akt-mediated phosphorylation potentiates the *Xenopus* and mouse oocytes maturation (Han et al. 2006).

2.43 pp25 and phosvitin

Functions of multiple vitellogenin (VgA, VgB, and VgC)-derived yolk products, e.g. lipovitellin/**phosvitin** were described during oocyte maturation and early embryos in various species, e.g. barfin flounder, *Verasper moseri*, a marine teleost (Matsubara et al. 1999; Sawaguchi et al. 2006), red seabream (*Pagrus major*), another marine teleost and gray mullet (*Mugil cephalus*) (Amano et al. 2008). A substrate **pp25** for protein serine/threonine kinases was derived from the precursor of pp43 that is consisting of a portion of the *Xenopus* VgB1 protein (Xi et al. 2003). pp25 may have a role as an inhibitory modulator of some protein phosphorylation mediated by CKII and PKC in *Xenopus* oocytes and embryos (Sugimoto and Hashimoto 2006). A differentially distributed pp25 was shown to localize at the surface just below the plasma membrane in oocyte and in embryogenesis a transition from beneath the outer surface of each germ layer to endoderm during tail budding from where it gradually decreased and disappeared at the tadpole stage in *Xenopus* (Nakamura et al. 2007).

2.44 Protein methyl transferase 5 (PRMT5)

Distinct protein/DNA methylation patterns were observed in developmental stages during genomic reorganization. The protein methylase activity was measured at mesenchymal blastula and at young gastrula of sea urchin embryonic development and lysine of histones H3 and H4 are the main target (Branno et al. 1983). A Janus-2 (JAK-2) binding protein, JBP1, acts as an arginine methyl transferase and is now designated as **PRMT5**. In *Xenopus* oocytes, PRMT5 inhibited the oncogenic/transformed $p21^{Ras}$ mediated maturation but not the insulin mediated maturation that involve the wild-type $p21^{Ras}$ (Chie et al. 2003). Decreased level of methylated H3K79 was observed soon after fertilization and the hypomethylated state was maintained at interphase (before the blastocyst stage) and variation in methylation was observed at M phase (Ooga et al. 2008) in mouse. DNA methyltransferase-1 might work during the late stage of oocyte differentiation, maturation and early embryonic development in mammals e.g. cow (Lodde et al. 2009).

2.45 Proline-rich inositol phosphate 5-phosphatase (PIPP)

Different types of inositol polyphosphate 5-phosphatases (IPP) selectively remove the phosphate from the 5-position of the inositol ring from both soluble and lipid substrates, i.e., inositol 1,4,5-trisphosphate, inositol 1,3,4,5-tetrakisphosphate, phosphatidylinositol 4,5-bisphosphate or phosphatidylinositol 3,4,5-trisphosphate and they have various protein modules probably responsible for specific cell organelle localization or recruitment e.g. SH2 domain, SH3-binding motif, proline-rich sequences, etc. (Erneux et al. 1998; Kong et al. 2000; Mochizuki and Takenawa 1999). They demonstrate the restricted substrate specificity and act downstream of various receptors by removing a phosphate. Proline-rich IPP (**PIPP**) had been studied in PI3K pathway for early development of fertilized mouse eggs. PIPP might affect development of fertilized mouse eggs by inhibition of level of phosphorylated Akt at Ser-473 and subsequent inhibition of downstream signal cascades resulting reduced cleavage rate of fertilized mouse eggs (Deng et al. 2011). In embryonic day 15.5 mice, SHIP2 a homologue of SHIP1 was strongly expressed in the liver, specific regions of the central nervous system, the thymus, the lung, and the cartilage perichondrium (Schurmans et al. 1999).

2.46 Protein phosphatase 1/2A (PP1/PP2A)

Numerous protein kinases and phosphatases have important functions during mitosis and meiosis. Protein phosphatase (PP) 1 (**PP1**) and 2A (**PP2A**) that preferentially dephosphorylate the β- and α-subunit of phosphorylase kinase had been identified in starfish oocyte (Pondaven and Cohen 1987). With the similar mechanism involved in mammals and *Drosophila*, PP4, a centrosomal protein, involved in the recruitment of pericentriolar material components to the centrosome from prophase to telophase, but not during interphase, and is essential for the activation of microtubule nucleation that promote spindle formation in *C. elegans* (Sumiyoshi et al. 2002). When the normal physiological function of PP1 and PP2A was blocked, premature separation of sister chromatids during meiosis I and aneuploidy in mouse oocytes was observed (Mailhes et al. 2003). In *Xenopus* oocyte, PP2A negatively regulates Cdc2 activation whereas Aurora-A activation is indirectly controlled by Cdc2 activity independent of either PP1 or PP2A activity (Maton et al. 2005). Constant cyclin B levels are maintained during a CSF arrest through the regulation of Emi2 activity that inhibits the anaphase-promoting complex (APC), an E3 ubiquitin ligase that targets cyclin B for degradation in vertebrates like *Xenopus* (Wu et al. 2007b). Rsk or Cdc2-mediated phosphorylation of Emi2 was antagonized by PP2A, which could bind to Emi2 and promote Emi2-APC interactions results CSF arrest (Wu et al. 2007a; Wu et al. 2007b). Cdk1/cyclin B (MPF) induced active Gwl promotes PP2A (B55 is the regulatory subunit) inhibition to enter and maintenance the M phase that would otherwise remove MPF-driven phosphorylations (Castilho et al. 2009; Vigneron et al. 2009).

2.47 Protein tyrosine phosphatase (PTP)

In the early steps of embryogenesis both the protein tyrosine phosphorylation and the protein tyrosine phosphatase (**PTP**) regulated activities are involved. In *Xenopus* MPF and progesterone but not insulin-induced oocyte maturation was retarded by PTPase 1B action (Tonks et al. 1990) whereas non receptor PTP13 activate the oocyte maturation (Nedachi and Conti 2004). PTP exert its role by different mechanism for example, PTP regulate the oocyte maturation in pig (Kim et al. 1999a), receptor-type PTP regulate Fyn in zebrafish egg fertilization (Wu and Kinsey 2002), Src homology-2 domain containing PTP (SHP2) regulate normal human trophoblast proliferation (Forbes et al. 2009), and pseudo-PTP (lack at least one key residue in the catalytic site) regulate oocyte-embryo transition in nematode (Heighington and Kipreos 2009) and antagonist of PTP reduced GVBD and MAPK/MPF activities in sea water treated marine nemertean worms oocytes (Stricker and Smythe 2006). Receptor type PTP and PTP are essential for convergence and extension cell movements to shape the body axis during vertebrate gastrulation e.g. for zebrafish in a signaling pathway parallel to non-canonical Wnt and upstream of Fyn, Yes and RhoA (van Eekelen et al. 2010).

2.48 Pumilio1/2

In *Xenopus*, the cytoplasmic polyadenylation element (CPE) in the 3′-untranslated region (UTR) of cyclin B1 mRNA is responsible for both the translational repression (masking) and activation (unmasking) of the mRNA where CPE is bound by a CPE-binding (CPEB) protein (Hake and Richter 1994; Hodgman et al. 2001; Mendez and Richter 2001). *Xenopus* **pumilio** (Pum) in coordination with CPEB-maskin complex acts as a specific regulator for timing translational activation of cyclin B1 mRNA first as repressor in mature oocyte by binding and as activator by its release from phosphorylated CPEB during oocyte maturation (Nakahata et al. 2003). Usually nemo-like kinase (NLK) that acts downstream of Mos, phosphorylate Pum1, Pum2 and CPEB and this phosphorylation is proceeded with translational activation of cyclin B1 mRNA stored in oocytes for maturation (Ota et al. 2011a; Ota et al. 2011b).

2.49 $p21^{Ras}$

In *Xenopus* oocytes, transformed/active **$p21^{Ras}$** increased the level of total cell protein phosphorylation that culminated with germinal vesicle breakdown (GVBD) in the absence of protein synthesis and the same pattern of phosphorylation was observed by hormone either progesterone or insulin treatment (Nebreda et al. 1993). Activated $p21^{Ras}$ and GTPase-activating protein (GAP) complex may promote MAPK activity by tyrosine phosphorylation followed by the activation of S6-kinase II (Nebreda et al. 1993; Pomerance et al. 1992). Later it was shown that Ras-GAP activity is required for Cdc2 activation and Mos induction independent of MAPK activation (Pomerance et al. 1996). It should be note that active Ras increased MAPK and S6K activities and sensitized the oocytes to insulin-stimulated maturation via IRS-1 (Chuang et al. 1994). T-Cell Origin protein Kinase (TOPK) and the nuclear kinase, DYRK1A are attractive candidates in insulin mediated wild-type $p21^{Ras}$-induced oocyte maturation independent of MAPK (Qu et al. 2006; Qu et al. 2007). Phospholipase D (PLD) activity induced MAPK and S6K II activity might constitute a relevant step in Ras-induced GVBD in *Xenopus* oocytes was also reported (Carnero and Lacal 1995). $p21^{Ras}$ did not appear to be ubiquitous in the rat conceptus prior to gastrulation but was found in embryos from 6.5 to 12 days of age (Brewer and Brown 1992).

2.50 Phosphatidylinositol 3-kinase (PI3K)

PI3K is a lipid kinase that phosphorylates 3′-position in the inositol ling structure of inositol phospholipids (e.g. phosphatidylinositol 4,5-bisphosphate). Inactive PI3K consists of a heterodimer of one catalytic subunit (e.g. p110) and one regulatory subunit (e.g. p85), a latter of which is known to be tyrosine-phosphorylated in response to a variety of extracellular signals (Vanhaesebroeck et al. 1997). The tyrosine-phosphorylated regulatory subunit releases the catalytic subunit so that PI3K becomes enzymatically active. Involvement of PI3K in oocyte maturation and fertilization has been examined with the use of specific inhibitors such as LY294002 and Wortmannin as well as expression of native or mutant PI3K proteins (Chuang et al. 1993a; Hoshino and Sato 2008; Hoshino et al. 2004; Mammadova et al. 2009). In starfish oocyte, 1-methyladenine-induced oocyte maturation involves a sequential activation of the hormone receptor on the cell surface, G-proteins attached to the receptor, and PI3K. The activated PI3K promotes Akt kinase activation through the production of PIP_3 and stimulation of PIP_3-dependent protein kinase PDK1 (Kishimoto 2011). In oocytes of *Xenopus* or other frog species, PI3K is suggested to be a component of progesterone-induced oocyte maturation (Bagowski et al. 2001; Ota et al. 2008). However, wortmannin promotes oocyte maturation in the absence of hormonal signal (Carnero and Lacal 1998), suggesting the possibility that this drug targets unknown factor(s) other than PI3K or that, as opposed to the case in starfish, PI3K is negative regulator of oocyte maturation. On the other hand, LY294002 has been shown to block sperm-induced egg activation (Mammadova et al. 2009). LY294002 also blocks sperm-induced Src activation and Ca^{2+} release, suggesting that PIP_3 production by PI3K plays a role in fertilization. Interestingly, however, tyrosine phosphorylation of p85 subunit of PI3K is not detected, suggesting that alternative pathway for PI3K activation (e.g. recruitment to membrane microdomains) is working in this system.

2.51 Phospholipase Cγ (PLCγ)

PLCγ is a member of PLC family proteins (other members are PLCβ, PLCδ, PLCε, PLCζ etc.) that hydrolyzes phosphatidylinositol 4,5-bisphosphate into DG and IP_3, both of which are second messenger to promote PKC activation and intracellular Ca^{2+} mobilization, respectively (Rhee 2001). PLCγ is the first example of non-tyrosine kinase protein, whose structure contains SH2 and SH3 domains (Stahl et al. 1988). PLCγ is also unique in its regulatory mechanism, where tyrosine phosphorylation of the protein can up-regulate the enzyme activity. Under this background, function of PLCγ in oocyte maturation and fertilization has been analyzed extensively in relation to tyrosine kinase signaling. In fact, tyrosine kinase-dependent activation of PLCγ at fertilization has been demonstrated in some vertebrate (e.g. fish, frog) and invertebrate species (e.g. ascidian, sea urchin, starfish) (Carroll et al. 1999; Carroll et al. 1997; Giusti et al. 1999; Giusti et al. 2000; Mehlmann et al. 1998; Runft et al. 2004; Runft and Jaffe 2000; Runft et al. 2002; Runft et al. 1999; Sato et al. 2002a; Sato et al. 2001; Sato et al. 2003; Sato et al. 2000b; Shearer et al. 1999; Tokmakov et al. 2002). It should be noted that Src-dependent activation of PLCγ involves a new function of PLCγ as GEF for small G-protein Ras (Bivona et al. 2003), suggesting that other means of cellular function contributes to egg activation in these species. On the other hand, Ca^{2+} release associated with mammalian fertilization does not seem to involve tyrosine kinase activity and PLCγ activation, probably because sperm-derived PLCζ activity is necessary and sufficient for sperm-induced Ca^{2+} release in these species (Kurokawa et al. 2004; Parrington et al. 2002; Saunders et al. 2002).

2.52 RNA polymerase II large subunit

RNA polymerase II (also called RNAP II or Pol II), a complex of twelve subunits (p550) is an enzyme that catalyzes the transcription of DNA to synthesize precursors of mRNA and most snRNA and microRNA (Kornberg 1999; Sims et al. 2004). A large subunit of RNAPII (p220) was shown to be phosphorylated at the onset of wheat germination that moderately increase the RNA polymerase activity (Mazus et al. 1980). In *C. elegans*, embryonically transcribed gene products are required for gastrulation initiation where a large subunit of RNAPII is involved (Powell-Coffman et al. 1996). In *Xenopus*, the largest subunit of RNA polymerase II (RPB1) accumulates in large quantities from previtellogenic early diplotene oocytes up to fully grown oocytes where the C-terminal domain (CTD) was essentially hypophosphorylated in growing oocytes from stage IV to VI (Bellier et al. 1997). Upon maturation, RPB1 is hyperphosphorylated dramatically and abruptly but dephosphorylated within 1 h after fertilization (Bellier et al. 1997). Metaphase II-arrested oocytes showed a much stronger CTD kinase activity than that of prophase stage VI and this kinase activity were attributed to the activated MAPK i.e. RPB1 could be a substrate of MAPKs (e.g. p42) during *Xenopus* oocyte maturation (Bellier et al. 1997).

2.53 Receptor for activated C kinase (RACK)

PKC, serine/threonine kinase, is a pivotal enzyme in a variety of signal transduction pathways that includes the maturation through actin cytoskeleton rearrangement and cortical granules exocytosis (CGE) to early stages of embryogenesis. The translocation of PKC is facilitated by receptor for activated C kinase (**RACK**). Activation of PKC exposes the RACK-binding site, enabling the association of the enzyme with its anchoring RACK (Ron and Mochly-Rosen 1995). Inhibition of binding the PKC to RACK blocks the function of PKC (Ron et al. 1995). During the activation of MII eggs, PKCα, βII and γ individually and RACK1 together with both PKCα and PKCβII translocate to the egg cortex (Haberman et al. 2011). The association of PKC and actin with RACK1 is known to be involved in CGE. Upon egg activation, increased level of RACK1 shuttles activated PKCs to the egg cortex, thus facilitating CGE (Haberman et al. 2011). The phytohormone abscisic acid promoted the expression level of RACK that is regulated by Gα-protein and plays an important role in a basic cellular process as well as in rice embryogenesis and germination (Komatsu et al. 2005).

2.54 Rho

The **Rho** family of small GTPases is known to organize and maintain the actin filament-dependent cytoskeleton, and rho is involved in the control mechanism of cytokinesis. Actin-depolymerizing factor (ADF)/coffilin, a key regulator for actin dynamics during cytokinesis, is suppressed and reactivated by phosphorylation and dephosphorylation respectively. Rho-induced dephosphorylation of ADF/coffilin is dependent on the XSSH (*Xenopus* homologue of Slingshot phosphatase) activation that is caused by increase in the amount of F-actin induced by Rho signaling (Tanaka et al. 2005). XSSH may reorganize actin filaments through dephosphorylation and reactivation of ADF/coffilin at early stage of contractile ring formation during *Xenopus* cleavage (Tanaka et al. 2005). In sea urchin egg, Rho is synthesized early in oogenesis in soluble form, associates with cortical granules in the end of maturation and after insemination secreted by cortical granules exocytosis and retained in the fertilization membrane indicate the involvement of Rho in Ca^{2+}-regulated exocytosis or actin reorganization that accompany the egg activation (Covian-Nares et al. 2004; Cuellar-Mata et al. 2000; Manzo et al. 2003). In ascidians Rho proteins are involved in egg deformation, ooplasmic segregation and cytokinesis downstream of the Ca^{2+} transients (Yoshida et al. 2003).

2.55 Ribosomal S6

In *Xenopus* oocytes 40S ribosomal protein **S6** becomes phosphorylated by S6K on serine residues in response to hormones or growth factors and following microinjection of the tyrosine-specific protein kinases associated with Rous sarcoma virus or Abelson murine leukemia virus. S6 is minimally phosphorylated in unstimulated oocytes and in progesterone induced *Xenopus* oocyte maturation: phosphorylation of S6 precedes germinal vesicle breakdown (GVBD) and is maximal at the time when 50% of the oocytes have undergone GVBD (Erikson and Maller 1985; Hanocq-Quertier and Baltus 1981; Nielsen et al. 1982). In *Xenopus* oocytes, Ras (p21, have GTPase activity) proteins activate the pathway linked to S6 phosphorylation and that PKC has a synergistic effect on the Ras-mediated pathway (Kamata and Kung 1990). Microinjection of purified $pp60^{v\text{-}Src}$ into *Xenopus* caused the phosphorylation of S6 and accelerated the time course of progesterone-induced oocyte maturation (Spivack et al. 1984).

2.56 RINGO

RINGO/Speedy (Rapid Inducer of G2/M transition in Oocytes) proteins can bind to and directly stimulate CDKs (CDK1 and CDK2) that regulate cell cycle transition although they do not have amino acid sequence homology with cyclins. In *Xenopus* oocytes RINGO (XRINGO) accumulates transiently during meiosis I entry and this process is directly stimulated by several kinases, including PKA and GSK3β, and contributes to the maintenance of G2 arrest (Gutierrez et al. 2006). Later XRINGO is down-regulated/degraded after meiosis I that is mediated by the ubiquitin ligase Siah-2, which probably requires phosphorylation of XRINGO on Ser-243 and important for the omission of S phase at the meiosis-I-meiosis-II transition in *Xenopus* oocytes and finally trigger G2/M progression (Gutierrez et al. 2006; Karaiskou et al. 2001). p42 MAPK (ERK2) activity and RINGO accumulation are also required for activating phosphorylation of CPEB by Cdk1.

RINGO/Speedy, is necessary for CPEB-directed polyadenylation-induced translation of Mos and cyclin B1 mRNAs in maturing *Xenopus* oocytes (Padmanabhan and Richter 2006). Recently, it was shown that XGef (a Rho family guanine nucleotide exchange factor) is involved in XRINGO/CDK1-mediated activation of CPEB and that an XGef/XRINGO/ERK2/CPEB complex forms in ovo to facilitate the maturation process (Kuo et al. 2011). In mammals for example in porcine RINGO A2 (SPDYA2) speed up the oocyte maturation (Kume et al. 2007) and in mouse RINGO efficiently triggers meiosis resumption of oocytes and induces cell cycle arrest in embryos (Terret et al. 2001).

2.57 Sam68 adaptor protein (Sam68)

Sam68 is a KH domain-containing, STAR (signal transduction and activation of RNA) family RNA-binding protein that has been originally identified as a mitosis-specific Src-phosphorylated protein of 68 kDa (Taylor et al. 1995; Taylor and Shalloway 1994). Sam68 has also a proline-rich sequence that would interact with SH3 domain-containing proteins, linking its possible function to Src-dependent signal transduction pathways. The RNA-binding ability of Sam68 contributes to, like hnRNP K, another KH-containing RNA-binding protein, posttranscriptional regulation of mRNAs (e.g. splicing, translation). While its physiological function in spermatogenesis has been well known to date (Sette et al. 2010), roles of Sam68 in the oocyte and/or egg system have just recently been shown in mammalian species: Sam68-deficient female mice are severely subfertile (Bianchi et al. 2010). Further studies demonstrated that Sam68 directly binds the mRNAs for the follicle-stimulating hormone (FSH) and the luteinizing hormone (LH) receptors (FSHR and LHR) and is involved in proper expression of these transcripts in pre-ovulatory follicles in adult ovary. Whether these Sam68 functions involve phosphorylation of Sam68 is not known.

2.58 Separase

The cysteine protease named **separase** is widely expressed in unicellular and multicellular organisms and is involved in a timely cleavage of the sister chromatid protein cohesins/SCC1 so that the separation of sister chromatids is made possible in the anaphase. The activity of separase can be negatively regulated by two mechanisms: one is the binding of securin, and the other is Cdc2-dependent phosphorylation on Ser-1126 and subsequent phospho-dependent binding of cyclin B (Nagao and Yanagida 2002; Nasmyth et al. 2000; Stemmann et al. 2001). In meiotic cell cycles in *Xenopus* oocytes, phospho-dependent inhibition of separase seems to occur: progesterone-induced oocyte maturation promotes firstly an accumulation of *Xenopus* homolog of securin, and then it undergoes degradation at the meiotic anaphase I and II in an APC/C-dependent manner (Fan et al. 2006; Holland and Taylor 2006). Mutation studies of the phosphorylation site in separase demonstrated that phospho-dependent regulation of this enzyme also works in germ cell developmental stages and early embryonic (8-cell and 16-cell) stages (Huang et al. 2009).

2.59 SHB

The adaptor protein **SHB** (Src homology 2 domain-containing adapter protein B) mediates certain responses in platelet-derived growth factor (PDGF) receptor-, fibroblast growth factor (FGF) receptor-, neural growth factor (NGF) receptor-, T cell (TC) receptor-, interleukin-2 (IL-2) receptor- and focal adhesion kinase- (FAK) signaling where in some cells the Src-like Fyn-related kinase (FRK/RAK) act upstream of SHB (Cross et al. 2002; Karlsson et al. 1998; Karlsson et al. 1995; Welsh et al. 1998).The absence of SHB enhanced ERK (extracellular-signal regulated kinase) and RSK (ribosomal S6K) signaling in mouse oocytes increasing the ribosomal protein S6 phosphorylation and activation (Calounova et al. 2010). SHB regulates normal oocyte and follicle development and that perturbation of SHB signaling causes defective meiosis I and early embryo development in mouse (Calounova et al. 2010). The SHB protein is required for normal maturation of mesoderm and efficient multilineage differentiation during in vitro differentiation of embryonic stem cells (Kriz et al. 2006; Kriz et al. 2003).

2.60 Shc adaptor protein (Shc)

Src homology and collagen (**Shc**) is an SH2-containing adaptor protein that has been identified as a mammalian proto-oncogene, whose overexpression in fibroblast cells leads to the malignant transformation (McGlade et al. 1992; Pelicci et al. 1992; Rozakis-Adcock et al. 1992). Shc consists of three isoforms (i.e. p46, p52, and p66) produced by alternative transcription and translation from one transcript and all isoforms also have an additional phosphotyrosine-binding domain in its amino-terminal region, named PTB domain. In some receptor/tyrosine kinase-mediated signal transduction pathway, Shc is recruited to the phosphotyrosine clusters of the activated receptor proteins, phosphorylated on its tyrosine residues (e.g. in mammals, Tyr-239/240 for Myc activation, Tyr-317 for MAPK/Fos activation), and recruit other SH2 and/or SH3-containing proteins (e.g. Grb2) to elicit downstream signaling cascade. In *Xenopus*, insulin-dependent oocyte maturation and egg fertilization seem to involve tyrosine kinase-dependent function of Shc (Aoto et al. 1999; Chesnel et al. 2003). Because two of three isoforms of Shc (p52 and p66) has been shown to be a direct activator of Src tyrosine kinase (Sato et al. 2002b), it is interesting to examine whether Shc-dependent Src activity contributes to these physiological events.

2.61 SNT/FRS2

Membrane anchored adaptor protein Suc1-associated neurotrophic target-1 or -2/fibroblast growth factor receptor substrate-2 or (**SNT**-1 or -2/FRS2), is implicated in the transmission of extracellular signals from several growth factor receptors e.g. fibroblast growth factor receptors (FGFRs) and neurotrophin receptors (Trks) through their N-terminal phosphotyrosine binding (PTB) domains to the mitogen-activated protein (MAP) kinase signaling cascade during embryogenesis. SNT-1 physically associates with the Src-like kinase Laloo, and SNT-1 activity is required for mesoderm induction by Laloo in *Xenopus* (Akagi et al. 2002; Hama et al. 2001). Activated FGFR and FRS2 induced Mek/MAPK activity for germinal vesicle breakdown (GVBD) and substantial H1 kinase activity might be through PI3 kinase activation for *Xenopus* oocyte maturation but not by progesterone (Mood et al. 2002). During progesterone-induced oocyte maturation Mek/MAPK activity is critical for the induction and/or maintenance of H1 kinase activity (Mood et al. 2002).

2.62 Sperm receptor/p350

During fertilization, sperm must first bind in a species-specific manner to the eggs thick extracellular coat, the zona pellucida or vitelline envelope and then undergo a form of cellular exocytosis, the acrosome reaction. Little is known about sperm-binding proteins in egg envelope of vertebrate/invertebrate species. In sea urchin the sperm receptor is phosphorylated by an egg cortical tyrosine kinase in response to sperm or purified ligand (bindin) binding within 20 sec (Abassi and Foltz 1994). In sea urchin egg, a protein (**p350**) was isolated as sperm receptor with the egg plasma membrane-vitelline layer complexes (Giusti et al. 1997) and another report have shown that EBR1 gene product serves a species-specific sperm-interacting protein on the egg vitelline envelope (Kamei and Glabe 2003). In Ascidians (*Halocynthia roretzi*), the sperm-egg binding is mediated by the molecular interaction between HrUrabin, a glycosylphosphatidylinositol-anchored CRISP (cysteine-rich secretory protein)-like protein on the sperm surface and HrVC70 on the polymorphic vitelline coat, but that HrUrabin per se is unlikely to be a direct allorecognition protein (Urayama et al. 2008). In *Xenopus* egg, gp69/64 glycoproteins are two glycoforms in the vitelline envelope and have the same number of N-linked oligosaccharide chains but differ in the extent of O-glycosylation, might serve as sperm receptor (Tian et al. 1999). In *bufo*, gp75 is expressed by previtellogenic oocytes and follicle cells and can be considered as a sperm receptor that undergoes N-terminal proteolysis during fertilization (Scarpeci et al. 2008). mZP3, a zona pellucida glycoprotein that serve as sperm receptor is unique to mammalian eggs, from mice to humans, although related glycoproteins are found in vitelline envelopes of a variety of non-mammalian eggs, from fish to birds (Wassarman and Litscher 2001).

2.63 STAT1/3

Signal transducer and activator of transcription (**STAT**) proteins are transcription factors that play the important roles in fertility and early embryonic development. STAT1 and STAT3 are known to interact with each other and the heterodimer complex enters the nucleus and controls the expression of specific genes. Several studies have reported the association of JAK/STAT signaling pathway with fertility traits in cattle. Genotype combinations of STAT1 and STAT3 are found to promote fertilization and embryonic survival in Holstein cattle (Khatib et al. 2009). Leptin that is secreted from granulosa and follicular cells through the binding of leptin receptor can trigger the phosphorylation of STAT3 during mouse oocyte maturation (Matsuoka et al. 1999). JAK-STAT signaling crucially contributes to early embryonic patterning (Baumer et al. 2011). It was reported that *Drosophila* STAT (STAT92E) in conjunction with Zelda (Zld; Zinc-finger early *Drosophila* activator), plays an important role in the transcription of the zygotic genome at the onset of embryonic development (Tsurumi et al. 2011).

2.64 Stomatin-like protein-2 (SLP-2/STML-2)

Stomatin is an integral membrane protein, which is widely expressed in many cell types. **Stomatin-like protein-2** (SLP-2; p42), a novel and unusual stomatin homologue, has been implicated in interaction with erythrocyte cytoskeleton and presumably with other integral membrane proteins. SLP-2 is overexpressed in human esophageal squamous cell carcinoma, lung cancer, laryngeal cancer, and endometrial adenocarcinoma (Zhang et al. 2006). SLP-2 is a mitochondrial protein, interact with the mitochondrial fusion mediator mitofusin 2 (Mfn2) and might be participate in mitochondrial fusion (Hajek et al. 2007). On the other hand, human erythrocytes and T-cells express plasma membrane-associated SLP-2, where it seems to act as a transmembrane signaling involving protein phosphorylation (Kirchhof et al. 2008; Wang and Morrow 2000). In *Xenopus* eggs, a 40-kDa SLP-2-like protein has been identified as a membrane microdomain-associated protein that becomes tyrosine-phosphorylated by Src in vitro and in vivo (our unpublished results), suggesting that it is a component of sperm-induced tyrosine kinase signaling at fertilization.

2.65 Transcription factor IIIA

In *Xenopus* oocytes, transcription factor IIIA (**TFIIIA**), was isolated from the cytoplasmic 7 S ribonucleoprotein complex and is phosphorylated on Ser by CKII (Westmark et al. 2002). Expression of the TFIIIA gene is differentially regulated in oogenesis, early embryos and in somatic cells in *Xenopus*. The incorporation of histone H1 into chromatin during *Xenopus* embryogenesis directs the specific repression of the TFIIIA-activated transcription of 5S rRNA genes (Bouvet et al. 1994). Phospho-form of TFIIIA may allow the factor to act as repressor for oocyte-type 5S rRNA genes (Ghose et al. 2004). TFIIIA favorably binds to the somatic nucleosome whereas H1 preferentially binds to the oocyte nucleosome, excluding TFIIIA binding in *Xenopus* oocyte (Panetta et al. 1998).

2.66 TPX2

TPX2, targeting protein for *Xenopus* kinesin-like protein (Xklp2), has multiple functions during mitosis, including microtubule nucleation around the chromosomes and the targeting of Xklp2 and Aurora A, a serine/threonine kinase, to the spindle. At the physiological conditions, TPX2 is essential for microtubule nucleation around chromatin (Brunet et al. 2004). TPX2 is required for spindle assembly and spindle pole integrity in mouse oocyte maturation (Brunet et al. 2008). In *Xenopus* oocyte, activation of the centrosomal Aurora A by TPX2 is required during spindle assembly (Sardon et al. 2008). Localized Aurora A kinase activity is required to target the factors involved in microtubule (MT) nucleation and stabilization to the centrosome, therefore promoting the formation of a MT aster (Sardon et al. 2008). In *Xenopus*, TPX2 is required for nearly all Aurora A activation and for full p53 synthesis and phosphorylation during oocyte maturation (Pascreau et al. 2009).

2.67 Tr-kit

The c-kit, a tyrosine kinase receptor, is consists of an extracellular ligand binding domain and an intracellular kinase domain. With the onset of meiosis c-kit expression ceases, but a truncated c-kit product, **Tr-kit**, is specifically expressed in post-meiotic stages of spermatogenesis, and is accumulated in mature spermatozoa (Rossi et al. 2000). Fyn is localized in the cortex region underneath the plasma membrane in mouse oocytes. The interaction of Tr-kit with Fyn, make the Fyn active and that phosphorylate PLCγ1 with the result of Ca^{2+} oscillation (Sette et al. 2002). The truncated c-kit protein is present in primary tumors and shows a correlation between Tr-kit expression and activation of the Src pathway in the advanced stages of human prostate cancer (Paronetto et al. 2004). Recently it was shown that Tr-kit is present in the equatorial region of human spermatozoa, which are the first sperm components that enter into the oocyte cytoplasm after fusion with the egg (Muciaccia et al. 2010).

2.68 Tubulin β

Several studies were carried out to reveal the function of **tubulin** in some species oocytes to embryo because the spindle of vertebrate eggs must remain stable and well organized during the second meiotic arrest. The transition of tubulin from the quiescent oocyte state to that competent to form spindle microtubules may involve the changes in the availability of microtubule and qualitative changes in tubulin mRNAs occurred between the early blastula and hatched blastula stages in sea urchin embryos (Alexandraki and Ruderman 1985). Tubulin β1 mRNA is evenly distributed during early embryogenesis but in later stages of embryogenesis is predominantly expressed in neural derivatives whereas tubulin β3 mRNA is restricted to the mesoderm in *Drosophila* (Gasch et al. 1988). Vg1 RBP is associated with microtubules and co-precipitated by heterologous, polymerized tubulin in *Xenopus* oocytes (Elisha et al. 1995). It was shown recently that Fyn and tubulin are closely associated where Fyn can phosphorylate tubulin and thus SFKs mediate significant functions during the organization of the MII spindle that involves possibly microtubules in rat eggs (Talmor-Cohen et al. 2004). Similarly, well-organized microtubule formation increased the GVBD and MII development in mouse oocytes (Mohammadi Roushandeh and Habibi Roudkenar 2009).

2.69 Ubiquitin-proteasome pathway

The **ubiquitin-proteasome** pathway (Schonfelder et al. 2006) is involved in the degradation of proteins e.g. cyclin B, a regulatory subunit of MPF that are related to oocyte meiotic maturation, fertilization and embryogenesis. Proteasome (26S) catalyzes the ATP- and ubiquitin-dependent degradation of Mos in an early stage of meiotic maturation of *Xenopus* oocytes and egg activation (Aizawa et al. 1996; Ishida et al. 1993). *Xenopus* RINGO/Speedy, a direct activator of Cdk1 and Cdk2, is limitedly processed by UPP to maintenance of G2 arrest and fully degraded by the ubiquitin ligase Siah-2 during MI-MII transition (Gutierrez et al. 2006). UPP is important for oocyte meiotic maturation, fertilization, and early embryonic mitosis and may play its roles by regulating cyclin B1 degradation and MAPK/p90^{Rsk} phosphorylation in pig (Huo et al. 2004a; Sun et al. 2004) and in mouse (Huo et al. 2004b; Karabinova et al. 2011; Tan et al. 2005a). UPP is required for meiotic maturation of rat oocyte (Tan et al. 2005b). In gold fish, cyclin B degradation is initiated by the ATP-dependent and ubiquitin-independent proteolytic activity of 26S proteasome and then the cyclin to be ubiquitinated for further destruction by ubiquitin-dependent activity of the 26S proteasome that leads to MPF inactivation (Tokumoto et al. 1997).

2.70 Uroplakin Ib/III (UPIb/UPIII)

Uroplakins (UP; UPIa, UPIb, UPII, UPIIIa and UPIIIb) were first identified in highly differentiated somatic cells plasma membrane called asymmetric unit membrane (AUM), which is believed to play a protective role. Recently, they were identified in genital tract (Kalma et al. 2009; Shapiro et al. 2000) and germ cells and their function has been described in *Xenopus* fertilization (Mahbub Hasan et al. 2011; Sakakibara et al. 2005; Sato et al. 2006), pathogen infection (Thumbikat et al. 2009a; Thumbikat et al. 2009b) and cancer (Matsumoto et al. 2008). In *Xenopus*, UPIIIa a single transmembrane protein is tyrosine phosphorylated transiently in the cytosolic domain by a tyrosine kinase Src and this tyrosine phosphorylation is required for sperm mediated egg activation. UPIIIa was shaded in the extracellular domain by cathepsin B like activity that is present in sperm and this activity are essential for egg activation and fertilization (Mahbub Hasan et al. 2005; Mizote et al. 1999). UPIIIa can serve as sperm receptor as the antibody against the extracellular domain of UPIIIa inhibited the fertilization (Sakakibara et al. 2005). UPIIIa is an interactive partner of UPIb, a tetraspanin and their interaction is required to negatively regulate the Src activity (Mahbub Hasan et al. 2007).

2.71 Vg1RBP

Xenopus **Vg1RBP** (RNA binding protein), also known as Vera or IMP3, is a member of the highly conserved IMP family of four KH (hnRNP K-homologous)-domain RNA binding proteins, with roles in RNA localization, translational control, RNA stability, and cell motility. *Xenopus* Vg1 mRNA is localized to the vegetal cortex during oogenesis for the regulation of germ layer formation and germ cell development where proteins e.g. Vg1RBP/Vera that specifically recognize the vegetal localization element (VLE) within the 3' untranslated region. It is reported that multiple KH domains are important in mediating RNA-protein and protein-protein interactions in the formation of a stable complex of Vg1RBP and Vg1 mRNA (Git and Standart 2002). PTB/hnRNP I (ribonucleo protein) is required for remodeling of the interaction between Vg1 mRNA and Vg1RBP/Vera in *Xenopus* oocytes (Lewis et al. 2008). Vg1RBP undergoes regulated phosphorylation by Erk2 MAPK during meiotic maturation in *Xenopus* (Git et al. 2009).

2.72 XEEK

The PAR-4 and PAR-1 kinases are necessary for the formation of the anterior-posterior (A-P) axis in *C. elegans*. The *Drosophila* PAR-4 homologue, LKB1, is required for the early A-P polarity of the oocyte, and for the repolarization of the oocyte cytoskeleton that defines the embryonic A-P axis in *Drosophila* (Martin and St Johnston 2003) and in mouse (Szczepanska and Maleszewski 2005). PKA phosphorylates *Drosophila* LKB1 on a conserved site that is important for its activity(Martin and St Johnston 2003). **LKB1/XEEK1** (*Xenopus* egg and embryo kinase 1) is found to exist in a complex with GSK3 and PKC, a known kinase for GSK3 and to regulate GSK3 phosphorylation resulting in increased Wnt-catenin signal in *Xenopus* embryonic development and mammalian cells (Clements and Kimelman 2003; Ossipova et al. 2003).

2.73 Xp95

In *Xenopus* oocytes, a protein **Xp95** is tyrosine-phosphorylated from the first through the second meiotic divisions during progesterone-induced oocyte maturation. The Xp95 protein sequence exhibited homology to mouse Rhophilin, budding yeast Bro1, and *Aspergillus* PalA, all of which are important in signal transduction (Che et al. 1999). Src kinase mediated phosphorylation of Xp95 was increased during oocyte maturation (Che et al. 1999). Xp95 is phosphorylated at multiple sites within the N-terminal half of the proline-rich domain (PRD) during *Xenopus* oocyte maturation and the phosphorylation may both positively and negatively modulate their interaction with partner proteins at different stage of cell cycle (Dejournett et al. 2007). Human homologue of Xp95, termed Hp95, induces G1 phase arrest in confluent HeLa cells when overexpressed (Wu et al. 2001).

2.74 Tyrosine 3-monooxygenase/tryptophan 5-monooxygenase activation protein (YWHA)/14-3-3

The tyrosine 3-monooxygenase/tryptophan 5-monooxygenase activation protein family (**YWHA**; also known as 14-3-3) are involved in the regulation of many intracellular processes. PKB, PKC and JNK target 14-3-3 to phosphorylate at different sites (Aitken 2006). YWHA might play the role regulating peptidylarginine deiminase type VI (PADI6), that undergo a dramatic developmental change in phosphorylation during mouse oocyte maturation until two cell stage (Snow et al. 2008). 14-3-3 protein binds to Cdc25C and inhibits dephosphorylation of Ser-287 by PP2A, allowing the arrest in the meiotic metaphase II in *Xenopus* oocytes (Hutchins et al. 2002). If 14-3-3 binding to Cdc25 is prevented while nuclear export is inhibited, the coordinate nuclear accumulation of Cdc25 that dephosphorylates Cdc2-cyclin B1 to make it active, which promotes oocyte maturation (Yang et al. 1999).

3. Conclusion

Since the discovery in the late 1800's of the gamete membrane interaction and fusion as an initial and indispensable process for the beginning of life, i.e. fertilization, a number of research have dealt with the molecular and cellular basis of fertilization. In this chapter, we have reviewed the structure and function of key molecules likely involved in the phospho-signaling at oocyte maturation, sperm-egg interaction and subsequent events for activation of development, collectively called "egg activation". This work is an updated version of the review paper that we published in 2000 (Sato et al. 2000a), and thus a special focus point in this chapter is the kinases (both tyrosine kinases and serine/threonine kinases, total number of 53) and their regulators and/or substrates expressed in oocytes/eggs and/or early embryos of animal species (including some algae, total number of 74). We have compiled the currently available knowledge in the molecular level to explore the general as well as the species-specific features of oocyte maturation and fertilization, which is widely employed as an only-one strategy to give rise to a newborn in the bisexual reproduction system. It seems that number of kinases and their regulators/substrates will still be growing from day to day, and we may miss some important molecules in this chapter: we would continue to update that information not cited here in a future. Although the phospho-signaling system is just one kind of the post-translational modifications of cellular proteins, other kinds of steps e.g. transcriptional regulations or post-transcriptional modifications would also contribute to oocyte maturation and fertilization. We hope that this chapter could be helpful and enthusiastic for the readers in any kind of research field that deals with molecular (in particular, cellular proteins') network involved in physiological and/or pathological features of biological system.

4. Acknowledgements

We apologize to those whose work was not cited or insufficiently cited. This work is supported by a Grant-in-Aid on Innovative Areas (22112522), and a grant for Private University Strategic Research Foundation Support Program (S0801060) from the Ministry of Education, Culture, Sports, Science and Technology, Japan to K.S.

5. References

Abassi YA, Foltz KR. 1994. Tyrosine phosphorylation of the egg receptor for sperm at fertilization. Dev Biol 164(2):430-443.

Abe H, Obinata T, Minamide LS, Bamburg JR. 1996. Xenopus laevis actin-depolymerizing factor/cofilin: a phosphorylation-regulated protein essential for development. J Cell Biol 132(5):871-885.

Acevedo N, Ding J, Smith GD. 2007. Insulin signaling in mouse oocytes. Biol Reprod 77(5):872-879.

Achour-Frydman N, Ledee N, Fallet C. 2010. [Secrets of proportions in follicular liquid]. J Gynecol Obstet Biol Reprod (Paris) 39(1 Suppl):2-4.

Aitken A. 2006. 14-3-3 proteins: a historic overview. Semin Cancer Biol 16(3):162-172.

Aizawa H, Kawahara H, Tanaka K, Yokosawa H. 1996. Activation of the proteasome during Xenopus egg activation implies a link between proteasome activation and intracellular calcium release. Biochem Biophys Res Commun 218(1):224-228.

Akagi K, Kyun Park E, Mood K, Daar IO. 2002. Docking protein SNT1 is a critical mediator of fibroblast growth factor signaling during Xenopus embryonic development. Dev Dyn 223(2):216-228.

Alexandraki D, Ruderman JV. 1985. Expression of alpha- and beta-tubulin genes during development of sea urchin embryos. Dev Biol 109(2):436-451.

Amano H, Fujita T, Hiramatsu N, Kagawa H, Matsubara T, Sullivan CV, Hara A. 2008. Multiple vitellogenin-derived yolk proteins in gray mullet (Mugil cephalus): disparate proteolytic patterns associated with ovarian follicle maturation. Mol Reprod Dev 75(8):1307-1317.

Aoto M, Sato K, Takeba S, Horiuchi Y, Iwasaki T, Tokmakov AA, Fukami Y. 1999. A 58-kDa Shc protein is present in Xenopus eggs and is phosphorylated on tyrosine residues upon egg activation. Biochem Biophys Res Commun 258(2):265-270.

Armant DR, Kilburn BA, Petkova A, Edwin SS, Duniec-Dmuchowski ZM, Edwards HJ, Romero R, Leach RE. 2006. Human trophoblast survival at low oxygen concentrations requires metalloproteinase-mediated shedding of heparin-binding EGF-like growth factor. Development 133(4):751-759.

Asano Y, Mabuchi I. 2001. Calyculin-A, an inhibitor for protein phosphatases, induces cortical contraction in unfertilized sea urchin eggs. Cell Motil Cytoskeleton 48(4):245-261.

Baessler KA, Lee Y, Sampson NS. 2009. Beta1 integrin is an adhesion protein for sperm binding to eggs. ACS Chem Biol 4(5):357-366.

Bagowski CP, Myers JW, Ferrell JE, Jr. 2001. The classical progesterone receptor associates with p42 MAPK and is involved in phosphatidylinositol 3-kinase signaling in Xenopus oocytes. J Biol Chem 276(40):37708-37714.

Bamburg JR, McGough A, Ono S. 1999. Putting a new twist on actin: ADF/cofilins modulate actin dynamics. Trends Cell Biol 9(9):364-370.

Barr KJ, Garrill A, Jones DH, Orlowski J, Kidder GM. 1998. Contributions of Na+/H+ exchanger isoforms to preimplantation development of the mouse. Mol Reprod Dev 50(2):146-153.

Baumer D, Trauner J, Hollfelder D, Cerny A, Schoppmeier M. 2011. JAK-STAT signalling is required throughout telotrophic oogenesis and short-germ embryogenesis of the beetle Tribolium. Dev Biol 350(1):169-182.

Bellier S, Dubois MF, Nishida E, Almouzni G, Bensaude O. 1997. Phosphorylation of the RNA polymerase II largest subunit during Xenopus laevis oocyte maturation. Mol Cell Biol 17(3):1434-1440.

Bergeron L, Perez GI, Macdonald G, Shi L, Sun Y, Jurisicova A, Varmuza S, Latham KE, Flaws JA, Salter JC, Hara H, Moskowitz MA, Li E, Greenberg A, Tilly JL, Yuan J. 1998. Defects in regulation of apoptosis in caspase-2-deficient mice. Genes Dev 12(9):1304-1314.

Bergink EW, Wallace RA. 1974. Precursor-product relationship between amphibian vitellogenin and the yolk proteins, lipovitellin and phosvitin. J Biol Chem 249(9):2897-2903.

Bianchi E, Barbagallo F, Valeri C, Geremia R, Salustri A, De Felici M, Sette C. 2010. Ablation of the Sam68 gene impairs female fertility and gonadotropin-dependent follicle development. Hum Mol Genet 19(24):4886-4894.

Bivona TG, Perez De Castro I, Ahearn IM, Grana TM, Chiu VK, Lockyer PJ, Cullen PJ, Pellicer A, Cox AD, Philips MR. 2003. Phospholipase Cgamma activates Ras on the Golgi apparatus by means of RasGRP1. Nature 424(6949):694-698.

Bolanos-Garcia VM, Blundell TL. 2011. BUB1 and BUBR1: multifaceted kinases of the cell cycle. Trends Biochem Sci 36(3):141-150.

Bomsztyk K, Denisenko O, Ostrowski J. 2004. hnRNP K: one protein multiple processes. Bioessays 26(6):629-638.

Bonilla AQ, Oliveira LJ, Ozawa M, Newsom EM, Lucy MC, Hansen PJ. 2011. Developmental changes in thermoprotective actions of insulin-like growth factor-1 on the preimplantation bovine embryo. Mol Cell Endocrinol 332(1-2):170-179.

Bouvet P, Dimitrov S, Wolffe AP. 1994. Specific regulation of Xenopus chromosomal 5S rRNA gene transcription in vivo by histone H1. Genes Dev 8(10):1147-1159.

Branno M, De Franciscis V, Tosi L. 1983. In vitro methylation of histones in sea urchin nuclei during early embryogenesis. Biochim Biophys Acta 741(1):136-142.

Brewer LM, Brown NA. 1992. Distribution of p21ras in postimplantation rat embryos. Anat Rec 234(3):443-451.

Brewis IA, Clayton R, Browes CE, Martin M, Barratt CL, Hornby DP, Moore HD. 1998. Tyrosine phosphorylation of a 95 kDa protein and induction of the acrosome reaction in human spermatozoa by recombinant human zona pellucida glycoprotein 3. Mol Hum Reprod 4(12):1136-1144.

Browaeys-Poly E, Broutin I, Antoine AF, Marin M, Lescuyer A, Vilain JP, Ducruix A, Cailliau K. 2007. A non-canonical Grb2-PLC-gamma1-Sos cascade triggered by lipovitellin 1, an apolipoprotein B homologue. Cell Signal 19(12):2540-2548.

Brunet A, Bonni A, Zigmond MJ, Lin MZ, Juo P, Hu LS, Anderson MJ, Arden KC, Blenis J, Greenberg ME. 1999. Akt promotes cell survival by phosphorylating and inhibiting a Forkhead transcription factor. Cell 96(6):857-868.

Brunet S, Dumont J, Lee KW, Kinoshita K, Hikal P, Gruss OJ, Maro B, Verlhac MH. 2008. Meiotic regulation of TPX2 protein levels governs cell cycle progression in mouse oocytes. PLoS One 3(10):e3338.

Brunet S, Sardon T, Zimmerman T, Wittmann T, Pepperkok R, Karsenti E, Vernos I. 2004. Characterization of the TPX2 domains involved in microtubule nucleation and spindle assembly in Xenopus egg extracts. Mol Biol Cell 15(12):5318-5328.

Bugner V, Aurhammer T, Kuhl M. 2011. Xenopus laevis insulin receptor substrate IRS-1 is important for eye development. Dev Dyn 240(7):1705-1715.

Bui HT, Van Thuan N, Kishigami S, Wakayama S, Hikichi T, Ohta H, Mizutani E, Yamaoka E, Wakayama T, Miyano T. 2007. Regulation of chromatin and chromosome morphology by histone H3 modifications in pig oocytes. Reproduction 133(2):371-382.

Burks DJ, Carballada R, Moore HD, Saling PM. 1995. Interaction of a tyrosine kinase from human sperm with the zona pellucida at fertilization. Science 269(5220):83-86.

Busch S. 1997. Cloning and sequencing of the cDNA encoding for a Na+/H+ exchanger from Xenopus laevis oocytes (X1-NHE). Biochim Biophys Acta 1325(1):13-16.

Busch S, Wieland T, Esche H, Jakobs KH, Siffert W. 1995. G protein regulation of the Na+/H+ antiporter in Xenopus laevis oocytes. Involvement of protein kinases A and C. J Biol Chem 270(30):17898-17901.

Buszczak M, Cooley L. 2000. Eggs to die for: cell death during Drosophila oogenesis. Cell Death Differ 7(11):1071-1074.

Cailliau K, Browaeys-Poly E, Broutin-L'Hermite I, Nioche P, Garbay C, Ducruix A, Vilain JP. 2001. Grb2 promotes reinitiation of meiosis in Xenopus oocytes. Cell Signal 13(1):51-55.

Cailliau K, Le Marcis V, Bereziat V, Perdereau D, Cariou B, Vilain JP, Burnol AF, Browaeys-Poly E. 2003. Inhibition of FGF receptor signalling in Xenopus oocytes: differential effect of Grb7, Grb10 and Grb14. FEBS Lett 548(1-3):43-48.

Calounova G, Livera G, Zhang XQ, Liu K, Gosden RG, Welsh M. 2010. The Src homology 2 domain-containing adapter protein B (SHB) regulates mouse oocyte maturation. PLoS One 5(6):e11155.

Capco DG, Tutnick JM, Bement WM. 1992. The role of protein kinase C in reorganization of the cortical cytoskeleton during the transition from oocyte to fertilization-competent egg. J Exp Zool 264(4):395-405.

Carnero A, Lacal JC. 1995. Activation of intracellular kinases in Xenopus oocytes by p21ras and phospholipases: a comparative study. Mol Cell Biol 15(2):1094-1101.

Carnero A, Lacal JC. 1998. Wortmannin, an inhibitor of phosphatidyl-inositol 3-kinase, induces oocyte maturation through a MPF-MAPK-dependent pathway. FEBS Lett 422(2):155-159.

Carroll DJ, Albay DT, Terasaki M, Jaffe LA, Foltz KR. 1999. Identification of PLCgamma-dependent and -independent events during fertilization of sea urchin eggs. Dev Biol 206(2):232-247.

Carroll DJ, Ramarao CS, Mehlmann LM, Roche S, Terasaki M, Jaffe LA. 1997. Calcium release at fertilization in starfish eggs is mediated by phospholipase Cgamma. J Cell Biol 138(6):1303-1311.

Castilho PV, Williams BC, Mochida S, Zhao Y, Goldberg ML. 2009. The M phase kinase Greatwall (Gwl) promotes inactivation of PP2A/B55delta, a phosphatase directed against CDK phosphosites. Mol Biol Cell 20(22):4777-4789.

Chao MV, Hempstead BL. 1995. p75 and Trk: a two-receptor system. Trends Neurosci 18(7):321-326.

Che S, El-Hodiri HM, Wu CF, Nelman-Gonzalez M, Weil MM, Etkin LD, Clark RB, Kuang J. 1999. Identification and cloning of xp95, a putative signal transduction protein in Xenopus oocytes. J Biol Chem 274(9):5522-5531.

Chen GC, Turano B, Ruest PJ, Hagel M, Settleman J, Thomas SM. 2005. Regulation of Rho and Rac signaling to the actin cytoskeleton by paxillin during Drosophila development. Mol Cell Biol 25(3):979-987.

Cheng KC, Klancer R, Singson A, Seydoux G. 2009. Regulation of MBK-2/DYRK by CDK-1 and the pseudophosphatases EGG-4 and EGG-5 during the oocyte-to-embryo transition. Cell 139(3):560-572.

Cheng Y, Yata A, Klein C, Cho JH, Deguchi M, Hsueh AJ. 2011. Oocyte-expressed interleukin 7 suppresses granulosa cell apoptosis and promotes oocyte maturation in rats. Biol Reprod 84(4):707-714.

Chesnel F, Bonnec G, Tardivel A, Boujard D. 1997. Comparative effects of insulin on the activation of the Raf/Mos-dependent MAP kinase cascade in vitellogenic versus postvitellogenic Xenopus oocytes. Dev Biol 188(1):122-133.

Chesnel F, Heligon C, Richard-Parpaillon L, Boujard D. 2003. Molecular cloning and characterization of an adaptor protein Shc isoform from Xenopus laevis oocytes. Biol Cell 95(5):311-320.

Chiba K. 2004. MI arrest and apoptosis in starfish oocytes. Zoolog Sci 21(12):1193.

Chie L, Cook JR, Chung D, Hoffmann R, Yang Z, Kim Y, Pestka S, Pincus MR. 2003. A protein methyl transferase, PRMT5, selectively blocks oncogenic ras-p21 mitogenic signal transduction. Ann Clin Lab Sci 33(2):200-207.

Chiu TT, Patel N, Shaw AE, Bamburg JR, Klip A. 2010. Arp2/3- and cofilin-coordinated actin dynamics is required for insulin-mediated GLUT4 translocation to the surface of muscle cells. Mol Biol Cell 21(20):3529-3539.

Choi M, Lee OH, Jeon S, Park M, Lee DR, Ko JJ, Yoon TK, Rajkovic A, Choi Y. 2010. The oocyte-specific transcription factor, Nobox, regulates the expression of Pad6, a peptidylarginine deiminase in the oocyte. FEBS Lett 584(16):3629-3634.

Chuang LM, Hausdorff SF, Myers MG, Jr., White MF, Birnbaum MJ, Kahn CR. 1994. Interactive roles of Ras, insulin receptor substrate-1, and proteins with Src homology-2 domains in insulin signaling in Xenopus oocytes. J Biol Chem 269(44):27645-27649.

Chuang LM, Myers MG, Jr., Backer JM, Shoelson SE, White MF, Birnbaum MJ, Kahn CR. 1993a. Insulin-stimulated oocyte maturation requires insulin receptor substrate 1 and interaction with the SH2 domains of phosphatidylinositol 3-kinase. Mol Cell Biol 13(11):6653-6660.

Chuang LM, Myers MG, Jr., Seidner GA, Birnbaum MJ, White MF, Kahn CR. 1993b. Insulin receptor substrate 1 mediates insulin and insulin-like growth factor I-stimulated maturation of Xenopus oocytes. Proc Natl Acad Sci U S A 90(11):5172-5175.

Chung E, Chen RH. 2003. Phosphorylation of Cdc20 is required for its inhibition by the spindle checkpoint. Nat Cell Biol 5(8):748-753.

Clements WK, Kimelman D. 2003. Wnt signalling gets XEEKy. Nat Cell Biol 5(10):861-863.

Coles MC, Veiga-Fernandes H, Foster KE, Norton T, Pagakis SN, Seddon B, Kioussis D. 2006. Role of T and NK cells and IL7/IL7r interactions during neonatal maturation of lymph nodes. Proc Natl Acad Sci U S A 103(36):13457-13462.

Coppola D, Ouban A, Gilbert-Barness E. 2009. Expression of the insulin-like growth factor receptor 1 during human embryogenesis. Fetal Pediatr Pathol 28(2):47-54.

Cormier P, Pyronnet S, Morales J, Mulner-Lorillon O, Sonenberg N, Belle R. 2001. eIF4E association with 4E-BP decreases rapidly following fertilization in sea urchin. Dev Biol 232(2):275-283.

Covian-Nares F, Martinez-Cadena G, Lopez-Godinez J, Voronina E, Wessel GM, Garcia-Soto J. 2004. A Rho-signaling pathway mediates cortical granule translocation in the sea urchin oocyte. Mech Dev 121(3):225-235.

Cross MJ, Lu L, Magnusson P, Nyqvist D, Holmqvist K, Welsh M, Claesson-Welsh L. 2002. The Shb adaptor protein binds to tyrosine 766 in the FGFR-1 and regulates the Ras/MEK/MAPK pathway via FRS2 phosphorylation in endothelial cells. Mol Biol Cell 13(8):2881-2893.

Cuellar-Mata P, Martinez-Cadena G, Lopez-Godinez J, Obregon A, Garcia-Soto J. 2000. The GTP-binding protein RhoA localizes to the cortical granules of Strongylocentrotus purpuratas sea urchin egg and is secreted during fertilization. Eur J Cell Biol 79(2):81-91.

Danial NN. 2008. BAD: undertaker by night, candyman by day. Oncogene 27 Suppl 1:S53-70.

Dawson IA, Roth S, Akam M, Artavanis-Tsakonas S. 1993. Mutations of the fizzy locus cause metaphase arrest in Drosophila melanogaster embryos. Development 117(1):359-376.

Dejournett RE, Kobayashi R, Pan S, Wu C, Etkin LD, Clark RB, Bogler O, Kuang J. 2007. Phosphorylation of the proline-rich domain of Xp95 modulates Xp95 interaction with partner proteins. Biochem J 401(2):521-531.

Deng X, Feng C, Wang EH, Zhu YQ, Cui C, Zong ZH, Li GS, Liu C, Meng J, Yu BZ. 2011. Influence of proline-rich inositol polyphosphate 5-phosphatase, on early development of fertilized mouse eggs, via inhibition of phosphorylation of Akt. Cell Prolif 44(2):156-165.

Detwiler MR, Reuben M, Li X, Rogers E, Lin R. 2001. Two zinc finger proteins, OMA-1 and OMA-2, are redundantly required for oocyte maturation in C. elegans. Dev Cell 1(2):187-199.

Ding J, Swain JE, Smith GD. 2011. Aurora kinase-A regulates microtubule organizing center (MTOC) localization, chromosome dynamics, and histone-H3 phosphorylation in mouse oocytes. Mol Reprod Dev 78(2):80-90.

Dreyfuss G, Kim VN, Kataoka N. 2002. Messenger-RNA-binding proteins and the messages they carry. Nat Rev Mol Cell Biol 3(3):195-205.

Du Pasquier D, Dupre A, Jessus C. 2011. Unfertilized Xenopus eggs die by bad-dependent apoptosis under the control of Cdk1 and JNK. PLoS One 6(8):e23672.

Dube F, Eckberg WR. 1997. Intracellular pH increase driven by an Na+/H+ exchanger upon activation of surf clam oocytes. Dev Biol 190(1):41-54.

Eberlin A, Grauffel C, Oulad-Abdelghani M, Robert F, Torres-Padilla ME, Lambrot R, Spehner D, Ponce-Perez L, Wurtz JM, Stote RH, Kimmins S, Schultz P, Dejaegere A,

Tora L. 2008. Histone H3 tails containing dimethylated lysine and adjacent phosphorylated serine modifications adopt a specific conformation during mitosis and meiosis. Mol Cell Biol 28(5):1739-1754.

Edgecombe M, Patel R, Whitaker M. 1991. A cyclin-abundance cycle-independent p34cdc2 tyrosine phosphorylation cycle in early sea urchin embryos. EMBO J 10(12):3769-3775.

Elisha Z, Havin L, Ringel I, Yisraeli JK. 1995. Vg1 RNA binding protein mediates the association of Vg1 RNA with microtubules in Xenopus oocytes. EMBO J 14(20):5109-5114.

Eliyahu E, Tsaadon A, Shtraizent N, Shalgi R. 2005. The involvement of protein kinase C and actin filaments in cortical granule exocytosis in the rat. Reproduction 129(2):161-170.

Erikson E, Maller JL. 1985. A protein kinase from Xenopus eggs specific for ribosomal protein S6. Proc Natl Acad Sci U S A 82(3):742-746.

Erneux C, Govaerts C, Communi D, Pesesse X. 1998. The diversity and possible functions of the inositol polyphosphate 5-phosphatases. Biochim Biophys Acta 1436(1-2):185-199.

Esposito G, Vitale AM, Leijten FP, Strik AM, Koonen-Reemst AM, Yurttas P, Robben TJ, Coonrod S, Gossen JA. 2007. Peptidylarginine deiminase (PAD) 6 is essential for oocyte cytoskeletal sheet formation and female fertility. Mol Cell Endocrinol 273(1-2):25-31.

Evans EK, Lu W, Strum SL, Mayer BJ, Kornbluth S. 1997. Crk is required for apoptosis in Xenopus egg extracts. EMBO J 16(2):230-241.

Evans T, Rosenthal ET, Youngblom J, Distel D, Hunt T. 1983. Cyclin: a protein specified by maternal mRNA in sea urchin eggs that is destroyed at each cleavage division. Cell 33(2):389-396.

Eyers PA, Maller JL. 2004. Regulation of Xenopus Aurora A activation by TPX2. J Biol Chem 279(10):9008-9015.

Fan HY, Sun QY, Zou H. 2006. Regulation of Separase in meiosis: Separase is activated at the metaphase I-II transition in Xenopus oocytes during meiosis. Cell Cycle 5(2):198-204.

Feller SM, Posern G, Voss J, Kardinal C, Sakkab D, Zheng J, Knudsen BS. 1998. Physiological signals and oncogenesis mediated through Crk family adapter proteins. J Cell Physiol 177(4):535-552.

Feller SM, Ren R, Hanafusa H, Baltimore D. 1994. SH2 and SH3 domains as molecular adhesives: the interactions of Crk and Abl. Trends Biochem Sci 19(11):453-458.

Finn RN. 2007. Vertebrate yolk complexes and the functional implications of phosvitins and other subdomains in vitellogenins. Biol Reprod 76(6):926-935.

Fissore RA, Longo FJ, Anderson E, Parys JB, Ducibella T. 1999. Differential distribution of inositol trisphosphate receptor isoforms in mouse oocytes. Biol Reprod 60(1):49-57.

Fleig UN, Gould KL. 1991. Regulation of cdc2 activity in Schizosaccharomyces pombe: the role of phosphorylation. Semin Cell Biol 2(4):195-204.

Forbes K, West G, Garside R, Aplin JD, Westwood M. 2009. The protein-tyrosine phosphatase, SRC homology-2 domain containing protein tyrosine phosphatase-2, is a crucial mediator of exogenous insulin-like growth factor signaling to human trophoblast. Endocrinology 150(10):4744-4754.

Gaffre M, Martoriati A, Belhachemi N, Chambon JP, Houliston E, Jessus C, Karaiskou A. 2011. A critical balance between Cyclin B synthesis and Myt1 activity controls meiosis entry in Xenopus oocytes. Development 138(17):3735-3744.

Gallego Melcon S, Sanchez de Toledo Codina J. 2007. Molecular biology of rhabdomyosarcoma. Clin Transl Oncol 9(7):415-419.

Gallo CJ, Hand AR, Jones TL, Jaffe LA. 1995. Stimulation of Xenopus oocyte maturation by inhibition of the G-protein alpha S subunit, a component of the plasma membrane and yolk platelet membranes. J Cell Biol 130(2):275-284.

Gasch A, Hinz U, Leiss D, Renkawitz-Pohl R. 1988. The expression of beta 1 and beta 3 tubulin genes of Drosophila melanogaster is spatially regulated during embryogenesis. Mol Gen Genet 211(1):8-16.

Ghose R, Malik M, Huber PW. 2004. Restricted specificity of Xenopus TFIIIA for transcription of somatic 5S rRNA genes. Mol Cell Biol 24(6):2467-2477.

Gilman AG. 1987. G proteins: transducers of receptor-generated signals. Annu Rev Biochem 56:615-649.

Git A, Allison R, Perdiguero E, Nebreda AR, Houliston E, Standart N. 2009. Vg1RBP phosphorylation by Erk2 MAP kinase correlates with the cortical release of Vg1 mRNA during meiotic maturation of Xenopus oocytes. RNA 15(6):1121-1133.

Git A, Standart N. 2002. The KH domains of Xenopus Vg1RBP mediate RNA binding and self-association. RNA 8(10):1319-1333.

Giusti AF, Carroll DJ, Abassi YA, Foltz KR. 1999. Evidence that a starfish egg Src family tyrosine kinase associates with PLC-gamma1 SH2 domains at fertilization. Dev Biol 208(1):189-199.

Giusti AF, Hoang KM, Foltz KR. 1997. Surface localization of the sea urchin egg receptor for sperm. Dev Biol 184(1):10-24.

Giusti AF, Xu W, Hinkle B, Terasaki M, Jaffe LA. 2000. Evidence that fertilization activates starfish eggs by sequential activation of a Src-like kinase and phospholipase cgamma. J Biol Chem 275(22):16788-16794.

Goud PT, Goud AP, Van Oostveldt P, Dhont M. 1999. Presence and dynamic redistribution of type I inositol 1,4,5-trisphosphate receptors in human oocytes and embryos during in-vitro maturation, fertilization and early cleavage divisions. Mol Hum Reprod 5(5):441-451.

Gu L, Wang Q, Wang CM, Hong Y, Sun SG, Yang SY, Wang JG, Hou Y, Sun QY, Liu WQ. 2008. Distribution and expression of phosphorylated histone H3 during porcine oocyte maturation. Mol Reprod Dev 75(1):143-149.

Gutierrez GJ, Vogtlin A, Castro A, Ferby I, Salvagiotto G, Ronai Z, Lorca T, Nebreda AR. 2006. Meiotic regulation of the CDK activator RINGO/Speedy by ubiquitin-proteasome-mediated processing and degradation. Nat Cell Biol 8(10):1084-1094.

Habelhah H, Shah K, Huang L, Ostareck-Lederer A, Burlingame AL, Shokat KM, Hentze MW, Ronai Z. 2001. ERK phosphorylation drives cytoplasmic accumulation of hnRNP-K and inhibition of mRNA translation. Nat Cell Biol 3(3):325-330.

Haberman Y, Alon LT, Eliyahu E, Shalgi R. 2011. Receptor for activated C kinase (RACK) and protein kinase C (PKC) in egg activation. Theriogenology 75(1):80-89.

Hajek P, Chomyn A, Attardi G. 2007. Identification of a novel mitochondrial complex containing mitofusin 2 and stomatin-like protein 2. J Biol Chem 282(8):5670-5681.

Hake LE, Richter JD. 1994. CPEB is a specificity factor that mediates cytoplasmic polyadenylation during Xenopus oocyte maturation. Cell 79(4):617-627.

Hama J, Xu H, Goldfarb M, Weinstein DC. 2001. SNT-1/FRS2alpha physically interacts with Laloo and mediates mesoderm induction by fibroblast growth factor. Mech Dev 109(2):195-204.

Han SJ, Vaccari S, Nedachi T, Andersen CB, Kovacina KS, Roth RA, Conti M. 2006. Protein kinase B/Akt phosphorylation of PDE3A and its role in mammalian oocyte maturation. EMBO J 25(24):5716-5725.

Hanocq-Quertier J, Baltus E. 1981. Phosphorylation of ribosomal proteins during maturation of Xenopus laevis oocytes. Eur J Biochem 120(2):351-355.

Hansen DV, Tung JJ, Jackson PK. 2006. CaMKII and polo-like kinase 1 sequentially phosphorylate the cytostatic factor Emi2/XErp1 to trigger its destruction and meiotic exit. Proc Natl Acad Sci U S A 103(3):608-613.

Heck MM. 1997. Condensins, cohesins, and chromosome architecture: how to make and break a mitotic chromosome. Cell 91(1):5-8.

Heighington CS, Kipreos ET. 2009. Embryogenesis: Degenerate phosphatases control the oocyte-to-embryo transition. Curr Biol 19(20):R939-941.

Hirose T, Izumi Y, Nagashima Y, Tamai-Nagai Y, Kurihara H, Sakai T, Suzuki Y, Yamanaka T, Suzuki A, Mizuno K, Ohno S. 2002. Involvement of ASIP/PAR-3 in the promotion of epithelial tight junction formation. J Cell Sci 115(Pt 12):2485-2495.

Hodgman R, Tay J, Mendez R, Richter JD. 2001. CPEB phosphorylation and cytoplasmic polyadenylation are catalyzed by the kinase IAK1/Eg2 in maturing mouse oocytes. Development 128(14):2815-2822.

Holland AJ, Taylor SS. 2006. Cyclin-B1-mediated inhibition of excess separase is required for timely chromosome disjunction. J Cell Sci 119(Pt 16):3325-3336.

Homer H, Gui L, Carroll J. 2009. A spindle assembly checkpoint protein functions in prophase I arrest and prometaphase progression. Science 326(5955):991-994.

Hoshino Y, Sato E. 2008. Protein kinase B (PKB/Akt) is required for the completion of meiosis in mouse oocytes. Dev Biol 314(1):215-223.

Hoshino Y, Yokoo M, Yoshida N, Sasada H, Matsumoto H, Sato E. 2004. Phosphatidylinositol 3-kinase and Akt participate in the FSH-induced meiotic maturation of mouse oocytes. Mol Reprod Dev 69(1):77-86.

Huang X, Andreu-Vieyra CV, Wang M, Cooney AJ, Matzuk MM, Zhang P. 2009. Preimplantation mouse embryos depend on inhibitory phosphorylation of separase to prevent chromosome missegregation. Mol Cell Biol 29(6):1498-1505.

Hunt T. 1989. Maturation promoting factor, cyclin and the control of M-phase. Curr Opin Cell Biol 1(2):268-274.

Huo LJ, Fan HY, Liang CG, Yu LZ, Zhong ZS, Chen DY, Sun QY. 2004a. Regulation of ubiquitin-proteasome pathway on pig oocyte meiotic maturation and fertilization. Biol Reprod 71(3):853-862.

Huo LJ, Fan HY, Zhong ZS, Chen DY, Schatten H, Sun QY. 2004b. Ubiquitin-proteasome pathway modulates mouse oocyte meiotic maturation and fertilization via regulation of MAPK cascade and cyclin B1 degradation. Mech Dev 121(10):1275-1287.

Hutchins JR, Dikovskaya D, Clarke PR. 2002. Dephosphorylation of the inhibitory phosphorylation site S287 in Xenopus Cdc25C by protein phosphatase-2A is inhibited by 14-3-3 binding. FEBS Lett 528(1-3):267-271.

Inzunza J, Danielsson O, Lalitkumar PG, Larsson O, Axelson M, Tohonen V, Danielsson KG, Stavreus-Evers A. 2010. Selective insulin-like growth factor-I antagonist inhibits mouse embryo development in a dose-dependent manner. Fertil Steril 93(8):2621-2626.

Ishida N, Tanaka K, Tamura T, Nishizawa M, Okazaki K, Sagata N, Ichihara A. 1993. Mos is degraded by the 26S proteasome in a ubiquitin-dependent fashion. FEBS Lett 324(3):345-348.

Ito J, Yoon SY, Lee B, Vanderheyden V, Vermassen E, Wojcikiewicz R, Alfandari D, De Smedt H, Parys JB, Fissore RA. 2008. Inositol 1,4,5-trisphosphate receptor 1, a widespread Ca2+ channel, is a novel substrate of polo-like kinase 1 in eggs. Dev Biol 320(2):402-413.

Ito J, Yoshida T, Kasai Y, Wakai T, Parys JB, Fissore RA, Kashiwazaki N. 2010. Phosphorylation of inositol 1,4,5-triphosphate receptor 1 during in vitro maturation of porcine oocytes. Anim Sci J 81(1):34-41.

Iwasaki T, Koretomo Y, Fukuda T, Paronetto MP, Sette C, Fukami Y, Sato K. 2008. Expression, phosphorylation, and mRNA-binding of heterogeneous nuclear ribonucleoprotein K in Xenopus oocytes, eggs, and early embryos. Dev Growth Differ 50(1):23-40.

Jelinkova L, Kubelka M. 2006. Neither Aurora B activity nor histone H3 phosphorylation is essential for chromosome condensation during meiotic maturation of porcine oocytes. Biol Reprod 74(5):905-912.

Jellerette T, He CL, Wu H, Parys JB, Fissore RA. 2000. Down-regulation of the inositol 1,4,5-trisphosphate receptor in mouse eggs following fertilization or parthenogenetic activation. Dev Biol 223(2):238-250.

Jensen JT, Zelinski-Wooten MB, Schwinof KM, Vance JE, Stouffer RL. 2005. The phosphodiesterase 3 inhibitor ORG 9935 inhibits oocyte maturation during gonadotropin-stimulated ovarian cycles in rhesus macaques. Contraception 71(1):68-73.

Joberty G, Petersen C, Gao L, Macara IG. 2000. The cell-polarity protein Par6 links Par3 and atypical protein kinase C to Cdc42. Nat Cell Biol 2(8):531-539.

Jones KT, Holt JE. 2010. BubR1 highlights essential function of Cdh1 in mammalian oocytes. Cell Cycle 9(6):1029-1030.

Jordan P, Karess R. 1997. Myosin light chain-activating phosphorylation sites are required for oogenesis in Drosophila. J Cell Biol 139(7):1805-1819.

Kalinowski RR, Berlot CH, Jones TL, Ross LF, Jaffe LA, Mehlmann LM. 2004. Maintenance of meiotic prophase arrest in vertebrate oocytes by a Gs protein-mediated pathway. Dev Biol 267(1):1-13.

Kalinowski RR, Jaffe LA, Foltz KR, Giusti AF. 2003. A receptor linked to a Gi-family G-protein functions in initiating oocyte maturation in starfish but not frogs. Dev Biol 253(1):139-149.

Kalma Y, Granot I, Gnainsky Y, Or Y, Czernobilsky B, Dekel N, Barash A. 2009. Endometrial biopsy-induced gene modulation: first evidence for the expression of bladder-transmembranal uroplakin Ib in human endometrium. Fertil Steril 91(4):1042-1049, 1049 e1041-1049.

Kamata T, Kung HF. 1990. Modulation of maturation and ribosomal protein S6 phosphorylation in Xenopus oocytes by microinjection of oncogenic ras protein and protein kinase C. Mol Cell Biol 10(3):880-886.

Kamei N, Glabe CG. 2003. The species-specific egg receptor for sea urchin sperm adhesion is EBR1, a novel ADAMTS protein. Genes Dev. 17(20):2502-2507.

Kang HJ, Feng Z, Sun Y, Atwal G, Murphy ME, Rebbeck TR, Rosenwaks Z, Levine AJ, Hu W. 2009. Single-nucleotide polymorphisms in the p53 pathway regulate fertility in humans. Proc Natl Acad Sci U S A 106(24):9761-9766.

Karabinova P, Kubelka M, Susor A. 2011. Proteasomal degradation of ubiquitinated proteins in oocyte meiosis and fertilization in mammals. Cell Tissue Res.

Karaiskou A, Cayla X, Haccard O, Jessus C, Ozon R. 1998. MPF amplification in Xenopus oocyte extracts depends on a two-step activation of cdc25 phosphatase. Exp Cell Res 244(2):491-500.

Karaiskou A, Perez LH, Ferby I, Ozon R, Jessus C, Nebreda AR. 2001. Differential regulation of Cdc2 and Cdk2 by RINGO and cyclins. J Biol Chem 276(38):36028-36034.

Karlsson T, Kullander K, Welsh M. 1998. The Src homology 2 domain protein Shb transmits basic fibroblast growth factor- and nerve growth factor-dependent differentiation signals in PC12 cells. Cell Growth Differ 9(9):757-766.

Karlsson T, Songyang Z, Landgren E, Lavergne C, Di Fiore PP, Anafi M, Pawson T, Cantley LC, Claesson-Welsh L, Welsh M. 1995. Molecular interactions of the Src homology 2 domain protein Shb with phosphotyrosine residues, tyrosine kinase receptors and Src homology 3 domain proteins. Oncogene 10(8):1475-1483.

Kawamura K, Kawamura N, Mulders SM, Sollewijn Gelpke MD, Hsueh AJ. 2005. Ovarian brain-derived neurotrophic factor (BDNF) promotes the development of oocytes into preimplantation embryos. Proc Natl Acad Sci U S A 102(26):9206-9211.

Kay C, Jeyendran RS, Coulam CB. 2006. p53 tumour suppressor gene polymorphism is associated with recurrent implantation failure. Reprod Biomed Online 13(4):492-496.

Kaziro Y, Itoh H, Kozasa T, Nakafuku M, Satoh T. 1991. Structure and function of signal-transducing GTP-binding proteins. Annu Rev Biochem 60:349-400.

Keady BT, Kuo P, Martinez SE, Yuan L, Hake LE. 2007. MAPK interacts with XGef and is required for CPEB activation during meiosis in Xenopus oocytes. J Cell Sci 120(Pt 6):1093-1103.

Khatib H, Huang W, Mikheil D, Schutzkus V, Monson RL. 2009. Effects of signal transducer and activator of transcription (STAT) genes STAT1 and STAT3 genotypic combinations on fertilization and embryonic survival rates in Holstein cattle. J Dairy Sci 92(12):6186-6191.

Kim JH, Do HJ, Wang WH, Machaty Z, Han YM, Day BN, Prather RS. 1999a. A protein tyrosine phosphatase inhibitor, sodium orthovanadate, causes parthenogenetic activation of pig oocytes via an increase in protein tyrosine kinase activity. Biol Reprod 61(4):900-905.

Kim SH, Li C, Maller JL. 1999b. A maternal form of the phosphatase Cdc25A regulates early embryonic cell cycles in Xenopus laevis. Dev Biol 212(2):381-391.

Kinoshita K, Noetzel TL, Pelletier L, Mechtler K, Drechsel DN, Schwager A, Lee M, Raff JW, Hyman AA. 2005. Aurora A phosphorylation of TACC3/maskin is required for centrosome-dependent microtubule assembly in mitosis. J Cell Biol 170(7):1047-1055.

Kirchhof MG, Chau LA, Lemke CD, Vardhana S, Darlington PJ, Marquez ME, Taylor R, Rizkalla K, Blanca I, Dustin ML, Madrenas J. 2008. Modulation of T cell activation by stomatin-like protein 2. J Immunol 181(3):1927-1936.

Kishimoto T. 2011. A primer on meiotic resumption in starfish oocytes: The proposed signaling pathway triggered by maturation-inducing hormone. Mol Reprod Dev 78(10-11):704-707.

Kitagawa R, Law E, Tang L, Rose AM. 2002. The Cdc20 homolog, FZY-1, and its interacting protein, IFY-1, are required for proper chromosome segregation in Caenorhabditis elegans. Curr Biol 12(24):2118-2123.

Kline D, Kopf GS, Muncy LF, Jaffe LA. 1991. Evidence for the involvement of a pertussis toxin-insensitive G-protein in egg activation of the frog, Xenopus laevis. Dev Biol 143(2):218-229.

Komaba S, Hamao H, Murata-Hori M, Hosoya H. 2001. Identification of myosin II kinase from sea urchin eggs as protein kinase CK2. Gene 275(1):141-148.

Komatsu S, Abbasi F, Kobori E, Fujisawa Y, Kato H, Iwasaki Y. 2005. Proteomic analysis of rice embryo: an approach for investigating Galpha protein-regulated proteins. Proteomics 5(15):3932-3941.

Kong AM, Speed CJ, O'Malley CJ, Layton MJ, Meehan T, Loveland KL, Cheema S, Ooms LM, Mitchell CA. 2000. Cloning and characterization of a 72-kDa inositol-polyphosphate 5-phosphatase localized to the Golgi network. J Biol Chem 275(31):24052-24064.

Kornberg RD. 1999. Eukaryotic transcriptional control. Trends Cell Biol 9(12):M46-49.

Kriz V, Agren N, Lindholm CK, Lenell S, Saldeen J, Mares J, Welsh M. 2006. The SHB adapter protein is required for normal maturation of mesoderm during in vitro differentiation of embryonic stem cells. J Biol Chem 281(45):34484-34491.

Kriz V, Anneren C, Lai C, Karlsson J, Mares J, Welsh M. 2003. The SHB adapter protein is required for efficient multilineage differentiation of mouse embryonic stem cells. Exp Cell Res 286(1):40-56.

Kume S, Endo T, Nishimura Y, Kano K, Naito K. 2007. Porcine SPDYA2 (RINGO A2) stimulates CDC2 activity and accelerates meiotic maturation of porcine oocytes. Biol Reprod 76(3):440-447.

Kume S, Yamamoto A, Inoue T, Muto A, Okano H, Mikoshiba K. 1997. Developmental expression of the inositol 1,4,5-trisphosphate receptor and structural changes in the endoplasmic reticulum during oogenesis and meiotic maturation of Xenopus laevis. Dev Biol 182(2):228-239.

Kuo P, Runge E, Lu X, Hake LE. 2011. XGef influences XRINGO/CDK1 signaling and CPEB activation during Xenopus oocyte maturation. Differentiation 81(2):133-140.

Kurokawa M, Sato K, Fissore RA. 2004. Mammalian fertilization: from sperm factor to phospholipase Czeta. Biol Cell 96(1):37-45.

Kushima S, Mammadova G, Mahbub Hasan AK, Fukami Y, Sato K. 2011. Characterization of Lipovitellin 2 as a tyrosine-phosphorylated protein in oocytes, eggs and early embryos of Xenopus laevis. Zoolog Sci 28(8):550-559.

Lambert H, Collazo I, Steinleitner A. 1992. IL-7 and IL-8 inhibit gamete interaction in the zona-free hamster egg sperm penetration assay. Mediators Inflamm 1(1):67-69.

Lane M, Bavister BD. 1999. Regulation of intracellular pH in bovine oocytes and cleavage stage embryos. Mol Reprod Dev 54(4):396-401.

Lapasset L, Pradet-Balade B, Lozano JC, Peaucellier G, Picard A. 2005. Nuclear envelope breakdown may deliver an inhibitor of protein phosphatase 1 which triggers cyclin B translation in starfish oocytes. Dev Biol 285(1):200-210.

Lapasset L, Pradet-Balade B, Verge V, Lozano JC, Oulhen N, Cormier P, Peaucellier G. 2008. Cyclin B synthesis and rapamycin-sensitive regulation of protein synthesis during starfish oocyte meiotic divisions. Mol Reprod Dev 75(11):1617-1626.

Lasko P. 2003. Gene regulation at the RNA layer: RNA binding proteins in intercellular signaling networks. Sci STKE 2003(179):RE6.

Lee B, Vermassen E, Yoon SY, Vanderheyden V, Ito J, Alfandari D, De Smedt H, Parys JB, Fissore RA. 2006. Phosphorylation of IP3R1 and the regulation of [Ca2+]i responses at fertilization: a role for the MAP kinase pathway. Development 133(21):4355-4365.

Lee MS, Kang SK, Lee BC, Hwang WS. 2005. The beneficial effects of insulin and metformin on in vitro developmental potential of porcine oocytes and embryos. Biol Reprod 73(6):1264-1268.

Levine AJ, Tomasini R, McKeon FD, Mak TW, Melino G. 2011. The p53 family: guardians of maternal reproduction. Nat Rev Mol Cell Biol 12(4):259-265.

Lewis RA, Gagnon JA, Mowry KL. 2008. PTB/hnRNP I is required for RNP remodeling during RNA localization in Xenopus oocytes. Mol Cell Biol 28(2):678-686.

Li X, Dai Y, Allen WR. 2004. Influence of insulin-like growth factor-I on cytoplasmic maturation of horse oocytes in vitro and organization of the first cell cycle following nuclear transfer and parthenogenesis. Biol Reprod 71(4):1391-1396.

Lim HJ, Dey SK. 2009. HB-EGF: a unique mediator of embryo-uterine interactions during implantation. Exp Cell Res 315(4):619-626.

Lin R. 2003. A gain-of-function mutation in oma-1, a C. elegans gene required for oocyte maturation, results in delayed degradation of maternal proteins and embryonic lethality. Dev Biol 258(1):226-239.

Littlepage LE, Ruderman JV. 2002. Identification of a new APC/C recognition domain, the A box, which is required for the Cdh1-dependent destruction of the kinase Aurora-A during mitotic exit. Genes Dev 16(17):2274-2285.

Liu H, Luo LL, Qian YS, Fu YC, Sui XX, Geng YJ, Huang DN, Gao ST, Zhang RL. 2009. FOXO3a is involved in the apoptosis of naked oocytes and oocytes of primordial follicles from neonatal rat ovaries. Biochem Biophys Res Commun 381(4):722-727.

Liu J, Maller JL. 2005. Calcium elevation at fertilization coordinates phosphorylation of XErp1/Emi2 by Plx1 and CaMK II to release metaphase arrest by cytostatic factor. Curr Biol 15(16):1458-1468.

Liu M, Oh A, Calarco P, Yamada M, Coonrod SA, Talbot P. 2005. Peptidylarginine deiminase (PAD) is a mouse cortical granule protein that plays a role in preimplantation embryonic development. Reprod Biol Endocrinol 3:42.

Liu XJ, Sorisky A, Zhu L, Pawson T. 1995. Molecular cloning of an amphibian insulin receptor substrate 1-like cDNA and involvement of phosphatidylinositol 3-kinase in insulin-induced Xenopus oocyte maturation. Mol Cell Biol 15(7):3563-3570.

Lodde V, Modina SC, Franciosi F, Zuccari E, Tessaro I, Luciano AM. 2009. Localization of DNA methyltransferase-1 during oocyte differentiation, in vitro maturation and early embryonic development in cow. Eur J Histochem 53(4):199-207.

Lutz RJ. 2000. Role of the BH3 (Bcl-2 homology 3) domain in the regulation of apoptosis and Bcl-2-related proteins. Biochem Soc Trans 28(2):51-56.

Mahbub Hasan AK, Fukami Y, Sato KI. 2011. Gamete membrane microdomains and their associated molecules in fertilization signaling. Mol Reprod Dev. 78(10-11):814-830.

Mahbub Hasan AK, Ou Z, Sakakibara K, Hirahara S, Iwasaki T, Sato K, Fukami Y. 2007. Characterization of Xenopus egg membrane microdomains containing uroplakin Ib/III complex: roles of their molecular interactions for subcellular localization and signal transduction. Genes Cells 12(2):251-267.

Mahbub Hasan AK, Sato K, Sakakibara K, Ou Z, Iwasaki T, Ueda Y, Fukami Y. 2005. Uroplakin III, a novel Src substrate in Xenopus egg rafts, is a target for sperm protease essential for fertilization. Dev Biol 286(2):483-492.

Mailhes JB, Hilliard C, Fuseler JW, London SN. 2003. Okadaic acid, an inhibitor of protein phosphatase 1 and 2A, induces premature separation of sister chromatids during meiosis I and aneuploidy in mouse oocytes in vitro. Chromosome Res 11(6):619-631.

Malcuit C, Knott JG, He C, Wainwright T, Parys JB, Robl JM, Fissore RA. 2005. Fertilization and inositol 1,4,5-trisphosphate (IP3)-induced calcium release in type-1 inositol 1,4,5-trisphosphate receptor down-regulated bovine eggs. Biol Reprod 73(1):2-13.

Maller JL. 1990. Xenopus oocytes and the biochemistry of cell division. Biochemistry 29(13):3157-3166.

Mammadova G, Iwasaki T, Tokmakov AA, Fukami Y, Sato K. 2009. Evidence that phosphatidylinositol 3-kinase is involved in sperm-induced tyrosine kinase signaling in Xenopus egg fertilization. BMC Dev Biol 9:68.

Manzo S, Martinez-Cadena G, Lopez-Godinez J, Pedraza-Reyes M, Garcia-Soto J. 2003. A Rho GTPase controls the rate of protein synthesis in the sea urchin egg. Biochem Biophys Res Commun 310(3):685-690.

Marangos P, Verschuren EW, Chen R, Jackson PK, Carroll J. 2007. Prophase I arrest and progression to metaphase I in mouse oocytes are controlled by Emi1-dependent regulation of APC(Cdh1). J Cell Biol 176(1):65-75.

Martin SG, St Johnston D. 2003. A role for Drosophila LKB1 in anterior-posterior axis formation and epithelial polarity. Nature 421(6921):379-384.

Martinez SE, Yuan L, Lacza C, Ransom H, Mahon GM, Whitehead IP, Hake LE. 2005. XGef mediates early CPEB phosphorylation during Xenopus oocyte meiotic maturation. Mol Biol Cell 16(3):1152-1164.

Maruyama R, Velarde NV, Klancer R, Gordon S, Kadandale P, Parry JM, Hang JS, Rubin J, Stewart-Michaelis A, Schweinsberg P, Grant BD, Piano F, Sugimoto A, Singson A. 2007. EGG-3 regulates cell-surface and cortex rearrangements during egg activation in Caenorhabditis elegans. Curr Biol 17(18):1555-1560.

Masciarelli S, Horner K, Liu C, Park SH, Hinckley M, Hockman S, Nedachi T, Jin C, Conti M, Manganiello V. 2004. Cyclic nucleotide phosphodiesterase 3A-deficient mice as a model of female infertility. J Clin Invest 114(2):196-205.

Masui Y. 2000. The elusive cytostatic factor in the animal egg. Nat Rev Mol Cell Biol 1(3):228-232.

Maton G, Lorca T, Girault JA, Ozon R, Jessus C. 2005. Differential regulation of Cdc2 and Aurora-A in Xenopus oocytes: a crucial role of phosphatase 2A. J Cell Sci 118(Pt 11):2485-2494.

Maton G, Thibier C, Castro A, Lorca T, Prigent C, Jessus C. 2003. Cdc2-cyclin B triggers H3 kinase activation of Aurora-A in Xenopus oocytes. J Biol Chem 278(24):21439-21449.

Matsubara T, Ohkubo N, Andoh T, Sullivan CV, Hara A. 1999. Two forms of vitellogenin, yielding two distinct lipovitellins, play different roles during oocyte maturation and early development of barfin flounder, Verasper moseri, a marine teleost that spawns pelagic eggs. Dev Biol 213(1):18-32.

Matsui M, Takahashi Y, Hishinuma M, Kanagawa H. 1995. Effects of supplementation of the maturation media with insulin on in vitro maturation and in vitro fertilization of bovine oocytes. Jpn J Vet Res 43(3-4):145-153.

Matsumoto K, Satoh T, Irie A, Ishii J, Kuwao S, Iwamura M, Baba S. 2008. Loss expression of uroplakin III is associated with clinicopathologic features of aggressive bladder cancer. Urology 72(2):444-449.

Matsuoka T, Tahara M, Yokoi T, Masumoto N, Takeda T, Yamaguchi M, Tasaka K, Kurachi H, Murata Y. 1999. Tyrosine phosphorylation of STAT3 by leptin through leptin receptor in mouse metaphase 2 stage oocyte. Biochem Biophys Res Commun 256(3):480-484.

Mattick JS. 2004. RNA regulation: a new genetics? Nat Rev Genet 5(4):316-323.

Mayer BJ, Hamaguchi M, Hanafusa H. 1988. A novel viral oncogene with structural similarity to phospholipase C. Nature 332(6161):272-275.

Mayer BJ, Hanafusa H. 1990. Mutagenic analysis of the v-crk oncogene: requirement for SH2 and SH3 domains and correlation between increased cellular phosphotyrosine and transformation. J Virol 64(8):3581-3589.

Mayes MA, Sirard MA. 2002. Effect of type 3 and type 4 phosphodiesterase inhibitors on the maintenance of bovine oocytes in meiotic arrest. Biol Reprod 66(1):180-184.

Mazus B, Szurmak B, Buchowicz J. 1980. Phosphorylation in vitro and in vivo of the wheat embryo RNA polymerase II. Acta Biochim Pol 27(1):9-19.

McGlade J, Cheng A, Pelicci G, Pelicci PG, Pawson T. 1992. Shc proteins are phosphorylated and regulated by the v-Src and v-Fps protein-tyrosine kinases. Proc Natl Acad Sci U S A 89(19):8869-8873.

McGuinness BE, Anger M, Kouznetsova A, Gil-Bernabe AM, Helmhart W, Kudo NR, Wuensche A, Taylor S, Hoog C, Novak B, Nasmyth K. 2009. Regulation of APC/C activity in oocytes by a Bub1-dependent spindle assembly checkpoint. Curr Biol 19(5):369-380.

Mehlmann LM. 2005. Stops and starts in mammalian oocytes: recent advances in understanding the regulation of meiotic arrest and oocyte maturation. Reproduction 130(6):791-799.

Mehlmann LM, Carpenter G, Rhee SG, Jaffe LA. 1998. SH2 domain-mediated activation of phospholipase Cgamma is not required to initiate Ca2+ release at fertilization of mouse eggs. Dev Biol 203(1):221-232.

Mehlmann LM, Saeki Y, Tanaka S, Brennan TJ, Evsikov AV, Pendola FL, Knowles BB, Eppig JJ, Jaffe LA. 2004. The Gs-linked receptor GPR3 maintains meiotic arrest in mammalian oocytes. Science 306(5703):1947-1950.

Meijer L, Arion D, Golsteyn R, Pines J, Brizuela L, Hunt T, Beach D. 1989a. Cyclin is a component of the sea urchin egg M-phase specific histone H1 kinase. EMBO J 8(8):2275-2282.

Meijer L, Azzi L, Wang JY. 1991. Cyclin B targets p34cdc2 for tyrosine phosphorylation. EMBO J 10(6):1545-1554.

Meijer L, Dostmann W, Genieser HG, Butt E, Jastorff B. 1989b. Starfish oocyte maturation: evidence for a cyclic AMP-dependent inhibitory pathway. Dev Biol 133(1):58-66.

Mendez R, Richter JD. 2001. Translational control by CPEB: a means to the end. Nat Rev Mol Cell Biol 2(7):521-529.

Meng XQ, Zheng KG, Yang Y, Jiang MX, Zhang YL, Sun QY, Li YL. 2006. Proline-rich tyrosine kinase2 is involved in F-actin organization during in vitro maturation of rat oocyte. Reproduction 132(6):859-867.

Miyamoto S, Yagi H, Yotsumoto F, Kawarabayashi T, Mekada E. 2006. Heparin-binding epidermal growth factor-like growth factor as a novel targeting molecule for cancer therapy. Cancer Sci 97(5):341-347.

Mizote A, Okamoto S, Iwao Y. 1999. Activation of Xenopus eggs by proteases: possible involvement of a sperm protease in fertilization. Dev Biol 208(1):79-92.

Mochida S, Hunt T. 2007. Calcineurin is required to release Xenopus egg extracts from meiotic M phase. Nature 449(7160):336-340.

Mochizuki Y, Takenawa T. 1999. Novel inositol polyphosphate 5-phosphatase localizes at membrane ruffles. J Biol Chem 274(51):36790-36795.

Mohammadi Roushandeh A, Habibi Roudkenar M. 2009. The influence of meiotic spindle configuration by cysteamine during in vitro maturation of mouse oocytes. Iran Biomed J 13(2):73-78.

Mood K, Friesel R, Daar IO. 2002. SNT1/FRS2 mediates germinal vesicle breakdown induced by an activated FGF receptor1 in Xenopus oocytes. J Biol Chem 277(36):33196-33204.

Morita Y, Tilly JL. 1999. Oocyte apoptosis: like sand through an hourglass. Dev Biol 213(1):1-17.

Muciaccia B, Sette C, Paronetto MP, Barchi M, Pensini S, D'Agostino A, Gandini L, Geremia R, Stefanini M, Rossi P. 2010. Expression of a truncated form of KIT tyrosine kinase in human spermatozoa correlates with sperm DNA integrity. Hum Reprod 25(9):2188-2202.

Muller AH, Gawantka V, Ding X, Hausen P. 1993. Maturation induced internalization of beta 1-integrin by Xenopus oocytes and formation of the maternal integrin pool. Mech Dev 42(1-2):77-88.

Nagao K, Yanagida M. 2002. Regulating sister chromatid separation by separase phosphorylation. Dev Cell 2(1):2-4.

Nakahata S, Kotani T, Mita K, Kawasaki T, Katsu Y, Nagahama Y, Yamashita M. 2003. Involvement of Xenopus Pumilio in the translational regulation that is specific to cyclin B1 mRNA during oocyte maturation. Mech Dev 120(8):865-880.

Nakamura H, Yoshitome S, Sugimoto I, Sado Y, Kawahara A, Ueno S, Miyahara T, Yoshida Y, Aoki-Yagi N, Hashimoto E. 2007. Cellular distribution of Mr 25,000 protein, a protein partially overlapping phosvitin and lipovitellin 2 in vitellogenin B1, and yolk proteins in Xenopus laevis oocytes and embryos. Comp Biochem Physiol A Mol Integr Physiol 148(3):621-628.

Nakaya M, Fukui A, Izumi Y, Akimoto K, Asashima M, Ohno S. 2000. Meiotic maturation induces animal-vegetal asymmetric distribution of aPKC and ASIP/PAR-3 in Xenopus oocytes. Development 127(23):5021-5031.

Nasmyth K, Peters JM, Uhlmann F. 2000. Splitting the chromosome: cutting the ties that bind sister chromatids. Science 288(5470):1379-1385.

Naz RK, Ahmad K. 1994. Molecular identities of human sperm proteins that bind human zona pellucida: nature of sperm-zona interaction, tyrosine kinase activity, and involvement of FA-1. Mol Reprod Dev 39(4):397-408.

Nebreda AR, Porras A, Santos E. 1993. p21ras-induced meiotic maturation of Xenopus oocytes in the absence of protein synthesis: MPF activation is preceded by activation of MAP and S6 kinases. Oncogene 8(2):467-477.

Nedachi T, Conti M. 2004. Potential role of protein tyrosine phosphatase nonreceptor type 13 in the control of oocyte meiotic maturation. Development 131(20):4987-4998.

Nielsen PJ, Thomas G, Maller JL. 1982. Increased phosphorylation of ribosomal protein S6 during meiotic maturation of Xenopus oocytes. Proc Natl Acad Sci U S A 79(9):2937-2941.

Nishi Y, Lin R. 2005. DYRK2 and GSK-3 phosphorylate and promote the timely degradation of OMA-1, a key regulator of the oocyte-to-embryo transition in C. elegans. Dev Biol 288(1):139-149.

Nishiyama T, Yoshizaki N, Kishimoto T, Ohsumi K. 2007. Transient activation of calcineurin is essential to initiate embryonic development in Xenopus laevis. Nature 449(7160):341-345.

Nishizuka Y. 1984. The role of protein kinase C in cell surface signal transduction and tumour promotion. Nature 308(5961):693-698.

Nishizuka Y. 1986. Studies and perspectives of protein kinase C. Science 233(4761):305-312.

Nogueira D, Albano C, Adriaenssens T, Cortvrindt R, Bourgain C, Devroey P, Smitz J. 2003a. Human oocytes reversibly arrested in prophase I by phosphodiesterase type 3 inhibitor in vitro. Biol Reprod 69(3):1042-1052.

Nogueira D, Cortvrindt R, De Matos DG, Vanhoutte L, Smitz J. 2003b. Effect of phosphodiesterase type 3 inhibitor on developmental competence of immature mouse oocytes in vitro. Biol Reprod 69(6):2045-2052.

Nogueira D, Cortvrindt R, Everaerdt B, Smitz J. 2005. Effects of long-term in vitro exposure to phosphodiesterase type-3 inhibitors on follicle and oocyte development. Reproduction 130(2):177-186.

Nutt LK, Margolis SS, Jensen M, Herman CE, Dunphy WG, Rathmell JC, Kornbluth S. 2005. Metabolic regulation of oocyte cell death through the CaMKII-mediated phosphorylation of caspase-2. Cell 123(1):89-103.

Oh JS, Han SJ, Conti M. 2010. Wee1B, Myt1, and Cdc25 function in distinct compartments of the mouse oocyte to control meiotic resumption. J Cell Biol 188(2):199-207.

Okumura E, Fukuhara T, Yoshida H, Hanada Si S, Kozutsumi R, Mori M, Tachibana K, Kishimoto T. 2002. Akt inhibits Myt1 in the signalling pathway that leads to meiotic G2/M-phase transition. Nat Cell Biol 4(2):111-116.

Olivier JP, Raabe T, Henkemeyer M, Dickson B, Mbamalu G, Margolis B, Schlessinger J, Hafen E, Pawson T. 1993. A Drosophila SH2-SH3 adaptor protein implicated in coupling the sevenless tyrosine kinase to an activator of Ras guanine nucleotide exchange, Sos. Cell 73(1):179-191.

Ooga M, Inoue A, Kageyama S, Akiyama T, Nagata M, Aoki F. 2008. Changes in H3K79 methylation during preimplantation development in mice. Biol Reprod 78(3):413-424.

Ossipova O, Bardeesy N, DePinho RA, Green JB. 2003. LKB1 (XEEK1) regulates Wnt signalling in vertebrate development. Nat Cell Biol 5(10):889-894.

Ostareck-Lederer A, Ostareck DH, Cans C, Neubauer G, Bomsztyk K, Superti-Furga G, Hentze MW. 2002. c-Src-mediated phosphorylation of hnRNP K drives translational activation of specifically silenced mRNAs. Mol Cell Biol 22(13):4535-4543.

Ota R, Kotani T, Yamashita M. 2011a. Biochemical characterization of Pumilio1 and Pumilio2 in Xenopus oocytes. J Biol Chem 286(4):2853-2863.

Ota R, Kotani T, Yamashita M. 2011b. Possible involvement of Nemo-like kinase 1 in Xenopus oocyte maturation as a kinase responsible for Pumilio1, Pumilio2, and CPEB phosphorylation. Biochemistry 50(25):5648-5659.

Ota R, Suwa K, Kotani T, Mita K, Yamashita M. 2008. Possible involvement of phosphatidylinositol 3-kinase, but not protein kinase B or glycogen synthase kinase 3beta, in progesterone-induced oocyte maturation in the Japanese brown frog, Rana japonica. Zoolog Sci 25(7):773-781.

Padmanabhan K, Richter JD. 2006. Regulated Pumilio-2 binding controls RINGO/Spy mRNA translation and CPEB activation. Genes Dev 20(2):199-209.

Pallen CJ, Wang JH. 1985. A multifunctional calmodulin-stimulated phosphatase. Arch Biochem Biophys 237(2):281-291.

Panetta G, Buttinelli M, Flaus A, Richmond TJ, Rhodes D. 1998. Differential nucleosome positioning on Xenopus oocyte and somatic 5 S RNA genes determines both TFIIIA and H1 binding: a mechanism for selective H1 repression. J Mol Biol 282(3):683-697.

Papin C, Rouget C, Lorca T, Castro A, Mandart E. 2004. XCdh1 is involved in progesterone-induced oocyte maturation. Dev Biol 272(1):66-75.

Paronetto MP, Farini D, Sammarco I, Maturo G, Vespasiani G, Geremia R, Rossi P, Sette C. 2004. Expression of a truncated form of the c-Kit tyrosine kinase receptor and activation of Src kinase in human prostatic cancer. Am J Pathol 164(4):1243-1251.

Parrington J, Brind S, De Smedt H, Gangeswaran R, Lai FA, Wojcikiewicz R, Carroll J. 1998. Expression of inositol 1,4,5-trisphosphate receptors in mouse oocytes and early embryos: the type I isoform is upregulated in oocytes and downregulated after fertilization. Dev Biol 203(2):451-461.

Parrington J, Jones ML, Tunwell R, Devader C, Katan M, Swann K. 2002. Phospholipase C isoforms in mammalian spermatozoa: potential components of the sperm factor that causes Ca2+ release in eggs. Reproduction 123(1):31-39.

Parry JM, Velarde NV, Lefkovith AJ, Zegarek MH, Hang JS, Ohm J, Klancer R, Maruyama R, Druzhinina MK, Grant BD, Piano F, Singson A. 2009. EGG-4 and EGG-5 Link Events of the Oocyte-to-Embryo Transition with Meiotic Progression in C. elegans. Curr Biol 19(20):1752-1757.

Pascreau G, Delcros JG, Cremet JY, Prigent C, Arlot-Bonnemains Y. 2005. Phosphorylation of maskin by Aurora-A participates in the control of sequential protein synthesis during Xenopus laevis oocyte maturation. J Biol Chem 280(14):13415-13423.

Pascreau G, Eckerdt F, Lewellyn AL, Prigent C, Maller JL. 2009. Phosphorylation of p53 is regulated by TPX2-Aurora A in xenopus oocytes. J Biol Chem 284(9):5497-5505.

Paul S, Pramanick K, Kundu S, Bandyopadhyay A, Mukherjee D. 2009. Involvement of PI3 kinase and MAP kinase in IGF-I- and insulin-induced oocyte maturation in Cyprinus carpio. Mol Cell Endocrinol 309(1-2):93-100.

Pelicci G, Lanfrancone L, Grignani F, McGlade J, Cavallo F, Forni G, Nicoletti I, Pawson T, Pelicci PG. 1992. A novel transforming protein (SHC) with an SH2 domain is implicated in mitogenic signal transduction. Cell 70(1):93-104.

Perdiguero E, Nebreda AR. 2004. Regulation of Cdc25C activity during the meiotic G2/M transition. Cell Cycle 3(6):733-737.

Perdiguero E, Pillaire MJ, Bodart JF, Hennersdorf F, Frodin M, Duesbery NS, Alonso G, Nebreda AR. 2003. Xp38gamma/SAPK3 promotes meiotic G(2)/M transition in Xenopus oocytes and activates Cdc25C. EMBO J 22(21):5746-5756.

Pesin JA, Orr-Weaver TL. 2008. Regulation of APC/C activators in mitosis and meiosis. Annu Rev Cell Dev Biol 24:475-499.

Phillips KP, Leveille MC, Claman P, Baltz JM. 2000. Intracellular pH regulation in human preimplantation embryos. Hum Reprod 15(4):896-904.

Pirino G, Wescott MP, Donovan PJ. 2009. Protein kinase A regulates resumption of meiosis by phosphorylation of Cdc25B in mammalian oocytes. Cell Cycle 8(4):665-670.

Pomerance M, Schweighoffer F, Tocque B, Pierre M. 1992. Stimulation of mitogen-activated protein kinase by oncogenic Ras p21 in Xenopus oocytes. Requirement for Ras p21-GTPase-activating protein interaction. J Biol Chem 267(23):16155-16160.

Pomerance M, Thang MN, Tocque B, Pierre M. 1996. The Ras-GTPase-activating protein SH3 domain is required for Cdc2 activation and mos induction by oncogenic Ras in Xenopus oocytes independently of mitogen-activated protein kinase activation. Mol Cell Biol 16(6):3179-3186.

Pondaven P, Cohen P. 1987. Identification of protein phosphatases-1 and 2A and inhibitor-2 in oocytes of the starfish Asterias rubens and Marthasterias glacialis. Eur J Biochem 167(1):135-140.

Powell-Coffman JA, Knight J, Wood WB. 1996. Onset of C. elegans gastrulation is blocked by inhibition of embryonic transcription with an RNA polymerase antisense RNA. Dev Biol 178(2):472-483.

Qian YW, Erikson E, Taieb FE, Maller JL. 2001. The polo-like kinase Plx1 is required for activation of the phosphatase Cdc25C and cyclin B-Cdc2 in Xenopus oocytes. Mol Biol Cell 12(6):1791-1799.

Qu Y, Adler V, Chu T, Platica O, Michl J, Pestka S, Izotova L, Boutjdir M, Pincus MR. 2006. Two dual specificity kinases are preferentially induced by wild-type rather than by oncogenic RAS-P21 in Xenopus oocytes. Front Biosci 11:2420-2427.

Qu Y, Adler V, Izotova L, Pestka S, Bowne W, Michl J, Boutjdir M, Friedman FK, Pincus MR. 2007. The dual-specificity kinases, TOPK and DYRK1A, are critical for oocyte maturation induced by wild-type--but not by oncogenic--ras-p21 protein. Front Biosci 12:5089-5097.

Quesnel H. 1999. Localization of binding sites for IGF-I, insulin and GH in the sow ovary. J Endocrinol 163(2):363-372.

Rasar M, DeFranco DB, Hammes SR. 2006. Paxillin regulates steroid-triggered meiotic resumption in oocytes by enhancing an all-or-none positive feedback kinase loop. J Biol Chem 281(51):39455-39464.

Rauh NR, Schmidt A, Bormann J, Nigg EA, Mayer TU. 2005. Calcium triggers exit from meiosis II by targeting the APC/C inhibitor XErp1 for degradation. Nature 437(7061):1048-1052.

Reddy P, Shen L, Ren C, Boman K, Lundin E, Ottander U, Lindgren P, Liu YX, Sun QY, Liu K. 2005. Activation of Akt (PKB) and suppression of FKHRL1 in mouse and rat oocytes by stem cell factor during follicular activation and development. Dev Biol 281(2):160-170.

Reddy VR, Rajeev SK, Gupta V. 2003. Alpha 6 beta 1 Integrin is a potential clinical marker for evaluating sperm quality in men. Fertil Steril 79 Suppl 3:1590-1596.

Reimann JD, Freed E, Hsu JY, Kramer ER, Peters JM, Jackson PK. 2001a. Emi1 is a mitotic regulator that interacts with Cdc20 and inhibits the anaphase promoting complex. Cell 105(5):645-655.

Reimann JD, Gardner BE, Margottin-Goguet F, Jackson PK. 2001b. Emi1 regulates the anaphase-promoting complex by a different mechanism than Mad2 proteins. Genes Dev 15(24):3278-3285.

Reimann JD, Jackson PK. 2002. Emi1 is required for cytostatic factor arrest in vertebrate eggs. Nature 416(6883):850-854.

Reverte CG, Yuan L, Keady BT, Lacza C, Attfield KR, Mahon GM, Freeman B, Whitehead IP, Hake LE. 2003. XGef is a CPEB-interacting protein involved in Xenopus oocyte maturation. Dev Biol 255(2):383-398.

Rhee SG. 2001. Regulation of phosphoinositide-specific phospholipase C. Annu Rev Biochem 70:281-312.

Richard FJ, Tsafriri A, Conti M. 2001. Role of phosphodiesterase type 3A in rat oocyte maturation. Biol Reprod 65(5):1444-1451.

Rime H, Huchon D, De Smedt V, Thibier C, Galaktionov K, Jessus C, Ozon R. 1994. Microinjection of Cdc25 protein phosphatase into Xenopus prophase oocyte activates MPF and arrests meiosis at metaphase I. Biol Cell 82(1):11-22.

Rogers E, Bishop JD, Waddle JA, Schumacher JM, Lin R. 2002. The aurora kinase AIR-2 functions in the release of chromosome cohesion in Caenorhabditis elegans meiosis. J Cell Biol 157(2):219-229.

Ron D, Luo J, Mochly-Rosen D. 1995. C2 region-derived peptides inhibit translocation and function of beta protein kinase C in vivo. J Biol Chem 270(41):24180-24187.

Ron D, Mochly-Rosen D. 1995. An autoregulatory region in protein kinase C: the pseudoanchoring site. Proc Natl Acad Sci U S A 92(2):492-496.

Rossi P, Sette C, Dolci S, Geremia R. 2000. Role of c-kit in mammalian spermatogenesis. J Endocrinol Invest 23(9):609-615.

Rozakis-Adcock M, Fernley R, Wade J, Pawson T, Bowtell D. 1993. The SH2 and SH3 domains of mammalian Grb2 couple the EGF receptor to the Ras activator mSos1. Nature 363(6424):83-85.

Rozakis-Adcock M, McGlade J, Mbamalu G, Pelicci G, Daly R, Li W, Batzer A, Thomas S, Brugge J, Pelicci PG, et al. 1992. Association of the Shc and Grb2/Sem5 SH2-containing proteins is implicated in activation of the Ras pathway by tyrosine kinases. Nature 360(6405):689-692.

Rudner AD, Murray AW. 2000. Phosphorylation by Cdc28 activates the Cdc20-dependent activity of the anaphase-promoting complex. J Cell Biol 149(7):1377-1390.

Runft LL, Carroll DJ, Gillett J, Giusti AF, O'Neill FJ, Foltz KR. 2004. Identification of a starfish egg PLC-gamma that regulates Ca2+ release at fertilization. Dev Biol 269(1):220-236.

Runft LL, Jaffe LA. 2000. Sperm extract injection into ascidian eggs signals Ca(2+) release by the same pathway as fertilization. Development 127(15):3227-3236.

Runft LL, Jaffe LA, Mehlmann LM. 2002. Egg activation at fertilization: where it all begins. Dev Biol 245(2):237-254.

Runft LL, Watras J, Jaffe LA. 1999. Calcium release at fertilization of Xenopus eggs requires type I IP(3) receptors, but not SH2 domain-mediated activation of PLCgamma or G(q)-mediated activation of PLCbeta. Dev Biol 214(2):399-411.

Sakakibara K, Sato K, Yoshino K, Oshiro N, Hirahara S, Mahbub Hasan AK, Iwasaki T, Ueda Y, Iwao Y, Yonezawa K, Fukami Y. 2005. Molecular identification and characterization of Xenopus egg uroplakin III, an egg raft-associated transmembrane protein that is tyrosine-phosphorylated upon fertilization. J Biol Chem 280(15):15029-15037.

Sakamoto I, Takahara K, Yamashita M, Iwao Y. 1998. Changes in cyclin B during oocyte maturation and early embryonic cell cycle in the newt, Cynops pyrrhogaster: requirement of germinal vesicle for MPF activation. Dev Biol 195(1):60-69.

Salaun P, Pyronnet S, Morales J, Mulner-Lorillon O, Belle R, Sonenberg N, Cormier P. 2003. eIF4E/4E-BP dissociation and 4E-BP degradation in the first mitotic division of the sea urchin embryo. Dev Biol 255(2):428-439.

Saling PM. 1991. How the egg regulates sperm function during gamete interaction: facts and fantasies. Biol Reprod 44(2):246-251.

Santella L, Ercolano E, Lim D, Nusco GA, Moccia F. 2003. Activated M-phase-promoting factor (MPF) is exported from the nucleus of starfish oocytes to increase the sensitivity of the Ins(1,4,5)P3 receptors. Biochem Soc Trans 31(Pt 1):79-82.

Sardon T, Peset I, Petrova B, Vernos I. 2008. Dissecting the role of Aurora A during spindle assembly. EMBO J 27(19):2567-2579.

Sasseville M, Cote N, Guillemette C, Richard FJ. 2006. New insight into the role of phosphodiesterase 3A in porcine oocyte maturation. BMC Dev Biol 6:47.

Sasseville M, Cote N, Vigneault C, Guillemette C, Richard FJ. 2007. 3'5'-cyclic adenosine monophosphate-dependent up-regulation of phosphodiesterase type 3A in porcine cumulus cells. Endocrinology 148(4):1858-1867.

Sato K, Iwasaki T, Ogawa K, Konishi M, Tokmakov AA, Fukami Y. 2002a. Low density detergent-insoluble membrane of Xenopus eggs: subcellular microdomain for tyrosine kinase signaling in fertilization. Development 129(4):885-896.

Sato K, Nagao T, Kakumoto M, Kimoto M, Otsuki T, Iwasaki T, Tokmakov AA, Owada K, Fukami Y. 2002b. Adaptor protein Shc is an isoform-specific direct activator of the tyrosine kinase c-Src. J Biol Chem 277(33):29568-29576.

Sato K, Ogawa K, Tokmakov AA, Iwasaki T, Fukami Y. 2001. Hydrogen peroxide induces Src family tyrosine kinase-dependent activation of Xenopus eggs. Dev Growth Differ 43(1):55-72.

Sato K, Tokmakov AA, Fukami Y. 2000a. Fertilization signalling and protein-tyrosine kinases. Comp Biochem Physiol B Biochem Mol Biol 126(2):129-148.

Sato K, Tokmakov AA, He CL, Kurokawa M, Iwasaki T, Shirouzu M, Fissore RA, Yokoyama S, Fukami Y. 2003. Reconstitution of Src-dependent phospholipase Cgamma phosphorylation and transient calcium release by using membrane rafts and cell-free extracts from Xenopus eggs. J Biol Chem 278(40):38413-38420.

Sato K, Tokmakov AA, Iwasaki T, Fukami Y. 2000b. Tyrosine kinase-dependent activation of phospholipase Cgamma is required for calcium transient in Xenopus egg fertilization. Dev Biol 224(2):453-469.

Sato K, Yoshino K, Tokmakov AA, Iwasaki T, Yonezawa K, Fukami Y. 2006. Studying fertilization in cell-free extracts: focusing on membrane/lipid raft functions and proteomics. Methods Mol Biol 322:395-411.

Saunders CM, Larman MG, Parrington J, Cox LJ, Royse J, Blayney LM, Swann K, Lai FA. 2002. PLC zeta: a sperm-specific trigger of Ca(2+) oscillations in eggs and embryo development. Development 129(15):3533-3544.

Sawaguchi S, Ohkubo N, Matsubara T. 2006. Identification of two forms of vitellogenin-derived phosvitin and elucidation of their fate and roles during oocyte maturation in the barfin flounder, Verasper moseri. Zoolog Sci 23(11):1021-1029.

Scarpeci SL, Sanchez ML, Cabada MO. 2008. Cellular origin of the Bufo arenarum sperm receptor gp75, a ZP2 family member: its proteolysis after fertilization. Biol Cell 100(4):219-230.

Schonfelder EM, Knuppel T, Tasic V, Miljkovic P, Konrad M, Wuhl E, Antignac C, Bakkaloglu A, Schaefer F, Weber S. 2006. Mutations in Uroplakin IIIA are a rare cause of renal hypodysplasia in humans. Am J Kidney Dis 47(6):1004-1012.

Schurmans S, Carrio R, Behrends J, Pouillon V, Merino J, Clement S. 1999. The mouse SHIP2 (Inppl1) gene: complementary DNA, genomic structure, promoter analysis, and gene expression in the embryo and adult mouse. Genomics 62(2):260-271.

Schwab MS, Roberts BT, Gross SD, Tunquist BJ, Taieb FE, Lewellyn AL, Maller JL. 2001. Bub1 is activated by the protein kinase p90(Rsk) during Xenopus oocyte maturation. Curr Biol 11(3):141-150.

Sen A, O'Malley K, Wang Z, Raj GV, Defranco DB, Hammes SR. 2010. Paxillin regulates androgen- and epidermal growth factor-induced MAPK signaling and cell proliferation in prostate cancer cells. J Biol Chem 285(37):28787-28795.

Sette C, Messina V, Paronetto MP. 2010. Sam68: a new STAR in the male fertility firmament. J Androl 31(1):66-74.

Sette C, Paronetto MP, Barchi M, Bevilacqua A, Geremia R, Rossi P. 2002. Tr-kit-induced resumption of the cell cycle in mouse eggs requires activation of a Src-like kinase. EMBO J 21(20):5386-5395.

Shapiro E, Huang HY, Wu XR. 2000. Uroplakin and androgen receptor expression in the human fetal genital tract: insights into the development of the vagina. J Urol 164(3 Pt 2):1048-1051.

Shearer J, De Nadai C, Emily-Fenouil F, Gache C, Whitaker M, Ciapa B. 1999. Role of phospholipase Cgamma at fertilization and during mitosis in sea urchin eggs and embryos. Development 126(10):2273-2284.

Shen SS. 1989. Na+-H+ antiport during fertilization of the sea urchin egg is blocked by W-7 but is insensitive to K252a and H-7. Biochem Biophys Res Commun 161(3):1100-1108.

Shilling FM, Carroll DJ, Muslin AJ, Escobedo JA, Williams LT, Jaffe LA. 1994. Evidence for both tyrosine kinase and G-protein-coupled pathways leading to starfish egg activation. Dev Biol 162(2):590-599.

Shimada M, Yokosawa H, Kawahara H. 2006. OMA-1 is a P granules-associated protein that is required for germline specification in Caenorhabditis elegans embryos. Genes Cells 11(4):383-396.

Shimizu T. 1997. Reorganization of the cortical actin cytoskeleton during maturation division in the Tubifex egg: possible involvement of protein kinase C. Dev Biol 188(1):110-121.

Shirayama M, Soto MC, Ishidate T, Kim S, Nakamura K, Bei Y, van den Heuvel S, Mello CC. 2006. The Conserved Kinases CDK-1, GSK-3, KIN-19, and MBK-2 Promote OMA-1 Destruction to Regulate the Oocyte-to-Embryo Transition in C. elegans. Curr Biol 16(1):47-55.

Shteinberg M, Protopopov Y, Listovsky T, Brandeis M, Hershko A. 1999. Phosphorylation of the cyclosome is required for its stimulation by Fizzy/cdc20. Biochem Biophys Res Commun 260(1):193-198.

Sims RJ, 3rd, Mandal SS, Reinberg D. 2004. Recent highlights of RNA-polymerase-II-mediated transcription. Curr Opin Cell Biol 16(3):263-271.

Smith JJ, Evans EK, Murakami M, Moyer MB, Moseley MA, Woude GV, Kornbluth S. 2000. Wee1-regulated apoptosis mediated by the crk adaptor protein in Xenopus egg extracts. J Cell Biol 151(7):1391-1400.

Snow AJ, Puri P, Acker-Palmer A, Bouwmeester T, Vijayaraghavan S, Kline D. 2008. Phosphorylation-dependent interaction of tyrosine 3-monooxygenase/tryptophan 5-monooxygenase activation protein (YWHA) with PADI6 following oocyte maturation in mice. Biol Reprod 79(2):337-347.

Spivack JG, Erikson RL, Maller JL. 1984. Microinjection of pp60v-src into Xenopus oocytes increases phosphorylation of ribosomal protein S6 and accelerates the rate of progesterone-induced meiotic maturation. Mol Cell Biol 4(8):1631-1634.

Stahl ML, Ferenz CR, Kelleher KL, Kriz RW, Knopf JL. 1988. Sequence similarity of phospholipase C with the non-catalytic region of src. Nature 332(6161):269-272.

Standart N, Minshull J, Pines J, Hunt T. 1987. Cyclin synthesis, modification and destruction during meiotic maturation of the starfish oocyte. Dev Biol 124(1):248-258.

Stefanello JR, Barreta MH, Porciuncula PM, Arruda JN, Oliveira JF, Oliveira MA, Goncalves PB. 2006. Effect of angiotensin II with follicle cells and insulin-like growth factor-I or insulin on bovine oocyte maturation and embryo development. Theriogenology 66(9):2068-2076.

Stemmann O, Zou H, Gerber SA, Gygi SP, Kirschner MW. 2001. Dual inhibition of sister chromatid separation at metaphase. Cell 107(6):715-726.

Stith BJ, Woronoff K, Espinoza R, Smart T. 1997. sn-1,2-diacylglycerol and choline increase after fertilization in Xenopus laevis. Mol Biol Cell 8(4):755-765.

Stitzel ML, Cheng KC, Seydoux G. 2007. Regulation of MBK-2/Dyrk kinase by dynamic cortical anchoring during the oocyte-to-zygote transition. Curr Biol 17(18):1545-1554.

Stitzel ML, Pellettieri J, Seydoux G. 2006. The C. elegans DYRK Kinase MBK-2 Marks Oocyte Proteins for Degradation in Response to Meiotic Maturation. Curr Biol 16(1):56-62.

Stricker SA, Smythe TL. 2006. Differing mechanisms of cAMP- versus seawater-induced oocyte maturation in marine nemertean worms II. The roles of tyrosine kinases and phosphatases. Mol Reprod Dev 73(12):1564-1577.

Sugimoto I, Hashimoto E. 2006. Modulation of protein phosphorylation by Mr 25,000 protein partially overlapping phosvitin and lipovitellin 2 in Xenopus laevis vitellogenin B1 protein. Protein J 25(2):109-115.

Sumara I, Vorlaufer E, Stukenberg PT, Kelm O, Redemann N, Nigg EA, Peters JM. 2002. The dissociation of cohesin from chromosomes in prophase is regulated by Polo-like kinase. Mol Cell 9(3):515-525.

Sumiyoshi E, Sugimoto A, Yamamoto M. 2002. Protein phosphatase 4 is required for centrosome maturation in mitosis and sperm meiosis in C. elegans. J Cell Sci 115(Pt 7):1403-1410.

Sun L, Haun S, Jones RC, Edmondson RD, Machaca K. 2009. Kinase-dependent regulation of inositol 1,4,5-trisphosphate-dependent Ca2+ release during oocyte maturation. J Biol Chem 284(30):20184-20196.

Sun QY, Fuchimoto D, Nagai T. 2004. Regulatory roles of ubiquitin-proteasome pathway in pig oocyte meiotic maturation and fertilization. Theriogenology 62(1-2):245-255.

Swain JE, Ding J, Brautigan DL, Villa-Moruzzi E, Smith GD. 2007. Proper chromatin condensation and maintenance of histone H3 phosphorylation during mouse oocyte meiosis requires protein phosphatase activity. Biol Reprod 76(4):628-638.

Swan A, Schupbach T. 2007. The Cdc20 (Fzy)/Cdh1-related protein, Cort, cooperates with Fzy in cyclin destruction and anaphase progression in meiosis I and II in Drosophila. Development 134(5):891-899.

Swann K, Igusa Y, Miyazaki S. 1989. Evidence for an inhibitory effect of protein kinase C on G-protein-mediated repetitive calcium transients in hamster eggs. EMBO J 8(12):3711-3718.

Swann K, Whitaker M. 1985. Stimulation of the Na/H exchanger of sea urchin eggs by phorbol ester. Nature 314(6008):274-277.

Szczepanska K, Maleszewski M. 2005. LKB1/PAR4 protein is asymmetrically localized in mouse oocytes and associates with meiotic spindle. Gene Expr Patterns 6(1):86-93.

Talmor-Cohen A, Tomashov-Matar R, Tsai WB, Kinsey WH, Shalgi R. 2004. Fyn kinase-tubulin interaction during meiosis of rat eggs. Reproduction 128(4):387-393.

Tan X, Peng A, Wang Y, Tang Z. 2005a. The effects of proteasome inhibitor lactacystin on mouse oocyte meiosis and first cleavage. Sci China C Life Sci 48(3):287-294.

Tan X, Peng A, Wang YC, Wang Y, Sun QY. 2005b. Participation of the ubiquitin-proteasome pathway in rat oocyte activation. Zygote 13(1):87-95.

Tanaka K, Okubo Y, Abe H. 2005. Involvement of slingshot in the Rho-mediated dephosphorylation of ADF/cofilin during Xenopus cleavage. Zoolog Sci 22(9):971-984.

Tang ED, Nunez G, Barr FG, Guan KL. 1999. Negative regulation of the forkhead transcription factor FKHR by Akt. J Biol Chem 274(24):16741-16746.

Tang W, Wu JQ, Guo Y, Hansen DV, Perry JA, Freel CD, Nutt L, Jackson PK, Kornbluth S. 2008. Cdc2 and Mos regulate Emi2 stability to promote the meiosis I-meiosis II transition. Mol Biol Cell 19(8):3536-3543.

Tang Z, Shu H, Oncel D, Chen S, Yu H. 2004. Phosphorylation of Cdc20 by Bub1 provides a catalytic mechanism for APC/C inhibition by the spindle checkpoint. Mol Cell 16(3):387-397.

Tarone G, Russo MA, Hirsch E, Odorisio T, Altruda F, Silengo L, Siracusa G. 1993. Expression of beta 1 integrin complexes on the surface of unfertilized mouse oocyte. Development 117(4):1369-1375.

Taylor SJ, Anafi M, Pawson T, Shalloway D. 1995. Functional interaction between c-Src and its mitotic target, Sam 68. J Biol Chem 270(17):10120-10124.

Taylor SJ, Shalloway D. 1994. An RNA-binding protein associated with Src through its SH2 and SH3 domains in mitosis. Nature 368(6474):867-871.

Tchang F, Gusse M, Soussi T, Mechali M. 1993. Stabilization and expression of high levels of p53 during early development in Xenopus laevis. Dev Biol 159(1):163-172.

Tchang F, Mechali M. 1999. Nuclear import of p53 during Xenopus laevis early development in relation to DNA replication and DNA repair. Exp Cell Res 251(1):46-56.

Terret ME, Ferby I, Nebreda AR, Verlhac MH. 2001. RINGO efficiently triggers meiosis resumption in mouse oocytes and induces cell cycle arrest in embryos. Biol Cell 93(1-2):89-97.

Thomas RE, Armstrong DT, Gilchrist RB. 2002. Differential effects of specific phosphodiesterase isoenzyme inhibitors on bovine oocyte meiotic maturation. Dev Biol 244(2):215-225.

Thumbikat P, Berry RE, Schaeffer AJ, Klumpp DJ. 2009a. Differentiation-induced uroplakin III expression promotes urothelial cell death in response to uropathogenic E. coli. Microbes Infect 11(1):57-65.

Thumbikat P, Berry RE, Zhou G, Billips BK, Yaggie RE, Zaichuk T, Sun TT, Schaeffer AJ, Klumpp DJ. 2009b. Bacteria-induced uroplakin signaling mediates bladder response to infection. PLoS Pathog 5(5):e1000415.

Tian AG, Deng WM. 2008. Lgl and its phosphorylation by aPKC regulate oocyte polarity formation in Drosophila. Development 135(3):463-471.

Tian J, Gong H, Lennarz WJ. 1999. Xenopus laevis sperm receptor gp69/64 glycoprotein is a homolog of the mammalian sperm receptor ZP2. Proc Natl Acad Sci U S A 96(3):829-834.

Tokmakov AA, Sato KI, Iwasaki T, Fukami Y. 2002. Src kinase induces calcium release in Xenopus egg extracts via PLCgamma and IP3-dependent mechanism. Cell Calcium 32(1):11-20.

Tokumoto T, Yamashita M, Tokumoto M, Katsu Y, Horiguchi R, Kajiura H, Nagahama Y. 1997. Initiation of cyclin B degradation by the 26S proteasome upon egg activation. J Cell Biol 138(6):1313-1322.

Tonks NK, Cicirelli MF, Diltz CD, Krebs EG, Fischer EH. 1990. Effect of microinjection of a low-Mr human placenta protein tyrosine phosphatase on induction of meiotic cell division in Xenopus oocytes. Mol Cell Biol 10(2):458-463.

Totsukawa G, Himi-Nakamura E, Komatsu S, Iwata K, Tezuka A, Sakai H, Yazaki K, Hosoya H. 1996. Mitosis-specific phosphorylation of smooth muscle regulatory light chain of myosin II at Ser-1 and/or -2 and Thr-9 in sea urchin egg extract. Cell Struct Funct 21(6):475-482.

Tse AC, Ge W. 2009. Differential regulation of betacellulin and heparin-binding EGF-like growth factor in cultured zebrafish ovarian follicle cells by EGF family ligands. Comp Biochem Physiol A Mol Integr Physiol 153(1):13-17.

Tsurumi A, Xia F, Li J, Larson K, LaFrance R, Li WX. 2011. STAT is an essential activator of the zygotic genome in the early Drosophila embryo. PLoS Genet 7(5):e1002086.

Tung JJ, Hansen DV, Ban KH, Loktev AV, Summers MK, Adler JR, 3rd, Jackson PK. 2005. A role for the anaphase-promoting complex inhibitor Emi2/XErp1, a homolog of early mitotic inhibitor 1, in cytostatic factor arrest of Xenopus eggs. Proc Natl Acad Sci U S A 102(12):4318-4323.

Tunquist BJ, Maller JL. 2003. Under arrest: cytostatic factor (CSF)-mediated metaphase arrest in vertebrate eggs. Genes Dev 17(6):683-710.

Tunquist BJ, Schwab MS, Chen LG, Maller JL. 2002. The spindle checkpoint kinase bub1 and cyclin e/cdk2 both contribute to the establishment of meiotic metaphase arrest by cytostatic factor. Curr Biol 12(12):1027-1033.

Turner CE. 1991. Paxillin is a major phosphotyrosine-containing protein during embryonic development. J Cell Biol 115(1):201-207.

Urayama S, Harada Y, Nakagawa Y, Ban S, Akasaka M, Kawasaki N, Sawada H. 2008. Ascidian sperm glycosylphosphatidylinositol-anchored CRISP-like protein as a binding partner for an allorecognizable sperm receptor on the vitelline coat. J Biol Chem 283(31):21725-21733.

van Eekelen M, Runtuwene V, Overvoorde J, den Hertog J. 2010. RPTPalpha and PTPepsilon signaling via Fyn/Yes and RhoA is essential for zebrafish convergence and extension cell movements during gastrulation. Dev Biol 340(2):626-639.

Vanderheyden V, Wakai T, Bultynck G, De Smedt H, Parys JB, Fissore RA. 2009. Regulation of inositol 1,4,5-trisphosphate receptor type 1 function during oocyte maturation by MPM-2 phosphorylation. Cell Calcium 46(1):56-64.

Vanhaesebroeck B, Leevers SJ, Panayotou G, Waterfield MD. 1997. Phosphoinositide 3-kinases: a conserved family of signal transducers. Trends Biochem Sci 22(7):267-272.

Vesela J, Cikos S, Hlinka D, Rehak P, Baran V, Koppel J. 1995. Effects of impaired insulin secretion on the fertilization of mouse oocytes. Hum Reprod 10(12):3233-3236.

Vigneron S, Brioudes E, Burgess A, Labbe JC, Lorca T, Castro A. 2009. Greatwall maintains mitosis through regulation of PP2A. EMBO J 28(18):2786-2793.

Visintin R, Prinz S, Amon A. 1997. CDC20 and CDH1: a family of substrate-specific activators of APC-dependent proteolysis. Science 278(5337):460-463.

Wakai T, Vanderheyden V, Yoon SY, Cheon B, Zhang N, Parys JB, Fissore RA. 2011. Regulation of inositol 1,4,5-trisphosphate receptor function during mouse oocyte maturation. J Cell Physiol.

Wang Q, Wang CM, Ai JS, Xiong B, Yin S, Hou Y, Chen DY, Schatten H, Sun QY. 2006. Histone phosphorylation and pericentromeric histone modifications in oocyte meiosis. Cell Cycle 5(17):1974-1982.

Wang Y, Li J, Ying Wang C, Yan Kwok AH, Leung FC. 2007. Epidermal growth factor (EGF) receptor ligands in the chicken ovary: I. Evidence for heparin-binding EGF-like growth factor (HB-EGF) as a potential oocyte-derived signal to control granulosa cell proliferation and HB-EGF and kit ligand expression. Endocrinology 148(7):3426-3440.

Wang Y, Morrow JS. 2000. Identification and characterization of human SLP-2, a novel homologue of stomatin (band 7.2b) present in erythrocytes and other tissues. J Biol Chem 275(11):8062-8071.

Wasielak M, Bogacki M. 2007. Apoptosis inhibition by insulin-like growth factor (IGF)-I during in vitro maturation of bovine oocytes. J Reprod Dev 53(2):419-426.

Wassarman PM, Litscher ES. 2001. Multiple functions of mouse zona pellucida glycoprotein mZP3, the sperm receptor. Ital J Anat Embryol 106(2 Suppl 2):21-32.

Watts JL, Etemad-Moghadam B, Guo S, Boyd L, Draper BW, Mello CC, Priess JR, Kemphues KJ. 1996. par-6, a gene involved in the establishment of asymmetry in early C. elegans embryos, mediates the asymmetric localization of PAR-3. Development 122(10):3133-3140.

Weber GM, Moore AB, Sullivan CV. 2007. In vitro actions of insulin-like growth factor-I on ovarian follicle maturation in white perch (Morone americana). Gen Comp Endocrinol 151(2):180-187.

Weber GM, Sullivan CV. 2005. Insulin-like growth factor-I induces oocyte maturational competence but not meiotic resumption in white bass (Morone chrysops) follicles in vitro: evidence for rapid evolution of insulin-like growth factor action. Biol Reprod 72(5):1177-1186.

Wei L, Liang XW, Zhang QH, Li M, Yuan J, Li S, Sun SC, Ouyang YC, Schatten H, Sun QY. 2010. BubR1 is a spindle assembly checkpoint protein regulating meiotic cell cycle progression of mouse oocyte. Cell Cycle 9(6):1112-1121.

Weinstein J. 1997. Cell cycle-regulated expression, phosphorylation, and degradation of p55Cdc. A mammalian homolog of CDC20/Fizzy/slp1. J Biol Chem 272(45):28501-28511.

Welsh M, Songyang Z, Frantz JD, Trub T, Reedquist KA, Karlsson T, Miyazaki M, Cantley LC, Band H, Shoelson SE. 1998. Stimulation through the T cell receptor leads to interactions between SHB and several signaling proteins. Oncogene 16(7):891-901.

Westmark CJ, Ghose R, Huber PW. 2002. Phosphorylation of Xenopus transcription factor IIIA by an oocyte protein kinase CK2. Biochem J 362(Pt 2):375-382.

Wiersma A, Hirsch B, Tsafriri A, Hanssen RG, Van de Kant M, Kloosterboer HJ, Conti M, Hsueh AJ. 1998. Phosphodiesterase 3 inhibitors suppress oocyte maturation and consequent pregnancy without affecting ovulation and cyclicity in rodents. J Clin Invest 102(3):532-537.

Wiles MV, Ruiz P, Imhof BA. 1992. Interleukin-7 expression during mouse thymus development. Eur J Immunol 22(4):1037-1042.

Williams CJ, Mehlmann LM, Jaffe LA, Kopf GS, Schultz RM. 1998. Evidence that Gq family G proteins do not function in mouse egg activation at fertilization. Dev Biol 198(1):116-127.

Wright PW, Bolling LC, Calvert ME, Sarmento OF, Berkeley EV, Shea MC, Hao Z, Jayes FC, Bush LA, Shetty J, Shore AN, Reddi PP, Tung KS, Samy E, Allietta MM, Sherman NE, Herr JC, Coonrod SA. 2003. ePAD, an oocyte and early embryo-abundant peptidylarginine deiminase-like protein that localizes to egg cytoplasmic sheets. Dev Biol 256(1):73-88.

Wu JQ, Hansen DV, Guo Y, Wang MZ, Tang W, Freel CD, Tung JJ, Jackson PK, Kornbluth S. 2007a. Control of Emi2 activity and stability through Mos-mediated recruitment of PP2A. Proc Natl Acad Sci U S A 104(42):16564-16569.

Wu JQ, Kornbluth S. 2008. Across the meiotic divide - CSF activity in the post-Emi2/XErp1 era. J Cell Sci 121(Pt 21):3509-3514.

Wu Q, Guo Y, Yamada A, Perry JA, Wang MZ, Araki M, Freel CD, Tung JJ, Tang W, Margolis SS, Jackson PK, Yamano H, Asano M, Kornbluth S. 2007b. A role for Cdc2- and PP2A-mediated regulation of Emi2 in the maintenance of CSF arrest. Curr Biol 17(3):213-224.

Wu W, Kinsey WH. 2002. Role of PTPase(s) in regulating Fyn kinase at fertilization of the zebrafish egg. Dev Biol 247(2):286-294.

Wu Y, Pan S, Che S, He G, Nelman-Gonzalez M, Weil MM, Kuang J. 2001. Overexpression of Hp95 induces G1 phase arrest in confluent HeLa cells. Differentiation 67(4-5):139-153.

Xi J, Sugimoto I, Yoshitome S, Yasuda H, Ogura K, Mori N, Li Z, Ito S, Hashimoto E. 2003. Purification and characterization of Mr 43,000 protein similar to Mr 25,000 protein, a substrate for protein Ser/Thr kinases, identified as a part of Xenopus laevis vitellogenin B1. J Protein Chem 22(6):571-583.

Yamamoto-Honda R, Honda Z, Ueki K, Tobe K, Kaburagi Y, Takahashi Y, Tamemoto H, Suzuki T, Itoh K, Akanuma Y, Yazaki Y, Kadowaki T. 1996. Mutant of insulin receptor substrate-1 incapable of activating phosphatidylinositol 3-kinase did not mediate insulin-stimulated maturation of Xenopus laevis oocytes. J Biol Chem 271(45):28677-28681.

Yang J, Winkler K, Yoshida M, Kornbluth S. 1999. Maintenance of G2 arrest in the Xenopus oocyte: a role for 14-3-3-mediated inhibition of Cdc25 nuclear import. EMBO J 18(8):2174-2183.

Yoshida M, Horiuchi Y, Sensui N, Morisawa M. 2003. Signaling pathway from [Ca2+]i transients to ooplasmic segregation involves small GTPase rho in the ascidian egg. Dev Growth Differ 45(3):275-281.

Yu Y, Halet G, Lai FA, Swann K. 2008. Regulation of diacylglycerol production and protein kinase C stimulation during sperm- and PLCzeta-mediated mouse egg activation. Biol Cell 100(11):633-643.

Yuan J, Li M, Wei L, Yin S, Xiong B, Li S, Lin SL, Schatten H, Sun QY. 2009. Astrin regulates meiotic spindle organization, spindle pole tethering and cell cycle progression in mouse oocytes. Cell Cycle 8(20):3384-3395.

Zhang L, Ding F, Cao W, Liu Z, Liu W, Yu Z, Wu Y, Li W, Li Y. 2006. Stomatin-like protein 2 is overexpressed in cancer and involved in regulating cell growth and cell adhesion in human esophageal squamous cell carcinoma. Clin Cancer Res 12(5):1639-1646.

Zhang L, Liang Y, Liu Y, Xiong CL. 2010. The role of brain-derived neurotrophic factor in mouse oocyte maturation in vitro involves activation of protein kinase B. Theriogenology 73(8):1096-1103.

Zhang Y, Zhang Z, Xu XY, Li XS, Yu M, Yu AM, Zong ZH, Yu BZ. 2008. Protein kinase A modulates Cdc25B activity during meiotic resumption of mouse oocytes. Dev Dyn 237(12):3777-3786.

Zhao Y, Haccard O, Wang R, Yu J, Kuang J, Jessus C, Goldberg ML. 2008. Roles of Greatwall kinase in the regulation of cdc25 phosphatase. Mol Biol Cell 19(4):1317-1327.

Ziyyat A, Rubinstein E, Monier-Gavelle F, Barraud V, Kulski O, Prenant M, Boucheix C, Bomsel M, Wolf JP. 2006. CD9 controls the formation of clusters that contain tetraspanins and the integrin alpha 6 beta 1, which are involved in human and mouse gamete fusion. J Cell Sci 119(Pt 3):416-424.

23

Morphometry as a Method of Studying Adaptive Regulation of Embryogenesis in Polluted Environments

Elena A. Severtsova, David R. Aguillón Gutiérrez and Aleksey S. Severtsov
Lomonosov Moscow State University
Russian Federation

1. Introduction

Amphibians- one of the most convenient natural objects to study the effect of various pollutants (Dawson et al, 1985). They are very sensitive to changes in the environment. Larval and adult specimens have a high permeable skin and their life cycle takes place in water and in terrestrial ecosystems, depending on the stage of the life cycle; they have different types of food; their special reproduction allows monitoring of development and the quantity to conduct representative research (Cooke, 1974; Greenhouse, 1976; Sparling et al, 2001).

In addition, some amphibian species are laboratory animals with a well-studied biology and genetics, for example the clawed frog (*Xenopus laevis*), which is the biological model in the FETAX project (Fort et al, 2004; Morgan et al, 1996) and *Xenopus* metamorphosis assay (XEMA) (Opitz et al, 2005) which conducted test of various chemical pollutants. Applied nature of these programs involves testing the impact on the embryogenesis of each substance alone (FETAX, 1991), although in nature, in the embryo affects a complex of pollutants of the lake. Therefore, in recent years, within the confines of FETAX system, are conducted analyzes of the synergistic complex of pollutants (Orton et al., 2006; Ettler et al., 2008), which allows to evaluate the natural biotoxicity and anthropogenic pollutants.

However, being just test models, laboratory animals because of its unsuitability to the full range of factors in nature, can not be regarded as indicators of ecosystem pollution. Thus, the experimental exposure to pesticides (particularly DDT [dichlorodiphenyltrichloroethane] and HCH [Hexachlorocyclohexane]) on eggs of Clawed and Moor frogs, showed significantly more sensitive reaction in *Xenopus laevis* than natural populations of *Rana arvalis*, making an incorrect comparative analysis (Voronova et al, 1983).

Therefore, to study the effects of pollution in natural habitats are more informative the representatives of natural populations (Stroganov, 1971). Field studies are conducted on widely distributed amphibian species: *Rana pipens* (Allran & Karasov, 2000, 2001), *Rana arvalis* (Andren et al, 1989), *Rana temporaria* (Leontieva & Semenov, 1997; Dunson et al, 1992; Johansson et al, 2001), *Bufo americanus* (Hecnar, 1995) and other species which by 1992 had already been tested 211 types of pollutants in 45 amphibian species (Hall & Henry, 1992). Among these works dominates the studies on tadpoles or adult animals (Vershin, 1997; Freda, 1986; Horne & Dunson, 1995). Typically, field studies are limited to the proportion of those who died and/or are abnormal embryos (Beattie et al, 1991). This is certainly an important indicator of overall population status, but, in our view, insufficient because they do not reflect the actual adaptation processes in natural populations under the action of a new environmental evolutionary factor (Vershinin, 1997; Severtsova, 2002), and is an indicator of only a fraction of genotypes who dropped out of population diversity. More informative is the method of morphometric evaluation of the nature of variability (Severtsova & Severtsov, 2005).

2. Morphometric analysis of early development

The object of developmental studies is the development of the individual, whereas the subject of population studies - the aggregate of individuals united in a population. These two lines of research have traditionally developed independently. In the analysis of specimens is estimated the condition of the body at a certain stage of development and its dynamics in time and space. The study of ontogeny itself, which often is limited to embryonic development and identify differences between individuals.

In the study of population is estimated the populations status in a determinate moment and also its dynamics in time and space, it means the assessment of population dynamics and detection of inter and intrapopulation differences. This is usually not taken into account that each individual is ontogeny, and the population estimate is a slice of the trajectories of individual development. In those cases where this is taken into account the possible ontogenetic change as something that interferes with population estimate, and the problem usually comes down to their elimination by the analysis of individuals of the same age. At the same time as a special analysis of individual ontogeny is not only necessary for the correct assessment of populations and their dynamics in time and space, but also for understanding the mechanisms of the stability of population processes.

Stabilized development is one of the most common characteristics of the developing organism. It was shown that high stability is maintained on the basis of genetic coadaptation under optimal conditions of development (Zakharov, 1989; Moller & Swaddle, 1997). A growing number of studies of developmental stability and incessant debate about the significance of such studies to characterize the state of the population determines the need to assess the possibility of using developmental stability as a measure of environmental stress for monitoring populations. In this case, the most convenient is the morphometric method based on an evaluation of morphological variability. Themselves morphometric methods for assessing variability are used frequently, including to assess the variability of synanthropic populations of animals and plants (see "Intraspecific variation ..." 1980; "Animals in ...", 1990, "Structure and functional role ...", 2001).

Assessment of variability in the earliest stages of development in this aspect was not carried out, although the method of study of their variability exists. Apparently, the quantitative study of the variability of morphogenetic traits was a Gurwitsch's idea (Gurwitsch, 1922: in Cherdantsev, 2003). The idea is that by studying the relation between the average and the variance of quantitative traits of the embryo or its parts, you can get a fairly accurate idea of the nature of interactions corresponding to the morphogenetic field. Specific studies on the Gurwitsch's planned program are very few (Cherdantsev & Scobeyeva, 1994; Glukhova & Cherdantsev, 1999; Severtsova, 2002), although this method can be used to study the variability of embryogenesis during the development in different contexts, including the anthropogenic pollution condition.

The model of some-like research is the most convenient anuran eggs at the stage of mid-late gastrula (Cherdantsev & Scobeyeva, 1994), since the earlier stages are not enough informative, and the analysis of later stages must take into account a large number of complex processes, including those related to organogenesis. Gastrula stage is best studied in terms of morphogenetic processes and the genetic basis of regulation of these processes (Beetschen, 2001). In particular, revealed that in the analysis of morphological variability of gastrulation, in some amphibian species (*Rana temporaria, Rana lessonae* and *Pelobates fuscus*) there is huge value of the coefficients of variation of characters in the embryos that are genetically homogeneous (from the same clutch of eggs), developing in quite the same conditions, and the most importantly, developing normally in terms of the final result of embryonic development. It may be more than 50%, ie almost an order of magnitude higher than normal variability of quantitative traits in definitive stages of development of the phenotype (see Falconer, 1981). In addition, is shown that this is the stage in early development of amphibians most sensitive to environmental effects (Saber & Dunson, 1978; Beattie et al., 1992; Severtsova, 2005), that allows us to estimate the variability in the development stages, when the abnormality of the morphogenetic processes have not yet discernible to the naked eye.

For morphometric analysis, we selected the most popular anuran species in Moscow: Common frog (*Rana temporaria* L.), Moor frog (*Rana arvalis* Nills.) and the Marsh frog (*Pelophylax ridibundus* Pallas). In fixed eggs of these species were removed all the membranes, including the vitelline, made by standard embryological methods, divided sagittal and measured under a binocular microscope with eyepiece micrometer (accurate to 1 division of ocular micrometer; 20 divisions of ocular micrometer range – 1mm) following features (Fig. 1A): *D1* - total diameter of the gastrula, *D2* - diameter of yolk plug, *ArthG* - roof height of gastrocele, *vh* - the maximum height of the yolk duct, *LbalD* - the depth of the dorsal lip of blastopore screwing, *LbalV* - the depth of the ventral lip of blastopore screwing, *G* - the distance between the deepest dorsal screwing and ventral blastopore lip, *preg* - the distance between the cavities of gastrocele and blastocele, *ArthB* - blastocoel roof height. The choice of these features provides a fairly complete description of gastrulation - one of the most important stages of embryogenesis (Slack et al., 1992; Gilbert, 1993; Cherdantsev, 2003). Such signs as *LbalD, LbalV* and *G* are key indicators of advanced gastrulation processes, as they reflect the extent and nature of the blastopore lip formation. *ArthG* - roof height of gastrocele - describes the process of forming chordomesoderm in the investigates development stage. Signs *preg* and *ArthB* are closely related to the previous stage of embryogenesis - blastulation, as they mark the location of the reducing blastocoel, and thus may serve, in conjunction with *ArthG* an index of "looseness" of the embryo. "Loose", commonly referred to the gastrula with non-dense intercellular contacts, or with abnormally large cells that do not allow because of the physical features of morphogenesis to form cavities or even to continue the further development (Cherdantsev, 2003).

1A

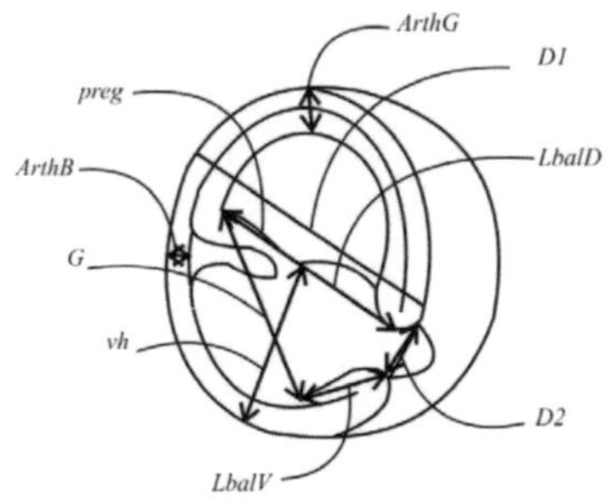

1B

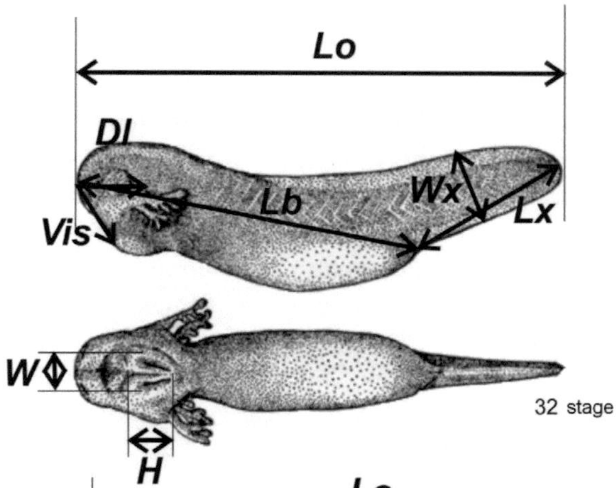

1C

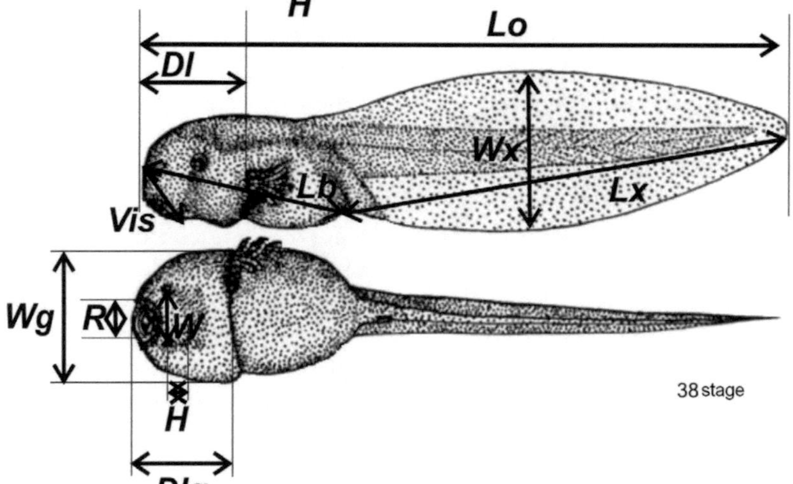

Fig. 1. Research of morphometrical signs. See notation in text.

Assessment of variability is possible at later stages of embryogenesis, for example at the stage of hatching larvae from the eggs (Fig. 1B). This stage of development is longer in comparison with gastrulation, but also allows to evaluate representatively the intra-population and intra-egg mass variability. Signs for the morphometric analysis are indicators such as: *Lo*- tadpole total length (from the outermost point of the snout to the tip of the tail plate); *Lx* - the length of the tail plate (from the cloaca to the tip of the tail plate); *Dl* - the length of the muzzle (from the base of the gill filaments to the outermost point of the muzzle); *Vis* - the height of the muzzle (from oral sucker to the outermost point of the muzzle); *W* - width of oral sucker, *H* - height of the oral sucker; *G* - the number of gill filaments, summarized on the left and right sides of the embryo. In the analysis of development assessment is possible also include indices that reflect the proportional development of larvae. Correlation *Lx* / *Lo* - index of proportion of the tail plate's size relative to the total body length. Correlation *Dl* / *Vis* is a measure of proportionality of head structures development. We considered the area of the oral sucker (*W* * *H*) / 2, as an indicator of the reliability of attachment when the tadpole had just hatched from the egg, where it is some time before moving on to the stage of free swimming. An indicator of the symmetry of the gill filaments development was like a asymmetry coefficient . At tadpole stages of development, including at the stage prior to the commencement of metamorphosis, the number of features can be extended (Fig. 1C), introducing measures such as the maximum width of the tail plate (*Wx*), head width (*Wg*) - the distance measured along the line of gill slits in the tadpole; the length of the head (*Dlg*) – the distance measured from the ventral surface of the tadpole through gills slits to the outermost point of the snout; sucker width (*W*) – the distance between the sucker rollers; sucker heigh (*H*) in the sagittal direction; mouth opening width (*R*) - the distance between the corners of the mouth opening; the distance between the pupils of the eyes (*eye*). Evaluation of these indicators reflect the two most important processes: growth and differentiation. The same measurements can be made even in vivo, without damaging the tadpoles and without exerting a strong influence on the course of development. Last is the most valuable in studies aimed to studying the dynamics of development, including passing under the influence of various pollutants.

3. Variability and correlation of early development

One of the main parameters, with which operates the morphometric analysis - is the concept of "variability". From a biological point of view, it implies the diversity of individuals in the study group. Expressed mathematically in such quantities as the variance, standard deviation or coefficient of variation. The latter parameter is used in our studies because, as a dimensionless quantity allows the comparison of mixed-signs. No less important is the concept of "correlation", i.e. consistency of the emerging structures of the developing organism. Mathematically, the nature and strength of this mutual influence is expressed through the correlation coefficient calculated for the signs in the role of characteristics of structures.

The results of morphometric research of gastrula stage in three species of anurans: Common frog (*Rana temporaria* L.), Moor frog (*Rana arvalis* Nills.) and Marsh frog (*Pelophylax ridibundus* Pallas, «*Rana ridibunda* in fig. 2»), inhabiting the territory of Moscow (Russia) show the ratio between the variability and the correlation of the processes of morphogenesis, as a response to environmental degradation (Severtsova, Severtsov, 2005, 2007). At the same time such a change occurs in different areas in different ways. In the district of Ramenki, in the Moor frog is observed a high variability and low correlation of morphogenetic processes (Fig. 2).

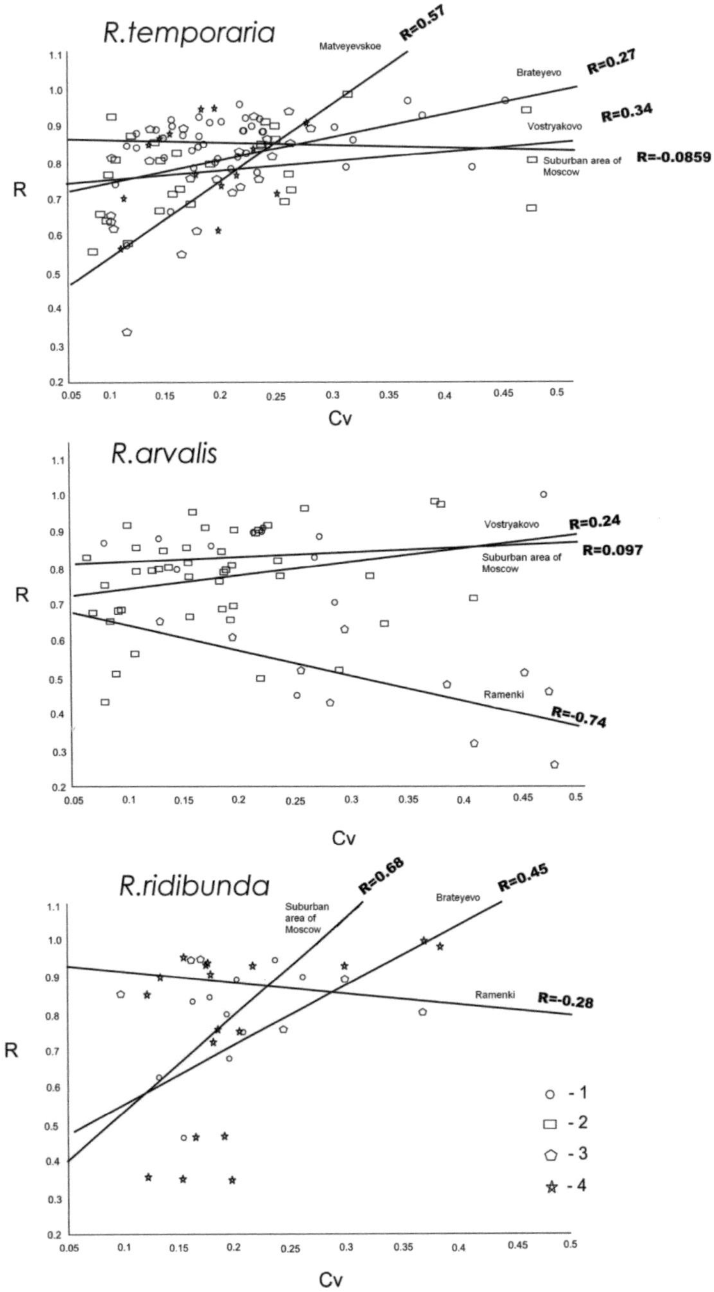

Fig. 2. Dependence of developmental variability (Cv) of general correlation (R^2) for clutches from: 1 – Suburban areas of Moscow; 2 – Vostryakovo area; 3 – Ramenky area or Matveyevskoe area; 4 – Brateyevo area.

In the first place at the end of gastrulation comes the preparation for the neurulation processes, up to heterochronies, when the yolk plug has not disappeared yet, but it's not just the formation of the neural plate, but the rise of the neural crest (Fig. 3).

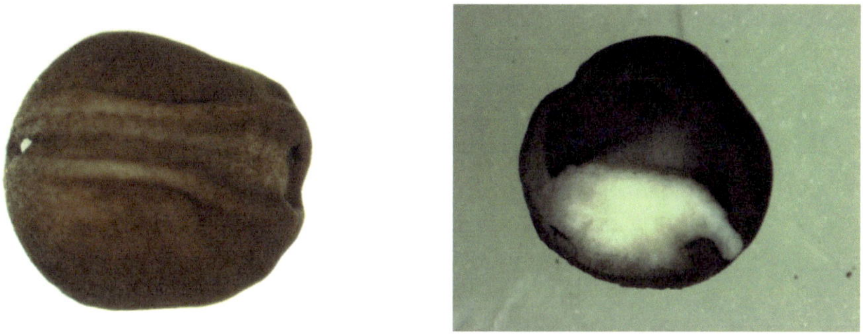

Fig. 3. Embryos of Common frog in 22nd stage with unclosed blastopore.

However, this accelerated development of high variability and miscorrelation leads to high mortality (about 5 times more in Moscow, compared with the population living outside the city of Moscow, which is characterized by low levels of anthropogenic pollution). In the Marsh frog in the district of Ramenki, the low overall correlation of development, compensates the large number of weakly inter-dependent processes. In the district Brateevo, in the Marsh frog is observed a combination of low variability and a high correlation (see Fig. 2), which allows embryos to grow more consistently and leads to low mortality. A somewhat different picture from Moor frog, living in the same area: with very low overall correlation of development, the key role is played by the ventral lip of blastopore screwing. A similar pattern was observed in embryos of the Common frog, which clutches were fixed from the pond, located 5 km downstream of the Setun river - in the district of Matveevskoe. In the Common frog gastrula, with high variability of the gastrulation processes, is observed a significant increase of the correlation among morphogenetic processes, ie with a correlation coefficient of less than 0.6 in the relationship between developing structures. This ensures the integrity of the eggs with the predominant role of the process of screwing in the ventral lip of blastopore.

The development of Common and moor frogs in the district of Vostryakovo varied. In the Common frog with a relatively low correlation of the general development, as well as in the district of Brateevo, an important role played the processes of changes in the diameter of eggs associated with the beginning of the neural elongation of the embryo. In the moor frog with a very high proportion of significance, but not high correlation coefficients between the studied traits is observed as a characteristic of gastrulation the predominance of the role on the ventral lip of blastopore invagination. In the eggs in gastrulation from nests near Moscow also significantly affects the overall high correlation of development in conjunction with their low variability (see Fig. 2). However, for the eggs of the Common frog populations near Moscow, the dimensional characteristics are closely related to the amount of yolk in the eggs. To Moor and Marsh frogs, fixed at 17th stage, the predominant role is played by processes of the screwing of the ventral lip of blastopore.

As can be seen from the above analysis the changing nature of morphogenetic processes during early development in anurans is due to changes in the correlation of variability and correlation of the emerging structures. This is manifested by increasing the total number of interrelated features that allows to keep and maintain the integrity of the embryo and thus provide a clearer differentiation of developing structures, despite their high variability. The second possible way of regulating early ontogenesis is realized in the amplification of correlative linked structures formed precisely at the stage of investigation, coupled with the increasing variability of morphogenetic processes. As a result, the development of this structure is accelerated. An extreme version of such correlation of variability and correlation of development is the emergence of heterochronies, i.e. situation where the structures of the embryo is formed, advancing the general process of development. Our data show that the occurrence of heterochrony changes may occur as a result of a sharp drop of the general correlation of development, against the backdrop of significantly increased variability in the emerging structures. This leads to a significant increase in mortality and in the case of the population of the Ramenki district to its extinction, aside from the small number of this population.

No less important is the conclusion that, in spite of interspecific ecological and morphological differences between Common and Marsh frogs, the mechanisms of regulation of early development occur in a general scheme. This indicates a non-specific reactions of early embryogenesis. The differences in overall mortality between them, apparently due to a later spawning, characteristic of the Marsh frog. Its embryogenesis is under more favorable terms than those with Common frogs against a background of lower concentrations of pollutants.

4. Adaptation of embryogenesis to a new environmental evolutionary factor – Is it possible?

Modern concepts are based on the division of any sign of variability into three components: genetic, paratypic (environmental) and epigenetic. As the name implies, genetic variability is formed due to the work of the genotype, paratypic - is the result of the impact of external environmental factors on the ontogeny, and epigenetic variability appears as a result of interactions among cells, tissues, organs developing, so changes in one element leads to changes of many interacting structures and functions (Cherdantsev & Scobeyeva, 1994; Horder, 2006, 2008). As shown by the few experimental data, the proportion of the genetic components of the total variability in the early stages of embryogenesis is not large and varies considerably in the investigated characteristics, depending on experimental conditions (Surova, 1988a; Travis, 1980, 1981; Berven, 1982; Berven & Gill, 1983).

For example, in tadpoles of *Rana silvatica* of populations of the plains of Maryland, the mountains of Virginia and tundra of northern Canada, the heritability of growth rate is 0.08, 0.58 and 0.27, respectively (Berven & Gill, 1983). Our own calculation of the coefficient of heritability (in the broadest sense of the term) of a number of morphometric characters of Common frog embryos at the stage of hatching, showed that the average proportion of the genetic component is about 10%. This allows us to consider the overall variability of the early embryonic stages as a combination of paratypic and epigenetic components of variability and to assess their contribution to the variability in development. To do this, we performed an experiment using the cross-combinations of two environmental factors: water chemistry and density of embryos per unit volume of water. At the same time as the other parameters are aligned (temperature, light, etc.). Eggs, collected in the natural ponds of Moscow, has evolved in the water from their home pond and water from the ponds, which are located outside the city of Moscow in an area with low anthropogenic load. Eggs from the ponds that are located outside Moscow has evolved in the water of the native ponds and water from the city's ponds. Because in the experiment were used clutches of Common frogs from Moscow ponds, placing these eggs in ponds from outside Moscow, for the chemical composition that is different from that in which live and breed frogs of urban populations for many generations, should not be considered as a control or optimal conditions. The second environmental factor - tadpoles density - is no less important. Of course, its impact is more significant in the later stages of development, when begins to operate the so-called "group effect" (Schwartz et al, 1976; Severtsov, 1996). However, even at stages of development before hatching, the cluster of eggs is also important because is a regulator of oxygen inside the cluster (Surova & Severtsov, 1985). The results of factor analysis performed on the results of this experiment, allow us to conclude that the effect of the chemical composition of water and different densities of tadpoles have little impact on the overall morphogenesis. Plays a fundamental role the tempo of growth characteristics: an increase in the overall size of the larvae, depending on the stage of development that allow us to demonstrate that in the early development plays an important role the epigenetic component of variability.

The idea of epigenetic effect is to shape the developing embryo belongs to Huxley (1942) and developed by Waddington (1956). All stages of the development are potentially open to evolutionary changes, but as epigenetic interactions is so fundamental, early evolutionary stages are stable (Horder, 2006). These stages are called critical (Svetlov, 1978), nodal (Cherdantsev 2003), or even Phylotypic (Sander, 1983), as this stages may coincide with the conservative Haeckel's stages (Hall, 1997; Richardson, 1998). But is possible find a name such as "Korpergrundestalt" (Seidel, 1960), "Phyletic stage" (Cohen, 1977) "Zootip / Phylotype" (Slack et al., 1993), "Phylotypic period" (Richardson, 1995) "Hounglass model" (Duboule, 1994). However, the critical stages (or even critical periods of development) do not always coincide with the phylogenetic stages. Allocation of such stages in the development, usually is based on the idea of laying new structures of the embryo at this stage and determination of the fact that it is at these stages when is observed a high mortality of embryos.

Morphometric analysis of several successive stages of development showed that the duration of the critical stages may be limited to one or several consecutive stages - a critical period in development (Severtsova & Severtsov, 2011). During these stages (period) value of the estimated coefficients of variation of traits in embryos from different nests are not significantly different. Between the critical periods, the variability can have high or low significance, characteristic of the critical period. This is clearly seen in the analysis of changes in the values of the coefficients of variation in egg, died during the experiment. To them were characteristic the values of the coefficients of variation above or below the critical value. Among the survivors clutches in the critical period of development was observed an increase in mortality and the occurrence of anomalies incompatible with life, but the proportion of those embryos was low and the clutch continues the development. The earliest nodal stage can be seen from 18 to 20 stage of development.

The second critical period in early embryogenesis involves stage after hatching, i.e. 32 - 33rd stage of development. This period is critical for the formation of the overall length of the embryo (*Lo*) and the length of the tail plate (*Lx*). At the same time, critical for the formation of the caudal plate width (*Wx*) is the stage 34, where there is a transition of tadpoles from attached to embryonic jelly coat (gallert) to free-swimming lifestyle. 36th stage of development is critical for the formation of signs of "length of the body» (*Lb*) and "long tail plate» (*Lx*), but not for the sign " total length of the embryo» (*Lo*). For the features that characterize the differentiation of the embryo were selected the following nodal stages: " length of the muzzle " (*Dl*) and "width of the head" (*Wg*) - 36th stage, for the feature "length of the head" (*Dlg*) - 34th stage, and for the feature "width of the sucker" (*W*) - 33th stage of development. For other characters, *Vis, H, R,* and *eye,* - the allocation of nodal stages in the investigated interval of development is difficult. Perhaps, all the investigated features of the critical period are present even in the 39th stage of development, but to confirm this fact, studies should be undertaken at more advanced stages of development. Thus, in the development the critical periods can be distinguished, but these periods are critical not only for the development of the embryo as a whole, but also for the process of formation of its individual structures. In some cases, these periods can be the same for different structures and then a group is formed ("modules") signs, that changes the correlation between "variability - correlation" which is similar. Thus, the signs of the first group, *Lo, Lb, Lx* and *Wx,* describing the growth processes exhibit insignificance, with the development, reduced the general variability with a significant increase of the correlation (Fig. 4).

At the same correlation of growth processes sharply increases from 29 to 32 stage and 34 to 36th, i.e. just to pre-nodal and nodal stages. Signs that do not have the segment of the nodal stage (*Vis, H, R,* and *eye*) are characterized by an increase in the variability of development and low coherence. In signs (*Dl, Dlg, Wg, W*), for which was isolated nodal stage, with low variability increases, anyway there is an increase in the coherence of development. Our findings are confirmed by other researchers, which also showed that the so-called Phylotypic stages of development increases the level of morphological interactions by a decline in variability (Irmler et al., 2004), and such stage is also characterized by modularity (Raff & Sly, 2000; Galis & Metz, 2001; Galis & Sinervo, 2002).

It is shown that modularity acts as a buffer mechanism for deviant development in extreme environments (Schmidt & Starck, 2010). Thus, influencing on the signs themselves, the environment does not change the modularity of its structure. Only when the impact causes an increase in the variability of development, there is either independent development units (up to the emergence of heterochronies (Richardson, 1995), or the emergence of new correlation coefficients between the modules and, consequently, the formation of a unified system of non-rigid correlation interactions. (Severtsova & Severtsov, 2011).

In a variety of environmental conditions the extent to which you can change a sign, is limited by its norm of reaction. This term was proposed by I. I. Schmalhausen (1969) and is special an individual characteristic, reflecting the breadth of variability in body shape in response to exposure to the environment and the ongoing without changing its genotype (Severtsov, 2004).

In the english-language evolutionary studies, the concept of norm of reaction criterion is close to the concept of "phenotypic plasticity" (Gordon, 1992; Via et al., 1995; Pigliucci, 2005; Garland & Kelly, 2006). As wider is the norm of reaction of genotype, wider is the variation of sign limits and is wider the range of environmental conditions in which this feature ensures the survival of the individual. It is in unstable conditions where the individual with the most wide norm of reaction will get a selective advantage (Severtsov, 1985; Severtsov & Surova, 1981).

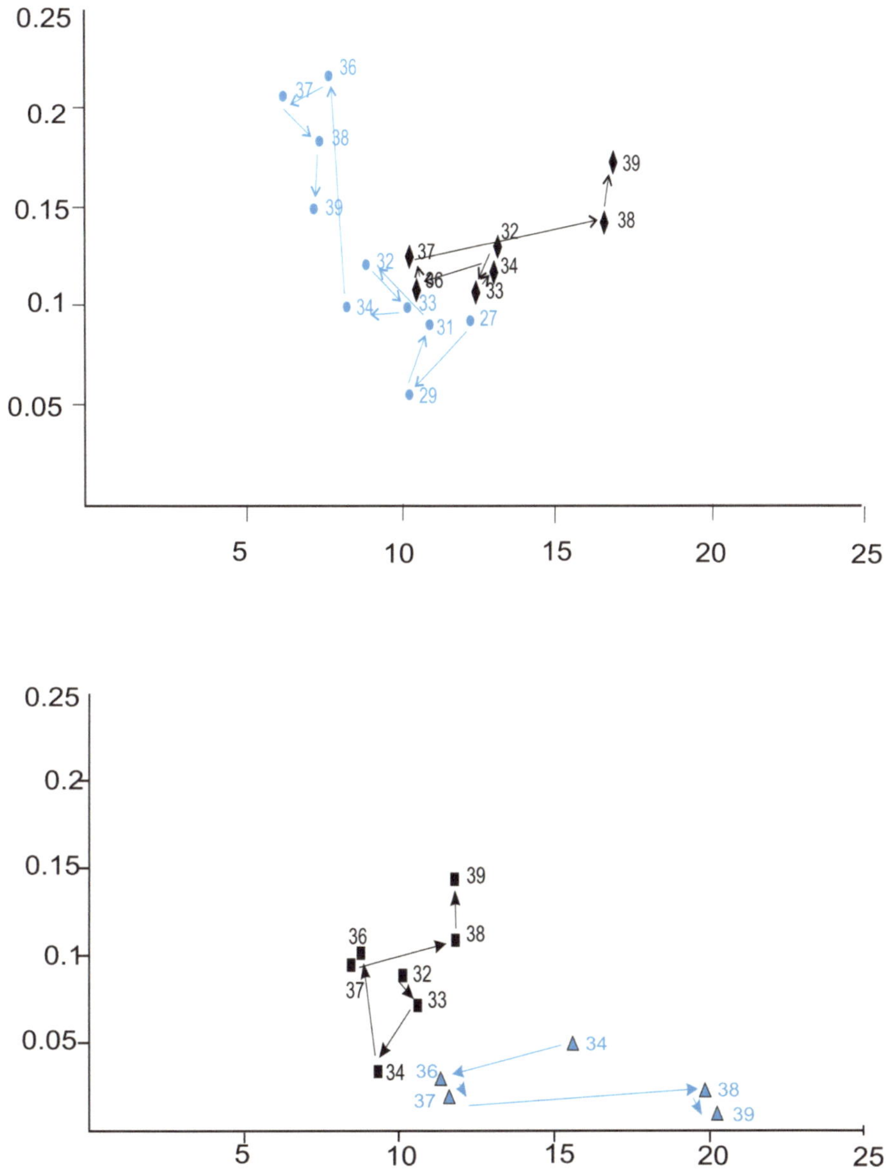

Fig. 4. Stepwise analysis of change in values of a generalized coefficient of determination ($Cv_{\text{общ}}$) (axis X) from determination coefficient (R^2) (axis Y). Numbers means the stage number. For signs: ● - *Lo, Lb, Lx, Wx* and ♦ - *Dl, Vis, Wg, Dlg, W, H, R, eye*. For signs: ■ - for signs *Dl, Wg, W, Dlg* and ▲ -for signs *Vis, H, R, eye*.

Mechanisms of "retention" of the formation of character in this framework for early embryogenesis practically have not been studied. In our works we have considered as a possible regulatory mechanism the changing of the correlation of the variability and consistency (correlation) of the formed structures. This is manifested by increasing the total number of interrelated features that allows to keep and maintain the integrity of the embryo's development and thus provide a clearer differentiation of developing structures, despite their high variability. The second possible way of regulating early ontogenesis is realized by the amplification of correlative linked structures, formed precisely at the stage of investigation, coupled with the increasing variability of morphogenetic processes. As a result, the developmental process of this structure is accelerated up to the emergence of heterochronies. Perhaps this way of regulation can be illustrated by a moving ball in the trench chreod in the model of epigenetic landscape proposed by Waddington (1947) (Shishkin, 1984).

If we consider the ball as a separate character state, not as a body (in the original model) then the path traveled by the ball-sign would be the way of development for this sign. In a stable environment occurs the moving of the ball on the bottom of the "trench" and we, analyzing the variability of this path, will see that it is not high. In the case of "interference" occurs "swing" of the ball in the trench chreod and thus an increase in the variability of the characteristic (Fig. 5). In this case we need constant adjustment the path of development that holds "the ball" in the trench, which will be implemented by changing the consistency of development of a specific sign with other signs of the developing embryo. But we should not forget that epigenomics has no additive genetic component, so the variability in developing systems is characterized by stability and equifinality (Schmalhausen 1942; Shishkin, 1984; Cherdantsev, 2003).

In this form of organization of morphogenetic variability the direct action of natural selection on early signs of morphogenesis is hampered. By itself, the variability of development can not be used as material for selection, because it´s basically epigenomic and also is lost on the nodal stages of development. However, this does not mean that the adaptive evolution of the early stages of ontogeny to the effects of pollutants is not possible (Holloway et al., 1990; Forbes & Calow, 1997), although in many cases, the rate of environmental change might be too quick to create adaptations (Lynch & Lande, 1993; Burger & Lynch, 1997). However, published data show an increase in resistance to pollutants (Hesnar, 1995; Forbes & Calow, 1997; Gu et al., 2000; Johanson et al., 2001) and even the direct effects of environment on gene expression (Morozova et al., 2006; Wittkopp, 2007).

In some cases, is shown the stability of embryogenesis to the action of pollutants in amphibians from populations living in conditions of water pollution by organic substances (Hecnar, 1995; Johansson et al., 2001; Severtsova, 2002) or strong acidification (Andren et al., 1989). Comparison of resistance to pollution by nitrates of two populations of *Bufo americanus* showed a higher tolerance for this type of pollution in populations that spends a long time under the action of nitrates (Hecnar, 1995). Studies in Sweden have shown that the more resistant to prolonged exposure to a solution of ammonium nitrate are frog eggs from the southern regions, where the concentration of nitrate in nature is higher than in the northern (Johansson et al., 2001).

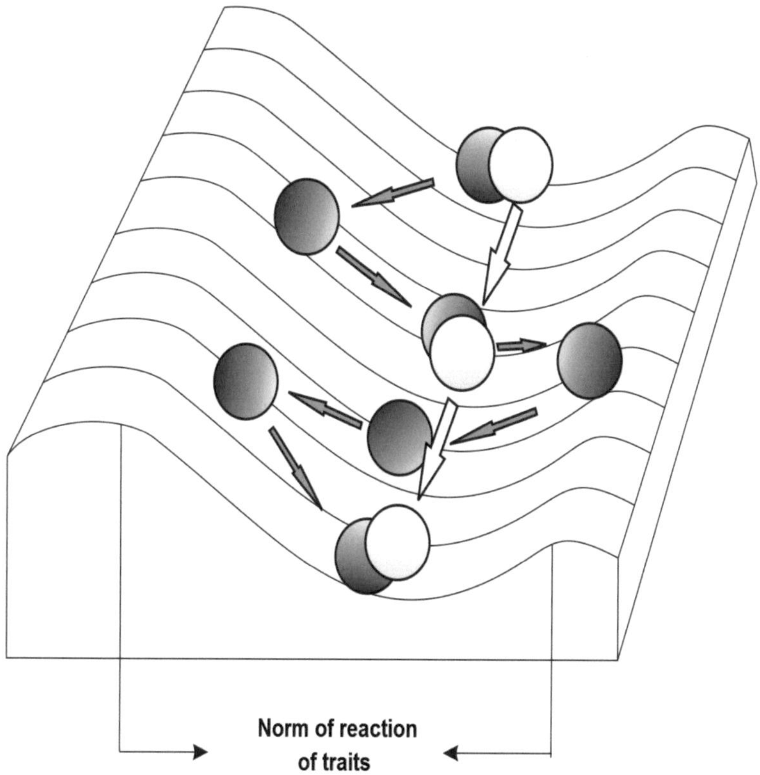

Fig. 5. Model of epigenetic landscape of Waddington (Shishkin, 1984)with changes. Plot of epigenetic landscape of the valley (chreod) which moves the ball, which symbolizes the path of the trait development. The chreoda's width is determinate by the norm of reaction of a trait, the depth, by the genetic determinism. Moving the light ball in the chreoda symbolizes the development of a trait in the right conditions, the dark ball, under adverse conditions that requiring regulation of development.

All these data indicate the possibility of adaptive evolution. Certainly, the formation of such adaptations are in all stages of the life cycle. However, as shown by the results, the factor analysis carried by us, according on the results of experiments with cross-coupling conditions for the development of tadpoles, response to exposure to the environment occurs individually for each clutch in each year of analysis (Severtsova, 2009). Consequently, the evolutionary transformation will occur at the level of change in the way of individual development of each clutch, driving changes in the way of development of each trait (West-Eberhard, 2003).

5. Conclusion

In conclusion, we emphasize that our approach using morphometric analysis of early embryogenesis allow us to evaluate the general condition of the population, living in conditions of anthropogenic pollution of the environment and to answer the important question of the possible adaptations of early embryogenesis in this new evolutionary environmental factor. Variability- an inherent property of life. Variability is the material for natural selection and, therefore, the methodological approaches to the study of variability in understanding the degree of diversity and mechanisms of evolutionary changes have been well worked. Embryological studies dealing with the investigation of the features of ontogeny or evolutionary change of early development use morphometric approach for the study of variability in a lower grade.

6. References

Animals in conditions of anthropogenic landscape. (1990). Sverdlovsk ASUSSR UrO pp. 125. (Russ.).

Intraspecific variation in animal ontogenesis. (1980) M.: Nauka. pp 226 (Russ.).

Structure and functional role of animal populations in natural and transformed ecosystems. (2001) Abstract: I International Conference 17-20 September. Dnepropetrovsk. pp. 247. (Russ).

Allran, J. & Karasov, W. (2000). Effects of atrazine and nitrate on northern leopard frog (*Rana pipience*) larvae exposed in the laboratory from posthatch through metamorphosis. *Environ. Toxicol. Chem.* V. 19, №.11, pp. 2850-2855.

Allran, J. & Karasov, W. (2001) Effects of atrazine on embryos, larvae and adults of anuran amphibians. *Environ. Toxicol. Chem.* V. 20, №. 4, pp. 769-775.

Andren C., Marden M. & Nilson G. (1989). Tolerance to low pH in a population of moor frogs, *Rana arvalis*, from an acid and a neutral environment: a possible case of rapid evolutionary response to acidification. *Oikos.* V. 56, pp. 215-223.

Beattie R.C., Aston R.J. & Milner A.G .P. (1991)A Field-Study of Fertilization and Embryonic-Development in the Common Frog (*Rana temporaria*) with Particular Reference to Acidity and Temperature. *J. of Applied ecology.* V. 28, № 1, pp. 346-357.

Beattie R.S., Tyler-Jones R. & Baxter M.J. (1992). Influence of pH, aluminum, temperature on embryonic development of *Rana temporaria*. *J. Zool.* V. 228. № 4. pp.557-570.

Beetschen, J.C. (2001). Amphibian gastrulation: history and evolution of a 125 year-old concept. *Int J Dev Biol.* V. 45, pp. 771-795.

Berven K.A. (1982). The genetic basis of altitudinal variation in the wood frog, *Rana sylvatica*. 1. An experimental analysis of larval development. *Oecologia.* v. 52. № 3. pp. 360-369.

Berven K.A. & Gill D.E. (1983). Interpreting geographic variation in life-history traits. *Amer. Zool.* v. 23. № 1. pp. 85-97.

Burger R. & Lynch M. (1997). Adaptation and extinction in changing environments. In: Environmental stress, Adaptation and Evolution. Bijlsma R.; Loeschcke V. Springer Verlag, pp. 209–240.

Cherdantsev, V.G. & Scobeyeva, V.A. (1994). The morphological basis of self-organization. Developmental and evolutionary aspects. *RiVista di Biologyca- Biology forum.* v. 87. № 1. pp. 57-85.

Cherdantsev, V. G. (2003). *Morphogenesis and evolution.* M. KMK. pp. 359 (Russ.).

Cohen, J. (1977) *Reproduction.* London: Butterworths.

Cooke A.S. (1974). The effect of pp'-DDT on adult frog (*Rana temporaria*). *Brit. J. Herp.* №4. pp. 647-652.

Dawson, D.A., McCormick, C.A. & Bantle, J.A. (1985). Detection of teratogenic substances in acidic mine water samples using the frog embryo teratogenesis assay - *Xenopus* (FETAX). *J. Appl. Toxicol.* V. 5. № 4. pp. 234-44.

Duboule, D. (1994) Temporal colinearity and the phylotipic progression: a basis for the stability of a vertebrate Bauplan and the evolution of morphologies through heterochrony. *Dev Suppl* pp. 135-142.

Dunson, W.A., Wyman, R.L. & Corbett, E.S. (1992) A symposium of amphibians declines and habitat acidification. *J. Herpetol.* V.26. pp. 349-352.

Ettler, V., Mihaljevič, M., Matura, M., Skalová, M., Šebek, O. & Bezdička P. (2008). Temporal Variation of Trace Elements in Waters Polluted by Municipal Solid Waste Landfill Leachate. *Bulletin of Environmental Contamination and Toxicology*. V. 80, №3, pp. 274-279.

Falconer, D. (1981) *Introduction to qualitative genetics*. M.: Agropromizdat. pp. 486 (Russ).

Fetax. (1991). Standard guide for conduction the frog embryo teratogenesis assays- Xenopus (Fetax). *Amer. Soc.for test. and mat.* pp. 1-11.

Forbes, V.E. & Calow, P. (1997). Responses of aquatic organisms to pollutant stress: theoretical and practical implications. In: Environmental stress, Adaptation and Evolution. Bijlsma R. & Loeschcke V. B: Springer Verlag. pp. 25-42.

Fort, D.J., Guiney P., Weeks, J., Thomas J., Rogers, R., Noll, A. & Spaulding, C. (2004). Effect of Methoxychlor on Various Life Stages of Xenopus laevis. Toxicological sciences. V. 81, pp. 454–466.

Freda, J. (1986). The influence of acidic ponds water on amphibians: A review. *Water Air Soil Poll.* V. 20. pp. 439-450.

Galis, F. & Metz, J.A. (2001). Testing the vulnerability of the phylotipic stage: on modularity and evolutionary conservation. *J exp Zool (Mol Dev Evol).* V. 291, pp. 195-204.

Galis, F., & Sinervo, B. (2002). Divergence and convergence in early embryonic stages of metazoans. *Contrib Zool.* V. 71, pp. 101–113.

Garland, T. & Kelly, S. A. (2006). Phenotypic plasticity and experimental evolution. J. Exp. Biol. V. 209. pp. 2344-2361.

Gilbert, S. (1993).*Developmental Biology*. T. 1. M.:Mir. pp. 110-144. (Russ.).

Glukhova, E.V. & Cherdantsev V.G. (1999) Microfolds in suprablastopore zone o frog´s gastrula and its relation to mechanics and geometrics of the gastrula. *Ontogenez.* V. 30. № 6. pp. 369-379. (Russ.).

Gordon, D.M. (1992). *Phenotypic plasticity*. In keywords in evolutionary biology. Cambridge, MA: Harvard University Press. pp. 255-262.

Greenhouse, G. (1976). The evaluation of toxic effects of chemicals in fresh water by using frog embryos and larval. *Environ. Poll.* V.11. №4. pp. 303-315.

Gu, Y.Z., Hogenesch, J.B. & Bradfield C.A. (2000). The PAS superfamily: sensors of environmental and developmental signals. *Annu. Rev. Pharmacol. Toxicol.* V.40. P.519–561.

Hall, R.J. & Henry P.F.P. (1992). Assessing effects of pesticides on amphibians and reptiles: status and needs. *Herpetol. J.* V. 2. pp. 65-71.

Hall, B.K. (1997). Phylotypic stage or phantom: is there a highly conserved embryonic stage in vertebrates? *Trends Ecol Evol.* V. 12. pp. 461–463.

Hecnar, S.J. (1995). Acute and chronic toxicity of ammonium nitrate fertilizer to amphibians from southern Ontario. *Environ. Tox. and Chem.* V.14. pp. 2131-2137.

Holloway, G.J., Sibly, R.M. & Pover, S.R. (1990). Evolution in toxic stress environments. *Funct. Ecology.* V. 4. pp. 289-294.

Horder, T.J. (2006). Gavin Rylands de Beer: how embryology foreshadowed the dilemmas of the genome. *Nat Rev Genet.* V. 7. pp. 892–898.

Horder, T. (2008). A history of evo-devo in Britain. Theoretical ideals confront with biological complexity. *Ann Hist Phil Biol.* V. 13 pp. 101–174.

Horne, M.T. & Dunson W.A. (1995). Toxicity of metals and low pH to embryos and larvae of the Jefferson salamander, *Ambystoma jeffersonianum. Arch. Environ. Contam. Toxicol.* V. 29. pp. 110-114.

Huxley, J.S. (1942). *Evolution: The modern synthesis.* London, pp. 74.

Irmler, I., Schmidt, K. & Starck, J.M. (2004). Developmental variability during early embryonic development of zebra fish, *Danio rerio. J exp Zool B: Mol Dev Evol.* V. 302 pp. 446-457.

Johansson, M., Rasanen, K. & Merila J. (2001). Comparison of nitrate tolerance between different populations of the common frog, *Rana temporaria. Aquatic Toxicol.* V. 54. pp. 1-14.

Leontieva, O. A. & Semenov D. V. (1997). Amphibians as bioindicators of anthropogenic change in environment. *Uspeji Sobrem. Biologii.* T. 117. No. .6. pp. 726-736. (Russ.).

Lynch, M. & Lande, R. (1993). Evolution and extinction in response to environmental change In *Biotic Interactions and Global Change.* Eds. Kareiva P.; Kingsolver J. & Huey R.Sinauer Associates, Inc. Sunderland. MA. pp. 234–250.

Moller, A.P. & Swaddle, J.P. *Asymmetry, developmental stability, and evolution.* Oxford: University Press, pp. 1997. 291.

Morgan, M. K., Scheuerman, P.R., Bishop, C.S. & Pyles, R.A. (1996) Teratogenic potential of atrazine and 2,4-D using FETAX. *J. Toxicol Environ Health.* V. 48(2). pp. 151-168.

Morozova, T. V., Anholt, R. R. & Mackay, T. F. (2006). Transcriptional response to alcohol exposure in *Drosophila melanogaster. Genome Biol.* V. 7. pp. 95.

Opitz, R., Braunbeck, T., Bögi, C., Pickford, D.B., Nentwig, G., Oehlmann, J., Tooi, O., Lutz, I. & Kloas, W. (2005). Description and initial evaluation of a Xenopus metamorphosis assay for detection of thyroid system-disrupting activities of environmental compounds. *Environ Toxicol Chem.* V. 24(3) pp.653-64.

Orton, F., Carr, J.A. & Handy, R.D. (2006). Effects of nitrate and atrazine on larval development and sexual differentiation in the northern leopard frog *Rana pipiens. Environ Toxicol Chem.* V. 25(1) pp. 65-71.

Pigliucci, M. (2005). Evolution of phenotypic plasticity: where are we going now? *Trends Ecol. Evol.* V. 20. pp. 481-486.

Raff, R.A. & Sly, B.J. (2000). Modularity and dissociation in the evolution of gene expression territories in development. *Evol Dev.* V. 2 pp. 102-113.

Richardson, M.K. (1995). Heterochrony and the phylotypic period. *Dev Biol.* V. 172, pp. 412–421.

Richardson, M.K., Minelli, A., Coates, M. & Hanken J. (1998). Phylotypic stage theory. *Tree.* V. 13. № 4. pp. 158.

Saber, D.A. & Dunson W.A. (1978). Toxicity of bog water to embryonic and larval anuran amphibians. *J. Exp. Zool.* V. 204. № 1. pp. 33-34.

Sander, K. (1983) The evolution of patterning mechanism: gleaning from insect embryogenesis and spermatogenesis. In: *Development and Evolution.* Goodwin, B.C.; Holder, N. & Wylie, C.C. editors. Cambridge University Press, Cambridge. pp. 123-159

Schmalhausen I. I. (1942) Organism as a whole in individual and hitorical development. M.; L. AS USSR. pp. 212. (Russ.).

Schmalhausen, I. I. (1969) Problems of Darwinism.L. Nauka. pp. 492. (Russ.).

Schmidt, K. & Starck, J.M.. (2010). Developmental plasticity, modularity, and heterochrony during the phylotypic stage of the zebra fish, *Danio rerio*. *J Exp Zool B Mol Dev Evol*. V. 15 № 314(2), pp. 166-78.

Schwartz, S.S., Pyastolova, O.A., Dobrininskaya, A.A. & Runova, G.G. (1976). *Group effect in populations of aquatic animals and chemical ecology*. M.:Nauka. pp. 1-152 (Russ.).

Seidel, F. (1960). Korpergrundgestalt und Keimstruktur. Eine erorterung uber die Grundlagen der vergleichenden und experimentellen Embryologie und deren Gultigkeit bei phylogenetischen Uberlegungen. *Zool Anz*. V. 164 pp. 245-305.

Severtsov, A.S. (1985). Emergence of plastic features in phenotype under selection. *Zhurnal obshei biologii*. T. 46. № 5. pp. 579-589. (Russ.).

Severtsov, A.S. (1996). Group selection as a cause of emergence group adaptations. *Zoologichesky zhurnal*. T 75, No. 10, pp. 1525-1540. (Russ.).

Severtsov, A.C. (2004) *Theory of evolution*. Vlados. pp. 380. (Russ.).

Severtsov, A.S. & Surova, G.S. (1981). Individual variability o norm of reaction and adaptation of population. *Zhurnal obshei biologii* T XLII, №2, pp. 181-192. (Russ.).

Severtsova, E.A. (2002) *Adaptive processes and variability of embryogenesis of anuran amphibians in urban populations*. Synopsis PhD thesis M.: MSU. 2002. 24 p russ.

Severtsova, E.A. (2005). Adaptation of Amphibian gastrulating embryos to an influence of anthropogenic pollution. *10th congress European Society for Evolutionary Biology*. Poland. 15-20.08.2005. pp.514.

Severtsova, E.A. (2009). Experimental work on the correlation of variability components of development of Common frog tadpoles (*Rana temporaria*, Anura, Amphibia) in hatching stage. *Zoologichesky zhurnal* T 88, №1, pp. 1-10. (Russ.).

Severtsova, E.A. & Severtsov, A.C. (2005). Interpopulation comparison of variability o gastrulation of Common frog embryos living in conditions of anthropogenic polluted ponds. *Ontogenez*. T. 36. №2. p. 110-122. (Russ.).

Severtsova, E.A. & Severtsov, A.C. (2007). Interpopulation comparison of gastrula of Moor and Marsh frogs living in conditions of anthropogenic polluted ponds. *Ontogenez*. T. 38. № 1. pp. 1-14. (Russ.).

Severtsova, E.A. & Severtsov A.C. (2011). Crucial stages of embryogenesis of *R.arvalis* Part 1: Linear Measurements of Embryonic structures. *Russian Journal of Developmental Biology*. Vol. 42, № 5, pp. 331-341.

Shishkin. (1984). Individual development and natural selectionp. *Ontogenez*. T. 15. № 2. pp. 115-136. (Russ.).

Slack, J.M.., Isaacs, H.V., Johnson, G.E., Lettice, L.A., Tannahill, D. & Thompson J. (1992). Specification of the body plan during Xenopus gastrulation: dorsoventral and anteroposterior of the mesoderm. *Dev. Suppl*. V. 1. pp.143-149.

Slack, J.M.., Holland, P.W. & Graham C.F. (1993). The zootype and the phylotypic stage. *Nature*, V. 361, pp. 490–492.

Sparling, D.W., Linder, G. & Bishop C.A. (2001). *Ecotoxicology of amphibian and reptiles*. SETAC press. Pensacola. FL.

Stroganov, N.N. (1971). Methods for determinate the toxicity in aquatic environments . In *Methods for biological research in aquatic toxicology*. M.: Nauka.. pp. 14-60.

Svetlov. (1978). *Physiology (mechanics) of development.* L.: Nauka, T.1. Processes of morphogenesis in cellular and organismic levels. 279 p. T.2. Internal and external actors of development. 263 p.

Surova, G. (1988). Interaction of tadpoles of Common frog in natural conditions. *Ekologiya* № 4. pp. 49-54.

Surova, G. (1988a). Environmental and hereditary components of periods of ontogenesis of Common (*Rana temporaria*) and Moor (*R. arvalis*) frog tadpoles. *Zool Zhur* T. 67.No. 3. pp. 396-405. (Russ.).

Surova, G. & Severtsov A.C. (1985). Death in Common frog (*Rana temporaria* L.) in early ontogenesis and factors of it cause. *Zool. Zhur*. T. 44. No. 1, pp. 61-71. (Russ.).

Travis, J. (1980). Genetic variation for larval specific growth rate in the *Hyla gratiosa. Growth.* V. 44. № 3. pp. 167-181.

Travis, J. (1981). Control of larval growth variation in a population of *Pseudacris triseriata* (Amura:Hylidae). *Evolution*. V. 35. № 3. pp. 424-432.

Vershin, V.L. (1997) *Ecological features in amphibian populations of urban territories*. Synopsis: Doctoral degree thesis. Ekaterinburg: Institute of plant and animal ecology UrORAS pp. 47.

Via, S., Gomulkiewicz, R., De Jong, G., Scheiner, S. M., Schlichting, C. D. & Van Tienderen, P. H. (1995). Adaptive phenotypic plasticity: consensus and controversy. *Trends Ecol. Evol.* V. 10. pp. 212-217.

Voronova, L.D., Golichenkov, V.A., Popov, D.V., Kalistratova, E.N. & Sokolova Z.A. (1983). Reaction of pigmentary system of amphibian tadpoles in lower concentrations of some pesticides. In *Problems of ecological monitoring and ecosystem model.* L. Gidmeteoizdat . T. VI. pp. 77-90. (Russ.).

Waddington, C.H. (1947). *Organizers and genes.* M.: Gos. Izdat. Inostran. Lit. pp. 240. (Russ).

Waddington, C.H. (1956). *Principles of Embryology.* Allen & Unwin, London.

West-Eberhard. (2003). *Developmental Plasticity and Evolution.* N. Y.: Oxford University Press. pp. 794.

Wittkopp. (2007) Variable gene expression in eukaryotes: a network perspective. *J. Exp. Biol.* V. 210. pp. 1567-1575.

Zakharov, V.M. (1989). Future prospects for population phenogenetics. *Sov. Sci. Rev. Physiol. Gen. Biol.* V.4. pp.1-79.

24

Microspore Embryogenesis

Tara D. Silva
University of Colombo
Sri Lanka

1. Introduction

Microspores are the precursors of the male gametes of plants and are equivalent to spermatids of animals. Microspores develop into pollen grains within the anthers of a flower in angiosperms. Mature pollen grains are the male gametophytes. The function of the male gametophyte is to participate in the sexual reproduction of plants.

Quite separate from this intended pathway of gametogenesis, a microspore can also be induced to assume sporophytic development. "Totipotency", which is unique to plant cells, allows a microspore that is already destined to develop into a male gametophyte, to re-direct its development pathway so that a haploid sporophyte is regenerated under specified conditions. The cellular totipotency displayed by the microspore is considered an adaptive mechanism for survival that is brought about under stressful environmental conditions (Bonet et al. 1998). The process that leads to the development of a sporophyte from a microspore is referred to as microspore embryogenesis (or pollen embryogenesis). It is also commonly termed androgenesis.

Androgenesis rarely occurs in nature, but is relatively easily induced in several plant species under in vitro conditions. The first report on regeneration of androgenic plants was in the Solanaceous species, *Datura innoxia,* where Guha and Maheshwari (1964) demonstrated that the anthers cultured in vitro yielded haploid plants. Following this initial discovery, many attempts have been made to repeat the success in other plant species. Early studies were mostly empirical and were directed at identifying suitable culture media, pre-treatment conditions that are required for inducing sporophytic development in microspores, and other such practical considerations. Since then, much progress has been made, particularly toward the understanding of the basic processes that occur at cellular level with the switching of developmental pathway of the microspore, from gametogenesis to microspore embryogenesis. Concerted efforts on many different plants have resulted in the documentation of the microspore embryogenesis process in over 250 species (Maluszynski et al. 2003), even though achieving success with androgenesis is still restricted to annuals and herbaceous or non-woody plants mostly. The two main techniques that are employed to generate androgenic plants in vitro are the anther culture and the microspore (pollen) culture methods. Anther culture is the more widely applied, where the excised immature anthers dissected out from flower buds are cultured whole on suitable growth media under appropriate in vitro conditions. The microspores inside the anther develop into plants through a process by which their normal gametophytic development is stalled and sporophytic development is initiated. As the microspores are endowed with only one set of chromosomes instead of the two sets present in the somatic cells of the diploid plant, the pollen-derived plants are haploid. In the anther culture method, even though the goal is to produce plants of microspore origin, there is a danger of plants regenerating from somatic tissue of the anther wall rather than from the haploid microspore cells. In the microspore culture technique, individual pollen cells isolated from anther tissue are placed directly in culture. It is possible to isolate microspores by mechanical means such as crushing of anthers and release into medium by magnetic stirring. They can also be isolated as naturally shed microspores in the culture medium after pre-culture of anthers. Although microspore culture is technically more demanding and is less efficient in some plant species than the culture of whole anthers, it has several advantages over anther culture. Mainly it eliminates the danger of plant development from anther wall tissue. As individual plants develop from separate pollen cells, the chance of chimera production is also low. Further, the culture of individual microspores makes possible the tracing of events that occur from microspore initiation through to embryogenic development, by cell tracking studies allowing for the greater understanding of the process of androgenesis in plants.

Haploid plants are weak and sterile and have no regular means to produce sexual progeny. Therefore, haploid plants by themselves serve no useful purpose. However, haploid plants regenerated from cultured anthers or microspores can afterwards be brought back to the normal diploid state by duplicating their chromosome number through application of chemicals such as colchicine, or other in vitro techniques. The resulting plants will have two identical chromosome sets and be perfectly homozygous, and therefore will give rise to fertile homogenous progenies. Thus, the usefulness of the technique is not in deriving haploid plants but in producing doubled haploids or dihaploids. The great interest in androgenesis among the scientific community, particularly among those involved in practical plant breeding, is this perceived potential of the technique to rapidly develop homozygous lines in the breeding material, which otherwise would require several generations of inbreeding through conventional procedures. The effectiveness of the technique depends on the efficiency of haploid plant regeneration from microspores contained within the anthers, and the conversion of these haploids to doubled haploid plants either spontaneously during the tissue culture phase or induced thereafter. With this method, true-breeding lines are produced in the immediately succeeding generation, and thus the technique has immense utility for developing homozygous breeding lines in a relatively short period.

The objective of this Chapter is to detail out the process of microspore embryogenesis in plants and discuss the factors that influence its induction, particularly with reference to the recent progress made in the understanding of molecular events that occur during the re-programming of the microspore development pathway.

2. Gametogenesis versus embryogenesis

In normal gametogenesis, the diploid microsporocytes or pollen mother cells in the anther undergo meiotic division to yield haploid microspores. Each uni-nulceate microspore then divides mitotically to produce a cell with two haploid nuclei, which is the bi-nucleate state of pollen. Cytokinesis that follows produces two cells that are of unequal size. The larger cell is termed the vegetative cell and the smaller one is known as the generative cell. The generative nucleus divides again by mitosis to produce two haploid sperm nuclei. The vegetative nucleus remains without further division. Thus a mature male gametophyte at the time of affecting fertilization is often bi-cellular (and sometimes tri-cellular) with three haploid nuclei of which two nuclei of the generative cell origin participate in the "double fertilization" that is characteristic of angiosperm reproduction, producing the diploid zygote and the triploid endosperm of the seed.

In contrast, the embryogenic development of a uni-nucleate microspore that is induced in vitro, is usually initiated by a symmetric mitotic division that results in two equal-sized cells. Further mitotic divisions result in a group of undifferentiated cells, and their rapid proliferation gives rise to a multi-cellular mass. Depending on the in vitro conditions provided, the multi-cellular structures may become embryogenic or remain meristematic. Embryogenic cells, following further division and pattern-formation, are able to develop into structures referred to as somatic embryos. The microspore-derived somatic embryos are initiated as globular structures, and become heart-shaped, and with further morphogenesis become torpedo-shaped and finally develop into cotyledonary embryos with bipolar embryo axes, mimicking closely the zygotic embryo development process. Under some in vitro conditions, regeneration of shoots and roots may occur directly from proliferating callus through a process of organogenesis without producing somatic embryos. The regenerated plants may possess a haploid chromosome complement, similar to the microspore cell of origin, or the chromosome number may have doubled during cycles of cell division, to give rise to doubled haploid plants that are completely homozygous.

3. Conditions under which microspore embryogenesis can be induced

To deviate from the normal pathway of gametogenesis and for re-direction towards a pathway of embryogenesis, a microspore has to be subjected to specific conditions. The conditions that are required to induce such developmental reprogramming will obviously vary with the species, and often within a species among its genotypes or varieties also. Nevertheless, several key factors have been recognized that positively influence the microspore embryogenesis induction in a variety of plant species. In Table 1 these various

Broad categorization of factors influencing microspore embryogenesis	Specific effects
Of the anther donor plant	Genotype, variety or species
	Physiological status - influenced by the growth condition, including seasonal effects such as day length, light, temperature etc.
Of the microspore	Developmental stage, pollen genotype
Of the pre-culture environment	Pre-treatments
Of the in vitro culture conditions	Culture media
	Incubation conditions

Table 1. Factors affecting microspore embryogenesis

biotic and abiotic factors, that have a strong bearing on the ability of a microspore to undergo embryogenesis, are grouped into factors of the anther donor plant, the microspore, pre-culture environment and of the in vitro culture condition.

3.1 Genotype

Often, the in vitro androgenic response is genotype-dependent, and culture conditions may have to be optimized for each genotype. Even of the same species, different varieties and genotypes respond vastly differently to induction attempts. For example, in rice, japonica varieties are known to be more responsive than indica types (Yan et al. 1996), while within each ecotype considerable variation exists between varieties in their anther culture responsiveness (Silva and Ratnayake 2009). Plant regeneration occurs from cultured microspores usually in two stages. Initially the microspore divides and proliferates into an undifferentiated cell mass, followed by pattern formation and morphogenesis that lead to shoot regeneration which occurs through embryogenesis (or sometimes organogenesis). Inheritance studies on anther culture ability have shown that in many species these two processes are genetically determined independent events, and whether any of the two processes or both would occur during anther culture is determined to a large extent by the genetic makeup of the cells. The stimulation of these two events often requires different conditions, and is likely controlled by different genes. Experimental evidence suggests that the mode of inheritance is quantitative in nature (Silva 2010 and references therein). No sustained efforts have been made to actually breed the trait, anther culture ability into anther culture-recalcitrant genotypes, perhaps due to the complexities of the genetic control of in vitro response. Nevertheless the possibility of transferring the trait through sexual hybridization remains a viable prospect. On the other hand, the existence of a large non-genetic component of variation for anther culture ability suggests that there is sufficient scope for improving anther culture efficiency through the manipulation of these non-genetic factors that include the culture media components and pre- and post-culture conditions.

3.2 Physiological status of the anther donor plant

The number and the vigor of microspores found within the anther, the nutritional status of the tissues of the anther, the endogenous levels of growth regulators, may to some extent be influenced by the physiological age and growth condition of the donor plant, which in turn will have a bearing on microspore embryogenic competence. Seasonal variations in anther response have been observed in wheat and barley (Datta 2005). Differences in competence of the cultured microspores to assume embryogenic development when anthers are collected from field grown plants and when harvested from pot plants bear further testimony to the influence of the parent plant growth condition on their microspore embryogenic competence (Datta 2005, Silva 2010). It is common practice in anther culture to use anthers from the first or early flush of flowers rather than anthers from buds in later branches or tillers of the plant. The physiology of the donor plant can be altered, and the androgenic response improved, when the donor plant is carefully nurtured and grown under favorable environmental conditions, although pest control measures may have a detrimental effect on in vitro microspore response. Critical environmental factors include light intensity, photoperiod, temperature, nutrition and carbon dioxide concentration. Seasonal variations in the anther response have also been observed, which is probably also related to the overall growth of the donor plant.

3.3 Microspore development stage

The microspore development stage is a complex factor that has a strong influence on the success of anther culture. The exact stage of the microspore that responds to inductive treatment varies with the species, and is restricted to a relatively narrow developmental window. Only microspores that are at a stage sufficiently immature can be induced to change course from a gametophytic pre-programme to embryogenic re-programming leading to sporophytic development. Even though all microspores within an anther would be roughly of a similar age, the incremental differences in the stages of development of individual microspores can be considered significant, in setting each apart with regard to their embryogenic competence. Therefore, even within the same anther only a percentage of pollen cells would undergo divisions leading to their embryogenic development. For many species, the most amenable stage is either the uni-nucleate stage of the microspore or, at or just after the first pollen mitosis, which is the early bi-nucleate stage. At this time the transcriptional status of the microspore may still be proliferative and not yet fully differentiated (Malik et al. 2007). More mature microspores are considered irreversibly committed to gametogenesis and are at points of no return in their programme of maturation into male gametophytes.

In the practical implementation of the anther culture technique, it is necessary to identify easily, the flower buds that need to be harvested in order to collect microspores at the correct stage of maturity that is appropriate for in vitro culture. In many species, a maturity gradient is observed in flower buds within the inflorescence that displays either an acropetal or basipetal developmental succession. Therefore, a series of buds taken from different positions on the inflorescence (or in the case of individual flowers, buds of different sizes) need to be pre-examined in order to identify the stage of microspore development within their anthers. This is done by squashing anthers to release pollen, and staining with acetocarmine to observe the nuclei under the light microscope. DAPI (4', 6-diamidino-2-phenylindole) may be also used to stain the nuclear DNA, which can then be visualized using a fluorescent microscope. Such pre-examination will be very useful to establish a correlation between an easily observable morphological trait, (e.g. the petal to sepal length ratio in tobacco) with the pollen development stage, to be used as a quick guide to identify flowers that would have anthers carrying microspores at the required stage of maturity.

3.4 Pre-treatment stresses

For almost all the plant species in which anther culture has been attempted, it is common to include a physical or chemical pre-culture treatment that is applied to excised flower buds, whole inflorescences or separated anthers. The pre-treatment is required to trigger the induction of the sporophytic pathway, thereby preventing the development of fertile pollen through the gametophytic pathway. A variety of microspore pre-treatment stresses have been tested and found to enhance pollen embryogenesis, although the type, duration and the time of application of these pre-treatments may vary with the species or even the variety. The more commonly used anther or microspore pre-treatment conditions are temperature (cold or heat shock), sucrose and nitrogen starvation, centrifugation, as well as the use of microtubili disruptive agents such as colchicine. Lesser known stress-treatments include irradiation, use of high humidity, anaerobic treatment, electro-stimulation, high medium pH, ethanol and heavy metal treatment. These pre-treatments may be classified into three categories based on their application as widely used, neglected and novel (Shariatpanahi et al. 2006). The more notable stress treatments that promote androgenesis are discussed below.

Temperature pre-treatment: A commonly used pre-treatment to induce androgenesis in microspores is the low temperature shock. Cold pre-treatment is usually carried out at 4 - 10 ^{0}C for a few days up to several weeks. For example in rice, for many varieties, a 10 ^{0}C pre-treatment of harvested panicles for 10 – 30 days is sufficient to trigger androgenesis. Several other cereal species including barley, wheat, oat and triticale require low temperature treatment of the excised spikes or flower buds in order to induce microspore embryogenesis. Different views exist on how cold pre-treatment affects the development of the microspore, some or all of which may be relevant to a given species. It is believed that the cold treatment delays the degeneration of anther wall tissues thereby protecting the microspores within, from toxic compounds released by the degenerating maternal tissues. It has also been suggested that at cold temperatures there is greater survival of embryogenic pollen grains leading to enhanced levels of embryogenesis than would occur without pre-treatment. A further explanation is that microspores in the cold pre-treated anthers disconnect from the tapetum resulting in starvation, causing them to switch from gametophytic pathway to embryogenic development. Also, it has been noted that in cold pre-treated anthers the total content of free amino acids is increased, which is suggestive of metabolic re-programming that a microspore needs to undergo, in preparation for embryogenesis induction. Following cold treatment, small heat shock protein genes have been shown to be expressed in tomato and it has been argued that this is possibly to protect cells against chilling injury. The different explanations (Shariatpanahi et al. 2006 and references therein) are based on observations and experiences with different plant species, and the exact mode of action (or actions) is still to be unraveled convincingly.

High temperature has been also used to trigger microspore embryogenesis in certain species. The method is applied routinely with the isolated microspore culture of rapeseed. Embryogenesis is induced efficiently and synchronously in rapeseed microspores subjected to 32 ^{0}C heat shock for about 8 hours, whereas normal gametogenesis occurs at 18 ^{0}C under otherwise similar conditions. High temperature induced microspore embryogenesis does also occur in wheat (Touraev et al. 1996b) and tobacco (Touraev et al. 1996a). As with cold shock, different mechanisms have been proposed to explain the basis of microspore induction through high temperature treatment. It is known that several heat shock proteins (HSPs) are synthesized in various plant tissues in response to elevated temperatures, which have a role in protecting cells from thermo-damage (Schoffl et al. 1996). This is considered an adaptive mechanism since plants are unable to escape extreme environmental conditions due to their immobility. Amongst the HSPs, members of HSP 70 are the most abundant and evolutionarily conserved while HSP 90 is also abundant and is constitutively expressed in eukaryotes with a specific role in heat stress (Chug and Eudes 2008). Synthesis of HSPs has been observed in heat-stressed microspores also, and HSP 70 was suggested to inhibit apoptosis (Jaattela et al. 1998). Even though much significance was attached earlier to the HSPs, for their considered role in enabling microspore embryogenesis (Cordewener et al. 1995, Zarsky et al. 1995, Touraev et al. 1996), subsequent studies have proved that embryogenesis can be induced in rapeseed microspores even when HSPs are not synthesized. For example, embryogenesis can be induced in rapeseed microspores that are stressed with microtubule de-polymerizing agent, colchicine also (Zhao et al. 2003) and this proves that HSPs are not essentially required. Since plants reportedly produce HSPs in response to a variety of other environmental stresses such as cold, drought, heavy metal stress, and starvation (Schoffl et al. 1998, Zarsky et al. 1995), it is more likely that HSPs have an overall protective role that allows the cells to survive during the periods of adverse environment conditions, and embryogenesis may simply be the consequence of blocked pollen development (Zhao et al. 2003). In rapeseed microspores, the heat shock is believed to also cause microtubule and cytoskeleton rearrangements that lead to altered cell cycle events during microspore culture (Simmonds and Keller 1999).

Nitrogen and sugar starvation: Nutrient starvation, particularly of nitrogen and sugar, has been effective in enhancing the in vitro anther response in some species. Nitrogen starvation may be applied to the anther donor plant or the excised anthers and microspores. The mother plant can be nitrogen-stressed by restricting the application of nitrogen fertilizer to the plant. Excised anthers can be starved of nitrogen by withdrawing or limiting the inorganic and organic nitrogen sources in the initial culture media. In several species, isolated microspores have shown a better embryogenic response with nitrogen starvation. For example, with tobacco pollen, a high rate of embryogenic induction was achieved from starving the microspores of glutamine, by an initial period of growth on glutamine free medium (Kyo and Harada 1986). Also in tobacco, sucrose and nitrogen starvation of pollen of the mid bi-cellular stage resulted in embryogenic induction and yielded a high number of embryos when transferred to a simple medium containing sucrose and nitrogen (Touraev et al.1997). Similarly sucrose starvation at 25 ^{0}C resulted in the efficient formation of embryogenic microspores in tobacco when transferred to sugar containing medium (Touraev et al. 1996a). In wheat, the culture of excised anthers under starvation and heat shock conditions induced the formation of embryogenic microspores at high frequency (Touraev et al. 1996b). During starvation, cytoplasmic and nuclear changes have been observed in the microspores including de-differentiation of plastids, changes in chromatin and nuclear structure, changes in the level of RNA synthesis and protein kinase activity, and the activation of small heat shock protein genes (Shariatpanahi et al. 2006 and refereces therein).

Centrifugation: Subjecting anthers to centrifugation pre-treatment has been useful to improve the efficiency of microspore embryogenesis. In tobacco anthers, a four-fold increase in the regeneration of haploid plants was reported following centrifugation of the anthers prior to culture, although the maturity stage of the microspores determined the degree of success (Tanaka 1973). Experiments with chick pea (*Cicer arietinum*) also appear to suggest that centrifugation may have a positive impact on embryo initiation from cultured anthers, even though the response is variety specific (Grewal et al. 2009). Because the appropriate centrifugal force and the duration of treatment vary with the microspore development stage and variety, it is difficult to standardize protocols for centrifugation pre-treatment.

Colchicine: The use of colchicine for microspore pre-treatment has been reported to be effective in enhancing microspore embryogenesis in rapeseed (Zaki and Dickinson 1991, Zhao et al. 1996), wheat (Barnabas 2003a), coffee (Herrera et al. 2002) and maize (Obert and Barnabas 2004). Colchicine acts by binding to α- and β-tubulin heterodimers thereby inhibiting further dimer addition to microtubules, which causes de-polymerization of the microtubule (Sternlicht et al. 1983). During normal gametogenesis of pollen, the peripheral position of the nucleus is maintained by microtubules and actin filaments (Hause et al. 1992). The de-polymerization of the microtubules causes a shift in the nuclear position from the cell periphery to cell center leading to altered cell polarity. This may eventually result in a symmetric division in place of the asymmetric division that is the standard for first pollen mitosis (Zhao et al. 1996), and maybe the trigger that directs microspores onto the sporophytic pathway. It is also suggested that when colchicine prevents dimer addition to α- and β-tubulin heterodimers, the excess of free tubulins that remain in the cell will inhibit the synthesis of new molecules, some of which may be specifically required for pollen development (Carpenter et al. 1992). Thus, normal gametogenesis is suppressed and embryogenesis is initiated.

From the above account it becomes clear that the microspores can be induced to become embryogenic under a variety of different stresses. The kind of stress to be applied will depend on the plant species. However, more than one stress treatment will work with microspores of some species, particularly in relation to the stage of microspore development at the time of induction. For example, in rapeseed, severe heat stress (41 ^{0}C) is required to induce efficient embryogenic development in late bi-nucleate microspores (Binarova et al. 1997), mild heat stress (32 ^{0}C) to induce late uni-nucleate to early bi-nucleate staged microspores (Ferrie and Keller 1995), whereas uni-nucleate microspores at an earlier stage of development corresponding to vacuolated stage are induced more effectively with colchicine (Zhao et al. 1996). Similarly, in tobacco bi-cellular pollen is easily induced under sucrose and nitrogen starvation pre-treatment conditions (Garrido et al. 1995, Kyo and Harada 1986) whereas microspores at the uni-nucleate stage are induced under heat shock (Touraev et al. 1996a), and centrifugal pre-treatment (Tanaka 1973), although the latter two pre-treatments have little influence in inducing embryogenesis from bi-cellular pollen. Accordingly, through careful experimentation and judicious choice of pre-treatments, it would be possible to induce microspores of a wider developmental range than anticipated before, towards successful embryogenic re-programming.

3.5 Culture medium

As with all other in vitro culture systems, successful induction of embryogenesis from cultured microspores or anthers depends to a large extent on the composition of the culture medium. The requirements of a given species are identified mainly through an empirical process of trial and error. The source of carbon, macronutrients (particularly the form in which nitrogen is supplied in the medium) and micronutrients may determine if embryogenesis will be initiated or not. The type and concentration of the growth regulators, particularly the auxins and cytokinins, as well as their interactive presence can be the deciding media factor that would influence pollen embryogenesis. Standard media have been developed for different species although specific genotypes may have their individual requirements. The more widely used basal media for anther culture are the N6 (Chu 1978), Nitsch and Nitsch (1969), MS (Murashige and Skoog 1962) and B 5 (Gamborg et al. 1968). These media are used often in their original form, but sometimes modified by supplementing or subtracting one or more components to better suite a given plant species or genotype. With more recalcitrant species, new media will have to be formulated that are tailor-made to address their specific requirements.

Carbon source: The carbon source is an important component in tissue culture media that provides the energy required for the growth of the cultured explants. The most frequently used carbon source in tissue culture media is sucrose. Sugars also play a significant role in regulating the osmotic pressure in the culture media, although this would be secondary to its main role as the source of energy. Plants belonging to the families Poaceae and Brassicaceae require fairly high sucrose levels (6 - 17%) for the induction of microspore embryogenesis (Dunwell and Thurling 1985), whereas more regular lower concentrations (2 - 5%) are used with Solanaceous species (Dunwell 2010). Since of late, maltose has come to replace sucrose as the major carbon source in cereal anther culture, usually at 6% in the induction medium and at half this strength in the regeneration medium (Wedzony et al. 2009). Maltose in the anther culture medium is degraded more slowly than sucrose and yields only glucose upon hydrolysis whereas sucrose is metabolized very rapidly into glucose and fructose. Fructose is known to have a detrimental effect on embryoid production in wheat anther culture (Last and Brettell 1990, Navarro-Alvarez et al. 1994). The reduced efficiency of androgenesis observed in the presence of sucrose as the carbon source maybe due to the sensitivity of microspores to fructose that is generated from the hydrolysis of sucrose in the culture medium. Further, the superiority of maltose over other sugars such as glucose, fructose and mannitol, has also been proven with rice anther culture (Bishnoi et al. 2000, Lentini et al. 1995). Exogenously supplied carbohydrates in the culture medium may also in part fulfill the osmotic requirements of the cells growing in vitro. Nevertheless, results indicate that the type of sugar to be used is more important as an energy source rather than in osmotic regulation of the medium. On the other hand, certain sugar alcohols such as mannitol and sorbitol have been used in microspore culture media purely for their role in osmo-regulation. Both mannitol (Raina and Irfan 1998) and sorbitol (Kishore and Reddy 1986) have had beneficial effects on rice anther culture.

Nitrogen source: Nitrogen can be supplied to the culture medium in the inorganic or organic form. The inorganic nitrogen is usually introduced in the form of nitrate or ammonium ions while nitrogen in the organic form can be supplied as vitamins and amino acid supplements. Often, anther cultures may require more than one form of the nitrogen and the correct balance of the different sources of nitrogen may be very important for successful androgenesis. For example, Chu (1978) demonstrated that the level of nitrogen in the form of ammonium ions was critical for androgenesis in rice, on which basis he developed the N6 medium with appropriate concentrations of $(NH_4)_2SO_4$ and KNO_3. While the N6 medium has become the most widely used for rice anther culture, particularly of the japonica types, the nitrogen requirement of the indica rice varieties was proved to be somewhat different. For indica rices, lowering the level of $(NH_4)_2SO_4$ and increasing the concentration of KNO_3 was shown to produce better anther response and green plant regeneration from anther-derived callus (Raina and Zapata 1997).

Micronutrients: Micronutrients play an important and sometimes a crucial role in normal plant growth and development. Deficiency symptoms arise in plants that are grown under sub-optimal levels of micronutrients. As such, the tissue culture media are also formulated with the inclusion of essential micronutrients. However, in depth studies of their influence on in vitro cell culture, particularly microspore embryogenesis, are limited. This neglect is in spite of their absolute requirement for many physiological and biochemical cellular processes, including the catalysis of enzymatic reactions. Two of the micronutrients that have been investigated for their influence on microspore embryogenesis are copper and zinc. The addition of copper sulphate in the anther pre-treatment medium allowed green plant regeneration from an otherwise exclusively albino plant producing recalcitrant barley cultivar (Jacquard et al. 2009, Wojnarowiez et al. 2002).

3.6 Incubation conditions

The temperature at which the cultures are incubated, light / dark conditions, the density of anthers or microspores in a culture vessel and other such post culture environmental conditions may have a subtle effect on the success of microspore embryogenesis, depending on the plant species or genotype. The temperature at which anther cultures are incubated has been shown to be an important factor in rice (Okamoto et al. 2001). However, very few investigations have been carried out to manipulate culture temperatures for enhanced anther culture efficiency. Light is another environmental factor that has a bearing on anther culture success because it is a stimulus that influences in vitro pollen morphogeneis (Reynolds and Crawford 1997). Generally, anther or microspore cultures are maintained in the dark during the initial phase of culture, particularly when regeneration occurs through callus, and transferred to illuminated conditions at a later stage. For some plant species diurnal alternation of incubation for several hours in the light and then darkness has been beneficial (Germana et al. 2005, Sunderland 1971). However, optimal conditions need to be determined for each system.

4. Cellular changes that occur at the initiation of microspore embryogenesis

Basic studies on microspore embryogenesis have been dealt with in detail in a few plant species only, that are considered model systems for generating haploid plants from cultured microspores. The following descriptions pertaining to the changes that occur in the microspores under induction conditions are therefore based largely on the work carried out on these model plant systems, namely; *Brassica napus* (rapeseed), *Hordeum vulgare* (barley), *Nicotiana tobaccum* (tobacco) and *Triticum aestivum* (wheat).

A microspore in which embryogenic development is initiated will display characteristic features that will distinguish it from a normal microspore that is developing into a male gametophyte. These distinguishing features have been observed to be common among many of the plant species that have been subjected to detailed study, and therefore may be adopted as cellular markers of pollen embryogenesis, allowing the development of a unified model for the microspore embryogenic induction process. The changes associated with the de-differentiation process of the microspore include changes in cellular morphology and biochemical processes as well as changes in gene expression profiles.

4.1 Changes in the cellular landscape of microspores during embryogenic induction

Following stress treatment, microspores that have been induced to become embryogenic become enlarged. The enlargement of stress-induced microspores in comparison to the relatively smaller size of the normal microspores is generally taken to be associated with their acquisition of embryogenic competence (Maraschin et al. 2005a), although all the cells that enlarge may not continue in the embryogenic pathway of development.

During early development, a normal microspore that is released from the tetrad has its nucleus located in the center of a cytoplasm–rich cell. Subsequently a vacuole develops and expands to occupy a large part of the cell, which pushes the cytoplasm with the embedded nucleus to the periphery of the cell. In the young microspores that are induced to assume embryogenic development, there is re-positioning of the nucleus from its peripheral location to the center of the cell and the large vacuole gets broken up by radial strands of cytoplasm creating several smaller vacuoles giving the cell a star-like appearance. This stellar morphology of the cell is considered to be one of the early markers that portend re-programming of the microspore for switching from gametogenesis to embryogenic development and has been observed during the embryogenic induction in the four androgenic model systems; barley, wheat, rapeseed and tobacco irrespective of whether the embryogenic induction occurs in the uni- or bi-nuclear stage microspores (Zaki and Dickinson 1991, Touraev et al. 1996, Indrianto et al. 2001, Maraschin et al. 2005).

4.2 Cytoskeletal rearrangements and changes to division symmetry

During normal development of the uni-nucleate microspore, the peripheral position of the pollen nucleus is maintained by cytoskeletal components; the microtubules and actin filaments (Hause et al. 1992). In stress-induced microspores, the re-positioning of the nucleus from the periphery of the cell to its center is considered to be associated with cytoskeletal re-arrangements. The fact that the destruction of the cytoskeleton by colchicine can induce pollen embryogenesis, of which process an initial manifestation is the migration of the nucleus, supports this proposition (Zaki and Dickinson 1991, Zhao et al. 1996, Gervais et al. 2000, Obert and Barnabas 2004). The central nuclear positioning is believed to confer radial polarity in the cell, initiating a symmetric division that results in two equal-sized cells. The plane of division is equatorial and is similar to what is observed in mitotically activated somatic cells (Segui-Simarro and Nuez 2008). Further subsequent divisions eventually lead to the formation of a multi-cellular pro-embryo. This is in contrast to what occurs during the normal process of gametogenesis. In normal pollen development the peripheral nucleus of the uni-nucleate microspore undergoes the first pollen mitosis which is an asymmetric division yielding two cells of distinctly different sizes. The vegetative cell is large and contains bulk of the pollen cytoplasm allowing its nucleus to assume a more central position in the pollen grain. The smaller generative cell, with its arch-shaped cytoplasm, remains close to the intine wall surrounded by the vegetative cell cytoplasm. The nucleus of the smaller generative cell undergoes a second mitotic division to yield the two fertilizing nuclei that carry out the double-fertilization event characteristic of the angiosperms.

However, it must be noted that the division symmetry is not a mandatory requirement for embryogenesis initiation in the microspore. For example, treating maize pollen with colchicine, although allows embryogenic induction, does not result in division symmetry (Barnabas et al. 1999). This appears to suggest that the role of cytoskeletal inhibitors on embryogenic induction in microspores is not confined to the triggering of symmetric divisions alone. Also in some plant species, stress-induced pollen embryogenesis occurs at the bi-nucleate stage, at which time the pollen cell has already undergone an initial asymmetric division, resulting in two very unequal-sized cells. This does not preclude embryogenic development in bi-nucleate *B. napus* microspores when subjected to heat shock at 32 ^{0}C (Custers et al. 1994) and in late bi-nucleate pollen by an extra heat shock treatment at 41 ^{0}C (Binarova et al, 1997).

As with colchicine pre-treatment, heat and cold shock have been identified to produce cytoskeletal rearrangements in microspores leading to the migration of the nucleus to the cell center, with resultant initiation of embryogenic development (Binarova et al. 1997, Wallin and Stromberg 1995). Several other stress treatments that have the ability to induce embryogenesis also affect cytoskeletal rearrangements in the microspore and the migration of the nucleus to the center of the cell.

4.3 Biochemical changes and cytoplasmic re-modeling

In normal pollen development following the first pollen mitosis, the large vacuole gets re-absorbed. The larger vegetative cell accumulates food reserves such as carbohydrates (starch), lipids and proteins, as well as RNA (Touraev et al. 1997) that powers the pollen tube's growth during its passage through the style to reach the female gametophyte. The generative cell contains much less stored products and fewer organelles. With embryogenic induction, changes occur in the cytoplasm. The cytoplasm becomes more alkaline in contrast to the slightly acidic pH that is observed in the normal microspores (Pauls et al. 2006). There is destruction of cellular organelles such as the plastids, and a decline in the synthesis of ribosomes along with a decrease in the accumulation of starch grains and lipid bodies. Thus there is an overall clearing of the cytoplasm which is suggestive of a state of de-differentiation of the microspore in preparation for the re-programming events that would follow with the initiation of embryogenic development.

Based on these observations it has been proposed that stress leads to the dedifferentiation of microspores by the repression of gametophytic development. It was believed that this re-programming was only possible in microspores that were still at a very early stage of development, and in many experimental systems this stage corresponded to the late uni-nucleate to the early bi-nucleate stage of the microspore. It was also generally accepted that androgenesis could no longer be triggered in bi-nucleate pollen cells in which starch and lipid accumulation has already occurred. The starch-filled cells were deemed irreversibly committed to gametogenesis. However, more recent evidence suggests that this window of opportunity could be made much wider than initially anticipated by precisely timing the application of the stress treatment and the type of stress (Touraev et al. 1997). For example, in *B. napus* an extra heat treatment allows even the late binucleate pollen to undergo embryogenic development.

There are two main pathways by which cytoplasmic remodeling occurs in normal eukaryotic cells. Autophagy is the process by which the destruction of cellular organelles occurs via lysosomes. The destruction of cellular molecules, both long- and short-lived ones, occurs through the ubiquitin 26S proteosomal pathway. Both these pathways are developmentally regulated, but maybe activated by subjecting cells to stress such as heat shock, cold shock and starvation. Autophagial activity mediated by lysosomes in which cellular organelles are destroyed, has been observed to occur in early embryogenesis of *N. tobaccum* microspores (Sunderland and Dunwell 1974). *H. vulgare* microspores in which embryogenic development has been induced by stress have shown expression of genes coding for enzymes of the ubiquitin 26S proteosomal pathway (Maraschin et al. 2005).

4.4 Nuclear rearrangements

In the normal microspores, at the two-celled stage, the vegetative and generative nuclei perform different functions. The vegetative cell concentrates on accumulating metabolites.

In keeping with this function, its nucleus shows high transcriptional activity and contains diffused chromatin. In contrast, the generative cell which is in preparation for a second mitotic division displays greater chromatin condensation in readiness for mitosis and is transcriptionally less active. Changes in the nuclear organization and content are observed in embryogenically induced microspores when compared with microspores that are developing into mature pollen grains. These include changes to patterns of chromatin condensation, nucleolar activity and transcriptional activity of the nucleus. Following the first symmetric division, the two cells of the embryogenic microspores typically display nuclear organization and function that are characteristic of mitotically active cells, such as condensed chromatin patches and compacted nucleoli (Germana 2011). With regard to nuclear DNA content, the doubling of the normal number of chromosomes may be observed. This appears to be a consequence of the in vitro culture conditions, and depending on the species or the genotype, may not compulsorily occur. In the event that chromosomal doubling does occur, the mechanism is believed to be nuclear fusion in the main, and this would normally occur at the initial stages of embryogenic divisions (Segui-Simarro and Nuez 2008).

5. Changes in gene expression

The microspore embryogenesis has been established to work precisely under defined conditions in four plant species, namely *Brassica napus* (rapeseed), *Hordeum vulgare* (barley), *Nicotiana tobaccum* (tobacco) and *Triticum aestivum* (wheat). The reliability with which these species lend themselves to the induction process and the unerring regularity and repeatability of success have allowed these plants to emerge as model systems on which basic studies of the microspore embryogenesis process has been pivoted. In the last decade or so, findings from the burgeoning expansion of genomic, proteomic and metabolomic research and their tools have been applied also to understand the fundamental processes leading to the switching of pathways in pollen development from gametogenesis to embryogenesis, and in the search for genes that are responsible for this turn-around.

Molecular and gene expression studies on microspore embryogenesis have been largely dealt with in the four model plants; wheat, barley, rapeseed and tobacco. This is mainly because of the repeatability and efficiency of the well-established protocols that are available in these plant species for embryogenesis induction from cultured microspores or anthers.

Early studies on molecular aspects have concentrated on identifying genes that are differentially expressed in embryogenic and non-embryogenic microspores. These studies have helped to understand the cellular processes that take place during the transition of the microspore to embryogenic development, from its original gametophytic developmental program. More recently, genomics and bioinformatics approaches have been implemented for gene discovery and functional characterization of candidate genes, whose expression appear to be associated with the embryogenic re-programming in the stress-induced microspores. Once elucidated, the genes that are identified to be expressed in common among different plant species during the initiation of embryogenesis and its progression towards embryo development, may be used as markers for early detection of the embryogenic induction process.

5.1 Genes expressed during barley microspore embryogenesis

In barley microspores, embryogenic induction can be achieved in up to 50% of the microspores by subjecting the cells to a combined mannitol stress and starvation treatment, and thus, the barley microspore embryogenic system provides a very good platform to study differential gene expression (Maraschin et al. 2005b).

In an early study by Vrinten et al. (1999), differential screening of a cDNA library prepared from mannitol-induced 3 day old barley microspores identified three genes that were expressed during embryogenesis initiation. The genes were functionally characterized as encoding a non-specific lipid transfer protein (ECLTP), glutathione-S-transferene (ECGST) and an arabinogalactan-like protein.

A more detailed study involving the screening of mRNA populations of uni-nucleate microspores about to undergo the first pollen mitosis, bi-cellular pollen, and stress-induced embryogenic microspores against microarrays of Expressed Sequence Tags (ESTs) derived from early stages of barley zygotic embryogenesis was carried out by Maraschin et al. (2006) in order to elucidate the gene expression profiles associated with each development programme. Following Principle Component Analysis (PCA) of the normalized gene expression data, it was revealed that in uni-nucleate pollen, mRNAs related to mitotic division and lipid biosynthesis were detected mainly. In bi-cellular pollen induction of genes involved in carbohydrate and energy metabolism were observed. In contrast, the embryogenic pollen displayed the expression of genes involved in protein degradation, starch and sugar hydrolysis, stress responses, inhibition of programmed cell death, metabolism and cell signaling. The gene expression profiles of stress-induced embryogenic microspores point to metabolic changes including proteolysis that appears to relate to the de-differentiation process of the induced microspores. Proteolysis is considered to play an important role in a regulatory mechanism in all cell differentiation and cell cycle progression in plant cells (Hellman and Estelle 2004) and is involved in many aspects of plant development including somatic and zygotic embryogenesis, germination, tissue re-modeling and programmed cell death (Beers et al. 2004). In microspore embryogenesis whether pollen specific proteins are degraded by the expression of genes coding for proteolytic enzymes, allowing the cells to deviate from pre-programmed gametogenesis to assume embryogenic development, remains to be proved.

5.2 Molecular basis of wheat microspore embryogenesis

Differential gene expression between stress-induced microspores and freshly isolated pollen has been studied in wheat using the Suppression Subtractive Hybridization of cDNA clones. These screens have yielded a number of differentially expressed genes (Hosp et al. 2007). Nearly one third of the genes that were differentially expressed could be assigned to functional categories based on similarity with database sequences, while the others were of unknown function or without significant matches to database sequences. A majority of the annotated sequences were found to have a metabolic function which again points to significant biochemical and physiological changes that occur during the switch from gametogenesis to embryogenesis.

A gene that has been identified to be differentially expressed between late-stage microspore derived embryos and mature pollen is one that encodes a cysteine-labeled metallothionine

(EcMt) (Reynolds and Crawford 1996). EcMt was thus indicated as a marker for microspore embryogenesis although it is also induced following Abscisic Acid (ABA) treatment in diverse tissue.

5.3 Tobacco microspore embryogenesis

In tobacco, genes encoding phosphoproteins (NtEP) have been isolated from embryogenic microspores which were shown to have selective expression in de-differentitating pollen (Kyo et al. 2002). In a subsequent study Kyo et al. (2003) isolated 16 cDNAs that were differentially expressed in embryogenic pollen of tobacco. Of these, 13 transcripts were expressed in de-differentiating pollen while the other three were observed in de-differentiating microspores as well as in cell populations undergoing active division. The genes whose expression was confined to de-differentiating pollen included the earlier observed gene coding for NtEP, stress induced genes including ABA-responsive genes, genes coding for Myb transcription factor, glucanase & chitinase, and some unknown genes. Genes that were expressed in both type of cells, the de-differentiating and dividing cells, coded for histones and a mini-chromosome maintaining protein.

Subtraction hybridization of cDNA derived from stress-induced microspores and normal pollen indicated that several genes, involved in metabolism, chromosome re-modeling, (transcription and translation) were up regulated in the induced microspores.

5.4 Rapeseed microspore embryogenesis

The discovery of genes involved in *B. napus* (rapeseed) microspore embryogenesis has relied to a great extent on the genomic data of its close taxonomic relative, *Arabidopsis thaliana*. *A. thaliana* is considered a model organism for genome and transcriptome studies since its genome is fully sequenced and a large number of its genes identified and functionally annotated. Transcriptome analysis of *A. thaliana* microspores has been carried out in detail and the genes involved in regulating the microspore development towards a male gametophyte have been characterized. However, in the absence of a protocol to initiate embryogenic development in *A. thaliana* microspores, there has not been the opportunity to leverage the wealth of genome and transcriptome data on normal gametogenesis, in establishing the genes that are differentially expressed during microspore embryogenesis. On the other hand, the availability of such a well-characterized genome resource, with a good deal of genome-wide similarity and identity among orthologous genes between the two species, *Arabidopsis* and *Brassica*, has meant that *A. thaliana* genome resource could be used as a reference database in the discovery of genes that are expressed during embryogenesis re-programming in rapeseed microspores, and differential screens of gene expression profiles between *Arabidopsis* and *Brassica* have produced fruitful interpretations.

An early study on differential gene expression between 4 day heat stressed embryogenic and non-embryogenic microspores of rapeseed identified five different cDNAs that were up regulated in the induced microspores (Boutilier et al. 2002). Two of these encoded BURP domain proteins with unknown function (Hattori et al. 1998), the third encoded an AP2/EREBP domain transcription factor which has since been named BABY BOOM (BBM), the fourth cDNA encoded the orthologue of the Arabidopsis AKT1 K^+ channel protein (Sentenac et al. 1992), while the last sequence was one to which no open reading frame had been assigned. Of these, the genes coding for BURP domain proteins were found to be expressed through out microspore and zygotic embryogenesis in rapeseed, with highest intensity during the initial period of storage product accumulation. BBM gene was found to be expressed in the early stages of microspore and zygotic embryogenesis. Over-expressing the BBM gene with a constitutive promoter resulted in the ectopic induction of somatic embryos from seedling tissue in rapeseed and *Arabidopsis*, suggesting a vital role for this gene in embryogenic induction. Further studies have successfully isolated a number of genes that are expressed during later stages of microspore embryo development, one of which is a gene encoding a CLAVATA3/ESR (CLE) family member, CLE 19. In zygotic and microspore embryogenesis the expression of this gene is restricted to globular and heart-shaped embryo development stages. This gene encodes a small secreted protein that is considered to promote cell differentiation and inhibit meristem formation in a range of plant organs (Fiers et al. 2004). Transcriptome analysis of different stages of microspore-derived embryo development has confirmed that there is gradual transition from pollen-dominated expression profiles to embryo-eclipsed profiles in mature cultures (Custers et al. 2001).

Genes that were differentially expressed during microspore embryogenesis in rapeseed have been isolated by subtractive hybridization, and a subtracted cDNA library constructed (Tsuwamoto et al. 2007). After sequencing over 2000 clones that showed differential expression in embryogenically-induced and non-embryogenic microspores, the non redundant sequences selected were searched against the well annotated Arabidopsis Munich Information center for Protein Sequences (MIPS) database to identify functional categories of the differentially expressed genes. When characterized, many sequences related to embryo-specific genes, the most frequent among them being the gene coding for Lipid Transfer Protein (LTP). Although the detailed function of LPTs is mostly unknown, several genes encoding LTPs have been found to be expressed in different embryogenic systems such as zygotic embryos in maize (Sossountzov et al. 1991), somatic embryos in carrot (Sterk et al. 1991), and microspore-derived embryos in barley (Vrinten et al. 1999), suggesting that it has a definite role in the embryogenesis process. In addition, ESTs of genes that code for napin and cruciferine (seed storage proteins in *Brassica*), oleosin (a major component of oil bodies) and phytosulfokine have been identified as being up-regulated during embryogenic induction. A detailed analysis of the expression patterns of 15 selected genes, determined by quantitative real-time reverse transcription-polymerase chain reaction (RT-PCR), found all of them to be highly expressed in the early stages of microspore embryogenesis, but poorly expressed in microspores when freshly isolated (before induction) or cultured under non-embryogenic induction conditions. The Principle Component Analysis based on the expression profiles of the 15 genes placed them in two groups; those having high expression during androgenic initiation and those expressed in the early to middle stage (globular to torpedo stage) of embryogenesis.

Malik et al. (2007) conducted a detailed examination of transcript profiles of embryogenic microspores and pollen-derived embryos in *B. napus* that represented a developmental series, starting from fresh pollen (0 d) to pollen after 3 d (induced), 5 d (dividing microspores), and 7 d stress treatments. Based on the *A. thaliana* information resource, they described ESTs that were most abundant at each stage. According to this study, microspores after a 3 d stress treatment have lost gene transcripts associated with protein synthesis (40 S and 60 S ribosomal proteins, initiation and elongation factors). These transcriptional changes may well relate to the cytoplasmic clearing of the de-differentiation process. In the cDNA libraries derived from microspore cultures following 3 d to 5 d stress treatments, a large number of pollen specific transcripts (pectinesterase, exopolygalactouronase, Bnm1, BP4) were isolated. However, it was not clear if these expression profiles were observed because the cultures may still have contained microspores that were not induced but were developing into mature pollen, or because during the period of transition, from pollen development to early stages of embryo induction, there was parallel expression of both pollen- and embryo-specific genes. A transcript that was abundant in all stages of development after induction (3 d, 5 d, and 7 d) was Bnm1 (invertase / pectin methylesterase inhibitor). This has been earlier shown to be expressed in the early stages of microspore embryogenesis in rapeseed up to globular stages (Treacy et al. 1997). In the 5 d and 7 d cultures, AGP gene transcripts were abundant. AGPs are a large multi-gene family coding for glycosylated Hyp-rich proteoglycans. While no specific function has been determined for AGPs, at least some AGPs have been implicated in the regulation of somatic embryogenesis (Chapman et al. 2000) and microspore embryogenesis (Letarte et al. 2006). In the 7 d microspore cultures, LTP were frequent. The LTP are able to transport phospholipids across cell membranes and are required for functioning of several biological processes such as embryogenesis, defense reaction, adaptations to stress and cutin formation (Kader 1996, Wang et al. 2005). LTPs are expressed in both somatic and zygotic embryos (Sterk et al. 1991). The cDNA libraries constructed from 5-day dividing and 7-day embryogenic microspores contained a number of ESTs for BnCYP78A whose functions are still not known.

From the various analyses of gene expression profiles carried out with stress induced microspores of the four model species, copious amount of data has been generated and is continued to be produced on the different types of genes that are found to be turned on or differentially expressed between the two developmental pathways of the microspore. Although a lot of concentration has been applied in trying to determine the genes that are involved in regulating the stress-induced embryogenic response in microspores and to understand the gene expression patterns that follow, the information gathered from the model species is far from complete at present, and thus elude a unified scheme whereby one could predict the expression of a common cascade of genes that would cause the switching of pathways from gametogenesis to embryogenesis that result in embryo development. Given the complexity of development re-programming that would have had to occur, and considering that there are different pathways by which embryogenesis is induced in microspores of different species, it is not surprising that a clear overall picture has not emerged yet.

However, the genes that have so far been identified as being specifically up-regulated during pollen embryogenesis have been broadly categorized into three main groups; stress responsive genes, gametogenesis-repressive genes and embryogenesis-related genes with functions identified as below.

5.5 Stress responsive genes

During microspore embryogenesis the up regulation of the Head Shock Protein (HSP) genes is observed, not only in response to heat stress but also other stresses applied on microspores such as starvation and colchicine. However, a distinct role for HSP on microspore embryogenesis has yet to be clearly established.

5.6 Gametogenesis repressive genes

Suppression of the gametophytic development must occur in the microspore before the genes for embryogenesis can be switched on (Hosp et al. 2007). Accumulation of starch in the microspore signifies that the cell has embarked on a gametophytic pathway of development where as the inhibition of starch accumulation portends the initiation of embryogenesis. The genes involved in starch synthesis and accumulation are seen to be down regulated during embryogenesis (Maraschin et al. 2006).

5.7 Embryogenesis related genes

Microspore embryogenesis occurs in a pattern of morphogenesis akin to zygotic embryo development. Based on this similarity, embryo pattern regulators such as members of the gene family 14-3-3 of barley have been observed to be up regulated, both in time and space (Maraschin et al. 2003).

6. Development of a multi-cellular pollen embryo

An induced microspore will undergo several rounds of mitotic divisions that result in a number of cells, contained together bounded by the exine or the outer wall of the microspore. There can be different pathways by which muli-cellular structures are produced from an initial star-like microspore. The four basic routes, based on the symmetry of the initial division of the microspore, as described by Razdan (2003) are as follows.

Pathway I: The initial division of the uni-nucleate microspore is symmetrical and results in two cells of equal size. Each of these cells undergoes further divisions producing a ball of cells within the exine.

Pathway II: An asymmetric initial division produces two cells of unequal size. The ball of cells may originate from the continued division of the larger vegetative cell while the smaller generative cell may divide a few times before degenerating.

Pathway III: Following an initial asymmetric division, the generative cell divides successively yielding the multi-cellular state. The vegetative cell remains arrested in division.

Pathway IV: Following an initial asymmetric division, both vegetative and generative cells will be equally active and divide to give rise to the multi-cellular structure.

The first pathway is considered to be the more common, and is observed in many species that are capable of embryogenic initiation from uni-nucleate microspores, prior to the first pollen mitosis (Smykal 2000). Apart from the stage of microspore development (uni- or bi-nucleate) at which it transits from gametogenesis to embryogenesis, it is also possible that the genotype or the plant species, as well as the stress conditions applied to induce embryogenesis in the microspore may also be factors that determine the pathway of cell division that leads to the development of multi-cellular structures from star-like microspores.

Irrespective of the above early pattern of microspore divisions, the embryogenic multi-cellular structures ultimately burst out through the restraining pollen wall, gradually assuming the form of a globular embryo akin to the globular stage of the zygotic embryo. A distinct outer layer of cells that surround a core of meristematic cells is the usual cellular anatomy that is observed in the microspore embryo at early stages of its development. The two types of cells differ in cellular morphology and metabolic processes that distinguish their developmental competences. The cells in the peripheral layer are vacuolated and filled with starch grains, which is suggestive of their differentiated nature, whereas cells to the interior are cytoplasm-filled and devoid of starch deposits which indicates their undifferentiated state and which are in fact capable of further meristematic activity (Barany et al. 2010a). Differences in the organization of cell wall components, particularly the distribution of polysaccharides, have also been noted and linked with the changes that occur in the cellular developmental processes. In microspore-derived embryos of *Capsicum annum* (pepper), cells in the peripheral layer contain a higher level of de-esterified pectins as wall components, a feature that is common with the cell wall of the mature pollen grain which is committed to normal gametogenesis. On the other hand esterified pectins are found in the cell walls of proliferating inner cells of the microspore embryo as with the walls of very young microspores prior to their gametophytic commitment (Barany et al. 2010b). Thus, the esterification of pectins in the cell walls may be considered as a cellular marker of their state of de-differentiation or meristematic activity, and therefore being capable of subsequent re-programming towards embryogenic development.

During further development, the microspore-derived globular embryos will follow the normal stages of post-globular embryogeny as seen in zygotic embryo development. As such, passage through heart-shaped and torpedo-shaped stages will culminate in the development of cotyledonary-staged mature somatic embryos that are ready to germinate into full-fledged sporophytic plants.

Alternatively, the multi-cellular mass that is liberated from the rupture of the microspore wall may proliferate to form a callus, from which organogenesis occurs by the regeneration of shoots and roots following transfer to culture media with appropriate growth regulators. It may sometimes be possible to obtain androgenic haploids either via embryo formation or organogenesis from callus in the same species by the manipulation of the chemical components of the culture medium.

7. References

Barany I, Fadon B, Risueno MC and Testillano PS. 2010a. Microspore reprogramming to embryogenesis induces changes in cell wall and starch accumulation dynamics associated with proliferation and differentiation events. Plant Signaling and Behavior 5(4):341 - 345.

Barany I, Fadon B, Risueno MC and Testillano PS. 2010b. Cell wall components and pectin esterification levels as markers of proliferation and differentiation events during pollen development and pollen embryogenesis in Capsicum annum L. Journal of Experimental Botany 61(4):1159 - 1175.)

Barnabas B. 2003a. Protocol for producing doubled haploid plants from anther culture of wheat (*Triticum aestivum* L.). In: Maluszynaki M, Kasha KJ, Forster BP, Szarejko I.

(eds.). Doubled haploid production in crop plants, a manual. Kluwer Academic Publishers, Dordrecht, The Netherlands, pp 65 - 70.

Barnabas B, Obert B, Kovacs G. 1999. Colchicine, an efficient genome doubling agent for maize (Zea mays L.) microspores cultured in anthero. Plant Cell Reports 18:858 - 862.

Beers EP, Jones AM, Dickerman AW. 2004. The S8 serine, C1A cysteine and A1 aspartic protease families in Arabidopsis. Phytochemistry 65:43 - 58.

Binarova P, Hause G, Cenklova V, Cordewener JHG, van Lookeren Campagne MM. 1997. A short severe heat shock is required to induce embryogenesis in late binuclear pollen of *Brassica napus* L. Sexual Plant Reproduction 10:200 - 208.

Bonet FJ, Azhaid L & Olmedilla A (1998). Pollen embryogenesis: atavism or totipotency? *Protoplasma* 202:115 - 121.

Boutilier K, Offringa R, Sharma VK, Kieft H, Ouellet T, Zhang L, Hattori J, Liu CM, van Lammeren AA, Miki BL, Custers JB, van Lookeren Campagne MM. 2002. Ectopic expression of BABY BOOM triggers a conversion from vegetative to embryonic growth. Plant Cell 14:1737 - 1749.

Carpenter IL, Ploense SE, Snustad DP, Silflow CD. 1992. Preferential expression of an α-tubulin gene of Arabidopsis in pollen. Plant Cell 4:557 - 571.

Chu C. 1978. The N6 medium and its application to anther culture of cereal crops. In: Proc Symp Plant Tissue Culture. Science Press, Peking, pp 43 - 50.

Chugh A and Eudes F. 2008. Isolated microspore embryogenesis in cereals: aspects and prospects. In: Recent advances in plant biotechnology and its applications. Ed. KH Neumann, A Kumar and SK Sopory. IK International Publishing House, Pvt. Ltd., New Delhi. p 205 - 226.

Cistue L, Riomas A, Castillo AM and Romagosa L. 1994. Production of a large number of doubled haploid plants from barley anthers protected with high concentration of mannitol. Plant Cell Report 13:709 - 712.

Cordewener JHG, Hause G, Gorgen E, Busink R, Hause B, Dons HJM, Van Lammeren AAM, Van Lookeren Campagne MM and Pechan P. 1995. Changes in synthesis and localization of members of the 70-kDa class of heat-shock proteins accompany the induction of embryogenesis in Brassica napus L. microspores. Planta 196:747 - 755.

Custers JBM, Cordewener JHG, Fiers MA, Maasen BTH, van Lookeren Campagne MM, Liu CM. 2001. Androgenesis in *Brassica*: a model system to study the induction of plant embryogenesis. In: Bhojwani SS, Soh WY (Eds). Current trends in the embryology of angiosperms. Kluwer Academic Publishers, Dordrecht. Pp. 451 - 470.

Custers JBM, Cordewener JHG, Nollen Y, Dons JJM, van Lookeren Campagne MM. 1994. Temperature controls both gametophytic and sporophytic development in microspore cultures of Brassica napus. Plant Cell Reports 16:267 - 271.

Datta SK. 2005. Androgenic haploids: factors controlling development and its application in crop improvement. Current Science 89(11):1870 - 1878.

Dunwell JM. 2010. Haploids in flowering plants: origins and exploitation. Plant Biotechnol. J. 8:377 - 424.

Dunwell JM and Thurling N. 1985. Role of sucrose in microspore embryo production in *Brassica napus* ssp. *Oleifera*. J. Exp. Bot. 36:1478 - 1491.

Fiers M, Hause G, Boutilier K, Casamitjana-Martinez E, Weijers D, Offringa R, van der Geest L, van Lookeren Campagne M, Liu CM. 2004. Mis-expression of the CLV3/ESR-like gene CLE 19 in *Arabidopsis* leads to a consumption of root meristem. Gene 18:37 - 49.

Herrera JC, Moreno LG, Acuna JR, Pena MD, Osorio D. 2002. Colchicine-induced microspore embryogenesis in coffee. Plant Cell Tiss Org Cult 71:89 - 92.

Gamborg OL, Miller RA, Ojima K. 1968. Nutrient requirement suspension cultures of soybean root cells. Exp Cell Res 50:151 - 158.

Garrido D, Vicente O, Heberle-Bors E, Isabel Rodriguez-Garcia M. 1995. Cellular changes during the acquisition of embryogenic potential in Nicotiana tobaccum. Protoplasma 186:220 - 230.

Germana MA. 2011. Anther culture for haploid and doubled haploid production. Plant Cell Tissue and Organ Culture 104:283 - 300.

Germana MA, Chiancone B, Iaconia C, Muleo R. 2005. The effect of light quality on anther culture of Citrus clementina Hort. Ex Tan. Acta Physiol Plant 27(4B):717 - 721.

Gervais G, Newcomb W, Simmonds DH. 2000. Re-arrangement of actin filament and microtubule cytoskeleton during induction of microspore embryogenesis in Brassica napus L. cv. Topas. Protoplasma 213:194 - 202.

Grewal RK, Lulsdorf M, Croser J, Ochatt S, Vandenberg A and Warkentin TD. 2009. Doubled haploid production in chick pea (Cicer arietinum L.): role of stress treatments. Plant Cell Rep 28:1289 - 1299.

Guha S. and Maheshwari SC. 1964. In vitro production of embryos from anthers of *Datura*. Nature 204:497.

Hause G, Hause B, van Lammeren AAM. 1992. Microtubular and actin filament configurations during microspore and pollen development in Brassica napus cv. Topas. Canadian Journal of Botany 70:1369 - 1376.

Hattori j, Boutilier K, van Lookeren Campagne MM, Miki BL. 1998. A conserved BURP domain defines a novel group of plant proteins with unusual primary structures. Mol Gen Genet 259:424 - 428.

Hellmann H and Estelle M. 2004. Plant development: regulation by protein degredation. Science 297(5582):793 - 797.

Hoekstra S, van Zijderveld MH, Louwerse JD, Heidekamp F, van der Mark F. 1992. Anther and microspore culture of *Hordeum vulgare* L. cv. Igri. Plant Science 86:89 - 96.

Hosp J, Maraschin SF, Touraev A and Boutilier K. 2007. Functional genomics of microspore embryogenesis. Euphytica 158:275 - 285.

Indrianto A, Barinova I, Touraev A, Heberle-Bors E. 2001. Tracking individual wheat microspores in vitro: identification of embryogenic microspores and body axis formation in the embryo. Planta 212:163 - 174.

Jaattela M, Wissing D, Kokholm K, Kallunki T, and Egeblad M. 1998. HSP70 exerts its anti-apoptic function downstream of capsase-3-like proteases. EMBO J. 17:6124 - 6134.

Kishor PBK and Reddy GM. 1986. Retention and revival of regenerating ability by osmotic adjustment in long-term cultures of four varieties of rice. J. Plant Physiol. 126:49 - 54.

Kyo M and Harada H. 1986. Control of the developmental pathway of tobacco pollen in vitro. Planta 168:427 - 432.

Kyo M, Yamaji N, Yuasa Y, Maeda T, and Fukui H. 2002. Isolation of cDNA coding for NtEPb1-b3 marker proteins for pollen de-differentiation in a tobacco pollen culture system. Plant Sci 163:1055 - 1062.

Kyo M, Hattori S, Yamaji N, Pechan P and Fukui H. 2003. Cloning and characterization of cDNAs associated with the embryogenic de-differentiation of tobacco immature pollen grains. Plant Sci 164(6):1057 - 1066.

Malik MR, Wang F, Dirpaul JM, Zhou N. Polowick PL, Ferrie AMR, Krochko JE. 2007. Transcript profiling and identification of molecular markers for early microspore embryogenesis in *Brassica napus*. Plant Physiology 144:134 - 154.

Maluszynski M, Kasha KJ, Szarejko I 2003. Published double haploid protocols in plant species. In: Maluszynski M, Kasha K, Forster BP, Szarejko I (eds.). Doubled haploid production in crop plants. A manual. Kluwer, Dordrecht, pp 309 - 335.

Maraschin SF, Priester W de, Spaink HP and Wang M. 2005a. Androgenic switch: an example of plant embryogenesis from the male gametophyte perspective. Journal of Experimental Botany 56:1711 - 1726.

Maraschin SF, Vennik M, Lamers GEM, Spaink HP, Wang M. 2005b. Time-lapse tracking of barley androgenesis reveals position-determined cell death within pro-embryos. Planta 220:531 - 540.

Maraschin SF, Caspers M, Potokina E, Wulfert F, Graner A, Spaink HP and Wang M. 2006. cDNA array analysis of stress-induced gene expression in barley androgenesis. Physiologia Plantarum 127:535 - 550.

Murashige T and Skoog F. 1962. A revised medium for rapid growth and bioassays with tobacco tissue cultures. Physiol. Plantarum 15:473 - 497.

Nitsch JP and Nitsch C. 1969. Haploid plants from pollen grains. Science 163:85 - 87.

Obert B, Barnabas B. 2004. Colchicine induced embryogenesis in maize. Plant Cell Tissue and Organ Culture 77:283 - 285.

Okamoto Y, Kinoshita A, Satake T. 2001. Enhancement of the frequency of callus formation and plant regeneration from rice anther culture by alternating temperature. Breed Res 3:87 - 94 (in Japanese).

Palmer CED and Keller WA. 2005. Overview of haploidy. In: Haploids in Crop Improvement II. Ed. CE Palmer, WA Keller and KI Kasha. Biotechnology in Agriculture and Forestry Vol. 56, Springer Verlag, Berlin, Heidelberg pp: 3 - 7.

Pauls KP, Chan J, Woronuk G, Schulze D, Brazolot J. 2006. When microspores decide to become embryos - cellular and molecular changes. Can J Bot Rev Can Bot 84:668 - 678.

Raina SK and Irfan ST. 1998. High frequency embryogenesis and plantlet regeneration from isolated microspores of indica rice. Plant Cell Rep. 17:957 - 962.

Raina SK and Zapata FJ. 1997. Enhanced anther culture efficiency in indica rice (*Oryza sativa* L.) through modification of the culture media. Plant Breed 116(4):305 - 315.

Razdan MK. 2003. Introduction to plant tissue culture. 2nd Ed. Science Publishers Inc. Enfield, NH, USA.

Reynolds TL and Crawford RL. 1997. Effects of light on the accumulation of abscisic acid and expression of an early cysteine-labeled metallothionein gene in microspores of *Triticum aestivum* during induced embryogenic development. Plant Cell Rep 16(7):458 - 463.

Schoffl F, Prandl R and Reindl A. 1998. Regulation of heat shock response. Plant Physiology 117:1135 - 1141.

Segui-Simarro JM and Nuez F. 2008. How microspores transform into haploid embryos: changes associated with embryogenesis induction and microspore-derived embryogenesis. Physiologia Plantarum 134:1 - 12.

Sentenac H, Bonneaud N, Minet M, Lacroute F, Salmon JM, Gaymard F, Grignon C. 1992. Cloning and expression of a plant potassium ion transport system. Science 256:663 - 665.

Shariatpanahi ME, Bal U, Heberle-Bors E, and Touraev A. 2006. Stresses applied for the re-programming of plant microspores towards in vitro embryogenesis. Physiologia Plantarum 127:519 - 534.

Silva TD. 2010. Indica rice anther culture: can the impasse be surpassed? Plant Cell Tissue and Organ Culture 100:1 -11.

Silva TD and Ratnayake WJ. 2009. Anther culture potential of indica rice varieties, Kurulu thuda and Bg 250. Tropical Agricultural Research and Extension 12(2):53 - 56.

Simmonds DH and Keller WA. 1999. Significance of preprophase bands of microtubules in the induction of microspore embryogenesis in *Brassica napus*. Planta 208:383 - 391.

Smykal P. 2000. Pollen embryogenesis - the stress mediated switch from gametophytic to sporophytic development. Current status and future prospects. Biol. Plant. 43:481 - 489.

Sternlicht H, Ringel I, Szasz J. 1983. Theory for modeling the copolymerization of tubulin and tubulin-colchicine complex. Biophys J 42:255 - 267.

Sunderland N. 1971. Anther culture: a progress report. Sci Prog (Oxford) 59:527 - 549.

Tanaka M. 1973. The effect of centrifugal treatment on the emergence of plantlets from cultured anther of tobacco. Japan J Breed 23:171 - 174.

Toureav A, Illham A, Vincente O, Heberle-Bors E (1996a). Stress induced microspore embryogenesis from tobacco microspores: an optimized system for molecular studies. Plant Cell Reports 15:561 - 565.

Toureav A, Indrianto A, Wratschko I, Vincente O, Heberle-Bors E (1996b). Efficient microspore embryogenesis in wheat (*Triticum aestivum* L.) induced by starvation at high temperatures. Sex Plant Reprod 9:209 - 215.

Touraev A, Pfosser M, Vicente O, Heberle-Bors E. 1996. Stress as the major signal controlling the developmental fate of tobacco microspores: towards a unified model of induction of microspore/pollen embryogenesis. Planta 200:144 - 152.

Touraev A, Vicente O and Heberle-Bors E. 1997. Initiation of micropsore embryogenesis by stress. Trends in Plant Science 2(8):297 - 302.

Vrinten PL, Nakamura T, Kasha KJ. 1999. Characterization of cDNAs expressed in the early stages of microspore embryogenesis in barley (*Hordeum vulgare* L.). Plant Mol. Biol. 41(4):455 - 463.

Wallin M, Stromberg E. 1995. Cold-stable and cold-adapted microtubules. International Review of Cytology 157:1 - 31.

Wedzony M, Forster BP, Zur I, Golemiec E, Szechynska-Hebda M, Dubas, Gotebiowska G. 2009. Progress in doubled haploid technology in higher plants. In: Touraev A, Forster BP, Jain SM, (eds.). Advances in haploid production in higher plants. Springer, Berlin, pp 1 - 34.

Yan J, Xue Q and Zhu J. 1996. Genetic studies of anther culture ability in rice (*Oryza sativa*). Plant Cell Tissue and Organ Culture 45:253 - 258.

Zaki MAM, Dickinson HG. 1991. Microspore-derived embryos in *Brassica*: the significance of division symmetry in pollen mitosis I to embryogenic development. Sexual Plant Reproduction 4: 48 - 55.

Zarsky V, Garrido D, Eller N, Tupy J, Vicente O, Schoffl F and Heberle-Bors E. 1995. The expression of a small heat shock gene is activated during induction of tobacco pollen embryogenesis by starvation. Plant Cell Environ. 18:139 - 147.

Zhao JP, Simmonds DH, Newcomb W. 1996. Induction of embryogenesis with colchicine instead of heat in microspores of *Brassica napus* L. cv. Topas. Planta 189:433 - 439.

25

Somatic Embryogenesis in Recalcitrant Plants

Laura Yesenia Solís-Ramos[1,2,*], Antonio Andrade-Torres[3,4],
Luis Alfonso Sáenz Carbonell[3], Carlos M. Oropeza Salín[3] and
Enrique Castaño de la Serna[1]
[1]*Unidad de Bioquímica y Biología Molecular de Plantas,
Centro de Investigación Científica de Yucatán, (CICY), Mérida, Yucatán,
Studies on habanero chilli biotechnology*
[2]*Escuela de Biología, Universidad de Costa Rica, San Pedro,
Genetic Plant Transformation and Biotechnology*
[3]*Unidad de Biotecnología, Centro de Investigación Científica de Yucatán, (CICY),
Mérida, Yucatán, Biotechnological studies on coconut*
[4]*INBIOTECA- Instituto de Biotecnología y Ecología Aplicada, Universidad Veracruzana,
Xalapa, Veracruz, México, Genetic Plant Transformation and Biotechnology*
[1,3,4]*México*
[2]*Costa Rica*

1. Introduction

There are two types of embryogenesis in plants: zygotic and somatic (Figure 1). Zygotic embryogenesis is one of the most important steps in the life cycle of plants. The process begins with double fertilization, followed by determination of the three axes of embryos (longitudinal, lateral, and radial) and morphologic changes of the embryos (globular, heart-shaped, and torpedo-shaped; Figure 1). Subsequently, seed storage proteins accumulate in the embryos, and finally, the embryos become desiccated and dormant. These processes are regulated by numerous factors, including phytohormones, enzymes, and other substances related to embryogenesis.

Somatic embryogenesis (SE) is the process by which somatic cells, under induction conditions, generate embryogenic cells, which go through a series of morphological and biochemical changes (Quiróz-Figueroa *et al.*, 2006), that result in the production of bipolar structure without vascular connection with the original tissue. The development of somatic embryos closely resembles the development of zygotic embryos both morphologically and physiologically (Figure 1). The process is feasible because plants possess cellular totipotency where by individual somatic cells can regenerate into a whole plant. Since the first reports on carrot in 1958 (Reinert 1958; Steward *et al.*, 1958), somatic embryogenesis has been reported in various plant species.

In addition to natural *in vivo* forms embryogenesis (apomixis), there exist at least three ways to induce embryo development from *in vitro* cultured plant cells: *in vitro* fertilization, from

* Corresponding Author

microspores and *in vitro* somatic embryogenesis (Féher *et al.*, 2003). *In vitro* SE can develop either from callus (indirect SE) or directly from the explant without any intermediate callus stage (direct SE). Somatic embryogenesis is also induced directly, or through callus, in the culture of somatic embryos, and this process is called secondary SE in contrast to primary SE induced from explant cells (Gaj, 2004).

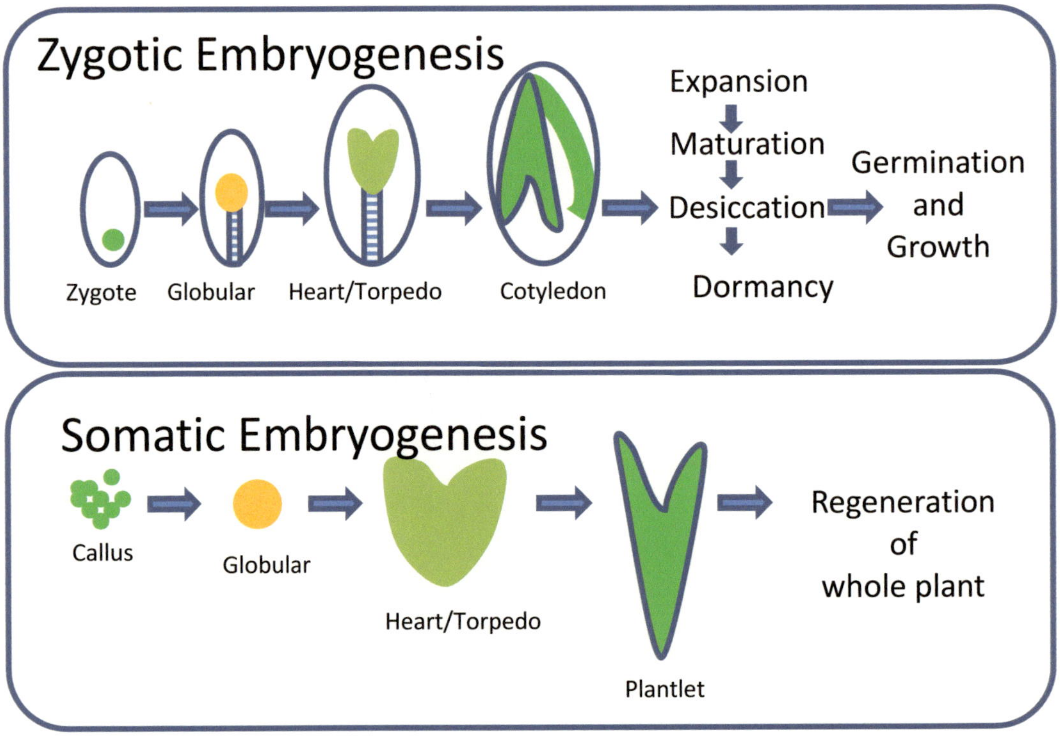

Fig. 1. Zygotic vs somatic embryogenesis. Modified from Zimmerman, 1993.

Somatic embryos originate by two pathways, unicellular or multicellular. When embryos have a unicellular origin, coordinated cell divisions are observed and the embryo sometimes connected to the maternal tissue by a suspensor-like structure. In contrast, multicellular-origin embryos are initially observed as a protuberance, with no coordinated cell divisions observable, and those embryos in contact with the basal area are typically fused to the maternal tissue (Quiroz-Figueroa *et al.*, 2006).

Somatic embryogenesis with a low frequency of chimeras, a high number of regenerates and a limited level of somaclonal variation (Ahloowalia, 1991; Henry *et al.*, 1998) is more attractive than organogenesis as a plant regeneration system (e.g., in genetic transformation, *in vitro* mutagenesis and selection). However there are several factors that influence the initiation of somatic embryogenesis in plants.

In the context of this paper, *in vitro* plant recalcitrance is defined as the inability of plant tissue cultures to respond to *in vitro* manipulations. In its broadest terms, tissue culture recalcitrance also concerns the time-related decline and/or loss of morphogenetic competence and totipotent capacity (Benson, 2000).

2. Some factors influencing somatic embryogenesis induction

The process of acquisition of embryogenic competence by somatic cells must involve reprogramming of gene expression patterns as well as changes in the morphology, physiology, and metabolism of plant cells. Studies on factors controlling *in vitro* plant morphogenesis are highly important not only for the development of improved regeneration systems, but also for the analysis of molecular mechanisms underlying plant embryogenesis.

In vitro development of cells and tissues depends on different factors such as: genotype, type of plant, age and developmental stage of an explant, physiological state of an explant-donor plant, and the external environment which includes composition of media and physical culture conditions (light, temperature) (Gaj, 2004).

The embryogenic potential is largely defined by the developmental program of the plant as well as by environmental cues (Féher, 2005). The key role of endogenous hormone metabolism affected by genetic, physiological and environmental cues is well accepted in the induction phase of somatic embryogenesis (Jiménez, 2005).

The cells which represent an intermediate state between somatic and embryogenic cells are called competent. Cellular competence is associated with the dedifferentiation of somatic cells that allows them to respond to new developmental signals. It is well accepted that embryogenic competent cells can be morphologically recognized as small, rounded cells with rich cytoplasm and small vacuoles. In this respect they are very similar to meristematic cells or zygotes and this similarity is further emphasized by their asymmetric division (Féher, 2005).

Wounding, high salt concentration, heavy metal ions or osmotic stress positively influenced somatic embryo induction in diverse plant species (reviewed by Dudits *et al.*, 1995). These procedures were accompanied by increased expression of diverse stress-related genes, evoking the hypothesis that somatic embryogenesis is an adaptation process of *in vitro* cultured plant cells (Dudits *et al.*, 1995).

Endogenous hormone levels however can be considered as major factors in determining the specificity of cellular responses to these rather general stress stimuli (Féher *et al.*, 2003). The temporal and spatial changes in endogenous auxin levels are important factors controlling the embryogenic cell fate (Féher *et al.*, 2003).

Among different external stimuli that induce an embryogenic pathway of development plant growth regulators (PGRs) such as auxins and cytokinins used for *in vitro* media have been the most frequently considered, as they regulate the cell cycle and trigger cell divisions (Francis and Sorrell, 2001). The high efficiency of 2,4-dichlorophenoxy acetic acid (2,4-D) for induction of embryogenic response found in different *in vitro* systems and plant species indicates a specific and unique character of this PGR. This synthetic growth regulator and an auxinic herbicide appear to act not only as an exogenous auxin analogue but also as an effective stressor (Gaj, 2004).

The polar transport of auxin in early globular embryos is essential for the establishment of bilateral symmetry during plant embryogenesis. Interference with this transport causes a failure in the transition from axial to bilateral symmetry and results in the formation of embryos with fused cotyledons (Liu *et al.*, 1993).

The chromatin remodelling plays two major roles during the early stages of somatic embryogenesis. Differentiation requires unfolding of the supercoiled chromatin structure, in order to allow the expression of genes inactivated by heterochromatinization during differentiation, and subsequent chromatin remodelling can result in the specific activation of a set of genes required for embryogenic development (Féher *et al.*, 2003).

Also a wide and complex variety of molecules can now be enlisted, including polysaccharides, amino acids, growth regulators, vitamins, low molecular weight compounds, polypeptides, etc. (Chung *et al.*, 1992). Some such compounds are derived from the cell wall, whereas others originate inside the cells (Quiroz-Figueroa *et al.*, 2006).

3. Some genes related to somatic embryogenesis

3.1 *WUSCHEL* (WUS)

WUS is a homeobox gene which encodes a transcription factor that regulates the pool of stem cells in the shoot meristem and is regulated by a feedback loop involving the CLAVATA (CLV) genes (Weigel and Jurgens, 2002; Bhalla and Singh, 2006). WUS expression can be first localized to the shoot meristem in the heart stage embryo, and the shoot meristem of the plant by regulating the stem cell pool can continue to produce organs throughout the life of the plant. The stem cells are specified by a WUS-dependent signal produced in the organizing center cells, which lie below the stem cell niche of the central zone and CLV3 is in turn produced by the stem cells of the central zone (Baurle and Laux, 2005; Reddy and Meyerowitz, 2005). Increases in the number of stem cells lead to an increasing amount of the secreted CLV3 protein, which acts via the CLV1/CLV2 receptor complex to reduce WUS expression and the number of stem cells, thus maintaining a constant pool of stem cells (Weigel and Jurgens, 2002).

3.2 *Baby Boom* (BBM)

The Baby Boom (BBM) gene, which was isolated from microspore embryo cultures of *Brassica napus* (Boutilier *et al.*, 2002), encodes a transcriptional factor belonging to the AP2/ERF family. BBM expression was observed during zygotic and pollen-derived somatic embryogenesis. The ectopic expression of BBM and *Arabidopsis* BBM (AtBBM) in transgenic plants induced the formation of somatic embryo-like structures on the edges of cotyledons and leaves, as well as additional pleiotropic phenotypes, including neoplastic growth, phytohormone-free plant regeneration from explants, and abnormal leaf and flower morphology. Therefore, BBM is likely to promote cell proliferation and morphogenesis during embryogenesis (Boutilier *et al.*, 2002).

3.3 *SERK* (Somatic Embryogenesis Receptor Kinase)

Among the genes involved in somatic embryogenesis, Somatic Embryogenesis Receptor Kinases (SERKs) genes has been detected in the early stages of the process, which form a subgroup in the Leucine-Rich Repeat-Receptor-Like Kinases (LRR-RLKs) comprising the largest subfamily of RLKs in plants and are also related to key processes in plant growth (Sharma *et al.*, 2008).

The first SERK gene was identified in competent cells of carrot (*Daucus carota*) *in vitro* cultured (Schmidt *et al.*, 1997), this gene encodes a transmembrane receptor kinase type with leucine-rich repeat (LRR). DcSERK has been considered as a marker of cells competent to form embryos in culture (Schmidt *et al.*, 1997). DcSERK has been found be expressed in somatic and zygotic embryos but in no other plant tissues at very early stages of somatic embryo development, i.e., from the single-cell stage to the globular stage (Schmidt *et al.*, 1997). Genes homologous to DcSERK were isolated from *Arabidopsis* (AtSERK1), maize (ZmSERK1, ZmSERK2), *Medicago truncatula* (MtSERK1) (Nolan *et al.*, 2003), *Hieracium* (HpSERK), *Helianthus annuus* (Thomas *et al.*, 2004), *Oryza sativa* (Hu *et al.*, 2005), *Theobroma cacao* (Santos *et al.*, 2005), Citrus unshui (Shimada *et al.*, 2005), y *Solanum tuberosum* (Sharma *et al.*, 2008) suggesting the ubiquity of a small family of SERK in all species of plants, in addition to the functional conservation of a specific role in embryogenesis. Their expressions were detected during somatic embryogenesis (Somleva *et al.*, 2000; Baudino *et al.*, 2001; Hecht *et al.*, 2001; Shah *et al.*, 2002; Nolan *et al.*, 2003; Tucker *et al.*, 2003; Thomas *et al.*, 2004), as well as in developing ovules and early-stage embryos of *Arabidopsis*, *Hieracium* and maize.

4. Genetic transformation to abate recalcitrance

Genetic transformation has proven to be an alternative to abate recalcitrance to *in vitro* morphogenesis and to increase resistance to pathogenic microorganisms (Cai *et al.*, 2003; Shin *et al.*, 2002; Zuo *et al.*, 2002; Herrera-Estrella *et al.*, 2004). This has been achieved by insertion and over-expression of genes related to the control of morphogenesis, such as the heterologous gene WUSCHEL in *Arabidopsis thaliana* and *Coffea canephora* cultures that promoted the transition from vegetative to embryogenic state, and eventually led to somatic embryo formation (Zuo *et al.*, 2002; Arroyo-Herrera *et al.*, 2008). In *Capsicum chinense*, the induced expression of WUSCHEL in segments of transformed stems began to form globular structures, suggesting that heterologous WUSCHEL was active and involved in the process of morphogenesis (Solís-Ramos *et al.*, 2009). It has been demonstrated in *Arabidopsis*, that over-expression of a SOMATIC EMBRYOGENESIS RECEPTOR-like KINASE (SERK) gene (AtSERK1) increases the embryogenic competence of callus derived from transformed seedlings 3 to 4-fold when compared with the wild-type callus (Hecht *et al.*, 2001).

Most of the important crops and grasses are recalcitrant for *in vitro* culturing, which hampers the development of reliable regeneration techniques. This document is focused in the somatic embryogenesis of recalcitrant plants, showing the particular cases of two plant species: habanero chili (*Capsicum chinense* Jacq.) and coconut palm (*Cocos nucifera* L.).

5. Studies in habanero chili (*Capsicum chinense* Jacq.)

5.1 Introduction

All chili peppers belong to the genus *Capsicum* of the Solanaceae family and are important horticultural crops. Members of the *Capsicum* genus have been shown to be recalcitrant to differentiation and plant regeneration under *in vitro* conditions, which in turn makes it very difficult or inefficient to apply recombinant DNA technologies via genetic transformation aimed at genetic improvement against pests and diseases (Ochoa-Alejo and Ramírez-Malagón, 2001). *Capsicum chinense* Jacq. (habanero chili) (Fig. 2-G), a species of economic importance for Mexico is no exception (Santana-Buzzy *et al.*, 2005; López-Puc *et al.*, 2006), and no efficient, reproducible somatic embryogenesis regeneration system has yet been developed for this species. A dependable system is indispensable for their genetic improvement and regeneration of transformed tissue (Solís-Ramos *et al.*, 2009).

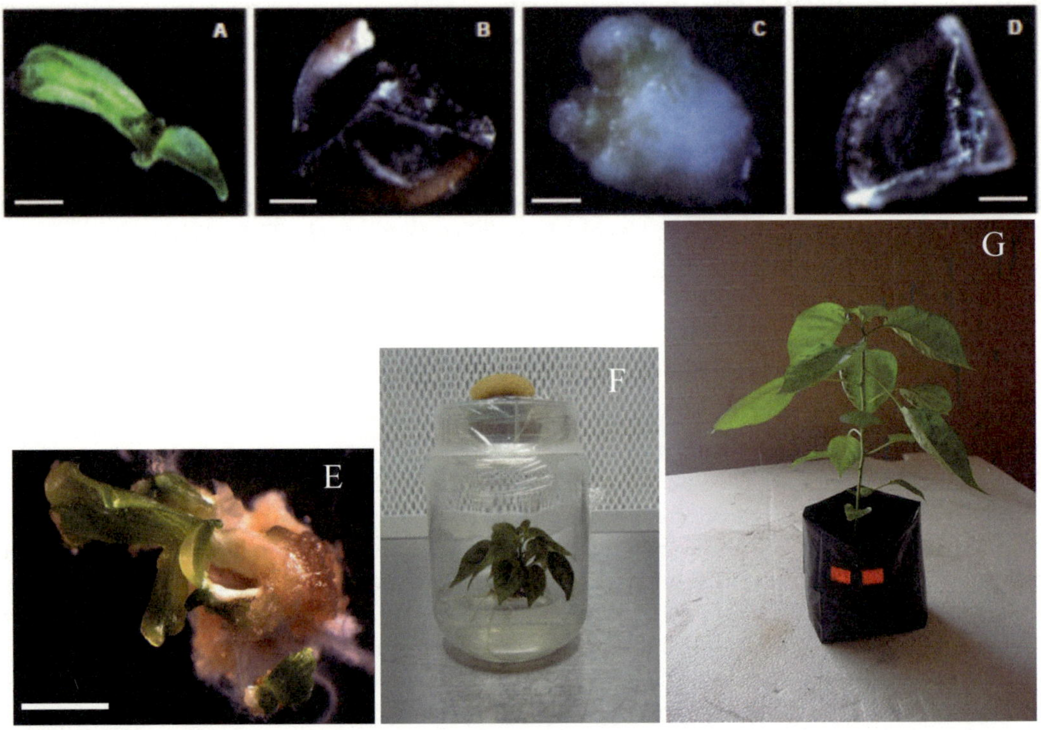

Fig. 2. A to G: Different responses of *C. chinense* explants after induction: A, cotyledon. Bar= 1mm; B, Zygotic embryo segment with radicle; C, Zygotic embryo segment forming callus; D, Zygotic embryo segment without embryogenic response. Bar= 0.5mm. E: somatic embryo germinating. Bar= 1mm. F: seedling obtained from somatic embryo. G: seedling after acclimatization under greenhouse conditions.

5.2 Indirect somatic embryogenesis protocol

Direct organogenesis has been the most frequently used morphogenic route for *in vitro* regeneration of *Capsicum* plants; however, the major problem faced to achieve this goal has been the failure of elongation of the induced shoot buds (Ochoa-Alejo and Ramírez-Malagón, 2001). Shoot buds and rosettes are not well formed during the induction step, perhaps because of a lack of true apical meristems (Binzel *et al.*, 1996; Ochoa-Alejo and Ramírez-Malagón 2001; Steinitz *et al.*, 2003).

In recent years, a number of investigators have developed methods in order to increase the efficiency of the somatic embryogenesis process for chili pepper micropropagation via direct somatic embryogenesis (DSE) (Harini and Sita 1993; Binzel *et al.*, 1996; Khan *et al.*, 2006) and indirect somatic embryogenesis (ISE) (Binzel *et al.*, 1996; Buyakalaca and Mavituna, 1996, Kintzios *et al.*, 2001, Zapata-Castillo *et al.*, 2007, Solís-Ramos *et al.*, 2010b). *Capsicum chinense* Jacq. is a recalcitrant species for *in vitro* morphogenesis, and up to date there is no efficient system for genetic transformation and regeneration of this species via somatic embryogenesis. However an ISE protocol was developed using mature *C. chinense* zygotic embryo segments (ZES) (Solís-Ramos *et al.*, 2010b) (Figure 2 C, E-G). The ZES cultured in semi-solid MS-3R medium (MS medium with 8.9 μM NAA, 11.4 μM IAA and 8.9 μM BAP) developed an embryogenic callus and 8% of these explants developed somatic embryos (Figure 2-E). Torpedo-stage somatic embryos were detached from the callus and subcultured in semi-solid MS medium without growth regulators, producing a 75% conversion rate to plantlets with well-formed root tissue. Histological analysis showed the developed structures to have no vascular connection to the source tissue and to be bipolar, confirming that this protocol induced formation of viable somatic embryos from mature *C. chinense* zygotic embryo segments, and seedlings can be obtained (Figure 2 F-G).

5.3 Endogenous GUS-like activity in *C. chinense* tissues

The gene *uidA* codes for β-glucuronidase which is utilized as a reporter in plant genetic transformation because it is generally believed that higher plants do not show GUS-like endogenous activity (Jefferson *et al.*, 1987; Martin *et al.*, 1991; Sudan *et al.*, 2006). However, several studies have demonstrated that some plant species show endogenous GUS-like activity in vegetative tissues as well as reproductive organs (Cervera, 2005; Sudan *et al.*, 2006). Therefore, in order to avoid undesirable effects in interpreting genetic transformation results, it is recommended to evaluate potential endogenous GUS-like activity in tissues that will be targeted to genetic transformation by using *uidA* as a reporter. The pH of the assay buffer is very critical for detection of the GUS activity in plants. The *E. coli*-derived GUS has optimum activity at pH 7.0 and hence plant tissues are assayed at neutral pH after transformation (Sudan *et al.*, 2006).

Segments of mature zygotic embryos of *C. chinense* were used as explants for transient transformation with *Agrobacterium tumefaciens* LBA4404 (pCAMBIA2301) and C58C1 (pER10W-35S Red) (Solís-Ramos *et al.*, 2010a, Solís-Ramos *et al.*, 2010b). T-DNA in pCAMBIA2301 (Center for the Application of Molecular Biology to International Agriculture, Canberra, Australia) includes a copy of *Escherichia coli uidA* gene under the control of CaMV35S promoter and the NOS terminator. In this binary vector, *uidA* gene coding sequence is interrupted by a Castor Bean catalase intron, which has to be removed for eukaryotic expression and prevents bacterial transcriptions of the gene coding sequence. Transient transformation of *C. chinense* explants and plant regeneration were carried out following the protocol previously described by Solís-Ramos *et al.* (2009). In addition, as a positive control leaves explants of *Nicotiana tabacum* were transient transformed via *A. tumefaciens* LBA4404 (pCAMBIA2301), to verify that the protocol used for GUS activity was done properly. Histochemical staining of *C. chinense* explants was carried out following a protocol reported by Jefferson (1987). Presence of blue spots was recorded and interpreted as transient GUS expression (Figure 3). Also the transient expression of red fluorescent protein was detected using a Leica MZFLIII stereoscopic microscope equipped with appropriate filtres (546/10 nm, 600/40 nm).

Successful transient transformed *C. chinense* zygotic embryo explants were achieved with *A. tumefaciens* LBA4404 (pCAMBIA2301) and the bacteria were eliminated with 1 g/L cefotaxime and 500 mg/L timentin (Solís-Ramos *et al.*, 2009). The calli of *C. chinense* transient transformed with pER10W-35S Red (used as control for transformation efficiency) expressed the red fluorescent protein (DsRFP), but not the non-transformed calli (data not shown) (Solís-Ramos *et al.*, 2010a). A screening for endogenous GUS-like activity in *C. chinense* tissues was performed in phosphate buffer adjusted to pH 6, 7, 7.5 and 8. At pH 6 and 7 the 100% of all samples (vegetative and reproductive tissues) presented endogenous GUS-like activity (Figure 3-C) (Solís-Ramos *et al.*, 2010a). At pH 7.5 no GUS-like activity was observed in all of the petals, root, stem or leaves. However, in septum, stamen and calli some GUS-like activity was observed. A substantial decrease, or even a total absence, of GUS-like activity was observed in phosphate buffer pH 8 in almost all tissue analyzed with an exception for a slight activity in stamens (Figure 3-A) (Solís-Ramos *et al.*, 2010a). Our results of histochemical staining in phosphate buffer pH 8, suggest that *uidA* gene was introduced in regenerants of *C. chinense* and *N. tabacum* and the gene was transcriptional active as it can be inferred from the blue stain observed in tissues of regenerated plantlets. The main problem during initial steps of transformation is just to get an assay conditions which can provide an initial screening. This problem has been solved by adjusting the pH to 8 for *C. chinense* (Solís-Ramos *et al.*, 2010a).

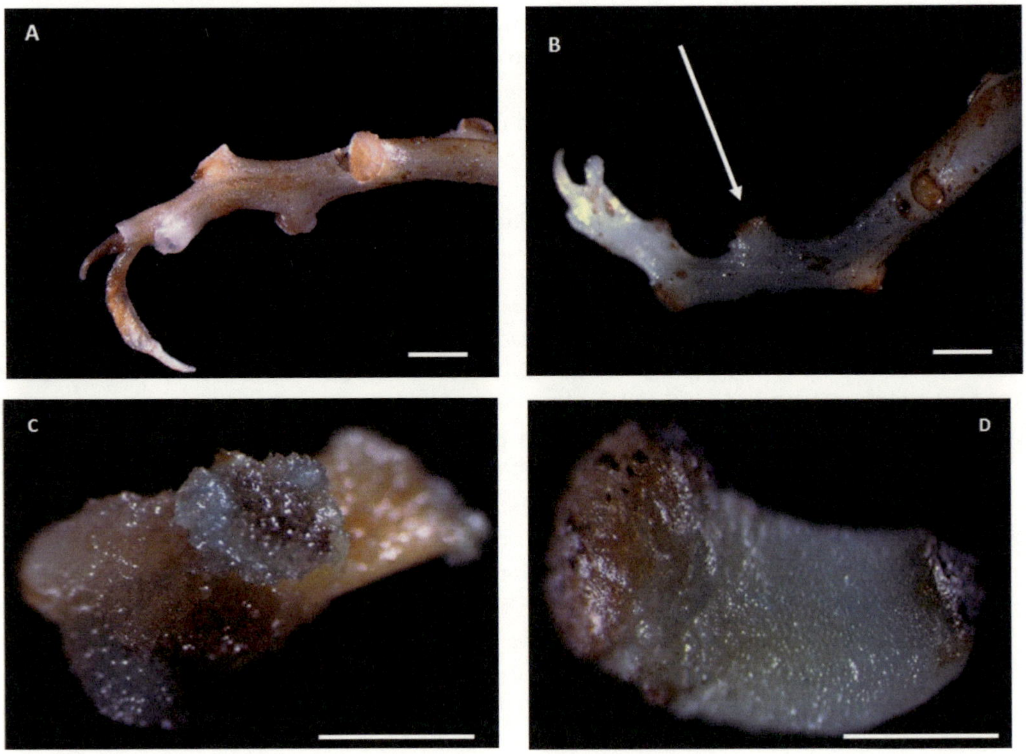

Fig. 3. *C. chinense* explants showing endogenous GUS-like activity at pH 7 (C), and without endogenous GUS-like activity at pH 8 (A). B and D transformed explants showing GUS expression. A, B bar= 5mm. C, D bar= 1mm.

5.4 Protocol for genetic transformation

Habanero chili plants were transformed via *Agrobacterium tumefaciens* co-cultivation with reporter genes: *uiDA, DsRFP,* and *WUSCHEL* (Solís-Ramos *et al.*, 2009, Solís-Ramos *et al.*, 2010a, Solís-Ramos *et al.*, 2010b). *WUSCHEL* (WUS) has been shown to promote the transition from vegetative to embryogenic state when overexpressed in *Arabidopsis thaliana* (Zuo *et al.*, 2002). The hypothesis tested is that the genetic transformation of Habanero chili and overexpression of heterologous gene *WUS* will promotes an embryogenic response in this species (Solís-Ramos *et al.*, 2009). The transformed chimeric plants where used for induction of expression of heterologous gene *WUS*. After 15 days of induction, the segments of transformed stems begun to form globular structures, and the wild type did not show development, suggesting that heterologus *WUS* was active and involved in the process of morphogenesis. The induced transformed explants showed the expression of *WUS* by Northern reverse analysis, and none *WUS* transcripts had detectable in the wild type. The histological analysis of induced transformed stems showed the development of meristematic nodules and the formation of globular somatic embryos, which presented necrosis after 45 days of in vitro culture, which did not continue development into other embryonic stages or in plants. The results showed that overexpression of gene *WUS* in stems of Habanero chili promote the formation of embryogenic structures but these stagnate in their growth suggesting that other signals may be need it for induction of proper development in this species (Solís-Ramos *et al.*, 2009). In addition this suggests that *WUS* encourages the development of undifferentiated tissue in species that may help as an alternative to solve the recalcitrance from this plant species (Solís-Ramos *et al.*, 2009).

6. Studies for coconut (*Cocos nucifera* L.) somatic embryogenesis

6.1 Introduction

Coconut (*Cocos nucifera* L.) is widely distributed throughout the humid tropics where it is cultivated over an estimated twelve million ha. It is a very important perennial crop, since it significantly contributes to food security, improved nutrition, employment and income generation. Coconut is a monospecific palm species consisting of numerous ecotypes and hybrids all possessing desirable agronomic properties. There is a great ethnic diversity in the ways that various coconut resources are produced and used (Foale, 2005). It is often referred to as "the tree of life" because of the many uses that have been developed for all parts of the palm. More recent uses of economic importance include fibre-derived products for the automobile industry; activated charcoal; virgin oil; bottled water; and oil for production of coco-biodiesel. In the Philippines, an industrial plant was launched in 2006 for the production of 75 million liters / year of coco-biodiesel where it is being used as a fuel additive (Lao, 2009). A blend at 2% coconut oil with diesel has been shown to reduce harmful exhaust emissions (opacity, K value) by as much as 63% (Lao, 2008).

However, most coconut groves require replanting because of loss due either to palm senescence or to diseases such as lethal yellowing in America (Harrison and Oropeza, 2008), the lethal diseases in Africa (Eden-Green, 1997) and cadang-cadang in Asia (Hanold and Randles, 1991). Unfortunately, improved disease resistant planting materials are scarce and seed propagation does not yield sufficient material to satisfy the rapidly growing demands.

Therefore, alternative approaches for the propagation of improved planting materials must be considered and *in vitro* propagation or micropropagation *via* somatic embryogenesis seems to provide a convenient alternative for the future due to its potential for massive propagation.

Several explants have been tested with diverse results, being the most responsive immature infloresencenes and plumules in increasing order (Blake and Hornung, 1995; Chan *et al.*, 1998; Pérez-Nuñez *et al.*, 2006). For this reason plumules have been more extensively used to improve on the different developmental changes in the process: callogenesis, embryo formation, germination and conversion.

6.2 *In vitro* culture of coconut palm

6.2.1 Coconut micropropagation using plumule explants

In order to increase the efficiency of somatic embryogenesis in coconut, two different approaches were evaluated, secondary somatic embryogenesis and multiplication of embryogenic callus. Primary somatic embryos obtained from plumule explants were used as explants and formed both embryogenic callus and secondary somatic embryos. The embryogenic calluses obtained after three multiplication cycles were capable of producing somatic embryos. The efficiency of the system was evaluated in a stepwise process beginning with an initial step for inducing primary somatic embryogenesis followed by three steps for inducing secondary somatic embryogenesis followed by three steps for embryogenic callus multiplication, and finally production of somatic embryos from callus (Pérez-Nuñez *et al.*, 2006). The actual process of somatic embryogenesis by embryogenic callus multiplication and secondary somatic embryogenesis is shown in Figure 4. The total calculated yield from one plumule was 98,000 somatic embryos (SEs). Comparing this to the yield obtained from primary somatic embryogenesis results in about a 50,000-fold increase (Pérez-Nuñez *et al.*, 2006).

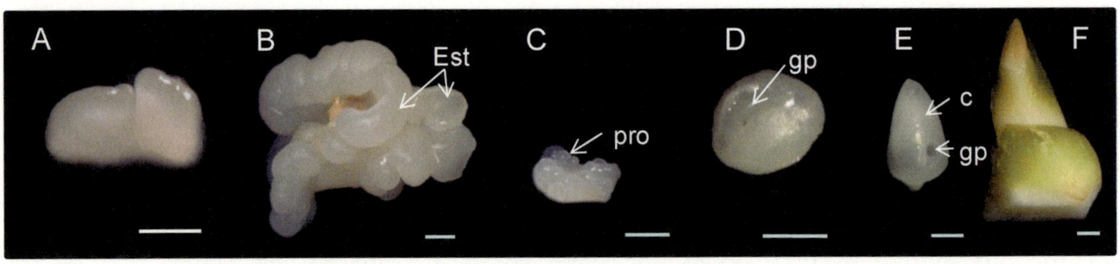

Fig. 4. An embryogenic structure derived from an embryogenic callus used as explant (A), developed an embryogenic callus (B) after 90 days of culture in medium I. After transferring embryogenic callus to medium II, callus with somatic embryos at different stages occurred. Piece of callus with pro-embryos (C), globular embryo (D), coleoptilar embryo (E) and germinating embryo (F). Bar= 1mm. Coleoptile: [c], germinative pore: [gp], pro-embryo [pro]

This protocol represented an important progress towards practical application by showing a way to improve the efficiency of coconut somatic embryo production. However has still some bottlenecks, as the relative low percentage of formation of embryogenic calli (40-

60%) and calli with somatic embryos (12-24%) and the low number of somatic embryos formed (2-10) per callus. In order to increase these figures and optimize this protocol to avoid many steps of multiplication, different plant growth regulators and compounds has been tested.

6.3 Exogenous plant growth regulators

6.3.1 Brassinosteroids

The effect of the brassinosteroid 22(S), 23(S)-homobrassinolide on initial callus, embryogenic callus and somatic embryo formation in coconut plumule explants was tested. The explants were exposed (during a 3 or 7 d pre-culture) to different concentrations (0.01, 0.1, 1, 2 and 4 μM) of the brassinosteroid. The explants responded favorably to the brassinosteroid increasing their capacity to form initial callus, embryogenic callus and somatic embryos. The largest amount of somatic embryos formed, 10.8 somatic embryos / explant, was obtained exposing the explants for 3 d to the brassinosteroid at 0.01 or 0.1 μM, whereas 3.8 somatic embryos / explant were obtained from untreated explants. Efficiency-wise the overall effect of HBr increases the total amount of somatic embryos formed per explant 2.8 times (Azpeitia *et al.* 2003).

6.3.2 Gibberellic acid

In some reports of coconut the GA_3 is added into the culture medium to promote the germination of somatic embryos (Perera *et al.*, 2009). However the effect of addition of this phytohormome had not been tested on the formation of somatic embryos. The results obtained with GA_3 were positive at 0.5 μM using the protocol of embryogenic calli multiplication from plumule explants. This concentration promoted 1.5 fold the number of the embryogenic calli forming somatic embryos. The number of somatic embryos per callus also increased, about 5 fold at day 30 (globular embryos) and 2 fold afterwards (coleptilar embryos). Also when the effect of GA_3 was evaluated on the germination of somatic embryos, the results were positive. The proportion of calli with germinating embryos was 2 fold higher than in the control treatment with no phytohormone. The number of germinating somatic embryos *per* callus was also higher under phytohormone treatment, also a 2 fold increase in relation to the control treatment. Therefore, a combined 4 fold increase in the overall number of germinating embryos (Montero-Cortés *et al.*, 2010). Then altogether, the use of GA_3 was positive both for the formation of somatic embryos and on their germination, so this could be a very useful approach to improve the performance of coconut micropropagation.

6.3.3 Uptake of auxins

6.3.3.1 Uptake of 2, 4-D

As previously reported for inflorescence coconut explants (Oropeza and Taylor, 1994), ^{14}C-2,4-D was taken up by plumular explants. The rate was faster during the first week of culture, and then reduced until reaching a plateau at day 90. The ^{14}C-2,4-D concentration in the explants reached its maximum values within the first 20 d of culture, prior to the appearance of any morphogenic response. It is interesting to note that when radioactivity was steadily taken up, calli were formed and once the calli started to form embryogenic structures, uptake practically stopped. This result suggests that the uptake of 2,4-D may be related to the induction of these morphogenic responses.

6.4 Characterization of genes related to somatic embryogenesis

6.4.1 Shoot apical meristem formation and maintaining (*KNOX* family genes)

The expression the class I *KNOX* (KNOTTED-like homeobox) genes seem to play an important role during somatic embryogenesis. In *Picea abies* overexpression of *HBK3,* a class I *KNOX* homeobox gene improves the development of somatic embryos and lines in which *HBK3* was down-regulated had reduced ability to produce immature somatic embryos and were not able to complete the maturation processes (Belmonte *et al.*, 2007).

The complete sequences of two *KNOX* like genes were obtained *CnKNOX1* and *CnKNOX2.* The deduced aminoacid sequence of both showed the highly conserved domains characteristic of *KNOX* genes. *CnKNOX1* showed high homology with KNOX class I proteins. *CnKNOX1* expression was detected throughout the embryogenesis process except in somatic embryos at the pro-globular stage, becoming highest in somatic embryos at the coleoptilar stage. No detection of *CnKNOX1* expression occurred in calli with aberrant embryos. The addition of gibberellic acid stimulated the expression of *CnKNOX1* earlier and the relative expression at all stages was higher. *CnKNOX2* expression occurred at all stages peaking at globular stage but gibberellic acid treatment decreased expression (Montero-Cortés *et al.*, 2010).

6.4.2 Somatic embryogenesis (Somatic Embryogenesis Related Kinase-*SERK*)

Somatic embryogenesis involves different molecular events including differential gene expression and various signal transduction pathways for activating or repressing numerous genes sets (Chugh and Khurana, 2002). Genes involved in somatic embryogenesis are stage specific and one of the genes identified in early somatic embryogenesis is SOMATIC EMBRYOGENESIS RECEPTOR-LIKE KINASE (DcSERK) that was originally isolated from embryogenic cells in suspension cultures of the dicot *Daucus carota* (Schmidt *et al.*, 1997). It was found to be expressed in embryogenic but not in non-embryogenic cultures, in cells predicted to be embryogenic, in tissue explants induced by placing them under embryogenic culture conditions, and during somatic embryogenesis up the globular stage. During *D. carota* zygotic embryogenesis, SERK expression occurred up to the early globular stage, but no expression was found in any other plant tissues, and cells transformed with a SERK promoter-luciferase reporter gene were able to form somatic embryos (Schmidt *et al.* 1997). Similar findings have been obtained in other dicots. In *A. thaliana,* the *AtSERK1* gene was expressed during the formation of embryogenic cells in culture, early embryogenesis, and in plant in developing ovules, specifically in all cells of the embryo sac up to fertilization, and in all cells after fertilization of the developing embryo until the heart stage (Hecht *et al.*, 2001). *A. thaliana* seedlings overexpressing AtSERK1 exhibited a three- to fourfold increase in efficiency for initiation of somatic embryogenesis; therefore, an increase in the level of the AtSERK1 conferred embryogenic competence in culture (Hecht *et al.*, 2001).

The complete sequence one *SERK* like gene was obtained and referred as *CnSERK.* Predicted sequence analysis showed that CnSERK encodes a SERK protein with the domains reported in the SERK proteins in other species. These domains consist of a signal peptide, a leucine zipper domain, five LRR, the Serine- Proline-Proline domain, which is a distinctive domain of the SERK proteins, a single transmembrane domain, the kinase domain with 11 subdomains and the C terminal region. Analysis of its expression showed that it could be detected in embryogenic tissues before embryo development could be observed. In contrast it was not detected or at lower levels in non-embryogenic tissues, thus suggesting that *CnSERK* expression is associated with induction of somatic embryogenesis and that it could be a potential marker of cells competent to form somatic embryos in coconut tissues cultured *in vitro* (Pérez-Nuñez *et al.*, 2009).

6.5 Protocol for genetic transformation

We have developed a protocol for genetic transformation of this palm species (Andrade-Torres *et al.*, 2011); evaluating reporter genes, transformation methods, and conditions for the use of antibiotics to select transformed plant cells. The gene *uidA* was first used for *A. tumefaciens* mediated transformation of coconut embryogenic calli. However, endogenous GUS-like activity was found in calli not co-cultured with bacteria. Then essays for *Agrobacterium*-mediated transformation were developed using green and red fluorescent genes. Both genes are suitables as reporter genes for coconut transformation. In order to establish a protocol for coconut genetic transformation, an approach was used that combined biobalistics to generate micro-wounds in explants, vacuum infiltration and co-culture with *A. tumefaciens* (C58C1+ pER10W-35SRed containing the embryogenesis related gene *WUSCHEL*). Calli treated with the combined protocol showed red fluorescence with greater intensity and greater area than calli treated with either biobalistics or infiltration, followed by bacteria co-culture. PCR amplification of DNA extracts from transformed embryogenic callus produced a band with the expected size using *WUSCHEL* primers (862 bp). No band was obtained using the *Vir*E2 primers. This is the first report of transient genetic transformation of *C. nucifera* and it is the first step toward a protocol that will be useful for the study of the role of genes of interest and for practical applications, such as the improvement of coconut micropropagation via somatic embryogenesis (Andrade-Torres *et al.*, 2011).

7. Conclusions and perspectives

The majority of the mechanisms that regulate plant embryogenesis still remain to be clarified. In the higher plants, some genes and factors related to important mechanisms of embryogenesis are plant-specific. The availability of model systems of plant somatic embryogenesis has created effective tools for examining the details of plant embryogenesis. However, studies that used no model plants for somatic embryogenesis systems also revealed the molecular mechanisms in charge of controlling the expression of some genes during somatic embryogenesis, and with practical applications. So the molecular mechanisms of plant embryogenesis might be clarified by experiments using somatic and zygotic embryogenesis either from model or not model plants.

Numerous protocols on successful somatic embryogenesis induction and plant regeneration in different plant species, published last years, suggest that nowadays SE can be achieved for any plant provided that the appropriate explant and culture treatment are employed

(Gaj, 2004). A prerequisite for the successful establishment of a SE system is a proper choice of plant material -the explants being a source of competent cells, and, on the other hand, determination of physical and chemical factors which switch on their embryogenic pathway of development (Gaj, 2004).

The process of acquisition of embryogenic competence by somatic cells must involve reprogramming of gene expression patterns as well as changes in the morphology, physiology, and metabolism (Namasivayam, 2007). These alterations reflect dedifferentiation, activation of cell division and a change in cell fate.

Although few genes have been associated with embryogenesis induction, the search for genes involved in embryogenesis, such as SERK (Hecht *et al.*, 2001), LEC (Lotan *et al.*, 1998; Stone *et al.*, 2001), BABY BOOM (Boutilier *et al.*, 2002), WUSCHEL (Zuo *et al.*, 2002), and PICKLE (Ogas *et al.*, 1999), is a major field of research today (Quiroz-Figueroa *et al.*, 2006).

The characterization and functional analysis of protein markers for somatic embryogenesis offer the possibility of determining the embryogenic potential of plant cells in culture long before any morphological changes have taken place, and of gaining further information on the molecular basis of induction and differentiation of plant cells (Tchorbadjieva *et al.*, 2005).

The genetic transformation is certainly an important goal to facilitate genetic improvement against several diseases caused by phytopathogenic fungi, bacteria, and viruses, as well as for improvement against different pests (Ochoa-Alejo and Ramírez-Malagon, 2001). However, development of a reproducible tissue culture regeneration protocol is the first step in utilizing the power and potential of this new technology. The system established for *Capsicum chinense* is a promising alternative for cell or transformed plant regeneration through indirect somatic embryogenesis, and may contribute to genetic improvement of *C. chinense* Jacq. by incorporating reporter and interest genes (Solís-Ramos *et al.* 2009; Solís-Ramos *et al*, 2010a; Solís-Ramos *et al.*, 2010b).

The protocol for micropropagation of coconut from plumule explants based on embryogenic callus multiplication provides an option not available before for massive propagation of coconuts (Figure 5). However, although it allows the propagation of the progenie of known selected palms, it cannot be used for the cloning of palm individuals with known desirable agronomic traits. On the other hand, the recent developments to obtain embryogenic callus and somatic embryos from immature ovary and anther explants (Perera *et al.*, 2007; 2008; 2009), provide an opportunity to try to use these calli as a source of explants (the embryogenic structures) an integrate them into the callus multiplication scheme used with plumule explants. This has already been attempted in CICY using also floral tissue explants, but in this case rachillae slices from immature inflorescences (Oropeza and Chan, unpublished results). The callus obtained was tested for multiplication and although it responded poorly at the beginning though a series of multiplications the percentage of callus formation from embryogenic structure explants was above 40%. Therefore, although preliminary, this is a very promising result that shows that massive propagation from somatic tissue explants from adult plants is attainable in the near future. Finally we should continue with the studies to understand somatic embryogenesis in coconut. The study of genetic control is central for this purpose; therefore it is very important to learn more about the role of those genes that have been isolated and to extend the study to other genes and components of the genetic control of somatic embryogenesis. The study of these processes, will allow us not only to understand a phenomenon but it might open new avenues of opportunity for further improvement for a more efficient and better quality clonal propagation of coconuts.

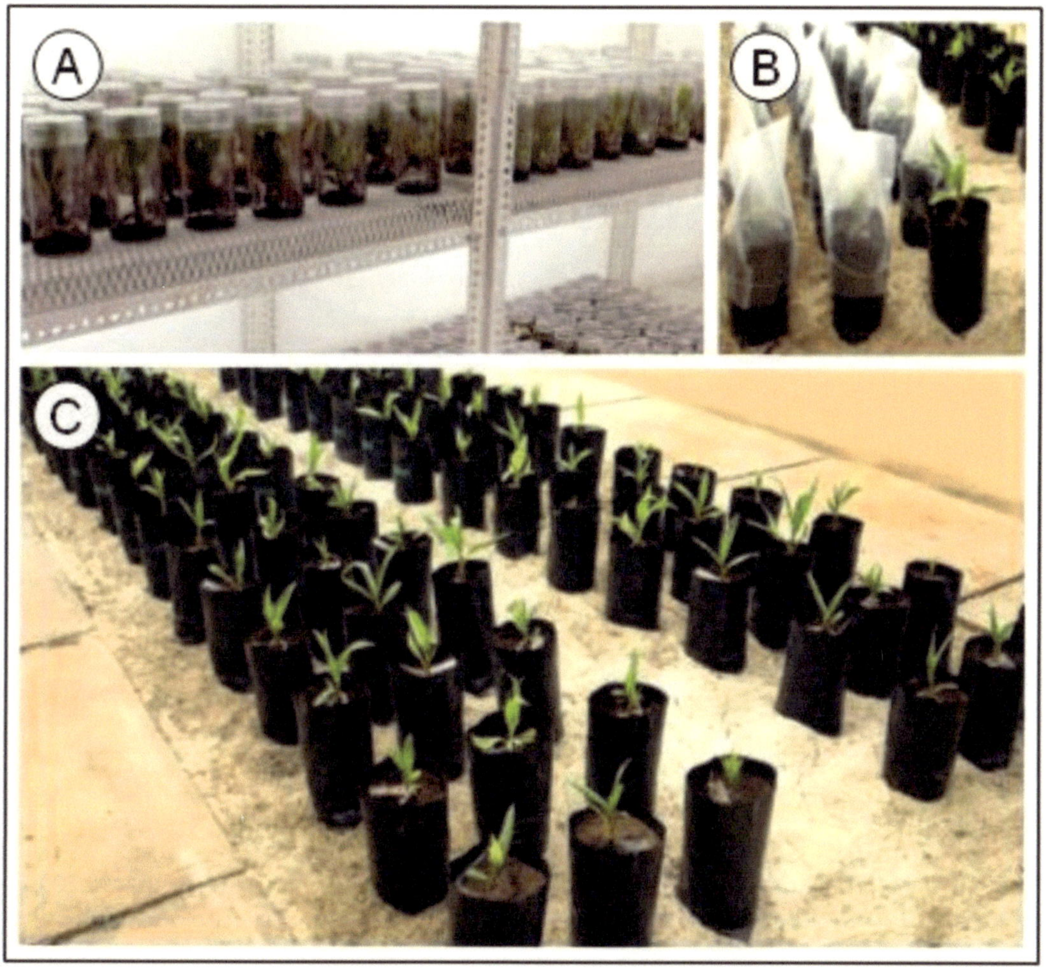

Fig. 5. Final stages of micropropagation process of coconut palm. (A) *In vitro* plantlets ready to be transferred to *ex-vitro* conditions. (B) Acclimatization of plantlets in greenhouse covered with transparent perforated bags and (C) plantlets ready to be transferred to field conditions.

8. Acknowledgments

Laura Solís-Ramos thanks the Ph.D. fellowship from Dirección de Intercambio Académico de la Secretaría de Relaciones Exteriores (SRE), Mexico (Academic Exchange Office of the Secretariat of Foreign Affairs, Mexico) and Centro de Investigación Científica de Yucatán

(CICY) for facilities and laboratory support. A. Andrade-Torres thanks to CONACYT for the Ph.D. scholarship (204774), and Universidad Veracruzana for the support through the Dirección General de Desarrollo Académico (DGDA) and PROMEP (UV-491). The authors would like to thank to V. Hocher and J-L. Verdeil IRD/CIRAD Montpellier, France respectively, where the isolation of *CnKNOX* was carried out. Partial funding of the research reported here was from CONACyT, México (Grant no. 43834-Z).

9. Abbreviations

SE: somatic embryogenesis

ZES: zygotic embryo segments.

MS: Murashige & Skoog medium (1962)

BAP, 6-benzylaminopurine

NAA: naphthaleneacetic acid

IAA: indoleacetic acid

ISE: indirect somatic embryogenesis

MS-3R: MS medium with BAP+IAA+NAA

DsRFP: Red fluorescent protein

GUS: β-glucuronidase (gene *uidA*)

pH: hydrogen potential

2, 4-D: 2, 4-dichlorophenoxyacetic acid

GA_3: gibberellic acid

10. References

[1] Andrade-Torres, A., C. Oropeza, L. Sáenz, T. González-Estrada, J. E. Ramírez-Benítez, K. Becerril, J. L. Chan, and L. C. Rodríguez-Zapata. 2011. Transient genetic transformation of embryogenic callus of *Cocos nucifera* L. Biologia. 66 (5):790-800.

[2] Ahloowalia BS. 1991. Somatic embryos in monocots. Their genesis and genetic stability. Rev. Cytol. Biol. Veget-Bot. 14: 223-235.

[3] Arroyo-Herrera A. Ku-González A. Canche-Moo R. Quiróz-Figueroa F.R. Loyola Vargas V. Rodríguez Zapata L.C. Burgeff D'Hondt C. Suárez-Solís V.M. & Castaño E. 2008. Expression of WUSCHEL in *Coffea canephora* causes ectopic morphogenesis and increases somatic embryogenesis. Plant Cell Tiss. Org. Cult. 94: 171-180.

[4] Azpeitia A, Chan J L, Sáenz L, Oropeza C. 2003. Effect of 22(S), 23(S)-homobrassinolide on somatic embryogenesis in plumule explants of *Cocos nucifera* (L.) Cultured *in vitro*. J of Hort Sci and Biotech. 78: 591-596.

[5] Baudino S, Hansen S, Brettschneider R, Hecht VRG, Dresselhaus T, Lorz H, Dumas C, Rogowsky PM. 2001. Molecular characterization of two novel maize LRR receptor-like kinases, which belong to the SERK gene family. Planta 213:1-10.
[6] Baurle, I. and Laux, T. 2005. Regulation of WUSCHEL transcription in the stem cell niche of the *Arabidopsis* shoot meristem. Plant Cell 17: 2271-2280.
[7] Belmonte MF, Tahir M, Schroeder D, Stasolla C. 2007. Overexpression of *HBK3*, a class I *KNOX* homeobox gene, improves the development of Norway spruce (*Picea abies*) somatic embryos. J Exp Bot 58: 2851-2861.
[8] Benson, E. 2000. Special Symposium: *In vitro* Plant recalcitrance do free radicals have a role in plant tissue culture recalcitrance. In vitro Cell. Dev. Biol.-Plant. 36: 163-170.
[9] Bhalla, P. L. and Singh, M. B. 2006. Molecular control of stem cell maintenance in shoot apical meristem. Plant Cell Rep. 25:249–256.
[10] Binzel ML, Sankhla N, Joshi S, Sankhla D. 1996. Induction of direct somatic embryogenesis and plant regeneration in pepper (*Capsicum annuum* L.). Plant Cell Reports 15: 536-540.
[11] Blake J and Hornung R. 1995. Somatic embryogenesis in coconut (*Cocos nucifera* L.) In: Jain S, Gupta P, Newton R (eds). Somatic Embryogenesis in Woody Plants, v. 2. Kluwer Academic Publishers Dordrecht pp 327-340.
[12] Boutilier, K.; Offringa, R.; Sharma, V. K.; Kieft, H.; Ouellet, T.; Zhang, L. M.; Hattori, J.; Liu, C. M.; van Lammeren, A. A. M.; Miki, B. L. A.; Custers, J. B. M.; Campagne, M. M. V. 2002. Ectopic expression of BABY BOOM triggers a conversion from vegetative to embryonic growth. Plant Cell 14:1737-1749.
[13] Buyukalaca S, Mavituna F. 1996. Somatic embryogenesis and plant regeneration of pepper in liquid media. Plant Cell, Tissue and Organ Culture 46: 227-235.
[14] Cai, W-Q, Fang, X., Shang, HS, Wang, X. and Mang, K.Q. 2003. Development of CMV- and TMV resistant transgenic chilli pepper: field performance and biosafety assessment. Molecular Breeding. Vol: 11. pp: 25-35.
[15] Cervera M. 2005. Histochemical and fluorometric assays for *uidA* (GUS) gene detection. Chapter 14. In: PEÑA, Leandro ed. Transgenic plants: Methods and protocols. Humana Press. 286: 203-213.
[16] Chan JL, Sáenz L, Talavera C, Hornung R, l Robert M, Oropeza C. 1998. Regeneration of coconut (*Cocos nucifera* L.) from plumule explants through somatic embryogenesis. Plant Cell Rep 17:515–521
[17] Chugh A. and P. Khurana. 2002. Gene expression during somatic embryogenesis - recent advances. Current Science. 83 (6): 715-730.
[18] Chung W, Pedersen H, Chin C-K. 1992. Enhanced somatic embryo production by conditioned media in cell suspension cultures of Daucus carota. Biotechnol Lett. 14: 837-840
[19] Dudits D, Gyugyey J, Bugre L, Bakó L. 1995. Molecular biology of somatic embryogenesis. In: Thorpe TA (ed) *In vitro* Embryogenesis in Plants. pp: 267-308. Kluwer Academic Publisher, Dordrecht.
[20] Eden-Green SJ. 1997. History and World distribution of lethal yellowing-like diseases of palms. In: Eden-Green SJ, Ofori F (eds). Proceeding of an International

Workshop on Lethal Yellowing Diseases of Coconut, Elmina, Ghana, November, 1995. Natural Resources Institute, Chatham, UK. pp 9-25.

[21] Fehér A, Pasternak TP, Dudits D. 2003. Review of Plant Biotechnology and Applied Genetics. Transition of somatic plant cells to an embryogenic state. Plant Cell, Tissue and Organ Culture 74: 201-228.

[22] Fehér A. 2005. Why Somatic Plant Cells Start to form Embryos? In. Mujib A., Samaj J. (eds). Plant Cell Monographs (2). Somatic Embryogenesis. Springer-Verlag Berlin Heidelberg. 85-101.

[23] Foale M. 2005. An introduction to the coconut palm. In: Batugal P, Ramanatha V, Rao GP, Oliver J (eds.). Coconut Genetic Resources. International Plant Genetic Resources Institute - Regional Office for Asia, the Pacific and Oceania (IPGRI-APO), Serdang, Selangor DE, Malaysia. pp 1-8.

[24] Francis D. and Sorrell D.A. 2001. The interference between the cell cycle and plant growth regulators: a mini review. Plant Growth Regul. 33: 1-12.

[25] Gaj MD. 2004. Factors influencing somatic embryogenesis induction and plant regeneration with particular reference to Arabidopsis thaliana (L.) Heynh. Plant Growth Regulation 43: 27-47.

[26] Hanold D and Randles JW. 1991. Detection of coconut cadang-cadang viroid-like sequences in oil and coconut palm and other monocotyledons in the south-west Pacific. Ann of Appl Biol 118: 139-151.

[27] Harini I, Sita L. 1993. Direct somatic embryogenesis and plant regeneration from inmature embryos of chilli (*Capsicum annuum* L.). Plant Science 89: 107-112.

[28] Harrison NA and Oropeza C. 2008. Phytoplasmas associated with coconut lethal yellowing. In: Harrison NA, Rao GP and Marcone C (eds). Characterization, Diagnosis and Management of Phytoplasmas. Studium Press LLC, Houston, USA pp: 219-248.

[29] Hecht V, Vielle-Calzada J-P, Hartog MV, Schmidt Ed DL, Boutilier K, Grossniklaus Ueli, de Vries SC. 2001. The *Arabidopsis* SOMATIC EMBRYOGENESIS RECEPTOR KINASE 1 Gene is expressed in developing ovules and embryos and embryo and enhances embryogenic competence in culture. Plant Physiol 127:803-816.

[30] Hecht V, Vielle-Calzada JP, Hartog MV, Schmidt DL, Boutilier K, Grossniklaus U, Vries SC. 2001. The *Arabidopsis* SOMATIC EMBRYOGENESIS RECEPTOR KINASE 1 Gene is expressed in developing ovules and embryos and enhances embryogenic competence in culture. Plant Physiology, november. 127: 803-816.

[31] Henry RJ. 1998. Molecular and biochemical characterization of somaclonal variation. In: Jain SM, Brar DS & Ahloowalia BS (eds) Somaclonal Variation and Induced Mutations in Crop Improvement (pp 485-499). Kluwer Academic Publishers, Dordrecht.

[32] Herrera-Estrella, L., Simpson, J., and Martínez-Trujillo, M. 2004. Transgenic Plants. An historical perspective. In: Peña, L. Transgenic Plants. Methods and Protocols. Humana Press. 286. Pp.: 3-31.

[33] Hu H, Xiong L, Yang Y. 2005. Rice SERK1 gene positively regulates somatic embryogenesis of cultured cell and host defense response against fungal infection. Planta 222:107–117.

[34] Jefferson R. 1987. Assaying chimeric genes in plants: the GUS gene fusion system. Plant Molecular Biology Reporter, December 5 (4): 387-405.
[35] Jiménez VM. 2005. Involvement of plant hormones and plant growth regulators on in vitro somatic embryogenesis. Plant Growth Regulation. 47:91–110.
[36] Khan H., Siddique I, Anis, M. 2006. Thidiazuron induced somatic embryogenesis and plant regeneration in *Capsicum annuum*. Brief communication. Biologia Plantarum, 50 (4): 789-792.
[37] Kintzios S., Drossopoulos J, Lymperopoulos CH. 2001. Effect of vitamins and inorganic micronutrients on callus growth and somatic embryogenesis from leaves of chilli pepper. Plant Cell, Tissue and Organ Culture, 67: 55-62.
[38] Lao DA. 2008. Coco-biodiesel more than a diesel replacement. Bioenergy Forum, Bangkok, April 2008.
[39] Lao DA. 2009. Coco-biodiesel in the Philippines. In: Coconut Philippines published by Asia Outsourcing
[40] Liu C, Xu Z, Chua Nh. 1993. Auxin Polar Transport is essential for the establishment of bilateral symmetry during early plant embryogenesis. The Plant Cell. 5: 621-630.
[41] López-Puc G, Canto-Flick A, Barredo-Pool F, Zapata-Castillo P, Peniche-Montalvo M, Barahona-Pérez F, Iglesias-Andreu, Santana-Buzzy N. 2006. Direct somatic embryogenesis: a highly efficient protocol for in vitro regeneration of habanero pepper (*Capscium chinense* Jacq.). HortScience 41(7):1645–1650.
[42] Lotan T, Ohto M, Yee MK, West MA, Lo R, Kwong RW, Yamagishi K, Fischer RL, Goldberg RB, Harada JJ. 1998. Arabidopsis LEAFY COTYLEDON 1 is sufficient to induce embryo development in vegetative tissue. Cell. 93: 1195-1205.
[43] Martin T, Wohner RV, Hummel S, Willmitzer L and Frommer WB.1991. The GUS reporter system as a tool o study plant gene expression. In: GALLAGER, S. ed. GUS protocols. Academic Press, Inc. California. pp. 23-43.
[44] Montero-Córtes M, Sáenz L, Córdova I, Quiroz A, Verdeil J-L, Oropeza C 2010. GA_3 stimulate the formation and germination of somatic embryos and the expression of a KNOTTED-like homeobox gene of *Cocos nucifera* (L.) Plant Cell Rep 29: 1049-1059
[45] Namasivayam P. 2007. Acquisition of embryogenic competence during somatic embryogenesis. Review paper. Plant Cell Tiss Organ Cult. 90: 1-8. DOI 10.1007/s11240-007-9249-9
[46] Nolan KE, Irwanto RR, Rose RJ. 2003. Auxin up-regulates MtSERK1 expression in both Medicago truncatula root-forming and embryogenic cultures. Plant Physiol 133:218–230.
[47] Ochoa-Alejo N and Ramírez-Malagon, R. 2001. In vitro chili pepper biotechnology. Invited review. In vitro Cell. Dev. Biol-Plant. 37: 701-729. DOI: 10.1079/IVP2001216.
[48] Ogas J, Kaufmann S, Henderson J, Somerville C. 1999. PICKLE is a CHD3 chromatin-remodeling factor that regulates the transition from embryogenic to vegetative development in *Arabidopsis*. Proc Natl Acad Sci USA. 96: 13839-13844.
[49] Oropeza C and Taylor HF. 1994. Uptake of 2,4-D in coconut (*Cocos nucifera* L.) explant. In: Lumsden PJ, Nicholas JR, Davies WJ (eds). Physiology, growth and development of plant in culture. Kluwer Academics Publishers, The Netherlands pp 284-288.

[50] Perera PIP, Hocher V, Verdeil JL, Doulbeau S, Yakandawala DMD, Weerakoon LK. 2007. Unfertilized ovary: a novel explant for coconut (*Cocos nucifera* L.) somatic embryogenesis. Plant Cell Rep 26: 21-28.

[51] Perera PIP, Perera L, Hocher V, Verdeil JL, Yakandawala DMD, Weerakoon LK. 2008. Use of SSR markers to determine the anther-derived homozygous lines in coconut. Plant Cell Rep 27: 1697-1703.

[52] Perera PIP, Yakandawala DMD, Hocher V, Verdeil J-L, Weerakoon LK. 2009. Effect of growth regulators on microspore embryogenesis in coconut anthers. Plant Cell Tiss Org Cult 96:171-180.

[53] Pérez-Nuñez MT, Chan JL, Sáenz L, González T, Verdeil JL, Oropeza C. 2006. Improved somatic embryogenesis from *Cocos nucifera* (L.) plumule explants. *In Vitro* Cell Dev Biol Plant 42:37-43.

[54] Pérez-Núñez MT. Souza R. Sáenz L. Chan J.L. González T. Zúñiga J.J. & Oropeza C. 2009. Detection of a *SERK*-like gene in coconut in vitro cultures and analysis of its expression during the formation of embryogenic callus and somatic embryos. Plant Cell Rep. 28: 11–19.

[55] Quiroz-Figueroa F., Rojas-Herrera R, Galaz-Avalos RM, Loyola-Vargas VM. 2006. Embryo production through somatic embryogenesis can be used to study cell differentiation in plants. Review paper. Plant Cell Tiss Organ Cult. 86: 285-301. DOI 10.1007/s11240-006-9139-6

[56] Reddy, G. V. and Meyerowitz, E. M. 2005. Stem-cell homeostasis and growth dynamics can be uncoupled in the *Arabidopsis* shoot apex. Science 310:663–667.

[57] Reinert J. 1958. Untersuchungen über die Morphogenese an Gewebekulturen. Ber Dtsch Bot Ges 71: 15.

[58] Santana-Buzzy N, Canto-Flick A, Barahona-Pérez F, Montalvo-Peniche MC, Zapata-Castillo P, Solís-Ruíz A, Zaldívar-Collí A, Gutiérrez-Alonso O, Miranda-Ham L. 2005. Regeneration of habanero pepper (*Capsicum chinense* Jacq) via organogenesis. HortScience 40(6): 1829–1831.

[59] Santos MD, Romano E, Yotoko KSC, Tinoco MLP, Dias BBA, Aragao FJL. 2005. Characterization of the cacao somatic embryogenesis receptor-like kinase (SERK) gene expressed during somatic embryogenesis. Plant Sci 168:723–729.

[60] Schmidt EDL, Guzzo F, Toonen MAJ, de Vries SC. 1997. A leucine rich repeat containing receptor-like kinase marks somatic plant cells competent to form embryos. Development 124:2049–2062.

[61] Schmidt EDL, Guzzo F, Toonen MAJ, de Vries SC. 1997. A leucine-rich repeat containing receptor-like kinase marks somatic plant cell competent to form embryos. Development 124:2049-2062.

[62] Shah, K.; Russinova, E.; Gadella, T. W. J.; Willemse, J.; de Vries, S. C. 2002. The Arabidopsis kinase-associated protein phosphatase controls internalization of the somatic embryogenesis receptor kinase 1. Genes Dev. 16:1707–1720.

[63] Sharma, S.K., S. Millam, I. Hein and G.J. Bryan. 2008. Cloning and molecular characterization of a potato SERK gene transcriptionally induced during initiation of somatic embryogenesis. Planta. 228: 319-330.

[64] Shimada T, Hirabayashi T, Endo T, Fujii H, Kita M, Omura M. 2005. Isolation and characterization of the somatic embryogenesis receptor-like kinase gene homologue (CitSERK1) from *Citrus unshui* Marc. Sci Hortic 103: 233-238.
[65] Shin R., Han J-H., Lee G.J., and Peak, K.H. 2002. The potencial use of viral coat protein genes as transgene screening marker and multiple virus resistance of pepper plants coexpressing coat proteins of cucumber mosaic virus and tomato mosaic virus. Transgenic Reseach. 11: 215-219.
[66] Solís-Ramos L.Y., González-Estrada T., Nahuath-Dzib S., Rodríguez-Zapata, L., Castaño E. 2009. Overexpression of WUSCHEL in *C. chinense* causes ectopic morphogenesis. Plant Cell, Tissue and Organ Culture. DOI: 10.1007/s11240-008-9485-7. 96:279-287.
[67] Solís-Ramos LY, González-Estrada T, Andrade-Torres A, Godoy-Hernández G, Castaño de la Serna E. 2010a. Endogenous GUS-like activity in *Capsicum chinense* Jacq. Electronic Journal of Biotechnology. July 15, 13 (4). DOI: 10.2225/vol13-issue4-fulltext-3.
[68] Solís-Ramos LY, Nahuath-Dzib S, Andrade-Torres A, Barredo-Pool F, González-Estrada T, Castaño de la Serna E. 2010b. Indirect somatic embryogenesis and morphohistological analysis in *Capsicum chinense*. Section Cellular and Molecular Biology. Biologia. 65(3): 504-511. DOI: 10.2478/s11756-010-0049-z.
[69] Somleva MN, Schmidt EDL, de Vries SC. 2000. Embryogenic cells in *Dactylis glomerata* L. (Poaceae) explants by cell tracking and by SERK expression. Plant Cell Rep 19:718–726.
[70] Steinitz B., Kusek M., Tabib Y., Paran I. & Zelcer A. 2003 Pepper (*Capsicum annuum* L.) regenerates obtained by direct somatic embryogenesis fail to develop a shoot. In vitro Cell. Dev. Biol. Plant 39: 296-303.
[71] Steward FC, Mapes MO, Mears K .1958. Growth and organized development of cultured cells. II. Organization in cultures grown from freely suspended cells. Am J Bot 45: 705–708
[72] Stone SL, Kwong LW, Yee KM, Pelletier J, Lepiniec L, Fischer RL, Goldberg RB, Harada JJ (2001) LEAFY COTYLEDON2 encodes a B3 domain transcription factor that induces embryo development. Proc Natl Acad Sci USA 98: 11806-11811.
[73] Suda Ch, Prakash S, Bhomkar P, Jain S and Bhalla-Sarin, N. 2006. Ubiquitous presence of β-glucuronidase (GUS) in plants and its regulation in some model plants. Planta, September 224 (4): 853-864.
[74] Tchorbadjieva M, Kalmukova R, Pantchev I, Kyurkchiev S. 2005. Monoclonal antibody against a cell wall marker protein for embryogenic potential of *Dactylis glomerata* L. suspension cultures. Planta 222:811–819.
[75] Thomas C, Meyer D, Himber C, Steinmetz A. 2004. Spatial expression of a sunXower SERK gene during induction of somatic embryogenesis and shoot organogenesis. Plant Physiol Biochem 42:35–42.
[76] Tucker, M. R.; Araujo, A. -C. G.; Paech, N. A.; Hecht, V.; Schmidt, E. D. L.; Rossell, J. -B.; de Vries, S. C.; Koltunow, A. M. G. 2003. Sexual and apomictic reproduction in *Hieracium subgenus* Pilosella are closely interrelated developmental pathways. Plant Cell 15:1524–1537.
[77] Weigel, D. and Jurgens, G. 2002. Stem cells that make stems. Nature 415: 751–754.

[78] Zapata-Castillo P, Canto-Flick A, López-Puc G, Solís-Ruíz A, Pérez-Barahona F, Iglesias-Andreu L, Santana-Buzzy N. 2007. Somatic embryogenesis in Habanero pepper (*C. chinense* Jacq.) from cell suspensions. Hort Science.

[79] Zuo J, Niu QW, Frugis G, Chua N.H. 2002. The WUSCHEL gene promotes vegetative-to-embryonic transition in *Arabidopsis*. The plant Journal 30(3): 349-359. doi: 10.1046/j.1365-313X.2002.01289.x.

26

Presumed Paternal Genome Loss During Embryogenesis of Predatory Phytoseiid Mites

Shingo Toyoshima[1] and Hiroshi Amano[2]
[1]*NARO Institute of Vegetable and Tea Science,*
[2]*Graduate School of Agriculture, Kyoto University,*
Japan

1. Introduction

Predatory phytoseiid mites are classified into the family Phytoseiidae (Acari: Mesostigmata), the most diverse group of mesostigmatic mites (Kranz & Walter, 2009). More than 2000 species of phytoseiid mites have been described (Chant & McMurtry, 2007), almost all of which are small (0.3 mm–0.4 mm; Fig. 1a) and eat other mites, insects, pollen, and fungi. Since they also prey upon pest insects and mites in agricultural fields, they are considered to be a key agent in an integrated pest management system (Gerson et al., 2003). To understand their role in agriculture, their morphology (external and internal), life history characteristics, and behavioral traits have been studied for more than 50 years (e.g., Helle & Sabelis, 1985). Several species of phytoseiid mites, mentioned below, are useful agents and are the most studied species (the recent name is given in parentheses). Because of their small size, they are not considered as an experimental animal in anatomical analyses examining their life cycle characteristics.

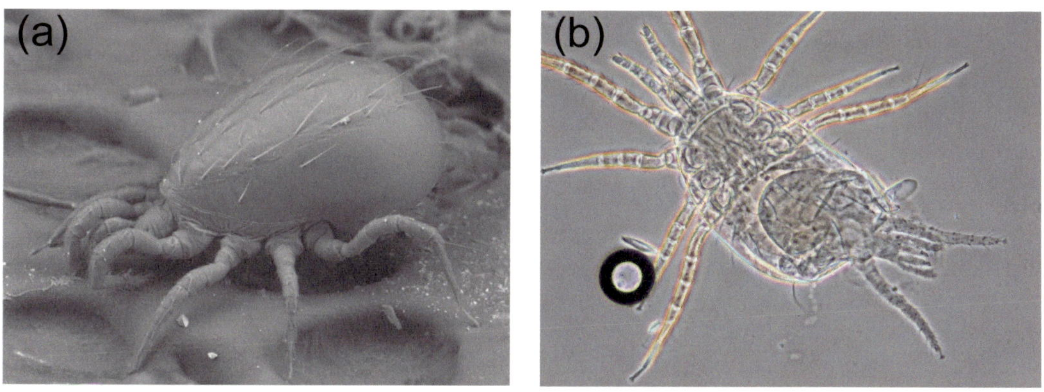

Fig. 1. External and internal appearance of phytoseiid mites. (a) *Neoseiulus womersleyi*. Body length is ca. 400 µm (scanning electron microscope image). (b) An example of delayed oviposition in *N. womersleyi*. Embryonic development proceeds regardless of the nutritional condition of the mother, and the larvae hatch in the mother's body (phase contrast microscope image).

The reproductive system of predatory phytoseiid mites has interested scientists for many years. While adult females start oviposition only after copulation, males and females were found to be haploids and diploids, respectively, by the karyotyping of eggs (Wysoki, 1985). Heterochromatinization in the part of the chromosomes was observed in eggs just after deposition (Nelson-Rees et al., 1980). Although cytological evidence is insufficient, this has been presented as pseudo-arrhenotoky: male-destined oocytes need to be fertilized to begin embryogenesis, and the heterochromatinization of the paternal genomes occurs in male-destined eggs, inducing the elimination of paternal genomes during embryogenesis, resulting in functionally haploid males (Schulten, 1985). This system was also described as "parahaploidy" in previous studies (e.g., Hoy, 1979) and was recently investigated as a form of "paternal genome loss" presented in several insects (Burt & Trivers, 2006). An explanation of several terms in relation to the reproductive system of phytoseiid mites is presented below.

"Pseudo-arrhenotoky" is described as a mode of reproduction, differing from true "arrhenotoky" in which haploid males in the arrhenotokous insects and mites are emerged parthenogenetically from unfertilized eggs. "Deuterotoky" and "thelytoky" are also known as parthenogenetic reproductive modes whereby mothers produce offspring of both sexes from unfertilized eggs (deuterotoky) and only female offspring from unfertilized eggs (thelytoky) (Bell, 1982; Norton et al., 1993). "Thelytoky" is also known in a few species of phytoseiid mites. "Parahaploidy" is described as a ploidy of the chromosomes, differing from true "haploidy" in males, which the haploid males are derived from haploid eggs (Hartl & Brown, 1970). "Paternal genome loss (PGL)" is a phenomenon of chromosome behavior and is divided into two classes, embryonic PGL and germ-line PGL (Ross et al., 2010b). In embryonic PGL, the paternal genome is eliminated during early embryonic development of males and is found in some armored scale insects. In germ-line PGL, the paternal genome is deactivated during male embryogenesis and is eliminated from the germline during or just before spermatogenesis. Germ-line PGL is found in most scale insects, sciarid flies, and in the coffee borer beetle. Since the prefixes "pseudo-" and "para-" are ambiguous, one may better describe the reproductive system of phytoseiid mites in terms of "PGL in diploid arrhenotoky," as in the case of scale insects (Ross et al., 2000a). Although "paternal genome elimination (PGE)" is a more accurate description of the same phenomenon (Herrick & Seger, 1999; Ross et al., 2010a, b), PGL is used in this article. Other terms should be referred to Bell (1982).

PGL in mites is known in three families: Anoetidae (phoretic with insects), Dermanyssidae (blood-feeding ectoparasites), and Phytoseiidae (Oliver, 1983). PGL in Anoetidae and Dermanyssidae has not been well studied and additional information is not available. In phytoseiid mites, although cytological evidence for PGL is insufficient to understand it thoroughly, elaborate hypotheses were developed to investigate their evolutionary significance (e.g., Nagerkerke & Sabelis, 1998). PGL in mites is believed to be an intermediate step from diplodiploid bisexual reproduction to haplodiploid arrhenotoky (Bull, 1983), as noted previously for PGL in scale insects (Schrader & Hugher-Schrader, 1931). Also, the evolutionary constraint of PGL in phytoseiid mites was examined from the viewpoint of sex ratio control (Sabelis et al., 2002). In recent studies, the evolution of PGL in scale insects was considered a consequence of genetic conflict between males and females, as well as between parents and offspring (Ross, 2010a). More genetic and cytological evidence of PGL in mites is needed to incorporate it into the general framework of genetic conflict in scale insects to better understand the mechanisms of sex determination and evolutionary significance of PGL in mites.

In this article, previous researches and additional evidence in relation to PGL in phytoseiid mites are briefly reviewed with a plenty of literatures, in order to interest scientists working on the different research fields. Authors hope that these scientists will contribute new ideas toward the completion of the reproductive biology of phytoseiid mites. Further understanding of the PGL in phytoseiid mites will make a contribution, hopefully, to the comprehensive researches on the reproductive biology and embryogenesis of various creatures.

2. Experimental evidence for the notion, pseudo-arrhenotoky

Recent knowledge of PGL in phytoseiid mites, referred to by many scientists working on reproductive biology, is based upon experimental evidence published in the 1970s and reviewed in the 1980s. Almost all data are well documented and reliable. For instance, behavioral observation established some basic information as follows: (1) Phytoseiid females need to copulate with males to produce female and male offspring. (2) After copulation, they drastically change their prey-search activity and prey consumption. (3) Around 24–36 h after copulation, they start oviposition when fed abundant prey under comfortable conditions (Fig. 2). Karyotyping revealed that males are haploid and females are diploid. However, these data and experimental evidence are insufficient to support the mechanism of pseudo-arrhenotoky. In this section, the experimental evidence to support pseudo-arrhenotoky is summarized, and problems are pointed out.

2.1 Indirect evidence for insemination in male eggs

Based upon the idea that sperm only serve to activate the ovary to start egg production, a belief was held that all eggs are deposited with a male-biased sex ratio even when a few sperms are accepted by females during copulation. However, Amano and Chant (1978) and Schulten et al. (1978) showed that the amount of egg production is correlated with the amount of sperm accepted by females during copulation in *Phytoseiulus persimilis*, *Amblyseius andersoni*, and *Amblyseius* (= *Neoseiulus*) *bibens*. For instance, in a study of *P. persimilis*, in which copulation was artificially interrupted (Amano & Chant, 1978), the average number of eggs deposited gradually increased from 2.7 to 66.3 when the duration of copulation increased from 30 min to 130 min. It was experimentally confirmed in advance that the duration of copulation was nearly correlated with the amount of sperms accepted by females.

These experimental results suggest not only that insemination activates the ovary for egg production, but also that each egg requires fertilization for its embryonic development. However, the presumption is made that the role of sperm is similar to what is known as "pseudogamy" or "gynogenesis." In pseudogamy or gynogenesis, eggs only develop after penetration by sperm, but the sperm nucleus degenerates without fusing with the egg nucleus so that it makes no genetic contribution to the developing embryo (White, 1973). It may be partially true that such "borrowed sperms" help to produce male offspring in phytoseiid mites, because male offspring were produced by crossbreeding between closely related species, and these individuals (sons) had only maternal characters (Congdon & McMurtry, 1988; Ho et al., 1995).

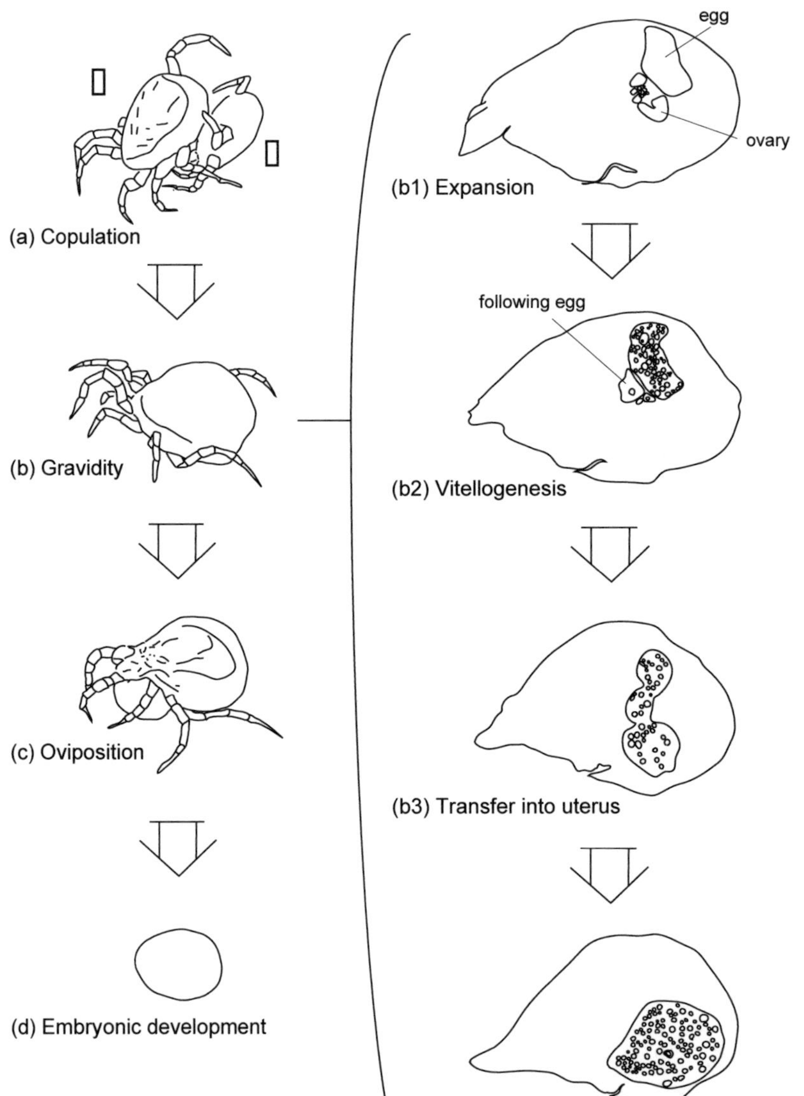

Fig. 2. Schematic illustration of reproductive events and the egg forming process during the gravid period. **Schematic flow on the left (a–d)**: A virgin female copulates for 2–3 h with a male. Mated females consume more prey than virgin females and become fat with a roundish body. Gravid females lay an egg 24–36 h after copulation and continue deposition of eggs, one by one, at intervals of ca. 8 h during which they consume large amounts of prey under ideal conditions. The egg is laid in the middle of embryogenesis. **Schematic flow on the right (b1–b4)**: After copulation, an oocyte expands toward the dorsal region from an ovary located in the center of the body; it is fertilized there and begins vitellogenesis. After expansion of other eggs, the first egg moves into the uterus in the ventral region and forms an eggshell there.

It was also shown at the almost same time that X-ray irradiation on adult males (fathers) induced sterility in male offspring (sons) in *P. persimilis*, *A. bibens* (Helle et al., 1978), and *Metaseiulus* (= *Galendromus*) *occidentalis* (Hoy, 1979). No daughters emerged, and total developing offspring was low in these experiments. A significant reduction in the expected number of sons was also seen. Many died in the early embryonic stages, while the survivors were sterile, even though mortality is not expected in the case of arrhenotoky. Thus, the irradiated paternal genomes are presumed to affect insemination and/or embryogenesis of daughters and sons, also suggesting that male offspring (sons) possess paternal genomes in their germ plasma, since the effect of radiation on the paternal genomes was seen in the male offspring as sterility.

2.2 Chromosome observations

According to studies on the karyotyping of many phytoseiid species (Hansell et al., 1964; Wysoki & Swirski, 1968; Wysoki, 1973; Blommers-Schlosser & Blommers, 1975; Wysoki & McMurtry, 1977; Wysoki & Bolland, 1983), most have a haploid number of 4 and a diploid number of 8 chromosomes, and 3 thelytokous species have 8 chromosomes, except for 3 (haploid) and 6 (diploid) chromosomes in 5 species (Wysoki, 1985). The chromosomes are generally acrocentric except for some metacentric one in a few species, and differ from each other only in size (1–4 μm). Since the ratio of haploid to diploid eggs was equal to that of males to females (Hansell et al., 1964), a haplodiploid genetic system was presumed in phytoseiid mites except for the thelytokous species. Although male diploidy was not confirmed in the karyotype investigations, heterochromatinized (heteropicnotic) chromosomes were observed in eggs immediately after deposition in *M. occidentalis* (Nelson-Rees et al., 1980).

Based on chromosome observation, pseudo-arrhenotoky was proposed (Schulten, 1985). According to this proposal, all eggs start their development from syngamy (2n = 6). The process of heterochromatinization starts within 24 h after egg deposition by arrangement of the 6 chromosomes into 2 groups: 3 heterochromatic chromosomes and 3 euchromatic chromosomes. The following stage strongly resembles the formation of bivalents, which is normally found at the diplotene stage in meiotic division. The heterochromatic chromosomes (n = 3) are eliminated from some or all cells, but almost certainly from the germ line. Thereafter, the male germ line and most somatic cells are haploid. Spermatogenesis in deutonymphs (immature stage) starts with a single equatorial mitotic division, and 2 sperm are produced.

Unfortunately, several events in the proposal have not been elucidated cytologically. In addition, the observation of heterochromatic chromosomes was not conducted in male eggs (the sexes of eggs were not specified), and the number of eggs observed was not sufficient to confirm diploidy in the early embryonic stages of deposited eggs. Furthermore, *M. occidentalis* is not a common species with regard to its chromosome number. Wysoki (1985) reported that 47 of 55 species examined have a basic number of n = 4 and that *M. occidentalis* has n = 3, which is exceptional and known in only 5 species. Therefore, further cytological evidence in a species with the common number of chromosomes (n = 4) is required to confirm the existence of pseudo-arrhenotoky or PGL in phytoseiid mites. In addition, no observations were made of the internal process of egg formation (Fig. 2b1–4) and embryogenesis in the proposal.

3. Presumed Paternal Genome Loss (PGL) in phytoseiid mites

In this section, the unrecognized and unpublished evidence for PGL in phytoseiid mites is briefly reviewed. The fusion of pronuclei and the elimination of the paternal genome during the early stages of embryogenesis in eggs destined to be male are shown as histological evidence for PGL. Inheritance of genetic markers from father to son is also explained as evidence for PGL. To clarify the evidence, the internal morphology, process of egg formation, and embryogenesis in phytoseiid mites are summarized. Hereafter, the eggs destined to be males and females are referred to as "male eggs" and "female eggs," respectively.

3.1 Internal morphology, process of egg formation and embryogenesis

The female genital system consists of a pair of spermathecae, a lyrate organ, an ovary, an oviduct, a uterus, a vagina, and a genital opening (see details in Di Palma & Alberti, 2001), which was determined by morphological comparisons between female and male specimens, as well as previous findings (Michael, 1892; Alberti & Hänel, 1986; Alberti, 1988). The spermathecae are a temporal storage of sperms just after copulation. The transfer of sperm from spermathecae into the ovary and the shape of sperm in the ovary have not yet been clearly elucidated (Di Palma & Alberti, 2001). It is hard to believe that the spermatozoa can find their opening and pass through the duct, since a lumen is hard to detect (G. Alberti, personal communication).

The morphology of the large lyrate organ consists of paired, distinct flattened arms separated indistinctly into several segments. The function of the lyrate organ is as a trophic (nutrimentary) tissue to support the rapid growth of oocytes and vitellogenesis. A nucleus and many mitochondria are distinguished in each segment. The lyrate organ is distinct in dermanyssid mites (Alberti & Hänel, 1986) and also in *P. persimilis* (Alberti, 1988). The ovary is located at the center of the two arms of the lyrate organ. The oocytes in the ovary are connected via nutritive cords (fusomes) to the nutritive tissue of the lyrate organ (Alberti & Hänel, 1986), although such connections are difficult to detect.

One of among several oocytes in the ovary expands toward the dorsal region of the body just after copulation (Fig. 2b) and starts vitellogenesis in the dorsal region (also see details in Toyoshima et al., 2000). Although the exact timing has not been confirmed, the penetration of sperm into the oocyte seems to occur when the oocyte occupies the dorsal region (Toyoshima et al., 2009). Following the completion of vitellogenesis (Fig. 2b2), the egg (an inseminated oocyte) passes via the short oviduct into the uterus (Fig. 2b3) and remains there, forming an eggshell and starting embryonic development (Fig. 2b4). Subsequently, the next oocyte expands and enters vitellogenesis in the dorsal region.

Superficial cleavage occurs in the centrolecithal egg cell in the early stages of ontogenesis. However, 2-, 4-, 8-, 16-, 32-cell stages are not well discriminated in the following steps because the egg in the uterus forms chorion of poor permeability, preventing the penetration of fixative solution for histological observation. After several nuclear divisions, spindle-shaped blastodermal cells are spherically distributed to form a continuous layer. The process of germinal band formation begins on the ventral surface of the periblastula. Entodermal cells have a rather loose distribution. Details of subsequent stages of embryogenesis are given in Yastrebtsov (1992).

The eggs, in the blastula stage, are deposited one by one (Fig. 3). Young females deposit an average of one to five eggs daily at 25°C (Sabelis, 1985a). The degree of embryonic development in deposited eggs depends upon internal and external factors (Sanderson & McMurtry, 1984). As an extreme case, a hatched larva was seen in a female body (Fig. 1b).

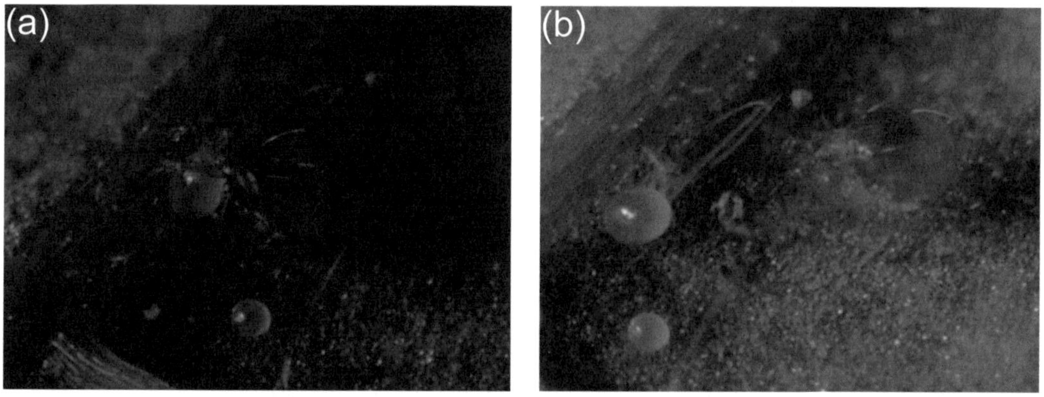

Fig. 3. Ovipositional behavior of *Phytoseiulus persimilis*. The first (a) and the second (b) eggs are laid, one by one, at 6-h intervals. As with all small phytoseiid mites, the egg is huge relative to the size of the gravid female. The rapid growth of large eggs may be supported by the lyrate organ, which is also large relative to the body.

3.2 Fusion of two pronuclei

As a first step in observing the insemination of male eggs, male eggs should be selected from the continuum of egg production during rearing experiments. The first egg should be the focus as a male egg candidate because over 90% of the first eggs develop into males (Toyoshima & Amano, 1998). According to the process of egg formation described above, the first egg in females just after copulation is determined easily and precisely by internal observation of the female. In contrast, unambiguously discriminating sperm in the ovary and recognizing their penetration into the oocyte (the first egg) are difficult (Di Palma & Alberti, 2001), because the sperms in the ovary have not yet been detected with full evidence.

Therefore, eggs with two pronuclei were sought thoroughly (Toyoshima et al., 2000). Then, two pronuclei were detected in the first egg before it had completed its expansion (at ca. 8 h after the end of copulatory behavior). The pronuclei were different in size, which was confirmed in a series of sliced specimens, and joined at the center of the egg. While yolk granules were developing and accumulating gradually around the joining pronuclei, the pronuclei were discriminated precisely by the double-membrane structure. When yolk granules filled the egg (at ca. 10.7 h after the end of copulatory behavior), the joining pronuclei began to change shape and finally fused. This observation was indirect evidence for insemination of male eggs, but histologically elucidated that the paternal genome fuses with the maternal genome in male eggs before embryogenesis.

After a period of time, the first egg moves into the uterus in the ventral region of the body (Fig. 2). A nucleus appears at the center of the egg and it later divides at the same position. The process of nuclear division following embryogenesis was not observed histologically because the eggshell prevented the fixation of the interior of the egg. Therefore, eggs were extracted from the female body for observation of chromosomal behavior, as described below.

3.3 Elimination of paternal genome during early embryogenesis

While male diploidy was confirmed in the first egg during vitellogenesis in *P. persimilis*, male diploidy has not been detected in eggs after deposition. By karyotyping just deposited eggs, the first and the following (presumed) male eggs were haploid in *P. persimilis* and in *Amblyseius* (=*Neoseiulus*) *womersleyi* determined from a previous study (Toyoshima & Amano, 1999). The time needed for the elimination of chromosomes differed from that of *M. occidentalis*, as reported by Nelson-Rees et al. (1980). Therefore, male diploidy in the early embryonic stages must be confirmed by extracting the first egg (male egg) from the female body cavity. In the first egg extracted from females of *P. persimilis*, diploid cells were observed in an early stage of embryogenesis (the exact stage was not confirmed), and the coexistence of haploid and diploid cells in the same egg was also seen at a later stage of embryogenesis (Toyoshima & Amano, 1999). Finally, only haploid cells were observed in eggs just before deposition. Although heterochromatinized chromosomes were not identified in this experiment, paternal genomes in male eggs were confirmed to be eliminated during the early stages of embryogenesis just before deposition. The stage of embryogenesis was not determined for the extracted eggs.

The difference in timing for chromosome elimination between *M. occidentalis* and *P. persimilis* seems to be due to the difference in the number of chromosomes: *M. occidentalis* has three whereas *P. persimilis* has four. In other words, one *speculates* that one of the three chromosomes in *M. occidentalis* is a result of the combination of two of the four chromosomes. If the total DNA content in the haploid genome appears to be equal among all species, one of the three chromosomes in *M. occidentalis* must be larger than those in other species with the basic number. Since the DNA C-value affects cell cycles (Cavalier-Smith, 1978), the size of chromosomes may also affect cell cycles. As a result, the chromosome elimination in male eggs of *M. occidentalis* seems to occur at a later stage of embryogenesis, which is observed at the time the egg is deposited. This speculation should be confirmed experimentally in the future.

3.4 Inheritance of genetic markers from father to sons

Inheritance of paternal genetic elements from father to son was partially elucidated in *Typhlodromus pyri* by the random amplified polymorphic DNA (RAPD) markers (Perrot-Minnot & Navajas, 1995) and in *Neoseiulus californicus* by the direct amplification of length polymorphism (DALP) markers (Perrot-Minnot et al., 2000). Of two RAPD markers, one marker (330 base pairs: bp) was paternally transmitted to male and female offspring, and the other (990 bp) was paternally transmitted to all females and to some male offspring. Although RAPD markers sometimes showed ambiguous inheritance, the conclusion was made that obligate fertilization could account for the inheritance of nuclear genetic material from father to son, and the *speculation* was made that the paternal genomes were partially retained in some tissues. On the other hand, the inheritance of codominant genetic markers, which is detected by DALP, provided evidence for selective elimination of the paternal genome among male tissues (Perrot-Minnot et al., 2000), also suggesting that sperm contained exclusively maternal genes whereas some male somatic tissues retained most paternal chromosomes.

The inheritance of a genetic marker from father to son was also confirmed in *N. womersleyi* (Toyoshima & Hinomoto, unpublished data). The sequence characterized amplified region (SCAR)-PCR marker was designed from a fragment amplified by using arbitrary primers (ca. 20 bases long) and used to confirm the inheritance of this marker. When a genetic marker was amplified from the extracted DNA of two populations of *N. womersleyi* with a primer set (Awa18A1&Awa18B3) by PCR and was digested by a restriction enzyme (*EcoR*I), the inheritance of paternal genetic material by sons was confirmed (Fig. 4). Since the paternal band was relatively weak in sons, only a small amount of template DNA was available for the primers in the extracted DNA solution. Whether the paternal genetic material is retained in a specific tissue or if the heterochromatinized fragments of paternal genomes are randomly dispersed in the entire body has not yet been clarified. According to the X-ray experiments mentioned above, as well as the weak presence of genetic markers, entire paternal genomes are probably retained only in the germ plasma of male offspring. Further investigation is necessary to confirm the maintenance of the effective paternal genomes in spermatocytes of male offspring.

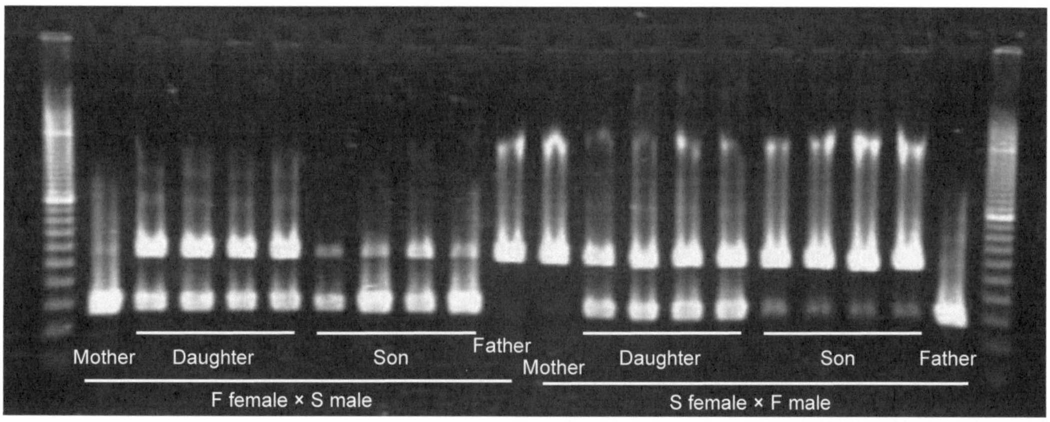

Fig. 4. An electropherogram of a SCAR-PCR marker in an agarose gel (Toyoshima & Hinomoto, unpublished data). A female of a strain of *Neoseiulus womersleyi* with a marker that ran fast on the gel (F) was crossed with a male with a slow marker (S), and vice versa. Daughters and sons have markers from both parents, but the paternal marker in the sons of both crosses is thin.

4. Presumed mechanisms of sex determination in phytoseiid mites

The sex of an individual is *determined* by an initial set of factors (genotypic or environmental). Then, sex *develops* (or *differentiates*) during an integrated series of genetic and physiological steps (Bull, 1983). The sex becomes *fixed* at a certain step during development. The initial set of factors (or "primary sex-determining signal") should be the focus in understanding the relationship between sex determination and PGL in phytoseiid mites.

The sex determination of phytoseiid mites was initially investigated by inbreeding experiments. While Poe and Enns (1970) indicated strong depression by inbreeding in two phytoseiid species, Hoy (1977) indicated weak or scant depression in *M. occidentalis*, and suggested that sex determination in *M. occidentalis* was not based on the multiple allele mechanism (complementary sex determination: CSD) that has been demonstrated for parasitoid wasps and the sawfly (e.g., Cook & Crozier, 1995). Although the sex of an individual is determined and fixed at fertilization in hymenopteran insects, sex may not be determined at fertilization in phytoseiid mites. Therefore, the elimination of the paternal genome in male eggs is not caused by the combination of alleles from the parents. Sex may be controlled by the mother and determined by the accumulation of certain substances in male eggs. In this section, a resultant phenomenon of maternal control is shown with a presumed mechanism of sex control.

4.1 Maternal control of offspring sex

Maternal control of offspring sex was demonstrated by sex ratio control under certain conditions. While the mother deposits eggs with female-biased sex ratios when prey is abundant, she deposits eggs with an even sex ratio (♀:♂=1:1) when prey abundance is insufficient (Friese & Gilstrap, 1982; Momen, 1996). Even in a prey patch with abundant prey, mothers also adjust the sex ratio of offspring in a manner that fits the sex ratio to the prediction of sex allocation theories (Hamilton, 1967). While the mother deposits eggs with a female-biased sex ratio when in isolation in a prey patch, she deposits eggs with an even sex ratio when in a crowd with abundant prey (Dinh et al., 1988; Nagerkerke & Sabelis, 1991). To estimate the mechanism to control the sex of the offspring by mothers, the nutritional condition of mothers should be considered as a proximate mechanism rather than the mating structure as a relatively ultimate (evolutionary) mechanism.

Female and male eggs deposited by gravid females of phytoseiid mites can be lined up in a sequence because the females deposit eggs one by one (Fig. 5). Several female eggs were shown to exist between male eggs in a sequence when gravid females deposit eggs with a female-biased sex ratio under abundant prey conditions. The number of female eggs between male eggs in a sequence decreased when gravid females adjusted the sex ratio of offspring in relation to the number of prey items available. Finally, only one female egg was present between male eggs in a sequence when gravid females deposited eggs with an even sex ratio under insufficient prey conditions (Toyoshima & Amano, 1998). It should now be presumed how to determine the sex of eggs.

The female eggs produced under abundant prey conditions may be changed into phenotypic males in response to the nutritional condition when produced. Paternal genomes would remain in the phenotypic males if PGL were genetically controlled but flexible. However, phenotypic sex is consistent with genetic sex (karyotype) in eggs produced with an even sex ratio under minimal prey conditions (Fig. 5; see also Toyoshima & Amano, 1999). Actually, the number of male eggs is similar among different prey conditions, although the total number of eggs decreased gradually in relation to the number of prey items available to gravid females (Toyoshima & Amano, 1998). The number of female eggs may have decreased rather than having changed into phenotypic males.

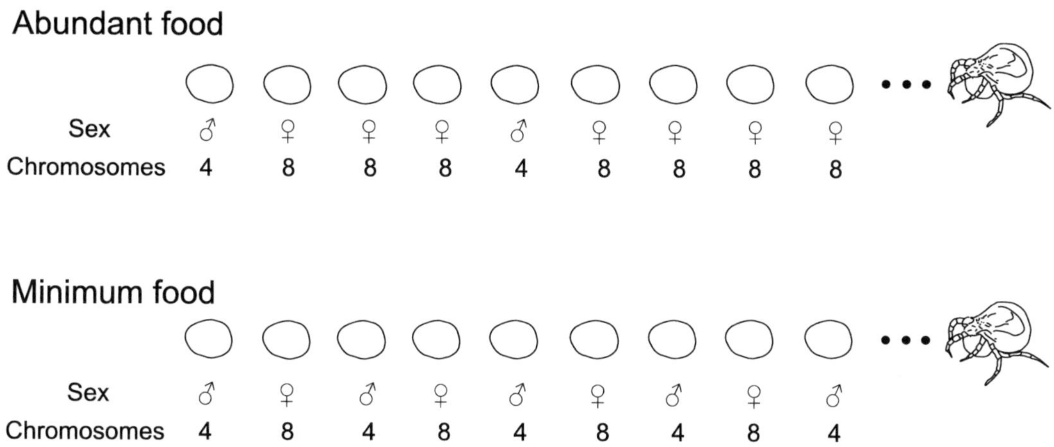

Fig. 5. Relationship between karyotypes of eggs and sex of offspring produced by mothers under abundant and minimum food condition.

Mothers may be able to choose sperm with a gene for maleness at a certain locus to control sex ratios under poor nutritional conditions. In this case, the paternal genomes are eliminated after the maleness of the egg is determined genetically. On the basis of genomic conflict between mother and father (e.g., Ross et al., 2010a), however, the utilization of sperm for maleness under poor prey conditions is a great disadvantage to the father because the genetic material in the sperm is eliminated during embryogenesis, and as a result does not contribute to the son's characteristics. Therefore, fathers probably do not produce sexually dimorphic sperm. Unfortunately, it is completely difficult to elucidate, anatomically, the sexual dimorphism of sperms in the ovary or to discriminate, genetically, the sperm with a gene for maleness. Detecting sperm for maleness modified by the mother in her ovary also presents a problem.

The possibility exists that the control of oocytes or eggs by the mother (without paternal contribution) is a simple process for maternal control of offspring sex. Mothers may be able to absorb female eggs under poor prey conditions, known as oosorption (resorption of oocytes), which is an effective mechanism to save resources on eggs in various insect species (Bell & Bohm, 1975). This is based on the idea that the sex of oocytes is already determined in the ovary upon emergence. According to this idea, mothers do not choose a male-destined oocyte for fertilization to develop into a male egg but absorbs female eggs when encountering a poor prey patch.

Gravid mothers under starvation were observed at 12-h intervals to confirm the absorption of female oocytes and/or eggs in the mother's body (Toyoshima et al., 2009). When gravid mothers just after depositing the first (male) egg were restricted to no prey items, the mothers did not hold an egg in the uterus but held 1–2 eggs in the dorsal region (refer to Fig. 2). Since mothers laid an average of 1.8 eggs during starvation, the 1–2 eggs in the dorsal region were transferred into the uterus, one by one, to form an eggshell and were deposited regardless of the nutritional condition of the mothers. An oocyte expanded during the deposition of the eggs and was maintained for at least 72 h in the dorsal region after vitellogenesis (Fig. 6). Two pronuclei were conjugated at first but later fused when the egg was in the dorsal region. The egg was deposited as a female egg when abundant prey items were provided for the starving mothers. According to this starvation experiment, female eggs may not be absorbed to control the sex ratio during food limitation. The confirmation was also made that oocyte expansion and vitellogenesis, as well as embryogenesis in the eggshell, advances until the nutrients in the starving mother are depleted. In this case, fertilization occurred after the sex of oocytes was determined, and the sex of the oocytes (and eggs) in the body was not influenced by the nutritional condition of the mothers. Paternal genomes in the egg may be eliminated during early embryonic development if the sex of the egg has been determined as male.

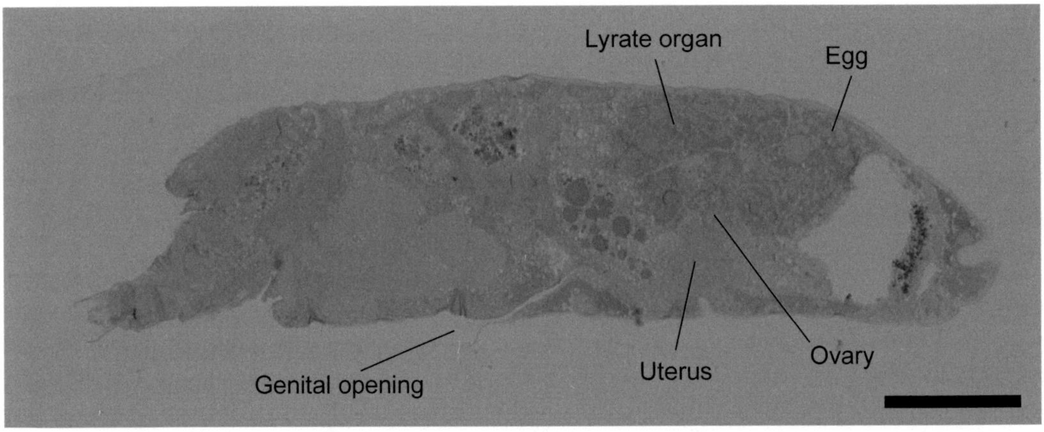

Fig. 6. Sagittal section of an adult female *Neoseiulus californicus* starved for 36 h. The starved female holds an egg in the dorsal region even after depositing an average of 1.8 eggs. The female is facing left (light microscope image). Bar = 50 μm.

4.2 Female-biased nutritional allocation in eggs

Mothers change their investment of nutrients into eggs in relation to the sex of eggs, as well as the prey consumption rate and their own age (Toyoshima & Amano, 1998). They produce larger eggs when consuming abundant prey, and gradually decrease egg size when aged and when prey consumption is restricted. In addition, they produce larger female eggs and smaller male eggs, and maintain the difference in size between sexes even when prey consumption is restricted. Although the evolutionary significance of sexual size dimorphism was discussed in a previous study, the sex determining mechanism of eggs was not yet determined from the size difference between sexes because of insufficient evidence.

The difference in egg size between sexes may be determined before fusion of the paternal and maternal pronuclei in the egg. According to an internal observation of starving females (Toyoshima et al., 2009), the vitelline membrane forms around the egg in the body of a starving female (Fig. 7c). The envelope was still not complete but interrupted. The adjacent, but not fused, pronuclei were visible in the egg enveloped with the vitelline membrane (Fig. 7a & 7b). The membrane is usually formed in oogenesis at the end of vitellogenesis. Since the size of the egg is determined when the vitelline membrane is formed, the combination of maternal and paternal genetic material did not influence size determination. In turn, the size of eggs was determined only by maternal control. More precisely, the size of eggs was influenced by sex, which was determined in response to the nutritional condition of the mothers.

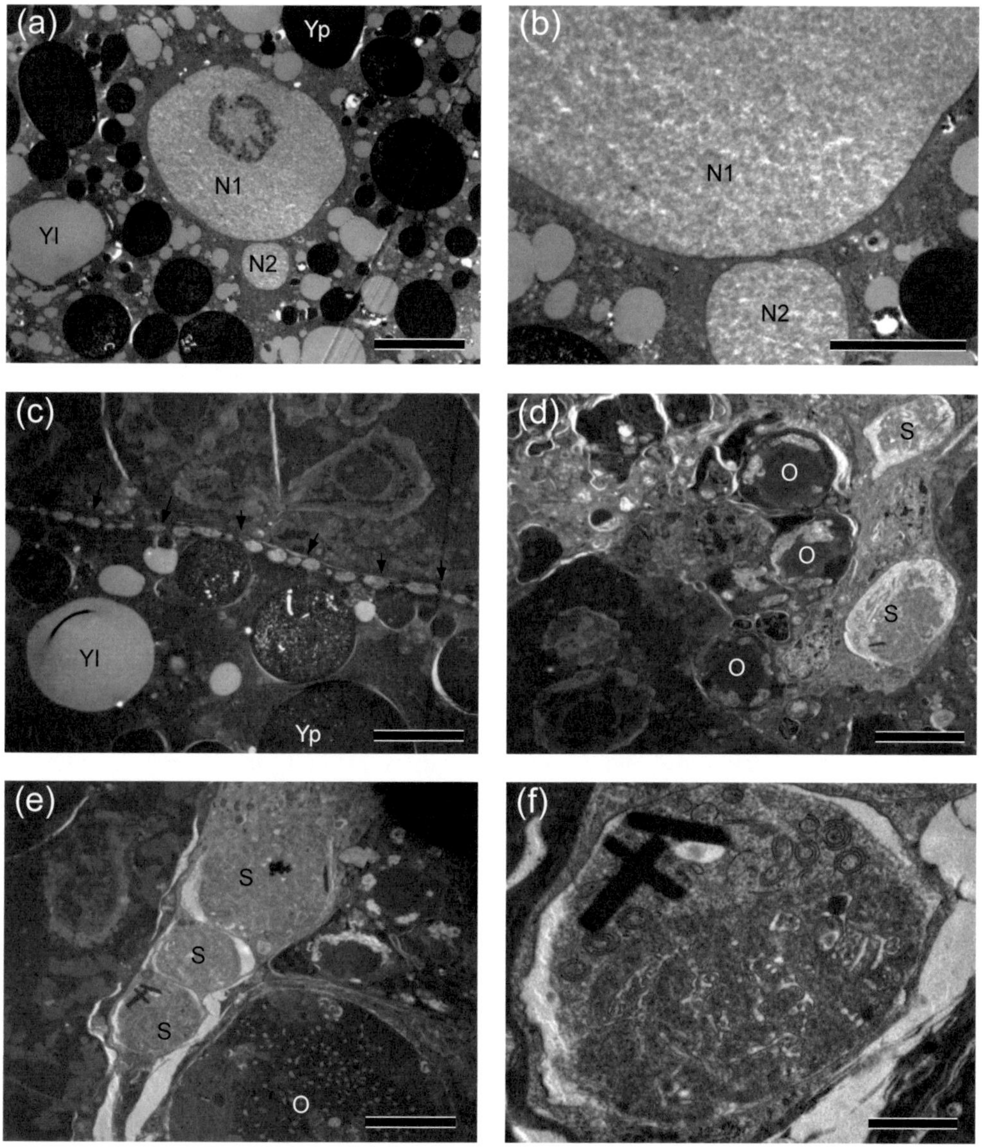

Fig. 7. Fine structures in the egg and around the ovary revealed by transmission electron microscopy. (a) Adjacent pronuclei in an egg filled with yolk granules. Bar = 10 µm. (b) Adjacent part of the pronuclei in (a). Bar = 5 µm. (c) The vitelline membrane (indicated by seven arrows). The envelope is still not completed, but interrupted. The vitelline membrane separates the egg with yolk granules (below) from the lyrate organ (above). Bar = 5 µm. (d) Ovary with several oocytes. Presumed sperms are visible around the ovary. Bar = 5 µm. (e) Presumed sperms between an oocyte and lyrate organ. Bar = 5 µm. (f) Detailed structure of a presumed sperm of (e). The detailed structure in the sperm cell is different from that shown in Di Palma & Alberti (2001). Black bars are not a staining artifact but an unknown structure. Bar = 1 µm. Abbreviations: N1, N2, nuclei; O, oocyte; S, presumed sperm; Yl, lipid-yolk granule; Yp, protein-yolk granule (unpublished micrographs by Toyoshima & Alberti).

How nutrition is invested into the eggs of each sex is still unclear. When female eggs are significantly different in size from male eggs, the size of eggs should be influenced only by the sex of the offspring. Thus, the sex of the eggs should be converted from male to female at a certain level of nutritional accumulation in the eggs. However, the size of the eggs is influenced not only by the sex but also the age and the nutritional condition of the mothers (Toyoshima & Amano, 1998). Female eggs deposited by mothers under poor prey conditions are smaller than male eggs deposited under abundant prey conditions, although the difference of egg size between the sexes (female eggs are larger than male eggs) is maintained at each prey condition. The switch from one sex to the other occurs at a relative criterion rather than an absolute criterion. The accumulation of a certain nutritional substance in addition to the minimum requirement of nutrition may lead to conversion of eggs from male to female. However, how the ratio of female to male is controlled in the ovary also remains unclear.

Sexual size dimorphism of eggs is also observed in an arrhenotokous phytophagous mite, *Tetranychus urticae* (Mache et al., 2010; Toyoshima, 2010), in which virgin mothers of this species lay only haploid male eggs, and fertilized mothers lay female (diploid) and male (haploid) eggs with female-biased sex ratios under good conditions on host plants. Male eggs produced by fertilized mothers are smaller not only than female eggs but also than male eggs produced by virgin females. If the sex of eggs produced by fertilized mothers is ignored, the eggs of fertilized females are not different from that of virgin females. From this comparison between eggs of fertilized and virgin females, virgin females are suspected to also produce concealable cytologically female eggs, which would be fundamentally destined as females but developed to males when not fertilized. This idea is not yet supported by data, but, if this is true, the evolutionary position of PGL in phytoseiid mites and arrhenotokous gynogenesis in certain animals may be understood in the course of the evolutional succession of sexual reproduction.

5. Future perspective

PGL in phytoseiid mites is still wrapped in mystery, although cytological and genetic evidence has accumulated since the 1980s. To understand the *evolutionary process* and *significance* of PGL in phytoseiid mites, we should clarify several events during oogenesis and embryogenesis (Fig. 8), as well as similar reproductive systems in closely related groups. The sex determining mechanism in eggs during oogenesis, sperm behavior in the ovary, and sperm penetration into oocytes are important events in the early reproductive process, which may lead to insights when exploring the signals for PGL. According to Di Palma & Alberti (2001), putative sperm cells extend a thick projection for insertion into an oocyte, and projections are visible around oocytes in the ovary (Fig. 7d–f). However, more investigation is necessary to determine when the sperm inserts into the oocyte and how the sperm nucleus behaves in the oocyte. Sperm behavior in the ovary and oocytes may also be influenced by the qualitative and/or quantitative differences between female-destined and male-destined oocytes. The difference in oocytes at the starting point in the ovary should be investigated histologically and genetically.

Thelytokous species are also known in phytoseiid mites. The thelytokous reproductive system is presumed to be derived from PGL because the number of thelytokous species is small compared to those with PGL. Comparative morphology of oogenesis and oocyte expansion in the ovary between thelytokous and PGL species will shed new light on the *evolutionary flexibility* and *constraints* of PGL in phytoseiid mites.

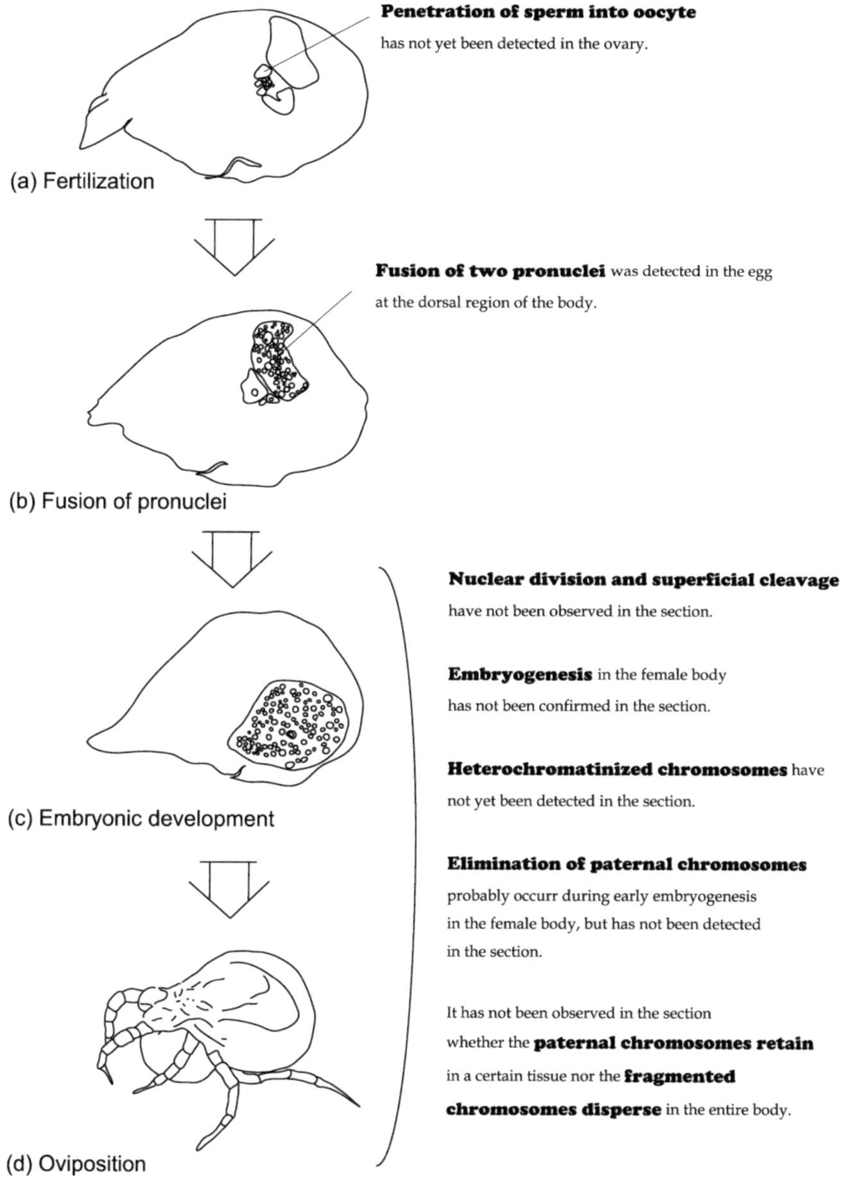

Fig. 8. Unknown events during oogenesis and embryogenesis of phytoseiid mites.

The process of the elimination of paternal genomes during embryonic development should be visualized to better understand the events of PGL. It is difficult, but not impossible, to penetrate the fixatives into the egg when wrapped in an eggshell in the female body. It is most important that the chromosome behavior in each cell during the blastula stage be observed to follow the heterochromatinized chromosomes, as a central point of the study of PGL. It may be able to reveal when, where, and how genomic material is eliminated during the embryonic development of males. Finally, we can start to understand why the paternal genome is eliminated and why this reproductive system is maintained in phytoseiid mites.

6. Acknowledgment

We are really grateful to Prof. em. Dr. Dr. h.c. G. Alberti (Ernst-Moritz-Arndt-Universität Greifswald) for his corrections and thoughtful suggestions to our manuscript. We also thank Drs. J. Abe (Kanagawa University), N. Hinomoto (NARO Agricultural Research Center), H. Kishimoto (NARO Institute of Fruit Tree Science), and Y. Tagami (Shizuoka University) for their valuable comments to the manuscript. Finally, we are grateful to the Publishing Process Manager of InTech for giving us an opportunity to review our previous researches.

7. References

Alberti, G. (1988) Genital system of gamasida and its bearing on phylogeny. In: *Progress in Acarology,* Volume I, Basavanna, G. P. C. & Viraktmath, C. A. (Eds.), 479-490, Ellis Horwood, Chichester

Alberti, G. & Hänel, H. (1986) Fine structure of the genital system inthe bee parasite, Varroajacobsoni (Gamasida: Dermanyssina) with remarks on spermiogenesis, spermatozoa and capacitation. *Experimental & Applied Acarology,* Vol.2, pp. 63-104

Amano, H. & Chant, D. A. (1978) Mating behaviour and reproductive mechanisms of two species of predacious mites, *Phytoseiulus persimilis* Athias-Henriot and *Amblyseius andersoni* (Chant) (Acarina: Phytoseiidae). *Acarologia,* Vol.20 pp. 196-213

Bell, G. (1982) *Masterpiece of Nature: The Evolution and Genetics of Sexuality,* 635p., Croom Helm, London

Bell, W. J. & Bohm, M. K. (1975) Oosorption in insects. *Biological Reviews,* Vol.50, pp. 373-396

Blommers-Schlosser, R. & Blommers, L. (1975) Karyotypes of eight species of Phytoseiid mites (Acarina: Mesostigmata) from Madagascar. *Genetica,* Vol.45, pp. 145-148

Bull, J. J. (1983) *The Evolution of Sex-Determining Mechanisms,* 316p., Menlo Park, Benjamin Cummings

Burt, A. & Trivers, R. (2006) *Genes in Conflict: The Biology of Selfish Genetic Elements,* 602p., Belknap Press of Harvard Univ. Press, Cambridge.

Cavalier-Smith, T. (1978) Nuclear volume control by nucleoskeletal DNA, selection for cell volume and cell growth rate, and the solution of the DNA C-value paradox. *Journal of Cell Science,* Vol.34, 247-278

Chant, D. A. & McMurtry, J. A. (2007) *Illustrated Keys and Diagnoses for the Genera and Subgenera of the Phytoseiidae of the World,* 220p., Indira Publishing House, Michigan

Congdon, B. D. & McMurtry, J. A. (1988) Morphological evidence establishing the loss of paternal chromosomes in males of predatory phytoseiid mites, genus *Euseius. Entomologia Experimentalis et Applicata,* Vol.48, pp. 95-96

Cook, J. M. & Crozier, R. H. (1995) Sex determination and population biology in the Hymenoptera. *Trends in Ecology & Evolution,* Vol.10, pp. 281-286

Di Palma, A. & Alberti, G. (2001) Fine structure of the female genital system in phytoseiid mites with remarks on egg nutrimentary development, sperm access system, sperm transfer, and capacitation (Acari, Gamasida, Phytoseiidae). *Experimental & Applied Acarology,* Vol.25, pp. 525-591

Dinh, N. V., Janssen, A. & Sabelis, M. W. (1988) Reproductive success of *Amblyseius idaeus* and *A. anonymus* on a diet of two-spotted spider mites. *Experimental & Applied Acarology,* Vol.4, pp. 41-51

Gerson, U., Smiley, R. L. & Ochoa, R. (2003) *Mites (Acari) for Pest Control.* 539p., Blackwell Science Ltd., Oxford

Hamilton, W. D. (1967) Extraordinary sex ratios. *Science,* Vol.156, pp.477-488

Hansell, R. I. C., Mollison, M. M. & Putman, W. L. (1964) A cytological demonstration of arrhenotoky in three mites of the family Phytoseiidae. *Chromosoma (Berl.)*, Vol.15, pp. 562-567

Hartl, D. L. & Brown, S. W. (1970) The origin of male haploid genetic systems and their expected sex ratio. *Theoretical & Population Biology*, Vol.1, pp. 165-190

Helle, W., Bolland, H. R., van Arendonk, R., De Boer, R. & Schulten, G. G. M. (1978) Genetic evidence for biparental males in haplo-diploid predator mites (Acarina: Phytoseiidae). *Genetica*, Vol.49, pp. 165-171

Helle, W. & Sabelis, M. W. (1985) *Spider Mites Their Biology, Natural Enemies and Control, Volume 1B*. 458p., Elsevier, Amsterdam

Herrick, G. & Seger, J. (1999) Imprinting and paternal genome elimination in insects. In: *Genomic Imprinting*, R. Ohlsson, (Ed.), 41-71, Springer Verlag, Amsterdam

Ho, C.-C., Lo, K.-C. & Chen, W.-H. (1995) Comparative biology, reproductive compatibility, and geographical distribution of *Amblyseius longispinosus* and *A. womersleyi* (Acari: Phytoseiidae). *Environmental Entomology*, Vol.24, pp. 601-607

Hoy, M. A. (1979) Parahaploidy of the "arrhenotokous" predator, *Metaseiulus occidentalis* (Acarina: Phyotoseiidae) demonstrated by X-irradiation of males. *Entomologia Experimentalis et Applicata*, Vol.26, pp. 97-104

Krantz, G. W. & Walter, D. E. (2009) *A Manual of Acarology (3rd. ed.)*. 807p., Texas Tech University Press, Texas

Macke, E., Magalhaes, S., Khan, H. D.-T., Luciano, A., Frantz, A., Facon, B. & Olivieri, L. (2010) Sex allocation in haplodiploid is mediated by egg size: evidence in the spider mite *Tetranychus urticae* Koch. *Proceedings of the Royal Society B*, Vol.278, No.1708, pp. 1054-1063

Michael, A. D. (1892). On the variations in the internal anatomy of the gamasinae, especially in that of the genital organs, and on their mode of coition. *Transactions of the Linnean Society of London. 2nd Series: Zoology*, Vol.5, No.9, pp. 281-317

Nagerkerke, C. J. & Sabelis, M. W. (1991) Precise sex-ratio control in the pseudo-arrhenotokous phytoseiid mite *Typhlodromus occidentalis* Nesbitt. In: *The Acari, Reproduction, Development and Life-History Strategies*. Schuster, R. & Murphy, P. W. (Eds.), 193-207, Chapman and Hall, London

Nagerkerke, C. J. & Sabelis, M. W. (1998) Precise control of sex allocation in pseuso-arrhenotokous phytoseiid mites. *Journal of Evolutionary Biology*, Vol.11, pp. 649-684

Nelson-Rees, W. A., Hoy, M. A. & Roush, R. T. (1980) Heterochromatinization, chromatin elimination and haploidization in the parahaploid mite *Metaseiulus occidentalis* (Nesbitt) (Acarina: Phytoseiidae). *Chromosoma (Berl.)*, Vol.77, pp. 263-276

Norton, R. A., Kethley, J. B., Johnston, D. E. & OConnor, B. M. (1993) Phylogenetic perspectives on genetic systems and reproductive modes of mites. In: *Evolution and Diversity of Sex Ratio in Insects and Mites*, Wrensch. D. L. & Ebbert, M. A. (Eds.), 8-99, Chapman & Hall, New York

Oliver, J. H. (1983) Chromosomes, genetic variance and reproductive strategies among mites and ticks. Bulletin of the ESA, Vol.29, No.2, pp.8-17

Perrot-Minoot, M.-J., Lagnel, J., Migeon, J. & Navajas, M. (2000) Tracking paternal genes with DALP markers in a pseudoarrhenotokoys reproductive system: biparental transmission but haplodiploid-like inheritance in the mite *Neoseiulus californicus*. *Heredity*, Vol.84, pp. 702-709

Perro-Minnot, M.-J. & Najavas, M. (1995) Biparental inheritance of RAPD markers in males of the pseudoarrhenotokous mite *Typhlodromus pyri*. *Genome*, Vol.38, pp. 838-844

Ross, L., Pen, I. & Shuker, D. M. (2010a) Genomic conflicts in scale insects: the causes and consequences of bizarre genetic systems. *Biological Reviews*, Vol.85, pp. 807-828

Ross, L., Shuker, D. M. & Pen, I. (2010b) The evolution and suppression of male suicide under paternal genome elimination. *Evolution*, Vol.65, pp. 554-563

Sabelis, M. W. (1985) Development. In : *Spider Mites, Their Biology, Natural Enemies and Control, Volume 1B*, Helle, W. & Sabelis, M. W. (Eds.), 43-53, Elsevier, Amsterdam

Sabelis, M. W., Nagerkerke, C. J. & Breeuwer, J. A. J. (2002) Sex ratio control in arrhenotokous and pseudo-arrhenotokous mites. In: *Sex Ratios, Concepts and Research Methods*, Hardy, I. C. W. (Ed.), 235-253, Cambridge University Press, Cambridge.

Sanderson, J. P. & McMurtry, J. A. (1984) Life history studies of the predaceous mite *Phytoseius hawaiiesis*. *Entomologia Experimentalis et Applicata*, Vol.35, pp. 27-234

Schrader, F. & Hughes-Schrader, S. (1931) Haploidy of metazoan. *Quarterly Review of Biology*, Vol.6, pp. 411-438

Schulten, G. G. M. (1985) Pseudo-arrhenotoky. In: *Spider Mites, Their Biology, Natural Enemies and Control, Volume 1B*, Helle, W. & Sabelis, M. W. (Eds.), 67-71, Elsevier, Amsterdam

Schulten, G. G. M., van Arendonk, R. C. M., Russell, V. M., & Roorda, F. A. (1978) Copulation, egg production and sex-ratio in *Phytoseiulus persimilis* and *Amblyseius bibens* (Acari: Phytoseiidae). *Entomologia Experimentalis et Applicata*, Vol.24, pp. 145-153

Schultz, R. J. (1969) Hybridization, unisexuality, and polyploidy in the teleost *Poeciliopsis* (Poeciliidae) and other vertebrates. *The American Naturalist*, Vol.103, pp. 605-619

Toyoshima, S. (2010) Effects of fertilization status and age of gravid females on the egg size in *Tetranychus urticae* Koch. *Journal of the Acarological Society of Japan*, Vol.19, pp. 107-112

Toyoshima, S. & Amano, H. (1998) Effect of prey density on sex ratio of two predacious mites, *Phytoseiulus persimilis* and *Amblyseius womersleyi* (Acari: Phytoseiidae). *Experimental & Applied Acarology*, Vol.22, pp. 709-723

Toyoshima, S. & Amano, H. (1999) Cytological evidence of pseudo-arrhenotoky in two phytoseiid mites, *Phytoseiulus persimilis* Athias-Henriot and *Amblyseius womersleyi* Schicha. *Journal of the Acarological Society of Japan*, Vol.8, pp. 135-142

Toyoshima, S., Michalik, P., Talarico, G., Klann, A. E. & Alberti, G. (2009) Effects of starvation on reproduction of the predacious mite *Neoseiulus californicus* (Acari: Phytoseiidae). *Experimental & Applied Acarology*, 47: 235-247.

Toyoshima, S., Nakamura, M., Nagahama, Y. & Amano, H. (2000) Process of egg formation in the female body cavity and fertilization in male eggs of *Phytoseiulus persimilis* (Acari: Phytoseiidae). *Experimental & Applied Acarology*, Vol.24, pp. 441-451

White, M. J. D. (1973) *Animal Cytology and Evolution (3rd ed.)*. 961p., University Press, Cambridge

Wysoki, M. (1973) Further studies on karyotypes an sex determination of phytoseiid mites (Acarina: Mesostigmata). Genetica, 44: 139-145.

Wysoki, M. (1985) Karyotyping. In: *Spider Mites, Their Biology, Natural Enemies and Control, Volume 1B*, Helle, W. & Sabelis, M. W. (Eds.), 191-196, Elsevier, Amsterdam

Wysoki, M. & Bolland, R. (1983) Chromosome studies of phytoseiid mites (Acari: Gamasida). *International Journal of Acarology*, Vol.9, pp. 91-99

Wysoki, M. & McMurtry, J. A. (1977) Karyotypes of eight species of phytoseiid mites of the genus *Amblyseius* Berlese (Acarina: Mesostigmata). *Genetica*, Vol.47, pp. 237-239

Wysoki, M. & Swirski, E. (1968) Karyotypes and sex determination of ten species of phytoseiid mites (Acarina: Mesostigmata). *Genetica*, Vol.39, pp. 220-228

Yastrebtsov, A. (1992) Embryonic development of gamadis mites (Parasitiformes: Gamasida). *International Journal of Acarology*, Vol.18, pp. 121-141

27

Liquid-Crystal in Embryogenesis and Pathogenesis of Human Diseases

MengMeng Xu[1] and Xuehong Xu[2,3,4,*]
[1]*Medical Scientist Training Program, Duke University School of Medicine,*
[2]*Department of Physiology Center for Biomedical Engineering Technology,*
[3]*Center for Stem Cell Biology and Regenerative Medicine,*
University of Maryland School of Medicine,
[4]*Shaanxi Normal University School of Life Science,*
[1,2,3]*USA*
[4]*China*

1. Introduction

In 1979, a systematic publication summarizing the state of research on liquid-crystals in biological organisms was published [Brown GH *et al* 1979]. After this historic publication on liquid-crystals and biology, the field remained largely dormant for more than two decades. However in 1978 and 1979, Haiping He and Xizai Wu, who had continued pursuing this field despite international disinterest, reported their findings on liquid-crystal involvement during chicken development. For the first time, they revealed that massive quantities of liquid-crystals in the liver, yolk sac, blood, and many other developing tissues and organs of chicken during embryogenesis. Their later studies also reported similar liquid-crystalline structures during fish development. In 1988, another group reported the existence of vaterite $CaCO_3$ within the liquid-crystals found in yolk fluid, identifying the spherical calcified structures first reported in 1979 as one of three iso-forms of calcium carbonate [Feher G 1979, Li M *et al* 1988]. Subsequent studies have identified liquid-crystalline structures to be omnipresent in the liver during avian development [Xu XH *et al* 1995a, 1995b, 1997]. Recent studies have revealed that liquid-crystals play a critical role in the preservation of calcium and other trace elements required for embryo development [Xu MM *et al* 2009, 2010, 2011; Xu XH *et al* 2009, 2011a].

In recent years, more and more human diseases have been related to liquid-crystals. Amongst these diseases are genetic disorders, such as Age-related Macular Degeneration [Haimovici R *et al* 2001], steatohepatitis and atherosclerosis [Goldstein JL *et al* 2008], and Anderson-Fabry Disease [Xu MM *et al* 2009]. For Fabry patients, the accumulation of liquid-crystal or concentric lamellar bodies glycosphingolipids in neurons can cause severe neuroradiological abnormalities, including periventricular white-matter signal intensity abnormality and single/multiple lacunar infarction, large ischaemic cerebral infarct and

* Corresponding Author

posterior thalamic involvement [Ginsberg L *et al* 2006; Lidove O *et al* 2006; Moore DF *et al* 2003]. This accumulation also occurs in the cardiac vascular system, resulting in angina and varied complications, ranging from arrhythmia to myocardial infarction and heart failure [Pieroni M *et al* 2006; Linhart A *et al* 2007]. Although a large volume of publications indicate an irreplaceable role for liquid-crystals in both normal physiological development and pathogenesis, the exact function of liquid-crystal is uncertain.

In this chapter, we will summarize current research around liquid-crystal involvement in embryogenesis and how these normal embryonic events, when triggered at inappropriate times, can lead to pathogenic events. Current publications indicate that liquid-crystals are often involved in normal embryogenesis, but the appearance of liquid-crystals in post-natal development often heralds pathogenesis in mature tissue. Normally embryogenic events can be trigger by a variety of factors, such genetic predispositions or bacterial infection. As part of normal embryogenesis, the formation of liquid-crystals indicates erroneous initiation of normal growth, often leading to disease.

2. Methodology for liquid-crystal function in medical biology and embryogenesis

Liquid crystal is refers to a material's physical state. As the term suggests, liquid-crystals display both liquid and solid tendencies. This fluid characteristic perfectly matches the properties of a living organism. However, this same adaptability to life introduces some critical attention to experimental approaches when studying liquid-crystals *in vitro.* In this section, we will focus on research approaches used for studying liquid-crystals in biological embryogenesis and human pathogenesis. The preeminent combination of all procedures could perform excellent inspection on the liquid crystal [Xu XH et al 2011a].

2.1 Animal sample collection according to animal IACUC

In the United States, any research application involving laboratory animals is required to be approved by the Institutional Animal Care and Use Committee (IACUC) prior to experimentation, if the research is funded by a federal agency such as the National Institute of Health. All animal procedures must also follow guidelines approved by the home institution's Animal Care and Use department. For mouse tissue and organ harvest, mice must first be euthanized via CO2 asphyxiation followed by cervical dislocation. After the necessary tissues have been harvested, the mouse remains should be sealed within plastic bagging and frozen for temporal storage in the animal core facility. Permanent treatment of animal body will be carried out by the core.

In most instances of commercial mice, such as 129SvEv and DBA/2J breeds from the Jackson Laboratory (Bar Harbor, ME), Harland Laboratories (Indianapolis, IN), and other commercial sources were bred under standard conditions and sacrificed by cervical dislocation according to IACUC regulation. All tissues were harvested immediately and snap frozen with liquid nitrogen upon dissection. For timing experiments using mouse embryo, appearance of the vaginal plug was designated as embryonic day (E) 0.5, and embryos were either collected from the stage of interest, or pregnancies were allowed to reach term. For postnatal studies, newborn mice were collected at the day of birth (postnatal day, P).

For avian experiments, fertilized chick eggs such as White Leghorn (*Gallus domesticus L.*) are normally incubated at 37⁰C with relative air humidity of 60%. Experiments are conducted and samples harvested at time-points according to experimental procedure. The age of embryos is documented as day of incubation (D) and the postnatal age of chicks is documented as Postnatal (P). Collections of tissues and organs are the same as described above and can be found within references [Xu MM *et al* 2009, 2010, 2011; Xu XH *et al* 2009, 2010, 2011ab].

2.2 Cryo-section histology analysis

For purely biological studies of embryogenesis, both paraffin section and cry-section are good options for well-preserved tissue and organ samples. However, for liquid-crystal functional studies during embryo development and pathological events, cryo- or frozen-section are preferred over paraffin sections, as the cryo/frozen methods preserve more of the sample's original characteristics than the more chemically intensive paraffin preservation method. If possible, fresh sample smear-slides are also preferred. [Xu MM *et al* 2009, Xu XH *et al* 2009].

Though the previous methods allow for long term storage, fresh smear-slide preparation arguably retains the most fidelity to *in vivo* systems as the tissue is not processed in any way prior to observation. In smear-slide preparation, samples are harvest from the embryos at different stages. Each sample is then immediately smeared on a slide wetted with PBS (PH 7.4) buffer then mounted with a cover slip. This method is best observed by polarization microscopy, which can be conducted immediately following the sample smear preparations.

When in need of a method for long term storage or if retaining the physical structure of the tissue is desired, sryosection preparation is preferred. Embryo samples are submerged in the cryomatrix embedding agent (OCT) and placed in an aluminum foil basket or other suitable container to be dipped. The samples are then frozen by dipping the foil basket or the container into liquid nitrogen. The now frozen tissues embedded in the OCT block can now be placed on the cryostat microtome and sections cut for experimentation. Thicker cuts 10~30 mm are preferred for polarization microscopy and thinner cuts of ~5mm are preferred for H&E staining. The samples collected using these two procedures should be mounted with 20% of glycerol in PBS (PH 7.2) and sealed before proceeding to further analysis.

2.3 Immunohistochemistry and confocal microscopy

After collection and smear-section preparation, samples should be washed with PBS, fixed in 4% formaldehyde in phosphate-buffered saline (PBS), and permeabilized for 10 min in PBS containing 0.25% Triton X-100. Immunocytochemical staining can be perform performed by incubating the samples with primary antibodies in PBS/Tween (PBS containing 0.1% Tween 20 and 3% BSA) for 1–2 hr, followed by incubation with appropriate secondary antibodies diluted according to the manufacturer's recommendation in PBS/Tween solution for 1–2 hr. Stained samples can then be visualized with confocal microscope.

Immunohistochemistry is a powerful approach to unveil distribution of protein of interest, which can be used to locate liquid-crystal related proteins in tissues and organs. However, because this method requires the use of damaging solutions such as formaldehyde, Triton X-100, and Tween containing blocking buffer, results should be compared to smear-samples for confirmation of signal localization corresponding to liquid crystal.

2.4 Polarization microscopy and thermal phase-transition

Polarization or polarized microscopy is an irreplaceable tool for studying materials with refractory activity. In the case of liquid crystal study, two states of material, crystal and liquid crystal, have birefringent activity. In our studies, we have found microscopy to be an invaluable tool in examining the light activity of liquid crystals in animal tissue.

Natural light such as light from an ordinary light source is called non-polarized because it vibrates in random directions. Polarized light on the other hand, travels within a single plane and presents with vertical vibrations that can produce linear, circular, and elliptical polarized light. A polarizing plate or polarizing prism is often used as a polarizing filter to remove all but one wave with the same directional vibration.

Observing liquid-crystals under polarized light requires a basic understanding of light polarization. To create a polarized light, two devices, the primary and secondary polarizing devices, are oriented perpendicular to each other as crossed nicols to filter polarized light from normal lighting. The primary device will filter a polarized light from the light source, while the secondary device cuts the light depending on orientation of the two devices. These primary polarizing device and secondary polarizing device are called Polarizer (P) and Analyzer (A), respectively. In perpendicular nicols, the analyzer is rotated to be perpendicular to the polarizer. Since both nicols act as filters, the analyzer cancels out the polarized light from the polarizing lense, to yield no light to the observer (Figure 1A). In parallel nicols, the analyzer is rotated so that the direction of the transmitting polarized light is parallel with the polarizer. This allows polarized light transmitted via the polarizer to travel through the Analyser, maximizing the amount of light transmitance (Figure 1B).

The light bending ability of liquid crystals can be thought of as an additional nicol. When polarized light launching through a crystal or liquid crystal materials is divided into two linearly polarized light rays, these two rays possess mutually crossing vibration directions, called birefringence (double refraction). A crystal or liquid crystal that refracts in this way is called anisotropy. When an anisotropic crystal or liquid crystal is inserted between a polarizer and an analyzer in a crossed nicols state, the crystal or liquid crystal changes the state of the polarized light and the light to pass through partially (Figure 1C). These changes are different depending on various crystal or liquid crystal, which can be utilized to determine characteristics of an anisotropic material, liquid crystal in this case.

Using this light-bending property of liquid crystals, thermal-probe sample stage in conjunction with polarization microscope, can be used to monitor and record phase transition of liquid crystals. When a sample is observed with crossed-nicols, the anisotropic texture of crystal or liquid crystal will vanish once the temperature of stage reaches the point of phase transition from liquid crystal to isotropic states. This technique is an effective method for observing the liquid crystal properties of biological samples containing liquid crystals [Xu MM *et al* 2010, 2011; Xu XH *et al* 2011a].

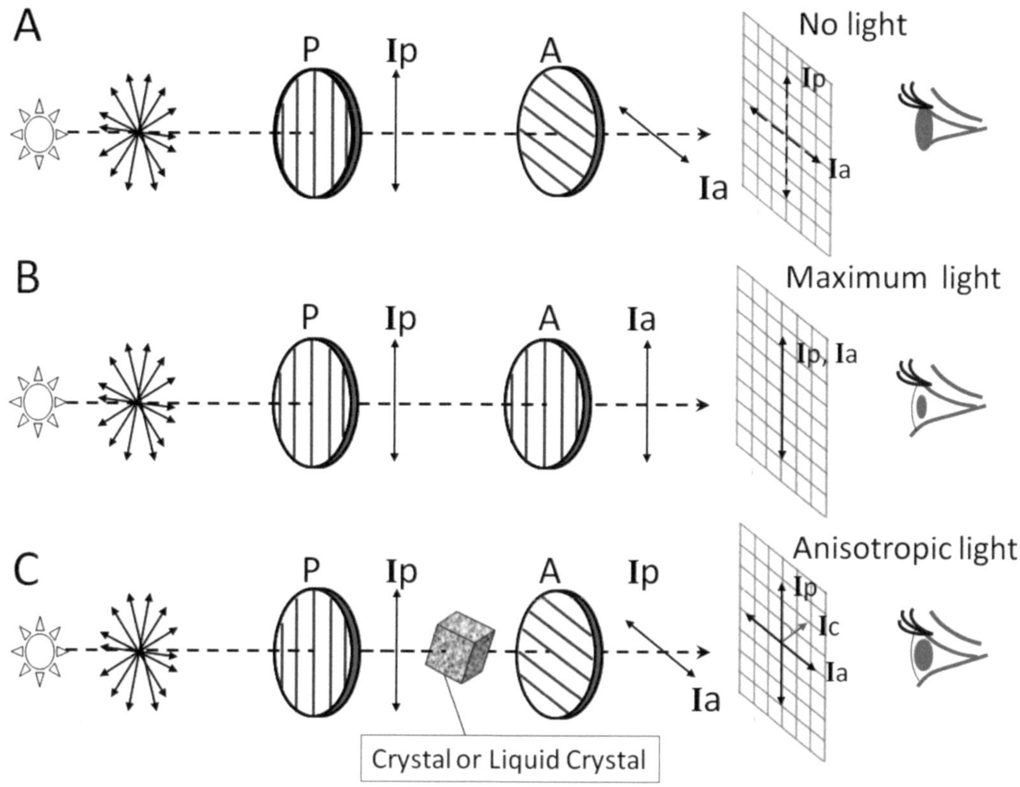

A. Crossed nicols;
B. Parallel nicols;
C. Anisotropy between crossed nicols.
P: polarizer
A: analyzer

Fig. 1. Light path of polarization and anisotropy

2.5 Small angle X-ray scattering (SAXS) and X-ray diffraction (XRD)

When X-ray beam of a particular wavelength diffracts from atoms in a crystalline structure, the wavelength of the x-ray (λ), scattering angle (θ), integer representing the order of the diffraction peak (n), and inter-plane distance (d), usually the distance between atoms, ions, molecules, follow the Bragg's Law (Figure 2A).

$$2d \sin\theta = n\lambda$$

This equation predicts that different layers of atoms in lattice planes will generate various distances corresponding to peaks. Crystal samples, multiple peaks will be present in a wide-spread diffraction angle (2θ, XRD; Figure 2B), while liquid crystal exhibit fewer peaks within an area of small scattering angles (2θ, SAXS; Figure 2C). For crystals or liquid-crystals within biological samples, once liquid-crystals or crystals have been isolated or extracted, temperature and other conditions must be tightly controlled to retain the original characteristics and diffraction pattern of samples.

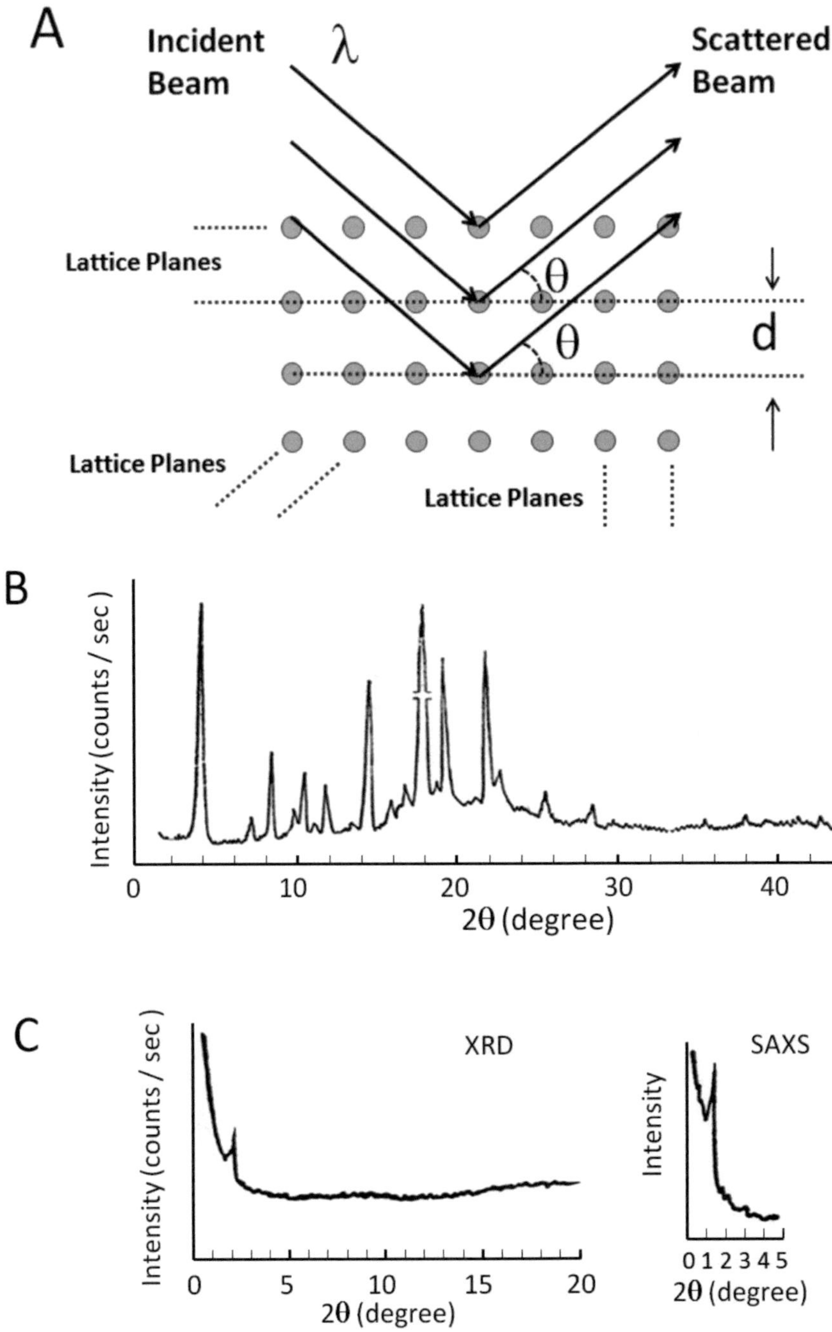

Fig. 2. Bragg's law and the diffraction patterns of crystal and liquid crystal. Relationship between wavelength, scattering angle, and distance of lattice planes (A). XRD pattern of crystal cholesteryl oleate within 50 degree of diffraction angle (2θ) (B), and SAXS pattern of liquid crystal in embryonic liver within 50 degree (2θ) (left in C) and within 5 degree of scattering angle degree (2θ) (right in C).

2.6 Generation of mouse model using daily diet procedure

Mice are obtained from Jackson Laboratories or another commercial facility. Male or female pups are split into two groups. Group one is fed on the standard chow diet (Harlan Teklad #2018 rodent chow) with 48% carbohydrate, 16% protein and 4% fat. Group two is on a low carbohydrate high protein diet with 15% carbohydrate, 58% protein and 26% fat, which we was designed to mimic the typical Western diet.

3. Comparative summary of liquid-crystals in embryonic tissue development and post-natal pathology

As discussed earlier in the chapter, embryonic tissues and organs of several animal models have exhibited traces of liquid-crystals during embryonic development stage that did not persist postnatally. In liver and yolk sac, massive liquid-crystals are present from embryogenesis to early post-natal development. In this section, we will summarize the characteristics of liquid-crystals in different tissues in comparison to the liquid-crystals found in human diseases (Table 1).

3.1 General characteristics of embryonic liquid-crystal

During embryogenesis, liquid crystals are widely distributed in the tissues of vertebrates and invertebrates, including Apis cerana chrysalis, fish, reptile, avian and mammal early embryo in vitro [X XH *et al* 1993, 2009, 2011a, Xu MM et al 2009 2011]. In chicken development, more than twenty different organs and tissues exhibit liquid crystal droplets including liver, meso- and metanephros, lungs, blood in heart, and brain. The presence of liquid crystal normally appears at different developmental stages depending on the tissue type, and lasts until early postnatal stages. The earliest liquid crystal droplets appear on the inner embryonic disc during the second day of development [He H et al 1978]. Regardless of their distribution, however, the liquid crystal droplets eventually vanish within three to four weeks into the postnatal period, also depending on tissue type maturation [X XH *et al* 2009, 2011a].

During chicken development, two particular organs, the liver and yolk sac, exhibit massive birefringent liquid crystal at higher levels than all over tissues in the developing embryo. The hepatic birefringent particles are mainly composed of cholesteryl oleate, cholesterol, lecithin and an unidentified component [Xu XH *et al* 1992, 1995a, 2011a]. These liquid crystal droplets are situated in hepatocytes of the hepatic cord region. In the kidney development, LC droplets can exist in the cytoplasm of epithelial cells and the lumen of proximal tubules in the mesonephros and metanephros. The existence of LC in two very different organs indicates that the liquid crystal likely plays many different roles during the development or a similar role in many tissues.

3.2 Decrease-rate dependent thermal phase transition

Under polarization microscope, liquid crystal exhibit Maltese-crosses optical textures, while crystals produced more angular (needle-like, rhombus, or dot-shape) diffraction patterns The two states also reacted differently to pressure experiments, with the liquid-crystals dividing into smaller Maltese-cross droplets, while crystals fractured uner duress [Xu XH et al 2009, 2011a].

Thermal phase transitions have also been revealed in liquid crystal obtained from various tissues (Table 1). Not surprisingly, with thermal stage temperature increase, the birefringent liquid crystal droplets transit to non-refracting isotropic droplets. With temperature decrease, the liquid crystal droplets transit into crystal. However, when the isotropic droplets cool, two different results, controllable by rate of temperature decrease, were possible. If the rate of temperature drop is fast (the slide is placed on a 4^{0}C plate), then the isotropic droplets will transition into liquid-crystals. However, if the rate of temperature decrease is slow (temperature is allowed to drop in step with the slowly cooling copper thermo-controller) then the isotropic droplets will transit to crystal (Figure 3). This finding

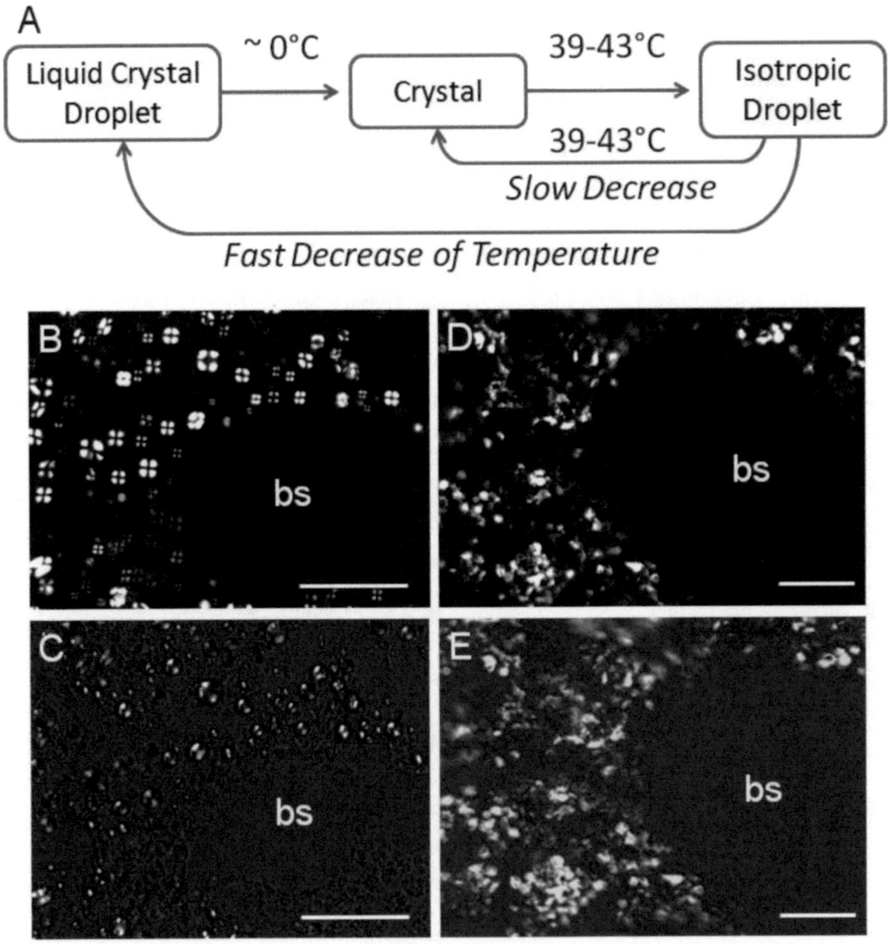

Fig. 3. Thermal phase transitions of liquid crystal droplet, crystal and isotropic droplet. The phase transition from isotropic droplet to crystal or liquid crystal depends on the rate of temperature decrease (A). B and C exhibit the hepatic liquid crystal droplets in crossed nicols with 90 degree of angle (B) and 45 degree (C). D and E show the hepatic crystal in crossed nicols at 90 degree of angle (D) and 45 degree (E), which transited from liquid crystals. Anisotropic liquid crystals locate in hepatocytes in the cords and are absent in the blood sinus (bs). Bars, 60 μm.

was initially established in embryonic hepatic liquid crystal then [Xu XH *et al* 1995] proven to be a general phenomenon in embryonic liquid crystal of other tissues and organs [Xu XH *et al* 2011 and Table 1].

Embryonic Tissue/Organ*		Temperature of Phase Transition (°C)			Liquid Crystal in Diseases	Ref.
		LC to Isotopic	Crystal to Isotopic	Isotopic to Crystal **		
Liver	E14	37.6 ~41.5	39.4~42.0	35.6~36.3	Steatohepatitis Gaucher disease	12, 13, 40, 43, 44, 51
Kidney Mesone-phros	E8	36.6~40.5	38.1~40.8	38.6~40.8	Fabry-Anderson	1, 6, 33, 36
Metane-phros	E14	36.2~40.2	37.9~41.1	38.6~40.7	disease	
Lung	E17	37.1~41.3	38.6~41.6	35.7~35.6	Gram-positive bacteria sputum	37
Aorta	E	37.8 ~41.1	NE	NE	Atherosclerotic lesions	10, 11, 19, 20
Vein	E	37.2 ~41.4	NE	NE	Foam cell abnormality	4, 5, 12, 13, 48
Heart	E	36.8 ~40.0	NE	NE	-	15
	P 10	Non-detectable	Non-detectable	Non-detectable		
Eye (retina)	E19	37.2 ~41.1	39.3~41.1	35.4~36.5	ARMD	14, 31, 32,34
	P6	Non-detectable	Non-detectable	Non-detectable		
York sac	E2~3	38.5~42.5	44.3~46.3	46.2~46.6	-	38, 47
	E17~9	38.9~42.3	44.1~46.3	46.3~47.2		
Blood	E9	NE	NE	NE	Gaucher disease	13, 26, 48

*The data from domestic fowl Taihe
**These temperatures are documented with slow decrease of thermal stage.
NE: Not examined

Table 1. Liquid-crystal characteristics in embryonic tissues/organs and post-natal diseases

3.3 SAXS and XRD measurements of liquid-crystal and crystal

SAXS pattern can be documented with massive hepatic liquid crystals. Within 50 degree of 2θ, only one scattering peak can be detected corresponding to 35 Å in small angle area, indicating the distance of molecular layers of liquid crystal droplets. Using this approach, the period distance of liquid crystal from the fat body of Apis cerana chrysalis [Xu XH *et al* 1994a] and hepatic liquid crystals of various avians have been documented [Xu XH et al

1995, 2009, 2011]. Crystals transited from liquid-crystals can generate many more diffraction peaks corresponding to more crystalgraphic planes. Oddly, XRD pattern reveals more orders on the hepatic crystals.

SAXS and XRD measurements elucidated significant differences between hepatic liquid crystals obtained from different species of avian. In Taihe fowl, the SAXS scattering of the hepatic liquid crystal expresses a strong peak at 2θ. But the peak is weak or absent in its crystal XRD diffraction. In pigeon, the SAXS hepatic liquid crystal peak does have a significant XRD diffraction pattern. This difference indicates that although liquid crystal can be found in the same tissues of the two avians, they likely contain different chemical components (Table 2).

3.4 Liquid crystals in human disease

Unlike during embryogenesis, no liquid crystals are found in postnatal development or in normal physiological systems. However, liquid crystalline structures have been reported in different tissues during pathological processes, including atherosclerosis, abnormal lipid depositions, Age-Related Macular Degeneration, and active monocytes.

In 95 patient samples of atherosclerotic lesions, liquid crystals composed of cholesterol, cholesterol ester, and phospholipid were observed [Lang PD *et al* 1970]. This data has been confirmed by another group [Goldstein JL et al 1977] and mimicked within *in vitro* systems [Goldstein JL et al 1979]. Maltese-crosses, indicating liquid-crystals, have also been found in lipid depositions accumulating in smooth muscle and foam cells [Kruth H 2001]. These liquid crystal depositions in the vascular wall were found to be low density lipoprotein-cholesteryl esters mediated by cell surface receptors [Goldstein JL et al 1977, 1979, 1997, 2008; Brown MS et al 1974, 1974].

Age-Related Macular Degeneration (ADM) is the leading cause of severe vision loss in adults over 50. The Center for Disease Control and Prevention estimates that 1.8 million people are suffering AMD and over 7 million are at substantial risk for vision loss from AMD in United State. Liquid crystal Maltese's-crosses and crystals structure were observed in the drusen of retina in ARMD patients [Small DM 1970, 1986, 1988; Haimovici R *et al* 2001]. In these patients, drusen are much bigger than normal and are filled with accumulated anisotropic structures.

Recently, cytoplasmic accumulation of liquid-crystal like droplets have also been found in monocytes, macrophages, and squamous epithelial cells of sputum from a patient affected with Gram-Positive Bacteria [MM Xu *et al* 2011]. In sputum collected during the recovery phase of respiratory infection, massive Maltese-crosses were fully loaded in host cells. Though the mechanism of formation for these liquid-crystal like droplets has discovered, further study could lead to new perspectives on post-infection removal of infectious agents.

In addition to Fabry-Anderson Disease [MM Xu *et al* 2009], birefringent particle accumulation are also observed in Gaucher disease [Goodman ZD *et al* 2009, Hillman RS *et al* 2005]. This disease is a lysosomal storage disorder, in which deficiency of glucocerebrosidase causes a buildup of fatty substance glucocerebroside in the monocyte and macrophages of certain organs. As the observations were made on biopsy samples, the birefringent fragments observed are likely crystals generated from native liquid crystals as an artifact of freezing. This birefringent accumulation was observed in liver and blood of the patients as well (Table 1).

Newborn Chicken				Newborn Pigeon			
Crystal from LC		Liquid Crystal		Crystal from LC		Liquid Crystal	
XRD		SAXS		XRD		SAXS	
I / I_0	d (Å)	I / I_0	d (Å)	I / I_0	d (Å)	I / I_0	d (Å)
-	-	100	37.0	46	38.10	100	38.02
100	19.55	-	-	32	19.48	-	-
5	17.63	-	-	11	12.10	-	-
1	10.59	-	-	10	10.71	-	-
6	9.44	-	-	30	7.21	-	-
1	7.70	-	-	17	5.89	-	-
2	5.90	-	-	12	5.38	-	-
1	5.22	-	-	100	5.13	-	-
1	5.12	-	-	33	5.01	-	-
18	4.91	-	-	56	4.82	-	-
2	4.60	-	-	22	4.48	-	-
3	4.08	-	-	43	4.39	-	-

Notes: No corresponding parameters between XRD and SAXS show with "-".

Table 2. SAXS and XRD comparison of liquid-crystal and crystal during avian development

4. Comparative study on mouse models of steatohepatitis and embryonic hepatic liquid crystal

4.1 High protein and fat diet mouse models

Using a diet high in protein and fat, a Steatohepatitis mouse model was generated. After three months, the liver of these animals turned light yellow and were larger in comparison to the liver of control animals. After 9 months, the livers were two to three times the size of mice being fed the normal diet. These livers also exhibited plaque and had significantly enlarged spleens. Using X-ray diffraction, small angle X-ray scattering, and phase transition, previous reports have characterized the distribution ultrastructure, and chemical composition of chicken hepatic LCLDs. Using this information and the well-established Steatohepatitis animal model, three conclusions were made: (1) The liquid-crystals in Steatohepatitis liver were produced in a pathological process similar to hepatic liquid-crystal formation in avian embryogenesis; (2) Small angle X-ray scattering revealed that liquid-crystal are distributed every 38Å in the hepatic tissue of Steatohepatitis animals. This distribution matched that reported in avian embryonic livers; (3) In Steatohepatitis animals, the liquid-crystals are distributed on the hepatic cords, which match the localization of liquid-crystals in embryonic liver.

4.2 Gene manipulation of related protein expression

Gene manipulation has become powerful tool for exploring gene function on molecular mechanisms of human diseases. In one instance, Shimano and colleges generated a transgenic mouse overexpressing truncated SREBP-1a (sterol-regulated proteolysis), a SREBP a membrane-bound transcription factor released by sterol-regulated proteolysis [Wang X *et al* 1994]. This gene abnormality resulted in lipid deposition in atherosclerotic lesions originating from liver accumulation of HLCDs [Shimano H *et al* 1996].

Stimulating a high level expression of the promoter in liver, the transgene was generated encoding the nuclear fragment of SREBP-1a, the most potent of the three SREBP isoforms. The truncated SREBP-1a is synthesized as a cytosolic protein instead of trafficking to cell surface, and it enters the nucleus without proteolysis, resulting in massive lipid overproduction. The livers of these transgenic mice dramatically enlarged and filled with fat, consisting of a cholesteryl esters and triglycerides mixture. The amounts of fat can be 5 to 25 25-fold higher than those observed in normal liver. The data on LDL receptors indicate that human steatohepatitis and atherosclerosis are linked diseases [Shimano H *et al* 1996]. Further studies have proven this biological mechanism to fit both alcoholic and non-alcoholic steatohepatitis within *in vitro* and *in vivo* studies [Horton JD *et al* 2002; Ji C *et al* 2006; You M *et al* 2002; Browning JD *et al* 2004].

4.3 Origins of fatty liver disease through hepatic liquid-crystals

In human, liver contains 4~6% fat, mostly made up of phospholipids, glycerides and cholesterol. When these fats accumulate in the liver, patients suffer from steatohepatitis or Hepatic steatosis (Fatty Liver Disease), which in turn causes liver enlargement, and abnormal liver function. Though Fatty Liver Disease is most common in overweight and diabetic patients [Hickman IJ et al 2007], a number of pathologic conditions such as excessive alcohol consumption or genetic disorder triggers this accumulation and will be followed by fibrosis and cirrhosis [Ban CR *et al* 2008; Preiss D *et al* 2008; Wilfred de Alwis *NM* et al 2008]. These associated illnesses make steatohepatitis a high mortality disease [El-Zayadi AR 2008; Xirouchakis E *et al* 2008]. Massive maltese-cross liquid-crystal droplets, like those found in embryonic liver, are observed in the biopsies of a large number of steatohepatitic patients. These hepatic liquid-crystal droplets (HLCDs) have been detected in large numbers of steatohepatitic patients through biopsy examination. Although their data has not yet been published, the phenomenon has been developed as a clinical examines procedure and filed for US documentation and invention disclosure.

4.4 Embryonic-like liquid-crystal linking steatohepatitis to atherosclerosis

Since the 1970s, liquid-crystalline structures have been observed in atherosclerotic lesions [Lang PD *et al* 1970, Saul S *et al* 1976]. The first investigation carried out on 95 individual atherosclerotic lesions obtained from 26 patients' classified thelesions into three groups, fatty streaks, fibrous plaques, and gruel (atheromatous) plaques. Using chromatography, the lipid composition of these legions was determined to be cholesterol, cholesterol ester, and phospholipid. Using polarizing microscopy and X-ray diffraction, these lesion lipids were revealed to accumulate as liquid-crystals in lesions composed of special smooth foam cells [Saul S *et al* 1976, Kruth HS *et al* 2001]. This phenomenon was further confirmed by another group [Goldstein JL *et al* 1977] and later mimicked *in vitro* [Joseph B et al 1984]. Analysis of familial hypercholesterolemia through *in vitro* fibroblast overloading experiments demonstrated that lipid deposition in the vascular wall is accomplished via low density lipoprotein-cholesteryl esters (LDL). These complexes are mediated by LDL receptors distributed on cell surfaces [Goldstein JL *et al* 2008; Brown MS *et al* 1974, 1975; Goldstein JL 1977 and 1979].

As discussed above, gain-of-function mutations containing overexpression of a truncated form of SREBP-1a links human steatohepatitis to atherosclerosis through LDL receptors. At this mutation results in liquid crystal depositions as part of the disease pathology, the finding directs a new prospect to exploring the biological function of liquid crystal. As a structure normally only found during embryogenesis, the existence of liquid crystals during disease biology suggests a new method approaching pathology from an embryological point of view. Further understanding of the role liquid crystals play in embryogenesis would doubtless reveal its role in pathogenesis of human diseases and help develop early diagnostics biophysics marker and more effective treatments.

5. Conclusion

Based on current discoveries obtained via XRD, SAXS, confocol microscope, and polarization microscopy in combination with cryo-section, push-release procedure for fluidity measurement, and thermal stage for phase transition progress has been made in the field of liquid crystal function in embryogenesis and pathogenesis of human diseases. With this methodology, the research has proved that, during the embryo development, liquid crystals are readily identifiable in the embryo through their Maltese Crosse birefringence texture. Liquid crystals with this configuration display strong fluidity accompanied with shape-changing properties under direct pressure conditions. XRD and SAXS analysis display a single-peak patterncorresponding to the Bragg distance of liquid crystal. Liquid crystals almost identical to those found in the developing embryo have been found in the affected tissue of multiple diseases.

Liquid crystal configuration within the embryo, animal disease models, and diseased human tissues are all cytoplasmic with Maltese-Crosses situated in cells of various tissues, especially in the luminal portion of kidney during diseases and embryonic blood. Further investigation into liquid crystal involvement in disease through its embryonic mechanisms is expected to generate new diagnostic protocols for liquid crystal related diseases, such as ARMD, Steatohepatitis, Atherosclerotic lesions, and Fabry-Anderson.

6. References

[1] Amico L, Visconti G, Amato A, Azzolina V, Sessa A, Li Vecchi M. Anderson-Fabry disease: a protean clinical behavior and a chance diagnosis. J Nephrol. 18(6):770-2 (2005)

[2] Ban CR, Twigg SM. Fibrosis in diabetes complications: pathogenic mechanisms and circulating and urinary markers. *Vasc Health Risk Manag.* 4(3):575-96 (2008)

[3] Brown GH and Wolken JJ, Liquid-crystals and Biological Structures. Academic Press, Inc. New York. 1979

[4] Brown MS, Goldstein JL. Familial hypercholesterolemia: defective binding of lipoproteins to cultured fibroblasts associated with impaired regulation of 3-hydroxy-3-methylglutaryl coenzyme A reductase activity. *Proc Natl Acad Sc. USA.* 71:788-92 (1974)

[5] Brown MS, Faust JR, Goldstein JL. Role of the low density lipoprotein receptor in regulating the content of free and esterified cholesterol in human fibroblasts. *J Clin Invest.* 55:783-93 (1975)

[6] Cho ME, Kopp JB. Fabry disease in the era of enzyme replacement therapy: a renal perspective. Pediatr Nephrol. 19(6):583-93 (2004)

[7] El-Zayadi AR. Hepatic steatosis: a benign disease or a silent killer. *World J Gastroenterol.* 14(26):4120-6 (2008)

[8] Fehér G. Yolk sac stones in domestic fowl. Anat Histol Embryol. 8(4):360-4 (1979)

[9] Ginsberg L, Manara R, Valentine AR, Kendall B, Burlina AP. Magnetic resonance imaging changes in Fabry disease. *Acta Paediatrica Suppl.* 451:57–62 (2006)

[10] Goldstein JL, Anderson RG, Buja LM, Basu SK, Brown MS. Overloading human aortic smooth muscle cells with low density lipoprotein-cholesteryl esters reproduces features of atherosclerosis in vitro. *J Clin Invest.* 59(6):1196–1202 (1977)

[11] Goldstein JL, Anderson RG, Brown MS. Coated pits, coated vesicles, and receptor-mediated endocytosis. *Nature.* 279:679-85 (1979)

[12] Goldstein JL, Brown, MS. The clinical investigator: bewitched, bothered, and bewildered--but still beloved *J Clin Invest*, 99, 2803-12 (1997)

[13] Goldstein JL, Brown MS. From fatty streak to fatty liver: 33 years of joint publications in the JCI. *J Clin Invest.* 118:1220-2 (2008)

[14] Haimovici R, Gantz DL, Rumelt S, Freddo TF, Small DM. The lipid composition of drusen, Bruch's membrane, and sclera by hot stage polarizing light microscopy. *IOVS.* 42:1592-9 (2001)

[15] He H, Zhou H, Wang G, Wu X. Liquid crystalline in yolk sac during chicken development. *J Wuhan Univ (Nature Science Ed.)* 4:32-46 (1978)

[16] Hickman IJ, Macdonald GA. Impact of diabetes on the severity of liver disease. A*m J Med.* 120(10):829-34 (2007)

[17] Horton JD, Goldstein JL, Brown MS. SREBPs: activators of the complete program of cholesterol and fatty acid synthesis in the liver. *J Clin Invest.* 109:1125-31 (2002)

[18] Ji C, Chan C, Kaplowitz N. Predominant role of sterol response element binding proteins (SREBP) lipogenic pathways in hepatic steatosis in the murine intragastric ethanol feeding model.Kruth HS. Lipoprotein cholesterol and atherosclerosis. *Cur Mol Med. 1:* 633-3 (2001)

[19] Kruth H. Lipoprotein cholesterol and atherosclerosis. *Curr Mol Med.* 1(6): 633-53 (2001)

[20] Lang PD, Insull W Jr. Lipid droplets in atherosclerotic fatty streaks of human aorta. *J Clin Invest.* 49:1479-88 (1970)

[21] Li M, Chao L. Structural study of lipid liquid crystal droplets in chicken development. *Acta Biophysica Sinica*, 12, 299-305(1988)

[22] Lidove O, Klein I, Lelièvre JD, Lavallée P, Serfaty JM, Dupuis E, Papo T, Laissy JP.Imaging features of Fabry disease. *Am J Roentgenol.* 186(4):1184-91 (2006)

[23] Linhart A, Kampmann C, Zamorano JL, Sunder-Plassmann G, Beck M, Mehta A, Elliott PM; European FOS Investigators. Cardiac manifestations of Anderson-Fabry

disease: results from the international Fabry outcome survey. *Eur Heart J.* 28(10):1228-35 (2007)

[24] Maruyama M*, BY Li*, HY Chen*. Xuehong Xu*, Long-Sheng Song, Wuqiang Zhu, Weidong Yong, Wenjun Zhang, Gui-Xue Bu, Shien-Fong Lin, Michael C. Fishbein, W. Jonathan Lederer, John H. Schild Loren J. Field, Michael Rubart, Peng-Sheng Chen, Weinian Shou. FKBP12 is a Critical Regulator of the Heart Rhythm and the Cardiac Voltage-Gated Sodium Current in Mice. *Circulation Research,* 108(9):1042-52 (2011) (*co-first author)

[25] Moore DF, Ye F, Schiffmann R, Butman JA. Increased signal intensity in the pulvinar on T1-weighted images: a pathognomonic MR imaging sign of Fabry disease. *Am J Neuroradiol.* 24: 1096–101 (2003).

[26] Pieroni M, Chimenti C, De Cobelli F, Morgante E, Del Maschio A, Gaudio C, Russo MA, Frustaci A.Pieroni M. Fabry's disease cardiomyopathy: echocardiographic detection of endomyocardial glycosphingolipid compartmentalization. *J Am Coll Cardiol.* 47(8):1663-71 (2006)

[27] Preiss D, Sattar N. Non-alcoholic fatty liver disease: an overview of prevalence, diagnosis, pathogenesis and treatment considerations. *Clin Sci (Lond).* 15(5):141-50 (2008)

[28] Robert S. Hillman, Kenneth A. Ault, Henry M. Rinder Hematology in clinical practice: a guide to diagnosis and management Chapter 26 McGraw-Hill Professional (2005)

[29] Shimano H, Horton JD, Hammer RE, Shimomura I, Brown MS, Goldstein JL. Overproduction of cholesterol and fatty acids causes massive liver enlargement in transgenic mice expressing truncated SREBP-1a. *J Clin Invest.* 98:1575–84 (1996)

[30] Small DM. Surface Chemistry of Biologic Systems. Plenum Press: New York, US. (1970)

[31] Small DM. The Physical Chemistry of Lipids. Plenum Press: New York, US. (1986)

[32] Small DM. George Lyman Duff memorial lecture. Progression and regression of atherosclerotic lesions. Insights from lipid physical biochemistry. Arteriosclerosis. 8(2):103-29 (1988).

[33] Utsumi K, Mitsuhashi F, Asahi K, Sakurazawa M, Arii K, Komaba Y, Katsumata T, Katsura K, Kase R, Katayama Y. Enzyme replacement therapy for Fabry disease: morphologic and histochemical changes in the urinary sediments. Clin Chim Acta.360(1-2):103-7 (2005)

[34] Wang X, Sato R, Brown MS, Hua X, Goldstein JL. SREBP-1, a membrane-bound transcription factor released by sterol-regulated proteolysis. *Cell.* 77:53–62 (1994).

[35] Wilfred de Alwis NM, Day CP. Genes and nonalcoholic fatty liver disease. *Curr Diab Rep.* 8(2):156-63 (2008)

[36] Xu MM, Xu XH, Cao G, Pan Y, Jones O, Bryant JL, Anthony DD, He H, Yan G, Zhang C. The liquid crystalline in normal renal development amplifies the comprehension for Anderson-Fabry disease. *Molecular Crystals and Liquid Crystals,* 508: 52-66 (2009)

[37] Xu MM, Jones OD, Chen X, Li YF , Yan G, Pan Y, Davis HG, Anthony DD, Xu Y, Zheng S, Bryant JL, Xu XH. Cytoplasmic Accumulation of Liquid-Crystal Like Droplets in Post-Infection Sputum Generated by Gram-Positive Bacteria. *Molecular Crystals and Liquid Crystals,* 547: 173-180 (2011)

[38] Xu MM, Jones OD, Cao G, Yan G, He H, Zhang C, Xu XH. Crystallization of calcium carbonate vaterite involves with another mechnisim associated with liquid crystal in embryonic yolk sacs. *Key Engineering Materials,* 428-9: 349-55 (2010)

[39] Xirouchakis E, Sigalas A, Manousou P, Calvaruso V, Pleguezuelo M, Corbani A, Maimone S, Patch D, Burroughs AK. Models for non-alcoholic fatty liver disease: a link with vascular risk. *Curr Pharm Des*. 14(4):378-84 (2008)

[40] Xu XH, Tang C, He H, Zhang X, The lipid components of hepatic liquid crystal lipoid droplets during developing chick embryo, *Acta Biochimica et Biophysica Sinica*, 24(4): 339-343 (1992)

[41] Xu XH, Tang C, Tang Z, Tong H, He H, The studies on otolith CaCO3 crystal structure of three species of fishes in *Sciaenidae*, *Acta Biophysica Sinica*, 9(1): 41-45, 1993

[42] Xu XH, Wang C, Ai X, Confirmation of liquid state of the trophocyte protein granules in the fat body of Chinese honeybee (*Apis cerana*) chrysalis, *Acta Biochimica et Biophysica Sinica*, 26(1): 105-110 (1994)

[43] Xu XH, Wang C, Wu X, He H. Comparative studies on the hepatic liquid crystal lipoid droplets of newborn ducks and newborn pigeons, *Molecular Crystal and Liquid Crystal*, 265: 659-668 (1995a)

[44] Xu XH, Wang C, Wang X, Lei X, He H, Comparative studies on liquid crystal lipoid droplets of livers from newborn birds (Domestic Fowl), *Acta Biochimica et Biophysica Sinica*, 27(5): 551-558 (1995b)

[45] Xu XH, Zhang C, He H, Lu Qand, Ji H, Construction of imitated liquid crystal lipoid droplets of chicken embryo liver, *Acta Biophysica Sinica*, 13(1): 29-34 (1997)

[46] Xu XH, Dong C, Vogel B, Hemicentin assemblies on diverse epithelia in the mouse, *Journal of Histochemistry and Cytochemistry*, 55(2):119-126 (2007)

[47] Xu XH, Xu MM, Cao G, Jones O, Zhao C, Cao L, Yan G, He H, Zhang C. Co-subsistence of liquid crystal droplets and calcium carbonate vaterite crystals reveals a molecular mechanism of calcium preservation in embryogenesis. *Molecular Crystals and Liquid Crystals*, 508:77–90 (2009)

[48] Xu XH, Xu MM, Jones O, Chen X, Li Y, Yan G, Pan Y, Davis HG, Xu Y, Bryant JL, Zheng S, Anthony DD, Liquid Crystal in Lung Development and Chicken Embryogenesis. *Molecular Crystals and Liquid Crystals*, 547: 164-172 (2011a)

[49] Xu XH, Vogel B. A Secreted Protein Promotes Cleavage Furrow Maturation during Cytokinesis. *Current Biology*, 21(2):114-119 (2011b)

[50] You M, Fischer M, Deeg MA, Crabb DW. Ethanol induces fatty acid synthesis pathways by activation of sterol regulatory element-binding protein (SREBP). *J Biol Chem*. 9;277(32):29342-7 (2002)

[51] Zachary D. Goodman and Hala R. Makhlouf,,Chapter 9, Hepatic Histopathology in Schiff's diseases of the liver Volume 2 (edited by Eugene R. Schiff), Lippincott Williams & Wilkins (2009)